Hydatidosis of the Central Nervous System: Diagnosis and Treatment

Mehmet Turgut
Editor

Hydatidosis of the Central Nervous System: Diagnosis and Treatment

Springer

Editor
Mehmet Turgut, MD, PhD
Department of Neurosurgery
Adnan Menderes University School
of Medicine
Aydın
Turkey

ISBN 978-3-642-54358-6 ISBN 978-3-642-54359-3 (eBook)
DOI 10.1007/978-3-642-54359-3
Springer Heidelberg New York Dordrecht London

Library of Congress Control Number: 2014938393

Printed on acid-free paper

Springer is part of Springer Science+Business Media (www.springer.com)

Foreword

It gives me great honor to write a prelude to this important work undertaken by Assistant Professor Mehmet Turgut, in collaboration with several other well-known specialists in hydatid disease from all over the world.

This parasitosis is a devastating but curable worldwide calamity, with a cosmopolitan predominance. Unfortunately, it is mainly found in the less resourced regions of the world, namely, the Mediterranean, African, and South American countries.

Throughout my entire more than 40-year-long career as a pediatric radiologist and biophysicist, I have had numerous opportunities to be involved in the diagnosis, prevention, vaccination, and treatment programs against this dreaded illness.

My personal interest in hydatid disease dates back to my medical school days. I was born in Thala, a small village in the center of Tunisia, an intensive sheep-farming but heavily hydatidosis-infested endemic region. I vividly remember a young lad, Houcine, employed on my father's farm, as shepherd, who presented with hemoptysis. I brought him to the small hospital in Thala where I did a chest conventional fluoroscopy, with a very old machine. I discovered that he had a large impressive opacity involving his entire right lung which turned out, at surgery, to be a pulmonary hydatid cyst (Hospital Ariana, Tunis).

Thanks to surgical and medical treatment, it is now 60 years after that incident but that lad, now an elderly man in his 80s, is still alive and enjoying perfect health.

That experience awakened a lifelong curiosity within me to do something about this devastating malady – a medical student dream.

On returning from Paris, as a recently graduated radiologist, biophysicist, and later on echographist, using my recently acquired skills in those fields, I straight away embarked on the hydatid disease fight.

I started diagnosing and mapping out the epidemiology of this illness and endeavored to find a remedy for it. I had the chance of collaborating with the greatest names of those days in radiology, parasitology, and gastroenterology fields in Tunisia, France, and Italy. Jointly we innovated a new strategy for treating hydatidosis. This involved the use of ultrasound to diagnose and guide a new mode of therapy which later came to be known as puncture-aspiration-injection-reaspiration (PAIR). This novel mode of staging was adopted by the World Health Organization and extended to other parasitic diseases, such as *Schistosoma haematobium* and *S. mansoni*.

Ultrasound imaging modality and PAIR are rarely used in cerebral hydatidosis (orbit), but they should contribute effectively to the eradication of this calamity and ought to be included in the strategy for the diagnosis and the treatment of cerebral hydatidosis.

It gives me great pleasure to appraise this great multidisciplinary undertaking by Dr. Turgut and his colleagues: radiologists, neurologists, neurosurgeons, pathologists, veterinarians, surgeons, orthopedists, ophthalmologists, psychologists, parasitologists, internists, and biologists. This book no doubt adds to and complements the existing armament in the fight against hydatidosis, more especially the disease's elusive cerebral location.

I am confident that this publication will be a great success and a landmark in the war against hydatidosis, eventually contributing to the ailment's total annihilation. Together, through a global effort, we can fight this and many other tropical parasitic diseases.

I am sure that this book will not only be academically and professionally inspiring but also an enjoyable piece of reading.

Congratulations Assistant Professor Turgut for this noble task.

Tunis, Tunisia Hassen A. Gharbi, MD

Professor of Radiology and Medical Biophysics
Honorary member of the International Association of Hydatidology
President elect of the World Federation for Ultrasound in Medicine and Biology, 2011–2013
Honorary President of the Tunisian Society of Radiology,
Honorary Fellow of the American College of Radiology,
Honorary Member of the Society for Pediatric Radiology

Preface

This book is designed to deliver succinct, up-to-date reference information to practicing physicians about imaging findings, differential diagnosis, pathology, clinical findings, and relevant surgical information of hydatidosis of central nervous system. Because of the fact that the problem is rare, no multidisciplinary information has been gathered from an exclusive source, although a significant amount of data is available on the care of patients with hydatidosis. The book is divided naturally into three major parts: the first section includes topics addressing epidemiological aspect of hydatidosis, the second section contains nonsurgical topics that affect decision-making in the patients, and the third section covers the topics on specific neurosurgical disorders. The relevant information given here is often very difficult for neurosurgeons to access elsewhere. The chapters in the book are written by authors who are world-renowned specialists in their respective fields of interest. The framework of each chapter has been designed according to their specific clinical and diagnostic considerations, but an identical format has been followed for all. It is believed that the information which is so crucial for the clinical neurosurgery practice is presented in this way. The detailed surgical information given in this book is intended to illustrate the basic techniques of the neurosurgical procedures and to give guidance which is expected to be useful for the execution of every operative approach. In fact, it should also give technical guidance to operations which are not specifically discussed. Apparently, all authors contributed to this book with their personal experience they have gained in their own institutions and with unusual images they have offered to illustrate each topic. At the end of each chapter, selected references are included for further review. I hope that the sections in which specific neurosurgical disorders are emphasized on an individual basis will prove helpful in surgical planning and in surgical management of patients for the individual neurosurgeon.

My particular thanks go to Dr. Inga von Behrens from Springer DE (Heidelberg, Germany) for his invaluable advice and support in the planning of the present book.

I would like to thank Professor Fuad Sami Haddad for his critical review and insightful supervision.

I owe thanks to my dear sons, Yaşar Barış and Ali Çağlar, for their devotion and constant support.

May I not forget Ms. Elise M. Paxson from Springer (New Jersey, USA) for her kindly assistance in the preparation of the figures for reproduction.

Aydın, Turkey Mehmet Turgut, MD, PhD

Contents

Contributors

Halil Arslan, MD Department of Radiology, Yıldırım Beyazıt University School of Medicine, Ankara, Turkey

Anita Arsovska, MD, PhD Department of Urgent Neurology, University Clinic of Neurology, Skopje, Macedonia

Zoran Arsovski, MD, Mr Sci Department of Allergy and Clinical Immunology, University Clinic of Pulmonology and Allergy, Skopje, Macedonia

Umit Yaşar Ayaz, MD Department of Radiology, Mersin Women's and Children's Hospital, Mersin, Turkey

Mohammed Benzagmout, MD Department of Neurosurgery, Clinical Neurosciences Laboratory, Faculty of Medicine and Pharmacy, University Hospital of Fez, Fez, Morocco

Branko Bobić, MD, PhD Centre for Parasitic Zoonoses, Institute for Medical Research, Serbian Center for Medical Research, University of Belgrade, Belgrade, Serbia

Claudia Borza, MD, PhD Department of Pathophysiology, Victor Babes University of Medicine and Pharmacy, Timisoara, Romania

Crenguta L. Calma, MD, PhD Department of Physiology and Immunology, Victor Babes University of Medicine and Pharmacy, Timisoara, Romania

Evangelia Chatzinasiou, PhD Laboratory of Microbiology and Infectious Diseases, Faculty of Veterinary Medicine, Aristotle University of Thessaloniki, Thessaloniki, Greece

Foteini Chatzinasiou, PhD Department of Dermatology, University of Athens Medical School, Athens, Greece

Klinik für Dermatologie und Venerologie CharitéUniversitätsmedizin Berlin, Berlin, Germany

Alexandru-Vlad Ciurea, MD, PhD, MSc Department of Neurosurgery, Sanador Medical Center Hospital, Bucharest, Romania

The National Center for Excellency in NeurosurgeryCarol Davila University School of Medicine, Bucharest, Romania

Alper Dilli, MD Department of Radiology, Dışkapı Yıldırım Beyazıt Training and Research Hospital, Ankara, Turkey

Olgica Djurković-Djaković, MD, PhD Centre for Parasitic Zoonoses, Institute for Medical Research, Serbian Center for Medical Research, University of Belgrade, Belgrade, Serbia

Sipho K. Dlamini, MBChB, FCF(SA) Department of Medicine, Groote Schuur Hospital, University of Cape Town, Cape Town, South Africa

Vikram S. Dogra, MD Department of Imaging Sciences, University of Rochester School of Medicine, Rochester, NY, USA

Sailike Duishanbai, MD, PhD Department of Neurosurgery, First Teaching Hospital of Xinjiang Medical University, Xinjiang, China

Victor Dumitrascu, MD, PhD Department of Biochemistry and Pharmacology, Emergency County Hospital, Victor Babes University of Medicine and Pharmacy, Timisoara, Romania

Omran Elshamam Department of Radiology, Tripoli Medical Center, Tripoli, Libya

Fatih Erdi, MD Department of Neurosurgery, Meram Faculty of Medicine, Necmettin Erbakan University, Konya, Turkey

Sunil V. Furtado, MS, MCh, DNB Department of Neurosurgery, Sri Sathya Sai Institute of Higher Medical Sciences, Bangalore, India

Claudia L. Gatta Department of Parasitology, Hospital de Clinicas, University of Buenos Aires, Buenos Aires, Argentina

Vaitsa Giannouli, BA, MSc, PhD Department of Cognitive Psychology and Neuropsychology, Aristotle University of Thessaloniki, Thessaloniki, Greece

Luis Gracia, PhD Department of Mechanical Engineering, University of Zaragoza, Zaragoza, Spain

Jorge A. Guisantes, MD, PhD Department of Immunology, Microbiology and Parasitology, Faculty of Pharmacy, University of the Basque Country, Vitoria, Spain

Fuad Sami Haddad, BA, MD, FRCS(C), FACS, ABNS Department of Surgery, American University of Beirut Medical Center, Beirut, Lebanon

Antonio Herrera, MD, PhD Department of Surgery, Medicine School, University of Zaragoza, Zaragoza, Spain

Department of Orthopaedic and Trauma Surgery, Miguel Servet University Hospital, University of Zaragoza Medical School, Zaragoza, Spain

Meryem Himmiche, MD Department of Neurosurgery, University Hospital of Fez, Fez, Morocco

Zahed Hossain, MD, MBBS, FCPS, MS Department of Neurosurgery, Rajshahi Medical College Hospital, Rajshahi, Dhaka, Bangladesh

Elena Ibarz, PhD Department of Mechanical Engineering, School of Engineering and Architecture, University of Zaragoza, Zaragoza, Spain

Erdal Kalkan, MD Department of Neurosurgery, Meram Faculty of Medicine, Necmettin Erbakan University, Konya, Turkey

Avinash K. Kanodia, MBBS, MD, DM Department of Radiology, Perth Royal Infirmary, Perth, Scotland, UK

Department of Radiology, Ninewells Hospitals, Dundee, Scotland, UK

Nidhameddine Kchir, MD Department of Pathology, La Rabta Hospital, Tunis, Tunisia

Fatih Keskin, MD Department of Neurosurgery, Meram Faculty of Medicine, Necmettin Erbakan University, Konya, Turkey

Chlodwig Kirchhoff, MD Klinik und Poliklinik für Unfallchirurgie, Klinikum Rechts der Isar, Technische Universitatet Muenchen, Muenchen, Germany

Faten Limaiem, MD Department of Pathology, Mongi Slim Hospital, Tunis, Tunisia

Antonio Lobo-Escolar, PhD Department of Orthopaedic and Trauma Surgery, Miguel Servet University Hospital, University of Zaragoza Medical School, Zaragoza, Spain

Jesus Mateo, PhD Department of Orthopaedic and Trauma Surgery, Miguel Servet University Hospital, University of Zaragoza Medical School, Zaragoza, Spain

Claudia I. Menghi, PhD Clinical Microbiology, Parasitology Division, Hospital de Clínicas, University of Buenos Aires, Buenos Aires, Argentina

Tropical Parasitic Diseases, University of Valencia, Valencia, Spain

Horatiu-Alexandru Moisa, MD Department of Neurosurgery, Sanador Medical Center Hospital, Bucharest, Romania

The National Center for Excellency in Neurosurgery, Carol Davila University School of Medicine, Bucharest, Romania

Roxana Moldovan, MD, PhD Department of Microbiology, Victor Babes University of Medicine and Pharmacy, Timisoara, Romania

Raul Neghina, MD, PhD Department of Infectious Diseases, Pneumology, Epidemiology and Parasitology, Discipline of Parasitology, Victor Babes University of Medicine and Pharmacy, Timisoara, Romania

Adriana M. Neghina, MD, PhD Department of Biochemistry and Pharmacology, Victor Babes University of Medicine and Pharmacy, Timisoara, Romania

Dan Aurel Nica, MD, PhD Department of Neurosurgery, St. Pantelimon Emergency University Hospital, Bucharest, Romania

Ntobeko B.A. Ntusi, MB, ChB, FCP(SA) Department of Cardiovascular Medicine, John Radcliffe Hospital, Oxford, UK

Department of Medicine, Groote Shuur Hospital, Cape Town, South Africa

Ante Popovski, MD, PhD Department of Neuropsychiatry, Private Neuropsychiatry Practice "Dr. A. Popovski", Skopje, Macedonia

Lukas L. Postl, Cand. Med Klinik und Poliklinik für Unfallchirurgie, Klinikum Rechts der Isar, Technische Universitaet Muenchen, Muenchen, Germany

Sucharitha Ramavath, MBBS, MS, FSIO Department of Oculoplasty, Vasan Eye Care, Bangalore, India

Ahmed Abdel Khalek Abdel Razek, MD Department of Diagnostic Radiology, Mansoura Faculty of Medicine, Mansoura University Hospital, Mansoura, Egypt

Deme Raja Reddy, MD, MBBS, FRCS (E), FRACS, FICS Department of Neurosurgery, Nizam's Institute of Medical Sciences, Hyderabad, India

Department of Neurosurgery, Apollo Hospital, Hyderabad, India

Sikó Barabási Sándor, DVM, Dr. Univ., MSc, PhD Department of Ecological and Biotechnological Systems, Faculty of Environmental Science, Babeş-Bolyai University Cluj-Napoca, Sfântu Gheorghe, Romania

Villiam Šnábel, PhD Department of Parasitic Zoonoses, Parasitological Institute, Slovak Academy of Sciences, Košice, Slovakia

Subrahmanyam Mallajosyula, MS, DO, FUBC, FUW Orbit and Ophthalmic Plastic Services, Sankar Foundation Eye Hospital, Vishakhapatnam, India

Hideki Sudo, MD, PhD Department of Advanced Medicine for Spine and Spinal Cord Disorders, Hokkaido University Graduate School of Medicine, Sapporo, Hokkaido, Japan

Nikolaos Syrmos, PhD, MSc, MD Department of Human Performance and Health, Aristotle University of Thessaloniki, Thessaloniki, Macedonia, Greece

Sumit Thakar, MCh Department of Neurosurgery, Sri Sathya Sai Institute of Higher Medical Sciences, Bangalore, India

Ahmet Tuncay Turgut, MD Department of Radiology, Ankara Training and Research Hospital, Ankara, Turkey

Mehmet Turgut, MD, PhD Department of Neurosurgery, Adnan Menderes University Hospital, Aydm, Turkey

Syeed Mehbub Ul Kadir, MS, FSIO Department of Oculoplasty, National Institute of Ophthalmology & Hospital, Dhaka, Bangladesh

Dimitar Vuchev, MD, PhD Department of Clinical Parasitology and Tropical Medicine, Medical University of Plovdiv, Plovdiv, Bulgaria

Department of Infectious Diseases, Parasitology and Tropical Medicine, St. George University Hospital, Plovdiv, Bulgaria

Hao Wen, MD, PhD Department of General Surgery, First Teaching Hospital of Xinjiang Medical University, Xinjiang, China

Historical Aspects of Hydatidosis of the Central Nervous System

1

Nikolaos Syrmos, Vaitsa Giannouli,
Evangelia Chatzinasiou, and Foteini Chatzinasiou

Contents

N. Syrmos, PhD, MSc, MD (✉)
Department of Human Performance and Health, Aristotle University of Thessaloniki, Papafi 159, Kato Toumba, Thessaloniki, Macedonia 54453, Greece
e-mail: milanako76@yahoo.gr

V. Giannouli, BA, MSc, PhD
Department of Cognitive Psychology and Neuropsychology, Aristotle University of Thessaloniki, Thessaloniki, Greece

E. Chatzinasiou, PhD
Laboratory of Microbiology and Infectious Diseases, Faculty of Veterinary Medicine, Aristotle University of Thessaloniki, Thessaloniki, Greece

F. Chatzinasiou, PhD
Department of Dermatology, University of Athens Medical School, Athens, Greece

Klinik für Dermatologie und Venerologie Charité, Universitätsmedizin Berlin, Berlin, Germany

Introduction

Echinococcosis could be characterized as a zoonotic infestation caused by cestode species of the genus *Echinococcus*. These parasites have life cycles that involve two mammalian hosts. The procedure is as follows: the adult cestode inhabits the small intestine of a carnivore (defined as definitive host) and produces eggs containing infective oncospheres. Cestode segments (proglottids) containing eggs or free eggs are released from the intestinal tract of the carnivore into the environment. After oral uptake of eggs by an intermediate host animal, a larval stage, the metacestode, develops in internal organs (Eckert and Deplazes 2004).

The complete life cycle of *Echinococcus* includes several carnivores, but humans are infected incidentally and usually in childhood by ingestion of the ova from contaminated hands or food. In case an embryo of *Echinococcus granulosus* lodges in the brain, a solitary cyst develops. Hydatid cysts are slow-growing lesions that do not invade the brain; they produce symptoms when the increasing size of the cysts exerts local pressure. Usually the late appearance of focal neurologic deficits follows a long history of epileptic attacks and general symptoms compatible with increased intracranial pressure (Abbassioun and Amirjamshidi 2001). The neuropsychological profile of each patient is mainly due to the differences in the affected brain structures and the possible relevant cognitive deficits (Luria and Karasseva 1968).

M. Turgut (ed.), *Hydatidosis of the Central Nervous System: Diagnosis and Treatment*,
DOI 10.1007/978-3-642-54359-3_1,

Geographic Range

Hydatidosis is mainly detected in areas such as the Middle East (Lebanon, Syria, Palestine, Kuwait, Egypt and Libya), Australia, New Zealand, Latin America (Argentina, Uruguay and Paraguay), Central Europe, South Africa and the Mediterranean countries (Spain, France, Italy, Greece and Turkey). The geographic range of hydatidosis is discussed in detail in Chaps. 2, 3 and 4.

Hydatid Disease in Humans

The three forms of echinococcosis occurring in humans—cystic echinococcosis caused by *E. granulosus*, alveolar echinococcosis caused *by E. multilocularis* and polycystic echinococcosis caused by *E. oligarthrus*—have special importance due to their wide geographic distribution and their medical and economic impact. The cystic echinococcosis and alveolar echinococcosis are statistically the most widespread, but polycystic echinococcosis is less frequent and is found only in Central and South America (Eckert and Deplazes 2004). The forms of hydatidosis are discussed in detail in Chaps. 2, 3, 4 and 24.

Historical Periods

The presence of hydatid cysts in both humans and animals was well known in ancient times (Prousalidis 2007; Syrmos 2007). In fact, the term "hydatid" is historically derived from Greek "ydatos" which means water (Abdennebi 2009).

"Hydatids" or watery vesicles seem to have been widely present since ancient times, discovered in the entrails of ritually slaughtered animals as well as those butchered for food. One hint that ruptured cysts located in human livers were invariably fatal appears in aphorisms attributed to Hippocrates (Foster 1965). According to Aristotelian ideas, these lumps were spontaneously generated in the afflicted organs themselves (Patterson 1993).

Egyptian Medicine

The ancient Egyptians suffered numerous epidemics and often tomb art described epidemics and parasitic infestations such as hydatidosis (Ruffer 1921a, b; Bryan 1930; Castiglioni 1936; Sullivan 1995).

We have a space occupying cranial lesion, maybe a tapeworm, cyst in mummy 22940 of the Manchester Museum Mummy Collection (Ruffer 1921a, b; Sullivan 1995).

Also we have the presence of "hydatid disease" in the lung cavity of the Mummy of Asru (Ruffer 1921a, b; Bryan 1930; Sullivan 1995).

The Ebers papyrus is an Egyptian medical papyrus dating to circa 1550 BC. Although the papyrus was written in about 1500 BC, it is believed to have been copied from earlier texts, perhaps dating as far back as 3400 BC (Ruffer 1921a, b; Bryan 1930; Castiglioni 1936; Sullivan 1995).

Ebers papyrus together with the Kahun Gynaecological papyrus (circa 1800 BC), the Edwin Smith papyrus (circa 1600 BC), the Hearst papyrus (circa 1600 BC), the Brugsch papyrus (circa 1300 BC) and the London Medical papyrus (circa 1300 BC) is among the oldest preserved medical documents (Ruffer 1921a, b; Bryan 1930; Castiglioni 1936; Sullivan 1995; Cox 2003).

In Ebers papyrus, we have the first written records of what are almost certainly parasitic infections such as hydatidosis that came from a period of Egyptian medicine from 3000 to 400 BC. We have the record that hydatid disease is caused by the larval stage of the dog tapeworm (Ruffer 1921a, b; Bryan 1930; Castiglioni 1936; Sullivan 1995; Cox 2003).

Greek Period

In ancient Greece, according to Galen, hydatidosis was described in the works of Hippocrates and Aretaeus (Castiglioni 1936; Prousalidis 2007; Syrmos et al. 2010).

Hippocrates of Kos (Ιπποκράτης) (460 BC–370 BC) (Fig. 1.1) was an ancient Greek

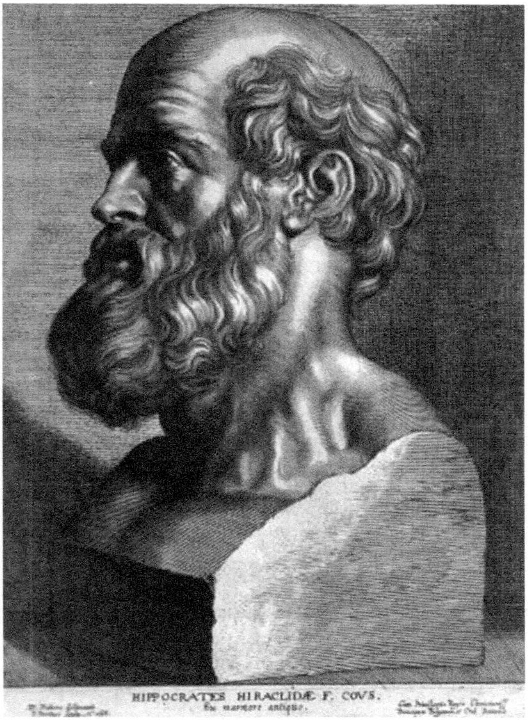

Fig. 1.1 Hippocrates of Kos (460 BC–370 BC)

physician of the Age of Pericles (The Golden Age, *Χρυσούς* Αιών) and is the most outstanding figure in the history of medicine worldwide (Castiglioni 1936; Syrmos 2007, 2009, 2011; Syrmos et al. 2010).

He is referred to as the father of modern medicine in recognition of his lasting contributions to the field as the founder of the Hippocratic School of Medicine. This intellectual school revolutionized medicine in ancient Greece, establishing it as a discipline distinct from other fields that it had traditionally been associated with (theurgy-θεουργία and philosophy- φιλοσοφία), thus establishing medicine as a profession (Castiglioni 1936; Syrmos 2007, 2009, 2011; Syrmos et al. 2010).

According to Galen, Hippocrates used the term "liver filled with water" for hydatid disease in a man (Pissiotis et al. 1972). In this earliest mention of hydatidosis, he suggested that "it breaks in the epiploon, when liver is distended with water; therefore the abdomen is full of water and the sick dies" (Pissiotis et al. 1972; Prousalidis 2007; Abdennebi 2009; Syrmos et al. 2010).

Hippocrates knew that rupture of the cyst meant the death of the patient, the disease represents the tumoral-vesicular growth of the *E. granulosus* larva into space occupying cysts, filled with an extremely allergenic fluid and the primordia of the worm, protoscoleces (Prousalidis 2007; Arseni et al. 1981; Lazar 2010; Syrmos et al. 2010).

Aretaeus of Cappadocia (Αρεταῖος) was also one of the most celebrated of the ancient Greek physicians (Haas 1991; Weber 1996; Syrmos et al. 2010). In the first century (AD), he wrote in Ionic Greek a general treatise on diseases such as hydatidosis, which is extant, and is certainly one of the most valuable relics of antiquity. Aretaeus had knowledge of hydatidosis and his consequences (Castiglioni 1936; Kudlien 1970; Weber 1996; Prousalidis 2007; Syrmos 2007, 2009, 2011; Syrmos et al. 2010).

Jewish Period

Hydatidosis was described in the Talmud (תַּלְמוּד) (Fig. 1.2), a central text of mainstream Judaism (Castiglioni 1936; Fielding 1966; Saidi 1976).

Talmud takes the form of a record of rabbinic discussions pertaining to Jewish medicine, ethics, law and culture. It has two components: the Mishnah (Hebrew: משנה), the first written compendium of Judaism's Oral Law, and the Gemara, an elucidation of the Mishnah and related Tannaitic writings that often ventures onto other subjects and expounds broadly on the Hebrew Bible (Castiglioni 1936; Fielding 1966; Saidi 1976).

In the Talmud, we have a primitive description about hydatidosis as bladder of water and his consequences (Castiglioni 1936; Fielding 1966; Saidi 1976).

Roman Period

Galen of Pergamon (Aelius Galenus or Claudius Galenus, Γαληνός, *Galēnos*) (Fig. 1.3) was an

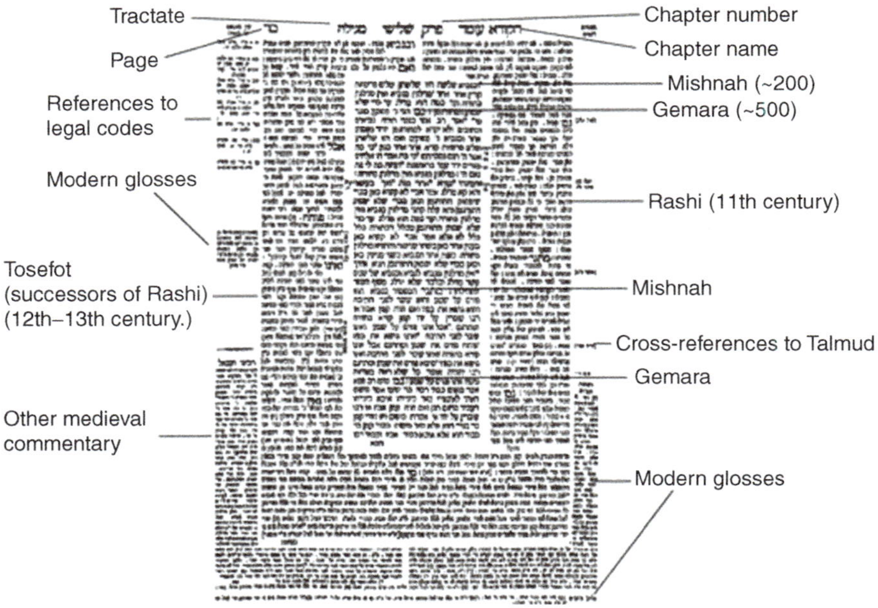

Fig. 1.2 Talmud

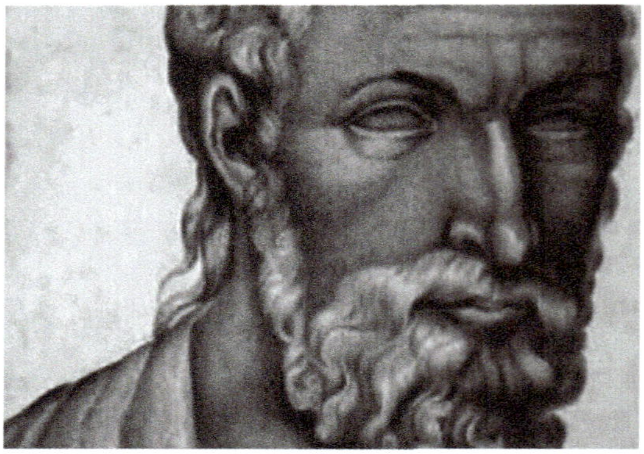

Fig. 1.3 Galen of Pergamon (129–199)

important Roman physician (of Greek ethnicity). In the second century (AD), Galen contributed greatly to the understanding of numerous scientific disciplines, including anatomy, physiology, pathology, pharmacology and neurology. He also describes hydatidosis in his works and he reported about Hippocrates and Aretaeus knowledge of the disease (Castiglioni 1936; Syrmos 2007, 2009, 2011; Syrmos et al. 2010).

According to Galen, Hippocrates used the term "liver filled with water" for hydatid disease in a man (Pissiotis et al. 1972).

Arabic Period

In the Arabic Period, the descriptions of infections such as hydatidosis became more accurate with the works of Jurjani, Rhazes and Avicenna (Ruffer 1921a, b; Bryan 1930; Castiglioni 1936; Sullivan 1995; Cox 2003; Proussalidis 2007; Syrmos et al. 2010).

Jurjani

Abu Sahl 'Isa ibn Yahya al-Masihi al-Jurjani (الجرجاني المسيحي يحيى بن عيسى ابوسهل) was a Persian Christian physician, from Gorgan, east of the Caspian Sea, in Iran. He was the teacher of Avicenna. He wrote an encyclopaedic treatise on medicine of one hundred chapters (*al-mā'a fi-l-sanā'a al-tabi'iyyah*; الطبيعية الصناعة في الماء), which is one of the earliest Arabic works of its kind and may have been in some respects the model for Avicenna's Qanun. In his work, he reported on human involvement by hydatidosis (Castiglioni 1936; Fielding 1966; Goichon et al. 1999).

Rhazes

Rhazes (الرازي بن زكريامحمد *Mohammad bin Zakariā- al Rāzi*) (860–932AD) was a Persian polymath, a prominent figure in Islamic Golden

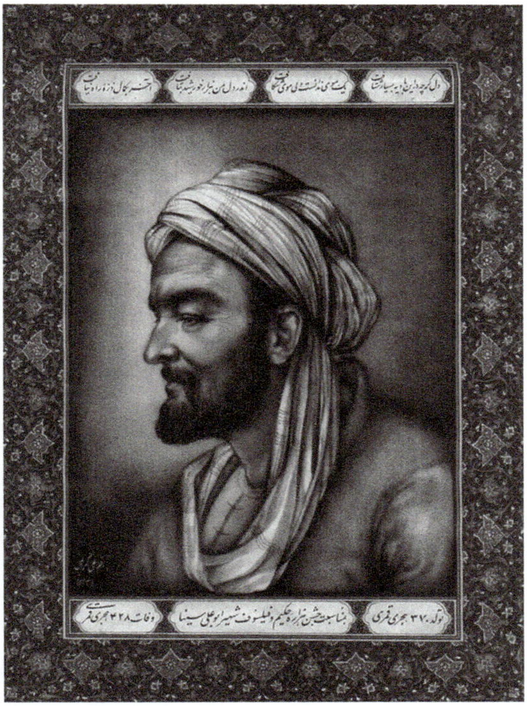

Fig. 1.4 Avicenna (980–1037) (From Aciduman et al. (2009); with permission)

Age. Edward Granville Browne considers him as "probably the greatest and most original of all the physicians and one of the most prolific as an author". He described hydatosis and its consequences (Castiglioni 1936; Fielding 1966; Goichon et al. 1999; Syrmos et al. 2010).

Avicenna

Avicenna (Ibn Sīnā, ابن سينا) (980–1037) (Fig. 1.4) was the most prominent philosopher in the Islamic tradition who wrote many works concentrated on medicine. He is regarded as the most famous and influential polymath of the Islamic Golden Age. Into his works (The Book of Healing and The Canon of Medicine), he made an attempt to describe hydatidosis. Ibn Sīnā's Canon of Medicine provides a complete system of medicine according to the principles of Galen and Hippocrates (Castiglioni 1936; Fielding 1966; Goichon et al. 1999; Cox 2003; Abdennebi 2009; Syrmos et al. 2010).

He reported on human involvement by hydatidosis and he wrote important medical works that contain a great deal of information about diseases clearly caused by parasites (Cox 2003; Abdennebi 2009).

The Seventeenth Century

By the seventeenth century, authors once more pointed out pathological similarities between the watery sacs in humans and those in domesticated animals, especially sheep and cattle (Patterson 1993).

The contribution of the animal factor of the hydatid disease was not suspected until the research in the seventeenth century by Redi, Tyson and Morgani (Castiglioni 1936; Fielding 1966; Goichon et al. 1999).

Redi

The first step towards figuring out the cause of echinococcosis occurred during the seventeenth century thanks to the studies of Francesco Redi (Fig. 1.5) (Castiglioni 1936; Fielding 1966; Goichon et al. 1999).

Francesco Redi (1626–1697) was an Italian physician, naturalist and poet. He is best known for his series of experiments, published in 1668 as Esperienze Intorno alla Generazione degl'Insetti (Experiments on the Generation of Insects), which is regarded as one of the first steps in refuting "spontaneous generation"—a theory also known as Aristotelian abiogenesis. As a physician, he became court physician to Ferdinando II de' Medici, Grand Duke of Tuscany, and, his successor, Cosimo III (Castiglioni 1936; Fielding 1966; Goichon et al. 1999).

He made a number of observations and experiments in rabbits regarding the presence of parasitic worms in cysts. With his studies, Redi demonstrated the animal origin of the disease, and his results were later confirmed by Edward Tyson and Philip Hartmann Redi (Castiglioni 1936; Fielding 1966; Goichon et al. 1999).

Tyson

Edward Tyson was a British scientist and physician, commonly regarded as the founder of modern comparative anatomy, which compares

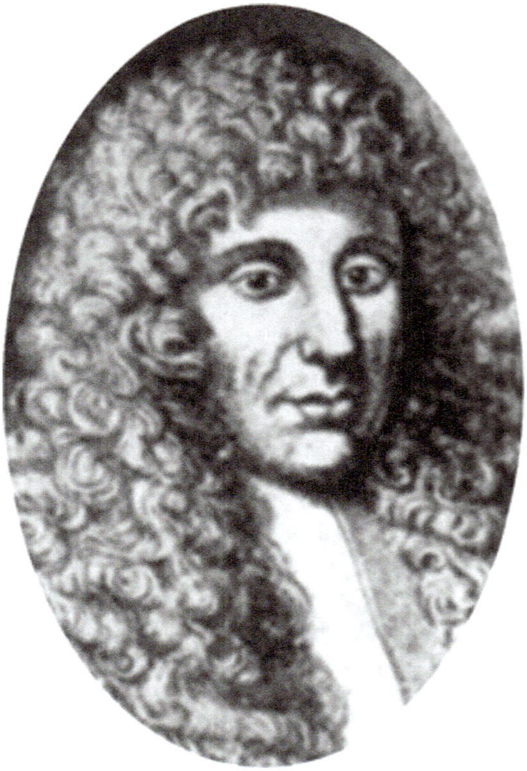

Fig. 1.5 Francesco Redi (1626–1697)

the anatomy between species. Edward Tyson and Philip Hartmann in Germany promoted the idea that hydatid cysts contained embryonic forms of insects or worms. Some of Tyson's dissections were carried out on "rotten sheep" (Castiglioni 1936; Risse 2005).

In 1680, he established that porpoises are mammals. In 1698, he dissected a chimpanzee and the result was the book, Orang-Outang, sive Homo Sylvestris: or, the Anatomy of a Pygmie Compared with that of a Monkey, an Ape, and a Man. In this book, he came to the conclusion that the chimpanzee has more in common with man than with monkeys, particularly with respect to the brain. This work was republished in 1894, with an introduction by Bertram C. A. Windle that includes a short biography of Tyson (Castiglioni 1936; Fielding 1966; Goichon et al. 1999).

Edward Tyson in 1687 suggested the parasitic nature of hydatid disease (Kattan 1997).

Morgagni

Giovanni Battista Morgagni (1682–1771) was an Italian anatomist, celebrated as the father of modern anatomical pathology. He reported a postmortem patient with a large hydatid cyst in the retroperitoneal tissue near the left kidney, containing many daughter cysts (Castiglioni 1936; Androutsos 2006). The spinal canal had been invaded through the intervertebral foramina, which was dilated (Castiglioni 1936; Androutsos 2006).

The Eighteenth Century

In the *eighteenth* century, the larva of *Echinococcus* and the similarity of the hydatid cysts in humans and other animals were described (Castiglioni 1936).

Bidloo

Govert Bidloo (1649–1713) was a Dutch Golden Age physician, anatomist, poet and playwright. He was the personal physician of William III of Orange-Nassau, Dutch stadholder and king of England (Castiglioni 1936). In 1708, Bidloo was the first to report osseous hydatidosis in a case involving the humerus (Işlekel et al. 1998a, b; Schnepper and Johnson 2004).

Peter Simon Pallas

Peter Simon Pallas was a famous German and Russian naturalist, scientist and traveller who became chief of Mineral cabinet (Fig. 1.6) (Castiglioni 1936; Fielding 1966; Goichon et al. 1999).

In 1760, Pallas noticed the similarities between hydatid diseases in humans and other mammals. In 1766, he was the first scientist to mention the similarity of the hydatid cysts in humans and other animals (Castiglioni 1936; Fielding 1966; Goichon et al. 1999).

John Hunter

John Hunter (1728–1793) was a Scottish surgeon regarded as one of the surgeons advocating of careful observation and scientific method in medicine. In 1773, he described the morphological picture the hydatid cyst (Abdennebi 2009).

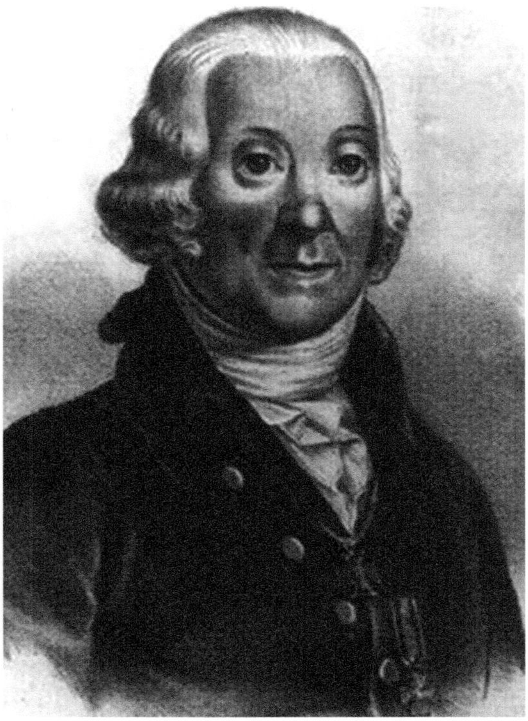

Fig. 1.6 Peter Simon Pallas (1741–1811)

Goeze

Johann August Ephraim Goeze was a German zoologist from Aschersleben. He did much work with aquatic invertebrates, particularly insects and worms. In 1773, he was the first to describe tardigrades which are commonly known as water-bears or moss piglets (Castiglioni 1936; Fielding 1966; Goichon et al. 1999).

In 1782, Goeze was the first to describe microscopically the scolices of the larva of *Echinococcus* (Castiglioni 1936; Fielding 1966; Goichon et al. 1999; Abdennebi 2009).

Edward Jenner

Edward Jenner (1749–1823) was an English naturalist and country physician. Famous for his cowpox vaccine, he recorded his dissections of numerous farm animals. Known to many as "the father of immunology", Edward Jenner made a lot of research and post-mortem studies in animals with hydatidosis and he gave his pioneer contribution to the first steps for the understanding of the disease (Castiglioni 1936; Prousalidis 2007).

Modern Era

In 1786 *E. granulosus* was introduced when it was discovered by Batsch (Eckert et al. 2001).

The French physician Cullerier, senior surgeon to the civil Parisian Venereal Hospital, was the first to describe a case of hydatid cyst of the bone in 1806 (Dew 1928; Dowling and Orlando 1929; Arana Iniguez 1978; Abdennebi 2009).

François Chaussier was a French anatomist. He reported a case of spinal hydatid disease in 1807. Initially he studied medicine in Besançon, and later returned to Dijon, where he worked as a hospital physician and performed pioneer research in forensic medicine. Later he became professor at the École Polytechnique and chief obstetrician at the Paris Maternité. In 1822, he was elected as a member of the Academy of Sciences. He performed early studies of neuralgia and introduced a procedure for revival of "near-dead" newborns. He also performed a descriptive survey of all muscles in the human body and developed a new system of designation for muscles (Dew 1928; Dowling and Orlando 1929; Arana Iniguez 1978; Benkhadra et al. 2008; Abdennebi 2009).

The term "echinococcus" was coined by Karl Asmund Rudolphi in 1808 (Craig and Faust 1970).

Rudolphi was a Swedish-born naturalist, who is credited with being the "father of helminthology". He worked widely across the fields of botany, zoology, anatomy and physiology. He investigated the anatomy of nerves, carried out studies of plant growth and was an early champion of the view that the cell is the basic structural unit of plants (Castiglioni 1936; Fielding 1966; Goichon et al. 1999) (Fig. 1.7).

In 1819, the first patient treated surgically for spinal hydatidosis was reported by Reydellet (Pamir et al. 2002; Abdennebi 2009). The patient was a 22-year-old lady who had a hydatid cyst in the lumbar spine, and the young lady died 12 months later from the occurrence of profuse suppuration in the sac (Maguire 1819; Castiglioni 1936; Ba'assiri and Haddad 1984; Pamir et al. 2002; Schnepper and Johnson 2004; Abdennebi 2009).

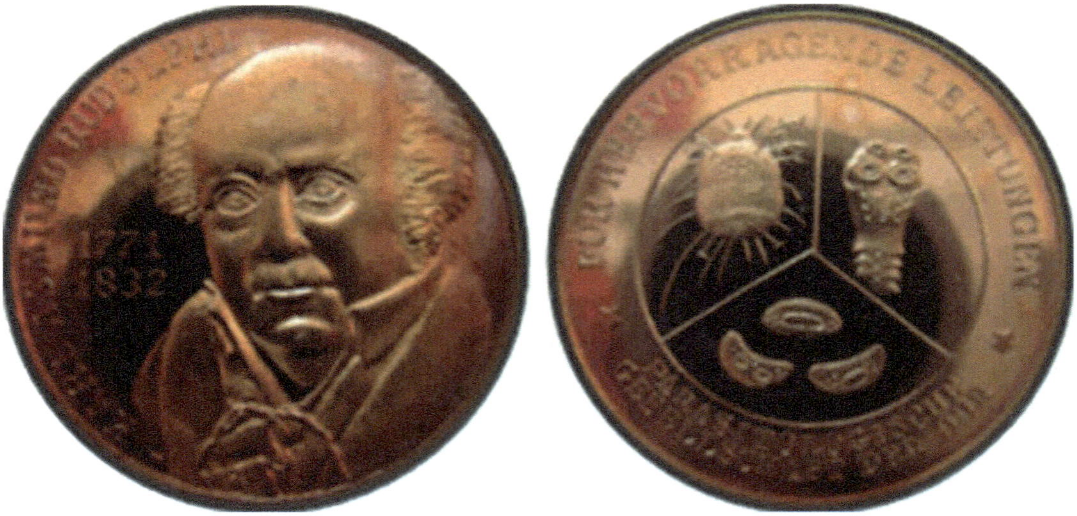

Fig. 1.7 Karl Asmund Rudolphi (1771–1832)

In 1827, Montansey described the brain of an idiot-epileptic woman containing a large number of cerebellar and cerebral hydatid cysts (Castiglioni 1936; Ba'assiri and Haddad 1984; Pamir et al. 2002; Schnepper and Johnson 2004; Abdennebi 2009).

In 1855, Rudolph Carl Virchow firstly suggested the helminthic nature of alveolar hydatid disease caused by *E. multilocularis*. Rudolph Carl Virchow (1821–1902) was a German doctor, anthropologist, pathologist, prehistorian, biologist and politician, known for his advancement of public health. Referred to as "the father of modern pathology", he is considered one of the founders of social medicine (Castiglioni 1936; Abdennebi 2009).

In 1863, two researchers stepped into the spotlight. Leuckart discovered *E. multilocularis* and Diesing *E. oligarthus* (Eckert et al. 2001).

In 1888, Naunyn, Krabbe, Finsen and Thomas proved that the definitive host of the disease is the dog (and its relatives, wolves, jackals, hyenas, dingo dogs), and starting with the year 1901 (with Felix Devè's thesis Secondary Echinococcosis), hydatidology was born as a "science" (Arseni et al. 1981).

Felix Devè continued his work and published an astonishing 325 papers which turned the city of Rouen (France) into the Mecca of hydatid disease researchers for 50 years (Arseni et al. 1981).

Surgeons and pioneer neurosurgeons led the way in clarifying the pathology and advising the correct treatment for cranial hydatid cyst (Webster and Cameron 1967; Anderson et al. 1975; De Villiers and Joubert 1975; Kune et al. 1983; MacPherson et al. 1984; Walters 1984; Syrmos et al. 2010).

Maunsell (1845–1895) was an Irish surgeon. He was initially educated in Ireland, where he worked hard both in experimental and also in natural science. In 1867, he became chief surgeon in Australia and there assisted William Gillbee with the application of the antiseptic principles advocated by Joseph Lister in Glasgow. Later he practiced surgery in New Zealand, until 1891 (Dew 1955).

Henry Widenham Maunsell in 1889 operated successfully on a case of probable subtentorial hydatid cyst in an 18-year-old boy in New Zealand (Dew 1955).

In 1890, the Australians Graham and Clubb were the first to report the successful removal of an undoubted hydatid cyst of the brain (Arana Iniguez 1978; Abdennebi 2009). Barnett in 1896 (from New Zealand) and Luis Morquio in 1901 (from Uruguay) reported, among others, their success in the medical treatment of hydatid cyst of the brain in children (Webster and Cameron 1967; Anderson et al. 1975; De Villiers and

Joubert 1975; Kune et al. 1983; MacPherson et al. 1984; Walters 1984).

Luis Morquio (1867–1935) was first qualified in medicine in Uruguay. Later he studied in Paris at the Pasteur Institute. He specialized in paediatrics. In 1894, he returned to Uruguay, where he became the director of a newly established paediatric clinic and professor of paediatrics in Montevideo. He studied the presence of intracranial hydatid cyst in children (Haas 2002).

The Australian professor of surgery, Sir Harold Robert Dew (1891–1962), in 1928 published the first classic book on hydatid disease (Dew 1928).

Harold Robert Dew was first educated at the Melbourne Continuation School and at Scotch College. In 1909, he entered Ormond College, University of Melbourne. After a year as resident medical officer at (Royal) Melbourne Hospital, he sailed for England where he was commissioned temporary lieutenant in the Royal Army Medical Corps. Later he served in France and in 1918 was officer commanding the cholera laboratory at the 3rd Egyptian Stationary Hospital, Kantara; there he also performed general and clinical pathology and surgery. He assembled a fine collection of pathological specimens of endemic Egyptian diseases, particularly those that illustrated dysentery and bilharziasis. The French government awarded him the médaille d'honneur des épidémies in August 1917. Later, Dew went to London for postgraduate study and hospital experience and in 1920 was admitted to the Royal College of Surgeons, England, as a fellow. After his European experience, he returned in Melbourne, and he became resident tutor in surgery and anatomy at Ormond College. As an honorary associate at the Walter and Eliza Hall Institute, he collaborated with Neil Fairley on such topics as dysentery, malaria and schistosomiasis and—in what was to become his outstanding work—hydatid disease and testicular tumours (Carmody 2012).

During the last century, Dowling and Arana-Iniguez described a perfect surgical procedure for hydatidosis of the brain, providing intact removal of the cyst, named as "hydatid birth", by irrigation with isotonic saline solution between cyst wall and the brain, called hydraulic method (Abdennebi 2009).

The Dowling-Orlando technique has been the main surgical choice for the intact removal of intracranial hydatid cysts. Dowling described his technique in 1929, well before the introduction of the microscope in neurosurgery. Using the operating microscope has not been reported in the removal of a large hydatid cyst (Balak et al. 2006).

Arana-Iniguez from Uruguay was Professor of Neurology Institute of Medical School; he had studied abroad, first next to Bailey and later at the Brain Research Institute at the University of California with Segundo JP, French J, Naquet R and Hernández-Peón R, and linked the growth of diverse basic disciplines with clinical disciplines and techniques over space and time (Azambuja 1977).

The last true discovery concerning the *Echinococcus* species occurred in 1972 when Rausch and Bernstein discovered *E. vogeli* (Eckert et al. 2001).

Conclusion

The presence of hydatid cysts in both humans and animals was well known in ancient times and was described in the works of Hippocrates in the fourth century AD and Aretaeus and Galen in the first and second centuries AD, respectively. However, it was not until the seventeenth century that the parasitic natures of these cysts were recognized by Francisco Redi. In 1766 German Pierre Simon Pallas formulated the hypothesis that hydatid cysts were the larval stages of tapeworms, and later in 1853 Carl von Siebold demonstrated that cysts from sheep lead to adult tapeworms in dogs. It was not until a decade later that Bernhard Naunyn recognized that the adult tapeworms directly develop from hydatid cysts. Full understanding of the clinical features of this disease came in the late 1800s, which progressed to the development of immunological diagnostic tests by the early 1900s. Surgical techniques to remove cysts were first attempted in the 1600s, which have proven to be an effective treatment which evolved with medical technology.

References

Abbassioun K, Amirjamshidi A. Diagnosis and management of hydatid cyst of the central nervous system: part 1: general considerations and hydatid disease of the brain. Neurosurg Q. 2001;11:1–9.

Abdennebi B. Parasitoses of the central nervous system. In: Sindou M, editor. Practical handbook of neurosurgery. From leading neurosurgeons. Wien/NewYork: Springer; 2009. p. 469–84.

Aciduman A, et al. What does Al-Qanun Fi Al-Tibb (The Canon of Medicine) say on head injuries? Neurosurg Rev. 2009;32:255–63.

Anderson M, Bickerstaff ER, Hamilton JG. Cerebral hydatid disease in Britain. J Neurol Neurosurg Psychiatry. 1975;38:1104–8.

Androutsos G. Giovanni-Battista Morgagni (1682-1773): creator of pathological anatomy. J BUON. 2006;11:95–101.

Arana Iniguez R. Echinococcus. In: Vinken PJ, Bruyn GW, editors. Handbook of neurology. Amsterdam: North Holland Publishing Co; 1978. p. 175–208.

Arseni C, Ciurea AV, Cristescu A, Horvath L, Marinescu V. Parasitoses of the central nervous system. Bucharest: The Scientific and Encyclopedic Publishing House; 1981.

Azambuja N. Román Arana Iñíguez R (1909-1977) (in Spanish). Acta Neurol Latinoam. 1977;23:1–6.

Ba'assiri A, Haddad FS. Primary extradural intracranial hydatid disease, CT appearance. AJNR Am J Neuroradiol. 1984;5:474–5.

Balak N, Cavumirza C, Yildirim H, Ozdemir S, Kinay D. Microsurgery in the removal of a large cerebral hydatid cyst: technical case report. Neurosurgery. 2006;59(4 Suppl 2):ONSE486.

Benkhadra M, Salomon C, Trouilloud P. François Chaussier (1746-1828). A vision of the anatomic nomenclature based on education (in French). Morphologie. 2008;92:195–8.

Bryan CP. The Papyrus Ebers (translated from the German). London: Geoffrey Bles; 1930.

Carmody J. Sir Harold Robert (1891-1962). Australian Dictionary of Biography, National Centre of Biography, Australian National University. 2012 http://adb.anu.edu.au/biography/dew-sir-harold-robert-9961/text17649. Accessed 4 June 2012.

Castiglioni A. Storia della Medicina. Milano: Edizioni Mondadori, Italia; 1936.

Cox FEG. History of human parasitology. Clin Microbiol Rev. 2003;16:174.

Craig CF, Faust EC. Craig & Faust's clinical parasitology. 8th ed. Holland: Lea & Feibiger; 1970.

Dew HR. Hydatid disease. Adelaide: Spiller; 1928.

Dew HR. Primary cerebral hydatid disease. Aust N Z J Surg. 1955;24:161–71.

De Villiers Hamman H, Joubert MJ. A review of hydatid disease of the brain. S Afr Med J. 1975;31:1163–7.

Dowling E, Orlando R. Quist hidatico del lobulo frontal derecho. Rev Espec Assoc Med Argent. 1929;4:209–17.

Eckert J, Deplazes P. Biological, epidemiological, and clinical aspects of echinococcosis, a zoonosis of increasing concern. Clin Microbiol Rev. 2004;17:107–35.

Fielding GH. History of medicine. Philadelphia: WB Saunders Company; 1966.

Foster WD. A history of parasitology. Edinburgh: Livingstone; 1965. p. 29–51.

Goichon AM. IBN SINA, Abu 'Ali al-Husayn b. 'Abd Allah b. Sina, known in the West as Avicenna. Encyclopedia of Islam. Brill Publishers; 1999.

Haas LF. Aretaeus of Cappadocia (130-200). J Neurol Neurosurg Psychiatry. 1991;54:203.

Haas LF. Luis Morquio (1867-1935) Neurological stamp. J Neurol Neurosurg Psychiatry. 2002;72:787.

Işlekel S, Erşahin Y, Zileli M, Oktar N, Oner K, Ovül I, Ozdamar N, Tunçbay E. Spinal hydatid disease. Spinal Cord. 1998a;36:166–70.

Işlekel S, Zileli M, Erşahin Y. Intradural spinal hydatid cysts. Eur Spine J. 1998b;7:162–4.

Kattan YB. Management of hydatid disease. Ann R Coll Surg Engl. 1997;59:108.

Kudlien F. Aretaeus of Cappadocia. Dictionary of Scientific Biography. 1. New York: Charles Scribner's Sons; 1970. p. 234–5.

Kune GA, Jones T, Sali A. Hydatid disease in Australia. Prevention, clinical presentation, and treatment. Med J Aust. 1983;2:385–8.

Lazar L. Synopsis of medical parasitology. Bucharest: Carol Davila University Press; 2010.

Luria AR, Karasseva TA. Disturbances of auditory-speech memory in focal lesions of the deep regions of the left temporal lobe. Neuropsychologia. 1968;6:97–104.

Maguire, ' Diet, des Sciences Medicales/t. xxxiii, art. Moelle/' 1819.

MacPherson CN, Zeykle E, Romig T. An Echinococcus pilot control program for north-west Turkana, Kenya. Ann Trop Med Parasitol. 1984;78:188–92.

Pamir MN, Ozduman K, Elmaci I. Spinal hydatid disease. Spinal Cord. 2002;40:153–60.

Patterson KD. Echinococcosis (hydatidosis). In: Kiple KF, editor. The Cambridge world history of human disease. New York: Cambridge University Press; 1993. p. 703.

Pissiotis CA, Wander JV, Condon RE. Surgical treatment of hydatid disease: prevention of complications and recurrences. Arch Surg. 1972;104:454–9.

Prousalidis I. Echinococcosis (in Greek). Thessaloniki, Macedonia; 2007.

Risse GB. Glimpses of a hidden burden: hydatid disease in eighteenth century Scotland. Bull Hist Med. 2005;79:534–43.

Ruffer MA. Studies in the palaeopathology of Egypt. Chicago: The University of Chicago press; 1921a.

Ruffer MA. The paleopathology of ancient Egypt. Chicago: Chicago University Press; 1921b.

Saidi F. Surgery of hydatid disease. London/Philadelphia/Toronto: WB Saunders; 1976.

Schnepper GD, Johnson WD. Recurrent spinal hydatidosis in North America. Case report and review of the literature. Neurosurg Focus. 2004;17:E8.

Sullivan R. A brief journey into medical care and disease in ancient Egypt. J R Soc Med. 1995;88:141–5.
Syrmos N. Historical back training in most important points of neurosurgery. Master thesis, Thessaloniki, Macedonia, 2007 (in Greek).
Syrmos N. Endoscopic anatomy of the upper part of the fourth ventricle (PhD thesis) (in Greek). Thessaloniki, Macedonia, 2009.
Syrmos N, Ampatzidis G, Fachantidou A, Mouratidis I, Syrmos C. Historical back training in most important points of neurosurgery. Ann Gen Psychiatry. 2010;9:S89.
Syrmos NC. Microcephaly in ancient Greece -the Minoan Microcephalus of Zakros. Childs Nerv Syst. 2011;27:685–6.
Walters TMH. Hydatid control scheme in South Powys, Wales, UK. Ann Trop Med Parasitol. 1984;78:183–7.
Weber G. Areteo di Cappadocia: interpretazioni e aspetti della formazione anatomo-patologica del Morgagni. Florence; 1996.
Webster GA, Cameron TW. Epidemiology and diagnosis of echinococcus in Canada. Can Med Assoc J. 1967;96:600–7.

Recommended Reading

Carmell A. Aiding Talmud study. New York: Feldheim Publishers; 1986.
Contributions of Professor Luis Morquio to the study of intracranial hydatid cyst in children (in undetermined language). Arch Pediatr Urug. 1950;21:235–7.
Eckert J, Gemmell MA, Meslin FX, Pawłowski ZS. WHO/OIE manual on echinococcosis in humans and animals: a public health problem of global concern. Paris: World Organization for Animal Health (Office International des Epizooties) and World Health Organization; 2001.
Hartmann P. Miscellanea curiosa (Nuremberg: Adelbulneri, 1705); see excerpts in English of Hartmann's "Vesicular Worms or Hydatids in the Omenta of Goats". In: Kean et al., Classic Investigations (n. 7), p. 619–20.

Hydatidosis of the Central Nervous System in Mediterranean Countries and the Middle East

2

Mohammed Benzagmout and Meryem Himmiche

Contents

M. Benzagmout, MD (✉)
Department of Neurosurgery, Clinical Neurosciences Laboratory, Faculty of Medicine and Pharmacy, University Hospital of Fez, 8589 Atlas, Fez 30003, Morocco
e-mail: benzagmout@hotmail.fr

M. Himmiche, MD
Department of Neurosurgery, University Hospital of Fez, BP.1893, Km 2.200 Sidi Hrazem Road, Fez 30000, Morocco

Introduction

Hydatidosis, also known as echinococcosis or hydatid disease, is a parasitic infection caused by the larval stages of taeniid cestodes of the genus *Echinococcus*. Six species have been identified, but four are of public health concern: *Echinococcus granulosus* (which causes cystic echinococcosis), *E. multilocularis* (which causes alveolar echinococcosis), and *E. vogeli* and *E. oligarthrus* (which cause polycystic echinococcosis) (Moro and Schantz 2009).

Both cystic echinococcosis (CE) caused by *E. granulosus* and alveolar echinococcosis (AE) caused by *E. multilocularis* have been reported in several countries of the Mediterranean region and Middle East. *E. granulosus* is the most common species present in the Mediterranean region, while *E. multilocularis* has been reported only sporadically in limited areas of France, Italy, Serbia and Montenegro, Tunisia, and Turkey (Dakkak 2010).

Hydatidosis has a wide geographical distribution affecting many countries of all continents. Indeed, hydatid disease affects about two to three million people living in endemic areas around the world, particularly in South America, the Mediterranean littoral, Middle East, Central Asia, Australia, New Zealand, and South Africa (Carrea et al. 1975; Altinörs et al. 1995; Khanfar 2004). This disorder is widespread in all mentioned countries, especially in rural communities, and continues to be a major public health problem in the entire Mediterranean zone and all

M. Turgut (ed.), *Hydatidosis of the Central Nervous System: Diagnosis and Treatment*,
DOI 10.1007/978-3-642-54359-3_2, © Springer-Verlag Berlin Heidelberg 2014

the Middle East countries (Anderson et al. 1997; Turgut 1997; Al Zain et al. 2002; Charrada-Ben-Farhat et al. 2006; Limaiem et al. 2010).

The liver and lung are the most frequently infected organs. The brain is involved in 2–3 % of all body localizations, whereas the spine in less than 1 %. Hence, central nervous system (CNS) involvement is fortunately rare compared to somatic localizations. However, it causes severe and permanent disabilities affecting functional and vital prognosis and gives rise to high economic losses.

Despite its morbidity and mortality and its perceived importance by the World Health Organization (WHO), prevention, early diagnosis, and treatment of hydatid disease still remain a serious health problem in developing countries of the world including South America, Australasia, the Mediterranean region, and the Middle East. In this review, we will focus on the epidemiological data of hydatidosis in the Mediterranean littoral and Middle East countries. Finally, we will stress the socioeconomic impact and control measures which should be applied to eradicate this parasitic infection.

Epidemiology

Countries of the north bank of the Mediterranean have more favorable socioeconomic conditions than those of the south bank and thus different prevalence of the disease. In fact, hydatidosis is endemic across the Mediterranean basin especially in the south bank and in all the west Asian countries of the Middle East (Anderson et al. 1997; Dar and Alkarmi 1997). The annual incidence of hydatidosis in these countries varies between 1 and 27 cases per 100,000 inhabitants with most being in the 5–10 cases per 100,000 ranges. It is estimated that close to half a million people across this endemic area are living with CE (Craig et al. 2007).

This geographical region is characterized by major shared affinities of a hot and dry climate; an arid, desert, or semiarid land mass; and linguistic and sociocultural ethnocentricity. It is well known that the rural population of the Mediterranean region and the Middle East has always depended on animals as sources of food, transport, labor, and companionship. Besides the rapid socioeconomic growth, agricultural and animal husbandry practices have great impact on the maintenance of the endemicity of CE in these regions (Dar and Alkarmi 1997).

In this chapter, we summarize the epidemiological status of hydatidosis in each country of the Mediterranean basin and the Middle East. The prevalence of hydatidosis in Mediterranean and Middle East countries could be divided in three different levels of endemicity: high, medium, and low. The geographical map shows the distribution of the disease in each country according to the strength of the endemicity (Fig. 2.1). However, various data are still missing considering the lack of complete epidemiological information about some countries allowing a better mapping of the disease.

Hydatidosis in Countries of the North Bank of the Mediterranean

Spain

Hydatidosis is still an endemic disease in Spain. The prevalence reached considerable rates up until a few years ago. Although specific control programs initiated in the 1980s have led to marked reductions in CE infection rates, the disease remains an important human and animal health problem in the northeastern, central, and western parts of Spain (Carmena et al. 2008). In the municipality of Madrid, hydatidosis affected 2.88 % of sheep (Rodrigo et al. 1997). In La Roja region, the overall prevalence reached 20.3 % of adult sheep and up to 23 % of sheep and cows (Jiménez et al. 2002).

The Spanish official statistics showed a decrease in the human incidence of CE from 2.52 (in 1982) to 1.01 cases per 100,000 inhabitants (in 1996) (Rojo-Vazquez et al. 2011). In the northeastern, central, and western parts of the country, human incidence rates are in the range of 1.1–3.4 cases per 100,000 inhabitants. However, in Salamanca, the incidence rate reached 10.8 per 100,000 inhabitants in the same period, twice

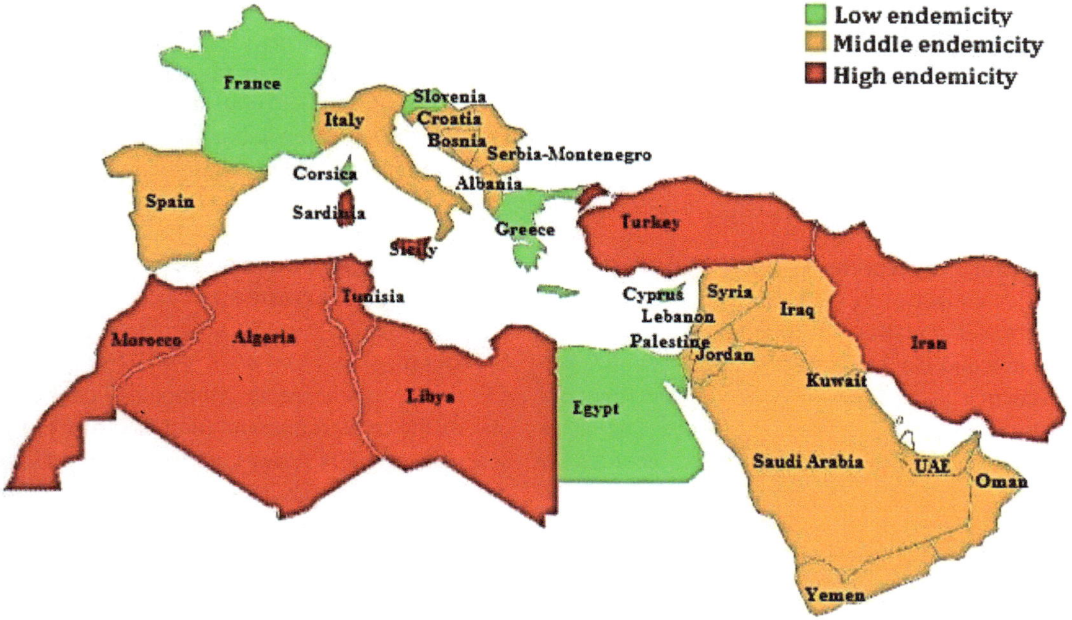

Fig. 2.1 The geographical map demonstrating the distribution of the disease according to the strength of endemicity in Mediterranean and Middle East countries

as many as previously reported, suggesting a potential reemergence of the disease (Pardo et al. 2005).

France

The prevalence of hydatidosis from 1994 to 1996 in the Midi-Pyrénées showed a marked decrease in livestock (2.5 %), while local human cases of hydatidosis were less than 0.28 per 100,000 inhabitants (Bichet and Dorchies 1998). From 1966 to 1970, the average annual incidence of human CE was 10 and 4.5 per 100,000 inhabitants in Corsica and in some eastern regions, respectively (Seimenis and Battelli 2003). In addition, AE has been reported in central France, while the Auvergne region represents the most south-western extension of this disease (Magnaval et al. 2004). Recently, the European Centre for Disease Prevention and Control reported 17 human cases of AE in 2005.

Cerebral occurrence of *E. multilocularis* disease is rare, accounting for only 1 % of cases. In a survey of 387 patients with AE, Piarroux et al. (2011) have showed that isolated extrahepatic locations of AE account for 4 % of the French cases with spinal and brain involvement in five cases and three cases, respectively (Piarroux et al. 2011).

Italy

Most cases of hydatidosis are recorded in the south of Italy and islands (Fabiani et al. 1980). In fact, the incidence of CE is considered high in Sardinia and Sicily, moderate in the central and southern regions, and low in the remaining areas of Italy (Garippa 2006). With over 1,000 cases requiring surgery each year, Italy is considered as a medium- to high-risk country for human hydatidosis (Dionigi et al. 2007).

The latest surveys on animal epidemiology have shown persistent high regional prevalence in sheep: 76 % in 1995–2000 and 68–75 % during the more recent 2004–2009 survey, ranging from 58 to 83 % in the different provinces, with 10–28 % of sheep harboring fertile cysts (Conchedda et al. 2010).

Human incidence rates in Sardinia was as high as 14.32 per 100,000 inhabitants in the 1940–1950s (Giromini and Granati 1954). Twenty years later, different surveys showed that the human incidence decreased from 14.6 per 100,000 inhabitants in 1969–1973 to 9.8 per 100,000 inhabitants in 1990–1995. During the period 2001–2005, CE still represents a serious health problem in Sardinia. Currently, the mean annual incidence is 6.62 per 100,000 inhabitants (Conchedda et al. 2010).

Former Yugoslavia-Affiliated Countries

CE is known to be endemic in these countries (Seimenis and Battelli 2003; Dakkak 2010). In Bosnia and Herzegovina, the disease is endemic particularly in the region of Herzegovina (Obradović et al. 2006). In Albania, 169 cases of unilocular echinococcosis were recorded in the country in 2010. Approximately 50 % of cases were aged between 16 and 40 years old (Berger 2010). Nevertheless, the AE incidence in Slovenia in 2001–2005 has been estimated at 0.45 per 100,000 inhabitants, with a mean annual incidence of 0.09 cases per 100,000 inhabitants (Logar et al. 2007).

Greece

CE remains a serious problem in Greece for both the public health and the livestock economy. The disease was widely prevalent long before the 1970s. The prevalence of infection in farm animals was as high as 82 % in cattle, 80 % in sheep, 24 % in goats, and 5 % in pigs. The surgical human cases reached 12.9 per 100,000 inhabitants in 1984 (Sotiraki et al. 2003). According to the National Statistical Service of Greece and the Greek Ministry of Health, the incidence of human CE in the period of 1977–1981 was estimated to be 10.9 per 100,000 inhabitants (Sotiraki et al. 2003).

Between 1969 and 1975, Karpathios et al. (1985) carried out a retrospective study to estimate the surgical incidence of hydatidosis among Greeks over 18 years old by collecting records from various communities and private hospitals (Karpathios et al. 1985). According to their findings, 4,202 adult patients were diagnosed with hydatidosis (600 per year) giving an annual incidence of 9.77 per 100,000 inhabitants while 3,397 (80.8 %) underwent surgery (485 patients per year or 7.9 surgical cases per 100,000 inhabitants). Recent data from reported cases indicate a further reduction in incidence. More precisely, the number of human cases reported was 46 (0.45 per 100,000 inhabitants) in 1999 and 0.3 per 100,000 inhabitants in 2008 (Sotiraki and Chaligiannis 2010).

Hydatidosis in Countries of the South Bank of Mediterranean

Morocco

CE is hyperendemic in Morocco, where it is one of the most important zoonoses, and represents a potentially serious public health and economic problem. Epidemiological studies have shown high prevalence rate both in humans and domestic animals, in most agropastoral regions. The first Moroccan series was reported in 1924 by Duckster including 24 cases from Cocard Hospital of Fez (Moroccan Ministry of Health 2007). The repartition of the disease is variable. The Atlas Mountains area is mostly infested compared to the Saharan regions. Indeed, 1.1 % of Berber people in the mid-Atlas mountain region are infested (Macpherson et al. 2004).

In Morocco, the disease is predominant in cow- and sheep-farming regions especially the region of Chaouia-Ouardigha, Meknes-Tafilalet, and Doukkala-Abda (Moroccan Ministry of Health 2007). Recently, Azlaf and Dakak (2006) conducted an epidemiological study aimed to update the prevalence of CE in different animal species living in the most important areas of the country. The global CE infection prevalence rates obtained were 10.58 % in sheep, 1.88 % in goats, 22.98 % in cattle, 12.03 % in camels, and 17.80 % in equines. The infection rates were high in middle Atlas in cattle (48.72 %) and in Northwest in cattle and sheep (37.61 % and 31.65 %, respectively).

In humans, the incidence of CE infection varies between 3.6 and 15.8/100,000 inhabitants (Anderson et al. 1997). Recently, 1,403 surgical human cases were recorded in the country in 2006, representing an annual rate of 4.55 cases per 100,000 inhabitants. Surgeries had to be repeated in 7–10 % and a mortality rate of 2–3 %

was observed (Moroccan Ministry of Health 2007). In addition, a human ultrasound screening performed in the middle Atlas Mountains showed much higher prevalence (1 %) than the surgery cases (Kachani et al. 2003).

Concerning CNS hydatidosis, most of the reports consisted of single case reports or small series (Ouboukhlik et al. 1994; Tizniti et al. 2000; El Quessar et al. 2001; Basraoui et al. 2010). These reports state that CNS hydatidosis is rare and constitutes 2 % of all locations (Tizniti et al. 2000). It mostly involves children and young adults (Basraoui et al. 2010; El Abbassi-Skalli et al. 2000) with a mean age of 30 years and male predominance (Ouboukhlik et al. 1994; El Abbassi-Skalli et al. 2000).

Algeria

CE is hyperendemic in Algeria essentially in the northeast of the country and constitutes an important public health problem. Several studies were performed at the beginning of the last century. A retrospective epidemiological study was made in 1979 by Larbaoui and Alloula and showed a clear predominance of cystic hydatidosis in rural areas (74 %). 75.3 % of the affected patients were younger than 40 years old (Larbaoui and Alloula 1979). Each year, more than 700 surgical cases are recorded by the Ministry of Health. Based on hospital records, the reported annual incidence was 3.6–4.6 per 100,000 inhabitants (Shambesh 1997).

Brain hydatidosis is a disease of childhood. This data was confirmed in a series of 99 patients operated for intracranial hydatidosis between 2000 and 2007 in four departments of neurosurgery in Algeria (two in Algiers, one in Annaba, and one in Constantine). 59.5 % of patients were 15 years old or younger (Abdennebi 2009).

Tunisia

CE is hyperendemic in Tunisia and represents a major public health problem due to its high prevalence, morbidity, and economic losses. It is a predominantly rural disease (80.3 % of patients). The annual human incidence of surgical cases of CE is approximately 15 cases per 100,000 inhabitants (Anon 1993). In central Tunisia, 3,986 cases of surgical echinococcosis were identified during 1982–1985, corresponding to an annual rate of 19.3 cases per 100,000 inhabitants (Bchir et al. 1989). Additionally, two autochthonous cases of *E. multilocularis* infection have been reported in humans from a mountainous region of northern Tunisia (Eckert et al. 2001).

Recently, Bellil et al. (2009) have analyzed the epidemiological features of 265 Tunisian cases of extrapulmonary hydatid cysts collected from 1990 to 2007 in the La Rabta Hospital, Bab Saâdoun, Tunis. They found that hydatidosis involved the CNS in 22.6 % of cases (Bellil et al. 2009). From the same hospital, Limaiem et al. (2010) reviewed retrospectively a series of 39 cases of primary CNS hydatid cysts operated between 1998 and 2007. They found that the disease involved mainly children (33.3 %). The mean age of all patients was 26.5 years old and the male/female ratio was equal. In this series, intracranial hydatid cysts represent 69.2 % (27 cases) and spinal hydatid cysts 30.8 % of cases (12 cases).

Libya

Echinococcosis is highly endemic in Libya. The incidence of surgically confirmed CE in eastern Libya was estimated to be at least 4.2 cases per 100,000 inhabitants, with a clear female predominance (Tashani et al. 2002). In addition, the ultrasound and serology investigations revealed that 1.6 % of population living in the northern Libya had the disease (Shambesh et al. 1999).

Hydatidosis in Western Middle East Countries

Turkey

Turkey is the typical example where echinococcosis is a common parasitic disease causing a serious public health and economic problem (Altinörs et al. 2000). Both CE and AE have been reported. CE is widespread throughout Turkey, whereas AE predominantly occurs in the eastern Anatolian region of the country (Altintas 2003).

According to the Ministry of Health records, 21,303 patients were operated for CE between

1987 and 1994; this corresponds to approximately 2,663 patients per year (Altintas 2003). The estimated surgical case rate ranged from 0.87 to 6.6 per 100,000 inhabitants in Turkey between 1987 and 1994 (Altintas 2003).

A retrospective study based on hospital, regional, and ministerial documents has shown that, from 2001 to 2005, a total of 14,789 CE surgical cases were recorded including 13.13 % that were diagnosed in the Marmara region, 16.94 % in the Aegean region, 16.09 % in the Mediterranean region, 38.57 % in the middle Anatolian region, 5.70 % in the Black Sea region, 6.80 % in the eastern Anatolian region, and 2.75 % in the southeastern Anatolian region (Yazar et al. 2008).

Brain hydatidosis represents 2 % of all space-occupying lesions in Turkish population (Engin et al. 2000). In 2001, Turgut reviewed a series of 276 Turkish cases of intracranial hydatidosis published since 1960. He noticed that most patients with intracranial hydatidosis were males (61 %), from rural areas (Turgut 2001). Cysts were generally located in the cerebral hemispheres and 18 % of patients had other organ infestation (Turgut 2001). He concluded that dimensions, localizations, and numbers of the cysts are the most important prognostic factors (Turgut 2001). The operative mortality rate in this series was 9 % (Turgut 2001). Similarly, Turgut (1997) have reviewed 28 reports of spinal hydatid disease from Turkey published between 1944 and 1996 (Turgut 1997). Turgut (2001) found a clear male predominance (73 %) and that 75 % of patients were aged between 30 and 50 years old. Cysts affecting the spine were commonly observed in the thoracic region and most patients had intraspinal extradural hydatid cysts associated with vertebral involvement (Turgut 2001). He concluded that spinal hydatid disease is still a life-threatening condition in Turkey despite all advances achieved in diagnostic procedures, surgical techniques, and antimicrobial therapeutics (Turgut 2001).

Cyprus

CE was widespread in Cyprus before the 1970s. It was a serious public health problem, with an annual surgical incidence rate of 12.9 per 100,000 inhabitants. In 1971, the first CE eradication campaign was implemented. After 1974, the control program was suspended in the north, while it continued in the southern part of Cyprus until 1985. At that time, the parasite was considered eradicated from both livestock and dogs, and the campaign was officially terminated. However, intermittent outbreaks discovered during slaughterhouse inspections led to reintroduction of the control program in 1993 (Economides and Christofi 2000). Currently, it is considered that echinococcosis transmission has been successfully interrupted in Cyprus as well as Iceland, New Zealand, and Tasmania (Eckert 2001).

Syria and Lebanon

CE is endemic in Syria, mainly in southern and northeastern provinces. Northern Syria, the main area of the country for livestock production, sheep rising, and nomadic tribal life, seems to be the most affected area. In Syria and Lebanon, the prevalence of *E. granulosus* infection in dogs appears to vary between 9 and 15 % (Seimenis and Battelli 2003), while in livestock, CE prevalence rates are estimated to be between 5 and 17 %, with the highest level in ruminants and donkeys (Seimenis and Battelli 2003).

In Lebanon, Abou-Daoud and Schwabe (1964) reported an incidence of 3.8 cases per 100,000 populations based on surgical records. The annual rate was estimated at 1.38 per 100,000 (1970–1985) (Berger 2010). However, there is no available published data on the current prevalence of human CE in these countries.

Palestine and Israel

Hydatidosis is endemic in Palestine. Abdel-Hafez and Kamhawi (1997) reported that the annual surgical prevalence of CE recorded from the Al-Maqased Hospital in Jerusalem was 1.76 per 100,000 inhabitants in 1995. Abu-Hassan et al. (2002) investigated the surgical incidence of the Palestinian West Bank hospitals between January 1990 and December 1997 (Abu-Hasan et al. 2002); he showed that the annual mean incidence was 3.1 per 100,000 inhabitants, with the highest rates of 4.9, 5.0, and 5.1 per 100,000 inhabitants found in Hebron, Jericho, and Bethlehem, respectively.

Epidemiological studies have reported a high prevalence of CE in both humans and animals in northern Israel (Shimshony 1997). In 2002, Youngster et al. conducted an epidemiological study in northern Israel and found a cumulative infection rate of 1.5 per 100,000 inhabitants, which is comparable to reports of worldwide endemic areas.

Jordan

Human CE is one of the most important endemic infectious diseases in Jordan. The annual rate of human infection was estimated to 2.9 per 100,000 in 1995 (Berger 2010). In serological study, serum samples from 2,388 subjects living in rural-agricultural, semi-Bedouin and Bedouin communities of Jordan showed 7.7 % positivity (Qaqish et al. 2003). Between January 1994 and September 2003, 65 patients from northern Jordan were treated for hydatid cyst in the Department of Surgery, Jordan University hospitals of Irbid. Forty-six percent of patients were below 40 years old and 57 % were females (Yaghan et al. 2004).

CNS hydatidosis is much more common in children than adults. The infant intracranial hydatid disease represents 50–75 % of total infection; the parietal lobe was mostly involved (Khanfar 2004). These data was in accordance with Al-Akayleh who prospectively analyzed five cases of intracranial hydatid cysts managed at the King Hussein Medical Centre, Amman, between 1993 and 2002. Al-Akayleh (2003) found that intracranial hydatidosis represented an incidence of 0.04 % of all space-occupying lesions operated during the studied period. All patients came from rural area and the average age of presentation was 9.4 years old (Al-Akayleh 2003).

Egypt

A survey for hydatidosis among slaughtered animals at two abattoirs in Ismailia and Cairo showed an infection rate of 4.8 % in sheep, 1.2 % in goats, 0.95 % in cattle, 0.46 % in buffalo, and 18.9 % in camels (Sadjjadi 2006). Although human CE is currently of low endemicity, this zoonotic disease may represent a public health concern in Egypt. A retrospective hospital study conducted by Kandeel et al. (2004) showed an annual surgical incidence varying between 1.34 and 2.60 per 100,000 inhabitants (Kandeel et al. 2004).

Hydatidosis in Eastern Middle East Countries

Iran

CE is highly prevalent in Iran, especially in sheep-grazing areas of East Azerbaijan and Kurdistan (Miabi et al. 2005). Cases of human hydatidosis are regularly reported from medical centers in different parts of the nation. Indeed, CE is responsible for approximately 1 % of admission to surgical wards and the rate of human infection is 0.6–1.2 (Rokni 2009). CNS involvement is seen in 2–3 % of patients and affects mainly young adults (Miabi et al. 2005). In addition, Iran is known as endemic areas of *E. multilocularis*. During a period of 3.5 years, 37 human cases of AE were diagnosed in various hospitals, most of them in the Ardabil province (Zariffard and Massoud 1998).

Iraq

Epidemiological studies on CE in Arbil province, northern Iraq, between 1990 and 1998 showed a human prevalence of 2/100,000 inhabitants (Saeed et al. 2000). In 2002, Al Zain et al. published a series of 34 patients with multiple intracranial hydatidosis collected from a retrospective study of intracranial hydatidosis cases managed at the Neurosurgical Hospital, Baghdad, and the Department of Neurosurgery, College of Medicine, Baghdad University, between 1976 and 1999. The age of patients varied between 3 and 55 years, with 26 patients under 20 years old (76.5 %) (Al Zain et al. 2002). There was a female predominance and the duration of symptoms was between 1 month and 3 years (Al Zain et al. 2002).

Hydatidosis in Arabic Persian Gulf Countries

CE is endemic in Kuwait, Yemen, Oman, Saudi Arabia, and some region of the United Arab Emirates (Sadjjadi 2006; Idris et al. 1999).

In Kuwait, the first report of human echinococcosis was published in 1962 (El Gazzar 1962). It concerned 51 cases of proved hydatidosis (including only five native Kuwaitis) admitted to the State hospitals from 1956 to 1960 inclusive. This represents an average of ten admissions per year and an incidence of 3.8 per 100,000 inhabitants. In 1990, an estimated incidence rate of 3.6 per 100,000 inhabitants has been reported (Shweiki et al. 1990; Dar and Alkarmi 1997). About 2 % of cases of hydatid disease have cerebral involvement (Rudwan and Khaffaji 1988).

In Saudi Arabia, echinococcosis is most common in southwestern province, followed by central province. Sixty-three percent of patients are women involved in sheep raising (Laajam and Nouh 1991). Besides, Malaika et al. (1981) reported that hydatidosis surgical cases represent 5 % of all major surgical operations performed in Saudi Arabia hospitals.

Socioeconomic Impact

Hydatidosis is highly prevalent in Mediterranean and Middle East countries; it continues to be a public health concern with negative impact on patients' health status on one hand and on financial resources of the nation (due to prolonged hospitalization periods and sick leaves and expensive treatment) on the other hand (Eckert et al. 2000). Benner et al. (2010) attempted to calculate the overall economic losses due to human and animal CE in Spain in 2005. They estimated the annual loss to approximately 149 million Euros (133 million Euros due to human ill health and 16 million Euros to animal health losses).

Economic evaluations have been undertaken also in Tunisia (Majorowski et al. 2005) and in Jordan (Torgerson et al. 2001). Results indicated that echinococcosis represents a substantial economic effect in relation to the respective countries' gross domestic product, probably up to 0.5 % of the total economic activity for these countries. Indeed in Turkey, the annual production losses due to CE in livestock have been estimated at 89 million dollars (Sariozkan and Yalcin 2009). These show a need to increase monitoring and control of CE in countries where the disease is widely distributed and still represents a considerable public health problem.

Control Program

During the last 20 years, considerable progress in the control of the disease has been recorded in countries of the northern Mediterranean littoral such as Spain, France, Italy, Greece, and Cyprus as a result of various implemented control measures. However, it should be reminded that the social, cultural, and economic conditions in these countries are more favorable for eradicating the hydatid disease.

In fact, the intersectorial collaboration and coordination between all competent authorities including the veterinary, medical, public health, and other governmental and nongovernmental organizations are the key to a successful control of echinococcosis (Seimenis 2003). However, prevention remains the best strategy of control and has been successful in many experienced countries, such as New Zealand, Australia, and China.

Unfortunately, effective control of hydatidosis has not yet been achieved in many countries of Mediterranean as well as Middle East regions despite extensive health education campaigns. Therefore, further efficient control programs are mandatory in order to reduce the incidence of this devastating parasitic disease (Limaiem et al. 2010).

Conclusion

Mediterranean and Middle East countries remain the predilection sites of hydatidosis. However, it is impossible to establish a precise hydatidosis epidemiological profile of each Mediterranean and Middle East countries. The current available data are very heterogeneous depending on each country and do not allow drawing equivalent epidemiological profiles based on the same epidemiological factors.

In addition, the human mass migration interferes considerably in determining the exact incidence of hydatidosis in concerned countries. Indeed, societies of Mediterranean and Middle East countries became more and more open to human and animal exchange. This makes individual country program less efficient and only collaborative programs between all involved countries including those "exporting" the disease might help to better eradicate the hydatid disease.

References

Abdel-Hafez SK, Kamhawi S. Cystic echinococcosis in the Levant countries (Jordan, Palestinian Authority, Israel, Syria, and Lebanon). In: Anderson FL, Ouheli H, Kachani M, editors. Compendium on cystic echinococcosis in Africa and Middle Eastern countries with special reference to Morocco. Pravo: Brigham Young University; 1997. p. 292–316.

Abdennebi B. Parasitoses of the central nervous system: hydatidosis. In: Practical handbook of neurosurgery, vol. 1. Wien: Springer; 2009.

Abou-Daoud K, Schwabe CW. Epidemiology of echinococcosis in the Middle East. III. A study of hydatid disease patients from the city of Beirut. Am J Trop Med Hyg. 1964;13:681–5.

Abu-Hasan N, Daragmeh M, Adwan K, Al-Qaoud K, Abdel-Hafez SK. Human cystic echinococcosis in the West Bank of Palestine: surgical incidence and seroepidemiological study. Parasitol Res. 2002;88:107–12.

Al-Akayleh A. Intracranial hydatid cysts: diagnosis and treatment. Bahrain Med Bull. 2003;25:91–4.

Altintas N. Past to present: echinococcosis in Turkey. Acta Trop. 2003;85:105–12.

Altinörs N, Bavbek M, Caner HH, Erdogan B. Central nervous system hydatidosis in Turkey: a cooperative study and literature survey analysis of 458 cases. J Neurosurg. 2000;93:1–8.

Altinörs N, Senveli E, Dönmez T, Bavbek M, Kars Z, Sanli M. Management of problematic intracranial hydatid cysts. Infection. 1995;23:283–7.

Al Zain TJ, Al-Witry SH, Khalili HM, Aboud SH, Al Zain Jr FT. Multiple intracranial hydatidosis. Acta Neurochir (Wien). 2002;144:1179–85.

Anderson FL, Ouhelli H, Kashani M. Compendium on cystic echinococcosis in Africa and in Middle Eastern countries with special reference to Morocco. Provo: Brigham Young University; 1997.

Annual report of fighting against hydatidosis/Echinococcosis: activities guide. Publication of the department of parasitical diseases. Direction of epidemiology and diseases fighting. Moroccan Ministry of Health, 2007.

Anon T. The surgical incidence rate of hydatidosis in Tunisia (1988-1992). Report of the D.S.S.B. (Direction de Santé et des Soins de base). Tunis: Ministry Public Health; 1993.

Azlaf R, Dakkak A. Epidemiological study of the cystic echinococcosis in Morocco. Vet Parasitol. 2006;137:83–93.

Basraoui D, El Idrissi I, Jalal H, Hiroual M, Essadki O, Ousehal A, Aniba K, Ghannane H, Lmejjati M, Ait Benali S. Intracranial hydatid cysts in children: a report of 9 cases. J Radiol. 2010;91:293–6.

Bchir A, Larouze B, Hamdi A, Bouden L, Letaiff R, Prazuck T, Dridi M, Gaudebout C, Rousset JJ, Jemmali M. Distribution of surgical hydatidosis in central Tunisia (1982-1985). Acta Trop. 1989;46:47–53.

Bellil S, Limaiem F, Bellil K, Chelly I, Mekni A, Haouet S, Kchir N, Zitouna M. Epidemiology of extrapulmonary hydatid cysts: 265 Tunisian cases. Med Mal Infect. 2009;39:341–3.

Benner C, Carabin H, Sánchez-Serrano LP, Budke CM, Carmena D. Analysis of the economic impact of cystic echinococcosis in Spain. Bull World Health Organ. 2010;88:49–57.

Berger S. Echinococcosis: global status. Amazon: Gideon Informatics; 2010.

Bichet H, Dorchies P. Estimation of the prevalence of bovine hydatid cyst in the south Pyrenees. Parasite. 1998;5:61–8.

Carmena D, Sanchez-Serrano LP, Barbero-Martinez I. Echinococcus granulosus infection in Spain. Zoonoses Public Health. 2008;55:156–65.

Carrea R, Dowling Jr E, Guevara JA. Surgical treatment of hydatid cysts of the central nervous system in the pediatric age (Dowling's technique). Childs Brain. 1975;1:4–21.

Charrada-Ben-Farhat L, Saïd W, Bouslama K, Oueslati S, Dridi L, Rezgui-Marhoul L, Hamzaoui S, Ben Dridi M, Hendaoui L. Vertebral and spinal cord hydatidosis: contribution of imaging. Med Mal Infect. 2006;36:58–61.

Conchedda M, Antonelli A, Caddori A, Gabriele F. A retrospective analysis of human cystic echinococcosis in Sardinia (Italy), an endemic Mediterranean region, from 2001 to 2005. Parasitol Int. 2010;59:454–9.

Craig PS, Budke CM, Schantz PM, Li T, Qiu J, Yang Y, Zeyhle E, Rogan MT, Ito A. Human echinococcosis: a neglected disease? Trop Med Health. 2007;35:283–92.

Dakkak A. Echinococcosis/hydatidosis: a severe threat in Mediterranean countries. Vet Parasitol. 2010;174:2–11.

Dar FK, Alkarmi T. Public health aspects of cystic echinococcosis in the Arab countries. Acta Trop. 1997;67:125–32.

Dionigi G, Carrafiello G, Recaldini C, Sessa F, Boni L, Rovera F, Dionigi R. Laparoscopic resection of a primary hydatid cyst of the adrenal gland: a case report. J Med Case Reports. 2007. doi:10.1186/1752-1947-1-61.

Eckert J. Echinococcosis: an emerging and re-emerging zoonoses. WHO Mediterranean Zoonoses Control Centre Information Circular. 2001;53:13–5. Review.

Eckert J, Conraths FJ, Tackmann K. Echinococcosis: an emerging or re-emerging zoonosis? Int J Parasitol. 2000;30:1283–94.

Eckert J, Deplazes P, Craig PS, Gemmell MA, Gottstein B, Heath D, Jenkins DJ, Kamiya M, Lightowlers M. Echinococcosis in animals: clinical aspects, diagnosis and treatment. In: Eckert J, Gemmel MA, Meslin FX, Pawlowski ZS, editors. WHO/OIE manual on echinococcosis in humans and animals: a public health problem of global concern. Paris: World Animal Health Organization (OIE) and World Health Organisation; 2001. p. 92–9.

Economides P, Christofi G. Evaluation of control programmes for echinococcosis/hydatidosis in Cyprus. Rev Sci Tech. 2000;3:784–92.

El Abbassi-Skalli A, Gharbi A, Adil A, Abdelouafi A, Kadiri R. Intracranial hydatid cyst: contribution of scanography. J Neuroradiol. 2000;27:196–9.

El Gazzar A. Hydatid disease in Kuwait. Br Med J. 1962;28:232–4.

El Quessar A, Jroundi L, Tizniti S, Cissé M, Chakir N, El Hassani MR, Benchaâboun H, Jiddane M. CT and MRI features of spinal hydatidosis. A report of 8 cases. J Radiol. 2001;82:917–21.

Engin G, Acunaş B, Rozanes I, Acunaş G. Hydatid disease with unusual localization. Eur Radiol. 2000;10:1904–12.

Fabiani A, Trebini F, Torta R. Brain hydatidosis: report of two cases. J Neurol Neurosurg Psychiatry. 1980;43:91–4.

Garippa G. Updates on cystic echinococcosis (CE) in Italy. Parasitologia. 2006;48:57–9.

Giromini M, Granati A. Studio su 5048 casi di Idatidosi verificatisi in Italia dal 1941 al 1952. Folia Med. 1954;37:746–70.

Idris MA, Ruppel A, Gehrig-Feistel H, Alansari AS, al-Rejaibi AK, Tageldin MH, el-Sinary K. The seroprevalence of cystic hydatidosis in Oman. Ann Trop Med Parasitol. 1999;93:259–63.

Jiménez S, Pérez A, Gil H, Schantz P, Ramalle E, Juste R. Progress in control of cystic echinococcosis in La Rioja, Spain: decline in infection prevalences in human and animal hosts and economic costs and benefits. Acta Trop. 2002;83:213–21.

Kachani M, Macpherson CN, Lyagoubi M, Berrada M, Bouslikhane M, Kachani F, El Hasnaoui M. Public health education/importance and experience from the field. Educational impact of community-based ultrasound screening surveys. Acta Trop. 2003;85:263–9.

Kandeel A, Ahmed ES, Helmy H, El Setouhy M, Craig PS, Ramzy RM. A retrospective hospital study of human cystic echinococcosis in Egypt. East Mediterr Health J. 2004;10:349–57.

Karpathios T, Fretzayas A, Nicolaidou P, Papadellis F, Vassalos M, Tselentis J, Thomaidis T, Matsaniotis N. Statistical aspects of hydatid disease in Greek adults. Am J Trop Med Hyg. 1985;34:124–8.

Khanfar N. Hydatid disease: a review and update. Curr Anaesth Crit Care. 2004;15:173–83.

Laajam MA, Nouh MS. Hydatidosis: clinical significance and morbidity patterns in Saudi Arabia. East Afr Med J. 1991;68:57–63.

Larbaoui D, Alloula R. Etude épidémiologique de l'hydatidose en Algérie: résultat de deux enquêtes rétrospectives portant sur 10 ans. Tunis Med. 1979;57:318–26.

Limaiem F, Bellil S, Bellil K, Chelly I, Mekni A, Khaldi M, Haouet S, Zitouna M, Kchir N. Primary hydatidosis of the central nervous system: a retrospective study of 39 Tunisian cases. Clin Neurol Neurosurg. 2010;112:23–8.

Logar J, Šoba B, Lejko-Zupanc T, Kotar T. Human alveolar echinococcosis in Slovenia. Clin Microbiol Infect. 2007;13:544–6.

Macpherson CN, Kachani M, Lyagoubi M, Berrada M, Shepherd M, Fields PF, El Hasnaoui M. Cystic echinococcosis in the Berber of the Mid Atlas mountains, Morocco: new insights into the natural history of the disease in humans. Ann Trop Med Parasitol. 2004;98:481–90.

Magnaval JF, Boucher C, Morassin B, Raoul F, Duranton C, Jacquiet P, Giraudoux P, Vuitton DA, Piarroux R. Epidemiology of alveolar echinococcosis in southern Cantal, Auvergne region, France. J Helminthol. 2004;78:237–42.

Majorowski MM, Carabin H, Kilani M, Bensalah A. Echinococcosis in Tunisia: a cost analysis. Trans R Soc Trop Med Hyg. 2005;99:268–78.

Malaika SS, Attayeb A, Sulaimani S, Reddy JJ. Human echinococcosis in Saudi Arabia. Saudi Med J. 1981;2:77–84.

Miabi Z, Hashemi H, Ghaffarpour M, Ghelichnia H, Media R. Clinicoradiological findings and treatment outcome in patients with intracranial hydatid cyst. Acta Med Iran. 2005;43:359–64.

Moro P, Schantz PM. Echinococcosis: a review. Int J Infect Dis. 2009;13:125–33.

Obradović Z, Zerem E, Beslagić Z, Susić A. Echinococcosis in Bosnia and Herzegovina. Med Arh. 2006;60:259–62.

Ouboukhlik A, Choukri M, Elazhari A, Elkamar A, Boucetta M. Cerebral hydatid cysts: apropos of 48 cases (in French). Neurochirurgie. 1994;40:242–6.

Pardo J, Muro A, Galindo I, Cordero M, Carpio A, Siles-Lucas M. Hydatidosis in the province of Salamanca (Spain): should we let down our guard? Enferm Infecc Microbiol Clin. 2005;23:266–9.

Piarroux M, Piarroux R, Giorgi R, Knapp J, Bardonnet K, Sudre B, Watelet J, Dumortier J, Gérard A, Beytout J, Abergel A, Mantion G, Vuitton DA, Bresson-Hadni S. Clinical features and evolution of alveolar echinococcosis in France from 1982 to 2007: results of a survey in 387 patients. J Hepatol. 2011;55:1025–33.

Qaqish AM, Nasrieh MA, Al-Qaoud KM, Craig PS, Abdel-Hafez SK. The seroprevalences of cystic echinococcosis, and the associated risk factors, in rural-agricultural, Bedouin and semi-Bedouin communities in Jordan. Ann Trop Med Parasitol. 2003;97:511–20.

Rodrigo MR, Canizares FJ, Nieto GA, Lopez FCR, Alcalde MS. Ovine hydatidosis in the community of Madrid (Spain). Rev Panam Salud Publica. 1997;5:376–9.

Rojo-Vazquez FA, Pardo-Lledias J, Francos-Von Hunefeld M, Cordero-Sanchez M, Alamo-Sanz R, Hernandez-Gonzalez A, Brunetti E, Siles-Lucas M.

Cystic echinococcosis in Spain: current situation and relevance for other endemic areas in Europe. PLoS Negl Trop Dis. 2011;5:e893.
Rokni MB. Echinococcosis hydatidosis in Iran. Iran J Parasitol. 2009;4:1–16.
Rudwan MA, Khaffaji S. CT of cerebral hydatid disease. Neuroradiology. 1988;30:496–9.
Sadjjadi SM. Present situation of echinococcosis in the Middle East and Arabic North Africa. Parasitol Int. 2006;55:S197–202.
Saeed I, Kapel C, Saida LA, Willingham L, Nansen P. Epidemiology of Echinococcus granulosus in Arbil province, northern Iraq, 1990-1998. J Helminthol. 2000;74:83–8.
Sariozkan S, Yalcin C. Estimating the production losses due to cystic echinococcosis in ruminants in Turkey. Vet Parasitol. 2009;163:330–4.
Seimenis A. Overview of the epidemiological situation on echinococcosis in the Mediterranean region. Acta Trop. 2003;85:191–5.
Seimenis A, Battelli G. Epidemiological situation and surveillance, Issue dedicated on Cystic Echinococcosis and the Mediterranean. WHO Mediterranean Zoonoses Control Centre Information Circular. 2003;57:6–8.
Shambesh MK. Human cystic echinococcosis in North Africa (excluding Morocco). In: Anderson FL, Ouheli H, Kachani M, editors. Compendium on cystic echinococcosis in Africa and Middle Eastern Countries with special reference to Morocco. Pravo: Brigham Young University; 1997. p. 223–44.
Shambesh MA, Craig PS, Macpherson CN, Rogan MT, Gusbi AM, Echtuish EF. An extensive ultrasound and serologic study to investigate the prevalence of human cystic echinococcosis in northern Libya. Am J Trop Med Hyg. 1999;60:462–8.
Shimshony A. Echinococcosis in Israel. Emerg Infect Dis. 1997;2:237.
Shweiki HM, Hira PR, Behbehani K. Cystic hydatid disease: aspects of the incidence in man in Kuwait Arabian Gulf. Eur J Epidemiol. 1990;6:15–9.
Sotiraki S, Chaligiannis I. Cystic echinococcosis in Greece. Past and present. Parasite. 2010;17:205–10.
Sotiraki S, Himonas C, Korkoliakou P. Hydatidosis-echinococcosis in Greece. Acta Trop. 2003;85:197–201.
Tashani OA, Zhang LH, Boufana B, Jegi A, McManus DP. Epidemiology and strain characteristics of Echinococcus granulosus in the Benghazi area of eastern Libya. Ann Trop Med Parasitol. 2002;96:369–81.
Tizniti S, Allali N, El Quessar A, Chakir N, El Hassani MR, Jiddane M. An unusual cerebral hydatid cyst. J Neuroradiol. 2000;27:200–2.
Torgerson PR, Dowling PM, Abo-Shehada MN. Estimating the economic effects of cystic echinococcosis. Part 3: Jordan, a developing country with lower-middle income. Ann Trop Med Parasitol. 2001;95:595–603.
Turgut M. Hydatid disease of the spine: a survey study from Turkey. Infection. 1997;25:221–6.
Turgut M. Intracranial hydatidosis in Turkey: its clinical presentation, diagnostic studies, surgical management, and outcome. A review of 276 cases. Neurosurg Rev. 2001;24:200–8.
Yaghan RJ, Bani-Hani KE, Heis HA. The clinical and epidemiological features of hydatid disease in Northern Jordan. Saudi Med J. 2004;25:886–9.
Yazar S, Ozkan AT, Hökelek M, Polat E, Yilmaz H, Ozbilge H, Ustün S, Koltaş IS, Ertek M, Sakru N, Alver O, Cetinkaya Z, Koç Z, Demirci M, Aktaş H, Parsak CK, Ozerdem D, Sakman G, Cengiz ZT, Ozer A, Keklik K, Yemenici N, Turan M, Daştan A, Kaya E, Tamer GS, Girginkardeşler N, Türk M, Sinirtaş M, Evci C, Kiliçturgay S, Mutlu F, Artiş T. Characterization of different isolates of Echinococcus granulosus in east and southeast regions of Turkey. Acta Trop. 2008;107:192–4.
Youngster I, Hoida G, Craig PS, Sneir R, El-On J. Prevalence of cystic echinococcosis among Muslim and Jewish populations in southern Israel. Acta Trop. 2002;82:369–75.
Zariffard MR, Massoud J. Study of echinococcus granulosus and echinococcus multilocularis infections in Canidiae in Ardabile province of Iran. Arch Razi Inst. 1998;48/49:47–52.

Hydatidosis of the Central Nervous System in South America

3

Claudia I. Menghi and Claudia L. Gatta

Contents

C.I. Menghi, PhD (✉)
Department of Parasitology, Hospital de Clínicas, University of Buenos Aires, Teodoro García 2350, 7 A, Buenos Aires, Argentina

University of Valencia, Valencia, Spain
e-mail: cmenghi@fibertel.com.ar, menghi.claudia@gmail.com

C.L. Gatta
Department of Parasitology, Hospital de Clínicas, University of Buenos Aires, Teodoro García 2350, 7 A, Buenos Aires, Argentina

Introduction

The most frequent species of *Echinococcus* in humans based on morphological criteria are *E. granulosus* and *E. multilocularis*; however, from the 1960s onward, two species from Central and South America, *E. vogeli* and *E. oligarthrus*, have been found (Gutiérrez 2000). The life cycle of these worms is similar to that of *E. granulosus*. Echinococcosis in animals is important because of the economic losses that the infection causes in livestock. Hydatidosis is endemic in several Latin American countries, such as Argentina, Bolivia, Brazil, Chile, Peru, and Uruguay. In the South American continent, *E. granulosus* is the most widespread parasite in dogs and sheep. There are no standard guidelines for case reporting, and methods differ by country. The main site of human infection is the liver. While secondary lesions mainly occur in the lungs, they can also affect the central nervous system (CNS) (Nourbakhsh et al. 2010). *E. granulosus* causes liver cysts in over half of the cases, with lung involvement in 10–40 % of the cases, while brain, periorbital tissue, kidney, and pericardium are affected in 5 % of cases. In contrast, *E. multilocularis* is almost invariably found in the liver but may also reach the lungs or the brain in 5–10 % of cases (Kammerer 1993). Table 3.1 shows the frequency of human cyst localization in Argentina (Guarnera 2009).

E. granulosus infection of the CNS has been estimated at below 2 % (Schantz 1972) and may be primary, often presenting as solitary

M. Turgut (ed.), *Hydatidosis of the Central Nervous System: Diagnosis and Treatment*, DOI 10.1007/978-3-642-54359-3_3, © Springer-Verlag Berlin Heidelberg 2014

Table 3.1 Frequency of location sites of human hydatid cysts in Argentina

Localization	Percentage (%)
Liver	68
Lung	23
Kidney	2
Brain	2
Bone	2
Striated muscle	1
Spleen	1
Multiple sites	1

Modified from Guarnera (2009)

parenchymal cysts, while intraventricular and meningeal locations are most exceptional (Arana Iñiguez et al. 1951). Secondary involvement is due to cyst rupture or hydatid fluid dissemination from a distant organ. CNS echinococcosis is more frequent in children up to 15 years of age with an estimated prevalence rate of 50–75 % (Dew 1955; Slim et al. 1971). A series of cerebral hydatid cysts in children describing diagnostic difficulties, surgical treatment, and possible complications have been reported (Krajewski and Stelmasiak 1991; Ersahin et al. 1993; Ozek 1994; Peter et al. 1994; Turgut 2002). Signs and symptoms include increased intracranial pressure, headache, vomiting, papilledema, and hemiparesis as well as occasional seizures, while meningeal or cranial nerve involvement is most unusual (Arana Iñiguez 1978; Kammerer 1993).

Epidemiology

Hydatidosis in South America

Hydatid disease is endemic in cattle- and sheep-raising regions of the world such as Central Europe, the Mediterranean countries (Tunisia, Spain), the Middle East (Turkey, Lebanon, Emirates), South America (Argentina, Peru, Uruguay, Brazil, Chile, and Bolivia), Australia, New Zealand, India, and South Africa (Carrea et al. 1975). South America is one of the regions of the world most affected by cystic echinococcosis.

Three of the four species of *Echinococcus*, *E. granulosus*, *E. vogeli*, and *E. oligarthrus*, have been described in South America (Fig. 3.1). However, *E. granulosus* presents transmission cycles in domestic animals, being sheep the principal intermediate hosts in this region. The reason for this fact is the great concentration of sheep in this part of the continent and the close relationship between this intermediate host and the definitive host, the dog. There are now approximately 65 million sheep in South America, out of which 63 million (97 %) are found in Argentina, Brazil, Chile, Peru, and Uruguay. These data turn nearly 9 % of the South American territory into a sheep-raising area (Organización Panamericana de la Salud [OPS] 2004). However, in certain regions, various animal species such as pigs, goats, and camelids have gained importance as intermediate hosts. In South America, a few described human cases of alveolar echinococcosis were due to *E. patagonicus* and *E. oligarthrus* (Taratuto and Venturiello 1997). The prevalence rate of infection in the asymptomatic human population obtained from ultrasonographic (US) screenings was 1.6 % in Tacuarembó, Uruguay; 1.6 % in Florida, Uruguay; 3.6 % in Durazno, Uruguay; and 5.1 % in Vichaycocha, Peru. In Argentina, the prevalence rate was 5.5 % in Rio Negro province and 14.2 % in Loncopue, Neuquen province (OPS 2004). Successful control programs based on systematic dog deparasitation with praziquantel have been developed in Uruguay, Chile, and Argentina.

In general, hydatid disease of the CNS is rare, with a reported incidence of 0.9–2.1 % of all cases of hydatidosis (Tamer et al. 2004). A differential diagnosis with other diseases such as abscesses, neoplasias, and other parasitoses such as coenurosis and congenital cysts should be determined (Mahadevan et al. 2011).

Hydatidosis in Argentina

In Argentina, *E. granulosus* is the most prevalent zoonotic helminth. It has been estimated that approximately 30 % of the Argentine territory harbors the domestic life cycle of *E. granulosus*. The provinces where sheep, goat, and cattle rear-

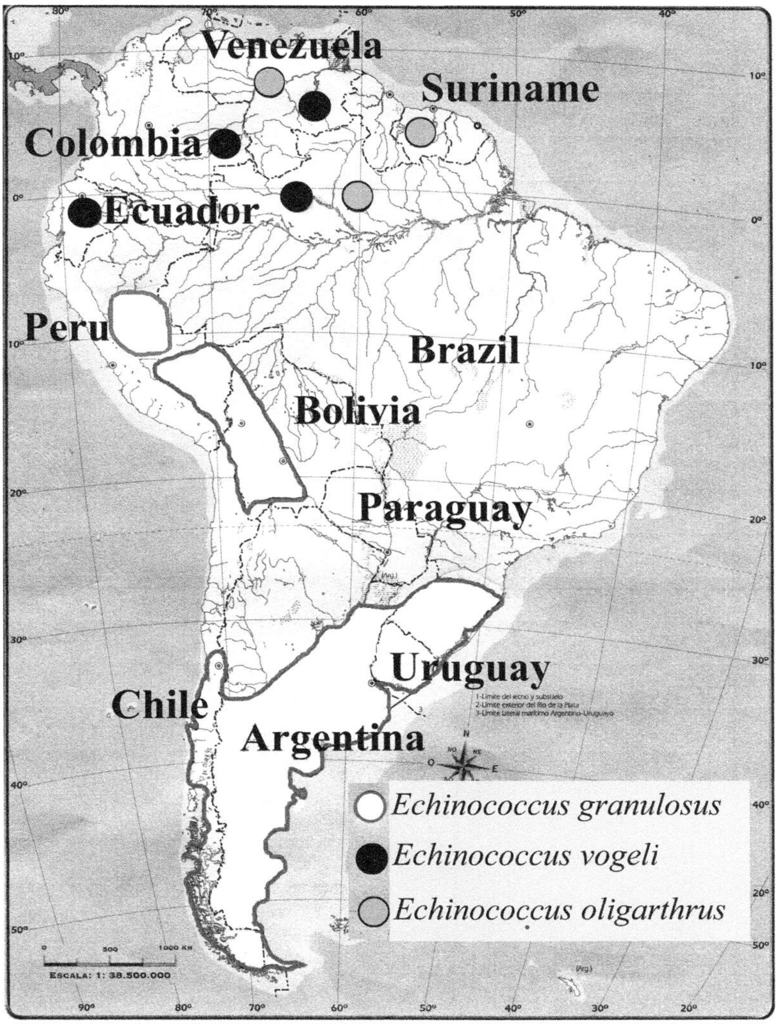

Fig. 3.1 Distribution of *Echinococcus granulosus*, *E. vogeli*, and *E. oligarthrus* in South America (Modified from OPS (Organización Panamericana de la Salud) 2004; with permission)

ing is quite common are the ones with the highest prevalence rates of infection. In particular, Neuquén is one of the provinces with the highest incidence (OPS 2004).

Although *E. granulosus* is widespread all over Argentina and hydatid disease is considered endemic in this country, the infection has a non-homogeneous geographic distribution (Fig. 3.2). The contribution of each kind of livestock (cattle, pig, sheep, etc.) to disease transmission depends on the region: for example, while sheep are the principal intermediate hosts in the Patagonian and Mesopotamic region, cattle are the prevalent hosts in the Pampas and northern regions of the country (Denegri et al. 2002). Particularly in the southeastern region of Buenos Aires province, echinococcosis is considered an important human and veterinary health problem, cattle being the main livestock involved in the transmission of this disease (Andresiuk et al. 2009). In a case-control study in Argentina, one of the risk factors for cystic echinococcosis was human exposure to a great number of dogs during the first years of life (Larrieu et al. 2002). In a survey of asymptomatic patients, Coltorti et al. (1988) found that 47 of 5,839 patients (80 %) were seropositive for *E. granulosus* antigens. These authors used antibodies against *E. granulosus* arc 5 antigens by the double diffusion arc 5 test (Coltorti et al. 1988).

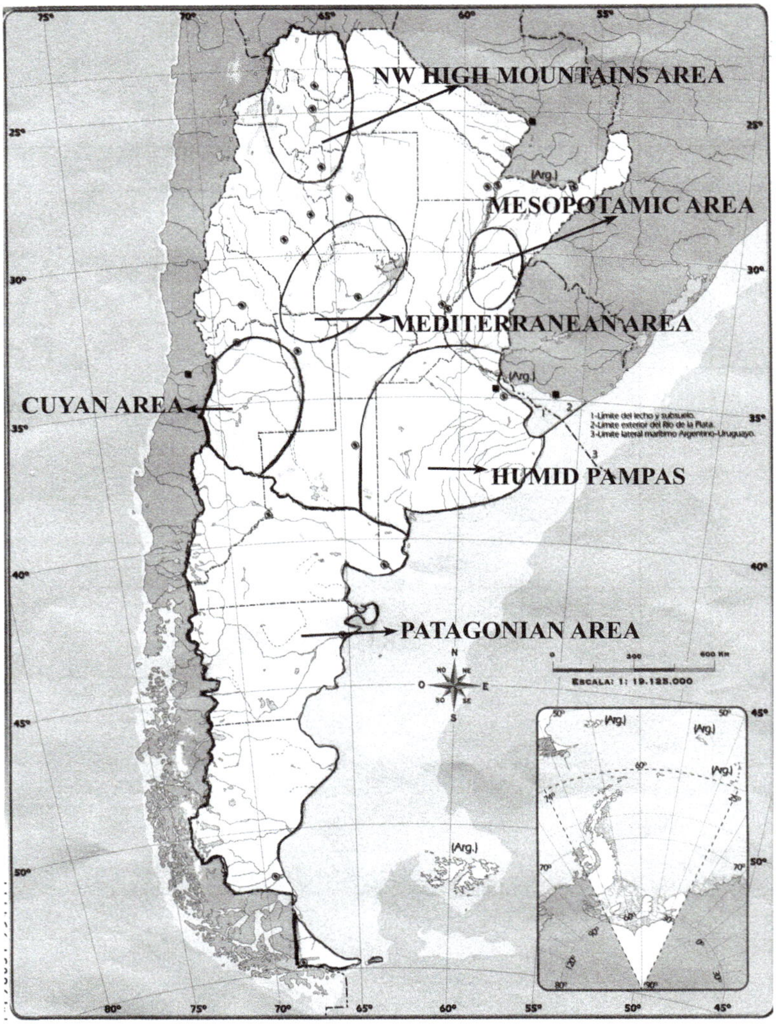

Fig. 3.2 Major endemic foci of echinococcosis in Argentina (Modified from OPS (Organización Panamericana de la Salud) 2004; with permission)

Argentine medicine has greatly contributed to the comprehension of hydatid cysts of the CNS. In Buenos Aires in 1889, Dr. Alejandro Castro performed a surgical operation for a cerebral hydatid cyst and introduced the new principles of surgical asepsis that had been previously developed in Europe. In 1895, Dr. Alejandro Posadas was the first surgeon to successfully treat hydatid cysts of the CNS in Argentina. In 1929, Dr. Ernesto Dowling performed his so-called "cyst delivery" method. The hydatid cyst is surgically removed intact. This technique (Dowling-Orlando technique) is mandatory in order to avoid further dissemination of the scolices (Obrador Alcalde 1964). In Buenos Aires, during the 1933–1974 period covering almost 42 years, 29 brain hydatid cysts and one of the spinal cord out of 35 pediatric cases of hydatidosis of the CNS were operated. No surgical mortality was reported in these cases (Carrea et al. 1975). The 20 patients who had their cysts removed unruptured with the Dowling technique (Dowling and Orlando 1939) remained alive, and only two patients suffered blindness as a sequela (Carrea et al. 1975). In Buenos Aires, in 1980, three patients (two adults and one child) were admitted to hospital with various neurological signs and symptoms. Although there was no evidence of cysts in the liver or lungs, hydatid disease was only suspected in the child, since he came from an endemic rural area in Buenos Aires province. A high degree of accuracy in identifying multiple supratentorial cysts by computed tomography (CT) scanning was obtained in all the cases, and the patients were followed by CT scans after surgery (Insausti et al. 1980). In Buenos Aires in 1998, Ure and Maegli reported a case of an adult patient born in Santiago del Estero province, who was admitted to a psychiatric hospital after surgery performed in Buenos Aires 1 year before (Ure and Maegli 1998). He suffered from alcoholism, diabetes mellitus, and Chagas trypanosomiasis. He had lived on a farm for several years and then moved to Buenos Aires. He presented with excruciating headache, vomiting, papilledema, left hemiparesis, somatic sensitivity in the left leg, slow mental activity, and urinary incontinence. A CT scan revealed a large right frontal cystic mass surrounded by a circular calcification. The mass turned out to be a hydatid cyst, which was opened and treated with formaldehyde. No extracerebral localizations were observed. Five years later, new CT scans revealed the bilateral and diffuse extension of the hydatid process with several small new cystic lesions unable to be treated by surgical reoperation. The patient died 2 months later (Ure and Maegli 1998).

In 2004, a case of a temporal hydatid cyst in a child was reported. The diagnosis was considered preoperatively on the basis of magnetic resonance imaging and magnetic resonance spectroscopy (MRS) findings. The MRS pattern appeared to be different from that seen in other cystic lesions of the CNS. Lactate, alanine, acetate, and a large pyruvate peak were observed. The cyst was surgically removed (Tamer et al. 2004).

Some orbital infections have been diagnosed in Turkey and Morocco (Turgut et al. 1992, 2004; Benazzou et al. 2009). A hydatid infection of the orbit recently diagnosed in Buenos Aires in a patient from Neuquén was characterized as an unusual localization of a hydatid cyst (Menghi and Gatta 2011).

Hydatidosis in Brazil

In Brazil, *Echinococcus* is widespread in an area of approximately 100,000 km^2, which is close to the Uruguayan and Argentinean borders. Several studies have shown that 14–50 % of farm dogs were infected with *E. granulosus* (de la Rue 1997). Particularly in the state of Rio Grande do Sul in southern Brazil as well as in other countries in South America, the habit of feeding sheep raw offal to dogs perpetuates the parasite's life cycle. The etiological agent found in dogs and other wild animals is predominantly *E. granulosus*.

In 1983, the first serological survey for echinococcosis was performed in seven municipal states near the border with Uruguay. A prevalence of 8.06/1,000 population was observed (OPS 2004). In 1999, another serological survey was conducted in 5 % of the total human population in rural areas of 18 municipal states of Brazil. The highest prevalence was observed in Municipio de Barra do Quaraí (89.44 %) and the lowest in Piratini (8.82 %) (Souza et al. 1999). To our knowledge, there have been no reported cases of hydatidosis of the CNS in the Brazilian literature.

Hydatidosis in Chile

In Chile, several serological surveys have been conducted throughout the country to document the prevalence of human echinococcosis from 1988 to 1997 (Nourbakhsh et al. 2010). The prevalence of human cases in apparently healthy people may reach up to 754.6/100,000 population in some regions of the country (Apt et al. 2000). Another serological survey reviewed 60,790 individuals and found that 82 had positive serological findings, resulting in a total incidence of 136/100,000 population. The calculated incidence rates for urban and rural regions were 87/100,000 and 241/100,000, respectively (Schenone et al. 1999). Pursuant to National Resolution N° 712/2000, echinococcosis is a disease of mandatory notification (OPS 2004) in Chile. Human echinococcosis is a prevalent disease in Chile with an incidence rate of 2–2.5/100,000 population. Considering the existing subdiagnoses, the incidence of this disease has been reported to be 10/100,000 (OPS 2004).

In Chile, dogs are the main definitive hosts for *E. granulosus*. Between 1977 and 1979, 71 % of dogs from the XII region were found to be infected with *Echinococcus* In 1984, after the control program, this prevalence decreased to 1.5 % (OPS 2004).

Between 1997 and 2000, of 15 patients studied at Dr. L. Calvo Mackenna Hospital in Santiago de Chile, only 2 had cerebral hydatid cysts, whereas the rest had other cyst localizations (Hauck et al. 2003). More recently, in March 2012, four cases of cysts located in the brain were reported. Three of the patients were admitted with intracranial hypertension, whereas the fourth one presented with left hemiparesis. Imaging studies of all intracerebral cysts showed features compatible with hydatidosis in all cases. All lesions were completely removed surgically, and the pathological study of the excised piece confirmed the diagnosis of hydatidosis (Tapia et al. 2012).

Hydatidosis in Peru

In Peru, echinococcosis is a major health problem in the central Peruvian Andes where sheep raising is widespread. In a Peruvian study, the prevalence of human hydatidosis has been reported to be 1.9 % by the enzyme-linked immunoelectrotransfer blot and double diffusion assays in endemic areas (Moro et al. 1994).

Studies in Peru have shown high prevalence of cystic echinococcosis in humans, particularly in the central and southern highlands (Gavidia et al. 2008). During 1997–1999, prevalence in the central Andes was 5.7–9.3 % according to US, radiography, or both studies and up to 18.2 % according to immunoblot testing (Moro et al. 1997, 1999). Portable US has facilitated the study and a more accurate reporting of cystic echinococcosis prevalence in endemic regions (Macpherson et al. 2003; Moro et al. 2005). Among the available serological tests, the immunoblot assay that uses bovine hydatid cyst fluid has been successfully applied in cystic echinococcosis in endemic areas of Peru (Moro et al. 1997, 2005).

Local control measures should focus primarily on decreasing dog and sheep infection. Cystic echinococcosis is a major public health problem in Peru, having a prevalence of 6–9 % in many areas of the country and numerous reported human cases every year. The Peruvian central highlands comprise approximately 70 % of the endemic areas for cystic echinococcosis in Peru (Santivañez et al. 2008).

By 1993, just one case of a 7-month evolution cerebral hydatid cyst was reported at Hospital Nacional Cayetano Heredia in a 12-year-old girl residing in Paracaos (Sierra de Lima). The patient presented with cephalalgia, progressive loss of strength in the right hemibody, and vomiting. She was diagnosed with cerebral and hepatic echinococcosis by CT and abdominal echography, respectively, and treated with albendazole. On the 7th day, the cyst was excised from the brain with no complications using the Dowling-Orlando technique. The cyst measured 9×6×7 cm. After 4 months, a hepatic cyst of similar size was removed. The patient is currently on anticonvulsant treatment and has remained asymptomatic, with no evidence of sequelae (Guillen et al. 1994).

Hydatidosis in Uruguay

Seroprevalence studies in rural communities using an enzyme-linked immunoassay test with crude sheep hydatid cyst fluid antigen to detect antibodies (total immunoglobulin) revealed an overall human seropositive rate of 1.2 % (Bonifacino et al. 1991). In 1990, in certain rural areas, 10.7 % of dogs were infected with *E. granulosus*. After the canine control program, the percentage of infected dogs had lowered from 10.7 to 0.74 %. Nevertheless, prevalence was 44.7 % in sheep and 64.8 % in cattle. By 2003, serological tests (enzyme-linked immunosorbent assay [ELISA]) had been performed on 41,004 school children with 20 positive cases (OPS 2004). The average annual morbidity for hydatid disease in Uruguay in 1969–1971, expressed as the incidence of all hospital cases (20.7/100,000 population) or only of new cases (17.7/100,000 population), is the highest yet reported for any country. Many Uruguayan health authorities now consider hydatid disease to be the most important rural health problem of specific etiology (Purriel et al. 1973). To our knowledge, there has been no reported case of hydatidosis of the CNS in the Uruguayan literature.

Hydatidosis in Bolivia

From January 1984 to February 1999, a total of 40 cases of hydatid cyst in 31 children were studied. Their medical histories were thoroughly checked, emphasizing all clinical aspects, cyst location, type of treatment, evolution, and readmission. Of the 31 children studied, 9 were admitted twice for the same reason, some of them with the cyst located in the same place as when they were first admitted and others in a different location. Most came from urban low-middle class neighborhoods in La Paz and El Alto. The most frequent cyst location was the lungs (25 cases), followed by the liver (10 cases); there were 8 cases with cysts in both organs; the rest had different and often unusual locations such as the peritoneum (3 cases). In the other six cases, the cysts were localized in the brain, parotid gland, spleen, posterior mediastinum, vertebral area, and retrovesical region. The only case of cerebral hydatidosis presented with meningeal signs and viable scolices in cerebral spinal fluid. Surgery was performed in all cases. From 1996 onward, albendazole was systematically administered before and after surgery following the confirmation of the diagnosis. This study reports an increasing frequency of this disease and confirms its high mortality rate as well as its high cost due to mandatory surgery, related infections, long hospital stays, and complications due to the disease. In 80 % of all cases, it was confirmed that patients lived in close proximity to dogs. The cysts excised from the children had an average size of 7 cm; the smallest ones were removed from the parotid gland and the vertebral area and measured 3 cm. The largest ones were lodged in the peritoneal cavity, lungs, and brain and measured 15 cm (Tamayo Meneses et al. 2004).

Control Program

In the Argentine province of Rio Negro, a control program including dog treatment with praziquantel (5 mg/kg of bodyweight) every 2 months for about 20 years (1979/1980 to 1999) reduced the prevalence of cysts in sheep from 61 to 18 % and of intestinal stages in rural dogs from an estimated 40 % to 2–3 % (Larrieu et al. 2001).

Conclusion

Based on our experience and the literature data upon hydatidosis of the CNS in South America, the following conclusions may be drawn from this chapter:

1. Argentina, Chile, Uruguay, Peru, Bolivia, and Brazil show the highest rates of incidence of human hydatidosis in South America. Nevertheless, the incidence of hydatid cysts of the CNS is very low.
2. The main reason for these high rates is, among others, the unawareness of risky behaviors, such as the regular habit of feeding raw sheep offal to dogs.
3. Since hydatidosis is most prevalent in cattle-raising areas, it is also an important veterinary problem leading to economic consequences.
4. The high morbidity in certain regions, the potential lethality if the disease is not adequately treated, the high incidence in young people, and the high costs involved in hospitalization and surgery highlight the epidemiologic importance of hydatidosis in South America.

References

Andresiuk MV, Gordo FP, Bandera CC, Elissondo MC, Dopchiz M, Denegri G. Echinococcus granulosus: biological comparison of cattle isolates from endemic regions of Argentina and Spain. Rev Argent Microbiol. 2009;41:218–25.

Apt W, Pérez C, Galdamez E, Campano S, Vega F, Vargas D, et al. Echinococcosis/hydatidosis in the VII Region of Chile: diagnosis and educational intervention. Rev Panam Salud Publica. 2000;7:8–16.

Arana Iñiguez R. Echinococcus. Infections of the nervous system. Part III. In: Vinken PJ, Bruyn GW, editors.

Handbook of clinical neurology. Amsterdam: North Holland Publishing; 1978.
Arana Iñiguez R, Rodriguez Barrios R, San Julian J. Nueva técnica para la extirpación del quiste hidático cerebral. Prensa Med Argent. 1951;38:891–7.
Benazzou S, Arkha Y, Derraz S, El Ouahabi A, El Khamlichi A. Orbital hydatid cyst: review of 10 cases. J Craniomaxillofac Surg. 2009;38:274–8.
Bonifacino R, Malgor R, Barbeito R, Balleste R, Rodríguez MJ, Botto C, Klug F. Seroprevalence of echinococcus granulosus infection in a Uruguayan rural human population. Trans R Soc Trop Med Hyg. 1991;85:769–72.
Carrea R, Dowling Jr E, Guevara J. Surgical treatment of hydatid cysts of the central nervous system in the pediatric age (Dowling's technique). Childs Brain. 1975;1: 4–21.
Coltorti E, Fernández E, Guarnera E, Lago J, Iriarte J. Field evaluation of an enzyme immunoassay for detection of asymptomatic patients in a hydatid control program. Am J Trop Med Hyg. 1988;38:603–7.
De la Rue ML. Epidemiology and transmission of cystic echinococcosis Brazil. Arch Int Hidat. 1997;32:48–50.
Denegri GM, Elissondo MC, Dopchiz MC. Situación de la hidatidosis-echinococcosis en la República Argentina. Mar del Plata\Buenos Aires: Editorial Martín; 2002.
Dew HR. Primary cerebral hydatid disease. Aust N Z J Surg. 1955;24:161–71.
Dowling E, Orlando R. Quiste hidático del lóbulo frontal derecho. Rev Espec Asoc Méd Argent. 1939;4:209–17.
Ersahin Y, Mutluer S, Guzelbag E. Intracranial hydatid cysts in children. Neurosurgery. 1993;33:219–24.
Gavidia CM, Gonzalez AE, Zhang W, McManus DP, Lopera L, Ninaquispe B, et al. Diagnosis of cystic echinococcosis, central Peruvian Highlands. Emerg Infect Dis. 2008;14:260–6.
Guarnera EA. Hidatidosis en Argentina: carga de enfermedad. Organización Panamericana de la Salud -OPS, Buenos Aires. 2009. http://publicaciones.ops.org.ar/publicaciones/otras%20pub/pubhidatidosis.pdf. Accessed 28 Aug 2011.
Guillen D, Campos P, Aguirre I, Noriega P, Noriega P, Alva M, Fuentes Dávila A, Alaba W. Quiste hidatídico cerebral en niños en el Hospital Nacional Cayetano Heredia: a propósito de un caso. Arq Neuropsiquiatr. 1994;52:266–8.
Gutiérrez Y. Diagnostic pathology of parasitic infections with clinical correlations. 2nd ed. New York: Oxford University Press; 2000.
Hauck IN, Viovy A, Zamorano R, Blanco A, Revello D, Vojkovic M, Cerva JL. Hidatidosis en la infancia: albendazol en su tratamiento médico y quirúrgico. Rev Chil Infect. 2003;20:229–34.
Insausti T, Ferreiro JL, Zamboni O. Tres casos de hidatidosis encefálica múltiple. Diagnóstico con tomografía computada cerebral. Pren Méd Arg. 1980;11:530–4.
Kammerer WS. Echinococcosis affecting the central nervous system. Semin Neurol. 1993;13:144–7.
Krajewski R, Stelmasiak Z. Cerebral hydatid cyst in children. Childs Nerv Syst. 1991;7:154–5.
Larrieu E, Costa MT, Cantoni G, Alvarez R, Cavagion L, Labanchi JL, Bigatti R, Araya D, Herrero E, Alvarez E, Mancini S, Cabrera P. Ovine Echinococcus granulosus transmission dynamics in the province of Rio Negro, Argentina, 1980–1999. Vet Parasitol. 2001;98:263–72.
Larrieu EJ, Costa MT, del Carpio M, Moguillansky S, Bianchi G, Yadón ZE. A case-control study of the risk factors for cystic echinococcosis among the children of Rio Negro province, Argentina. Ann Trop Med Parasitol. 2002;96:43–52.
Macpherson CN, Bartholomot B, Frider B. Application of ultrasound in diagnosis, treatment, epidemiology, public health and control of Echinococcus granulosus and E. multilocularis. Parasitology. 2003;127(Suppl):S21–35.
Mahadevan A, Dwarakanath S, Pai S, Kovoor JM, Radhesh S, Srinivas HV, Chandramouli BA, Shankar SK. Cerebral coenurosis mimicking hydatid disease -report of two cases from South India. Clin Neuropathol. 2011;30:28–32.
Menghi C, Gatta C. Unusual localization of an hydatid cyst: first reported case in Buenos Aires, Argentina. Braz J Infect Dis. 2011;15:81–2.
Moro PL, Guevara A, Verastequi M, Gilman RH, Poma H, Tapia B, Tsang VC, García HH, Pacheco R, Lapel C. The Cysticercosis Working Group in Peru (CWG). Distribution of hydatidosis and cysticercosis in different Peruvian populations as demonstrated by an enzyme-linked immunoelectrotransfer blot (EITB) assay. Am J Trop Med Hyg. 1994;51:851–5.
Moro PL, McDonald J, Gilman RH, Silva B, Verastegui M, Malqui V, Lescano G, Falcon N, Montes G, Bazalar H. Epidemiology of Echinococcus granulosus infection in the central Peruvian Andes. Bull World Health Org. 1997;75:553–61.
Moro PL, Bonifacio N, Gilman RH, Lopera L, Silva B, Takumoto R, Verastegui M, Cabrera L. Field diagnosis of Echinococcus granulosus infection among intermediate and definitive hosts in an endemic focus of human cystic echinococcosis. Trans R Soc Trop Med Hyg. 1999;93:611–5.
Moro PL, Garcia HH, Gonzales AE, Bonilla JJ, Verastegui M, Gilman RH. Screening for cystic echinococcosis in an endemic region of Peru using portable ultrasonography and the enzyme-linked immunoelectrotransfer blot (EITB) assay. Parasitol Res. 2005;96:242–6.
Nourbakhsh A, Vannemreddy P, Minagar A, Toledo EG, Palacios E, Nanda A. Hydatid disease of the central nervous system: a review of literature with an emphasis on Latin American countries. Neurol Res. 2010;32:245–51.
Obrador Alcalde S. Quistes hidatídicos encefálicos. Dia Med. 1964;58:1137–41.
OPS (Organización Panamericana de la Salud) (PAHO) (2004) Informe del proyecto subregional Cono Sur de control y vigilancia de la hidatidosis. Argentina, Brasil, Chile y Uruguay: primera reunión constitutiva. Reunión Constitutiva del Proyecto Regional Cono Sur de Control y Vigilancia de la Hidatidosis. Argentina, Brasil, Chile y Uruguay, 7–9 July 2004; Montevideo, Uruguay. Montevideo: OPS; 2004 OPS/DPC/VP/04.

http://www.bvsops.org.uy/pdf/equinoc.pdf. Accessed 29 Aug 2011.

Ozek MM. Complications of central nervous system: hydatid disease. Pediatr Neurosurg. 1994;20:84–91.

Peter JC, Domingo Z, Sinclair-Smith C, de Villiers JC. Hydatid infestation of the brain: difficulties with computed tomography diagnosis and surgical treatment. Pediatr Neurosurg. 1994;20:78–83.

Purriel P, Schantz PM, Beovide H, Mendoza G. Human echinococcosis (hydatidosis) in Uruguay: a comparison of indices of morbidity and mortality, 1962–71. Bull World Health Org. 1973;49:395–402.

Santivañez SJ, Gutiérrez AM, Rosenzvit MC. Human hydatid disease in Peru is basically restricted to Echinococcus granulosus genotype G1. Am J Trop Med Hyg. 2008;79:89–92.

Schantz PM. Localización de la hidatidosis en el sistema nervioso central. Bol Oficina Sanit Panam. 1972;73: 198–202.

Schenone H, Contreras MC, Salinas P, Sandoval L, Saavedra T, Rojas A. Human hydatidosis in Chile. Seroprevalence and estimate of the number of infected people. Bol Chil Parasitol. 1999;54:70–3.

Slim MS, Khayat G, Nasr AT, Jidejian YD. Hydatid disease in childhood. J Pediatr Surg. 1971;6:440–8.

Souza MAT, Mardini LBLF, Fernandes C, Tiecher F. Diagnostico sorologico de hidatidose humana na populacao rural de 18 municıpios do Rio Grande do Sul, Brasil. Presented at Brazilian Parasitology Congress, Pocos de Caldas, Brasil; 1999

Tamayo Meneses L, Pacheco Llerena R, Fernández Hinojosa R, Chungara Montaño J. Hidatidosis. Experiencia institucional. Rev Soc Boliv Ped. 2004;43:149–54.

Tamer I, Rugilo C, Cuccia V. Utilidad de espectroscopia protónica en el quiste hidatídico cerebral. Rev Neurol Arg. 2004;29:46–8.

Tapia O, Vidal A, Antonio L. Brain hydatidosis: report of four cases (in Spanish). Rev Méd Chil. 2012;140:358–63.

Taratuto AL, Venturiello SM. Echinococcosis. Brain Pathol. 1997;7:673–9.

Turgut M. Hydatidosis of central nervous system and its coverings in the pediatric and adolescent age groups in Turkey during the last century: a critical review of 137 cases. Childs Nerv Syst. 2002;18:670–83.

Turgut M, Saglam S, Ozcan OE. Orbital hydatid cyst. Report of a case followed by serial computed tomography. J Clin Neuroophthalmol. 1992;12:43–6.

Turgut AT, Turgut M, Koşar U. Hydatidosis of the orbit in Turkey: results from review of the literature 1963–2001. Int Ophthalmol. 2004;25:193–200.

Ure JA, Maegli JR. Alcmeon25. Hidatidosis cerebral atípica. 1998. http://www.alcmeon.com.ar/7/25/alc25_01.htm. Accessed 11 Apr 2011.

Hydatidosis of the Central Nervous System in Central and Eastern Europe

4

Raul Neghina, Villiam Šnábel, Branko Bobić, Olgica Djurković-Djaković, Roxana Moldovan, Claudia Borza, Victor Dumitrascu, Crenguta L. Calma, and Adriana M. Neghina

Contents

Introduction

Hydatidosis (also known as echinococcosis or hydatid disease) is one of Europe's neglected infections of poverty (Hotez and Gurwith 2011). Cystic echinococcosis (CE), which has *Echinococcus granulosus* as the pathogenic agent, is endemic to Southwestern and Eastern parts of Europe (Sotiraki and Chaligiannis 2010). Although alveolar echinococcosis (AE), produced by *E. multilocularis*, was considered to be rare in Central Europe, recent studies have shown its emerging nature and demonstrated that the endemic areas for this parasite are broader than previously thought (Kern 2010). The yearly disease incidence (cases per 100,000 inhabitants) in

R. Neghina, MD, PhD (✉)
Department of Infectious Diseases, Pneumology, Epidemiology and Parasitology, Discipline of Parasitology, Victor Babes University of Medicine and Pharmacy, 2 Eftimie Murgu Sq, 300041 Timisoara, Romania
e-mail: raul.neghina@gmail.com

V. Šnábel, RNDr., PhD
Department of Parasitic Zoonoses, Institute of Parasitology, Slovak Academy of Sciences, Košice, Slovakia

B. Bobić, MD, PhD
O. Djurković-Djaković, MD, PhD
Centre for Parasitic Zoonoses, Institute for Medical Research, University of Belgrade, Belgrade, Serbia

R. Moldovan, MD, PhD
Department of Microbiology, Victor Babes University of Medicine and Pharmacy, Timisoara, Romania

C. Borza, MD, PhD
Department of Pathophysiology, Victor Babes University of Medicine and Pharmacy, Timisoara, Romania

V. Dumitrascu, MD, PhD
Department of Biochemistry and Pharmacology, Emergency County Hospital, Victor Babes University of Medicine and Pharmacy, Timisoara, Romania

C.L. Calma, MD, PhD
Department of Physiology and Immunology, Victor Babes University of Medicine and Pharmacy, Timisoara, Romania

A.M. Neghina, MD, PhD
Department of Biochemistry and Pharmacology, Victor Babes University of Medicine and Pharmacy, Timisoara, Romania

M. Turgut (ed.), *Hydatidosis of the Central Nervous System: Diagnosis and Treatment*, DOI 10.1007/978-3-642-54359-3_4, © Springer-Verlag Berlin Heidelberg 2014

Europe's endemic areas has increased from a mean value of 0.1 (1993–2000) to 0.26 (2001–2005) (Moro and Schantz 2009; Sotiraki and Chaligiannis 2010). Farming was noted as an important risk factor for infected people. It has also been suggested that AE may be underdiagnosed in Europe because it is inadequately considered in the differential diagnosis. Regarding the location of lesions developed in AE, 34 % of the European patients had liver lesions with simultaneous involvement of other organs (Kern 2010).

This chapter aims to review and, at the same time, bring to light new epidemiological, clinical, and surgical information regarding hydatidosis of the central nervous system (CNS) in many countries in Eastern and Central Europe where data was available (Fig. 4.1). At the same time, it intends to shed light on particularly interesting cases reported in the literature. A special emphasis will be given to the casuistic from Romania, one of the countries with the highest prevalence of hydatidosis worldwide. Evidence regarding the status of the disorder in the former Soviet Union and Russia, considered Eurasian states, is also discussed in this chapter.

Epidemiological and Clinical Features Regarding Hydatidosis of the Central Nervous System in Central and Eastern European Countries

Hydatidosis in Romania

Epidemiology

In 1995, Romania was in the forefront of the European countries and among the first countries worldwide as regards the incidence of hydatid disease (Neghina et al. 2010, 2011a). Moreover, the severity of hydatidosis in Romania is emphasized by the fact that at least one person from 45.5 % of Romanian localities underwent surgery for this condition (Iacobiciu et al. 2005; Neghina et al. 2010, 2011b). Following the analysis of the available global data, Stefanoiu concluded in 2000 that the number of human cases of hydatidosis in Romania surpassed the number of cases from Lithuania, Belarus, Poland, Slovakia, Ukraine, Bulgaria, Czech Republic, and Latvia combined (Iacobiciu et al. 2005; Neghina et al. 2010). Nevertheless, hydatidosis is not a notifiable disease in Romania, and no cases were mentioned in the annals of the World Health Organization (WHO) during the period from 1996 to 2000 (Iacobiciu et al. 2005; Neghina et al. 2010). Studies performed in the entire country have shown that the incidence of the disease decreased from 5.6 cases per 100,000 inhabitants during the period 1953 to 1963 to 2.6 cases per 100,000 inhabitants from 1987 to 1991 (Neghina et al. 2010, 2011b; Calma et al. 2011). The most recent studies undertaken in four counties of western Romania indicated an average incidence between 2.4 and 4.4 cases per 100,000 inhabitants (Calma et al. 2011, 2012; Moldovan et al. 2012).

Hydatidosis of the Brain and Cranium

In 1900, Thoma Ionescu, considered the godfather of Romanian surgery, presented at the International Congress of Medicine and Surgery held in Paris a case of cerebral hydatidosis that he successfully operated on through temporal craniotomy, and at the same time, he emphasized the possible surgical risks. Two years later, he published in a reputable national journal new and useful data on the topic of cerebral hydatidosis with particular emphasis on the case he had previously managed (Arseni et al. 1988). In 1905, Antoniu reported for the first time in Romania a rare case of cranial hydatidosis. At that time, only seven such cases were registered in the medical literature worldwide. His paper, entitled "Hydatid Cyst of the Cranial Bones," represented a valuable starting point toward the knowledge of this pathology in Romania. The patient, hospitalized in Turnu Severin (southwestern Romania), presented with a single tumor that caused cerebral compression with epileptic crisis. Unfortunately, the patient died before the onset of any exterior signs suggesting cranial involvement (Arseni et al. 1988).

During the period of 1935–1968, there were 46 cases of cerebral hydatidosis reported in Romania (Arseni and Samitca 1957; Arseni et al. 1981)

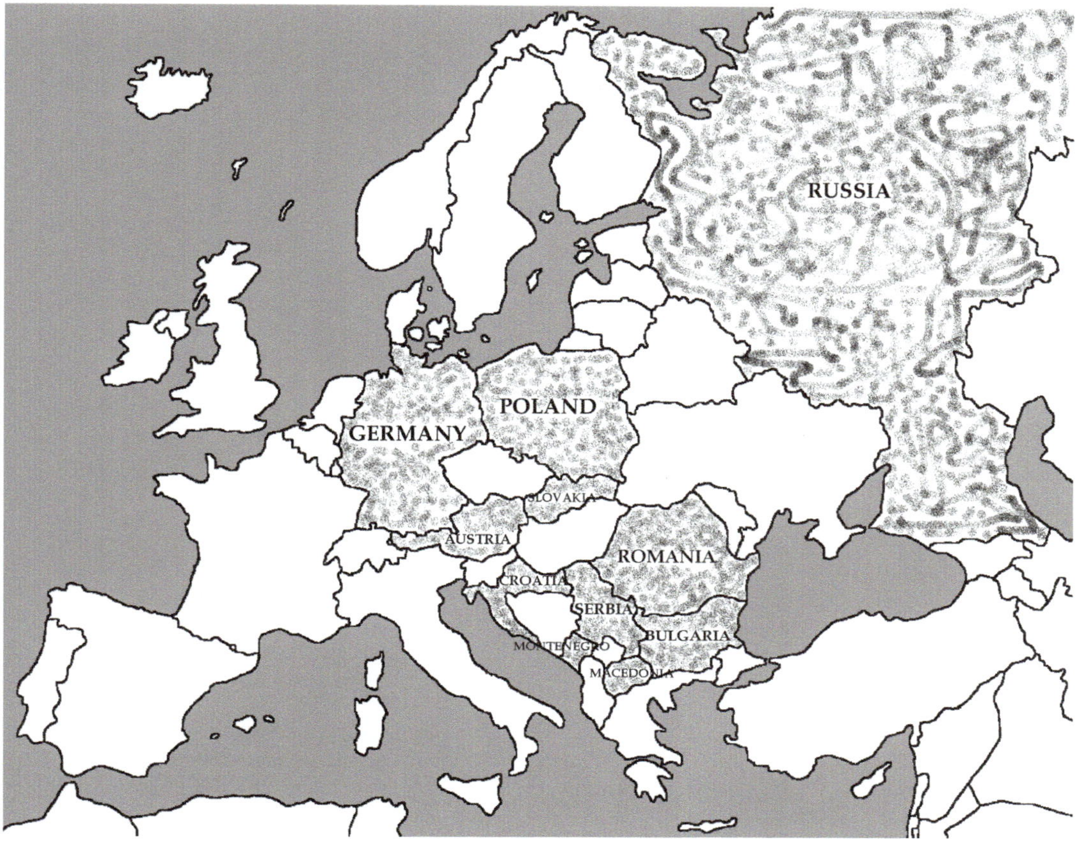

Fig. 4.1 Map of Europe. The status of central nervous system hydatidosis is discussed in the Eastern and Central European countries (sprayed on map) where data were available

(Table 4.1). Information that is more detailed was available for the cases managed during 1935–1955 in a Neurosurgery Clinic in Bucharest. Of 2,226 cases with intracranial space-occupying disorders, 36 patients (1.6 %) were found with cranial and intracranial hydatidosis (Arseni and Samitca 1957). The most significant epidemiological and clinical characteristics of this study group are summarized in Table 4.2.

Until 1980, the number of cases with cerebral involvement rose to 83 in the Neurosurgery Clinic in Bucharest. Of these patients, 55.4 % were males and more than 43 % were children. The youngest patient was 1.5 years old, and the oldest one was 65 years old (Arseni et al. 1981). A further study in the same clinic presented the characteristics of 27 pediatric cases who underwent surgery during the period from 1980 to 1992 (Ciurea et al. 1995). An additional 52 cases diagnosed during the same period were not discussed due to different reasons. The studied cases represented 2.8 % of the children with expansive nontraumatic lesions hospitalized in this clinic. The mean age of the study group was 8.2 years, and the youngest patient was 3.3 years old. A 67 % male prevalence was registered, and most of the patients (41 %) belonged to the age group 6–10 years. The most prevalent symptoms were headache and vomiting (96 %), followed by papillary edema (89 %) and hemiparesis (70.3 %). In the majority of patients (40.7 %), two cerebral lobes were affected. Recurrences occurred in 40.7 % of patients (in all the cases where total removal of the cysts could not be achieved). Another study undertaken at the same clinic included 76 patients who underwent surgery for

Table 4.1 Cases of cerebral hydatidosis in Romania during the period 1935–1968

Year(s)	Authors	Hospital, city	No. of cases	Specific comments	References
1935–1955	Arseni and Samitica	Neurosurgery Clinic, Bucharest	36	Presented in Table 4.2	Arseni et al. (1981), Arseni and Samitca (1957)
1954[a]	Marcovici and Steriade	Unspecified	1	Giant cerebral cyst, recidivated, with abscess	Arseni et al. (1981)
1957[a]	Russu	Unspecified	2	Study in children. The prevalence of cerebral hydatid cysts was 5.4 % of all locations One of the cysts (very voluminous) developed in a child who previously underwent surgery for a hepatic hydatid cyst	Arseni et al. (1981)
1960[a]	Waitsuk, Andrasofski, and Mera	Neurosurgery Clinic, Targu Mures	6	One of the cysts was situated in the right premotor cortex and had calcified walls	Arseni et al. (1981)
1968[a]	Theodorescu and Mitroi	Neurosurgery Clinic, Constanta	1	The cyst, about the size of a small fist, was located in the left parieto-occipital cortex At hospital admission, the patient was comatose with respiratory failure. Patient's condition worsened as a consequence of a lumbar puncture performed 1 month later The patient died	Arseni et al. (1981)
Total cases			46		

[a]Year when the cases were reported

cerebral hydatidosis during the period from 1981 to 2003 (Ciurea et al. 2006a). The main epidemiological and clinical characteristics of the study group were the following: 95.7 % of patients were children; the median age was 8.7 years in children and 29.3 years in adults; male patients prevailed (59.2 %); increased intracranial pressure was the most frequent symptom in children (91.1 %), while headache was the most prevalent finding in adults (88.9 %); 94.8 % of the cysts were supratentorial; rupture of the cysts during the surgery was reported in 26.3 % of cases; postsurgical complications occurred in 67.1 % of patients; relapses developed in 25 % of cases; the outcome (either at 6 months or at 2 years) showed a fatality rate of 5.3 %.

Hydatidosis of the Spine and Spinal Cord

The first documented information regarding vertebro-medullary hydatidosis dates from the period 1862 to 1865, when Kalenderu reported two cases with vertebral cysts (detected in the dorsolumbar muscles) (quoted from Arseni et al. 1981). In 1898, Botescu communicated a case of hydatid cyst located in the pelvis, and Tzaicu reported in 1930 a case with medullary compression whose starting point was in the musculature and presented a secondary rachidian invasion (quoted from Arseni et al. 1981). In 1927, Jianu detected a case of vertebral hydatidosis and later a case of thoracolumbar involvement without neurological symptomatology (cases communicated

Table 4.2 Main epidemiological and clinical characteristics of patients with cranial and intracranial hydatidosis managed during 1935–1955 in a Neurosurgery Clinic in Bucharest (Arseni and Samitca 1957)

Feature	Relevant statistics	Percent of total cases
Gender	Male	58
Age	<30 years	73
Inhabitance area	Rural	64
Duration of symptoms	<1 year	78
Type of cyst	Unilocular	81
Symptomatology onset	Insidious	92
Symptoms	Headache	59
	Epilepsy	50
Outcome	Immediate postsurgical mortality	9
	Late mortality (>18 months)	13
	Without neurological sequels (% of surviving patients)	40

in 1957) (quoted from Arseni et al. 1981). In 1946, the case of a patient with an epidural hydatid cyst was presented by Cosacescu and Vereanu. Later, in 1956, Horvath and Sandor presented their study on 14 patients with vertebro-medullary invasion (Arseni et al. 1981).

During the period from 1935 to 1957, a total of 20 cases of vertebro-medullary involvement due to hydatid cysts were noted in the Neurosurgery Clinic in Bucharest (Arseni et al. 1960). They account for approximately 3 % of cases with rachidian and intrarachidian tumors and approximately 0.06 % of all cases managed during this period. These cases represented about half the number of cases with cerebral hydatidosis. In most of the patients (40 %), the lesions were found in the lumbar region. The youngest patient was 14 years old and the oldest 66 years old. Male patients represented 55 % of the study group, and 80 % of the cases were rural inhabitants. It has been noticed that a high prevalence (25 %) of patients belonged to the 11- to 20-year-old age group. Radicular pain was the initial clinical symptom in most of the patients (70 %). However, syndrome of spinal cord compression was the most common finding (75 %) upon admission. The time span from the onset of the disease until hospital admission ranged between 0 and 6 months in the majority of the cases (40 %). Out of 19 cases who underwent surgery, the outcome was fatal in a single case; of the remaining patients who were operated and survived, relapses occurred in approximately 44 % of cases.

Throughout the time, other cases were also detected, as follows: a report on ten cases with bone involvement (of which four cases with vertebral involvement were diagnosed in the Department of Orthopedics of Brancovenesc Hospital, Bucharest) is presented by Negrea in 1957; in the same year, Vereanu reported four cases of bone involvement (including one case with vertebral location and one with sacral); in 1971, Marinescu reported 30 cases of vertebral hydatidosis (quoted from Arseni et al. 1981).

Craniospinal Hydatidosis

Lupascu and Panaitescu (1968) gave an overview in 1968, in their valuable treatise on hydatid disease, of the data reported by the National Cantacuzino Institute regarding involvement of different organs and systems in this disorder. According to this source, craniocerebral cases occurred with a prevalence of 1.4 %, and vertebral lesions were diagnosed in 0.7 % of patients.

A major epidemiological study performed in the entire country of Romania during the period from 1987 to 1991 (Iacobiciu et al. 2005), including 3,072 cases (2,701 adults and 371 children), provides valuable data on cerebral and vertebro-medullary involvement: 0.94 % of patients were diagnosed with the condition at first hospitalization, 0.16 % at the second admission, and 0.1 % at the third one (Table 4.3).

Further investigations in children up to 15 years old (407 patients, 1987–1992) indicated the following percentage of cerebral involvement according to age groups: 5.21 % (0–5 years), 5 % (6–10 years), and 1.8 % (11–15 years) (Iacobiciu et al. 2005). According to Gherman et al. (1991), the prevalence of cerebral hydatidosis was 1–2 % in 1991. In 1994, Stefanoiu and Vranceanu reported in their study a prevalence of 0.4 % for cerebral hydatidosis. In the same study, the prevalence of this condition was 4 % in 407

Table 4.3 Cerebral and vertebro-medullary involvement of hydatidosis in 3,072 patients hospitalized in all of the Romanian surgical sections between 1987 and 1991

Location of the hydatid cyst	Adults		Children		Total	
	No. of cases	% of adult cases ($n=2,701$)	No. of cases	% of children cases ($n=371$)	No. of cases	% of total cases ($n=3,072$)
First hospitalization						
Cerebral	11	0.41	15	4.04	26	0.85
Hepatic and vertebro-medullary	1	0.04	–	–	1	0.03
Thoracolumbar	1	0.04	–	–	1	0.03
Only vertebro-medullary	1	0.04	–	–	1	0.03
Total	14	0.53	15	4.04	29	0.94
Relapse, second hospitalization						
Cerebral	1	0.04	4	1.08	5	0.16
Relapse, third hospitalization						
Cerebral	–	–	3	0.81	3	0.1

For 1991, only partial data were available

pediatric cases (Stefanoiu and Vranceanu 1994; Iacobiciu 1999). A survey taken from 1994 to 1999 in a southern Romanian county (Dolj county) reported cerebral involvement in 1 out of 213 cases (0.5 %) (Iacobiciu et al. 2005).

In 2000, Plesamosca and his collaborators reported data on 14 pediatric cases of hydatidosis with less common locations. Of these cases, cerebral involvement coexisted with involvement of other organs in 14.3 % of patients (Iacobiciu et al. 2005). A major epidemiological survey of 1,004 cases with hydatidosis diagnosed between 1985 and 1997 in three southwestern Romanian counties (Timis, Arad, and Caras-Severin) indicated cerebral involvement in 0.1 % of the study group (Iacobiciu 1999). The most recent studies undertaken from 2004 to 2010 in Timis (182 patients) (Calma et al. 2011), Arad (79 patients) (Calma et al. 2012), Caras-Severin, and Hunedoara counties (190 patients) (Moldovan et al. 2012) detected no cases with CNS involvement.

Orbital Hydatidosis

Between 1883 and 1968, a total of 24 cases of orbital hydatidosis were reported in Romania (Arseni et al. 1981). More recently, in 2006, Ciurea et al. (2006b) described another two interesting pediatric cases in a 4-year-old boy and in a 15-year-old girl.

Hydatidosis in Former Yugoslavia and Countries Succeeding Former Yugoslavia

Yugoslavia

As reviewed in Arseni et al. (1981), in 1952, Stojanović and Vujadinović reported only a single case (2.3 %) with cerebral involvement out of 44 patients with hydatid disease (quoted from Arseni et al. 1981). Later, in 1957, Papo and Vrigisić found that of 200 cases in which patients underwent surgery, two patients (1 %) had hydatid cysts with cerebral location (quoted from Arseni et al. 1981). In the countries succeeding former Yugoslavia, data on cerebral echinococcosis are available for Serbia, Montenegro, Croatia, and Macedonia, whereas none are available for Slovenia and Bosnia and Herzegovina.

Serbia

Hydatidosis is a mandatory notifiable disease in Serbia, and consequently the relevant data on this topic are archived at the National Institute for Public Health (Tables 4.4 and 4.5). However, when comparing the official data to that published in the literature, it becomes obvious that cases are largely underreported to this institute. A clinical study on hepatic hydatidosis performed in the largest Serbian clinical center indicated that 1,016 adult patients underwent surgery for this illness between 1963 and 2006. Of this number of cases, 376 patients were managed between 1997 and 2006 (Basara 2007).

Although there are no specific surveys regarding CNS involvement of hydatidosis, the abovementioned extensive study on adult patients (Basara 2007) as well as another study on 149 children who underwent surgery for hydatid disease between 1990 and 2006 (Djuricic et al. 2010) evidenced no cases of CNS involvement. This suggests that the condition is probably extremely rare in Serbia. Nevertheless, a study performed from 2000 to 2004 analyzed the brain and meningeal biopsy samples from 4,987 patients with craniotomy. The results showed that hydatidosis was detected in three patients (0.06 % of the total cases) out of 23 cases with parasitic diseases. Two of them were adults (each presenting only a solitary cyst), and the third patient was a 12-year-old boy (who had two cysts) (Gazibara 2005).

Table 4.4 Cases of hydatidosis registered in Serbia during the period 1991–2010

Year	Cases per 100,000 inhabitants	Number of cases	Gender distribution: male (%)
1991	0.12	10	NA
1992	0.07	6	NA
1993	0.12	8	NA
1994	0.09	7	NA
1995	0.25	20	NA
1996	0.16	13	NA
1997	0.21	17	NA
1998	0.36	29	NA
1999	0.32	26	NA
2000	0.30	24	NA
2001	0.45	35	44.4
2002	0.36	27	31.4
2003	0.53	40	18.5
2004	0.28	21	37.5
2005	0.63	47	19
2006	0.51	38	29.79
2007	0.34	25	31.58
2008	0.50	37	32
2009	0.43	32	37.8
2010	0.38	28	28.6
Mean	0.32	24.5 (total: 490)	31.06

All data refers to Serbia only (without Kosovo) for the entire period 1991 to 2010 (from Reports on Infectious Diseases in Serbia, published annually by the Institute for Public Health in Serbia)
Abbreviations: *NA* not available

Montenegro

The data available for this country indicates the following incidence rates of hydatidosis (cases per 100,000 inhabitants): 0.48 in 2006, 0.32 in 2007, and no cases in 2008 (WHO Regional Office for Europe 2011). A recent report described two cases of cerebral hydatidosis in Montenegro. The first patient was a 16-year-old boy who had three independent cysts that were surgically removed. The outcome was favorable in this case, and no relapses were noticed 8 years after the surgical intervention. The second patient was a 22-year-old man previously operated on for a liver hydatid cyst. At admission, he presented multiple cysts detected by CT and MRI in the lungs, mediastinum, heart (left atrium), and brain (with cerebral infarction). He declined any surgical intervention, and no further information about the outcome is available (Asanin et al. 2008).

Table 4.5 Age groups and gender distribution of the cases of hydatidosis registered in Serbia during the period 2001–2010

	Age groups						
	0–9	10–19	20–29	30–39	40–49	50–59	60+
No. of cases	9	10	30	34	48	83	116
%	2.7	3.0	9.1	10.3	14.5	25.1	35.1
Males (no. of cases)	4	7	10	12	10	22	38
Males (%)	44.4	70.0	33.3	35.3	20.8	26.5	32.8

All data refers to Serbia only (without Kosovo) for the entire period 1991–2010 (from Reports on Infectious Diseases in Serbia, published annually by the Institute for Public Health in Serbia)

Croatia

In the Croatian region of Dalmatia, considered an endemic area for hydatidosis, a decrease of over 70 % in the incidence of this disorder was registered from the mid-1950s until 1997. Nevertheless, the relative proportions according to age, gender, and professional status distribution remained constant (Morovic 1997). According to the available data, the incidence of the disease (cases per 100,000 inhabitants) varied during the period from 1997 to 2010 between 0.23 (in 2010) and 0.81 (in 2004) (WHO Regional Office for Europe 2011).

CNS hydatidosis was diagnosed during the period from 1990 to 2000 in three patients (two males, ages 10 and 50 years, and a 20-year-old female with symptoms of elevated intracranial pressure who underwent surgery in Zagreb) (Negovetic et al. 1990; Talan-Hranilovic et al. 2002; Rumboldt et al. 2003), as well as in a 27-year-old male patient with brain involvement who was diagnosed in Sibenik in 2005 (Aleksic-Shihabi and Vidolin 2008).

Macedonia

From 1993 until 2009, the incidence of hydatidosis varied in this country between 0.15 and 1.9 cases per 100,000 inhabitants (WHO Regional Office for Europe 2011). In 1995, a case of vertebral hydatidosis presenting as paraplegic syndrome was reported in Germany in a 16-year-old child originally from Macedonia. The histological examination revealed multilocular cystic lesions (Druschky et al. 1995).

Hydatidosis in Bulgaria

In Bulgaria, the average annual number of surgical cases of hydatidosis increased by 60 % from the period 1971 to 1982 until 1983 to 1995. At the same time, the incidence increased from 2 to 3.3 cases per 100,000 inhabitants (Golemanov et al. 2011). During the period of 1985 to 2010, the average incidence (cases per 100,000 inhabitants) was approximately 6 (range: 2.3 in 1985 and 9.3 in 2002) (WHO Regional Office for Europe 2011). According to Golemanov et al. (2011), in some regions of southern Bulgaria, the incidence varied between 15 and 27 cases per 100,000 inhabitants during 1991 to 2000.

In 1966, Philippov reported 69 cases with hydatidosis and brain involvement that occurred over a 25-year period (Philippov 1966; Arseni et al. 1981). In 1988, Todorov et al. (1988) described the case of a 48-year-old male who had eight hydatid cysts localized in frontal, temporal, and parieto-occipital brain areas. Clinically, the patient presented with convulsive seizures, loss of consciousness, and headache. He was treated with albendazole, and the outcome was favorable.

Hydatidosis in the Former Soviet Union and Russia

During 2006 and 2010, the incidence rates of hydatidosis (cases per 100,000 inhabitants) ranged between 0.35 (in 2006) and 0.4 (in 2010) in the Russian Federation (WHO Regional Office for Europe 2011). A historical overview of cases of hydatid disease with CNS involvement is shown in Table 4.6.

Hydatidosis in Poland

Hydatidosis was and continues to be a rare disease in Poland (Arseni et al. 1981; WHO Regional Office for Europe 2011). Human cases of alveolar echinococcosis were detected as follows: one case in 1951, another one in 1958, and 22 cases during the period from 1994 to 2003 (Myjak et al. 2003). The data available for the period from 1998 to 2010 shows low incidence rates (cases per 100,000 inhabitants) of hydatidosis that ranged between 0.06 (in 2004) and 0.17 (in 2006) (WHO Regional Office for Europe 2011).

Regarding neurohydatidosis, Sokolowski and Mempel reported in a 1962 survey that only three patients were diagnosed with this condition during a 100-year period (Arseni et al. 1981). One of the cysts, the size of a bean, was clogged in the foramen of Magendie (Arseni et al. 1981). Another case with multiple cysts located in the posterior cranial fossa and in the spinal cord

Table 4.6 Reports on CNS hydatidosis in the former Soviet Union and Russia

Year(s)	Author(s)	Cyst location	No. of cases	Specific comments	References
1844	Reported by Grimberg in 1964	CNS	1	–	Arseni et al. (1981)
1959	Veselitskii	Brain	1	AE	Isik et al. (2007), Veselitskii (1959)
1962	Nikolski	Brain (frontoparietal)	1	Giant and calcified cyst Successful surgical removal	Arseni et al. (1981)
1963	Ogleznev	Vertebro-medullary	36	–	Arseni et al. (1981), Ogleznev (1963)
1965	Martyshin	Posterior fossa	1	AE Female patient	Isik et al. (2007), Martyshin (1965)
1966	Arutunov, Subina	CNS	108	28 cases (26 %) of AE	Arseni et al. (1981)
1966	Shubina and Timofeeva	Brain (frontal)	1	AE Female patient presenting seizures and mental disorder	Isik et al. (2007), Shubina and Timofeeva (1967)
1969	Kutniakov and Mitrofanov	Brain, cerebellum	5	AE Of 70 patients, brain metastases were noticed in 4 cases (5.7 %) and cerebellar metastasis in one case (1.4 %)	Arseni et al. (1981), Kutniakov and Mitrofanov (1969)
1977	Peresedov and Morgunov	Brain	1	Patient with a history of general epileptic seizures Association between primary calcified hydatid cyst of the left frontal wall and aneurysm of the supraclinoid portion of the left internal carotid artery with rupture of its wall The outcome was fatal because of massive subarachnoid hemorrhage due to rupture of the aneurysm	Arseni et al. (1981), Peresedov and Morgunov (1977)
1984	Kasumov and Nikonov	Sella turcica	1	AE Female patient	Isik et al. (2007), Kasumov and Nikonov (1984)
2011	Potapov et al.	Brain, heart, and kidneys	1	CE Male patient Removal of seven cysts without their rupture from the left parieto-occipital and right parietal area. Favorable postsurgical outcome	Potapov et al. (2011)

Abbreviations: *AE* alveolar echinococcosis, *CE* cystic echinococcosis, *CNS* central nervous system

Table 4.7 Single case reports on CNS hydatidosis in Germany

Year(s)	Author(s)	Cyst location	Specific comments	References
1934	Nachmacher	Brain (intraparenchymal, 2 hydatid cysts)	54-year-old female patient Rapid evolution to death	Arseni et al. (1981)
1941	Stieda	Brain (left cerebral hemisphere)	7-year-old child	Arseni et al. (1981)
1969	Bonis	Brain (parietal area)	AE Female Bavarian patient Disease evolution with epileptic seizures	Bonis and Sturm (1969), Isik et al. (2007)
1984	Bauer	Brain	AE Middle-aged female patient	Bauer et al. (1984), Isik et al. (2007)
1999	Hagemann et al.	Brain (left frontotemporal area, 2 hydatid cysts)	42-year-old male patient Recurrent headaches for 7 years The patient developed a severe meningeal inflammatory reaction to antihelminthic therapy	Hagemann et al. (1999)
2008	Spies et al.	Lumbar spine	18-year-old male patient Favorable outcome 1 year after surgical intervention	Spies et al. (2008)
2011	Nell et al.	Lumbar spine and psoas muscle	AE 80-year-old male patient Favorable postsurgical outcome	Nell et al. (2011)

Abbreviations: *AE* alveolar echinococcosis

(with favorable postsurgical outcome) was reported in 1973 by Mempel and Grochowski (Mempel and Grochowski 1973; Arseni et al. 1981).

Hydatidosis in Slovakia

During the period from 2000 to 2010, between 0 and 7 human clinical cases of CE were reported annually in Slovakia (except for the year 2000 when 31 cases were registered). The average incidence (cases per 100,000 population) was 0.098 (range: 0–0.58) (Czarkowski et al. 2008; Štefancíková and Dubinský 2010; Turceková et al. 2009). This figure was similar to the incidence found in the neighboring country of Poland (0.096) during the last decade (Czarkowski et al. 2008). Of the above-reported cases, cerebral hydatidosis was found in only one patient. In 2004, following neurological examination and CT screening, CNS hydatidosis was diagnosed in a woman treated for chronic obstructive pulmonary disease (Kinceková et al. 2008).

The first evidence of *E. multilocularis* in Slovakia was recorded in 1999 in a red fox (Dubinský et al. 1999), and since 2000, 16 human cases of AE have been registered. The average incidence rate was 0.027 cases per 100,000 inhabitants (Kinceková et al. 2011). Fourteen of these occurred in three endemic regions for *E. multilocularis* situated in the northern part of the country, where environmental conditions facilitated the overgrowth of the fox population and the parasite circulation (Miterpáková and Dubinský 2011). CNS involvement was not detected in any of these cases.

Hydatidosis in Germany

During 1999 to 2009, the incidence rates (cases per 100,000 inhabitants) of hydatidosis in Germany ranged between zero (in 1999) and 0.15 (in 2006) (WHO Regional Office for Europe 2011). Many interesting cases of CNS hydatidosis were reported in this country over time. A historical overview of particular single cases is provided in Table 4.7.

Of interest also are the findings of a survey undertaken from 1936 to 1960 on 600 cases of AE originating in Germany and Russia. Cerebral involvement was detected in 37 cases (6 %) (Bensaid et al. 1994; Clement et al. 1974; Isik et al. 2007). A retrospective study performed between 1985 and 1989 in Bavaria (situated in southern Germany and considered one of the main endemic regions for hydatidosis in Germany) reported an overall incidence (cases per 100,000 inhabitants) of 1.9 (1.5 for CE and 1.1 for AE). Of the 58 cases of AE included in the analysis, cerebral involvement was noted in 5.2 % of them. By contrast, none of the 123 cases with CE had CNS involvement (Nothdurft et al. 1995a, b).

Hydatidosis in Austria

Between 1854 and 1990, 128 cases of human AE were documented in this country; the average incidence was 0.94 cases per 100,000 inhabitants. None of these cases had CNS involvement (Auer and Aspock 1991). During 1999 to 2010, hydatidosis incidence (cases per 100,000 inhabitants) in Austria ranged between 0.04 (in 2006) and 0.59 (in 1999) (WHO Regional Office for Europe 2011). During 1995 and 2010, two cases with neurohydatidosis were reported in the literature: a 28-year-old female patient (AE of the liver, lungs, and brain) (Schmid et al. 1995, 1998; Reittner et al. 1996) and a 6-year-old girl originally from Bulgaria (CE of the spine involving T8–T9 vertebrae) (Thaler et al. 2010).

Conclusion

Although rare in Central and Eastern Europe, hydatidosis of the CNS should never be overlooked. It should be considered in the differential diagnosis of any patient who presents with seizures, focal neurological deficits, and symptoms of increased intracranial pressure (headache, nausea, vomiting, and papilledema), especially if that person comes from a region with a high prevalence of hydatid disease. Therefore, healthcare professionals should be aware of the disease epidemiology in order to identify at-risk patients.

References

Aleksic-Shihabi A, Vidolin EP. Cystic echinococcosis of the heart and brain: a case report. Acta Med Okayama. 2008;62:341–4.

Arseni C, Samitca DC. Cranial and cerebral hydatid disease. Acta Psychiatr Neurol Scand. 1957;32:389–98.

Arseni C, Horvath L, Sandor G. Compression of the spinal cord due to hydatid disease. Acta Psychiatr Scand. 1960;35:1–12.

Arseni C, Ciurea AV, Cristescu A, Marinescu V, Horvath L. Parazitoze ale sistemului nervos. Bucharest: Editura Stiintifica si Enciclopedica; 1981.

Arseni C, Aldea H, Obreja T, Ciurea AV, Tetraru C, Aldea A, Iacob M, Constantinescu AI. Momente din istoria neurochirurgiei romanesti. Bucharest: Editura Academiei Republicii Socialiste Romania; 1988.

Asanin B, Milic I, Milovic Z. Echinococcosis cerebri: report of two less common cases. Facta Universitatis, Ser Med Biol 2008;15:64–7.

Auer H, Aspock H. Incidence, prevalence and geographic distribution of human alveolar echinococcosis in Austria from 1854 to 1990. Parasitol Res. 1991;77: 430–6.

Basara D. Surgical treatment of liver echinococcosis and analysis of risk factors (in Serbian). Master thesis, University of Belgrade, School of Medicine, Belgrade. 2007.

Bauer WM, Obermuller H, Vogl T, Lissner J. Magnetic resonance in cerebral echinococcosis alveolaris (in German). Digitale Bilddiagn. 1984;4:129–31.

Bensaid AH, Dietemann JL, de la Palavesa MM, Klinkert A, Kastler B, Gangi A, Jacquet G, Cattin F. Intracranial alveolar echinococcosis: CT and MRI. Neuroradiology. 1994;36:289–91.

Bonis G, Sturm KW. Echinococcus alveolaris in the brain (in German). Med Klin. 1969;64:891–3.

Calma CL, Neghina AM, Vlaicu B, Neghina R. Cystic echinococcosis in the human population of a western Romanian county, 2004–2010. Clin Microbiol Infect. 2011;17:1731–4.

Calma CL, Neghina AM, Moldovan R, Dumitrascu V, Marincu I, Neghina R. Cystic Echinococcosis in Arad County, Romania. Vector Borne Zoonotic Dis. 2012; 12:333–5.

Ciurea AV, Vasilescu G, Nuteanu L, Carp N. Cerebral hydatid cyst in children. Experience of 27 cases. Childs Nerv Syst. 1995;11:679–85.

Ciurea AV, Fountas KN, Coman TC, Machinis TG, Kapsalaki EZ, Fezoulidis NI, Robinson JS. Long-term surgical outcome in patients with intracranial hydatid cyst. Acta Neurochir (Wien). 2006a;148:421–6.

Ciurea AV, Giuseppe G, Machinis TG, Coman TC, Fountas KN. Orbital hydatid cyst in childhood: a report of two cases. South Med J. 2006b;99:620–4.

Clement MD, Monange C, Miguet JP, Gisselbrecht H, Pageaut G, Garbillet JP. Cerebral localization of alveolar echinococcosis of the liver. Report of a case (in French). Rev Med Suisse Romande. 1974;94:11–4.

Czarkowski P, Cielebak E, Dacka P, Kondej B. Infectious diseases and poisonings in Poland in 2007. In: Bulletin of the National Institute of Hygiene, Warsaw; 2008, p. 165.

Djuricic SM, Grebeldinger S, Kafka DI, Djan I, Vukadin M, Vasiljevic ZV. Cystic echinococcosis in children – the seventeen-year experience of two large medical centers in Serbia. Parasitol Int. 2010;59:257–61.

Druschky KF, Niederstadt T, Jourdan W, Stoltze D, Heckl R. High-grade transverse syndrome caused by echinococcus cysts (in German). Nervenarzt. 1995;66: 136–9.

Dubinský P, Turekova L, Reiterova K, Svobodova V, Literak I, Klimes J, Martinek K, Kolarova L, Mrlik V. Echinococcus multilocularis in Slovak Republic: the first record in red foxes (Vulpes vulpes). Helminthologia. 1999;36:105–10.

Gazibara T. Parazitska oboljenja mozga i moždanica – analiza biopsija u periodu od 2000–2004. godine (Parasitic diseases of the brain and meninges – analysis of biopsies performed between 2000 and 2004). Medicinski podmladak. 2005;57:23–7.

Gherman I, Coman C, Fagarasanu D, Marinescu V. Boala hidatica. Bucharest: Editura Medicala; 1991.

Golemanov B, Grigorov N, Mitova R, Genov J, Vuchev D, Tamarozzi F, Brunetti E. Efficacy and safety of PAIR for cystic echinococcosis: experience on a large series of patients from Bulgaria. Am J Trop Med Hyg. 2011;84:48–51.

Hagemann G, Gottstein B, Witte OW. Isolated Echinococcus granulosus hydatid cyst in the CNS with severe reaction to treatment. Neurology. 1999;52:1100–1.

Hotez PJ, Gurwith M. Europe's neglected infections of poverty. Int J Infect Dis. 2011;15:e611–9.

Iacobiciu I. Aspecte imunoepidemiologice ale hidatidozei cu Echinococcus granulosus pe teritoriul Banatului. PhD thesis, Universitatea de Medicina si Farmacie Carol Davila, Bucharest; 1999.

Iacobiciu I, Stefanoiu V, Siko Barabasi S, Coroiu Z. Epidemiologia echinococozei-hidatidozei. Sfantu Gheorghe: SC Tipo Graf SRL; 2005.

Isik N, Silav G, Cerci A, Karabagli P, Elmaci I, Kalelioglu M. Cerebral alveolar echinococcosis. A case report with MRI and review of the literature. J Neurosurg Sci. 2007;51:145–51.

Kasumov RD, Nikonov AA. Alveolar echinococcosis of the cavity of the sella turcica (in Russian). Zh Vopr Neirokhir Im N N Burdenko1984;1:47–9.

Kern P. Clinical features and treatment of alveolar echinococcosis. Curr Opin Infect Dis. 2010;23:505–12.

Kinceková J, Pavlinová J, Dubinský Jr P, Bober J, Vrzgula A, Zachar M. Occurrence of echinococcosis and its clinical symptoms in humans – current status in Slovakia. Slovak Vet J. 2008;33:170–2.

Kinceková J, Dubinský P, Danová M, Bober J. Alveolar echinococcosis in humans in Slovakia in 2000–2010. In: Proceedings of Scientific Contributions and Abstracts from the 4th international scientific conference, infectious and parasitic diseases of animals, Košice, Slovakia; 2011. p. 141–3.

Kutniakov VE, Mitrofanov LN. Metastasis in human alveococcosis (in Russian). Med Parazitol (Mosk). 1969;38:325–8.

Lupascu G, Panaitescu D. Hidatidoza. Bucharest: Editura Academiei Republicii Socialiste Romania; 1968.

Martyshin NM. A case of alveolar cerebellar echinococcosis with favorable postoperative outcome (in Russian). Vopr Neirokhir. 1965;29:41–2.

Mempel E, Grochowski W. Multiple echinococcal cysts in posterior cranial fossa and spinal cord treated surgically (in Polish). Neurol Neurochir Pol. 1973;7:741–4.

Miterpáková M, Dubinský P. Fox tapeworm (Echinococcus multilocularis) in Slovakia – summarizing the long-term monitoring. Helminthologia. 2011;48:155–61.

Moldovan R, Neghina AM, Calma CL, Marincu I, Neghina R. Human cystic echinococcosis in two south-western and central-western Romanian counties: a 7-year epidemiological and clinical overview. Acta Trop. 2012;121:26–9.

Moro P, Schantz PM. Echinococcosis: a review. Int J Infect Dis. 2009;13:125–33.

Morovic M. Human hydatidosis in Dalmatia, Croatia. Epidemiol Infect. 1997;119:271–6.

Myjak P, Nahorski W, Pietkiewicz H, von Nickisch-Rosenegk M, Stolarczyk J, Kacprzak E, Felczak-Korzybska I, Szostakowska B, Lucius R. Molecular confirmation of human alveolar echinococcosis in Poland. Clin Infect Dis. 2003;37:e121–5.

Neghina R, Neghina AM, Marincu I, Iacobiciu I. Epidemiology and epizootology of cystic echinococcosis in Romania 1862–2007. Foodborne Pathog Dis. 2010;7:613–8.

Neghina R, Neghina AM, Marincu I, Iacobiciu I. Cystic echinococcosis in Romania: the pediatric approach. Vector Borne Zoonotic Dis. 2011a;11:993–9.

Neghina R, Neghina AM, Marincu I, Iacobiciu I. Epidemiology and history of human parasitic diseases in Romania. Parasitol Res. 2011b;108:1333–46.

Negovetic L, Lupret V, Smiljanic D, Arsenic B. Cranial vault and gigantic intracranial hydatid cyst in a young woman. Neurosurgery. 1990;27:480–1.

Nell M, Burgkart RH, Gradl G, von Eisenhart-Rothe R, Schaeffeler C, Trappe D, da Costa CP, Gradinger R, Kirchhoff C. Primary extrahepatic alveolar echinococcosis of the lumbar spine and the psoas muscle. Ann Clin Microbiol Antimicrob. 2011;15:10–3.

Nothdurft HD, Jelinek T, Mai A, Sigl B, von Sonnenburg F, Loscher T. Epidemiology of alveolar echinococcosis in southern Germany (Bavaria). Infection. 1995a; 23:85–8.

Nothdurft HD, Jelinek T, Mai A, Sigl B, von Sonnenburg F, Loscher T. Epidemiology of alveolar echinococcosis in Bavaria (in German). Dtsch Med Wochenschr. 1995b;120:1151–5.

Ogleznev KI. Echinococcosis of the spinal cord and spine (in Russian). Vopr Neirokhir. 1963;27:56–8.

Peresedov VV, Morgunov VA. Combination of aneurysm and primary echinococcosis of the brain (in Russian). Zh Vopr Neirokhir Im N N Burdenko. 1977;4: 49–51.

Philippov P. Clinical aspects and treatment of echinococcosis of the brain. Some peculiarities of echinococcosis of the brain (in German). Beitr Neurochir. 1966; 13:192–7.

Potapov AA, Goriainov SA, Okhlopkov VA, Kravchuk AD, Zakharova NE, Podoprigora AE, Kurnosov AB, Khit MA, Panina TN, Eliseeva NM. Multiple echinococcosis of brain, heart and kidneys (in Russian). Zh Vopr Neirokhir Im N N Burdenko. 2011;75:57–65.

Reittner P, Szolar DH, Schmid M. Case report. Systemic manifestation of Echinococcus alveolaris infection. J Comput Assist Tomogr. 1996;20:1030–2.

Rumboldt Z, Jednacak H, Talan-Hranilovic J, Rumboldt T, Kalousek M. Unusual appearance of a cisternal hydatid cyst. AJNR Am J Neuroradiol. 2003;24:112–4.

Schmid M, Samonigg H, Stoger H, Auer H, Sternthal MH, Wilders-Truschnig M, Reisinger EC. Use of interferon gamma and mebendazole to stop the progression of alveolar hydatid disease: case report. Clin Infect Dis. 1995;20:1543–6.

Schmid M, Pendl G, Samonigg H, Ranner G, Eustacchio S, Reisinger EC. Gamma knife radiosurgery and albendazole for cerebral alveolar hydatid disease. Clin Infect Dis. 1998;26:1379–82.

Shubina LP, Timofeeva AS. On mental disorders in alveolar echinococcosis of the brain (in Russian). Zh Nevropatol Psikhiatr Im S S Korsakova. 1967;67:755–7.

Sotiraki S, Chaligiannis I. Cystic echinococcosis in Greece. Past and present. Parasite. 2010;17:205–10.

Spies C, Weisskopf M, Ohnsorge JA. Intraspinal echinococcosis within the lumbar spine of an 18-year-old male patient (in German). Z Orthop Unfall. 2008; 146:463–7.

Štefancíková A, Dubinský P. Surveillance of zoonoses. Helminthozoonoses of the Slovak Republic [in Slovak]. In: State Veterinary and Food Administration of the Slovak Republic. Surveillance of Zoonoses: Slovak Republic 2009. Košice: Press Print; 2010. p. 18.

Stefanoiu V, Vranceanu L. Considerations on 407 cases of children hydatidosis. Rom J Parasitol. 1994;4:74–7.

Talan-Hranilovic J, Sajko T, Negovetic L, Lupret V, Kalousek M. Cerebral cysticercosis and echinococcosis: a preoperative diagnostic dilemma. Arch Med Res. 2002;33:590–4.

Thaler M, Gabl M, Lechner R, Gstottner M, Bach CM. Severe kyphoscoliosis after primary Echinococcus granulosus infection of the spine. Eur Spine J. 2010;19:1415–22.

Todorov T, Vutova K, Petkov D, Balkanski G. Albendazole treatment of multiple cerebral hydatid cysts: case report. Trans R Soc Trop Med Hyg. 1988;82:150–2.

Turceková L, Šnábel V, Dudinák V, Gašpar V, Dubinský P. Prevalence of cystic echinococcosis in pigs from Slovakia, with evaluation of size, fertility and number of hydatid cysts. Helminthologia. 2009;46:151–8.

Veselitskii SK. On the problem of remote results of operative treatment of alveolar echinococcosis of the brain (in Russian). Vopr Neirokhir. 1959;23:44–5.

World Health Organization (WHO) Regional Office for Europe. Centralized information system for infectious diseases (CISID). 2011. http://data.euro.who.int/CISID/. Accessed 3 Dec 2011.

Hydatidosis of the Skull

5

Zahed Hossain

Contents

Z. Hossain, MD, MBBS, FCPS, MS
Department of Clinical Neurosurgery,
National Institute of Neurosciences and Hospital,
Dhaka 1207, Bangladesh
e-mail: zaheddr@yahoo.com

Introduction

Cranial hydatid cyst is a relatively rare condition. In the world literature, many reports of cranial hydatid disease are available, but most of them are small series, and reports of skull hydatid cyst are very scarce. It is part of hydatidosis, which is a zoonotic disease. *Echinococcus granulosus* larva travels through systemic circulation from the gastric mucosa to the cranial cavity. Through this pathway it is filtered in the hepatic and pulmonary beds. Even after the pulmonary filtration, a few still make it to the systemic circulation and can lodge in almost any part of the body, including the brain, heart, and bones (Kovoor et al. 2007; Reddy 2009; Nemati et al. 2010). Cysts in the head and neck region, especially the skull base, can present with atypical clinical symptoms (Sureka et al. 2010). Intracranial extracerebral hydatid cysts are rare and may occur in three forms: (a) cranial, usually the bony spongiosa is the first to be involved; (b) cranial extradural, the extradural space may be infected by embolization of scolices or embryos via blood vessels, by extrusion of intracerebral cysts via healthy dura mater or by erosion of osseous hydatid into the extradural space; and (c) combined, there may be simultaneous intracerebral, extradural, and bony cysts. Of the three forms, extradural variety is extremely rare as the physiologic flow of blood to the brain is mainly through the internal carotid system, so the likelihood of the larvae traveling through the external carotid system is very low (Ravalji et al. 2006).

M. Turgut (ed.), *Hydatidosis of the Central Nervous System: Diagnosis and Treatment*,
DOI 10.1007/978-3-642-54359-3_5,

Incidence

Although hydatid cyst can occur in any organ or tissue of the body including brain and orbit, the bone and brain are the fourth common sites of involvement after the liver, lungs, and peritoneum (Mumtaz et al. 2009). Only 2 % of the hydatid cysts are located in the skeleton, and of these only 3–4 % are in the skull (Behari et al. 1997; Raynham et al. 2009). Recently, it has been reported that skull hydatidosis was firstly described by Guesnard in 1836, with the cranial vault (68.5 %) being more commonly involved than the skull base (Limaiem et al 2009). Skull base hydatid disease is extremely rare. Raynham et al. (2009) reported three cases of hydatid cyst of the skull base, the first of them involved the anterior cranial fossa and paranasal sinuses. The second was located in the infratemporal fossa. The last involved the temporal bone and posterior cranial fossa. Sureka et al. (2010) reported a case presenting with lower cranial nerve paresis, such as palatal and vocal cord palsy, mimicking a malignant mass. In 1992, Turgut et al. reported only three cases of orbital hydatidosis from their clinic, where non-orbital hydatidoses are frequently encountered. In 2004, Turgut et al. reported 25 cases of orbital hydatidosis in entire Turkey from 1963 to 2001 where hydatidosis is still a serious public health problem. A summary of the 38 reported cases of hydatidosis of the skull published in the world literature to date is given in Table 5.1 (Arseni and Samitca 1957; Orman and Le Roux 1968; Kanaka et al. 1970; Teymoorian and Bagheri 1976; Gokalp et al. 1979; Ozgen et al. 1984; Kanpolat et al. 1988; Gedikoglu et al. 1989; Benmoussa et al. 1990; Aydin et al. 1992; Rivierez et al. 1992; el Khamlichi 1993; Pasaoglu et al. 1998; Ennouri et al. 2000; Abbassioun and Amirjamshidi 2001; Erman et al. 2001; Turgut 2001; el Kohen et al. 2003; Taghipour et al. 2005; Lath et al. 2007; Limaiem et al. 2009; Raynham et al. 2009; Hossain et al. 2010; Siddiqui et al. 2010; Sureka et al. 2010; Yazdani et al. 2010).

Young males are most commonly affected (Teymoorian and Bagheri 1976). Because of the restricted geographic distribution of the echinococcal worms, persons of certain races are affected more commonly than others; however, the parasite has the capability of infecting persons of all races equally. No sexual predilection is recognized (Dandan 2008).

Pathology

Cranial hydatid cyst may occur in the skull bones (intraosseous) and in the intracranial space. In the skull, it may involve the cranial vault and skull base and may spread to the paranasal sinuses and orbit. Primary hydatid disease of bone due to *E. granulosus* occurs when a blood-borne scolex settles in the bone (Limaiem et al. 2009). It initially invades the diploe, and as it grows it widens the diploic space, and subsequently it extends in both directions (Dharkar 1996). The wall of the cyst consists of an inner endocyst (germinal layer) and outer ectocyst (laminated layer) (Nemati et al. 2010). In bone involvement, pericyst formation does not occur, thereby allowing aggressive proliferation in an irregular branching fashion along the line of least resistance, especially the bone canals. The parasite replaces the osseous tissue between trabeculae due to the slow growth of multiple vesicles. With time, the parasite reaches and destroys the cortex, with subsequent spread of the disease to surrounding tissues (Limaiem et al. 2009). Early cases present as an expansile osteolytic lesion in the diploe. The more advanced forms manifest as multilocular or unilocular destructive lesions with adjacent soft tissue masses (Teymoorian and Bagheri 1976). As the cyst grows, the bone undergoes pressure atrophy, and the inner or outer table of the skull ruptures. The inner table of the skull frequently ruptures, and the vesicular larva passes into the epidural space inducing symptoms of increased intracranial pressure. Less frequently, cysts may rupture the outer table of the skull at many spots and involve the scalp to produce prominence on the head (Aydin et al. 1992; Limaiem et al. 2009). When both outer table and inner table are destroyed, intra-cranial and extra-cranial spaces become communicated with each other (Fig. 5.1).

Table 5.1 Summary of the 38 reported cases of hydatidosis of skull published in the world literature to date

Author(s)	Country	Year of publication	No. of cases	Site of involvement	Radiological study	Outcome
Arseni and Samitca	Romania	1957	1	Skull	X-ray	NS
Orman and Roux	South Africa	1968	2	Vault—frontal (1) and base (1)	X-ray and angiogram	NS
Kanaka et al.	India	1970	1	Vault	X-ray	Behavior improved, recurrence after 6 mos
Teymoorian and Bagheri	Iran	1976	4	Base	X-ray	Complete recovery (2), died at 4 mos (1), well up to 2 yrs (1)
Gokalp et al.	Turkey	1979	1	Vault—Lt temporoparietal	X-ray	Complete recovery at postop 3 mos
Ozgen et al.	Turkey	1984	1	Intrasellar	X-ray and CT	Complete recovery at postop 10 mos
Kanpolat et al.	Turkey	1988	1	Base—cavernous sinus	CT	Unchanged ocular movement restriction at postop 12 mos
Gedikoglu et al.	Turkey	1989	1	Parasellar	CT	Complete recovery at postop 3 mos
Benmoussa et al.	Morocco	1990	2	Vault—parietal (1), occipital (1)	CT	Good (1), recurrence (1)
Aydin et al.	Turkey	1992	1	Vault—intradiploic, parietal, and occipital	X-ray, CT	Died at early postop
Rivierez et al.	France	1992	1	Base—cavernous sinus	CT, MRI	NS
el Khamlichi	Morocco	1993	1	Base—cavernous sinus	X-ray and CT	NS
Pasaoglu et al.	Turkey	1998	1	Base—infratemporal fossa	CT	Complete removal, No follow-up
Ennouri et al.	Tunisia	2000	1	Vault—Lt temporal	CT and MRI	Well at early postop
Abbassioun and Amirjamshidi	Iran	2001	7	Vault and base	X-ray, CT, and MRI	Well
Erman et al.	Turkey	2001	1	Vault—Rt parietal	CT	Complete recovery
Turgut[a]	Turkey	2001	3	Base	X-ray and CT	Complete recovery (2), unchanged (1)
el-Kohen et al.	Morocco	2003	1	Base—Lt jugular foramen	CT and MRI	Chemotherapy followed by motor improvement
Taghipour et al.	Iran	2005	1	Base—foramen magnum	MRI	Complete recovery
Lath et al.	India	2007	1	Base	CT	Well
Limaiem et al.	Tunisia	2009	1	Vault—Rt frontal	CT	Recurrence requiring second operation
Raynham et al.	South Africa	2009	3	Base	CT	Complete recovery
Hossain et al.	Bangladesh	2010	1	Vault—Rt temporal	CT	Complete recovery
Sureka et al.	India	2010	1	Base—posterior fossa	CT and MRI	Well at early postop
Yazdani et al.	Iran	2010	1	Base and orbit	CT	Recurrence
Siddiqui et al.	India	2010	1	Vault and orbit	CT	Complete recovery

Abbreviations: *NS* not stated, *Rt* right, *Lt* left, *CT* computed tomography, *MRI* magnetic resonance imaging, *mos* months, *yr(s)* year(s), *postop* postoperative

[a]Note that the number of cases was given within the brackets

The cases reported by the author had already been described by Ozgen et al., Kanpolat et al., and Gedikoglu et al. earlier

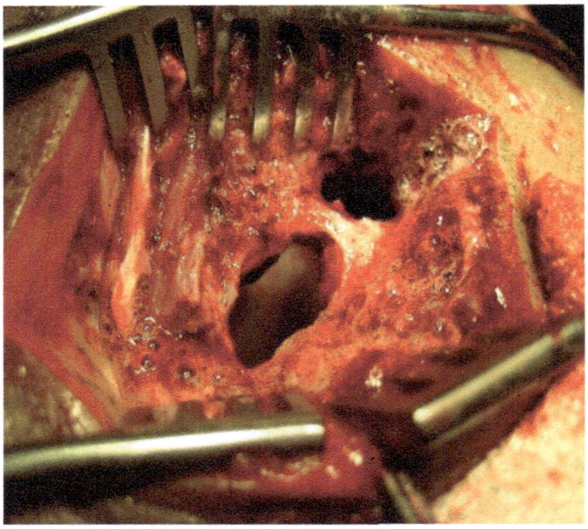

Fig. 5.1 Eroded bone seen perioperatively

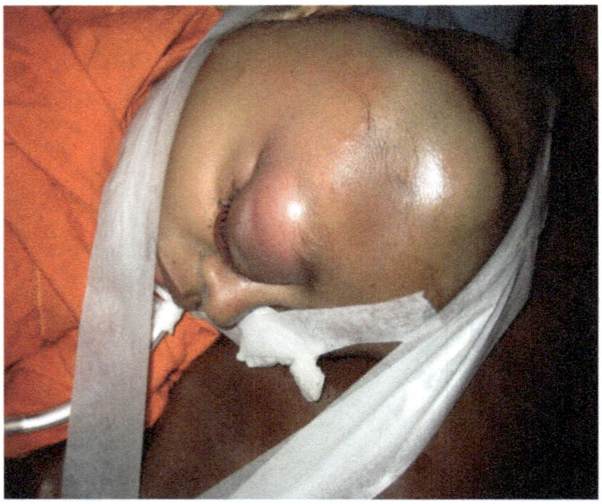

Fig. 5.2 Infected hydatid cyst (abscess) showing all the features of acute inflammation

Presentation

Cranial hydatid cysts present by their location in the skull. Nevertheless, if it ruptures, it may then show systemic features. Generally, four syndromes dominate the presenting clinical manifestations of cranial hydatid disease including increased intracranial pressure (48 %), skull deformity (48 %), cranial nerve palsies (42 %), and focal neurological disturbance (30 %) (Aydin et al. 1992; Limaiem et al. 2009).

When hydatid cyst involves the cranial vault, it may present with swelling on the head which causes the deformity of the head. It is usually painless and insidious in growth, but if it becomes infected, then it becomes painful. When frontal bone is involved, swelling is on the forehead and frontal region. When it involves the parietal bone, swelling will be on the parietal region. Accordingly, swelling may be on the temporal, occipital, or suboccipital region. The swelling is firm in consistency (Dharkar 1996). Scalp moves over the swelling if it is not ruptured externally. When it ruptures and involves the extra-calvarial soft tissues, swelling may be soft and cystic. If it becomes infected, all the features of acute inflammation may present in the form of swelling, redness, tenderness, and raised local temperature (Fig. 5.2).

Cranial hydatidosis may present with the features of intracranial space-occupying lesion. Presenting features may be classified as (a) features of raised intracranial pressure and (b) focal neurological signs. Intracranial pressure may increase due to its volume or it may obstruct the cerebrospinal fluid (CSF) pathway. These patients may also present with seizure (Al-Akayleh 2003). Features of raised intracranial pressure are headache, nausea and vomiting, papilledema, blurring of vision, gait disturbance/ataxia, vertigo, diplopia, bradycardia, and hypertension. In advanced conditions, respiratory irregularity and deterioration of level of consciousness may occur (Greenberg 2001). Focal neurological signs are according to the location of the cyst in the cranial vault, like hemiparesis, hemisensory deficit, cognitive disorder, and visual deficit. Diagnosis of a hydatid cyst can sometimes be confused with other space-occupying lesions of the brain, especially abscesses, neoplasms, and arachnoid cysts (Anvari et al. 2009; Bahloul et al. 2009; Nemati et al. 2010). Hydatid cyst in the skull base usually remains silent unless it involves the adjacent structures. It may involve the cranial nerves and may present with the features of cranial nerve palsies. Patient may present with anosmia if the cyst involves the olfactory nerve in the anterior cranial fossa at the cribriform plate. It may involve the optic nerve, and orbit

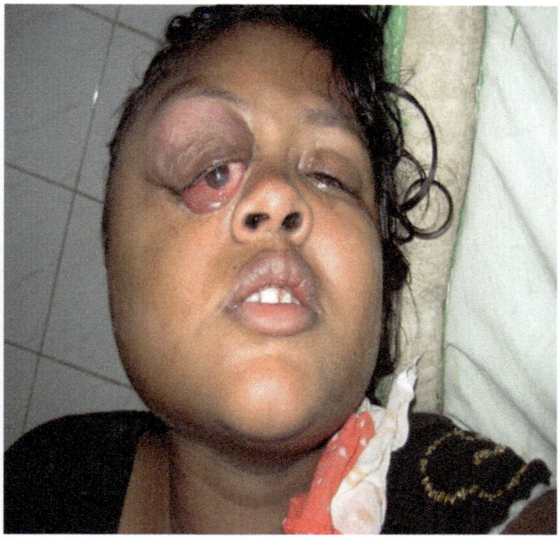

Fig. 5.3 Infected hydatid cyst involving orbit developing proptosis

may present with visual impairment and proptosis (Fig. 5.3). Third, fourth, and sixth cranial nerves may be involved in the cavernous sinus or at their exit from the cranial cavity with diplopia and/or ophthalmoplegia. Hydatid cyst of the anterior cranial fossa enters into the paranasal air sinuses, which may precipitate development of sinusitis. Hydatid cyst of the middle cranial fossa may present with third, fourth, fifth, and sixth cranial nerve palsy. It may enter into the infratemporal fossa. Hydatid cyst of the posterior cranial fossa may present with features of (a) lower cranial nerve palsy like facial asymmetry, vertigo, impaired hearing, tinnitus and ringing in the ear, and regurgitation on swallowing; (b) long tract signs like weakness of one or both upper and lower limbs; and also (c) cerebellar signs like speech difficulty (dysarthria), gait disturbance, and ataxia. Raynham et al. (2009) reported three cases of skull base hydatid cyst, among them one involving the paranasal air sinus and presenting with complicated sinusitis; a second one involving the infratemporal fossa and presenting with painless right facial swelling, lateral displacement of ramus of the mandible, and sensory impairment of maxillary and mandibular division of the fifth cranial nerve; and a third one involving the left temporal bone and posterior cranial

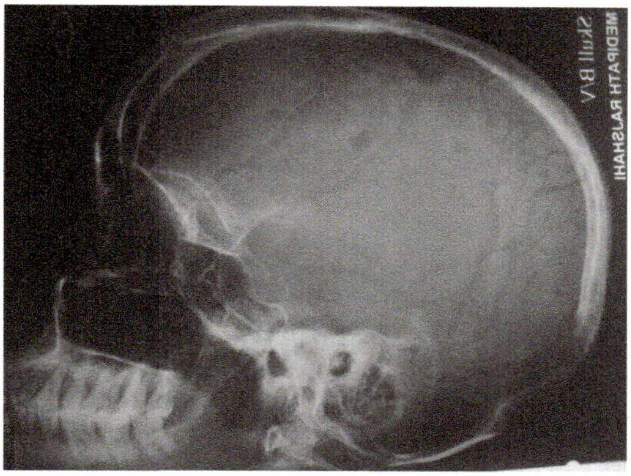

Fig. 5.4 Hydatid cyst involving the occipital bone

fossa and presenting with progressive weakness of legs, left arm, right face, and mixed sensorineural and conductive type of hearing loss.

Diagnosis

Diagnosis of echinococcosis is made by using imaging and serology techniques. Conventional radiography usually shows a variable-sized ill-delineated osteolysis (Figs. 5.4 and 5.5) without osteosclerosis (Limaiem et al. 2009). Computed tomography (CT) scan and magnetic resonance imaging (MRI) are valuable in the identification of cerebral and bone lesions and are helpful in surgical planning. CT scans obtained before and after contrast medium injection show the multivesicular pattern of the lesion and reveal its endo- and exocranial extensions (Ennouri et al. 2000; Limaiem et al. 2009) (Figs. 5.6, 5.7, and 5.8). Both CT and MRI are used frequently in diagnosing the cystic lesions (Tuzun and Hekimoglu 1998; Andronikou et al. 2002; el-Shamam et al. 2001; Ciurea et al. 2006; Kovoor et al. 2007; Anvari et al. 2009; Nemati et al. 2010). However, MRI is considered superior in demonstrating the cyst rim (Krajewski and Stelmasiak 1991; Tuzun and Hekimoðlu 1998; Altinörs et al. 2000; Pedrosa et al. 2001; Andronikou et al. 2002; Cavusoglu et al. 2009; Nemati et al. 2010). Contrast enhancement usually does not occur in cyst walls. But if cyst becomes infected, cyst wall may be enhanced faintly with contrast. Cyst fluid shows density and intensity similar to CSF on computed tomography (CT) and magnetic resonance imaging (MRI), i.e., hypodense on CT and hypointense on T1WI and hyperintense on T2WI in MRI.

The differential diagnosis of intraosseous hydatid cyst may be difficult especially in cases of pure skull involvement. The association of the intracranial cystic lesion to osteolysis of the inner and outer tables is highly suggestive of hydatid cyst (Limaiem et al. 2009). Pericyst formation does not occur in bone, and the cyst has a much thinner wall. Because of this fact and the rigid nature of bone, the cyst cannot assume its typical shape (sphere). The

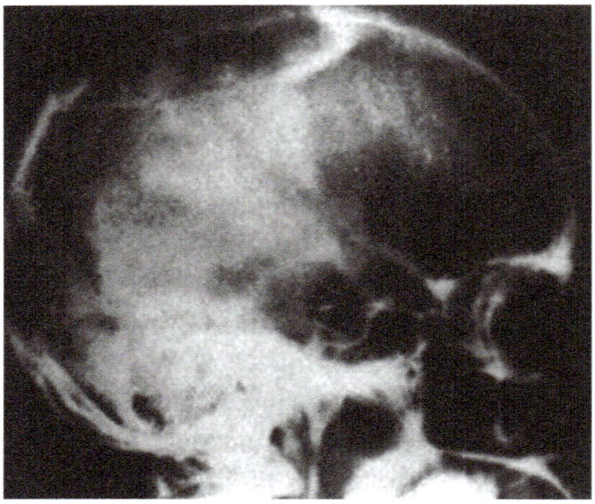

Fig. 5.5 Plain skull x-ray showing expansion of the parietal parasagittal bone due to an intradiploic hydatid cyst (Reproduced, with permission, from Abbassioun et al. 2003)

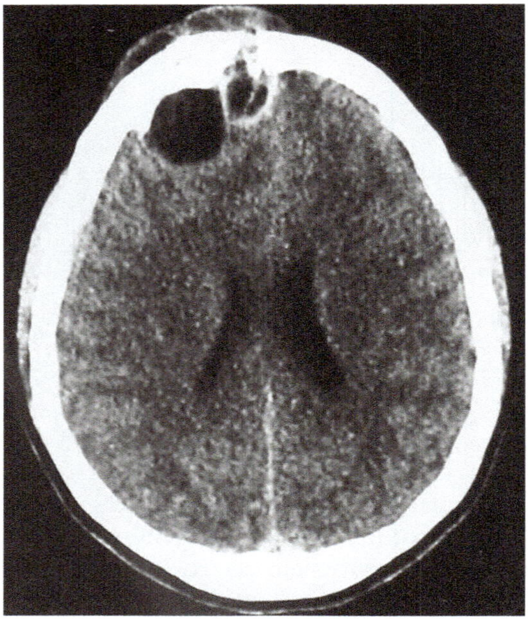

Fig. 5.7 Hydatid cyst of frontal bone on CT scan - axial view (Reproduced, with pemission, from Limaiem et al. 2009)

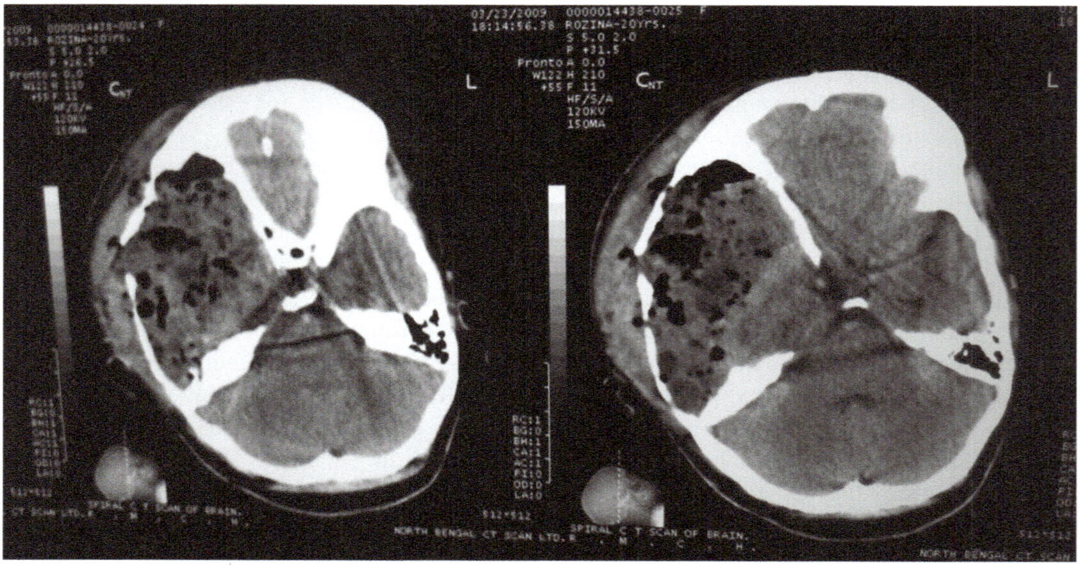

Fig. 5.6 Eroded bone with extracranial and intracranial extension of hydatid abscess seen on CT scan

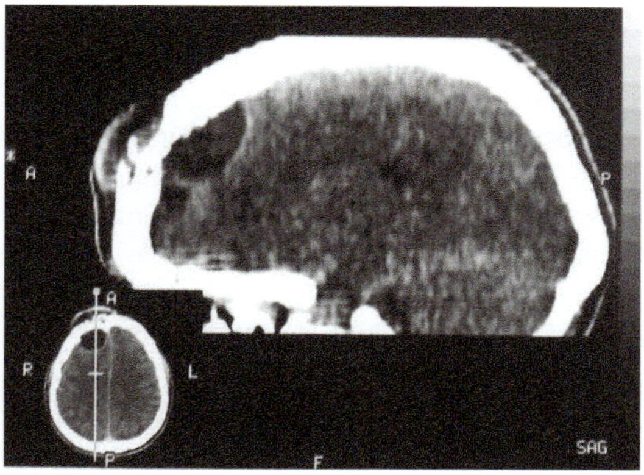

Fig. 5.8 Hydatid cyst of frontal bone on CT scan - sagittal view (Reproduced, with pemission, from Limaiem et al. 2009)

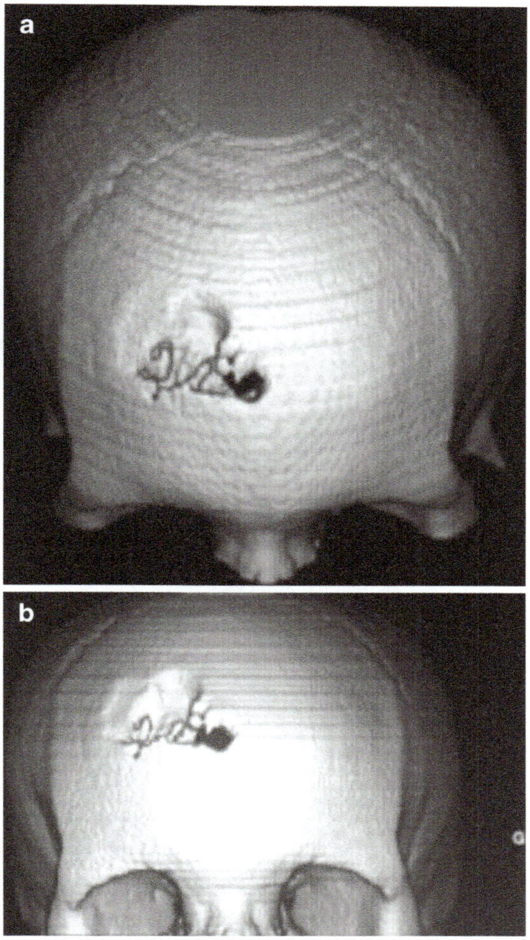

Fig. 5.9 (**a**, **b**) 3-D CT picture of hydatidosis of the cranial vault (Courtesy of F. Limaiem, MD)

cyst enlarges in an irregular branching fashion along the path of least resistance. Over time, the parasite replaces the osseous tissue and destroys the cortex (Fig. 5.9a, b). Extraosseous hydatid cysts may calcify (Fig. 5.10), whereas intraosseous hydatid cysts rarely show calcification (Polat et al. 2003). Ringlike calcification of the cyst wall and extensive calcification in the cyst have also been reported (Dharkar 1996) (Fig. 5.11). Parasitized bone has heterogeneous medium to low signal intensity on T1-weighted MRIs and high signal intensity on T2-weighted images. CT demonstrates the calcification in extraosseous hydatid cysts (Polat et al. 2003). When hydatid cyst grows internally, it causes compression over the subjacent brain, but there will be no perilesional brain edema. If cyst becomes infected, there may be perilesional edema and cyst wall may take the contrast. Imaging has an important role in making a diagnosis of hydatid cyst. Hydatid cysts in unusual anatomical locations are difficult to diagnose on imaging, even in patients from endemic regions. Therefore, familiarity with imaging findings is crucial to make a preoperative diagnosis. On CT, this multiloculated cystic skull base lesion mimicked a malignant mass. MRI is a more useful imaging modality when a complex cystic head and neck lesion is present. A cystic lesion with multivesiculated "bunch of grapes" appearance, a peripheral T_2 hypointense rim ("rim sign"), and separated collapsed membranes as irregular low-signal-intensity linear floating structures ("serpent sign") were considered diagnostic for hydatid disease (Sureka et al. 2010).

Bone and brain tissue evokes minimal or no immunological response to hydatidosis. The peripheral blood and cerebrospinal fluid eosinophilia tests may be helpful for the diagnosis of hydatid disease (Erman et al. 2001; Limaiem et al. 2009). Serologic tests are valuable when they are positive, but they are usually false negative for osseous hydatidosis (Arazi et al. 2005; Limaiem et al. 2009). The Casoni and Weinberg tests, indirect hemagglutination, eosinophilia, and ELISA are used in diagnosing hydatid cysts,

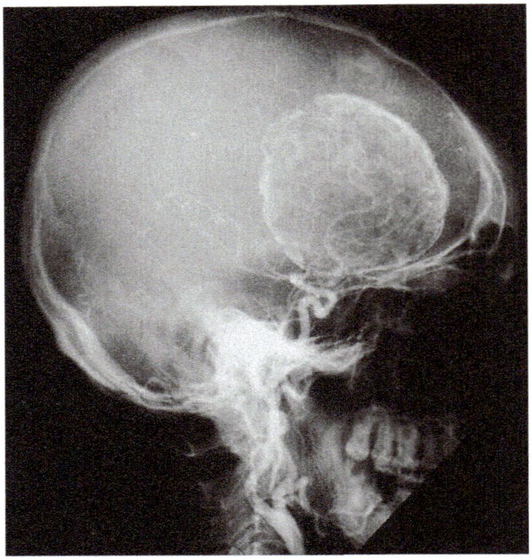

Fig. 5.10 Calcified hydatid cyst

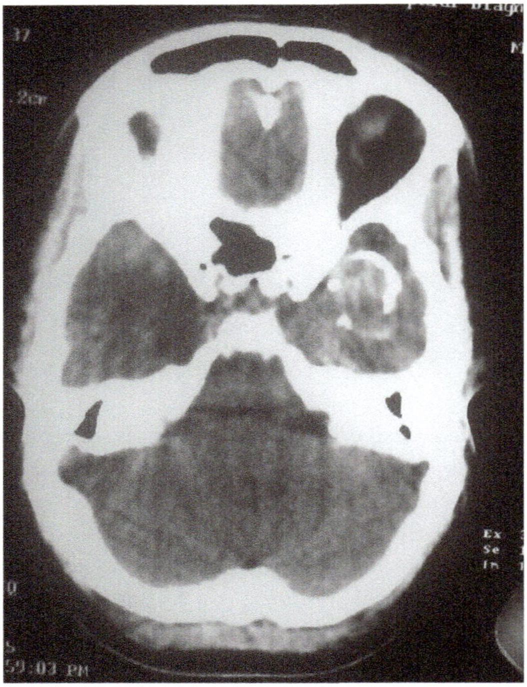

Fig. 5.11 Calcified cyst in the base of the skull (temporal)

but usually results tend to be false negatives (Khaldi et al. 2000; Andronikou et al. 2002; Cavusoglu et al. 2009; Reddy 2009; Nemati et al. 2010).

Differential Diagnosis

In particular, eosinophilic granuloma, cystic fibrous dysplasia, and calvarial epidermoid tumor/cyst must be considered in the differential diagnosis of intraosseous hydatid cyst. Eosinophilic granuloma is usually solitary and involves the diploe. CT scanning demonstrates a sharply marginated lytic skull defect more frequently involving the outer table than the inner table. The cystic form of fibrous dysplasia is usually homogeneously hypodense and typically has a smooth sclerotic border. An epidermoid tumor or cyst of the calvarium has a sclerotic rim and lacks inner trabeculae. Less likely considerations include solitary metastasis, brown tumor, and plasmacytoma. Metastases and brown tumors are rarely solitary, and they are characteristically poorly marginated. Plasmacytoma may be solitary; it usually has a septated, bubbly, and irregularly marginated appearance (Erman et al. 2001). Hydatid cyst growing internally causing compression over the brain can sometimes be confused with other space-occupying lesions of the brain, especially abscesses, neoplasms, and arachnoid cysts.

Treatment

Treatment of skull hydatid cyst should be aimed at the treatment of hydatidosis and skull defect caused by the cyst and treatment for the cyst (craniectomy). Both medical and surgical treatments are advocated for cranial hydatid disease. Medical therapy for small hydatid cysts has been promising. Albendazole alone or in combination with other compounds, such as praziquantel, has been reported with favorable results as an adjunct and, in certain circumstances, as the primary mode of treatment (Davis et al. 1989; Singounas et al. 1992; Todorov et al. 1992; Reddy 2009; Nemati et al. 2010). It is reported that albendazole results in the disappearance of up to 48 % of cysts and a substantial reduction in size of the cysts in another 28 % (Reddy 2009; Nemati et al. 2010). Albendazole therapy is given in a daily dose of 10 mg/kg, taken three times for 4 months (Al-Akayleh 2003).

The World Health Organization (WHO) recommendation on the duration of albendazole therapy is at least 3 months (Raynham et al. 2009). It is a broad-spectrum oral antihelminthic drug, which acts by blocking glucose uptake of the larva and adult worm. The glycogen storage is depleted, thereby decreasing the adenosine-5′-triphosphate formation resulting in death of the parasite (Al-Akayleh 2003).

Surgery is the mainstay of treatment for hydatid cyst of the skull. Total resection of the cyst along with the affected bone without rupture via the craniectomy is the recommended treatment; however, extradural hydatid cysts of intraosseous origin may be difficult to excise completely because of their adherence to dura and osseous trabeculae (Canbolat et al. 1994; Dharkar 1996; Erman et al. 2001; Limaiem et al. 2009). This, of course, is not possible when the disease affects the base of the skull (Dharkar 1996). During operation, the field of operation should be separated by hypertonic saline-soaked mop to minimize the spillage. After excision, the operative field should be generously irrigated with hypertonic saline solution. Chemotherapy should be continued postoperatively for 3–6 months (el Kohen et al. 2003; Raynham et al. 2009). Cysts in the base of the skull are aspirated by wide bore needle and injected with hypertonic saline or alcohol solution followed by partial or complete removal of the cyst. Then chemotherapy is continued for 3–6 months. Chemotherapy for hydatidosis of the central nervous system is discussed in Chap. 16.

Skull defect created by craniectomy is closed by cranioplasty with methyl methacrylate, i.e., bone cement or titanium plate. This can be done primarily if the surgeon is satisfied that the cyst is completely removed without any rupture or spillage. Steroids are helpful in relieving cranial nerve palsies (Dharkar 1996).

Complications

The most important complication of hydatid cyst is rupture with spillage of the hydatid fluid which is strongly immunogenic and may cause anaphylactic shock. This can happen during operation or due to head trauma which causes fracture of the skull bone. There has been repeated suggestion that coexistent bacterial infection of a liver hydatid cyst is possible, but suppuration of a hydatid cyst in the brain with daughter vesicles is an extremely rare occurrence. Erongun et al. (1994) found only two cases in the English literature from 1955 to 1991. Multiple infected cerebral hydatid cyst is uncommon entity and can be confused with other cystic brain lesions. Gana et al. (2008) described one case of infected hydatid cyst in the brain. Hossain et al. (2010) reported one case of abscess involving both intra- and extracranial spaces eroding the intervening bone. Complications of craniospinal hydatidosis are discussed in detail in Chaps. 17 and 18.

Conclusion

The following conclusions may be drawn from this chapter:

1. Hydatid disease of the skull is a rare entity.
2. Usually, it does not have any systemic sign unless it becomes ruptured or infected.
3. High index of clinical suspicion is required to diagnose the condition especially in the endemic areas. Painless swelling of the skull, unexplained features of raised intracranial pressure, focal neurological sign, or cranial nerve palsy should be investigated by CT scan or MRI as these are the most important tools for diagnosing the hydatidosis of the skull.
4. Bone and brain tissue evokes minimum or no immunological reaction to hydatidosis, so serologic tests are of little value in diagnosing the condition.
5. During operation, every effort should be made to prevent the spillage of the cyst fluid and to remove the cyst completely except in case of basal skull hydatidosis where complete removal of the cyst is not possible.

Acknowledgments I am expressing my heartfelt thanks and gratitude to Ass. Professor Mehmet Turgut, MD, PhD, the editor of this book who invited and encouraged me to write this chapter. I am indebted to my patient Mrs. Rozina Akhter who permitted me to use her photographs and CT scan report for publication and for any academic purpose.

References

Abbassioun K, Amirjamshidi A. Diagnosis and management of hydatid cyst of the central nervous system: part 2: hydatid cysts of the skull, orbit, and spine. Neurosurg Q. 2001;11:10–6.

Abbassioun K, Amirjamshidi A, Sabouri Deylamie M. Hydatid disease of the central nervous system: imaging characteristics and general features. Iran J Radiol. 2003;3–4:125–31.

Al-Akayleh A. Intracranial hydatid cysts: diagnosis and treatment. Bahrain Med Bull. 2003;25:91–4.

Altinörs N, Bavbek M, Caner HH, Erdogan B. Central nervous system hydatidosis in Turkey: a cooperative study and literature survey analysis of 458 cases. J Neurosurg. 2000;93:1–8.

Andronikou S, Welman C, Kader E. Classic and unusual appearances of hydatid disease in children. Pediatr Radiol. 2002;32:817–28.

Anvari M, Amirjamshidi A, Abbassioun K. Gradual and complete delivery of a hydatid cyst of the brain through a single burr hole, a wrong happening! Childs Nerv Syst. 2009;25:1639–42.

Arazi M, Erikoglu M, Odev K, Memik R, Ozdemir M. Primary echinococcus infestation of the bone and muscles. Clin Orthop Relat Res. 2005;432:234–41.

Arseni C, Samitca DC. Cranial and cerebral hydatid disease. Acta Psychiatr Neurol Scand. 1957;32:389–98.

Aydin Y, Aydin F, Turec U. Intradiploeic and cerebral hydatidosis: a case report and review of literature. Clin Neurol Neurosurg. 1992;94:229–33.

Bahloul K, Ouerchefani N, Kammoun B, Boudouara MZ. Unusual brain edema caused by an intracranial hydatid cyst: case report and literature review (in French). Neurochirurgie. 2009;55:53–6.

Behari S, Banerji D, Phadke RV. Multiple, infected, extradural, parasellar hydatid cysts. Surg Neurol. 1997;48:53–7.

Benmoussa H, Tamehmacht M, Bellakhdar F. Hydatidosis of the cranial vault. Two case reports (in French). Neurochirurgie. 1990;363:191–3.

Canbolat A, Onal C, Kaya U, Coban TE. Intracranial extradural hydatid cysts: report of three cases. Surg Neurol. 1994;41:230–4.

Cavusoglu H, Tuncer C, Ozdilmaç A, Aydin Y. Multiple intracranial hydatid cysts in a boy. Turk Neurosurg. 2009;19:203–7.

Ciurea AV, Fountas KN, Coman TC, Machinis TG, Kapsalaki EZ, Fezoulidis NI, Robinson JS. Long-term surgical outcome in patients with intracranial hydatid cyst. Acta Neurochir (Wien). 2006;148:421–6.

Dandan IS. Hydatid cysts. Medscape reference, http://emedicine.medscape.com updated on June 2008.

Davis A, Dixon H, Pawloski ZS. Multicentre clinical trials of benzimidazole-carbamates in human cystic echinococcosis (phase 2). Bull World Health Organ. 1989;67:503–8.

Dharkar SR. Hydatid disease. In: Ramamurthi B, Tandon PN, editors. Textbook of Neurosurgery. New Delhi: Churchill Livingstone; 1996. p. 535–44.

el Khamlichi A. Hydatid cyst of the cavernous sinus. A case (in French). Neurochirurgie. 1993;39:55–7.

el Kohen A, Benjelloun A, El Quessar A. Multiple hydatid cysts of the neck, the nasopharynx and the skull base revealing cervical vertebral hydatid disease. Int J Pediatr Otorhinolaryngol. 2003;67:655–62.

el-Shamam O, Amer T, El-Atta MA. Magnetic resonance imaging of simple and infected hydatid cysts of the brain. Magn Reson Imaging. 2001;19:965–74.

Ennouri S, Ayadi K, Ben Ali H, Mnif J. Hydatid cyst of the temporal bone. An exceptional location. AJR Am J Roentgenol. 2000;175:923–5.

Erman T, Tuna M, Göçer I, Ildan F, Zeren M, Çetinalp E. Intracranial intraosseous hydatid cyst. Case report and review of the literature. Neurosurg Focus. 2001;11:ECP1.

Erongun U, Özkal E, Acar O, Kocaogullar Y. Multiple and infected cerebral hydatid cysts. Case report. Neurosurg Rev. 1994;17:77–81.

Gana R, Skhissi M, Maaqili R, Bellakhdar F. Multiple infected cerebral hydatid cysts. J Clin Neurosci. 2008;15:591–3.

Gedikoglu Y, Colak A, Bertan V. Parasellar hydatid cyst. Case report. J Pediatr Neurosci. 1989;5:173–5.

Gokalp HZ, Kanpolat Y, Gokben B. Hydatid cyst of the skull. Neurosurgery. 1979;4:431–3.

Greenberg MS. Handbook of neurosurgery. 5th ed. New York: Thieme Medical Publishers; 2001. p. 389–92, 640–2.

Hossain MZ, Rahman MM, Badruddoza SM. Cranial hydatid abscess. Trop Doct. 2010;40:255–6.

Kanaka TS, Balasubramaniam V, Meenakshisundaram E, Varadarajan M. Hydatid of the skull. Indian J Surg. 1970;32:200–3.

Kanpolat Y, Mertol T, Şekerci Z, Kökeş F. Hydatid cyst of the cavernous sinus. Clin Neurol Neurosurg. 1988;90:175–6.

Khaldi M, Mohamed S, Kallel J, Khouja N. Brain hydatidosis: report on 117 cases. Childs Nerv Syst. 2000;16:765–9.

Kovoor JME, Thomas RD, Chandrashekhar HS, Jayakumar PN, Pillai S, Shankar SK. Neurohydatidosis. Australas Radiol. 2007;51:406–11.

Krajewski R, Stelmasiak Z. Cerebral hydatid cysts in children. Childs Nerv Syst. 1991;7:154–5.

Lath R, Ratnam BG, Ranjan A. Diagnosis and treatment of multiple hydatid cysts at the craniovertebral junction. Case report. J Neurosurg Spine. 2007;6:174–7.

Limaiem F, Bellil S, Bellil K, Chelly I, Mekni A, Kallel J, Haouet S, Zitouna M, Kchir N. Hydatid cyst of the cranial vault. J Infect Dev Ctries. 2009;3:807–10.

Mumtaz A, Mahmood K, Khan P. Hydatid cyst of the brain. J Ayub Med Coll Abbottabad. 2009;21:152–4.

Nemati A, Kamgarpour A, Rashid M, Nazari SS. Giant cerebral hydatid cyst in a child -a case report and review of literature. BJMP. 2010;3:338.

Orman DT, Le Roux AT. Cerebral hydatid disease: a radiological review. S Afr Med J. 1968;42:1048–51.

Ozgen T, Bertan V, Kansu T, Akalın S. Intrasellar hydatid cyst. Case report. J Neurosurg. 1984;60:647–8.

Pasaoglu E, Damgaci L, Tokoglu F, Yildirim N, Alp AO, Yüksel E. CT findings of hydatid cyst with unusual location: infratemporal fossa. Eur Radiol. 1998;8:1570–2.

Pedrosa I, Saiz A, Arrazola J, Ferreirós J, Pedrosa CS. Hydatid disease: radiologic and pathologic features and complications. Radiographics. 2001;20:795–817.

Polat P, Kantarci M, Alper F, Suma S, Bedel M, Koruyucu MB, Okur A. Hydatid disease from head to toe. Radiographics. 2003;23:475–94.

Ravalji M, Kumar S, Shah AK, Vaghela DU, Makwana GJ, Singh K. CT and MRI features of the typical and atypical intracranial hydatid cysts: report of five cases. Indian J Radiol Imaging. 2006;16:727–32.

Raynham OW, Mulwafu W, Fagan JJ. Hydatid disease of the skull base: report of three cases and a literature review. Skull Base. 2009;19:171–5.

Reddy DR. Managing cerebral and cranial hydatid disease. Neurol India. 2009;57:116–8.

Rivierez M, el-Azhari A, el Tantaoui M, Alaoui M. Hydatid cyst of the cavernous sinus. A case (in French). Neurochirurgie. 1992;38:46–9.

Siddiqui MA, Rizvi SW, Rizvi SA, Ahmad I, Ullah E. Atypical multifocal hydatid disease of cranial vault: simultaneous orbital and extradural meningeal involvement. Emerg Radiol. 2010;17:427–30.

Singounas EG, Leventis AS, Sakas DE, Hadley DM, Lampadarios DA, Karvounis PC. Successful treatment of intracerebral hydatid cyst with albendazole: case report and review of the literature. Neurosurgery. 1992;31:571–4.

Sureka J, Sarawagi R, Eapen A, Keshava SN, Vedantam R. Skull base hydatid cyst with intracranial extension presenting as vocal cord palsy: a case report. Br J Radiol. 2010;83:e67–9.

Taghipour M, Zamanizadeh B, Bagheri MH, Zare Z. Hydatid cyst of the foramen magnum. Case report. Neurosurg Q. 2005;15:110–2.

Teymoorian GA, Bagheri F. Hydatid cyst of the skull: report of four cases. Radiology. 1976;118:97–100.

Todorov T, Vutova K, Mechkov G, Tonchev Z, Georgiev P, Lazarova I. Experience in the chemotherapy of severe, inoperable echinococcosis in man. Infection. 1992;20:19–24.

Turgut M. Intracranial hydatidosis in Turkey: its clinical presentation, diagnostic studies, surgical management, and outcome. A review of 276 cases. Neurosurg Rev. 2001;24:200–8.

Turgut M, Saglum S, Ozkan OE. Orbital hydatid cyst -report of a case followed by serial computed tomography. J Clin Neuroophthalmol. 1992;12:43–6.

Turgut AT, Tugut M, Kosar U. Hydatidosis of the orbit in Turkey: results from review of the literature 1963–2001. Int Ophthalmol. 2004;25:193–200.

Tuzun M, Hekimoðlu B. Hydatid disease of the central nervous system imaging features. AJR Am J Roentgenol. 1998;171:1497–500.

Yazdani N, Basam A, Heidarali M, Kashani SS, Hasibi M, Mokhtari Z. Infratemporal hydatid cyst: a case presenting with blindness. J Laryngol Otol. 2010; 124:456–9.

Hydatidosis of the Brain

6

Faten Limaiem and Nidhameddine Kchir

Contents

Primary and Secondary Hydatidosis

Hydatid disease of the brain is a rare parasitic infestation which constitutes only 1–2 % of all intracranial space-occupying lesions (Mingde and Zheshang 1981; Micheli et al. 1987; Demir et al. 1991; Ciurea et al. 2006). Children are much more frequently affected than adults. In fact, 50–93 % of intracranial cysts are found in children younger than 17 years (Ciurea et al. 2006). In a previous study, this percentage was even higher, reaching 95.7 % (Ciurea et al. 2006). Characteristically, there is a predominance of males and children (Table 6.1) because these groups associate more closely with animals than do females and adults. In the meta-analysis of Turgut (2001), there were 67 male (56 %) and 52 female (44 %) patients. Conversely, in some series of brain hydatidosis (Tlili-Graiess et al. 2006; Ali et al. 2009), there was a slight female predominance. It has been suggested that an underlying ductus arteriosus patency during the neonatal period may be a cause of increased vulnerability of children by allowing passage of the parasites from the periphery to the brain (Lunardi et al. 1991; Onal et al. 2006).

In humans, intracranial hydatidosis can be associated with involvement of other organs such as liver or lung, or it may be an isolated infestation of the brain. Only embryos which succeed in passing through the filtering barrier systems in the liver and lung reach the brain by the systemic circulation. Once the hexacanth embryo has reached the brain, it will form a hydatid cyst

F. Limaiem, MD (✉)
Department of Pathology, Mongi Slim Hospital, La Marsa, Tunis 2046, Tunisia
e-mail: fatenlimaiem@yahoo.fr

N. Kchir, MD
Department of Pathology, La Rabta Hospital, Tunis, Tunisia

M. Turgut (ed.), *Hydatidosis of the Central Nervous System: Diagnosis and Treatment*,
DOI 10.1007/978-3-642-54359-3_6,

Table 6.1 Epidemiological characteristics of brain hydatidosis reported in some series between 1999 and 2012

Author(s)	Year	Number of cases	Sex ratio (M:F)	Mean age (years)
Gupta et al.	1999	5	3:2	13.4
Khaldi et al.	2000	117	Slight male predominance	7.2
Bükte et al.	2004	18	2:1	20.3 (7–50 years)
Ciurea et al.	2006	76	45:31	Children: 8.7 Adults: 29.3
Tlili-Graiess et al.	2006	25	0.78	14 (30 months–56 years)
Ali et al.	2009	21	1:1.3	7.42 ± 3.2
Duishanbai et al.	2010	30	21:9	11
Basraoui et al.	2010	9	1:1	7.5
Mohindra et al.	2012	9	7:2	7 (4–44 years)

because of the ideal growth conditions (Turgut 2001). Although hydatid disease may be located anywhere in the brain, it most frequently involves the cerebral hemispheres (90–95 % of the cases) (Abbassioun and Amirjamshidi 2001). Other reported sites of intracranial hydatid cysts include subarachnoid space, ventricles, pons, cerebellum, aqueduct of Sylvius, extradural space, and diploic space of skull bones (Gokalp and Erdogan 1988; Cemil et al. 2009; Furtado et al. 2009).

Brain hydatid cysts are most often localized supratentorially in the distribution of the terminal branches of the middle cerebral artery, usually temporo-parieto-occipitally (Behari et al. 1997; Tuzun and Hekimoglu 1998). Left hemispheral predominance has been noted in several series in the literature and is explained by the emergence of the left common carotid artery directly from the aortic arch (Ciurea et al. 2006). Three forms of intracranial hydatid disease occur: intracerebral, intracranial extradural, and a combined form (Samiy and Zadey 1965; Ba'assiri and Haddad 1984; Canbolat et al. 1994; Cemil et al. 2009). Intracranial epidural hydatid disease is extremely rare because the physiologic flow of blood to the brain is mainly through the internal carotid system, so the likelihood of the larvae traveling through the external carotid system is very rare (Samiy and Zadey 1965; Ba'assiri and Haddad 1984; Canbolat et al. 1994).

Multiple hydatid cysts of the brain are very rare. Primary multiple cysts of the brain resulting from arterial embolism and without any radiological or clinical evidence of hydatid disease elsewhere in the body are extremely rare (Iplikcioğlu et al. 1989; Gupta et al. 1991; Mancuso et al. 1997; Ozkan et al. 2001; Karadağ et al. 2004). In a review of the literature related to primary multiple intracranial cerebral hydatid cysts, we were able to find only 19 cases (Table 6.2). Secondary multiple hydatid cysts of the brain can result from spontaneous, traumatic, or surgical rupture of a primary solitary cerebral cyst or as a consequence of a cyst rupture elsewhere and embolization of hydatids to the brain (Nurchi et al. 1992; Martin Oterino et al. 1996; Mancuso et al. 1997; Anvari et al. 2009). Multiple hydatid cysts resulting from the rupture of a primary cyst are acephaloceles; they are infertile and have no brood capsule and scolices (Lunardi et al. 1991; Ciurea et al. 2006; Onal et al. 2006).

Primary hydatid infestation caused by embryos which escaped hepatic and pulmonary barriers is generally single and fertile. On the other hand, secondary hydatidosis caused by scolices from ruptured fertile cysts is usually multiple and sterile. It is usually caused by myocardial cysts rupturing into the left ventricle. In a review of 112 children with cerebral hydatid cysts, Carcassone et al. (1973) found only four cases of multiple cysts in the brain (4 %). In the meta-analysis of Turgut (2001), there were 53 cases of multiple cysts (19 %), and the source of secondary multiple cysts was the left ventricle of the heart in two patients. For this reason, in such cases the heart must be carefully investigated as the source of the secondary multiple intracranial cysts. There is no consensus on the growth rate of

Table 6.2 Summary of the previously reported primary multiple cerebral hydatid cysts

Author(s), year(s)	Age/sex	Localization	Treatment	Outcome
Sharma et al. (1982)	9/F	5 cysts in the right supratentorial region	Surgery	Good
Todorov et al. (1988)	45/M	8 cysts in the frontal, temporal, parieto-occipital regions	Albendazole	Good
Paşaoğlu et al. (1989)	15/M	3 cysts in the left frontoparietal and 1 cyst in the left occipital regions	Surgery	Good
İplikcioğlu et al. (1989)	7/F	3 cysts in the right frontal, 2 cysts in the left occipital, 1 cyst in the left frontal regions	Surgery	Good
Cataltepe et al. (1991)	8/M	2 cysts in both parieto-occipital regions	Surgery	Good
Gupta et al. (1991)	18/M	Multiple cysts in both cerebral and left cerebellar hemispheres	Surgery	Died
Nurchi et al. (1992)	9/M	30 cysts in the right parietal and occipital regions	Surgery	Good
Bilge et al. (1993)	37/M	2 cysts in the left frontoparietal and occipital regions	Surgery	Good
Martin Oterino et al. 1996	69/F	Multiple cysts in both cerebellar and temporal regions	Albendazole	Died
Mancuso et al. (1997)	62/M	1 cyst in the right frontal and 1 cyst in the left frontal regions	Surgery	Good
Baysefer et al. (1998)	20/M	20 cysts in the left frontoparietal regions	Surgery	Good
Popli et al. (1998)	20, M	Multiple cysts in the left temporoparietal region	Surgery + albendazole	Good
Ozkan et al. (2001)	8, M	More than 25 cysts in the left temporo-parieto-occipital region	Surgery	Good
Nowak et al. (2002)	46, F	2 cysts in the cerebral and cerebellar regions	Albendazole	Good
Karadağ et al. (2004)	45, F	2 cysts in the right parietal region	Surgery	Good
Yurt et al. (2007)	19, F	24 cysts in both cerebral hemispheres	Surgery + albendazole	Good
Erkutlu et al. (2008)	15, M	2 cysts in the right parietal and occipital regions	Surgery	Good
Cavusoglu et al. (2009)	15, M	19 hydatid cysts in the right parieto-occipital region	Surgery	Died

the hydatid cyst of the brain and has been variably reported between 1.5 and 10 cm per year. Importantly, hydatid cyst has been shown to grow faster in the cerebrum than in the liver by a ratio of 3:1 revealing that brain like the lung tissue facilitates growth of the cyst as it is a compressible organ (Abbassioun and Amirjamshidi 2001; Andronikou et al. 2002). According to a review by Duishanbai et al. (2010), supratentorial hydatid cysts tend to be larger than the infratentorial counterparts when causing symptoms.

Diagnostic Approach

Quite independently of the hydatid cyst localization and the circumstances of its discovery, the diagnostic approach is always the same based on epidemiological, clinical, biological, imaging, and pathological arguments.

Epidemiological Data

Patients are usually from rural areas; they may have hydatid contact and live in canine environment. Children are in close contact with dogs. People are not practicing proper sanitary procedures and eating raw and uncooked or improperly cooked vegetables contaminated with *Echinococcus ova*.

Clinical Data

Intracranial hydatid cyst presents with a wide range of clinical manifestations which mainly depend on the location and size of a given hydatid cyst (Altinörs et al. 2000). Cysts develop insidiously, usually being asymptomatic initially, and present with protean clinical and imaging features (Ersahin et al. 1993). Headache and vomiting due to raised intracranial tension are the most common presenting features (Carrea et al. 1975; Ersahin et al. 1993). Other manifestations of cerebral hydatid cysts are seizures, hemiparesis, visual disturbances, and ataxia. Papilledema is usually present at the time of presentation in children with cerebral hydatid cysts. Evidence of pyramidal tract dysfunction, appropriate to the location of the cyst, is noted in almost 90 % of patients. Mental changes are noted in 25 % of children and seizure activity in approximately 20 %. Other symptoms such as hemiparesis, seizures, visual field alteration, and gait disorders may vary with the location of the cyst (Paşaoğlu et al. 1989; Ozek 1994; Yuceer et al. 1998). According to some authors, clinical presentation of cerebral hydatidosis is somewhat different in children and adults (Micheli et al. 1987; Ersahin et al. 1993). Signs of increased intracranial pressure with papilledema dominate in the younger age group, whereas focal findings such as hemiparesis, speech disorders, and hemianopsia, sometimes associated with epileptic seizures, are more prevalent in the older age group (Micheli et al. 1987; Ersahin et al. 1993). The disparity between the size of the cyst and clinical presentation is an important feature of cranial hydatid cysts (Andronikou et al. 2002). In addition, duration time of symptoms is found to be an independent predictor of the outcome (Duishanbai et al. 2010).

Biological Diagnosis

Routine work-up of hydatid disease comprises blood investigations and serological tests. Blood investigations are abnormal in only few patients who demonstrate raised eosinophilic count. The serological tests are of little practical value in confirming the diagnosis of cerebral echinococcal disease (Popli and Khudale 1998). In systemic hydatidosis, serological test (Casoni skin test) is generally positive. However, in cerebral and intracranial hydatidosis, these serological tests are almost always negative (Baden and Elliot 2003).

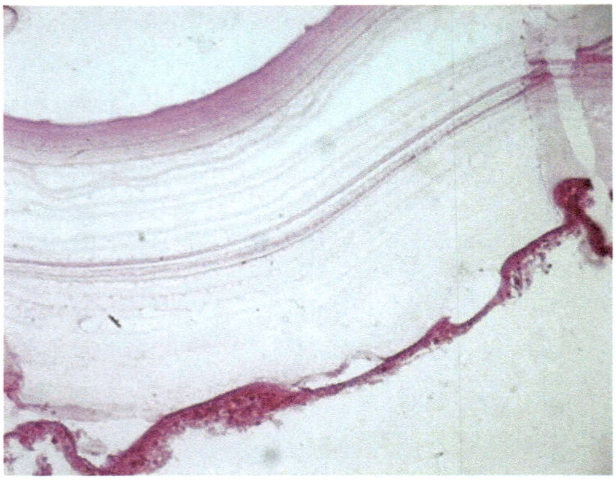

Fig. 6.1 Microscopic picture showing the laminated membrane and the germinal layer of the cyst (Haematoxylin and Eosin, magnification × 400)

Nonspecific Biology

The hemogram inconstantly shows hypereosinophilia.

Specific Biological Diagnosis of Hydatidosis

Direct Evidence of Parasitic Elements

Direct evidence of parasitic elements can be obtained from surgical samples. The parasitic elements to be sought are the cyst membranes, protoscolices, and hooklets. Although radiological investigations can be very helpful in identifying hydatid cysts preoperatively, their diagnosis is mainly based on histopathological examination (Figs. 6.1 and 6.2).

Histopathologically, the hydatid cyst has three layers: (a) First is the outer pericyst, composed of modified host cells. This layer is a dense fibrous zone in the liver and other organs. In the brain, however, there is only a shiny fine gliotic layer without any remarkable resistance surrounding the primary unruptured cysts. (b) The next layer is the middle laminated membrane which is acellular and allows the passage of nutrients. (c) The third is the inner germinal layer where the scolices (the larval stage of the parasite) and the laminated membrane are produced.

The middle laminated membrane and the germinal layer form the true wall of the cyst usually referred to as the endocyst. Daughter cysts are small spheres containing the protoscolices. The

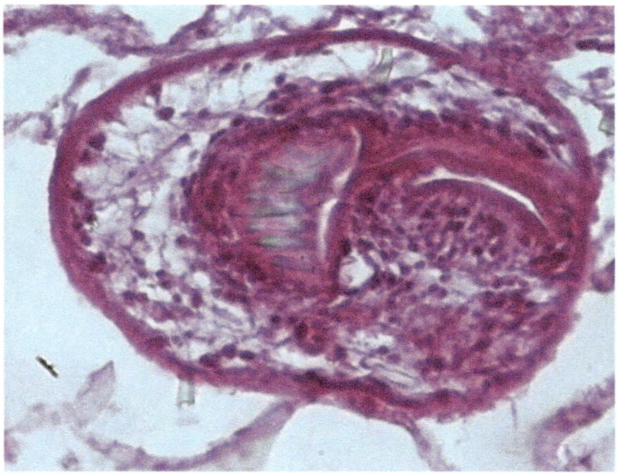

Fig. 6.2 Microscopic picture showing an enlarged view of a scolex. This section also includes the rostellar hooks (Haematoxylin and Eosin, magnification × 400)

innermost layer which is the germinative or fertile membrane performs two major functions: (a) production of the laminated membrane outward and (b) germination of a new generation of scolices inward. The formation of scolices takes place from the brood capsules attached to the germinative membrane. The pedicle of the brood cysts is very loosely attached to the germinal layer of the mother cyst. On gross examination, the vesicles resemble a bunch of grapes and may grow through the wall of the mother cyst. Cyst fluid, clear or pale yellow, has a neutral pH and contains sodium chloride, proteins, glucose, ions, and polysaccharides and is antigenic. When brood cysts and vesicles detach within the cyst, and pass into the cyst fluid, they form a white sediment known as "hydatid sand." Mild mononuclear cell infiltrates and occasional foreign body giant cells surround the cysts (Ameli and Abbassioun 1995).

Hydatid Serology

Serum is generally used for the detection of specific antibodies. Qualitative techniques include immunoelectrophoresis, electrosyneresis, and enzyme-linked immunoelectrodiffusion assay. Quantitative techniques include indirect hemagglutination and enzyme-linked immunosorbent assay, indirect immunofluorescence, and a review of the IgE level and of the immune complex.

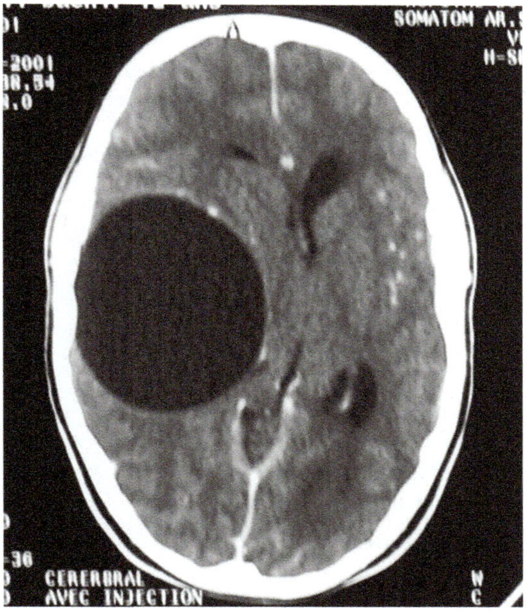

Fig. 6.3 Preoperative CT scan showing a right temporoparietal unilocular cyst with homogeneous fluid attenuation and midline shift toward left

Laboratory findings of patients with hydatidosis of central nervous system are discussed in Chap. 10.

Imaging Diagnosis

Imaging with CT and MRI are central to the diagnosis of cerebral hydatid cysts (Figs. 6.3, 6.4, 6.5, 6.6, 6.7, 6.8 and 6.9). Both are equally good for detection and localization of the cyst in brain. Whereas CT is better in demonstrating cyst wall calcification, MRI has an advantage in delineating the relationship of the cyst with adjacent structures (Bükte et al. 2004). Typical CT features of cerebral hydatid cyst include a spherical or oval homogenous fluid attenuation generally in the temporal and parietal lobes of cerebral hemispheres (Demir et al. 1991; Karak et al. 1992). Cystic lesion is usually large with significant mass effect in the form of ventricular compression and midline shift. Calcification in the cyst wall is very rare, seen in around 1 % of cases (McCorkell and Lewall 1985; Rudwan and Khaffaji 1988). No enhancement or perilesional

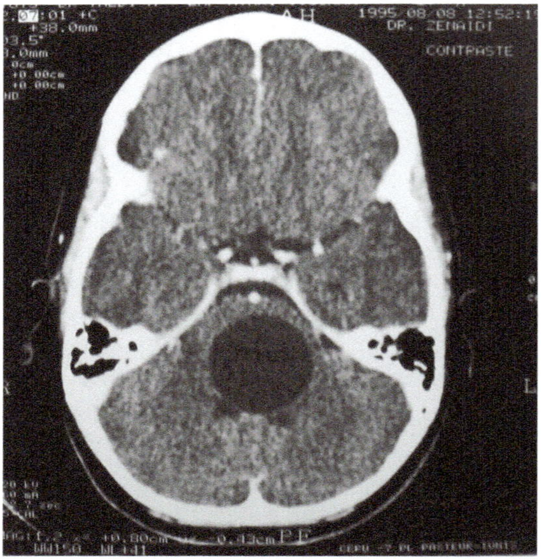

Fig. 6.4 Preoperative CT scan demonstrating a hydatid cyst of the brain stem with homogeneous fluid attenuation

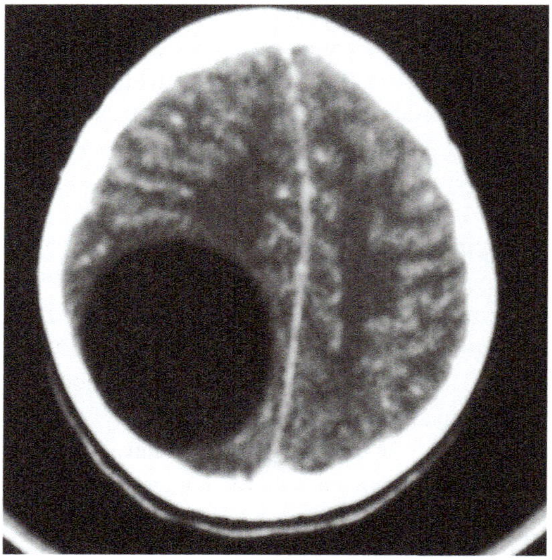

Fig. 6.5 Preoperative CT scan revealing a right univesicular occipitoparietal hydatid cyst

edema is seen in case of uncomplicated hydatid cysts. Enhancement of the cyst and perilesional edema in a case of cystic echinococcosis of brain indicates complications like rupture, hemorrhage, or infection in the cyst.

Although CT scan and MRI have greatly contributed to a correct early diagnosis, in a substantial

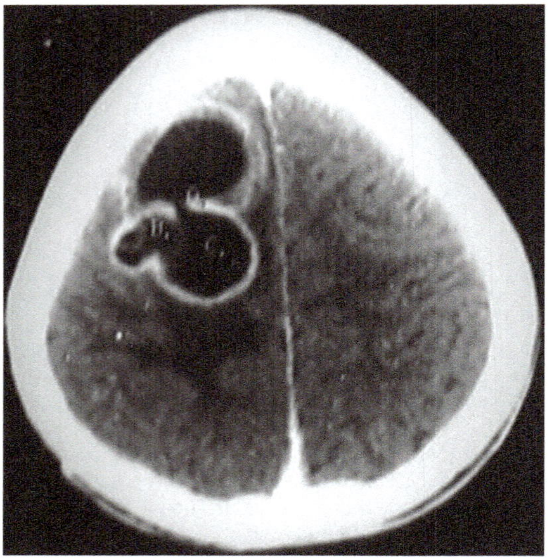

Fig. 6.6 Preoperative CT scan showing a thick-walled multivesicular, right frontal hydatid cyst

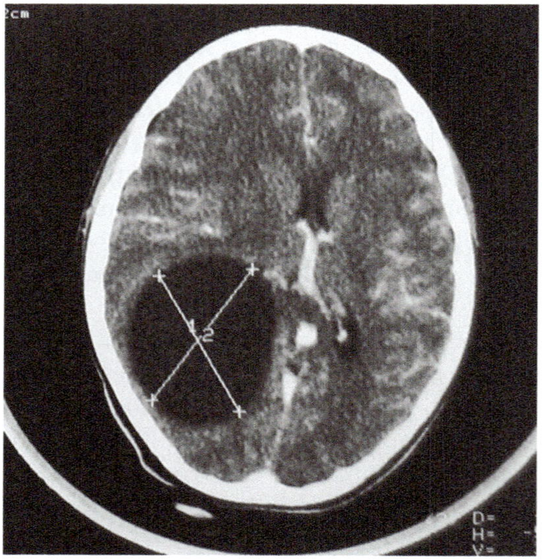

Fig. 6.7 Preoperative CT scan demonstrating a right parieto-occipital, spherical homogenous fluid attenuation mass with thin smooth wall and midline shift to left; no perilesional edema is seen. 1 and 2 are the two greatest diameters of the hydatid cyst

number of cases, diagnosis is obtained postoperatively. A high index of suspicion, when a cystic mass is found on CT or MRI, is therefore required in endemic areas, but also in non-endemic areas, since migration and frequent traveling have changed

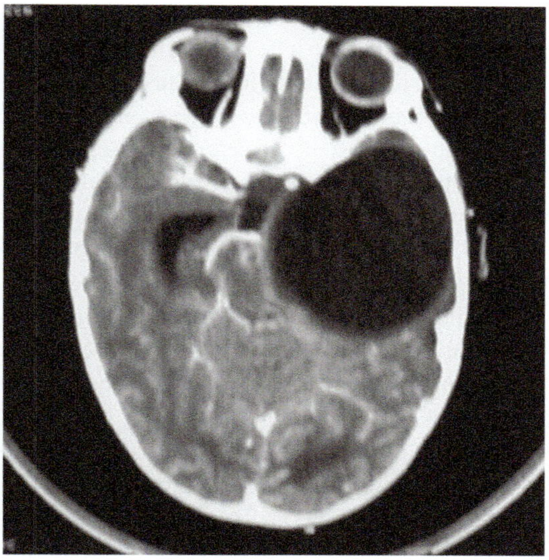

Fig. 6.8 Preoperative CT scan: unilocular left frontotemporal hydatid cyst with homogeneous fluid attenuation

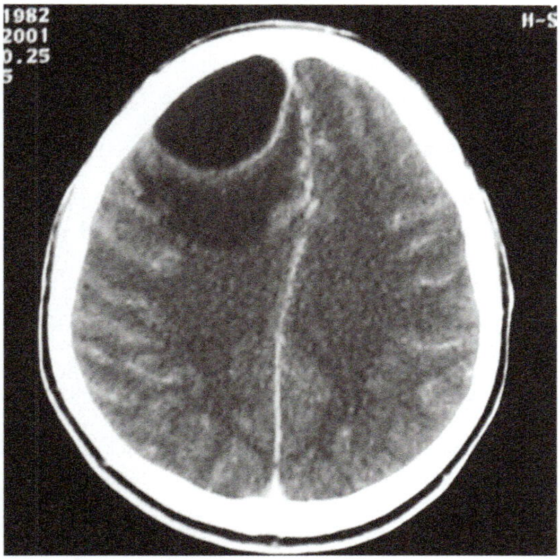

Fig. 6.9 Preoperative cerebral CT scan showing a right frontal univesicular hydatid cyst with perilesional edema

the worldwide occurrence. Newer imaging techniques, such as magnetic resonance spectroscopy and diffusion-weighted MRI, might further refine the diagnostic armamentarium (Ciurea et al. 2006).

The differential diagnosis of intracranial hydatid cysts includes cystic lesions such as porencephalic cyst, arachnoid cyst, cystic tumors of the brain, and pyogenic abscesses (Cataltepe et al. 1992; Sahin-

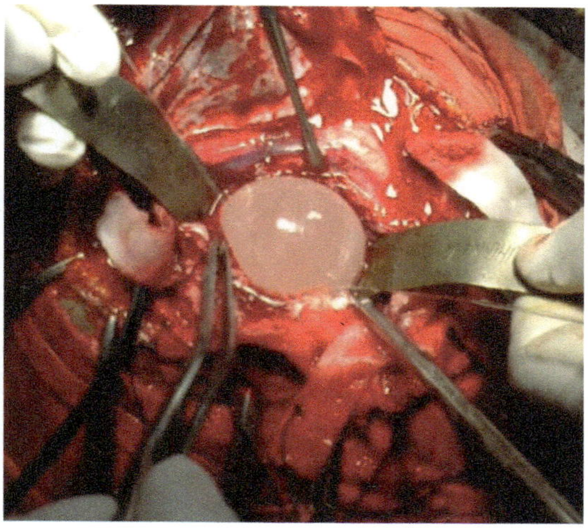

Fig. 6.10 Hydatid cyst being removed from brain (Courtesy of N. Khaled, M.D.)

Akyar 2002). In contrast to hydatid cysts, porencephalic cysts and arachnoid cysts are not spherical in shape and are not surrounded entirely by brain substance. Arachnoid cysts are extra-axial masses that may deform adjacent brain. Porencephalisc cysts result from insults to normal brain tissue and are lined by gliotic white matter that could easily be demonstrated with MRI (Topal et al. 1995; Tuzun et al. 2002).

Imaging of cerebral hydatid disease is discussed in detail in Chap. 11.

Treatment

In toto surgical removal of intracranial hydatid cysts remains the treatment of choice for cerebral hydatidosis (Figs. 6.10 and 6.11). The aim of surgery is to excise the cyst completely without rupture to prevent anaphylactic reaction and local recurrence. Preoperative diagnosis of cerebral hydatid cyst made on the basis of typical CT or MRI findings is an important component in the chain of events to prevent cyst rupture during surgery (Negovetic et al. 1990).

Subdural effusions and development of obstructive hydrocephalus are well-documented postoperative complications. Postoperative seizures (Abbassioun et al. 1978; Ersahin et al. 1993), development of porencephalic cysts, focal

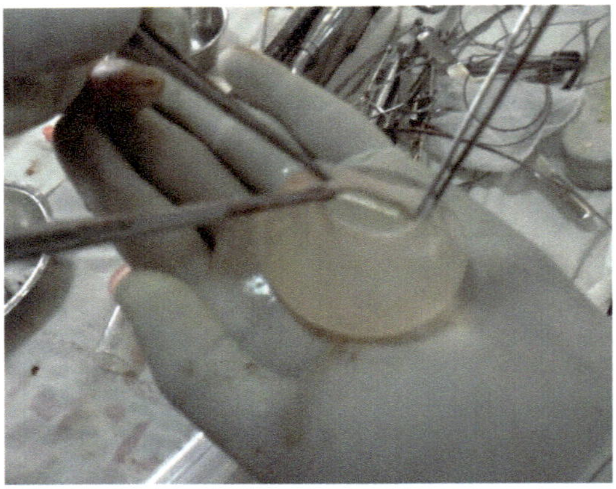

Fig. 6.11 Removed intact cyst being dissected (Courtesy of N. Khaled, M.D.)

signs (e.g., paresis), and nonbacterial meningitis have also been reported (Lunardi et al. 1991). Intraoperative rupture of the cyst may result in early death due to anaphylactic shock.

Chemotherapy is an adjunct treatment for patients with inoperable multiple cysts or deep-seated cysts and in those who are not good candidates for surgery or may be suffering from recurrent cysts (Yurt et al. 2007). Reported to be clinically effective, antihelminthic agents for the medical treatment of hydatid cyst are mebendazole and albendazole (Turgut 1998), but its effectiveness is still unclear.

Prognosis depends largely on accurate preoperative diagnosis, which is of extreme importance for the successful removal of an unruptured cyst. Long-term follow-up confirms that the outcome of intracranial hydatidosis without intraoperative cyst rupture remains excellent. Recurrence and multiplicity of cysts seem to be the most significant negative factors affecting the long-term outcome of patients with intracranial hydatid disease (Ciurea et al. 2006). Hydatid disease is generally a severe disease, with over 90 % mortality in untreated patients (Per et al. 2009).

Treatment of cerebral hydatid disease is discussed in detail in Chaps. 15 and 16.

Conclusion

Despite the introduction of modern surgical and pharmacological therapy, brain hydatid disease continues to be a substantial cause of morbidity and mortality in many parts of the world. New approaches to control and prevention of hydatidosis, including an effective livestock vaccine, potential dog vaccines against the tapeworm stage of *Echinococcus granulosus*, tailored educational programs, development of better diagnostics for definitive hosts and human beings (including dog coproantigen detection), more effective antiparasitic treatments, and the use of mathematical models to simulate best possible cost-effective interventions, will be expected to shorten the time of the attack phase and improve surveillance in the consolidation phase of hydatid control programs (Chabalgoity et al. 2000; McManus et al. 2003; Torgerson 2006).

References

Abbassioun K, Amirjamshidi A. Diagnosis and management of hydatid cyst of the central nervous system. Part 1. General considerations and hydatid disease of the brain. Neurosurg Q. 2001;11:1–9.

Abbassioun K, Rahmat H, Ameli NO, Tafazoli M. Computerized tomography in hydatid cyst of the brain. J Neurosurg. 1978;49:408–11.

Ali M, Mahmood K, Khan P. Hydatid cysts of the brain. J Ayub Med Coll Abbottabad. 2009;21:152–4.

Altinörs N, Bavbek M, Caner HH, Erdogan B. Central nervous system hydatidosis in Turkey: a cooperative study and literature survey analysis of 458 cases. J Neurosurg. 2000;93:1–8.

Ameli NO, Abbassioun K. Hydatid disease of the central nervous system. Tehran: Ketab Sara Co; 1995. p. 21–141. Chaps. 2–6.

Andronikou S, Welman CJ, Kader E. Classic and unusual appearances of hydatid disease in children. Pediatr Radiol. 2002;32:817–28.

Anvari M, Amirjamshidi A, Abbassioun K. Gradual and complete delivery of a hydatid cyst of the brain through a single burr hole, a wrong happening! Childs Nerv Syst. 2009;25:1639–42.

Ba'assiri A, Haddad FS. Primary extradural intracranial hydatid disease: CT appearance. AJNR Am J Neuroradiol. 1984;5:474–5.

Basraoui D, El idrissi I, Jalal H, Hiroual M, Essadki O, Ousehal A, Aniba K, Ghannane H, Lmejjati M, Ait Benali S. Intracranial hydatid cysts in children: a report of 9 cases. J radiol. 2010; 91:293–6.

Baden LR, Elliot DD. Case record of Massachusetts General Hospital: weekly clinicopathological exercises. Case 4–2003. A 42-year-old woman with cough, fever, and abnormalities on thoracoabdominal computed tomography. N Engl J Med. 2003;348:447–55.

Baysefer A, Erdoğan E, Gonul E, Kayali H, Timurkaynak E, Seber N. Primary multiple cerebral hydatid cysts: Case report with CT and MRI study. Minim Invasive Neurosurg. 1998; 41:35–7.
Behari S, Banerji D, Phadke RV, Shukla S, Krishnani N, Chhabra DK. Multiple infected extradural parasellar hydatid cysts. Surg Neurol. 1997;48:53–7.
Bilge T, Batur Ş, Bilge S, Aydın Y, Aksoy B, Şenol S. Primary multiple hydatid cysts of the brain: Case report. Surg Neurol. 1993; 39:377–9.
Bükte Y, Kemaloglu S, Nazaroglu H, Ozkan U, Ceviz A, Simsek M. Cerebral hydatid disease: CT and MR imaging findings. Swiss Med Wkly. 2004;134:459–67.
Canbolat A, Onal C, Kaya U, Coban TE. Intracranial extradural hydatid cysts. Report of three cases. Surg Neurol. 1994;41:230–4.
Carcassone M, Aubresby P, Dor V, Choux M. Hydatid cyst in childhood. Prog Pediatr Surg. 1973;5:1–35.
Carrea R, Dowling Jr E, Guevara JA. Surgical treatment of hydatid cysts of the central nervous system in pediatric age (Dowling's technique). Childs Brain. 1975;1:4–21.
Cataltepe O, Tahta K, Colak A, Erbengi A. Primary multiple cerebral hydatid cysts. Neurosurg rev. 1991; 14: 231–4.
Cataltepe O, Colak A, Ozcan OE, Ozgen T, Erbengi A. Intracranial hydatid cysts: experience with surgical treatment in 120 patients. Neurochirurgia (Stuttg). 1992;35:108–11.
Cavusoglu H, Tuncer C, Ozdilmac A, Aydin Y. Multiple intracranial hydatid cysts in a boy. Turk Neurosurg. 2009; 19: 203–7.
Cemil B, Tun K, Gurcay AG, Uygur A, Kaptanoglu E. Cranial epidural hydatid cysts: clinical report and review of the literature. Acta Neurochir (Wien). 2009;151:659–62.
Chabalgoity JA, Moreno M, Carol H, Dougan G, Hormaeche CE. Salmonella typhimurium as a basis for a live oral Echinococcus granulosus vaccine. Vaccine. 2000;19:460–9.
Ciurea AV, Fountas KN, Coman TC, Machinis TG, Kapsalaki EZ, Fezoulidis NI, Robinson JS. Long-term surgical outcome in patients with intracranial hydatid cyst. Acta Neurochir (Wien). 2006;148:421–6.
Demir K, Karsli AF, Kaya T, Devrimci E, Alkan K. Cerebral hydatid cysts: CT findings. Neuroradiology. 1991;33:22–4.
Duishanbai S, Jiafu D, Guo H, Liu C, Liu B, Aishalong M, Mijiti M, Wen H. Intracranial hydatid cyst in children: report of 30 cases. Childs Nerv Syst. 2010;26:821–7.
Erkutlu I, Buyukhatipoglu H, Alptekin M, Gok A. Where is the brain paranchyme? "Primary cerebral multiple cyst hydatid". Intern Med. 2008;47:333.
Ersahin Y, Mutluer S, Guzelbag E. Intracranial hydatid cysts in children. Neurosurgery. 1993;33:219–25.
Furtado SV, Visvanathan K, Nandita G, Reddy K, Hegde AS. Multiple fourth ventricular hydatidosis. J Clin Neurosci. 2009;16:110–2.
Gokalp HZ, Erdogan A. Hydatid cyst of the aqueduct of Sylvius: case report. Clin Neurol Neurosurg. 1988;90:83–5.
Gupta SK, Tandon SC, Khanna S, Asthana S. Case report: multiple intracranial hydatid cysts with post-operative dissemination. Clin Radiol. 1991;44:203–4.
Gupta S, Desai K, Goel A. Intracranial hydatid cyst : a report of five cases and review of the literature. Neurol india. 1999; 47: 214–7.
Iplikcioğlu AC, Ozer AF, Benli K, Işık N, Erbengi A. Multiple cerebral hydatid cysts: report of two cases. Br J Neurosurg. 1989;3:217–9.
Karadağ O, Gurelik M, Ozum U, Goksel HM. Primary multiple cerebral hydatid cysts with unusual features. Acta Neurochir (Wien). 2004;146:73–7.
Karak PK, Mittal M, Bhatia S, Mukhopadhyay S, Berry M. Isolated cerebral hydatid cyst with pathognomonic CT sign. Neuroradiology. 1992;34:9–10.
Khaldi M, Mohamed S, Kallel J, Khouja N. Brain hydatidosis report on 117 cases. Childs Nerv Syst. 2000;16:765–9.
Lunardi P, Missori P, Di Lorenzo N, Fortuna A. Cerebral hydatidosis in childhood: a retrospective survey with emphasis on long-term follow-up. Neurosurgery. 1991;29:515–7.
Mancuso P, Noubari BA, Gurusinghe NT. Multiple primary cerebral hydatid cysts: case report. Br J Neurosurg. 1997;11:248–9.
Martin Oterino JA, Chimpen Ruiz VA, Reviriego Jaen G, Sanchez Rodriguez A. Repeated strokes as a sign of multiple cerebral hydatid cysts. Neurologia. 1996;11:307–9.
McCorkell SJ, Lewall DB. Computed tomography of intracerebral echinococcal cysts in children. J Comput Assist Tomogr. 1985;9:514–8.
McManus DP, Zhang W, Li J, Bartley PB. Echinococcosis. Lancet. 2003;362:1295–304.
Micheli F, Lehkuniec E, Giannaula R, Caputi E, Paradiso G. Calcified cerebral hydatid cyst. Eur Neurol. 1987;27:1–4.
Mingde Q, Zheshang H. Echinococcosis of the central nervous system. Eur Neurol. 1981;20:125–31.
Mohindra S, Savardekar A, Gupta R, Tripathi M, Rane S. Varied types of intracranial hydatid cysts: radiological features and management techniques. Acta Neurochir (Wien). 2012;154:165–72.
Negovetic L, Lupret V, Smiljanic D, Arsenic B. Cranial vault and gigantic intracranial hydatid cyst in a young woman. Neurosurgery. 1990;27:480–2.
Nowak DA, Lucking MO, Böhmer RH, Schrenier R, Fuchs HH, Flügel KA. Isolated intracerebral cystic echinococcosis. Unusual presentation of a rare disease (in German). Dtsch Med Wochenschr. 2002;127:1638–42.
Nurchi G, Floris F, Montaldo C, Mastio F, Peltz T, Coraddu M. Multiple cerebral hydatid disease: case report with magnetic resonance imaging study. Neurosurgery. 1992;30:436–8.
Onal C, Erguvan-Onal R, Yakinci C, Karayol A, Atambay M, Daldal N. Can the requirement of a diversion procedure be predicted after an uncomplicated intracranial hydatid cyst surgery? Pediatr Neurosurg. 2006;42:383–6.
Ozek M. Complications of central nervous system hydatid disease. Pediatr Neurosurg. 1994;20:84–91.

Ozkan U, Kemaloğlu MS, Selcuki M. Gigantic intracranial mass of hydatid cyst. Childs Nerv Syst. 2001;17:623–5.
Paşaoğlu A, Orhon C, Akdemir H. Multiple primary hydatid cysts of the brain. Turk J Pediatr. 1989;31:57–61.
Per H, Kumandas S, Gümüs H, Kurtsoy A. Primary soliter and multiple intracranial cyst hydatid disease: report of five cases. Brain Dev. 2009;31:228–33.
Popli MB, Khudale B. Primary multiple hydatid cysts of the brain. Australas Radiol. 1998;42:90–1.
Rudwan MA, Khaffaji S. CT of cerebral hydatid disease. Neuroradiology. 1988;30:496–9.
Sahin-Akyar G. Computed tomography and magnetic resonance imaging findings in cerebral hydatid disease. Radiography. 2002;8:251–8.
Samiy E, Zadey FA. Cranial and intracranial hydatidosis with special reference to roentgen-ray diagnosis. J Neurosurg. 1965;22:425–33.
Sharma A, Abraham J. Multiple giant hydatid cysts of the brain : case report. J Neurosurg. 1982; 57:413–5.
Tlili-Graiess K, El Ouni F, Gharbi-Jemni H, Arifa N, Moulahi H, Mrad-Dali K, Guesmi H, Abroug S, Yacoub M, Krifa H. Cerebral hydatid disease: imaging features. J Neuroradiol. 2006;33:304–18.
Todorov T, Vutova A, Petrov D, Balkanski G. Albendazole treatment of multiple cerebral hydatid cysts : case report. Trans R Soc Trop Med Hyg. 1988; 82:150–2.
Topal U, Parlak M, Kilic E, Sivri Z, Sadikoglu MY, Tuncel E. CT and MRI findings in cerebral hydatid disease. Eur Radiol. 1995;5:244–7.
Torgerson PR. Mathematical models for the control of cystic echinococcosis. Parasitol Int. 2006;55: S253–8.
Turgut M. The role of mebendazole in the surgical treatment of central nervous system hydatid disease. Br J Neurosurg. 1998;12:289.
Turgut M. Intracranial hydatidosis in Turkey: its clinical presentation, diagnostic studies, surgical management and outcome, a review of 276 cases. Neurosurg Rev. 2001;24:200–8.
Tuzun M, Hekimoglu B. Hydatid disease of the central nervous system: imaging features. Am J Roentgenol. 1998;171:1497–500.
Tuzun M, Altinors N, Arda IS, Hekimoglu B. Cerebral hydatid disease CT and MR findings. Clin imaging. 2002; 26: 353–7.
Yuceer N, Guven MB, Yilmaz H. Multiple hydatid cysts of the brain: a case report and review of the literature. Neurosurg Rev. 1998;21:181–4.
Yurt A, Avci M, Selçuki M, Ozer F, Camlar M, Uçar K, Tasli F, Altinörs N. Multiple cerebral hydatid cysts. Report of a case with 24 pieces. Clin Neurol Neurosurg. 2007;109:821–6.

Intraventricular Hydatidosis

7

Sunil V. Furtado and Sumit Thakar

Contents

Introduction

Epidemiology

Hydatid disease caused by ingestion of eggs of the cestode *Echinococcus granulosus* is endemic in the Middle East, Mediterranean region, South America, North Africa, India, and Australia (Onal et al. 1997). Intracranial hydatid disease, seen in 1–2 % of all patients with hydatidosis, accounts for 0.02–0.22 % of all intracranial space-occupying lesions (Rahimizadeh and Hadadian 1984; Mohindra et al. 2012). Their growth rate has been reported to vary between 1.5 and 10 cm/year (Gupta et al. 1999). An exclusive intraventricular occurrence of the disease is rare.

Classification

Intracranial hydatid cysts may be classified as primary or secondary. Primary cysts are due to direct infestation of the brain by larvae, and secondary cysts result from spontaneous, traumatic, or surgical rupture of a primary intracranial hydatid cyst. The latter variety is infertile and lacks brood capsules and scolices. In one of our patient, the smaller cysts were probably seeded by rupture of the larger primary cyst, which was compressing them anteriorly against the brainstem (Figs. 7.1 and 7.2).

Primary and secondary hydatidoses of the brain are discussed in Chap. 6.

S.V. Furtado, MS, MCh, DNB (✉) • S. Thakar, MCh
Department of Neurosurgery,
Sri Sathya Sai Institute of Higher Medical Sciences,
EPIP Area, Whitefield, Bangalore, India
e-mail: sunilvf@gmail.com

M. Turgut (ed.), *Hydatidosis of the Central Nervous System: Diagnosis and Treatment*,
DOI 10.1007/978-3-642-54359-3_7, © Springer-Verlag Berlin Heidelberg 2014

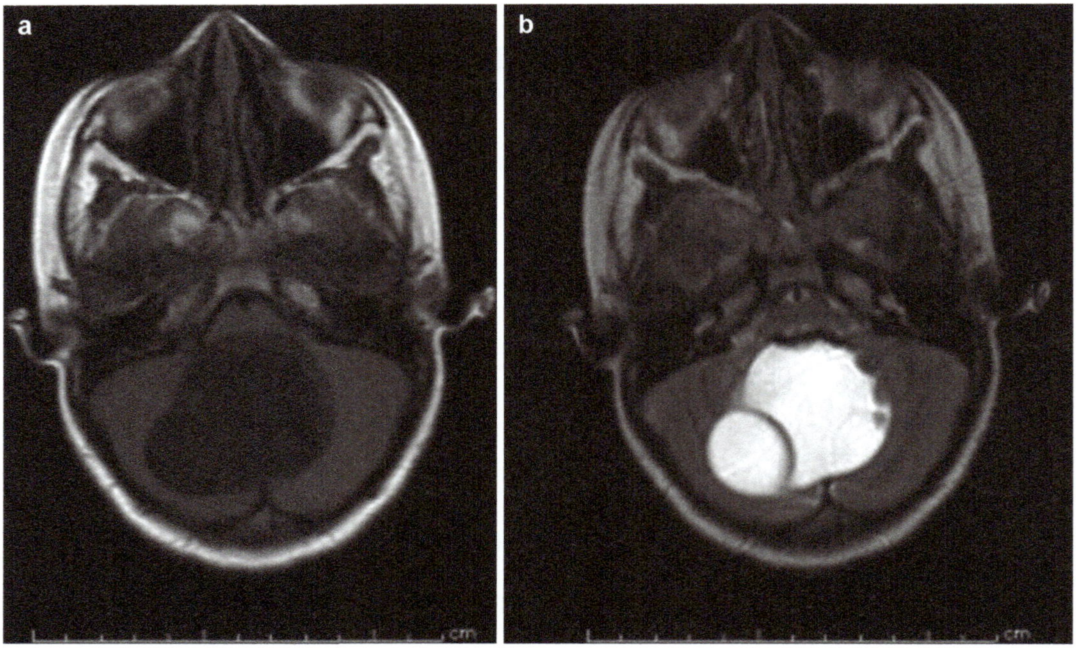

Fig. 7.1 (**a**) Axial T1-weighted image and (**b**) T2-weighted MRI showing two large hydatid cysts with the smaller cysts pushed anteriorly

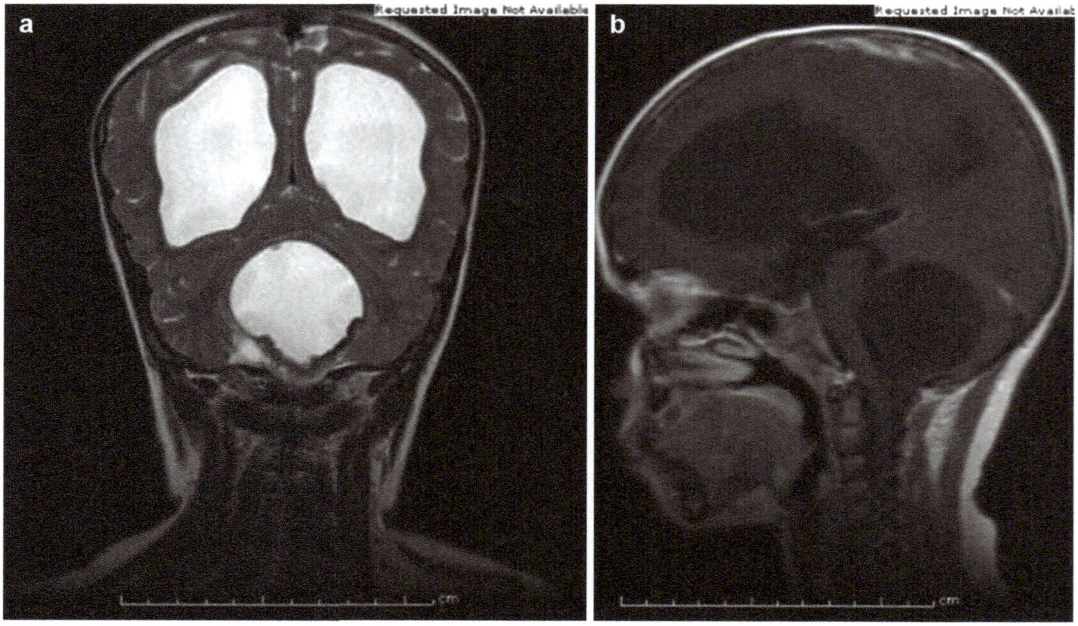

Fig. 7.2 (**a**) Coronal T2-weighted MRI showing a large cyst with daughter cysts filling the fourth ventricle. (**b**) Sagittal contrast image demonstrating no contrast enhancement

Intraventricular Hydatidosis

Multiple intracranial hydatid cysts are rare and are seen in about 10–15 % of intracranial hydatidosis (Ugur et al. 1998). Ruggiardo, in 1902, was the first to report the perforation of the ventricle by an intracerebral cyst (Valentino 1959). A literature search in PubMed revealed numerous reports of supratentorial intraventricular hydatid cysts (Negovetic et al. 1990; Lunardi et al. 1991; Peker et al. 1991; Cataltepe et al. 1992; Diren et al. 1993; Karadağ et al. 2004; Ciurea et al. 2006; Kamath et al. 2009; Mohindra et al. 2012) and only 9 reports of solitary cysts in the fourth ventricle (Rahimizadeh and Hadadian 1984; Pau et al. 1987; Gelabert Gonzalez et al. 1988; Singounas et al. 1992; Turgut 2001; Bukte et al. 2004; Furtado et al. 2009; Duishanbai et al. 2010; Mohindra et al. 2012). Turgut (2002) described a 13 % incidence of intraventricular hydatidosis based on a meta-analysis of all reported intracranial hydatidosis cases in the pediatric and adolescent group in Turkey. Table 7.1 provides a comprehensive list of all cases with intraventricular hydatidosis in indexed literature to date.

It has been postulated that oncospheres reach the ventricular cavity along the choroid plexus (Guzel et al. 2008). Another proposed mechanism is the spillage of ruptured primary cysts situated near the ependymal lining into the ventricle, causing multiple secondary cysts (Evliyaoglu and Keskil 2005). Like in other sites, surgery is the treatment of choice for intraventricular lesions, with cyst removal without spillage of fluid being the main prognostic factor (Altinörs et al. 2000; Furtado et al. 2009; Mohindra et al. 2012).

Presentation

Raised Intracranial Pressure

Intraventricular hydatidosis may either be asymptomatic or present with features of raised intracranial pressure, depending on the location of the cyst(s). Cysts in the posterior fossa, reportedly smaller than their supratentorial counterparts (Mohindra et al. 2012), and those in the posterior third ventricle or at the foramen of Monro are more likely to obstruct cerebrospinal fluid (CSF) pathways, causing hydrocephalus. All our patients reported headache and vomiting, while one patient with long-standing symptoms presented additionally with secondary optic atrophy and gait disturbances.

Incidental Pickups

In many cases, the lesions are incidentally picked up in the setting of multiple parenchymal cerebral lesions presenting with seizures or focal neurological deficits, or of systemic hydatidosis as seen in one of our patients with supernumerary seedling from a cardiac source with secondary intracranial cysts in the parenchyma and lateral and fourth ventricles (Fig. 7.3).

Unusual Symptoms

Location-specific symptoms include fluctuating signs of raised pressure like in one of our cases where the cyst was straddling the foramen of Monro, brainstem compression or cerebellar dysfunction like in one case involving the fourth ventricle (Figs. 7.1, 7.2, and 7.4), or third nerve paresis secondary to a trapped temporal horn (Choux et al. 1976; Onal et al. 1997; Evliyaoglu and Keskil 2005; Furtado et al. 2009; Mohindra et al. 2012).

Radiological Investigations

Computed Tomography Findings

Plain radiographs of the calvarium and cerebral angiography have lost their importance in the diagnosis of intracranial hydatidosis. On computed tomogram, unilocular cysts are often large, spherical, and homogenous lesions with sharply defined borders. There may be septations within the cysts, and these may occasionally be calcified. Less than 1 % of cases demonstrate calcification of the walls (Bukte et al. 2004). The thin

Table 7.1 Summary of selected cases with intraventricular hydatidosis published in indexed literature to date

Author(s)	Country	Year	Patient age (years), sex	Location	No. of cases/cysts	Presentation	Outcome
Filipov and Karag'ozov	Bulgaria	1955	NA	NA	NA	NA	NA
Djindjian and Porot	France	1957	NA	NA	NA	NA	NA
Valentino	Italy	1959	17, F	Lateral ventricle	1 case	Headache, vomiting	Favorable
Borne	France	1964	NA	NA	NA	NA	NA
Kaya et al.	Turkey	1975	21, F	Lateral ventricle	1 case	Headache, personality changes, papilledema	Multiple recurrences
	Turkey	1975	8, F	Lateral ventricle	1 case	Headache, papilledema, diplopia	Favorable
	Turkey	1975	12, M	Lateral ventricle	1 case	Headache, vomiting, papilledema	Favorable
	Turkey	1975	13, F	Lateral ventricle	1 case	Foster Kennedy syndrome, optic atrophy, seizure	Postoperative death
Rahimizadeh and Hadadian	Iran	1984	12, M	Fourth ventricle	1 case	Headache, vomiting, ataxia	Favorable
Pau et al.	Italy	1987	11, F	Lateral ventricle	Multiple	Hemiparesis	Favorable
	Italy	1987	58, M	Fourth ventricle	Multiple	Drowsiness, hemiparesis	Died
Gelabert Gonzalez et al.	Spain	1988	NA	Fourth ventricle	1 case	NA	A
Negovetic et al.	Yugoslavia	1990	20, F	Lateral ventricle	Multiple	Headache, seizure	Favorable
Peker et al.	Turkey	1991	15, M	Fourth ventricle and lateral ventricle	Multiple	Headache, nausea	Died
Cataltepe et al.[a]	Turkey	1992	NA	Lateral ventricle	12 cysts	NA	NA
	Turkey	1992	NA	Fourth ventricle	3 cysts	NA	NA
	Turkey	1992	NA	Aqueduct of Sylvius	1 cyst	NA	NA
	Turkey	1992	NA	Third ventricle	3 cysts	NA	NA
Copley et al.	South Africa	1992	12, F	Lateral ventricle	Multiple	Headache, dizziness	Favorable
	South Africa	1992	7, M	Lateral ventricle	1 case	Proptosis	Favorable

Singounas et al.	Greece	1992	33, F	Fourth ventricle	1 case	Headache, seizure	Favorable
Diren et al.	Turkey	1993	10, F	Lateral ventricle	1 case	Headache, visual deterioration	No follow-up
Altinörs et al.	Turkey	2000	NA	Intra- or periventricular	9 cases	NA	NA
	Turkey	2000	NA	Aqueduct of Sylvius	1 case	NA	NA
Onal et al.	Turkey	2001	NA	NA	5 cases	NA	NA
Turgut [b]	Turkey	2001	NA	Lateral ventricle	14 cases	NA	NA
	Turkey	2001	NA	Third ventricle	4 cases	NA	NA
	Turkey	2001	NA	Fourth ventricle	3 cases	NA	NA
	Turkey	2001	NA	Aqueduct of Sylvius	2 cases	NA	NA
	Turkey	2001	NA	Not specified	4 cases	NA	NA
Aydin et al.	Turkey	2002	18, M	Lateral ventricle	Multiple	Headache, blurred vision	Favorable
Karadag et al.	Turkey	2004	45, F	Lateral ventricle	2 cysts	Seizure	Favorable
Sherwani et al.	India	2003	10, F	Lateral ventricle	1 case	Headache, seizure	Favorable
Bukte et al.	Turkey	2004	7, F	Fourth ventricle	1 case	Cerebellar signs, ataxia	Favorable
Evliyaoglu and Keskil	Turkey	2005	7, F	Lateral ventricle	1 case	Headache, nausea, spasticity, cerebellar signs	Favorable
Iyigun et al.	Turkey	2004	2, M	Lateral ventricle	Multiple	Focal neurological deficit	Favorable
Ciurea et al.	Romania	2006	NA	Not specified	1 case	Raised intracranial pressure	Favorable
Guzel et al.	Turkey	2008	10, F	Lateral ventricle	1 case	Raised intracranial pressure	Favorable
Kamath et al.	India	2009	6, M	Lateral ventricle	1 case	Hemiparesis, headache	Favorable
Duishanbai et al.	China	2010	6, M	Fourth ventricle	1 case	Ataxia	Favorable
	China	2010	8, M	Fourth ventricle	1 case	Ataxia	Favorable
Guvenc et al.	Turkey	2011	33, F	Lateral ventricle	1 case	Headache, vomiting	Favorable

(continued)

Table 7.1 (continued)

Author(s)	Country	Year	Patient age (years), sex	Location	No. of cases/cysts	Presentation	Outcome
Mohindra et al.	India	2012	6, F	Lateral ventricle	1 case	Seizure	Favorable
	India	2012	5, M	Lateral ventricle	1 case	Increase in head size	Favorable
	India	2012	7, M	Lateral ventricle	3 cases	Headache, vomiting	Favorable
	India	2012	44, F	Fourth ventricle	4 cases	Headache, vomiting	Favorable
Majumdar et al.	India	2013	7, F	Lateral ventricle	1 case	Headache, vomiting	Favorable
Present series	India	2012	8, F	Fourth ventricle	Multiple	Headache, spasticity, visual disturbance, cerebellar signs	Favorable
	India	2012	9, M	Lateral ventricle and fourth ventricle	Multiple	Raised intracranial pressure	Recurrence

Abbreviations: *F* female, *M* male, *NA* not available data

[a]One of the cases reported by the authors had already been described by Peker et al. (1991)

[b]The cases reported by the author had already been described by Kaya et al. (1975), Peker et al. (1991), Cataltepe et al. (1992), and Diren et al. (1993)

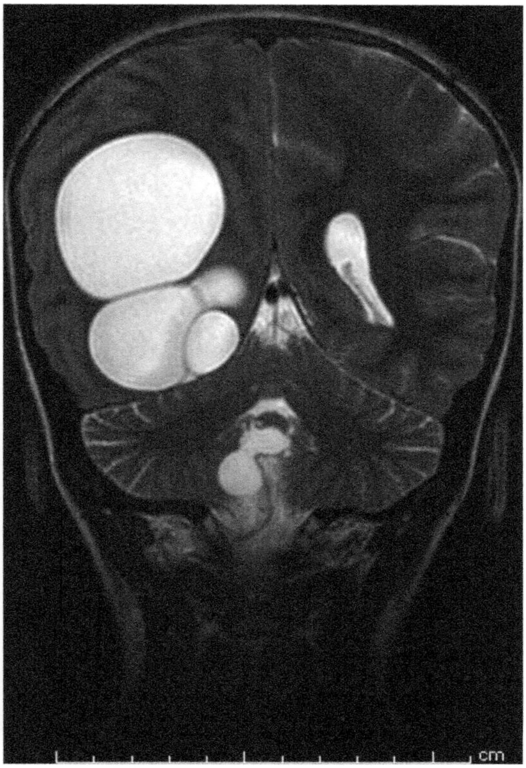

Fig. 7.3 Coronal T2-weighted MRI showing multiple cysts in the right occipital horn and fourth ventricle, extending outward through foramen of Luschka

membranes lining the cysts cannot be visualized as their density is similar to that of the adjacent brain tissue. Circular contrast enhancement and perifocal edema seen in multilocular cysts may result from active inflammation and must be differentiated from similar hallmarks of a brain abscess (Fig. 7.4) (Demir et al. 1991; Evliyaoglu and Keskil 2005).

Magnetic Resonance Imaging Findings

On magnetic resonance imaging (MRI), the lesions demonstrate CSF intensity with minimal or no enhancement in the simple cysts (Figs. 7.1, 7.2 and 7.3). Complicated cysts, viz., those with pericyst inflammation due to leakage of cyst content or infection, reveal intense contrast-enhancing rims with significant perilesional edema on T2-weighted images (Mohindra et al. 2012). Proton MR spectroscopy supplements diagnosis of these metabolically active lesions, with the cysts characteristically demonstrating elevated pyruvate, elevated succinate, acetate and alanine peaks, and a lipid-lactate peak at 1.33 ppm (Sreedhar 2006; Gupta et al. 2008).

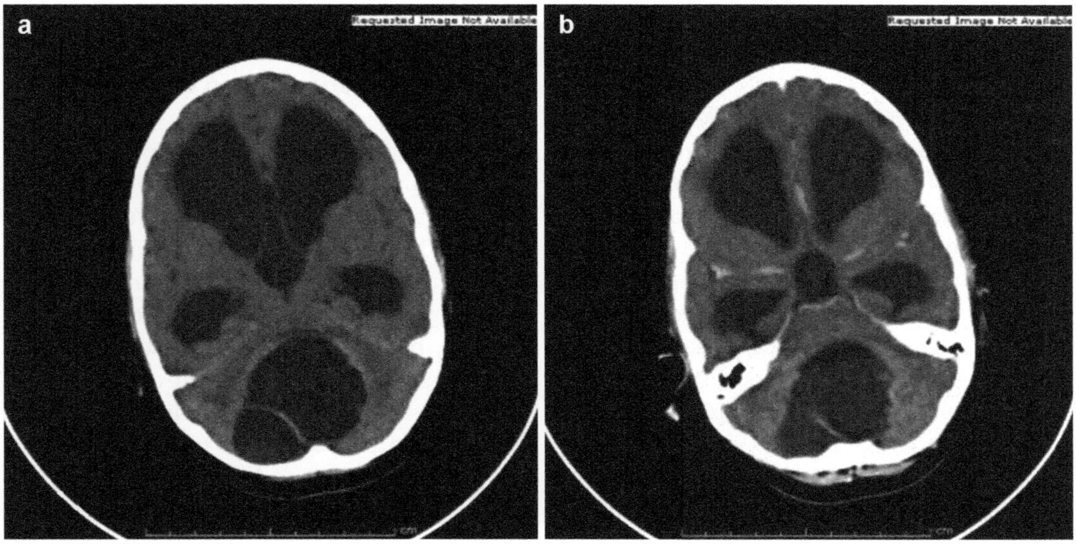

Fig. 7.4 (**a**) Plain and (**b**) contrast CT images of the cyst demonstrating no contrast enhancement with an added impression of septation

Differential Diagnoses

The radiological picture may be rendered complex by the presence of certain atypical features like intralesional nodular projections as seen in one of our patients (Figs. 7.1 and 7.2). In this case, the typical CSF signal intensities and lack of enhancement ruled out an astrocytoma, while the absence of preceding subarachnoid hemorrhage, infection, or congenital anomalies ruled out a trapped fourth ventricle (Zimmerman et al. 1978). Other close differentials that need exclusion are cysticercosis, arachnoid cysts, choroid plexus cysts, neoplastic cysts, infected or gliotic cysts, and colloid cysts (Handa et al. 1978; Zimmerman et al. 1978; Bukte et al. 2004). The final diagnosis, hence, is best arrived at by a combination of factors that include an appropriate clinical history, evidence of a primary hepatic focus, a high regional prevalence of hydatidosis, and laboratory findings.

Surgery

General Principles

In all cases, adequate anti-scolicidal measures need to be ensured by draping the brain with cotton strips soaked in scolicidal material like 10 % iodine or 1 % cetrimide (Altinörs et al. 2000; Furtado et al. 2009; Mohindra et al. 2012). Puncturing and aspiration of a large hydatid cyst followed by irrigation of the cyst with hypertonic solution and resection of the wall (puncture-aspiration-injection-reaspiration [PAIR] method) is not advisable because of the possibility of dissemination of cyst contents through the ventricular system (Altinörs et al. 2000). Complications that need to be anticipated with cyst rupture are the development of multiple daughter cysts, anaphylactic reaction, chemical meningitis, or ventriculitis induced by spillage of intracystic fluid (Altinörs et al. 2000).

Operative Technique

In the supratentorial compartment, a large frontoparietal craniotomy and a transcallosal transforaminal approach are used to deliver cysts at or near the foramen of Monro. A Cottonoid should be used at the foramen of Monro to prevent inferior migration of the cyst. Posterior fossa intraventricular cysts are approached by a midline suboccipital craniotomy in prone position with mild head elevation. We noticed that in these cases, the cerebral aqueduct, like the upper fourth ventricle, was enlarged by virtue of the proximal distension of ventricular system affected by the cyst. Care should thus be taken to prevent migration of the cyst into the third ventricle through an enlarged aqueduct (Fig. 7.5). This can be prevented again by the passage of Cottonoids under the cyst wall toward the aqueduct as the cyst is delivered (Fig. 7.6a). This prevents migration of smaller-sized primary and secondary cysts across the enlarged ventricular foramina. Cysts can be removed using the Dowling-Orlando water dissection technique through the foramen of Magendie. We used saline irrigation via a malleable ventricular catheter to prevent inadvertent cyst rupture and slow advancement of Cottonoids along with a Valsalva maneuver to deliver the cysts from the ventricle (Fig. 7.6b) (Furtado et al. 2009). These techniques and precautions facilitate the delivery of sizable unruptured ventricular cysts through narrow-sized foramina (Fig. 7.5).

Author's Experience and Case Studies

Of the two patients with intraventricular hydatid cysts we operated upon, the first (Figs. 7.1 and 7.2) was an 8-year-old girl from rural India who presented with occipital headache, vomiting, and deterioration of vision over a 1-year period. Her neurological deficits included secondary optic atrophy, poor visual acuity, coarse lateral gaze nystagmus, limb spasticity, and cerebellar dysfunction. At surgery via a midline suboccipital craniectomy, the vermis was found to be thinned out and the foramen of Magendie was enlarged. Three large and two small cysts were removed using Dowling's water dissection technique through the foramen. Abdominal MRI revealed a large hepatic hydatid cyst while MRI of the spine

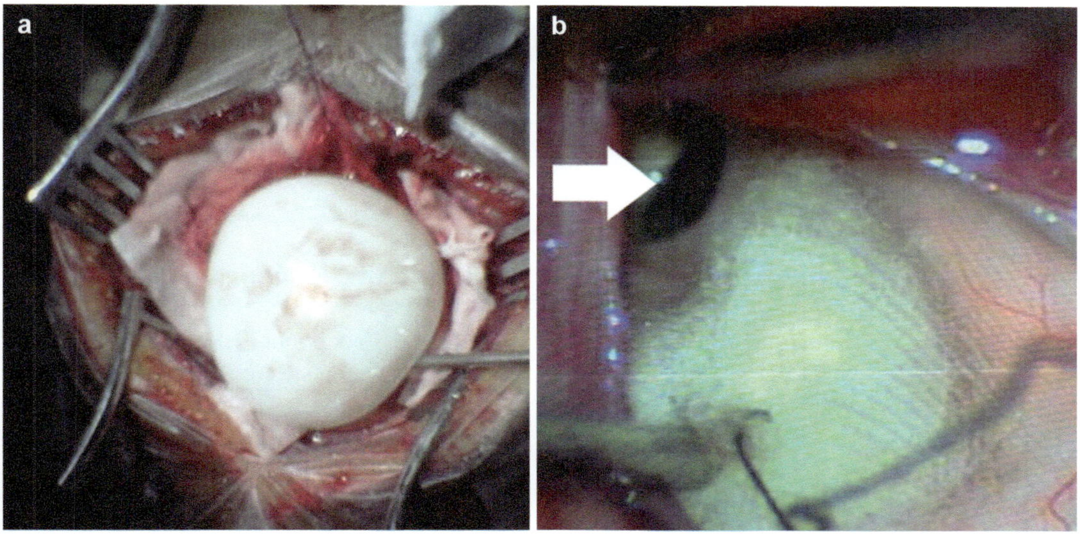

Fig. 7.5 (**a**) Large fourth ventricular cyst delivered in toto. (**b**) *Arrow* points to an enlarged cerebral aqueduct

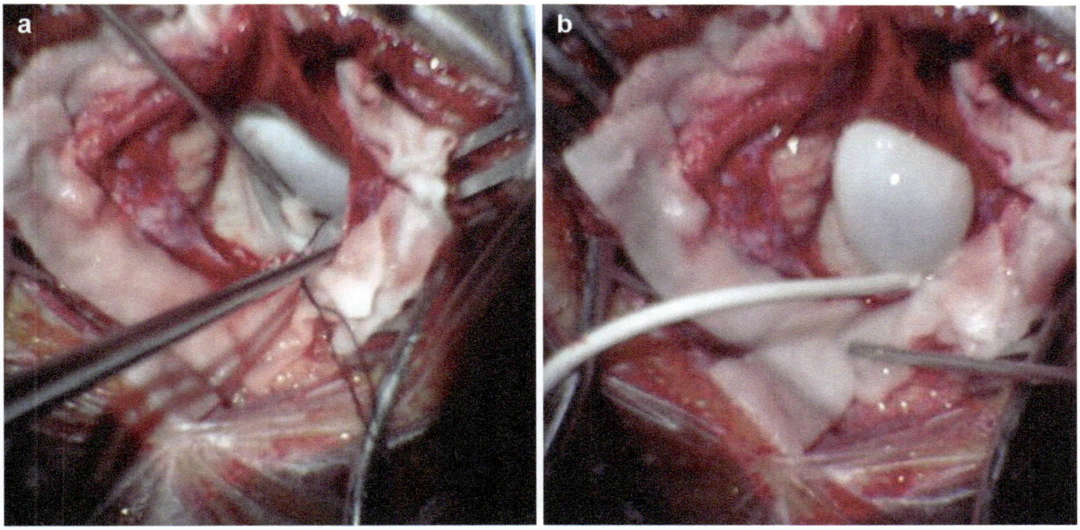

Fig. 7.6 (**a**) Cottonoids passed under the cyst wall toward the direction of the aqueduct. (**b**) Malleable ventricular catheter used to deliver the cyst

and heart were normal. Histopathological examination showed daughter cysts and a brood capsule within the large cyst. Hooklets were evident in the cytospin-prepared cyst fluid and absent in the smaller cysts (Furtado et al. 2009). At 1-year follow-up, she had no residual cyst(s) (Fig. 7.7) and her visual and cerebellar symptoms remained status quo.

The second case was a 9-year-old boy with holocranial (involving the whole head) episodic headache and vomiting of 3 months' duration (Fig. 7.3). Neurological examination revealed papilledema and a right sixth nerve palsy. He underwent bilateral parietal craniotomies and a midline suboccipital craniotomy for excision of multiple parenchymal, lateral ventricular cysts

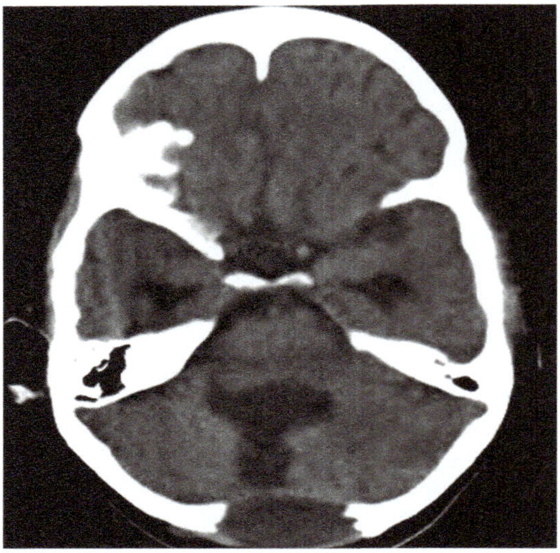

Fig. 7.7 Postoperative plain CT scan showing no residual cyst in the fourth ventricle

and fourth ventricular cysts, respectively. Postoperative imaging showed small residual parenchymal cysts which were treated with albendazole. He thereafter underwent cardiac surgery for removal of the cyst on the lateral wall of the left ventricle. These 2 representative cases were out of a total of 14 intracranial hydatid cysts operated over a 12-year period.

Endoscopy

Endoscopic removal of intraventricular hydatid cysts is an option which has to be weighed against the chances of complete removal of the cyst without spillage of contents. It has been performed in patients with an alternate diagnosis of colloid or arachnoid cysts, choroid plexus cysts, or neurocysticercosis (Husain et al. 2007).

Spillage of Cyst Contents

In case of spillage, irrigation with scolicidal agents such as 1 % cetrimide and 10 % formalin carries the risk of inducing ventriculitis (Furtado et al. 2009; Mohindra et al. 2012). A safer alternative is to administer antihelminthics like oral albendazole (10 mg/kg) for at least 2 months, a treatment regimen also indicated in cases of recurrence or systemic disease (Singounas et al. 1992; Gupta et al. 1999).

Postoperative Management

Based on the abdominal and cranial MRI findings, all our patients were administered albendazole (10 mg/kg per day) preoperatively and continued on the same postoperatively for a total duration of 2 months. Chemotherapy for hydatidosis of the central nervous system is discussed in Chap. 16.

Conclusion

Intraventricular hydatidosis can occur due to primary or secondary hydatid disease. A high index of suspicion is warranted for diagnosis especially when confronted with a smooth-walled, cystic intraventricular lesion of CSF intensity on MRI. This rare entity needs to be differentiated from cysts of gliotic, tumoral, or infective origins. Utmost caution needs to be exercised while delivering the cysts in order to prevent their rupture and subsequent dissemination, meningitis, or anaphylaxis.

References

Altinörs N, Bavbek M, Caner HH, Erdogan B. Central nervous system hydatidosis in Turkey: a cooperative study and literature survey analysis of 458 cases. J Neurosurg. 2000;93:1–8.

Aydin MD, Ozkan U, Altinors N. Quadruplets hydatid cysts in brain ventricles: a case report. Clin Neurol Neurosurg. 2002;104:300–2.

Borne G. A case of intraventricular cerebral hydatid cyst (in French). Bull Soc Pathol Exot Filiales. 1964;57: 28–32.

Bukte Y, Kemaloglu S, Nazaroglu H, Ozkan U, Ceviz A, Simsek M. Cerebral hydatid disease: CT and MR imaging findings. Swiss Med Wkly. 2004;134: 459–67.

Cataltepe O, Colak A, Ozcan OE, Ozgen T, Erbengi A. Intracranial hydatid cysts: experience with surgical treatment in 120 patients. Neurochirurgia. 1992;35:108–11.

Choux M, Pinsard N, Lehman G, Raybaud C, Vigouroux RP. Hydatid cyst of the fourth ventricle in a six-year-old child. Mod Probl Paediatr. 1976;18:273–5.

Ciurea AV, Fountas KN, Coman TC, Machinis TG, Kapsalaki EZ, Fezoulidis NI, Robinson JS. Long-term surgical outcome in patients with intracranial hydatid cyst. Acta Neurochir (Wien). 2006;148:421–6.

Copley IB, Fripp PJ, Erasmus AM, Otto DD. Unusual presentations of cerebral hydatid disease in children. Br J Neurosurg. 1992;6:203–10.

Demir K, Karsli AF, Kaya T, Devrimci E, Alkan K. Cerebral hydatid cysts: CT findings. Neuroradiology. 1991;33:22–4.

Diren HB, Ozcanli H, Boluk M, Kilic C. Unilocular orbital, cerebral and intraventricular hydatid cysts: CT diagnosis. Neuroradiology. 1993;35:149–50.

Djindjian R, Porot J. Voluminous intraventricular hydatic cyst; clinical particulars (in French). Sem Hop. 1957; 33:2065–8.

Duishanbai S, Jiafu D, Guo H, Liu C, Liu B, Aishalong M, Mijiti M, Wen H. Intracranial hydatid cyst in children: report of 30 cases. Childs Nerv Syst. 2010;26: 821–7.

Evliyaoglu C, Keskil S. Possible spontaneous "birth" of a hydatid cyst into the lateral ventricle. Childs Nerv Syst. 2005;21:425–8.

Filipov F, Karag'ozov L. Clinical observations on extradural and intraventricular distribution of echinococcosis (in Bulgarian). Khirurgiia (Sofiia). 1955;8: 337–9.

Furtado SV, Visvanathan K, Nandita G, Reddy K, Hegde AS. Multiple fourth ventricular hydatidosis. J Clin Neurosci. 2009;16:110–2.

Gelabert Gonzalez M, Bollar Zabala A, Garcia Allut A, Martínez Rumbo R. Hydatid cyst of the fourth ventricle. Rev Quir Esp. 1988;15:248–9.

Gupta S, Desai K, Goel A. Intracranial hydatid cyst: A report of five cases and review of literature. Neurol India. 1999;47:214–7.

Gupta K, Rajeswaran R, Joseph S, Ganesh K. Diagnosis of intracranial hydatid cyst by magnetic resonance spectroscopy. J Pediatr Neurosci. 2008;3:174–6.

Guvenc G, Özdemir N, Yildirim L. Successful treatment of hydatid cyst into the lateral ventricle with Dowling's technique in an adult patient. J Neurol Sci. 2011;28: 265–9.

Guzel A, Tatli M, Maciaczyk J, Altinors N. Primary cerebral intraventricular hydatid cyst: a case report and review of the literature. J Child Neurol. 2008;23:585–8.

Handa J, Nakano Y, Handa H. Computed tomography in the differential diagnosis of low-density intracranial lesions. Surg Neurol. 1978;10:179–85.

Husain M, Jha DK, Rastogi M, Husain N, Gupta RK. Neuro-endoscopic management of intraventricular neurocysticercosis (NCC). Acta Neurochir (Wien). 2007;149:341–6.

Iyigun O, Uysal S, Sancak R, Hokelek M, Uyar Y, Berney F, Ariturk E. Multiple organ involvement hydatid cysts in a 2-year-old boy. J Trop Pediatr. 2004;50: 374–6.

Kamath SM, Mysorekar VV, Rao SG, Varma RG. Intraventricular hydatid cyst in a child. Indian J Pathol Microbiol. 2009;52:571–2.

Karadağ O, Gürelik M, Ozüm U, Göksel HM. Primary multiple cerebral hydatid cysts with unusual features. Acta Neurochir (Wien). 2004;146:73–7.

Kaya U, Ozden B, Türker K, Tarcan B. Intracranial hydatid cysts. Study of 17 cases. J Neurosurg. 1975;42: 580–4.

Lunardi P, Missori P, Di Lorenzo N, Fortuna A. Cerebral hydatidosis in childhood: a retrospective survey with emphasis on long-term follow up. Neurosurgery. 1991;29:515–8.

Majumdar K, Saran RK, Sakhuja P, Jagetia A, Sinha S. Intact protoscolices and hooklets in cytospin preparation of intra-operative cyst fluid allow rapid confirmation of rare cerebral intraventricular hydatid infestation. Cytopathology. 2013;24:277–79.

Mohindra S, Savardekar A, Gupta R, Tripathi M, Rane S. Varied types of intracranial hydatid cysts: radiological features and management techniques. Acta Neurochir (Wien). 2012;154:165–72.

Negovetic L, Lupret V, Smiljanic D, Arsenic B. Cranial vault and gigantic intracranial hydatid cyst in a young woman. Neurosurgery. 1990;27:480–2.

Onal C, Barlas O, Orakdogen M, Hepgül K, Izgi N, Unal F. Three unusual cases of intracranial hydatid cysts in the pediatric age group. Pediatr Neurosurg. 1997;26: 208–13.

Onal C, Unal F, Barlas O, Izgi N, Hepgul K, Turantan MI, Canbolat A, Turker K, Bayindir C, Gokay HK, Kaya U. Long-term follow-up and results of thirty pediatric intracranial hydatid cysts: half a century of experience in the Department of Neurosurgery of the School of Medicine at the University of Istanbul (1952–2001). Pediatr Neurosurg. 2001;35:72–81.

Pau A, Brambilla M, Cossu M, Sehrbundt Viale E, Turtas S. Long term follow-up of the surgical treatment of the intracranial hydatid disease. Acta Neurochir (Wien). 1987;88:116–8.

Peker S, Celik H, Eryılmaz M, Gurcay O. Iohexol CT ventriculogram of multiple cerebral hydatid cysts. AJNR Am J Neuroradiol. 1991;12:797.

Rahimizadeh A, Hadadian K. Hydatid cyst of the fourth ventricle. Neurosurgery. 1984;14:787–8.

Sherwani RK, Abrari A, Jayrajpuri ZS, Srivastava VK. Intracranial hydatidosis. Report of a case diagnosed on cerebrospinal fluid cytology. Acta Cytol. 2003;47: 506–8.

Singounas EG, Leventis AS, Sakas DE, Hadley DM, Lampadarios DA, Karvounis PC. Successful treatment

of intracerebral hydatid cysts with albendazole: case report and review of the literature. Neurosurgery. 1992;31:571–4.
Sreedhar M. Disseminated hydatid disease a case report with mr spectroscopic correlation. Indian J Radiol Imaging. 2006;16:771–4.
Turgut M. Intracranial hydatidosis in Turkey: its clinical presentation, diagnostic studies, surgical management, and outcome. A review of 276 cases. Neurosurg Rev. 2001;24:200–8.
Turgut M. Hydatidosis of central nervous system and its coverings in the pediatric and adolescent age groups in Turkey during the last century: a critical review of 137 cases. Childs Nerv Syst. 2002;18:670–83.
Ugur HC, Attar A, Bagdatoglu C, Erdoğan A, Egemen N. Secondary multiple intracranial hydatid cysts caused by intracerebral embolism of cardiac echinococcosis. Acta Neurochir (Wien). 1998;140:833–4.
Valentino V. Combined intraventricular and intracerebral hydatid cysts: report of a case. Radiology. 1959;73: 250–2.
Zimmerman RA, Bilaniuk LT, Gallo E. Computed tomography of the trapped fourth ventricle. AJR Am J Roentgenol. 1978;130:503–6.

Hydatidosis of the Spinal Cord

8

Anita Arsovska, Ante Popovski, and Zoran Arsovski

Contents

A. Arsovska, MD, PhD (✉)
Department of Urgent Neurology,
University Clinic of Neurology,
Vodnjanska 17, Skopje 1000, Macedonia
e-mail: anita70mk@yahoo.com

A. Popovski, MD, PhD
Department of Neuropsychiatry,
Private Neuropsychiatry Practice "Dr. A. Popovski",
Skopje, Macedonia

Z. Arsovski, MD, MrSci
University Clinic of Pulmonology and Allergy,
Skopje, Macedonia

Introduction

Human echinococcosis, also known as hydatid (Greek for "watery cyst") disease or hydatidosis, is a rare but significant disease with a characteristic geographic distribution; it is mostly found in the sheep-raising regions of the world (Pamir et al. 1984; Morris and Richards 1992). Humans are infected with the larval form of the cyclozoonotic *Echinococcus* parasite, i.e., *Echinococcus granulosus* and less frequently *E. multilocularis*. Susceptibility of humans to infection varies, presumably because of individual differences in nutritional, immunologic, and genetic factors.

Etiology and Pathophysiology

Humans are incidental intermediate hosts. The infestation is mainly transmitted directly by contact with the infected animal or indirectly by feco-oral ingestion of the worm eggs from contaminated water or food (Prabhakar et al. 2005; Papanikolaou 2008). *E. granulosus* larvae develop slowly (usually over many years) into large unilocular, fluid-filled lesions—hydatid cysts. Incubation period may vary from months to years.

M. Turgut (ed.), *Hydatidosis of the Central Nervous System: Diagnosis and Treatment*,
DOI 10.1007/978-3-642-54359-3_8, © Springer-Verlag Berlin Heidelberg 2014

Hydatidosis of the Spinal Cord

Involvement of the epidural space with sparing of the vertebral column is rare (Desai et al. 1999; Mohamed et al. 2004; Kaen et al. 2009). There are some reports from the literature describing massive affection of the epidural space without involvement of the vertebral column. Medjek et al. (1991) reported an intradural spinal hydatid cyst in the thoracic region and Akhan et al. (1991) one in a child. The intradural and extramedullary involvement is extremely rare, especially in non-endemic countries (Goçer et al. 1994; Kaen et al. 2009; Lakhdar et al. 2009). It appears only sporadically worldwide. Table 8.1 summarizes a total of 144 selected cases of spinal hydatidosis in the world literature to date (quoted from Deve 1928; Bertrand et al. 1956; Boixados 1961; Carrea and Murphy 1964; Pierini et al. 1965; Baurand et al. 1970; Karvounis et al. 1977; Bettaieb et al. 1978; San Martin Sánchez et al. 1980; Sharma et al. 1981; Pamir et al. 1984; Akhan et al. 1991; Medjek et al. 1991; Fahl et al 1994; Haddad and Bitar 1997; Turgut 1997; Islekel et al. 1998; Kabbaj-El Kouhen et al. 1999; Chat et al. 2000; Pushparaj et al. 2001; Chakir et al. 2002; Onbas et al. 2004; Kahilogullari et al. 2005; Layadi et al. 2005; Prabhakar et al. 2005; Charrada-Ben-Farhat et al. 2006; Sapkas et al. 2006; Kalkan et al. 2007; Kotil et al. 2007, 2010; Secer et al. 2008; Arif and Zaheer 2009; Jaiswal et al. 2009; Kaen et al. 2009; Lakhdar et al. 2009; Midyat et al. 2009; Turan Süslü et al. 2009; Celik et al. 2010; Thaler et al. 2010; Ediz et al. 2011).

The disease usually spreads to the spine by direct extension from pulmonary, abdominal, or pelvic infestation and less often begins primarily in the vertebral body, affecting predominantly the dorsal region of the spine (Bhojraj and Shetty 1999; Garcia-Vicuna et al. 2000; Govender et al. 2000; Hamdan and Al-Kaisy 2000; Schnepper and Johnson 2004; Herrera et al. 2005; Prabhakar et al. 2005; Sapkas et al. 2006; Papanikolaou 2008; Spies et al. 2008). When hydatidosis begins in the spine, it usually begins in the marrow of a vertebral body and may progress around the neural arch, through adjacent ribs, reaching the spinal canal or the intervertebral discs; thus, spinal involvement is believed to occur through direct portovertebral venous shunts (Morshed 1977; Fiennes and Thomas 1982). The extradural disease may spread through the neural foramen into the surrounding soft tissues as in the upper thoracic involvement by direct extension from a pulmonary lesion. However, the main mechanism for the intradural extramedullary involvement is not yet clear. Primary hematic dissemination is regarded as the most plausible mechanism, but dural tearing during surgery or during an aggressive invasion of spinal space, like lumbar puncture, may have a role in the etiology of the spreading of the infestation into the intradural space. This mechanism is well known for bacterial dissemination, but not for parasite spread.

Mortality/Morbidity

Spinal cord hydatidosis causes serious and disabling symptoms. Occasionally, deaths occur because of anaphylactic shock.

Race

No racial predilection has been observed.

Sex

In some endemic regions, females are affected more than males because their lifestyle habits and practices bring them into contact with the parasite.

Age

Individuals of all ages are affected. In some endemic countries, children have higher infection rates because they are most likely to play with dogs.

Table 8.1 Summary of 144 selected cases of spinal hydatidosis in the world literature to date

Author(s), year	Country	Age and gender	Localization	Neurological status	Neuroimaging	Outcome
Bartel (1928)	France	NA	Cervical	NA	NA	NA
Deve (1928)	France	NA	Cervical, ID, EM	NA	NA	NA
Rauzier (1928)	France	NA	Cervical	NA	NA	NA
Vallè (1928)	France	NA	Cervico-thoraco-lumbar	NA	NA	NA
Bertrand et al. (1956)	Morocco	25, F	T11-T12 ID, EM	Paraplegia	Myelography	Recurrence after 13 mos
Boixados (1961)	Spain	4, F	T5 ID, EM	Paraplegia	Myelography	Partial recovery
Carrea and Murphy (1964)	Argentina	9, F	T4–T5 ID, EM	Paraplegia	Myelography	Total recovery
Pierini et al. (1965)	Argentina	NA	Cervical, ID	NA	Myelography	NA
Baurand et al. (1970)	North Africa	35, F	T6 ID, EM	Paraplegia	Myelography	Total recovery
Karvounis et al. (1977)	Greece	37, F	L5–S1 ID, EM	Sciatica	Myelography	Total recovery
Bettaieb et al. (1978)	Tunisia	4, M	Upper thoracic, ID, EM	Paraplegia	CT-myelography	Total recovery
	Tunisia	8, M	Upper thoracic, ID, EM	Paraplegia	CT-myelography	Total recovery
	Tunisia	8, M	Middle thoracic, ID, EM	Paraplegia	CT-myelography	Total recovery
San Martin Sánchez et al. (1980)	Spain	62, F	L2, ID, EM	Paraplegia	Myelography	Total recovery
Sharma et al. (1981)	India	14, M	T6–T10, ID, EM	Paraplegia	Myelography	Partial recovery
Pamir et al. (1984)	Turkey	34, F	L2, ID, EM	Paraplegia	Myelography	No change
Akhan et al. (1991)	Turkey	6, M	T9–T11, ID, EM	Paraplegia	CT-myelography	NA
Medjek et al. (1991)	Algeria	21, F	T12–L1, ID, EM	Paraplegia	CT-myelography	Total recovery
Fahl et al. (1994)	Lebanon	55, F	T12–L1	Paraparesis	CT-myelography, MRI	NA
Haddad and Bitar (1997)[a]	Lebanon	46, M	L4–S1	Sciatica	CT	Recovery
Turgut (1997)[b,c] Islekel et al. (1998)	Lebanon	7, M, and 7, F	Cervical (2), thoracic (11), lumbar (4), sacral (1)	Pain (13), urinary incontinence, weakness (5), sciatica (2)	Myelography (7), CT (4), MRI (2)	Death (2), total recovery (2), no change (1)
	Turkey	61, M, and 23, F (mean age: NA)	Cervical (3), thoracic (35), thoracolumbar (3), lumbar (28), sacral (1), cervical and lumbar (1)	Paraplegia and paraparesis (61), cauda equine syndrome (27)	Myelography (56), MRI (8), CT (6), US (1)	Death (2), total recovery (5), recurrence (15)
	Turkey	19, M	L2–L4, ID, EM	Paraplegia	Myelography	Partial recovery

(continued)

Table 8.1 (continued)

Author(s), year	Country	Age and gender	Localization	Neurological status	Neuroimaging	Outcome
Kabbaj-El Kouhen et al. (1999)	Morocco	6, M	L1–L3, ID, EM	Paraplegia	CT-myelography	Partial recovery
Chat et al. (2000)	Morocco	13, F	T5–T11, L4–L5, ID, EM	Paraplegia	CT-myelography, MRI	Partial recovery
Pushparaj et al. (2001)	India	40, F	T10–T11, ID, EM	Paraplegia	MRI	Total recovery
Chakir et al. (2002)	Morocco	18, M	L1–L2, ID, EM	Paraplegia	MRI	Subtotal recovery
Onbas et al. (2004)	Turkey	48, M	Cervicothoracic, ID, EM	Paraparesis	MRI	Recurrence
Kahilogullari et al. (2005)	Turkey	32, F	L5–S2, ID, EM	Paraparesis	MRI	Total recovery
Layadi et al. (2005)	Morocco	35, M	Sacral, ED	Cauda equina syndrome	MRI	NA
Prabhakar et al. (2005)	India	3, M, and 1, F (mean age, 40 yr)	T8–T10	Paraplegia	Myelography	Without recovery
	India		T5–T6	Paraplegia	Myelography	Without recovery
	India		L5–S1	ASIA Grade C	Myelography, CT, MRI with contrast	Complete recovery after 1 yr
	India		L2–L5 ED, ID	Cauda equina syndrome	Myelography, CT, MRI with contrast	Complete recovery after 1 yr
Charrada-Ben-Farhat et al. (2006)	Tunisia	40, M	T7–T8, ED	Paraplegia	MRI	Total recovery after discharge
Sapkas et al. (2006)	Greece	62, M	ED	NA	NA	NA
Kalkan et al. (2007)	Turkey	8, M	T7–T8, ID, EM	Paraparesis	MRI	Total recovery after 4 mos
Kotil et al. (2007)	Turkey	34, F	T11 ED	Paraplegia	MRI	NA
Secer et al. (2008)	Turkey	35, M	T12, ID, EM	Paraplegia	MRI	Total recovery after 8 mos
Arif and Zaheer (2009)	India	9, M	L1–L4, ID, EM	Paraparesis	MRI	Complete recovery after 6 mos
Jaiswal et al. (2009)	India	21, F	T10, ED	Paraplegia	MRI	Partial recovery after discharge
Kaen et al. (2009)	Spain	59, M	T6, T10–T12, ID, EM	Paraparesis	MRI	Without recovery

Lakhdar et al. (2009)	Morocco	22, M	T11	Paraparesis	MRI	Total recovery after 15 mos
	Morocco	5, M	T12–L2	Paraparesis	MRI	Total recovery after 15 mos
	Morocco	10, F	L2–L5, ID, EM	Paraparesis	MRI	Total recovery after 18 mos
Midyat et al. (2009)	Turkey	13, F	ID, EM	Paraparesis	NA	NA
Salduz et al. (2009)	Turkey	41, F	ED	Sciatica	MRI	Total recovery after 5.5 yr
Turan Süslü et al. (2009)	Turkey	34, M	T10–T11, ID	Paraparesis	MRI	Total recovery after 1 yr
Celik et al. (2010)	Turkey	34, M	Thoracic, ED	Paraplegia	MRI	Total recovery after 2 mos
Kotil et al. (2010)	Turkey	30, F	L4–L5, ED	Sciatica	MRI	Total recovery after 7 mos
Thaler et al. (2010)	Austria	6, F	T8–T9, ED	Paraplegia	CT, MRI	Total recovery after 18 mos
Ediz et al. (2011)	Turkey	25, F	T7–T12, ED	Paraplegia	MRI	Partial recovery

Abbreviations: *M* male, *F* female, *C* cervical, *T* thoracic, *TC* thoracolumbar, *L* lumbar, *S* sacral, *IM* intramedullary, *EM* extramedullary, *ID* intradural, *ED* extradural, *CT* computed tomography, *MRI* magnetic resonance imaging, *US* ultrasonography, *mos* months, *yr* year, *NA* not available

[a]Out of the cases reported by the authors, two cases had already been described by Fahl et al. earlier

[b]Except for 13 patients, all had data suggestive of the exact location of the cysts in the spine

[c]Out of the cases reported by the author, two cases had already been described by Pamir et al. and Akhan et al. earlier

Classification

Morphologically, spinal involvement has been classified by Braithwaite and Lees (1981) into five types: (1) primary intramedullary hydatid cysts, (2) intradural extramedullary hydatid cysts, (3) extradural intraspinal hydatid cysts, (4) vertebral hydatidosis, and (5) paravertebral hydatidosis (Fig. 8.1).

Symptoms and Signs

Before an individual exhibits any symptoms and signs, many months or years may pass, during which the destiny of *E. granulosus* cysts is variable. Some cysts may grow to a certain size and then persist without noticeable change for many years, while other cysts may rupture spontaneously or collapse and completely disappear. After a variable incubation period, infestation may become symptomatic if cysts are growing and exerting pressure on adjacent tissue and inducing other pathologic findings. Sudden symptomatology is usually due to spontaneous or traumatic cyst rupture.

The clinical features of spinal cord hydatidosis are variable. The spectrum of symptoms depends on the following:

- Which part of the spinal cord has been involved
- Size of cysts and their sites within the affected spinal cord
- Interaction between the expanding cysts and adjacent structures

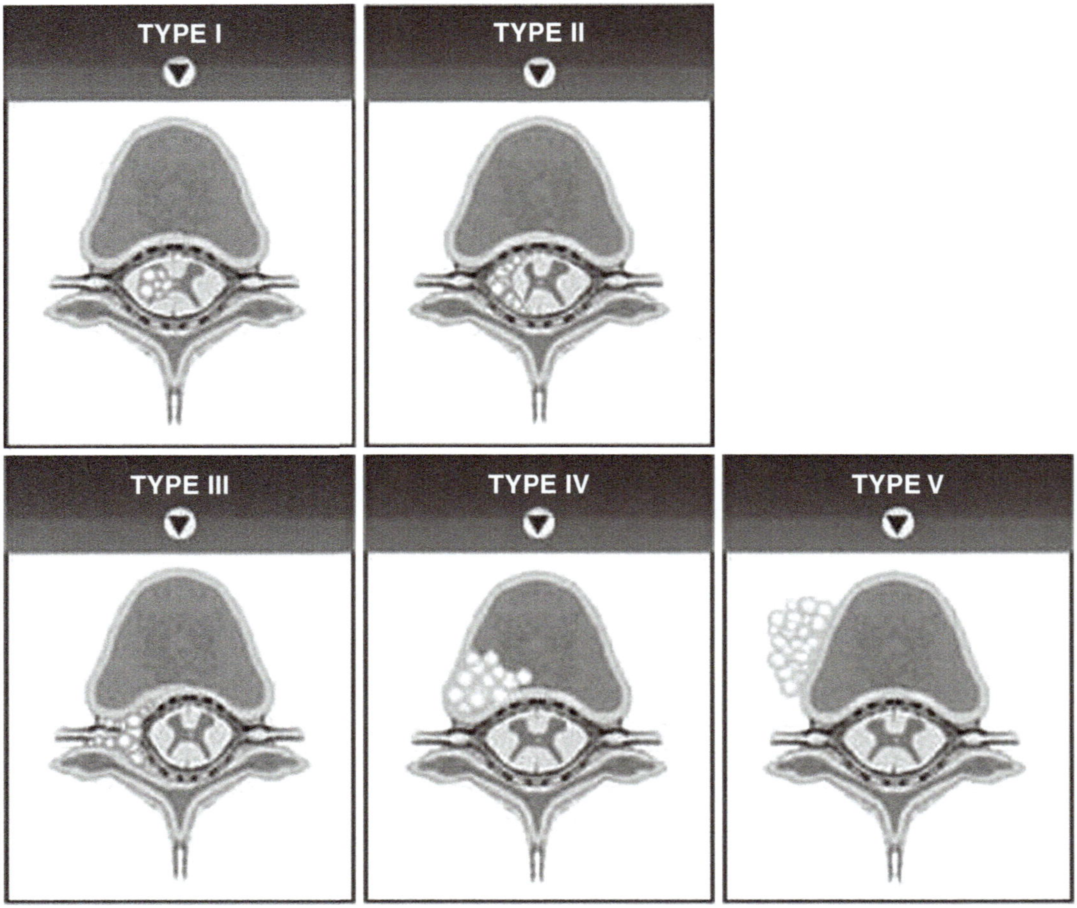

Fig. 8.1 Braithwaite and Lee's classification (Adapted from Braithwaite and Lees (1981))

- Complications caused by rupture of cysts
- Bacterial infection of cysts and spread of protoscolices and larval material into the blood vessels
- Immunologic reactions secondary to release of antigenic material

Physical

The initial clinical symptoms are usually nonspecific. In the beginning of the disease, the patient complaints of backache that lasts for a certain period of time (1–2 months). After disease-associated complications appear due to root and cord compression, the patients experience weakness in both lower limbs that gradually worsens, until the moment that the patients are unable to walk (Bilgic et al. 2009). The neurological complications are the result of invasive intradural and extradural growth of the cysts causing direct compression. This mixed picture poses a confusing picture for diagnosis and treatment planning.

Clinically, spinal cord echinococcosis manifests by radicular pain associated with objective sensory and motor disturbances. There are no pathognomonic signs and symptoms of this disease. For this reason it is often misdiagnosed initially as spinal tumor or disc herniation. The clinical presentation of spinal hydatidosis is variable, including paraparesis (62 %) or paraplegia (26 %), back pain or radicular pain (55 %), numbness or sensitivity loss (36 %), and sphincter disturbance (30 %) (Govender et al. 2000; Fares et al. 2003; Herrera et al. 2005; Papanikolaou 2008). The time period between the onset of the symptoms and medical consultation varies between 6 and 15 months (Khazim et al. 2003; Papanikolaou 2008).

Neurological Examination

Patients with spinal cord hydatidosis may present with one of three clinical syndromes: (1) a sensorimotor spinal tract syndrome, (2) a painful radicular spinal cord syndrome, or (3) rarely an intramedullary syringomyelic syndrome.

Sometimes, pain and stiffness of the back may antedate signs of spinal cord disease or dominate the clinical picture in some cases of extramedullary located cysts. The back pain usually worsens when the patient lies down and may be improved by sitting up. In the beginning, children experience severe back pain associated with spasm of paravertebral muscles; later in the course of the disease appear scoliosis and spastic weakness of the legs.

Sensorimotor Spinal Tract Syndrome

The signs of compression consist of (a) an asymmetrical spastic weakness of the arms and legs with cervical lesions and of the legs with thoracolumbar lesions, (b) reduced or lost sensory perception of pain and temperature below a certain level of the trunk, (c) signs of posterior column affection, and (d) a spastic bladder under weak voluntary control.

The onset of the compressive symptoms is usually gradual and the course progressive over a period of weeks and months, frequently with back pain. In patients with extradural cysts, paralysis usually develops over a period of days to several weeks, but the velocity of progression may vary. The initial disturbance may be motor or sensory and the distribution could be asymmetrical.

If the lesion is located in the low cervical segments and involves the anterior half of the spinal cord, the paralysis of the arms may be flaccid and areflexic in type and spastic of that of the legs. There is usually pain in the neck and shoulders and numbness of the hands; ataxia from posterior column lesions may accompany the paraparesis. In patients with cysts with high cervical location, a progressive syndrome of monoparesis, biparesis, and triparesis may be observed.

In thoracic lesions, one leg usually becomes weak and stiff before the other one. Subjective sensory symptoms of the dorsal column type (tingling paresthesias) may be present. Pain and thermal senses are more likely to be affected than tactile, vibration, and position senses.

The bladder and bowel usually become paralyzed coincident with the leg paralysis.

Radicular Spinal Cord Syndrome

Here, the syndrome of spinal cord compression is combined with radicular pain that is intensified by coughing or sneezing. It is described as knifelike or as a dull ache with superimposed sharp stabs of pain, which radiate in a distal direction. Besides the radicular pain, other usual symptoms include segmental sensory changes (paresthesias, impaired perception of pinprick and touch) and/or motor disturbances (cramp, atrophy, fascicular twitching, and loss of tendon reflexes) and an ache in the spine. Half of the patients experience tenderness of spinous processes over the growth by percussion. Sensory radicular symptoms often precede the signs of spinal cord compression by months.

Intramedullary Syringomyelic Syndrome

Intramedullary growths invade as well as compress and distort fasciculi in the spinal cord white matter. As the cord enlarges from the growing cyst, the free space around the cord is eventually consumed. No single symptom is unique to intramedullary cysts. Some degree of pain, sometimes minor, is common and is almost invariably present with lesions of the filum terminale. When the intramedullary cyst involves the central gray matter, a central cord or syringomyelic syndrome may result. The main symptoms are segmental or dissociated sensory loss, amyotrophy, early incontinence, and late corticospinal weakness. A sign of intramedullary lesion is a dissociation of thermal pain and tactile sensory loss over several segments on the trunk. Rarely, an extramedullary cyst may give rise to a syringomyelic syndrome, possibly by causing vascular insufficiency in the central portion of the cord.

Lesions at the level of the lowermost thoracic and the first lumbar vertebrae may result in mixed cauda equina and spinal cord symptoms. Positive Babinski sign indicates that the spinal cord is involved above the fifth lumbar segment. Lesions of the cauda equina alone, always difficult to separate from those of the lumbosacral plexuses and multiple nerves, are usually attended in the early stages by sciatic and other root pain and lumbar ache, which is variously combined with a bilaterally asymmetrical, atrophic, areflexic paralysis, radicular sensory loss, and sphincteric disorder. These must be distinguished from lesions of the conus medullaris, in which there are early disturbances of the bladder and bowel (urinary retention and constipation), back pain, symmetrical hypesthesia or anesthesia over the sacral dermatomes, a lax anal sphincter with loss of anal and bulbocavernosus reflexes, impotence, and sometimes weakness of leg muscles. Sensory abnormalities may precede motor and reflex changes by several months.

Complications

The primary cyst may contain daughter cyst and microruptures can give rise to secondary cysts. Spontaneous or traumatic cyst rupture and spillage of viable parasitic tissue during interventional procedures may result in secondary echinococcosis. Cysts may rupture into the blood vessels, leading to extraordinary manifestations and severe complications such as fever, urticaria, eosinophilia, and anaphylactic shock, as well as cyst dissemination.

Complications of spinal hydatidosis are discussed in detail in Chap. 18.

Diagnosis

Laboratory Studies

Routine laboratory tests should be obtained, but usually do not show specific values. Eosinophilia on cell blood count is absent or limited (<15 %). Indirect hemagglutination test and enzyme-linked immunosorbent assay are the most widely used methods for detection of anti-*Echinococcus* antibodies (immunoglobulin G). In spinal involvement, the serological sensitivity of antigens is 25 %, whereas it is 80–100 % in liver involvement (Kotil et al. 2007). Children aged 3–15 years may produce minimal serological reactions. No standard, highly sensitive, and specific serological test exists for cystic echinococcosis antibody detection.

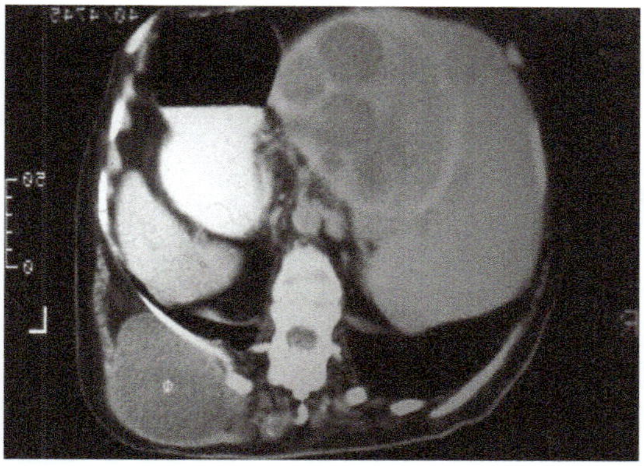

Fig. 8.2 Paravertebral hydatid cyst and hepatic cysts of a 49-year-old male patient with vertebral hydatid disease with destruction of two vertebral bodies (T12–L1) and paraplegia of 8 months of evolution. The patient was in a severe general state with sepsis, with fatal evolution (Courtesy of A. Herrera, M.D., Ph.D.)

Neuroimaging Studies

Imaging techniques such as plain radiographs, computed tomography (CT), and magnetic resonance imaging (MRI) of the spine should be obtained. They may be pathognomonic if daughter cysts and hydatid sand (protoscolices and debris) are present, but simple hydatid cysts may be difficult to differentiate from simple benign cysts, abscesses, Pott's disease, or benign or malignant tumors (Fahl et al. 1994; Turgut 1997). Imaging of spinal hydatid disease is discussed in detail in Chap. 12.

Radiographic Studies

Radiographic examination is useful for detecting calcified cysts.

Computed Tomography Studies

CT scanning can detect and locate smaller cysts precisely and sometimes differentiate parasitic from nonparasitic cysts (Fig. 8.2). Measurement of cyst density appears to be an additional tool to differentiate parasitic from nonparasitic cysts and for follow-up studies during chemotherapy.

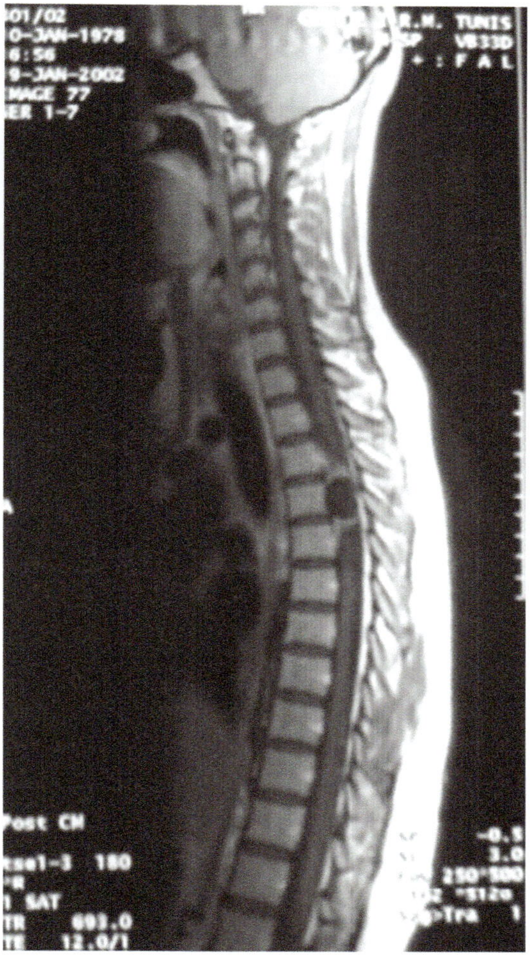

Fig. 8.3 MRI finding of a 24-year-old male patient showing extradural hydatid cyst at T4 vertebra corpus level (Courtesy of F. Limaiem, M.D.)

Magnetic Resonance Imaging Studies

MRI is the study of choice in the diagnosis of spinal echinococcosis since hydatid cysts have a unique appearance on MRI (Fahl et al. 1994; Mohamed et al. 2004; Lakhdar et al. 2009) (Fig. 8.3). Characteristic MRI findings of hydatid cysts are two dome-shaped ends, no debris in the lumen, and a "sausage-like" appearance with CSF-like signal intensities (Güneçs et al. 2009). The cysts are hypointense on T1W images. Intensity differences in T2W sequences of MRI can also determine the viability of the cyst (Jena et al. 1991). Viable cysts appear to contain a

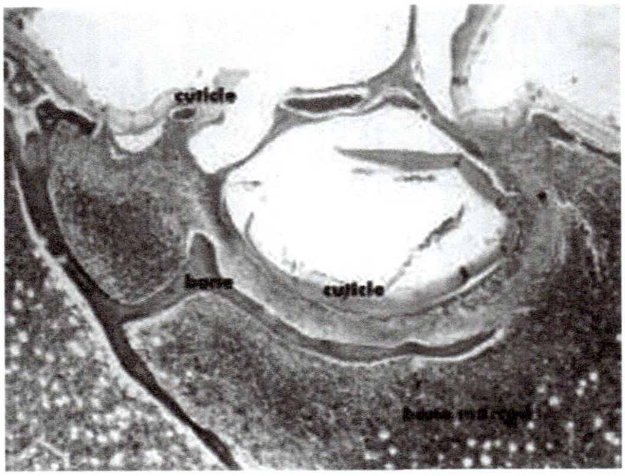

Fig. 8.4 Histopathological cross section of an excised hydatid cyst (Courtesy of A. Salduz, M.D.)

low-intensity fluid surrounded by an iso- to mildly hyperintense wall which on T2-weighted images appears as a low-intensity rim surrounding the high-signal cyst content (Tekkok and Benli 1993). Decrease in the intensity of the signal of the content and an increase of the signal of the cyst walls indicate a dying cyst. On T2W images they appear hyperintense with sharply defined, hypointense cyst wall which shows mild enhancement following intravenous gadolinium, reflecting the vascularity of the pericyst (Gupta et al. 2002).

Histopathological Diagnosis

The diagnosis can definitely be confirmed histopathologically by observing the allergic-type tissue reaction in the surrounding tissue and demonstration of the cyst wall histology and scolices (Salduz et al. 2009) (Fig. 8.4). Preoperative diagnosis is essential because the rupture and dissemination of cyst may result in anaphylaxis and recurrence.

Differential Diagnosis

The infection may be misdiagnosed initially as tuberculosis of the spine, which delays proper diagnosis and intervention. Other differential diagnostic possibilities include:

- Benign cysts
- Benign and malignant tumors
- Secondary tumors
- Abscesses
- Pyogenic infection of the spinal cord

Treatment

Despite the introduction of modern surgical and pharmacological therapy, the disease still continues to be difficult to cure and is highly prone to recurrence. Successful treatment of the spinal cord hydatidosis is challenging because of its invasiveness and its potentially severe complications.

Medical Care

The only antihelminthic agents that are effective against hydatidosis are albendazole and mebendazole (Turgut 1997; Brunetti et al. 2010). Praziquantel has recently been suggested; however, available data are limited (Bygott and Chiodini 2009). Medicamentous treatment should be applied before any surgical intervention in order to prevent the patient from a potentially lethal anaphylactic shock in case of a rupture of an active cyst (Hamdan and Al-Kaisy 2000). Chemotherapy for hydatidosis of the central nervous system is discussed in Chap. 16.

Surgical Treatment

Surgery is indicated if it is feasible, which depends on the size, location, and manifestation of the lesion (Prabhakar et al. 2005; Lakhdar et al. 2009; Salduz et al. 2009) (Figs. 8.4, 8.5, 8.6, 8.7, 8.8 and 8.9). Appropriate surgical treatment includes complete cyst resection without rupture of the wall (Bhojraj and Shetty 1999), appropriate decompression of the cord, correction of the deformity, and appropriate anterior and posterior instrumented stabilization techniques. Surgical treatment involves laminec-

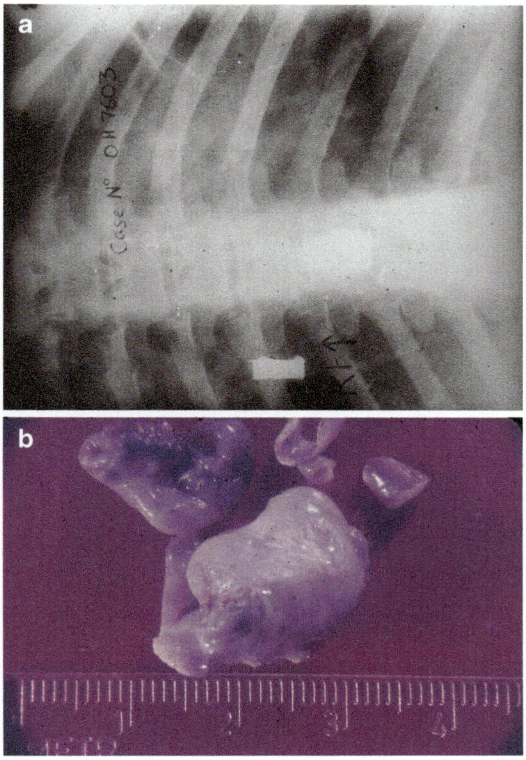

Fig. 8.5 Finding of spinal hydatidosis of a female patient, which did not recur (**a**, **b**) (Courtesy of F. S. Haddad, M.D.)

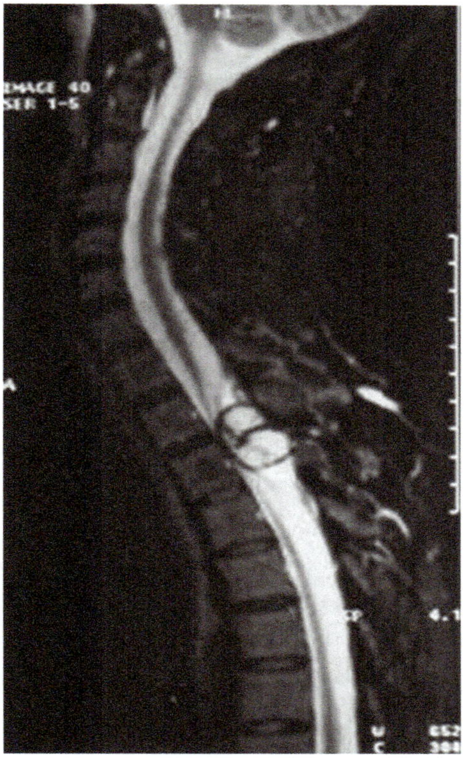

Fig. 8.6 Hydatidosis of L1. Anterior approach by thoracolaparotomy, extraction of cysts of the vertebral body (Courtesy of A. Herrera, M.D., Ph.D.)

tomy and decompression of the nerve elements/medulla. Difficulties in allocating of the intradural cyst(s) are due to the surrounding arachnoiditis, making them adhere to the arachnoid and difficult to remove. The principle is not to tear them apart in order to avoid spreading of the disease.

Generally, the patient should be in prone position, i.e., on the stomach, placed on a suitable bed or chair to release the abdomen that hangs freely in order to decrease the pressure in the paraspinal venous plexus to avoid excessive bleeding during the operation. Pillows are placed under the chest and both cristae spinae iliacae, or specially constructed frames, that support the chest and both cristae to release the abdomen.

Usually, the approach is made by a midline incision, along the line of the processus spinosus, at the appropriate level depending on the lesion localization. A standard procedure is applied to release the tendons of the paraspinal muscles and to display the rear aspects of spinous processes and lamina of the vertebrae. Laminectomy is performed at the levels of interest. Afterward, the dura is opened atraumatically in cases of intradural cysts; the surrounding operational area is coated with sterile material soaked with hypertonic 20 % NaCl for the isolation of the operative field (Turgut 1997). Then, the cysts are isolated from the surrounding nerve tissue (in cases of intradural extramedullary process). For intramedullary cysts, a medullotomy is carried out to open the medulla. This is performed with sharp instruments, such as diamond knife or microscissors, and the pia mater is cut in a substantial length (usually along the mid rear line of the medulla). Afterward, blunt microinstruments are used, usually two microdissectors. All procedures, starting from dura opening and finishing with its closure, are performed using an operating microscope.

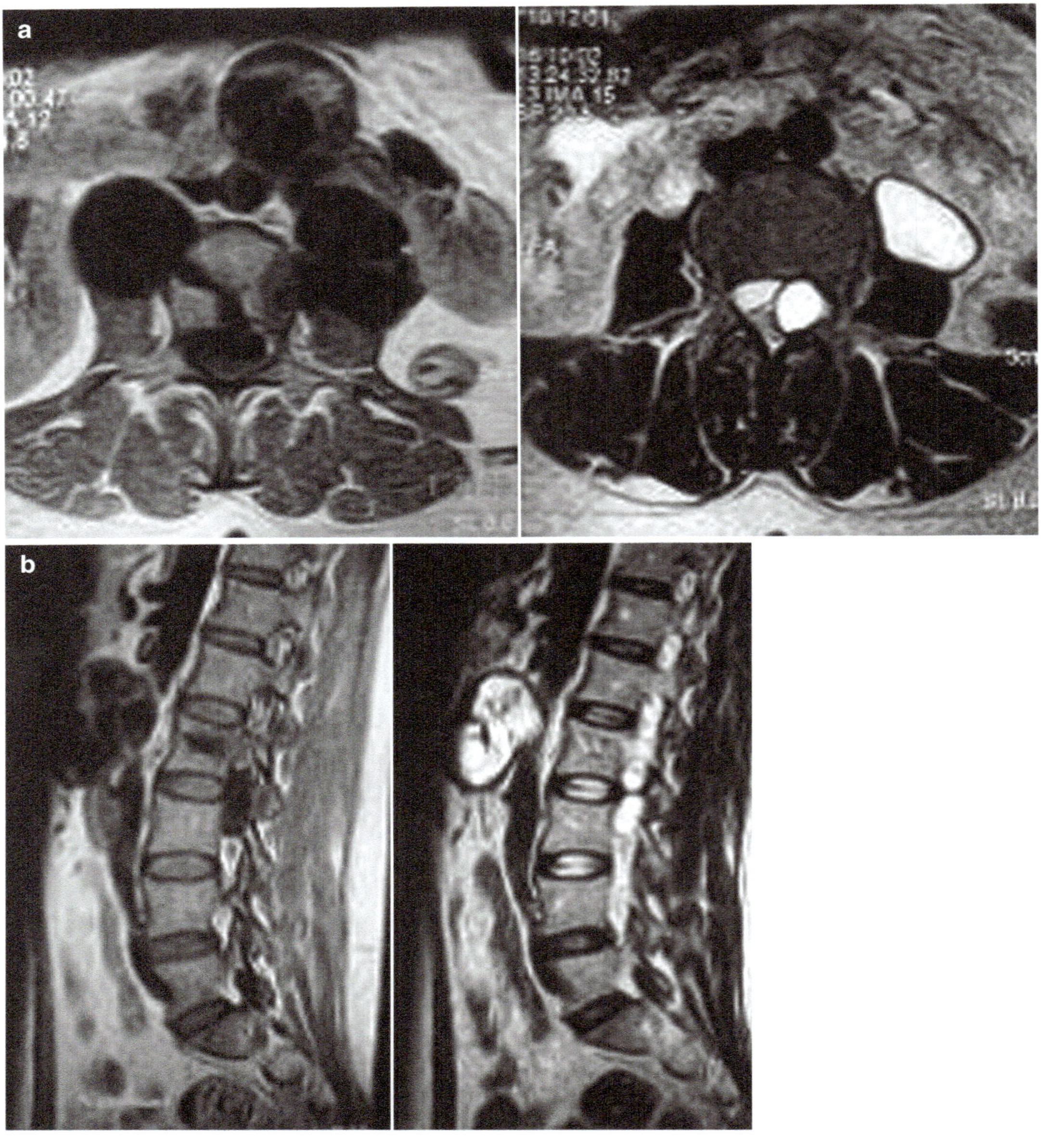

Fig. 8.7 Preoperative magnetic resonance images at (**a**) axial and (**b**) sagittal planes (Courtesy of A. Salduz, M.D.)

During the manipulation of the cyst(s), an irrigation with hypertonic 20 % NaCl solution and diluted Betadine is made (Turgut 1997). Some authors use 10 % formalin, but only when the dura is closed, never intradurally. Particular attention is made to avoid spreading of the disease intradurally or subarachnoidally and the surgeon has to avoid rupturing the cyst(s). For easier intraopera-

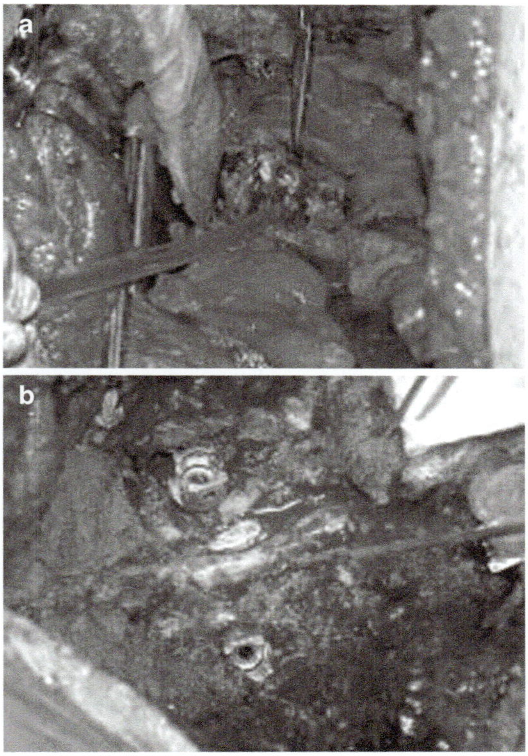

Fig. 8.8 (**a**) The image of the fistula at corpus of L2 vertebra extending posteriorly, (**b**) the image of the cyst after laminectomy (Courtesy of A. Salduz, M.D.)

tive navigation, it is possible to use intraoperative spinal monitoring with somatosensory and motor evoked potentials.

Complications related to intramedullary cysts removal are early (anaphylaxis, CSF fistula, wound infection, instability, delayed swelling of the medulla, and urinary tract infection) or late (dissemination of the cysts, instability of the spine, postsurgical myelopathy, postoperative syndrome of dysesthesia, and tethering of the spinal cord) (Turgut 1997).

Surgical treatment of spinal hydatidosis is discussed in detail in Chap. 14.

Conclusion

Hydatidosis of the spinal cord is a very serious condition with poor prognosis that has high morbidity and mortality. Long-term hydatidosis leads to persistent pain, secondary infections leading to sinuses and spinocutaneous fistulas, localized and remote recurrences, significant persistent neurological deficits, and spinal instability. Preventive measures should be taken in order to put the disease under control and eventually eradicate it, as has occurred in certain countries.

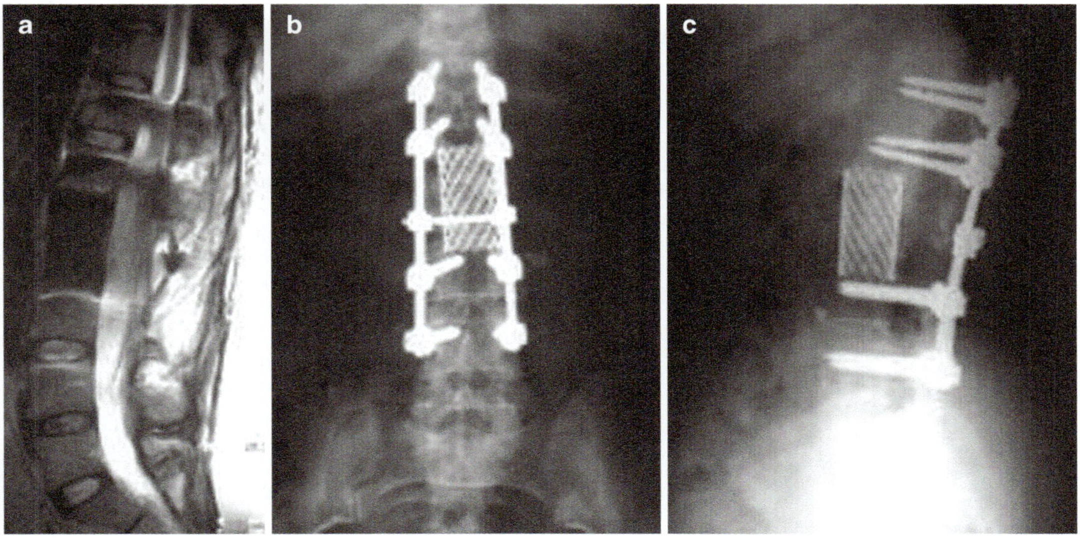

Fig. 8.9 (**a–c**) Magnetic resonance image and plain films after 5.5 years postoperatively (Courtesy of A. Salduz, M.D.)

References

Akhan O, Dinçer A, Saatçi I, Gulekin N, Besim A. Spinal intradural hydatid cyst in a child. Br J Radiol. 1991;64:465–6.

Arif SH, Zaheer S. Intradural extramedullary primary hydatid cyst of the spine in a child: a very rare presentation. Eur Spine J. 2009;18:179–82.

Baurand C, Daniel F, Guillermain P, Tournigand T, Gascard E. Spinal cord compression by an intra-dural hydatid cyst (apropos of a case) (in French). Mars Med. 1970;107:921–2.

Bertrand JL, Acquaviva R, Blavignanc F, Thevenot C. Medullar compression caused by arachnoid echinococcosis (in French). Maroc Med. 1956;35:320–4.

Bettaieb A, Khaldi M, Ben Rhouma T, Touibi S. Spinal echinococcosis; clinical study of 32 cases (in French). Neurochirurgie. 1978;24:205–10.

Bhojraj SY, Shetty NR. Primary hydatid disease of the spine: an unusual cause of progressive paraplegia: case report and review of the literature. J Neurosurg. 1999;91:216–8.

Bilgic S, Kose O, Sehirioglu A, Safaz I, Ozkan H. Primary paraspinal hydatid cyst treated with puncture, aspiration, injection and re-aspiration (PAIR) technique: a case report. Eur Spine J. 2009;18 Suppl 2:S165–7.

Boixados JR. Hidatidosis raqui-medular. Acta Neurochir (Wien). 1961;9:157–70.

Braithwaite PA, Lees RF. Vertebral hydatid disease: radiological assessment. Radiology. 1981;140:763–6.

Brunetti E, Kern P, Vuitton DA, Writing Panel for the WHO-IWGE. Expert consensus for the diagnosis and treatment of cystic and alveolar echinococcosis in humans. Acta Trop. 2010;114:1–16.

Bygott JM, Chiodini PL. Praziquantel: neglected drug? Ineffective treatment? Or therapeutic choice in cystic hydatid disease? Acta Trop. 2009;111:95–101.

Carrea R, Murphy G. Primary hydatid cyst of the spinal cord. Acta Neurol Latinoam. 1964;10:308–12.

Celik C, Sasmaz MF, Oktay F, Ucan H, Kaptanoglu E. Paraplegia associated with spinal hydatid cyst: a case report. Spine (Phila Pa 1976). 2010;35:E356–8.

Chakir N, Akhaddar A, El Quessar A, El Ouahabi A, El Hassani MR, El Khamlichi A, Jiddane M. Primary intradural extramedullary hydatidosis. Case report and review of the literature (in French). J Neuroradiol. 2002;29:177–82.

Charrada-Ben-Farhat L, Saïd W, Bouslama K, Oueslati S, Dridi L, Rezgui-Marhoul L, Hamzaoui S, Ben Dridi M, Hendaoui L. Vertebral and spinal cord hydatidosis: contribution of imaging (in French). Med Mal Infect. 2006;36:58–61.

Chat L, Akjouj M, Chellaoui M, Gueddari F, Alami D, Achaâban F, Najid A, Benamour-Ammar H. Spinal intradural hydatid cyst (in French). J Radiol. 2000;81:535–7.

Desai HJ, Bhatt CJ, Dave BA. Images-primary spinal echinococcosis. Indian J Radiol Imaging. 1999;9:73–6.

Deve F. Vertebral echinococcosis, pathogenic process and their lesions (in French). Ann Anat Pathol. 1928;5:841–59.

Ediz L, Tekeoglu I, Ceylan MF, Avcu S, Hiz O. Paraplegia due to spinal extradural hydatid disease and syringomyelia after surgical intervention: a case report. Turk J Phys Med Rehabil. 2011;57:182–5.

Fahl M, Haddad FS, Hubballah M, Kan'an S, Husheimi I, Azizi T. Magnetic resonance imaging in intradural and extradural spinal echinococcosis. Clin Imaging. 1994;18:179–83.

Fares Y, Khazim R, El Zaatari MM, Haddad GF, Bannes PR. Spinal hydatid disease and its neurological complications. Scand J Infect Dis. 2003;35:394–6.

Garcia-Vicuna R, Carvajal I, Ortiz-Garcia A, Lopez-Robledillo JC, Laffon A, Sabando P. Primary solitary echinococcosis in cervical spine. Postsurgical successful outcome after long-term albendazole treatment. Spine (Phila Pa 1976). 2000;25:520–3.

Goçer AI, Tuna M, Ildan F, Bagdatoglu H, Huaciyakupoglu S. Cervical intradural extramedullary hydatid cyst. Turk Neurosurg. 1994;4:169–71.

Govender TS, Aslam M, Parbhoo A, Corr P. Hydatid disease of the spine. A long-term follow-up after surgical treatment. Clin Orthop Relat Res. 2000;378:143–7.

Güneçs M, Akdemir H, Tuğcu B, Günaldi O, Gümüçs E, Akpinar A. Multiple intradural spinal hydatid disease: a case report and review of literature. Spine (Phila Pa 1976). 2009;34:346–50.

Gupta S, Rathi V, Bhargava S. Unilocular primary spinal extradural hydatid cyst-MR appearance. Indian J Radiol Imaging. 2002;12:271–3.

Hamdan TA, Al-Kaisy MA. Dumbbell hydatid cyst of the spine: case report and review of the literature. Spine. 2000;25:1296–9.

Herrera A, Martinez AA, Rodriguez J. Spinal hydatidosis. Spine. 2005;30:2439–44.

Islekel S, Zileli M, Ersahin Y. Intradural spinal hydatid cysts. Eur Spine J. 1998;7:162–4.

Jaiswal S, Jaiswal AK, Jain M, Behari S, Pandey R. Primary spinal extradural hydatid cyst causing paraplegia. Indian J Pathol Microbiol. 2009;52:432–3.

Jena A, Tripahti RP, Jain AK. Primary spinal echinococcosis causing paraplegia. Case report with MR and pathological correlation. AJNR Am J Neuroradiol. 1991;12:560.

Kabbaj-El Kouhen N, Dafiri R, el Ouahabi A, el Khamlichi A, Imani F. Isolated lumbar intradural hydatid cyst (in French). J Radiol. 1999;80:147–9.

Kaen A, Lagares A, Perez-Nuñez A, Rivas JJ, Ramos A, Lobato RD. Intradural extramedullary spinal hydatidosis: case report. Neurocirugia (Astur). 2009;20:282–7.

Kahilogullari G, Tuna H, Aydin Z, Colpan E, Egemen N. Primary intradural extramedullary hydatid cyst. Am J Med Sci. 2005;329:202–4.

Kalkan E, Cengiz SL, Cicek O, Erdi F, Baysefer A. Primary spinal intradural extramedullary hydatid cyst in a child. J Spinal Cord Med. 2007;30:297–300.

Karvounis PC, Singounas EG, Tsaprounis G. Intradural spinal echinococcus simulating lumbar disc protrusion. Neurochirurgia (Stuttg). 1977;20:58–60.

Khazim R, Fares Y, Heras-Palou C, Ruiz Barnes P. Posterior decompression of spinal hydatidosis: long

term results: Fundacion Jimenez Diaz, Madrid, Spain. Clin Neurol Neurosurg. 2003;105:209–14.
Kotil K, Tatar Z, Bilge T. Spinal hydatidosis accompanied by a secondary infection. Case report. J Neurosurg Spine. 2007;6:585–90.
Kotil K, Tari R, Savas Y. Medical treatment of primary extradural solitary lumbar hydatid disease. J Clin Neurosci. 2010;17:793–5.
Lakhdar F, Arkha Y, Rifi L, Derraz S, El Ouahabi A, El Khamlichi A. Spinal intradural extramedullary hydatidosis: report of three cases. Neurosurgery. 2009;65:372–7.
Layadi F, Boubrik M, Aït El Qadi A, Aït Benali S. Primary sacral epidural hydatid cyst: a case report (in French). J Radiol. 2005;86:1040–2.
Medjek L, Zenini S, Hammoum S, Hartani M. Intradural hydatidosis of the thoracic spine. Apropos of a case (in French). Ann Radiol. 1991;34:251–5.
Midyat L, Gökçe S, Onder A, Ozdemir Y, Mursalov G, Mir S. A very rare cause of childhood paraparesis: primary intradural extramedullary spinal hydatid cyst. Pediatr Infect Dis J. 2009;28:754–5.
Mohamed ZU, Agrawal M, Misra M, Jayaraj PA. Extradural compression of spinal cord caused by hydatid cyst. Internet J Anesth. 2004;8:2.
Morris DL, Richards KS. Hydatid disease. Oxford: Butterworth-Heinemann; 1992. p. 23.
Morshed AA. Hydatid disease of the spine. Neurochirurgia (Stuttg). 1977;20:211–5.
Onbas O, Kantarci M, Alper F, Sekmenli N, Okur A. Spinal widespread intradural extramedullary hydatidosis. Neuroradiology. 2004;46:310–2.
Pamir MN, Akalan N, Ozgen T, Erbengi A. Spinal hydatid cysts. Surg Neurol. 1984;21:54–7.
Papanikolaou A. Osseous hydatid disease. Trans R Soc Trop Med Hyg. 2008;102:233–8.
Pierini LD, Migliardi CD, Veppo AA. Hydatid compression of the cervical cord (in Spanish). Rev Asoc Med Argent. 1965;79:510–4.
Prabhakar M, Acharya A, Modi D, Jadav B. Spinal hydatid disease: a case series. J Spinal Cord Med. 2005;28:426–31.
Pushparaj K, Sundararajan M, Madeswaran K, Ambalavanan S. Primary spinal intradural hydatid cyst – a short report. Neurol India. 2001;49:203–4.
Salduz A, Koyuncu LO, Dikici F, Talu U. Long-term result of treatment for paraspinal and extradural hydatid cyst: a case report. Acta Orthop Traumatol Turc. 2009;43(3):267–71.
San Martin Sánchez L, López Zafra JJ, de la Riva Aguilar A, Oliva Alonso JM, Donnay Brisa G. Spinal subdural hydatidosis. A report on one case (in French). Neurochirurgie. 1980;26:235–8.
Sapkas GS, Machinis TG, Chloros GD, Fountas KN, Themistocleous GS, Vrettakos G. Spinal hydatid disease, a rare but existent pathological entity: case report and review of the literature. South Med J. 2006;99:178–83.
Schnepper GD, Johnson WD. Recurrent spinal hydatidosis in North America. Case report and review of the literature. Neurosurg Focus. 2004;17:E8.
Secer HI, Anik I, Celik E, Daneyemez MK, Gonul E. Spinal hydatid cyst mimicking arachnoid cyst on magnetic resonance imaging. J Spinal Cord Med. 2008;31:106–8.
Sharma A, Kashyap V, Abraham J, Kurian S. Intradural hydatid cysts of the spinal cord. Surg Neurol. 1981;16:235–7.
Tekkok IH, Benli K. Primary spinal extradural hydatid disease: report of a case with magnetic resonance characteristics and pathological correlation. Neurosurgery. 1993;33:320–3.
Thaler M, Gabl M, Lechner R, Gstöttner M, Bach CM. Severe kyphoscoliosis after primary Echinococcus granulosus infection of the spine. Eur Spine J. 2010;19:1415–22.
Turan Süslü H, Ceçen A, Karaaslan A, Börekçi A, Bozbuğa M. Primary spinal hydatid disease. Turk Neurosurg. 2009;19:186–8.
Turgut M. Hydatid disease of the spine: a survey study from Turkey. Infection. 1997;25:221–6.

Hydatidosis of the Spine

9

Antonio Herrera, Jesus Mateo,
Antonio Lobo-Escolar, Elena Ibarz, and Luis Gracia

Contents

A. Herrera, MD, PhD (✉)
Department of Surgery, Medicine School,
University of Zaragoza, Domingo Miral s.n,
Zaragoza 50009, Spain

Department of Orthopaedic and Trauma Surgery,
Miguel Servet University Hospital,
University of Zaragoza Medical School,
Zaragoza, Spain
e-mail: antonio.herrera@unizar.es

J. Mateo, PhD • A. Lobo-Escolar, PhD
Department of Orthopaedic and Trauma Surgery,
Miguel Servet University Hospital,
University of Zaragoza Medical School,
Zaragoza, Spain

E. Ibarz, PhD
Department of Mechanical Engineering,
School of Engineering and Architecture,
University of Zaragoza, Zaragoza, Spain

L. Gracia, PhD
Department of Mechanical Engineering, University
of Zaragoza, Zaragoza, Spain

Introduction

Hydatidosis is a rare parasitic disease that is considered prevalent in Mediterranean countries, the Middle East, Oceania, South Africa, and South America (Murray and Haddad 1959; Gemmell et al. 1987; Szypryt et al. 1987; Kern et al. 2003; Romig 2009). The incidence of hydatid disease in the northern hemisphere ranges from 0.03 to 1.2 per 100,000 (Kern 2003; Romig 2009). In Spain, the incidence was 2.6 per 100,000 in 1987, but it fell to 0.55 per 100,000 in 2007 (Carmena et al. 2010). A small rise in incidence of the hydatid disease has occurred in European countries. According to some authors, it is linked to an increase in the fox population, as a result of the increase in rabbit population after myxomatosis decline (Deplazes 2006; Romig 2009). In Spain, the increase in the number of North African immigrants could explain this rise in incidence. Regardless of the sanitary control measures, it has been proposed to use a vaccine to eradicate the disease (Craig and Larrieu 2006). Currently this vaccine is being implemented in some countries (Tan et al. 2012). The epidemiology of hydatidosis in the world is discussed in Chaps. 2, 3 and 4.

M. Turgut (ed.), *Hydatidosis of the Central Nervous System: Diagnosis and Treatment*,
DOI 10.1007/978-3-642-54359-3_9, © Springer-Verlag Berlin Heidelberg 2014

Bone involvement by hydatid disease is infrequent, ranging from 0.5 to 4 % of cases (Murray and Haddad 1959; Haddad and Bitar 1997; Merkle et al. 1997; Herrera and Martínez 2003; Bellil et al. 2009; Romig 2009). Spinal hydatidosis was first described by Chaussier in 1807 (Rayport et al. 1964). Vertebral bone location accounts for 50 % of cases of hydatid disease (Haddad and Bitar 1997; Turgut 1997; Govender et al. 2000; Martínez et al. 2001; Zlitni et al. 2001; Herrera and Martínez 2003; Herrera et al. 2005). The incidence of involvement in different areas of the spine varies from one author to another. By way of example, Rao et al. (1991) established that dorsal spine was involved in 50 % of cases, lumbar spine and sacrum in 20 % of cases, and cervical spine in 10 % of cases. Then, Haddad and Bitar (1997) found that multiple contagious vertebrae were affected in 11 of 14 cases with primary hydatid disease of the spine. In our experience, the lumbar spine is the most frequent location (34.61 %), followed by the dorsal spine (30.71 %), sacrum (26.9 %), and cervical spine (7.6 %). Nonetheless, these percentages vary widely.

Etiology

Several different species of *Echinococcus* have been described, but only two of them can parasitize humans: the *Echinococcus granulosus* species which causes cystic echinococcosis and the *E. multilocularis* species which causes alveolar echinococcosis. The *Echinococcus multilocularis* has a much lower incidence and never involves bone tissue (Szypryt et al. 1987). The *E. granulosus* species has been the etiologic agent in all of our cases. The species of *Echinococcus* are discussed in detail in Chap. 3.

Life Cycle

The life cycle of the tapeworm *Echinococcus* was not described until the nineteenth century (Lewis et al. 1975). Human hydatidosis is caused by the cystic (larval) stage of the tapeworm *E. granulosus*. Commonly, the intermediate host is sheep, and definitive hosts can be dogs, foxes, and other carnivores. Humans become the intermediate host by contact with an infected animal, usually a dog, or by eating vegetables contaminated by parasite eggs, which have come to them through the feces of an infected animal. Another source of infection is water pollution, a common vehicle in rural areas. The parasite passes through the intestinal wall and enters the portal circulation. It reaches the liver, which is the first filter, where most often it sets. The lung and the spleen may also be primarily colonized by the parasite. These primary visceral lesions behave as tumor nodes and transmit the parasite through the bloodstream to the bone tissue.

Pathogenesis

The larval parasite spreads through the circulatory system reaching the spine. The most usual site of infection is the metaphysis of a vertebral body, since this is the most vascularized area. A slower blood flow through the sinusoidal capillaries of the bone marrow and the fenestrations of the endothelium facilitate the deposition of the parasite.

Bone cysts in vertebral echinococcosis expand slowly with no development of the fibrous adventitious layer or pseudocapsule (pericyst) found in other locations (Fig. 9.1). On the contrary, the external layer (ectocyst) is an acellular membrane that allows the transfer of nutrients. The

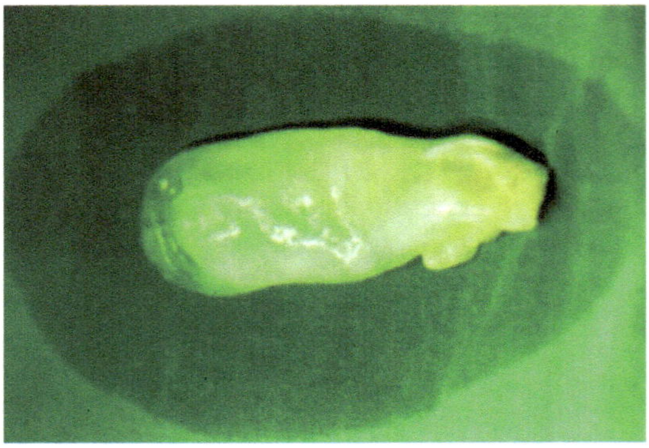

Fig. 9.1 Cyst removed from a vertebral body

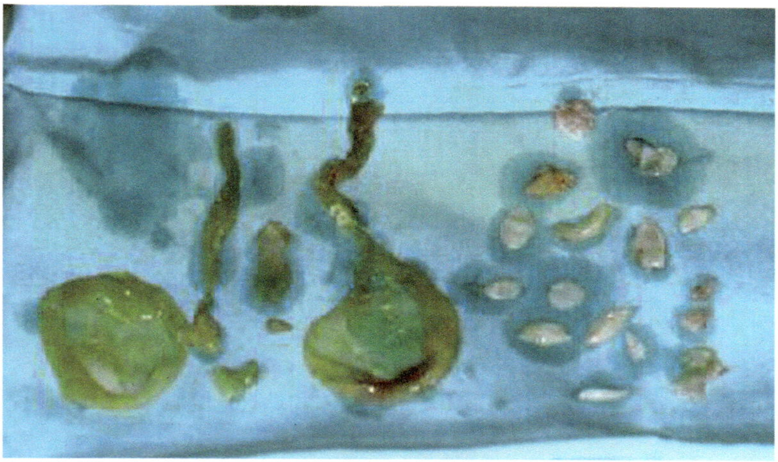

Fig. 9.2 Large open cyst with multiple daughter vesicles inside

internal layer, or germinal layer, usually shapes multiple compartments containing clear hydatid fluid and protoscoleces. These multiple vesicles remain attached to the germinal layer through a pedicle and resemble a bunch of grapes (Fig. 9.2). Sometimes these vesicles can grow through the external layer of the main cyst.

The clear, yellow hydatid fluid contains sodium chloride, proteins, lipids, polysaccharides, and ions, having a neutral pH. Breakage of a cyst can trigger an immunological reaction from the host, sometimes leading to an anaphylactic shock. Severe bone necrosis and inflammatory reaction may appear if bone lesions become infected, forming granulomas made up of lymphocytes, eosinophils, polymorphonuclears, and giant cells. Differential diagnosis with granulomatous infections might be very difficult.

Up until now it has been thought that disc space act as a barrier against infection. Colonization of several spinal levels at the same time, or spreading under the longitudinal ligaments from one vertebral body to the contiguous one, could explain the cases involving several spine levels. Nevertheless, Karantanas et al. (2003) have described a case of echinococcosis with cystic involvement of the disc space. Based on our experience with the hip joint, as well as the spread of the disease across the joint into the rib, our view is that the cartilage tissue is not an insuperable barrier against hydatid disease and parasite invasion through the joint surface is possible (Fig. 9.3).

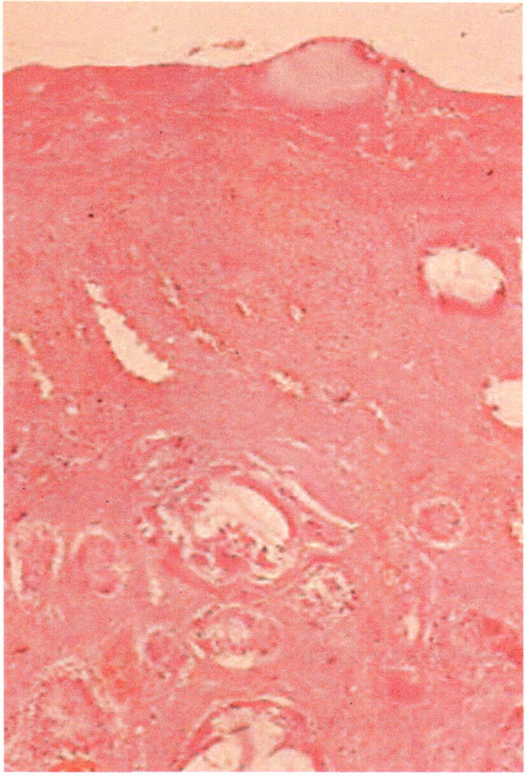

Fig. 9.3 Fibrous tissue on the surface of a femoral head. Hydatid membranes have replaced the cartilage

Bone cysts expand slowly and usually have a multilocular growth. Enlargement is achieved by local erosion of bone, and the pressure on the blood vessels of the marrow bone may result in a

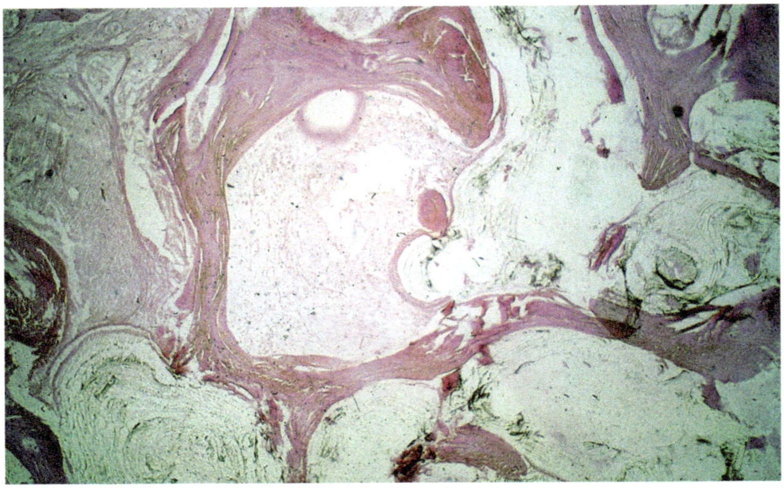

Fig. 9.4 Devitalized, eroded bone trabeculae by the growth of cysts

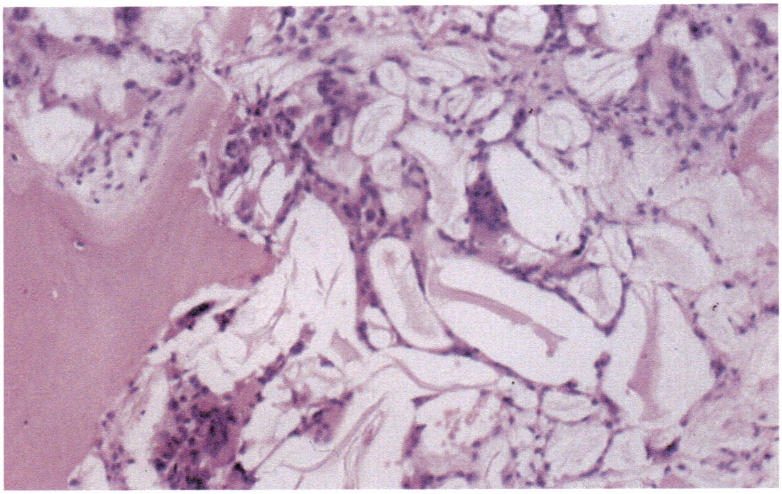

Fig. 9.5 Hydatid membranes with a giant-cell reaction next to an unstructured bone trabeculae

vascular necrosis (Fig. 9.4). Since trabecular destruction is complete (Fig. 9.5), infestation progresses toward the cortical bone and can spread through the anterolateral paravertebral area or into the spinal canal. Computed tomography (CT) scan or magnetic resonance imaging (MRI) may then show a pseudo-abscess (Fig. 9.6), and a differential diagnosis with spinal tuberculosis or vertebral pyogenic osteomyelitis is sometimes difficult.

Mechanical failure of the vertebrae can lead to compression fractures, even if cortical bone is preserved. The progression of the infection could lead to angular kyphosis and neural compression

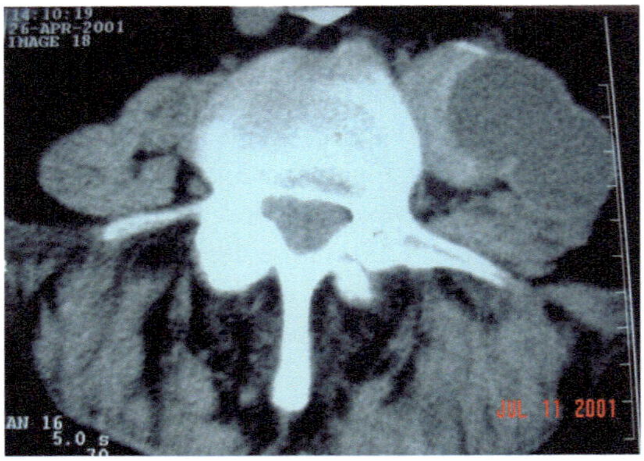

Fig. 9.6 CT: vertebral hydatidosis with large pseudo-extravertebral abscess

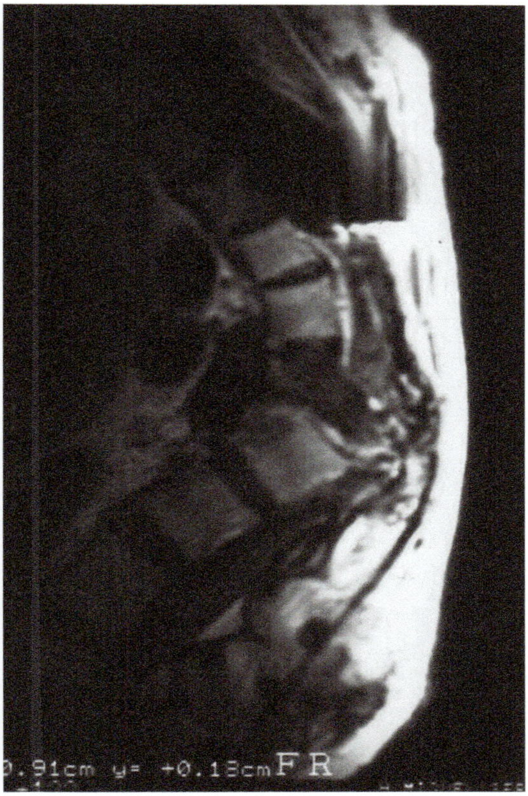

Fig. 9.7 Total destruction of two vertebrae producing severe kyphosis and cord compression

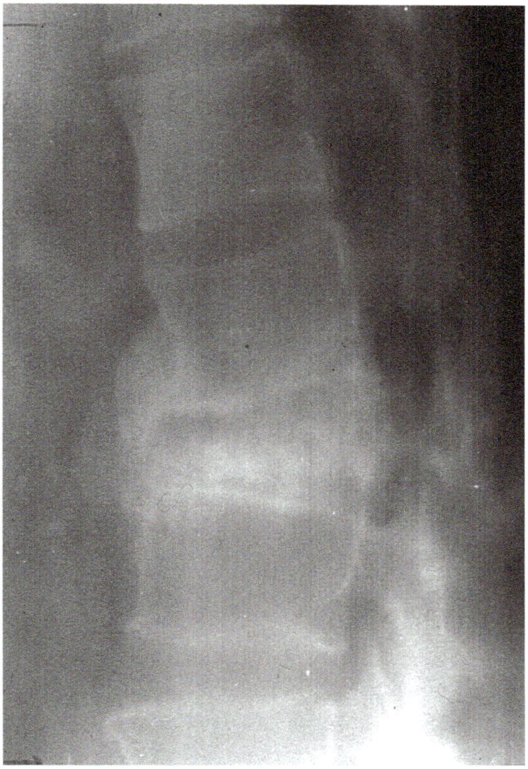

Fig. 9.8 Radiographic tomography: lumbar hydatidosis simulating a vertebral compression fracture

of the spinal cord (Fig. 9.7). In other cases, in which the infection progresses through the pedicles, the intervertebral foramina may be affected, and root compression symptoms could be present.

In this respect, the understanding of the mechanical strength properties of the vertebrae is necessary. Although the cortical bone is more resistant, cancellous bone plays a major role in the global mechanical strength of the spine, since its trabecular struts act as the internal scaffolding of the vertebral body. The damage to the cancellous bone leads to a loss of rigidity and to an initial loss of vertebral body height. If this damage progresses, the cortical bone remains as an empty eggshell, and it is not capable to withstand compressive loads, leading to a compression fracture (Fig. 9.8). If the infection involves also the cortical bone, the loss of resistance and the risk of fracture are then increased.

Clinical Presentation

Since 1807, when Chaussier described the first case of vertebral infection, there is a lack of published papers detailing accurately the clinical presentation of vertebral echinococcosis. This may be due to the unspecific presentation of the hydatid disease in the bone and to the long clinically silent period before the first symptoms (up to 40 years in some cases) (Murray and Haddad 1959; Zlitni et al. 2001; Song et al. 2007; Papanikolaou 2008). Echinococcosis in general, and that involving the spine in particular, is an adult disease, partly due to this long silent period. The youngest patient admitted to our service was 24 years old at the time of diagnosis, and the oldest one was 77 years old, with an average of 51.3 years at presentation.

Back pain is the most typical symptom of spinal hydatidosis, frequently associated with neurological deficits. Trabecular and cortical bone are progressively destroyed as bone cysts expand, and vertebral compression fractures may appear. An angular kyphosis could be present especially when several levels are affected. In severe cases, bone sequestrums extruded into the spinal canal from vertebral bodies cause neural compression. Neural compression can also be produced by cysts invading the extradural space. Usually, both facts (extradural cystic invasion and destruction of the vertebral body) are present when echinococcosis brings about neurological deficits.

If infection progresses through the vertebral pedicles, involving the foramina, root compression symptoms could appear. When the hydatid cysts destroy the anterior vertebral cortex, the infection spreads through the anterolateral vertebral area. In these cases, the appearance of a pseudo-abscess may resemble a pyogenic osteomyelitis or a granulomatous infection such as spinal tuberculosis.

Back pain is associated with vertebral collapse and compression fractures, occurring when the vertebral destruction is advanced. Pain is typically severe at the thoracic and cervical levels and mild at the lumbar and sacral segments. All the patients treated in our hospital service reported moderate to severe back pain for several weeks. Neurological symptoms were present in a high percentage of cases at the time of diagnosis.

In our experience, the clinical course is relatively fast since pain appears, and a worsening of the symptoms coincides with the onset of neurological deficits in a high percentage of cases. The most frequent presentation is a spinal cord compression associated with paraplegia or tetraplegia. Another type of neurological complaint is a root compression syndrome with severe pain and sensory and motor deficits or sphincter dysfunction, depending on the level affected.

Superinfection of the hydatid lesion is possible, but it is not as frequent as other complications. If this happens, a large abscess may spontaneously drain to the surrounding tissues or outside the body, as we have seen in two cases. The course of sacrum involvement is usually asymptomatic, and in some cases, posterior soft

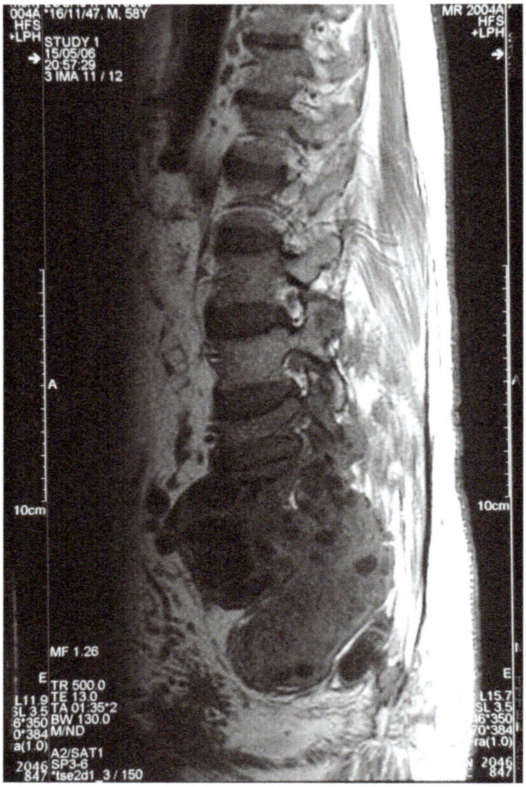

Fig. 9.9 Sacral hydatidosis with both extra- and intravertebral extensions

tissues or retroperitoneal invasion may be present without previous neurological complaints. Two of our patients initially presented with a posterior sacral tumor and rectal symptoms as the early presentation of hydatid disease of the lower spine (Fig. 9.9).

In conclusion, the clinical presentation of vertebral echinococcosis is totally unspecific and hardly suggests the diagnosis. Unfortunately, a progressive and severe back pain and the onset of neurological deficits are very common.

Complementary Tests

Imaging

Emergence of new imaging technologies has improved the diagnostic means of vertebral hydatidosis. CT was not available until the 1980s in

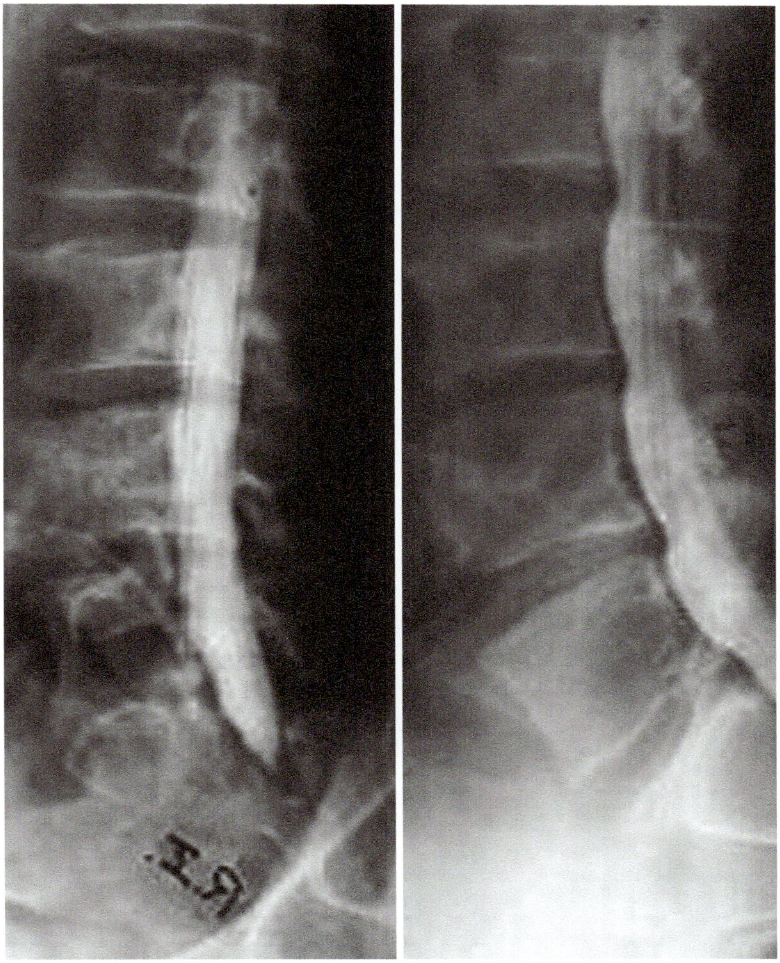

Fig. 9.10 Radiograph with contrast media

our hospital, and MRI was first used at the end of the same decade. MRI is the most reliable and useful method for diagnosis (Fahl et al. 1994; Işlekel et al. 1998; Singh et al. 1998) because it allows an excellent visualization of soft tissue injuries. Three-dimensional CT scan (3D CT) was also a breakthrough in identifying lesions and depicting its topography. Another technique ready to use is ultrasound, which has been applied to guide punctures of extravertebral injuries. But we consider most reliable, for this purpose, the CT-guided needle.

Taking advantage of modern methods of diagnosis, Braithwaite and Lees, in 1981, established five sets of column hydatid lesions which can lead to neurological problems: (a) primary intramedullary cyst, (b) intradural extramedullary cyst, (c) extradural intraspinal cyst, (d) hydatid disease of the vertebra, and (e) paravertebral hydatid disease. Currently, this classification is accepted by all the authors.

Our early experience with patients suffering from spinal hydatidosis began in the 1970s. At that time, the techniques at our disposal to diagnose neurological injuries were limited to conventional radiology and X-rays with contrast media (Fig. 9.10).

Images provided by conventional radiology are quite unspecific. Extensive osteolytic lesions affecting a vertebral body (Fig. 9.11) or the sacrum (Fig. 9.12) may be confused with tumor pathology. Likewise, plain radiography of a

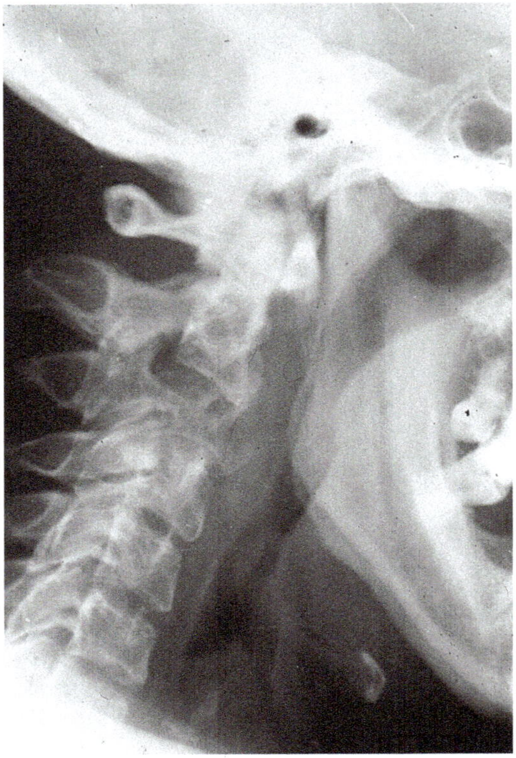

Fig. 9.11 Cervical hydatidosis: osteolysis of C3

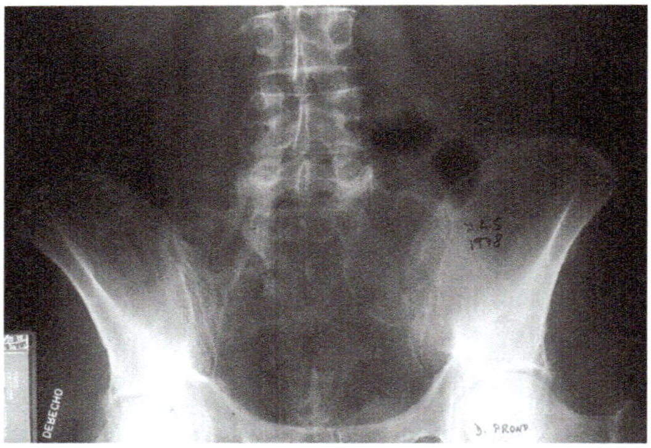

Fig. 9.12 Sacral hydatidosis: osteolytic lesion

crushed vertebral body (Fig. 9.13) may lead to the suspicion of a neoplastic etiology. In other cases, X-rays might suggest an infection of the spine, faced with reactive lesions simulating a vertebral osteomyelitis (Fig. 9.14). Only few skilled orthopedists or radiologists can suspect a hydatid injury on the basis of an X-ray, such as the case shown in Fig. 9.15, in which the diagnosis was suspected from an X-ray appearance showing little bony sequestrum, intervertebral disc integrity, and irregular osteolytic areas.

Radiographic tomography allows a more accurate identification of bone lesions. But its resolution is only slightly better than the X-ray; therefore, a tumor etiology is suspected in most cases. The introduction of CT scan in 1984 represented an inestimable help. It allowed us to establish which lesions are characteristic of hydatid disease in the vertebral body (Fig. 9.16): lytic lesions encircled with mild sclerosis, small bony sequestrum, and destruction of the cortex of the vertebra. In other cases, one may find an invaded spinal canal and vertebral pedicle destruction (Fig. 9.17) or small calcifications inside a lesion, which are typical of hydatid disease. The discovery of evident extravertebral, anterolateral lesions (Fig. 9.18), simulating a paravertebral abscess, should suggest a hydatid disease if they have a slight peripheral calcification. Other extra-spinal lesions can be located behind the spine (Fig. 9.19), resting on the rear face of the vertebral lamina. Sometimes, bony sequestrum fragments from the vertebral body might be seen occupying the spinal canal (Fig. 9.20). But most of these images can mislead to an infectious or tumor pathology. Therefore, knowledge of history, clinical signs, and laboratory tests of each patient must be the first step of the diagnostic process. CT scan may also lead to a false diagnosis in the cases when bone lesions resemble a neoplasm (aneurysmatic bone cysts) (Fig. 9.21). In short, CT scan has been a major contribution to the diagnostic process, but it should not be regarded as an infallible technique (Torricelli et al. 1990).

MRI and 3D CT scan allow a more refined diagnosis, particularly in the hands of a radiologist skilled in this disease and if one works in an area where vertebral hydatidosis is not unknown. MRI provides detailed pictures of both soft tissue and bone lesions. This technique usually gets an accurate identification of extravertebral cysts (Fig. 9.22), intravertebral lesions (Fig. 9.23), and extradural intraspinal cysts (Fig. 9.24). Sometimes, images may suggest a wrong infectious etiology. Careful observation will help rule

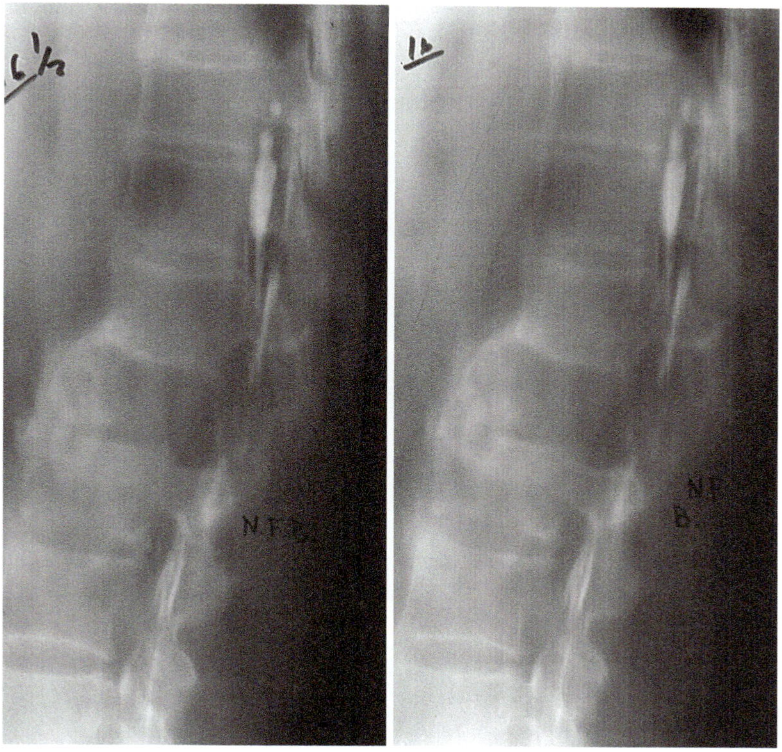

Fig. 9.13 Lumbar hydatidosis can be mistaken for tumor etiology

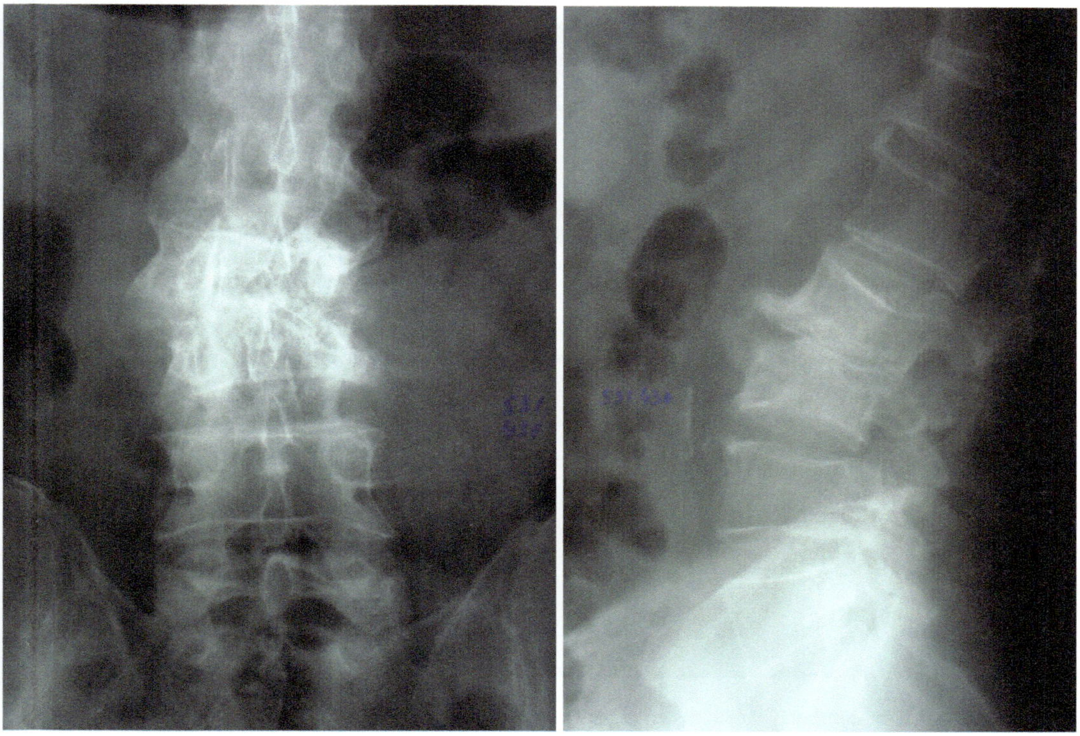

Fig. 9.14 (**a**, **b**) Radiographs of a lumbar hydatidosis can resemble a vertebral osteomyelitis

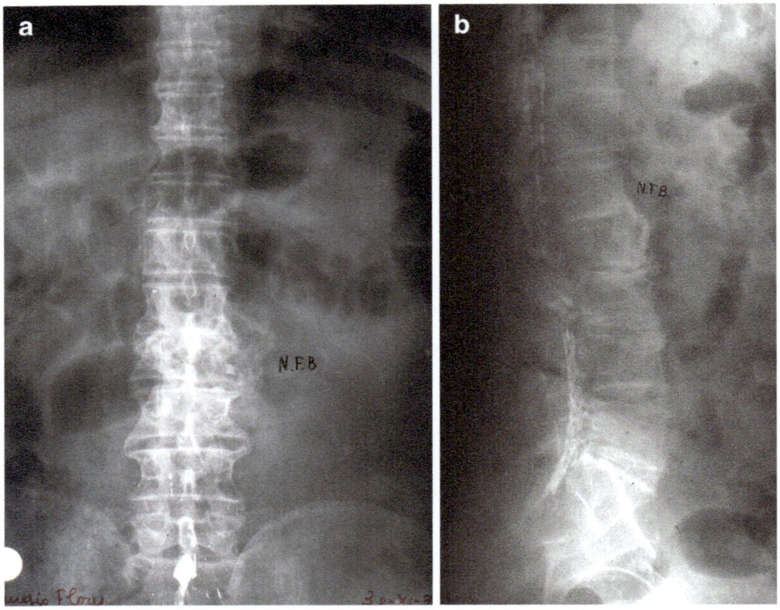

Fig. 9.15 (**a**, **b**) Lumbar hydatidosis

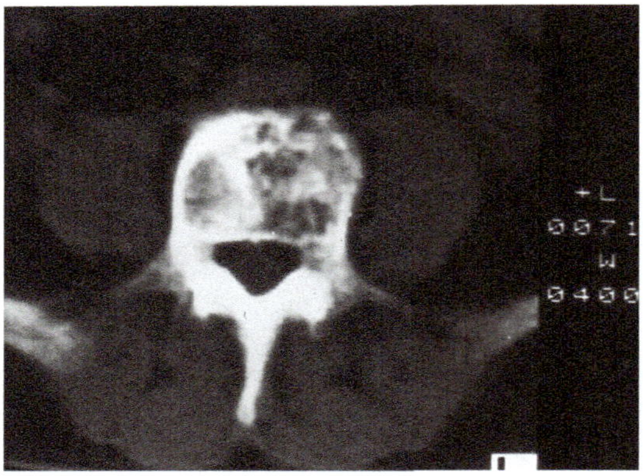

Fig. 9.16 CT: typical lesions of vertebral hydatidosis

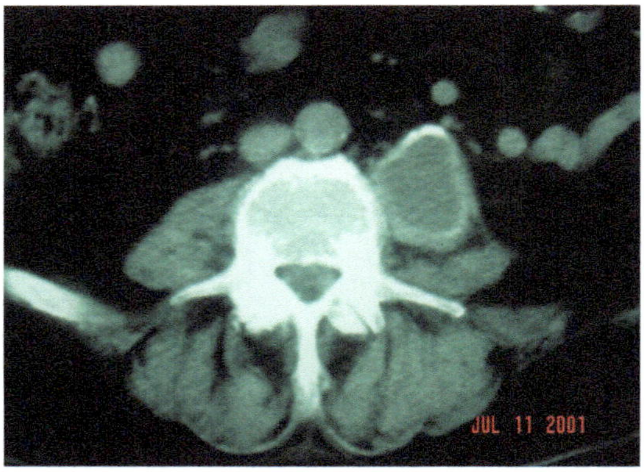

Fig. 9.18 CT: hydatid pseudo-abscess with peripheral calcification

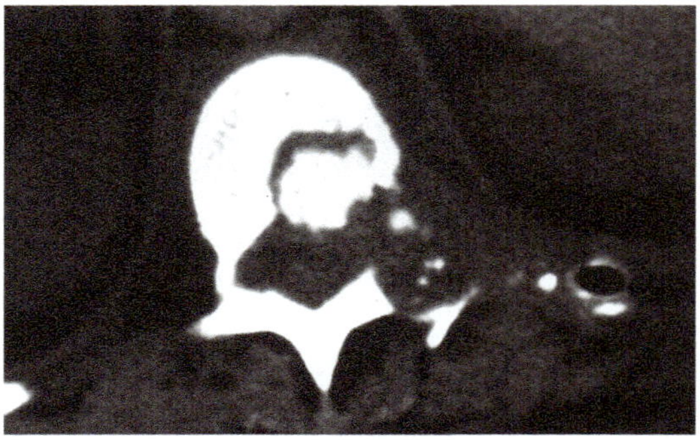

Fig. 9.17 CT: pedicle destruction and invasion of the spinal canal

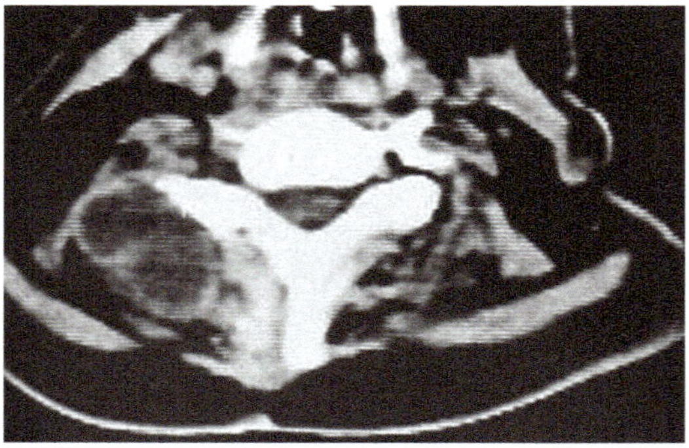

Fig. 9.19 Hydatid cysts on the rear face of a vertebral lamina

out a septic origin, based on the disc integrity and vertebral body images (Fig. 9.25). Another MRI possibility is the supervision of injuries evolution in patients undergoing medical or surgical treatment (Doganay and Kantarci 2009) (Fig. 9.26). 3D CT scan is another important aid in the diagnostic process, contributing to an accurate knowledge of the topography of the lesion (Fig. 9.27) and helping to determine the lesions etiology.

It may be concluded that the combination of different imaging techniques is essential for a diagnostic approach (Beggs 1985; von Sinner 1991), but we consider MRI as the most reliable mean. It is clear that modern imaging techniques have led to significant progresses in the diagnosis work-up, but accurate diagnosis of a lesion is not always possible. So, CT-guided puncture technique, or percutaneous biopsy technique guided by image intensifier or CT scan, is sometimes necessary to rule out different etiologies.

Laboratory Tests

Laboratory tests are useful tools in the diagnostic work. Some of these tests are not specific for

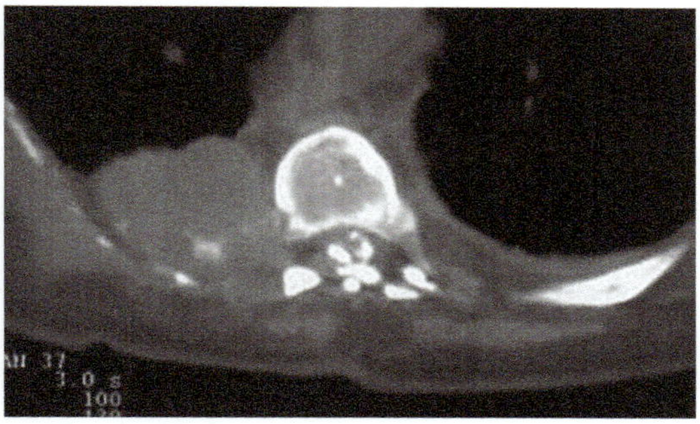

Fig. 9.20 Sequestrum fragments from the vertebral body occupying the spinal canal

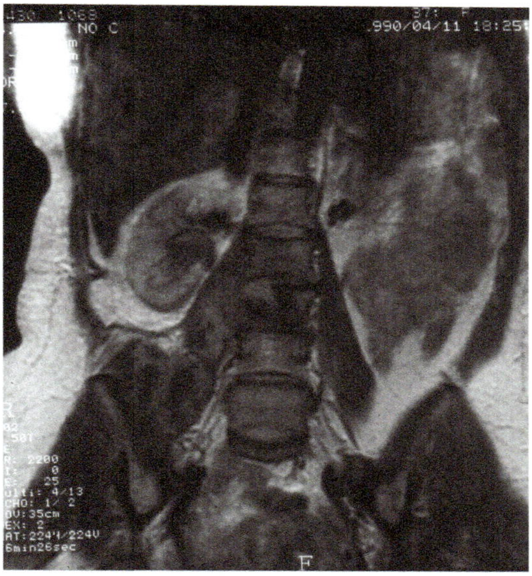

Fig. 9.22 MRI: extravertebral hydatid cysts in a lumbar hydatidosis

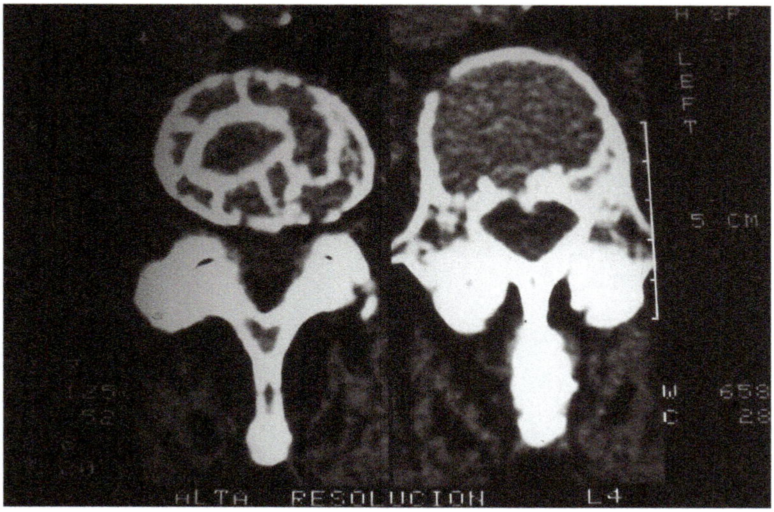

Fig. 9.21 CT: hydatid cyst simulating a vertebral aneurysmatic bone cyst

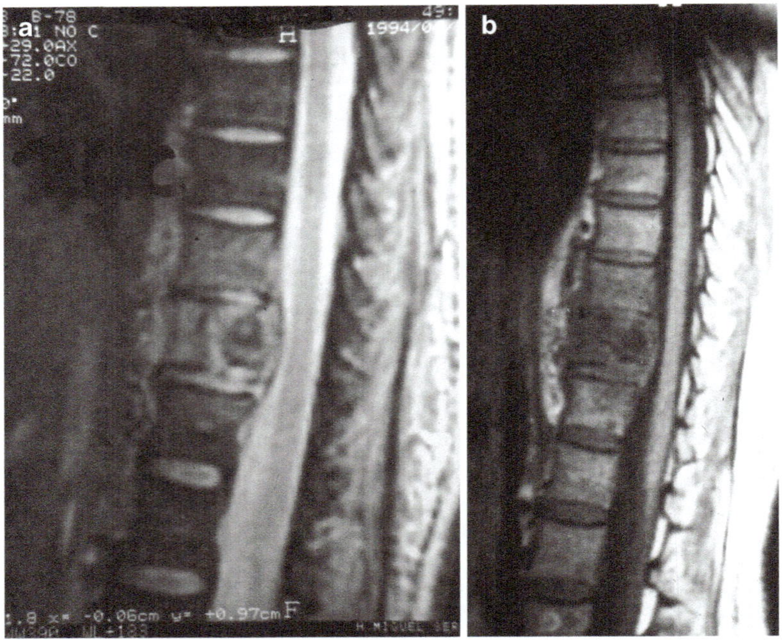

Fig. 9.23 Hydatid disease in a vertebral body: MRI images of thoracic spine in two planes (**a**, **b**)

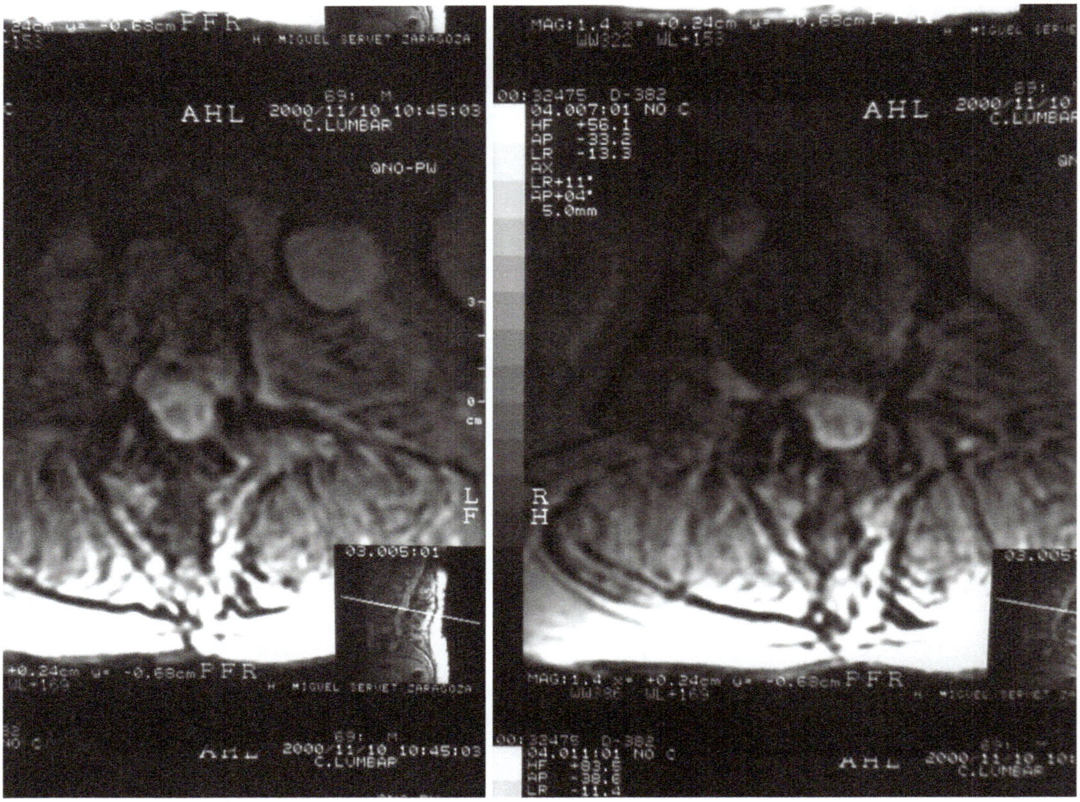

Fig. 9.24 Extradural intraspinal cysts

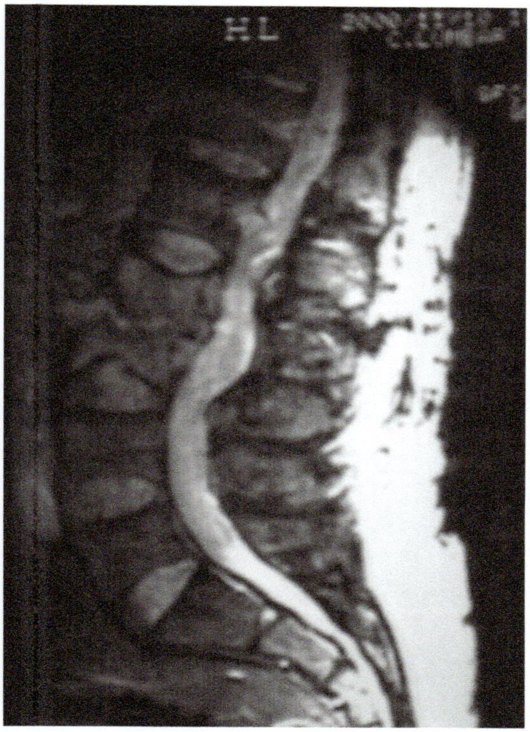

Fig. 9.25 Lumbar hydatidosis: involvement of two vertebral bodies, intraspinal cysts, and undamaged disc

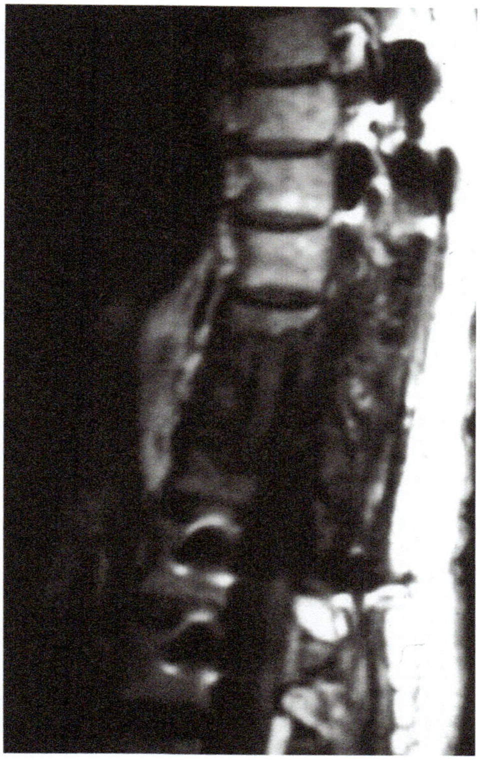

Fig. 9.26 MRI: follow-up in a case of partial corpectomy, bone graft, and posterior fixation

hydatidosis, but we use them routinely. White blood cell count is among these nonspecific tests. All of our patients had a slight leukocytosis, although a fair leukocytosis was found in two superinfection cases. Marked eosinophilia usually occurs in a high percentage of bone hydatid cases. In our experience, eosinophilia is found in 73.2 % of bone hydatidosis in any location and in 65.3 % of spine hydatidosis cases. All patients had an elevated erythrocyte sedimentation rate (ESR), ranging from 48 to73. ESR was higher in superinfection cases. The skin test, also known as Casoni's test, is clearly positive in a high percentage of cases, reaching an 88.7 % in our experience.

The application of enzyme-linked immunosorbent assay (ELISA) (Carmena et al. 2007) has been a breakthrough in the diagnostic process because of its greater precision and reliability. The most used technique is indirect ELISA. This test allows not only a qualitative diagnosis but also a quantitative one. Thus, the test can grade the intensity of the response and serves to determine the effectiveness of a surgical or medical treatment.

Significant levels of immunoglobulin G (IgG) can be detected using the purified antigen EM2 (Rausch et al. 1987). Likewise, high levels of IgG1 and IgG4 can be found using other antigens such as EM10 and Em18 (Wen and Craig 1994; Dreweck et al. 1997). We began using this test in the 1980s, and 82 % of our cases were positive. When the test was applied to monitoring the response to a surgery or chemotherapy treatment, a 40 % decline in total IgG values was detected. IgG2 determination was the most specific and better prognostic value test, which is consistent with the findings of Lawn et al. (2004). Laboratory findings of patients with hydatidosis of the central nervous system are discussed in Chap. 10.

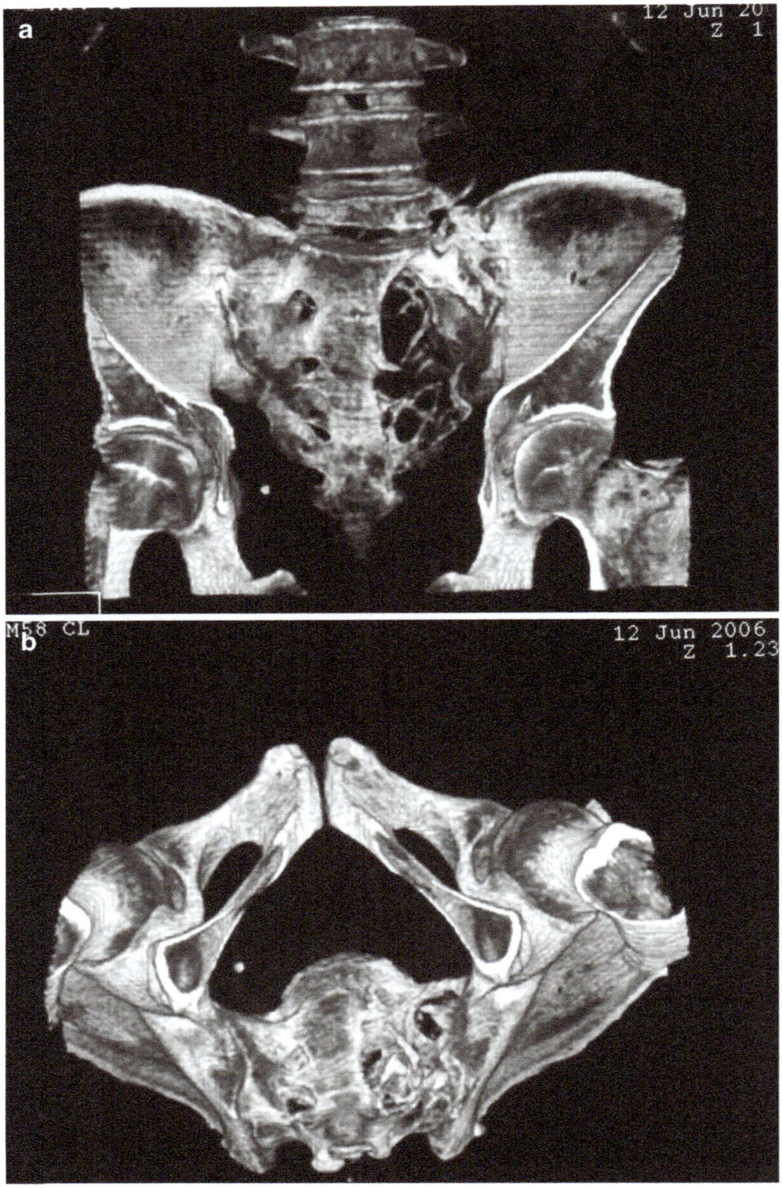

Fig. 9.27 (**a**, **b**) 3D CT of sacral hydatidosis

Diagnosis

The first step in the diagnosis is to suspect a vertebral echinococcosis in patients presenting with back pain, neurological deficits, and MRI or CT scan imaging findings suggesting spinal tumor or infection, especially in areas with high prevalence of hydatid disease. A detailed clinical interview is important, recording the medical history of the patient, region of origin, contact with farm or domestic animals or exposure to livestock, etc. History of echinococcal disease in other locations must be investigated. In our experience we found positive previous history of hydatid disease in 34.61 % of the patients with spinal echinococcosis. MRI and new laboratory tests

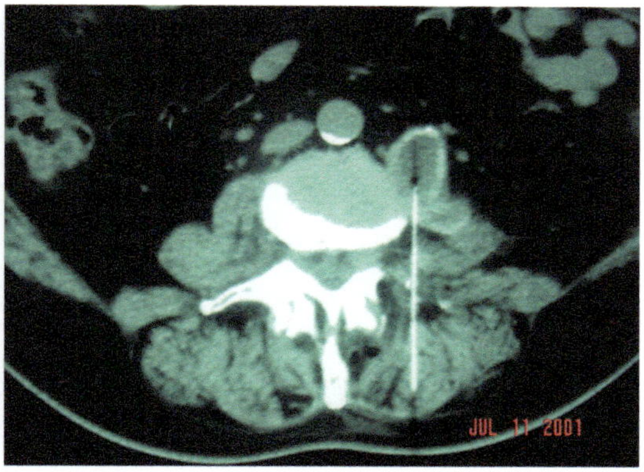

Fig. 9.28 CT-guided puncture of a hydatid pseudo-abscess

have provided a more precise diagnosis in the last years. CT scan images with 3D visualization of the spine can also be very helpful. In all cases under suspicion, we usually ask for a thoracoabdominal CT scan too.

While in the previous decades up to 40 % of the patients were diagnosed during the surgical procedure, nowadays 81.25 % of the diagnoses are made prior to the surgery. In our series, those cases resembling a vertebral pyogenic infection were the most challenging for the diagnosis. In two of them, we found a superinfection and the diagnosis was not made until the patients underwent surgery. In other two patients, a percutaneous CT scan-guided biopsy of a spinal abscess helped to clarify the diagnosis (Fig. 9.28).

Based on clinical findings, medical imaging, and laboratory tests, an early diagnosis must be made as an aid in surgical decision making, especially in patients with neurological deficit. The definitive diagnosis will be given by the surgical pathology analysis.

Treatment

Drug Treatment

Chemotherapy treatment of hydatid disease began in 1974 after the paper published by Heath and Chevis (1974). Within the benzimidazole drug group, mebendazole and albendazole have been the most widely used. We used mebendazole until 1986 with scarce effectiveness, possibly because of its poor absorption and subsequent low concentrations in serum and hydatid lesions (Bekhti et al. 1977). In 1986, we began to use albendazole, which has better absorption and achieves higher concentrations in serum by means of its active metabolite, albendazole sulfoxide (AlbSo) (Braithwaite and Lees 1981; Morris et al. 1983). Application rate of albendazole is 800 mg per day, in 28-day cycles, over a period of 6 months, with rest periods between cycles.

In our experience, chemotherapy can be considered as an adjunct to surgical treatment, but not as sole modality of treatment. Following the papers published at the end of the 1990s and early 2000 (Yasawy et al. 1993; Cobo et al. 1998; Urrea-Paris et al. 2000), we began to treat our patients with a combination of praziquantel, in doses between 25 and 50 mg/kg per day, and albendazole at 10 mg/kg per day. In our opinion, this association is more effective than albendazole alone, but the use of the combined chemotherapy has coincided with a more radical surgery, so it is difficult to assess the drug results. The fact is that we have treated several cases of spinal hydatidosis in recent years, and, currently, these patients are considered disease-free after a follow-up between 2 and 10 years post surgery. There were no major side effects, except for one patient with abnormal liver enzymes, who improved after discontinuation of therapy. Other drugs of the benzimidazole group have been used, such as oxfendazole and flubendazole (Morris and Gould 1982; Gavidia et al. 2010), but we have no experience with them. Other published studies talk about the use of substances that enhance the albendazole absorption or about the use of antimalarials such as mefloquine (Küster et al. 2011).

We believe that combined chemotherapy with praziquantel and albendazole is a good adjunct to surgical treatment. It is useful to limit the disease progression, but we don't believe that it must be

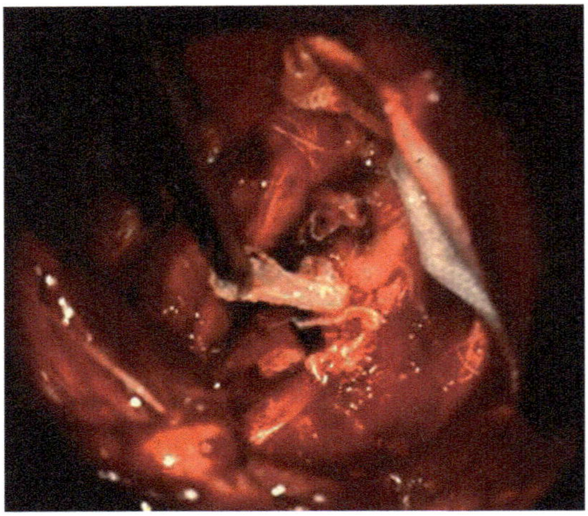

Fig.9.29 Removal of extradural cervical cysts

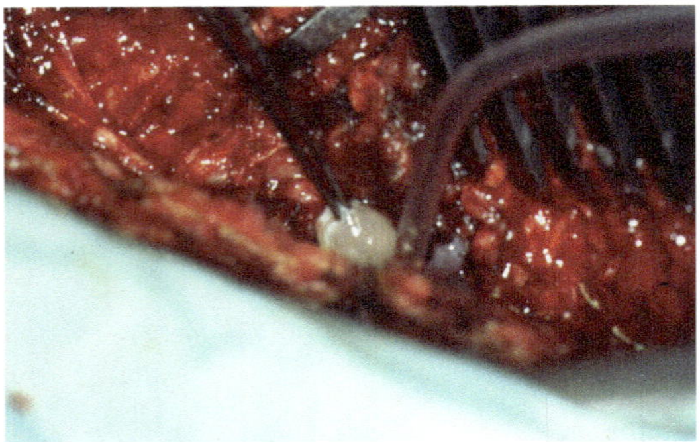

Fig. 9.30 Removal of extradural dorsal cyst

used as a sole treatment for bone hydatidosis. Our experience with two inoperable cases, located in the sacrum and the pelvis respectively, is that chemotherapy seems to stabilize the lesions. On the other hand, we do not take a month to complete one cycle of chemotherapy before spine hydatidosis surgery. Chemotherapy treatment is started if a firm diagnosis is available, and surgical treatment is carried out as soon as possible.

Surgical Treatment

An early surgical treatment is important when we suspect the diagnosis of vertebral echinococcosis. A delay in the diagnosis and treatment will result in a worse outcome of the surgery. In our hospital, which is the reference center for spine surgery in our region, a significant percentage of patients suffered of paraplegia or tetraplegia at the time of admission. Thirteen cases with spinal hydatid disease had severe neurological deficit. After surgery, although all patients improved, only one of them showed a complete neurological recovery.

Until the middle of the 1990s, the preferred operative treatment was an open debridement of the lesions and laminectomy with spinal cord decompression (Figs. 9.29 and 9.30). Continuous irrigation with hypertonic saline solution and formaldehyde was used during the surgery. This technique associated or not to an additional posterior fixation has been defended by many authors (Sami et al. 1996; Turgut 1997; Bhojraj and Shetty 1999; El Andaloussi et al. 2001). Nevertheless, in our experience, this surgical technique has shown suboptimal postoperative outcomes, especially a high percentage of infection recurrences.

From the 1990s onward, our approach to vertebral echinococcosis has become more aggressive, similar to that used for tumoral lesions (Herrera et al. 2005). When the infection is limited to the vertebral body, with or without involvement of the anterolateral aspect, we perform an excision of the cysts and a partial or complete corpectomy (Fig. 9.31) with anterior strut grafting (freeze-dried) through an anterior approach (Fig. 9.32). After that, a posterolateral spinal fusion is performed through a posterior approach (Figs. 9.33 and 9.34).

Sometimes the infestation spreads into the spinal canal through the extradural space. In these cases, when the cysts only affect the posterior aspect of the vertebral body or the pedicles, we use a posterior approach to perform a laminectomy, a

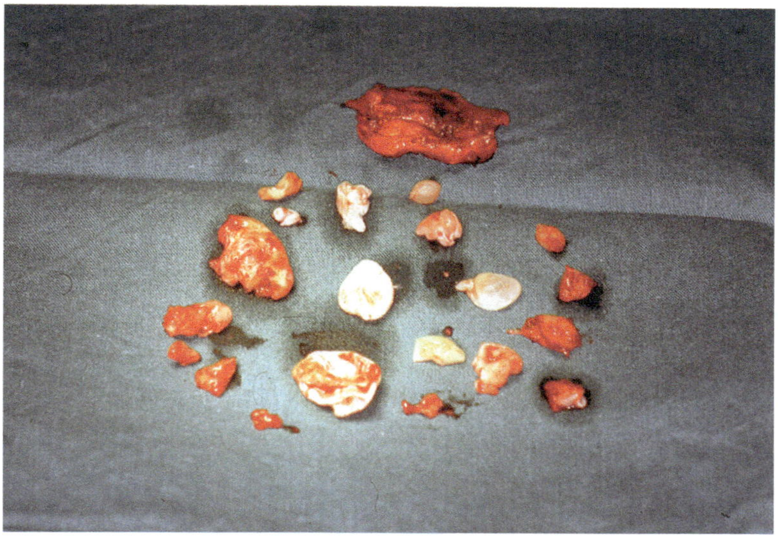

Fig. 9.31 Partial corpectomy: resected material

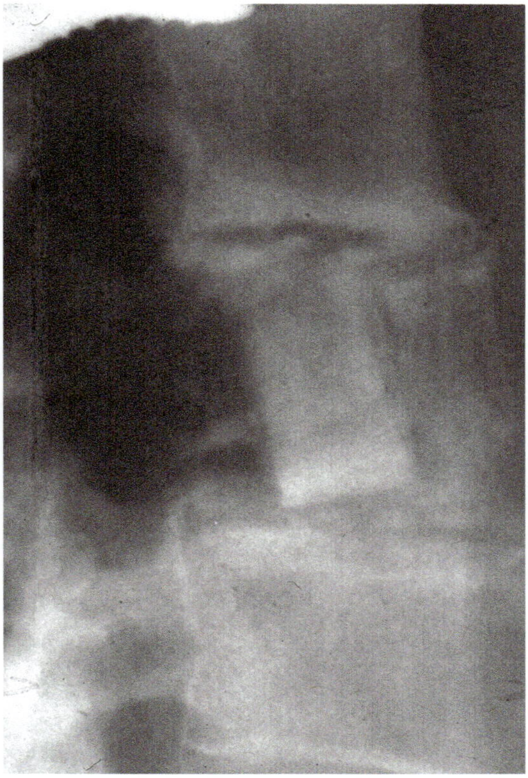

Fig. 9.32 Partial corpectomy: cryopreserved graft

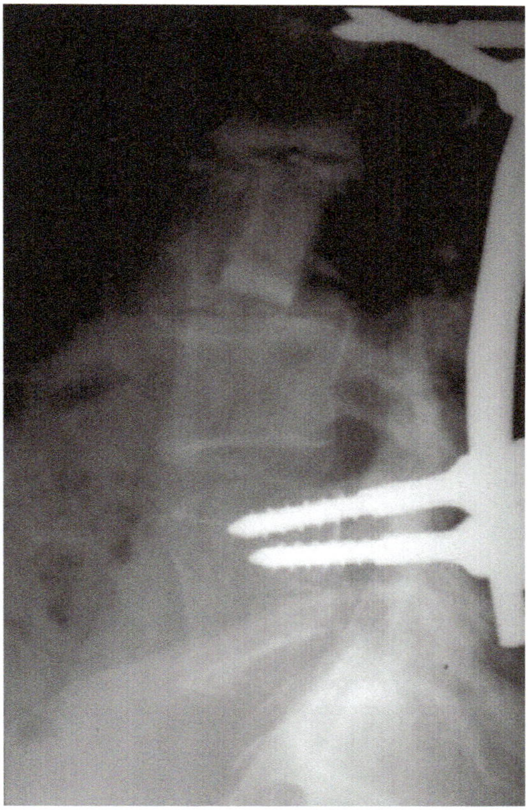

Fig. 9.33 Lateral radiograph: intersomatic graft and posterior fixation

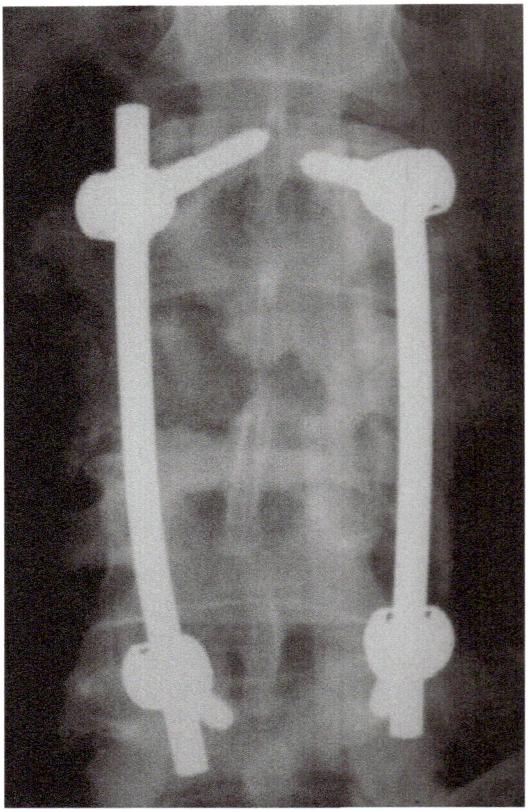

Fig. 9.34 AP radiograph of the case shown in Fig. 9.32

wide excision of the lesions, and a posterolateral instrumented fusion (Figs. 9.35 and 9.36).

But if the infection involves also the anterior part of the body, a combined approach will be necessary. We recommend performing first the decompression, curettage, and the instrumented posterior fixation through the posterior approach. Afterward, a partial or total corpectomy and grafting through the anterior approach are performed. With the combined radical surgery and a prolonged oral drug treatment, we have had good outcomes and absence of recurrences in the long-term follow-up in six of the eight patients treated with this protocol (Figs. 9.37 and 9.38). Those patients with paravertebral lesions or superinfection of the hydatid cysts had the worst outcomes, with the highest rates of recurrences that, in some cases, led to irresolvable infections. Surgical treatment of spinal hydatidosis is discussed in detail in Chap. 14.

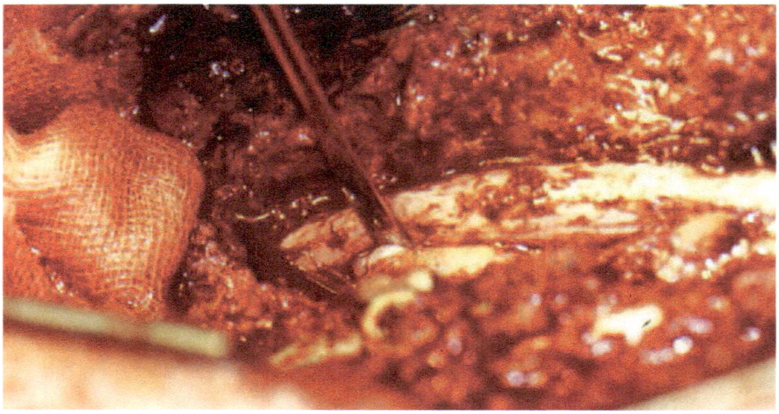

Fig. 9.35 Laminectomy and removal of extradural cysts

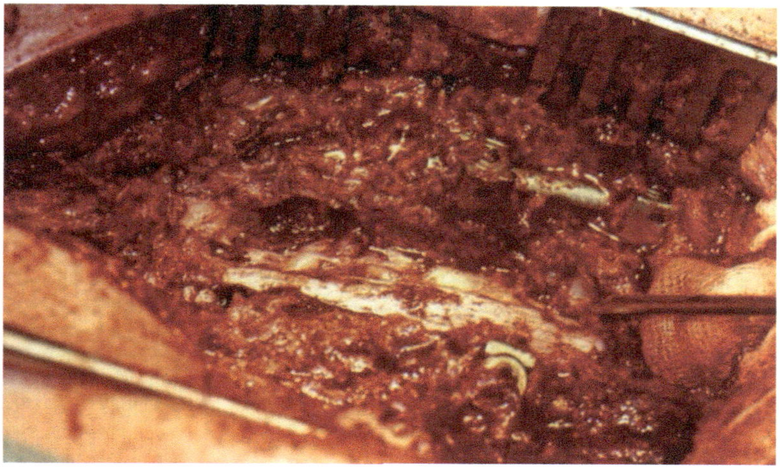

Fig. 9.36 Cyst removal in the case shown in Fig. 9.35. Note that pedicle screws placed

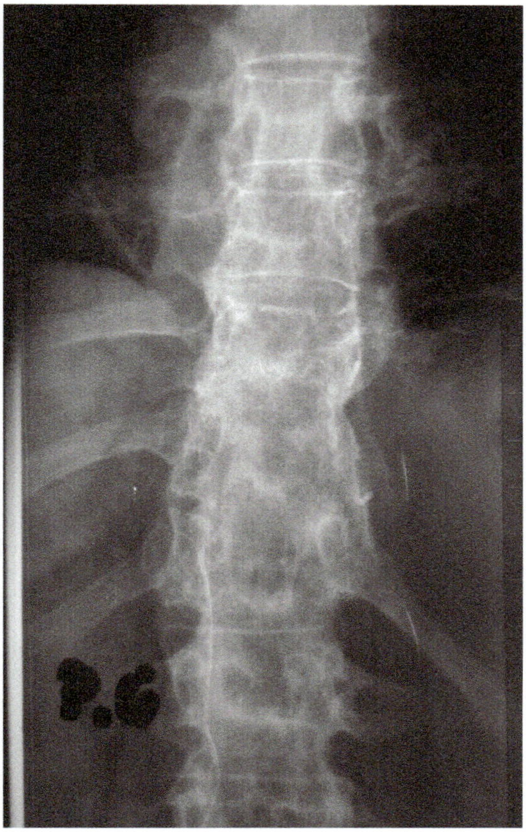

Fig. 9.37 AP radiograph at10-year follow-up: vertebral hydatidosis treated with partial corpectomy and posterior fixation. Note that the patient is disease-free

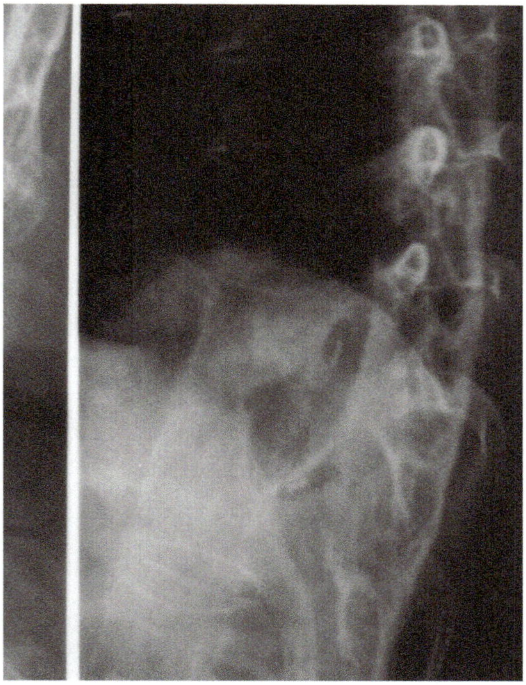

Fig. 9.38 Lateral radiograph of the same case shown in Fig. 9.37

Conclusion

Spinal echinococcosis is a severe disease with a technically demanding and challenging surgery. High migratory flows to the Western world might be associated with an upturn of the incidence of infectious diseases like this, previously eradicated in our country. New imaging techniques, CT scan with 3D visualization and especially MRI, and laboratory tests (ELISA) have allowed an early diagnosis and treatment of hydatid spinal disease. In our experience, an aggressive surgical treatment associated with the use of prolonged chemotherapy (albendazole and praziquantel) has improved the outcomes for patients with vertebral echinococcosis.

References

Beggs I. The radiology of hydatid disease. AJR Am J Roentgenol. 1985;145:639–48.

Bekhti A, Schaaps JP, Capron M, Dessaint JP, Santoro F, Capron A. Treatment of hepatic hydatid disease with mebendazole: preliminary results in four cases. Br Med J. 1977;ii:1047–51.

Bellil S, Limaiem F, Bellil K, Chelly I, Mekni A, Haouet S, Kchir N, Zitouna M. Descriptive epidemiology of extrapulmonary hydatid cysts: a report of 265 Tunisian cases. (in French). Tunis Med. 2009;87:123–6.

Bhojraj SY, Shetty NR. Primary hydatid disease of the spine: an unusual cause of progressive paraplegia. Case report and review of the literature. J Neurosurg. 1999;91(2 Suppl):216–8.

Braithwaite PA, Lees RF. Vertebral hydatid disease: radiological assessment. Radiology. 1981;140:763–7.

Carmena D, Benito A, Eraso E. The immunodiagnosis of Echinococcus multilocularis infection. Clin Microbiol Infect. 2007;13:460–75.

Carmena D, Benito-Pérez deMendiola A, Sánchez-Serrano LP. Reporting of human cystic echinococcosis in Spain: how effective is the epidemiological surveillance system? Enferm Infecc Microbiol Clin. 2010;28:135–6.

Cobo F, Yarnoz C, Sesma B, Fraile P, Aizcorbe M, Trujillo R, Diaz-de-Liaño A, Ciga MA. Albendazole plus praziquantel versus albendazole alone as a pre-operative treatment in intra-abdominal hydatisosis caused by Echinococcus granulosus. Trop Med Int Health. 1998;3:462–6.

Craig PS, Larrieu E. Control of cystic echinococcosis/hydatidosis: 1863–2002. Adv Parasitol. 2006;61:443–508.

Deplazes P. Ecology and epidemiology of Echinococcus multilocularis in Europe. Parassitologia. 2006;48:37–9.

Doganay S, Kantarci M. Role of conventional and diffusion-weighted magnetic resonance imaging of spinal treatment protocol for hydatid disease. J Spinal Cord Med. 2009;32:574–7.

Dreweck CM, Lűder CGK, Soboslay PT, Kern P. Subclass-specific serological reactivity and IgG4-specific antigen recognition in human echinococcosis. Trop Med Int Health. 1997;2:779–87.

El Andaloussi M, Yousri B, Aboumaarouf M. Vertebral hydatidosis: three case reports (In French). Rev Chir Orthop Reparatrice Appar Mot. 2001;87:392–6.

Fahl M, Haddad FS, Huballah M, Kana'an S, Husheimi I, Azizi T. Magnetic resonance imaging in intradural and extradural spinal echinococcosis. Clin Imaging. 1994;18:179–83.

Gavidia CM, Gonzalez AE, Barron EA, Ninaquispe B, Llamosas M, Verastegui MR, Robinson C, Gilman RH. Evaluation of oxfendazole, praziquantel and albendazole against cystic echinococcosis: a randomized clinical trial in naturally infected sheep. PLoS Negl Trop Dis. 2010;4:e616.

Gemmell MA, Lawson JR, Roberts MG. Towards global control of cystic and alveolar hydatid diseases. Parasitol Today. 1987;3:144–51.

Govender TS, Aslam M, Parbhoo A, Corr P. Hydatid disease of the spine. A long-term follow up after surgical treatment. Clin Orthop. 2000;378:143–7.

Haddad FS, Bitar E. Primary hydatid disease of the spine: report of 14 cases and review of the literature. Pan Arab J Neurosurg. 1997;1:46–52.

Heath DD, Chevis RAF. Mebendazole and hydatid cysts. Lancet. 1974;2:218–9.

Herrera A, Martínez AA. Extraspinal bone hydatidosis. J Bone Joint Surg Am. 2003;85:1790–4.

Herrera A, Martínez AA, Rodríguez J. Spinal hydatidosis. Spine. 2005;30:2439–44.

Işlekel S, Erşahin Y, Zileli M, Oktar N, Oner K, Ovül I, Ozdamar N, Tunçbay E. Spinal hydatid disease. Spinal Cord. 1998;36:166–70.

Karantanas AH, Paterakis K, Karavelis A. Intervertebral disk hydatid cysts: MR imaging findings. AJR Am J Roentgenol. 2003;180:1739–40.

Kern P, Bardonnet K, Renner E, Auer H, Pawlowski Z, Ammann RW, Vuitton DA, Kern P, European Echinococcosis Registry. European echinococcosis registry: human alveolar echinococcosis, Europe, 1982–2000. Emerg Infect Dis. 2003;9:343–9.

Küster T, Stadelmann B, Hermann C, Scholl S, Keiser J, Hemphill A. In vitro and in vivo efficacies of mefloquine-based treatment against alveolar echinococcosis. Antimicrob Agents Chemother. 2011;55:713–21.

Lawn SD, Bligh J, Craig PS, Chiodini PL. Human cystic echinococcosis: evaluation of post-treatment serologic follow-up by IgG subclass antibody detection. Am J Trop Med Hyg. 2004;70:329–35.

Lewis Jr JW, Koss N, Kerstein MD. A review of echinococcal disease. Ann Surg. 1975;181:390–6.

Martínez AA, Herrera A, Cuenca J, Herrero L. Hydatidosis of the pelvis and hip. Int Orthop. 2001;25:302–4.

Merkle EM, Schulte M, Vogel J, Tomczak R, Rieber A, Kern P, Goerich J, Brambs HJ, Sokiranski R. Musculoskeletal involvement in cystic echinococcosis: report of eight cases and review of the literature. AJR Am J Roentgenol. 1997;168:1531–4.

Morris DL, Gould SE. Serum and cyst concentrations of mebendazole and flubendazole in hydatid disease. Br Med J (Clin Res Ed). 1982;285:175.

Morris DL, Dykes PW, Dickson B, Marriner SE, Bogan JA, Burrows FG. Albendazole in hydatid disease. Br Med J (Clin Res Ed). 1983;286:103–4.

Murray RO, Haddad FS. Hydatid disease of the spine. J Bone Joint Surg Br. 1959;41-B:499–506.

Papanikolaou A. Osseous hydatid disease. Trans R Soc Trop Med Hyg. 2008;102:233–8.

Rao S, Parikh S, Kerr R. Echinococcal infestation of the spine in North America. Clin Orthop Relat Res. 1991;271:164–9.

Rausch RL, Wilson JF, Schantz PM, McMahon BJ. Spontaneous death of Echinococcus multilocularis: cases diagnosed serologically (by Em2 ELISA) and clinical significance. Am J Trop Med Hyg. 1987;36: 576–85.

Rayport M, Wisoff HS, Zaiman H. Vertebral echinococcosis: report of case of surgical and biological therapy with review of the literature. J Neurosurg. 1964;21: 647–60.

Romig T. Echinococcus multilocularis in Europe-state of the art. Vet Res Commun. 2009;33 Suppl 1:31–4.

Sami A, Elazhari A, Ouboukhlik A, Elkamar A, Jiddane M, Boucetta M. Hydatid cyst of the spine and spinal cord. Study of 24 cases (in French). Neurochirurgie. 1996;42:281–7.

Singh S, Korah IP, Gibikote SV, Shyam NK, Nair A, Korula A. Sacral hydatidosis: value of MRI in the diagnosis. Skeletal Radiol. 1998;27:518–21.

Song XH, Ding LW, Wen H. Bone hydatid disease. Postgrad Med J. 2007;83:536–42.

Szypryt EP, Morris DL, Mulholland RC. Combined chemotherapy and surgery for hydatid bone disease. J Bone Joint Surg Br. 1987;69:141–4.

Tan JL, Ueda N, Heath D, Mercer AA, Fleming SB. Development of virus as a bifunctional recombinant vaccine: surface display of Echinococcus granulosus antigen EG95 by fusion to membrane structural proteins. Vaccine. 2012;30:398–406.

Torricelli P, Martinelli C, Biagini R, Ruggieri P, De Cristofaro R. Radiographic and computed tomographic findings in hydatid disease of bone. Skeletal Radiol. 1990;19:435–9.

Turgut M. Hydatid disease of the spine: a survey study from Turkey. Infection. 1997;25:221–6.

Urrea-Paris MA, Moreno MJ, Casado N, Rodriguez-Caabeiro F. In vitro effect of praziquantel and albendazole combination therapy on the larval stage of Echinococcus granulosus. Parasitol Res. 2000;86:957–64.

von Sinner WN. New diagnostic signs in hydatid disease; radiography, ultrasound, CT and MRI correlated to pathology. Eur J Radiol. 1991;12:150–9.

Wen H, Craig PS. IgG subclass responses in human cystic alveolar echinococcosis. Am J Trop Med Hyg. 1994; 51:741–8.

Yasawy MI, al Karawi MA, Mohamed AR. Combination of praziquantel and albendazole in the treatment of hydatid disease. Trop Med Parasitol. 1993;44:192–4.

Zlitni M, Ezzaouia K, Lebib H, Karray M, Kooli M, Mestiri M. Hydatid cyst of bone: diagnosis and treatment. World J Surg. 2001;25:75–82.

Laboratory Findings of Patients with Hydatidosis of the Central Nervous System

10

Dimitar Vuchev

Contents

D. Vuchev, MD, PhD
Department of Clinical Parasitology and Tropical Medicine, Medical University of Plovdiv, Blvd. Vassil Aprilov 15A, BG-4002 Plovdiv, Bulgaria

Department of Infectious Diseases, Parasitology and Tropical Medicine, St. George University Hospital, Plovdiv, Bulgaria
e-mail: dvutchev@yahoo.com

Introduction

The diagnosis of hydatidosis, caused by the larval stage of *Echinococcus granulosus* and *E. multilocularis*, respectively cystic echinococcosis (CE) and alveolar echinococcosis (AE), localized within different organs, including of the central nervous system (CNS), is very difficult to make during the primary stage of invasion because of the asymptomatic development until the appearance of morbid symptoms, which may not be specific. During the last three decades, new technologically acquired methods for diagnostic imaging, ultrasound, computed tomography (CT), and magnetic resonance imaging (MRI) have considerably facilitated the diagnostic process. Such diagnostic imaging requires expert diagnosis to differentiate benign and malignant tumors, nonparasitic cysts, and tuberculosis (Turgut 2002).

In practice, the parasitic nature of hydatidosis is established directly through laboratory diagnostic morphological methods (observation of protoscoleces, hooklets, parasitic cysts and their fragments, and histological preparations) or indirectly through immunologic methods which specify the parasitic nature of the disease in the primary stage; the findings are

M. Turgut (ed.), *Hydatidosis of the Central Nervous System: Diagnosis and Treatment*, DOI 10.1007/978-3-642-54359-3_10, © Springer-Verlag Berlin Heidelberg 2014

confirmed by diagnostic imaging (Taratuto and Venturiello 1997).

The clinical evaluation of laboratory information in the diagnosis of CNS hydatidosis is complex and is based on results from parasitological, histological, immunological, and other examinations. Specific clinicolaboratory examinations for the etiological diagnosis of this condition are unknown.

Hematologic Examinations

Clinicolaboratory hematologic tests for CNS hydatidosis are not specific in most cases, show considerable variation, and are not indicative of the disease. The reason is probably that the early appearance of serious clinical symptoms leads to seeking of early medical help (Turgut 2002).

In spite of that, hematological examinations are prescribed as a possibility for obtaining additional information for clinical diagnosis. Eosinophilia and leucocytosis in the full blood count, possibly anemia, and raised erythrocyte sedimentation rate (ESR) are kept under observation (Abbassioun and Amirjamshidi 2001a, b).

Eosinophilia

Examinations for eosinophilia in leucocytic formula (over 5 %) and in blood (exceeding 700/μL) should be conducted carefully, because they are signs of the pathological processes. Notwithstanding, this is not a permanent and reliable sign for diagnosis of CNS hydatidosis although it is accepted as an indication of live parasites. After death, calcification, or suppuration of hydatid cysts the hypereosinophilia disappears. It is found in one-third of patients and rarely reaches above 12 %, especially in multiple hydatidosis (Donovan et al. 1995; Turgut et al. 1997; Turgut 2002).

After successful surgical treatment the eosinophilia gradually returns to normal within a few months. If it remains elevated for more than 6 months, it is indicative of a postoperative recurrence or of residual cyst(s). The examination is a subsidiary method, very useful in the postoperative period (Reittner et al. 1996).

Leucocytosis, Anemia, Raised Erythrocyte Sedimentation Rate

Leucocytosis is usually observed in cases of suppuration, as well as necrosis in *E. multilocularis*. It has a subsidiary diagnostic meaning. Hypochromic anaemia is relatively rare (in up to 15 % of the patients) - the haemoglobin decreases to 60 %. The raised ESR is observed almost always in patients with hydatidosis (Herrera et al. 2005). These indexes – leucocytosis, anemia, and elevated ESR – are usually due to hydatic complications or to other accompanying diseases. Changes detected by clinical, laboratory, and hematologic examinations are infrequent and they are accepted only as additional indications. However, it is necessary to carry out these tests because, in many cases, they may help in specifying the diagnosis.

Examination of the Cerebrospinal Fluid

Examination of cerebrospinal fluid (CSF) obtained through lumbar puncture is important for the diagnosis of CNS hydatidosis. The most important contraindication is an increased intracranial pressure, which occurs in the course of the disease and should be checked in advance (Reittner et al. 1996; Turgut 2002). One looks for eosinophilic cells, hydatid protoscoleces, and hooklets in the CSF or, in case of unclear or negative results from the parasitological examination, an immunological examination should be made of the liquor for hydatidosis (Tappe et al. 2008).

Hydatid Protoscoleces

If fertile hydatid cysts rupture in the ventricles, parasitic scoleces and hooklets flood the CSF. These appear in the centrifuged CSF sediment under the microscope at a magnification of 100× for the protoscoleces and 400× for the hooklets.

Eosinophilia in Cerebrospinal Fluid

An important diagnostic finding is the presence of eosinophilc cells in the centrifuged sediment of a CSF sample. This is best seen under Giemza staining. In CNS hydatidosis an abundant eosinophilic infiltrate collects around the cyst in the cerebral tissue. These cells penetrate the CSF channels. These cells are not always found in the CSF of patients suffering from CNS hydatidosis. In these cases the CSF reveals hyperproteinemia, with moderate pleocytosis, with a presence of eosinophilic cells.

Parasitological Morphodiagnostics

The most certain and precise diagnosis results from histopathological study of tissue removed at surgery.

Macroscopic Examination

A careful inspection of the presented operative material for presence of hydatid membranes, fragments of membrane, or daughter cysts is in order. The removed hydatid cyst is cut with sharp pointed scissors. The internal surface is scraped for "hydatid sand" (protoscoleces, hooklets, brood capsules) and small daughter cysts. These are removed and put into a glass container with water. The collected material is washed several times and is fixed in 70° ethanol and 10 % formalin for 1 h and is then kept in 70° ethanol.

Microscopic Examination

Protoscoleces

These are observed in native preparations. The collected hydatid fluid is centrifuged and a drop of sediment is put on a slide. The sediment is examined microscopically under a cover glass (magnification 100×). The protoscoleces have a characteristic structure and are agile. They have an oval form, sharply lined. Inside, a line of hooklets is observed, grouped around elongated axis in the middle of the protoscolex and forming a crown. Its dimensions are about 110/150 μm. From the sediment covering the slide a fixed stable preparation can be prepared for demonstration and training after Giemza staining.

Hooklets

Free hooklets can also be observed under the microscope in hydatid fluid sediment (magnification 400×). The hooklets of *E. multilocularis* are larger than those of *E. granulosus*. This comparison is possible when a single sample has hooklets from both species. They differ from one other in that the *E. granulosus* hooklets root has a bend while that of *E. multilocularis* has a more acute arc shaped bend (Vogel 1978).

Biological Method

The biological involves laboratory mice, inoculated with material suspected of hydatidosis.

Echinococcus granulosus

A specimen cyst, or fragments of it, should be washed with a saline solution and then placed into a laboratory conical glass container. After precipitation over 1 h the separated scolex sediment is washed several times with saline solution, drawn out into a syringe, and injected intraperitoneally into test animals. After 3–5 months an autopsy is performed. If in the examined material (hydatid cyst and hydatid fluid) there were viable scolices, new cysts are observed in the peritoneal cavity.

Echinococcus multilocularis

Cyst viability is investigated through test animals. Small pieces of surgically resected parasitic cysts are subjected to intraperitoneal or intrahepatic inoculation. If they do not increase in the animals, it is confirmed that the cysts are dead.

Determination of Protoscolex Vitality

This examination is particularly important to determine the prognosis by examining the operative specimen from *E. granulosus* cysts with protoscoleces, and for advice as far as non-recurrent conservative treatment is concerned. By heating the hydatid fluid (37–38 °C) the viable protoscoleces are desinvaginated, the crown with hooks comes out, and they begin to move actively. The staining method for determining the vitality of hydatid protoscoleces is easy. A hot, saturated methylene blue solution is used, which is put on a slide to obtaining an azure color. The solution is left to dry. For examination, a cover glass covered with protoscoleces is laid on the dye. The coloring agent penetrates only the dead protoscoleces and the viable ones do not absorb paint and remain unstained.

Morphological, Pathological, and Histological Examinations

Echinococcus granulosus

Primary localization of hydatid cysts in the CNS is rare. These cysts may be found in the hemispheres, ventricles, extradural and subcortical, and very rarely in the cerebellum and spinal cord. Children are more often and more severely affected and have an increased intracranial pressure. The hydatid cyst is normally single, spherical or oval, and filled with clear fluid (hydatid fluid). In some cases they appear as a "cluster." The pathological alterations in the surrounding tissues depend on the localization, size, and changes in the cyst itself: whether it is intact, ruptured, suppurated, or calcified (Abbassioun and Amirjamshidi 2001a, b; Haddad and Haddad 2005).

The appearance of the hydatid cyst is typical and it can be easily recognized visually. They consist of three layers: (1) an outer fibrous (adventitial) layer out of the real parasite, with different thicknesses and even absent – the pericyst; (2) an acellular (multilayered, laminated) membrane, easy to separate from the fibrous capsule and having a whitish color – the ectocyst; and (3) a very fine germinative membrane with numerous brood germinal capsules fastened to its internal surface – the endocyst. In larger cysts there can be "daughter cysts," swimming in hydatid fluid as well as "hydatid sand" in the sediment, formed from hydatid protoscoleces and hooklets which are visible under the microscope (Taratuto and Venturiello 1997).

The tissue reaction around the cyst is minimal, with infiltration of mononuclear cells. Degenerated and calcified cysts have similar infiltrates. In the case of bacterial infection there is a considerable inflammatory reaction with polynuclears, mainly eosinophils, and granulomatous inflammation with histocytes, giant cells, and connective tissue surrounding the cyst (Kars et al. 1982; Taghipour et al. 2008).

Histological diagnostics is best when made on material obtained by surgical operation or autopsy. All fragments from the obtained specimen have to be examined for laminated membranes, presence of daughter cysts, and viability. The dead cysts are necrotic, with semi-fluid content. The calcified cysts are also dead and they are removed surgically only if they are infected. In incompletely calcified cysts there are viable scolices. The viable cysts have the characteristic three-layer membrane (Kars et al. 1982; Özek et al 1993; Taratuto and Venturiello 1997).

The laminated membrane of the hydatid cyst is stained with the periodic acid (Schiff reaction), or PAS stain which is a histological marker for hydatid cyst. It is ten times thicker than the germinative layer which consists only of two cell layers. The protoscoleces are easily discernible with their characteristic hooklets; even if they are degenerated the hooklets remain (Taratuto and Venturiello 1997). Sediment from the hydatid fluid mixed with formalin is examined parasitologically; depend on where the sample is obtained, hooklets can be found as well as protoscoleces and fragments from laminated membrane. The hydatid cyst within bones (for example in the vertebral column) has no fibrous capsule, and in the intra-trabecular areas numerous small cysts develop. In the spinal cord the hydatidosis is a secondary invasion.

Echinococcus multilocularis

Clinically this looks like a malignant tumor, slowly increasing in size in the liver which can metastasize to the CNS: also occurs in the brain and, very rarely, in the orbit and spinal cord. The resected parasitical cysts look like a gray whitish mass, a conglomerate of small bladders connected with connective tissue. They have an exogenic growth and infiltrate the surrounding tissue (Craig 2003).

Around the cysts there is no fibrous layer and the germinative and laminated membrane of small cysts (2–3 mm) have a cellular appearance. They contain gelatinous material and only in some of them are protoscoleces found. (Taratuto and Venturiello 1997). The surrounding tissue reveals an inflammatory reaction, with infiltrates of polynuclears and many eosinophils, lymphocytes, histiocytes, and giant cells. The laminated membrane is stained for hydatidosis with PAS (Toussaint et al. 2001; Craig 2003; Yang et al. 2005).

Immunodiagnostics of Hydatidosis

Introduction

Early detection of the disease by immunodiagnostic methods is of considerable importance. It leads to early and adequate treatment and prevents the formation of serious complications, which can even lead to a fatal outcome.

Hydatid immunology investigations have developed considerably during the last few decades, but certain immunodiagnostic methods date from the very beginning of the last century: Gedhin, Weinberg test (1906, 1908), Casoni test (1911).

Characteristic of the *E. granulosus* antigen structure is the presence of heterogeneous antigens, which cross react with host antigens as well as with antigens of *E. multilocularis* and some other helminthes. As a result ,immunologic false results may be reported. False negative results are observed, too, in different organ localizations of hydatidosis, including the brain, orbit, as well as lungs, spleen, etc. Negative results are observed in new, small, dead, and calcified cysts.

False-positive and false-negative results are met less and less due to the introduction of new immunologic methods. They allow for an early diagnosis, because immune antibodies are detected 2–3 weeks after the primary invasion, even before clinical symptoms appear.

Evidences of Application

The immunological diagnosis of hydatidosis by different methods is used under the following circumstances.

Clinical Evidence

This is based on the detection of antibodies in the patient's blood, which are produced by the cysts while they are still very small – up to 1.0/1.5 cm. It differentiates hydatidosis from other diseases. Through repeated measurement it evaluates the efficiency of surgical treatment and of its successful outcome. In the case of decreasing specific antibody titers or negative diagnostic reaction, it reveals a good prognosis. In the case where the diagnostic titer remains at the same level or rises in level, this shows a postoperative recurrence. The clinical efficiency is evaluated by analogy to conservative therapy.

Epidemical and Prophylactic Evidences

Immunodiagnostic methods find application by large-scale diagnostic screening-seroepidemiologic surveys among the population at risk from different professional, social, and age groups. This is done for detection of epidemic foci, investigation of epidemiology, epizootiology, and infection risk degree. Of great importance here is the prophylactic diagnosis of family members of hydatidosis sick patient, where the diagnosis of so-called "family hydatidosis" is possible. Immunodiagnostic reactions by indirect hemagglutination (IHA) and enzyme-linked immunosorbent assay (ELISA) are suitable for large-scale investigations, in which reactions are highly sensitive and very specific. There are preprepared immunodiagnostic preparations, suitable for differential diagnostics–specific for *E. granulosus* and *E. multilocularis* invasion, respectively.

Contemporary National Programs

Contemporary national programs for control of hydatidosis include the early diagnosis of asymptomatic forms as one of their basic measures. It is realized by making large-scale screening examinations as a first diagnostic means or combined with diagnostic imaging methods. The combination of two tests is recommended, for example ELISA and Western blot (Craig and Larrien 2006). Such examinations are carried in some endemic countries on different continents.

Immunity and Diagnostics

The *E. granulosus* species is genetically heterogeneous and consists of ten strains (G1 to G10), defined through molecular biological methods such as polymerase chain reaction (PCR) and differences in antigen content as well as in basic intermediate and end hosts. The most widespread is the sheep strain (G1). Because of antigen differences of the irregularly spread genotypes, it is recommended that antigens of *E. granulosus* isolates are used, which are specific for a particular geographic area (Eckert and Dephazes 2008; Rosenvit et al. 2006; Gihan et al. 2009). By chronic invasion of *E. granulosus* and *E. multilocularis*, the interaction between parasite and host leads to considerably expressed humoral and cellular immune response.

Humoral Immune Response

B lymphocytes produce specific antibodies – a process conditioned by antigens passing through the parasitic cyst membrane. The immune response is influenced by the cyst structures, individual genetic host differences, invasion duration, etc. In serum of hydatidosis sick patients specific antibodies of IgG, IgE, IgA, and IgM types may be detected.

Antibodies of IgG type: these immunoglobulins are basic antibody types, which are produced by *E. granulosus* invasion and consist of four subclasses, respectively IgG1 to IgG4. Having most expressed sensitivity and specificity are IgG1, cross reactions are mostly due to IgG2, those with protective functions are IgG3, and specific and without cross reactions are IgG4 (the last mentioned are detected only in two-thirds of the cases of invasion) (Ramzy et al. 1999).

Depending on organ localization, the humoral immune response differs in diagnostic value. Those by parasitic cysts in brain and orbits IgG antibodies are quite often specific. The immune response also depends on the parasite morphology. In injured cyst membrane it is elevated and in suppurated cysts it is reduced and can even be missing. In secondary echinococcosis the immune response is more elevated in comparison with primary echinococcosis. After successful treatment the immune antibodies decrease and eventually disappear.

Antibodies of IgE Class: these are involved with the pathogenesis of allergic reactions of the first type (IgE mediated reaction of hypersensitivity). The specific IgE are tissue antigens, liberated under the influence of parasitic metabolic products. In *E. granulosus* invasion they are detected in the serum specific IgE antibodies in 25–90 % of cases, but allergic reactions of a quick type appear very rarely in intact cysts. The reason is the presence of IgG4, which blocks the anaphylactic reactions. Fixed in the skin, antiparasitic IgE explains the Casoni test effect. The common and specific IgEs are present more in multiple hydatidosis and in the presence of daughter cysts, but their level depends on the organ localization. In calcified cysts the IgEs decrease gradually. After effective treatment for up to 1 year they are detected only in a half of the cases (Ortona et al. 2003).

Antibodies of IgA and IgM Class: these are rarely examined. Antiparasitic antibodies of these classes are detected in serum of low parasite content antibodies – IgA to 54 % and IgM to 37.5 %, but with high specificity –100 % and 95.7 % respectively. After effective treatment they persist for some years and are unsuitable for evaluating post treatment tracing patients (Doiz et al. 2002).

Cell-Mediated Immune Response

T-lymphocytes decrease in the blood as does their functional activity. An immunosuppression develops as a result of cytotoxic effects of low molecular *E. granulosus* fractions, T-sub-spherical activation (CD8+), and unbalance between subpopulations Th1 and Th2 of T-helper cells (CD4+). In fertile cysts the activity of Th2 increases, becoming apparent with increased values of IL-4 and IL-10 and IFN-γ decreasing. After effective treatment the IL-4 and IL-10 generating decreases and IFN-γ increases. The examination results of these markers in various dynamics are indicative, but they are unsuitable for routine practice because of high cost and difficult execution (Ortona et al. 2003).

Now we will briefly discuss the basic routine immunodiagnostic tests, applied in practice as described below.

Routine Immunological Diagnostic Tests

According to the purpose of immunological tests in routine diagnostic practice, they are classified as either primary diagnostic and screening tests or secondary confirming tests, after WHO. Until now no absolutely specific and sensitive tests for hydatidosis diagnosis have been developed.

Primary Diagnostic and Screening Tests

Primary diagnostic and screening tests are of high sensitivity and limited specificity. The ELISA, IHA, latex agglutination test (LAT), and bentonite flocculation test (BFT) reactions and immunoelectrophoresis are the most often used in practice. It is recommended to use a minimum of two primary tests in each case under diagnosis.

Secondary Confirming Tests

Secondary confirming tests are usually less sensitive than the primary ones, but with higher specificity. These are the Western blot reactions, agar double-diffusion (DD5), and IgG subclass determination.

Antigens Used in Immunological Tests

Hydatid cyst liquid, which contains two important diagnostic antigens (Ag5 and AgB), is most often used for diagnosis (Biffin et al. 1993). Ag5 is a thermolabile lipoprotein complex which has two compound parts molecular masses of 57 and 67 kDa, respectively. It disintegrates into two fractions with molecular masses of 20/22 and 38/39 kDa (Gonsales-Sapiensa 2000). The second fraction can also be detected in healthy people. Cross reactions may occur with other helminthoses and in people with blood group antigen P1 (Gadea et al. 1999). AgB is a thermostable lipoprotein with a molecular mass of 120/160 kDa and is detected by all four Echinococcus species. Five forms of AgB with five different genes are detected in different strains. Basic, purified, and recombinant antigens are used in scientific investigations (Ortona et al. 2000). Besides hydatid liquid antigens, larva extracts as well as histological cuts of protoscolices are used in immunological reactions, being subjected to fluorescent antibody tests.

Immunological Methods Proving the Anti-Echinococcus IgG

Complement Fixation (CF, Weinberg–Ghedini Test)

Complement fixation was first used in Echinococcus diagnosis by Ghedini in 1906 and improved by M. Weinberg in 1908. Its sensitivity reaches 60–70 %. It is applied in parallel with the fluorescent antibody test (FAT) and indirect hemagglutination assay (IHA). The serological titer decreases quickly after successful therapy. However, if it remains elevated for 6–12 months this indicates a recurrence. This test is not very specific – it is complicated in execution and has now almost fell into disuse as a routine practice (Kagan 1968).

Agglutination Reactions

Agglutination reactions as immunological methods providing the anti-Echinococcus IgG are described below.

Indirect Hemagglutination Assay (IHA): introduced in 1957 and is still often used in practice. Erythrocytes loaded with Echinococcus antigens are used. The reaction sensitivity varies from 62 to 100 % and the specificity from 92 to 100 % depending on the diagnostic kit quality. It gives cross reactions with other helminthoses as well as nonparasitic diseases (Kagan 1968; Zhang and McManus 2006).

Latex Agglutination Test (LAT): introduced in 1960. Latex particles loaded with Echinococcus antigens are used. The sensitivity is between 50 and 92 % and the specificity is 95 %. Cross reactions are also observed in 10 % of cases (Kagan 1968). The test is easy and rapid in execution and suitable for the practice.

Bentonite Flocculation Test (BFT): applied for echinococcosis in 1959 by Norman, Sadun, and Allain. Inert bentonite particles loaded with parasitic antigens are used. The test sensitivity is 70–100 % and the specificity 94 %. Cross reactions with other diseases are observed in 3–27 % of cases (Kagan 1968).

Precipitation Reactions

Precipitation reactions as immunological methods providing the anti-Echinococcus IgG are described below.

Scolex Precipitation: first used by Schulz and Ismailov, 1962. Rarefied scolices are used in saline solution. On adding serum of patient, microscopic precipitates are observed on the scolex cuticular surface. The sensitivity is very high, 82–94 % and the specificity is 88–100 %. This is not applied in routine practice because live scolices are used.

Double Diffusion Arc 5 (DD5): arc 5 fraction – which is identical to Ag5 – is found in echinococcic liquid (Porreti et al. 1999; Zhang and McManus 2006). It is an agar reaction and the immune complexes are observed on a precipitation strip. The sensitivity is 47 % and specificity 93–100 %. Cross reactions occur with alveococcosis and cysticercosis.

Immunoelectrophoresis: used especially for investigation of the composition of antigens in echinococcic liquid. Antibodies and antigens form in the electric field on an agar precipitation strip. The sensitivity is 63–80 % and specificity 97 % (Zhang et al. 2003). It is unsuitable for seroepidemiologic investigations and is only used in clinical diagnosis.

Reactions with Participation of Marked Antibodies

Reactions with participation of marked antibodies as immunological methods produced by the anti-Echinococcus IgG are described below.

Fluorescent Antibody Test (FAT): introduced for echinococcosis diagnosis in 1963. Antibodies are proved through indirect immunofluorescence. Hydatid protoscolices or histological slices containing the antibodies are fixed on a slide. On contact with serum the antibodies combine with the parasite antigens. The reaction is visualized by addition of anti-human antibodies, conjugated with fluorochrome, which fluoresces specifically under ultraviolet light. The sensitivity is high – 82–100 % (Kagan 1968). It is often applied in parallel with IHA.

Enzyme-Linked Immunosorbent Assay (ELISA): applied to echinococcosis in 1974. A total echinococcic liquid is used as antigen. Methods have been developed with purified antigens – Ag5, AgB, and recombinant antigens (Gonzalez Sapienza et al. 2000; Siles-Lucas and Gottstein 2001; Ortona et al. 2003). The reaction sensitivity is 44–100 % and specificity 65–100 %. In rarer echinococcosis localizations, such as in brain and orbit, the sensitivity is lower –25–56 %. Cross reactions with other helminthoses (fasciolosis, schistosomiasis) and some malignant diseases are rarely observed. It is also applied to diagnosis of *E. multilocularis* invasion and the antigen used is from a parasite larva secretion, purified and recombinant antigens.

Enzyme-Linked Immunoelectrotransfer Blot (Immunoblot, Western blot, EITB): different antigen fractions are used. They are divided by molecular mass through electrophoresis and are transferred on a membrane, which undergoes an immunoenzymatic reaction. The presence of antibodies against antigen fractions is visualized as a strip with definite molecular mass. It is accepted that the 8/12 kDa fraction, which derives from AgB, is of diagnostic importance for the echinococcosis. The sensitivity is variable – 65–100 % – and the specificity is high – 94–100 %. Cross reactions with alveococcosis are met in 53–84 % of cases. The test is a reliable confirmatory diagnostic method with a high sensitivity and specificity index (Verastegui et al. 1992; Gadea et al. 1999; Porreti et al. 1999; Makni et al. 2007).

Immunological Tests for Investigation of Anti-Echinococcus IgE

Casoni Intradermal Test

This is a method for echicoccosis diagnosis and is applied "in vitro" and through allergic reaction. An echinoccocic liquid is injected intradermally and the erythema size is measured every 30 min. The use of unstandardized antigen often leads to false positive results. The sample sensitivity is 75–95 % and the specificity is low – 55–82 % (Kagan 1968). After a Casoni intradermal test the treatment efficiency cannot be determined with this test, because sensitization occurs, and remains positive so the humoral antibodies produced make the serological tests positive. At present it is not recommended by WHO because of the risk of serious allergic reactions and low specificity.

Basophil Degranulation Test

Concerns detection of anti-Echinococcus IgE, fixed on basophil cells. The developed degranulation test has a high sensitivity – 93% and specificity – 97–100 %.

Serologic Method

Recombinant antigens and monoclonal antibodies – called the Western blot – are investigated for IgE antibodies, which react with AgB. The sensitivity is low – 50–52 % – but the specificity is high – 95–100 %. The surveys for specific IgE are not enough and there are no diagnostic tests in routine practice. They are confirmatory tests because of their high specificity and low cross reactivity (Ortona et al. 2003).

Molecular Biological Method

The polymerase chain reaction (PCR) is used for species identification of *E. granulosus* and *E. multilocularis* in areas where both diseases are spread. By means of PCR a strain identification of *E. granulosus* is made from G1 to G10 (Weiss 1995; Yang et al. 2006).

Conclusion

The introduction of immunological methods and techniques in suitable combination leads to an optimal diagnostic conclusion. By means of other diagnostic possibilities such as imaging diagnostics and laboratory-clinical examinations it is possible to exclude other diseases. The use of at least two tests for routine immunological testing in hydatidosis of CNS, orbit, and spinal column is recommended. The suitable combinations are IHA with FAT as well as IHA with ELISA or ELISA with Western blot confirmation (Force et al. 1992; Doiz et al. 2001). In the post treatment period (surgical, conservative) we have accepted a minimum time limit of 5–10 years. Periodically we evaluate the antibody titer with immunological examination on ELISA and IHA. Following effective treatment it usually decreases progressively down to non-diagnostic values in 3–5 years. While FAT becomes negative quite quickly, the IHA remains positive for a long time (as long as one to two decades), but at low levels. High titers, as well as increasing after operation, indicate the presence of residual cysts or postoperative recurrences.

Figure 10.1 shows in bold characters the use of laboratory diagnostic methods on patients with hydatidosis of CNS.

Acknowledgments Thanks are due to Mr. Georgy Kerelov and Dr. Irina Marinova for operative collaboration in preparing the text and references. I would especially like to send my sincerest thanks to Fuad Sami Haddad for his critical comments and English language revision of the text.

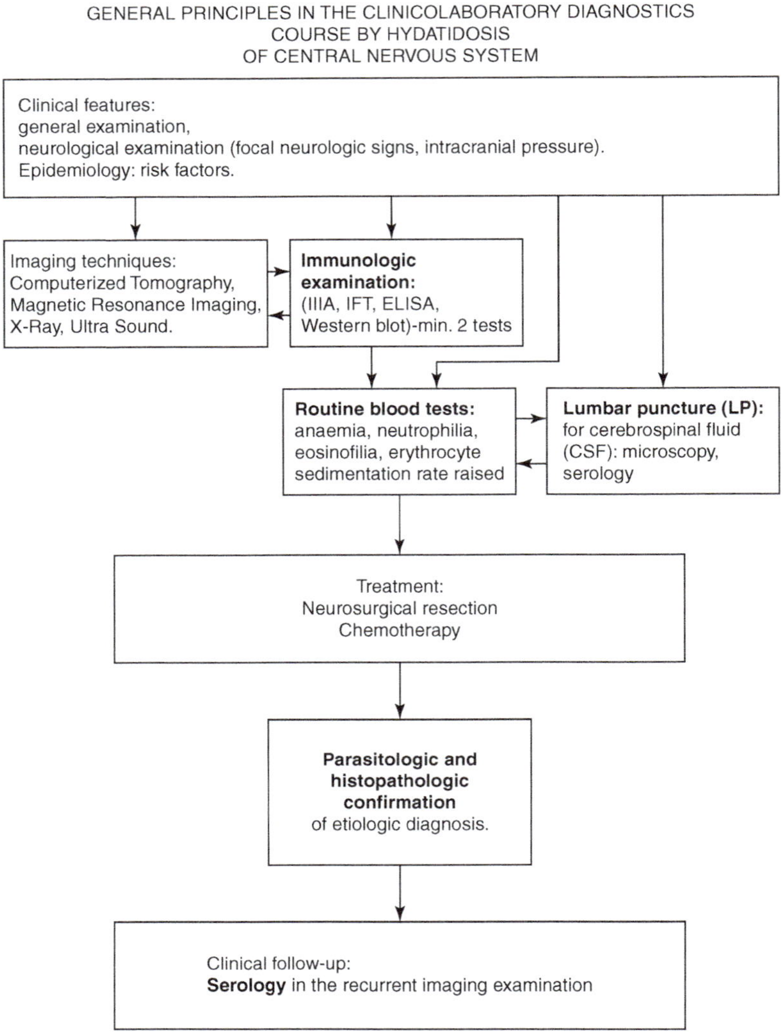

Fig. 10.1 General principles in the clinico-laboratory diagnosis course in hydatidosis of central nervous system (*Echinococcus granulosus* and *E. multilocularis*)

References

Abbassioun K, Amirjamshidi A. Diagnosis and management of hydatid cyst of the central nervous system: part 1: general consideration and hydatid disease of the brain. Neurosurg Q. 2001a;11:1–9.

Abbassioun K, Amirjamshidi A. Diagnosis and management of hydatid cyst of the central nervous system: part 2: hydatid cyst of the skull, orbit and spine. Neurosurg Q. 2001b;11:10–6.

Biffin A, Jones M, Palmer S. Human hydatid disease: evaluation of an ELISA for diagnosis, population screening and monitoring of control programmes. J Med Microbiol. 1993;39:48–52.

Craig P. Echinococcus multilocularis. Curr Opin Infect Dis. 2003;16:437–44.

Craig P, Larrien E. Control of cystic echinococcosis/hydatidosis: 1863–2002. Adv Parasitol. 2006;61:443–508.

Doiz O, Benito R, Sbihi Y, Osuna A, Clavel A, Gomez-Lus R. Western blot applied to the diagnosis and post-treatment monitoring of human hydatidosis. Diagn Microbiol Infect Dis. 2001;41:139–42.

Doiz O, Benito R, Gil J, Rojas A, Rubio MC, Osuna A. Pre- and postsurgical detection of IgG, IgM and IgA specific to hydatidosis by ELISA with purified antigen enriched with the 5/B antigen complex. J Clin Lab Anal. 2002;16:295–8.

Donovan SM, Mickiewicz N, Meyer RD, Panosian CB. Imported echinococcosis in southern California. Am J Trop Med Hyg. 1995;53:668–71.

Eckert J, Dephazes P. Biological, epidemiological and clinical aspects of echinococcosis, a zoonosis of increasing concern. Clin Microbiol Rev. 2004;17:107–35.

Force L, Torres J, Carrillo A, Busca J. Evaluation of eight serological tests in the diagnosis of human echinococcosis and follow-up. Clin Infect Dis. 1992;15:473–80.
Gadea I, Ayala G, Diago M, Cunat A, de Lomas JG. Immunological diagnosis of human cystic echinococcosis: utility of discriminant analyses applied to the enzyme linked immunoelectrotransfer blot. Clin Diagn Lab Immunol. 1999;6:504–8.
Gihan M, Hala S, Nabil S, Lalla E, Hala ST, Rania M, Samar K, Wagida A. Genetic variability of Antigen B among Echinococcus granulosus Egyptian isolates. Korean J Parasitol. 2009;4:250–64.
Gonzalez Sapienza G, Lorenzo C, Nieto A. Imported immunodiagnosis of cystic hydatid disease by using a synthetic peptide with higher diagnostic value than that of its parent protein, Echinococcus granulosus antigen B. J Clin Microbiol. 2000;38:3979–83.
Haddad FS, Haddad G. Hydatid disease of the central nervous system. Personal experience: its appearance, management, and outcome in the brain and the spine. Neurosurg Q. 2005;15:33–40.
Herrera A, Martinez A, Rodrigues J. Spinal hydatidosis. Spine (Phila Pa 1976). 2005;30:2439–44.
Kagan IG. A review of serological tests for diagnosis of hydatid disease. Bull World Health Organ. 1968;39:25–37.
Kars Z, Kansu T, Ozcan OE, Erbengi A. Orbital echinococcosis. Report of two cases studied by computerized tomography. J Clin Neuroophthalmol. 1982;2:197–9.
Makni F, Hachicha L, Mseddi F, Hammami H, Cheikhrouhou F, Sellami H, Mzali R, Boujelbene S, Rebai R, Beyrouti I, Ayadi A. Contribution of Western blotting to the diagnosis of hydatidosis. Bull Soc Pathol Exot. 2007;100:171–3.
Ortona E, Rigano R, Margutti P. Native and recombinant antigens in the immunodiagnosis of human cystic echinococcosis. Parasite Immunol. 2000;22:553–9.
Ortona E, Rigano R, Buttari B, Delunardo F, Ioppolo S, Margutti P, Profumo E, Teggi A, Vaccari S, Siracusano A. An update on immunodiagnosis of cystic echinococcosis. Acta Trop. 2003;85:165–71.
Özek MM, Pamir MN, Sav A. Spontaneous rupture of an intraorbital hydatid cyst. J Clin Neuroophthalmol. 1993;13:135–7.
Porreti D, Felleisen E, Grimm F, Pfister M, Teuscher F, Zuercher C, Reichen J, Gottstein B. Differential immunodiagnosis between cystic hydatid disease and other cross-reactive pathologies. Am J Trop Med Hyg. 1999;60:193–8.
Ramzy R, Helmi H, Zayyat E, Rifaat M, Hameed D, Abdel-Baki M. An enzyme-linked immunosorbent assay for detection of IgG1 antibodies specific to human cystic echinococcosis in Egypt. Trop Med Int Health. 1999;4:616–20.
Reittner P, Szolar D, Schmid M. Case report. Systemic manifestation of Echinococcus alveolaris infection. J Comput Assist Tomogr. 1996;20:1030–2.
Rosenvit M, Camicia F, Kamenetzky L, Musulin P, Gutierrez A. Identification and intra-specific variability analysis of secreted and membrane-bound proteins from Echinococcus granulosus. Parasitol Int. 2006;55:63–7.
Siles-Lucas M, Gottstein B. Review: molecular tools for the diagnosis of cystic and alveolar echinococcosis. Trop Med Int Health. 2001;6:463–75.
Taghipour M, Zamanizadeh B, Haghnegahdar A, Zare Z. Vertebral hydatidosis. Neurosurg Q. 2008;18(3):163–71.
Tappe D, Weise D, Ziegler U, Muller A, Mullges W, Stichr A. Brain and lung metastasis of alveoral echinococcosus in a refugee from a hyperendemic area. J Med Microbiol. 2008;57:1420–3.
Taratuto AL, Venturiello S. Echinococcosis. Brain Pathol. 1997;7:673–9.
Toussaint F, Pere P, Chaffotec L, Grandhaye P, Pourel J. Alveolar Echinococcosis of the spine. J Clin Rheumatol. 2001;7:448–51.
Turgut M. Hydatidosis of central nervous system and its coverings in the pediatric and adolescent age groups in Turkey during the last century: a critical review of 137 cases. Childs Nerv Syst. 2002;18:670–83.
Turgut M, Benli K, Eryilmaz M. Secondary multiple intracranial hydatid cysts caused by intracerebral embolism of cardiac echinococcosis: an exceptional case of hydatidosis. J Neurosurg. 1997;86:714–8.
Verastegui M, Moro P, Guevara A, Rodrigues T, Miranda E, Gilman R. Enzyme-linked immunoelectrotransfer blot test for diagnosis of human hydatid disease. J Clin Microbiol. 1992;30:1557–61.
Vogel H. How does the alveolar echinococcus grow (in German). Tropenmed Parasitol. 1978;29:1–11.
Weiss JB. DNA probes and PCR for diagnosis of parasitic infection. Clin Microbiol Rev. 1995;8:113–30.
Yang Y, Sun T, McManus D. Molecular confirmation of a case of multiorgan cystic echinococcosis. J Parasitol. 2006;92:206–8.
Yang Y, Vuitton D, Jones M, Craig P, McManus D. Brain metastasis of alveolar echinococcosis in hyperendemic focus of Echinococcus multilocularis infection. Trans R Soc Trop Med Hyg. 2005;99:937–41.
Zhang W, McManus D. Recent advances in the immunology and diagnosis of echinococcosis. Immunol Med Microbiol. 2006;47:24–41.
Zhang W, Li J, McManus D. Concepts in immunology and diagnosis of hydatid disease. Clin Microbiol Rev. 2003;16:18–36.

Imaging of Cerebral Hydatid Disease

11

Ahmed Abdel Khalek Abdel Razek and Omran Elshamam

Contents

A.A.K.A. Razek, MD
Department of Diagnostic Radiology, Mansoura Faculty of Medicine, Elgomheryia Street, Mansoura 35512, Egypt
e-mail: arazek@mans.edu.eg

O. Elshamam
Tripoli Medical Center, Tripoli, Libya

Introduction

In humans, the two main types of hydatid disease are cystic echinococcus (CE) and alveolar echinococcosis (AE) that are caused by *Echinococcus granulosus* and *E. multilocularis*, respectively (da Rocha et al. 2005; Foerster et al. 2007; Aiken 2010).

Classification

There are different classifications of CE. It may be classified as simple, complex, or infected cysts or as unilocular or multilocular cysts (Abdel Razek et al. 2009; Brunetti et al. 2010). The World Health Organization Informal Working Group on Echinococcus of CE follows the natural history of the cyst and classifies CE according to its viability into active fertile (CE1 and CE2); transitional (CE3); and degenerated, inactive, and infertile cysts (CE4 and CE5). The use of such classifications facilitates the application of uniform standards and principles of treatment for each cyst type in different parts of the world. The presence of protoscoleces and scoleces at histopathological examination is helpful in the evaluation of viability of the CE and serves as a guide for radiologists working in a multidisciplinary committee with clinicians, surgeons, and pathologists (Abdel Razek et al. 2009; Brunetti et al. 2010).

M. Turgut (ed.), *Hydatidosis of the Central Nervous System: Diagnosis and Treatment*,
DOI 10.1007/978-3-642-54359-3_11, © Springer-Verlag Berlin Heidelberg 2014

Methods of Examination

Routine pre- and post-contrast magnetic resonance imaging (MRI) is commonly used for diagnosis, localization, and classification of cerebral CE. Advanced MRI techniques such as magnetic resonance spectroscopy (MRS), diffusion-weighted MRI (DW-MRI), and perfusion-weighted MRI may help in the diagnosis of cerebral hydatid cyst. Multidetector computed tomography (CT) scan has also been used for the diagnosis of intracranial hydatid cysts, especially the calcified lesions (Demir et al. 1991; Topal et al. 1995; Tüzün and Hekimoglu 1998; El-Shamam et al. 2001; Sqahin-Akyar 2002; Bukte et al. 2004; Ravalji et al. 2006; Basraoui et al. 2010; Wani et al. 2010, 2011; Bartosch et al. 2011).

Imaging Appearance

The cystic lesion (CL) appears as a simple cyst without a discernible wall. This form must be considered in the differential diagnosis of cystic lesions of the brain. CL are active lesions, as they represent an early stage of cyst development (Abdel Razek et al. 2009, 2011).

The CE1 cyst: It is the most common type of CE and represents the active form of the disease. At CT scan, it appears as a large well-defined thin-walled hypodense cyst with marginal calcification along the wall in some cases (Bartosch et al. 2011; Basraoui et al. 2010; Bukte et al. 2004; Ravalji et al. 2006; Wani et al. 2010). On MRI, it appears as a spherical or oval and well-defined, smooth, thin-walled, homogeneous cerebrospinal fluid-isointense cystic lesion, which may reach up to 15 cm in size. Cerebral edema around the cyst is not a common finding, but may occur infrequently. The hypointense rim on T2-weighted MRIs represents the outer, host-derived pericyst, middle laminated membrane, and inner germinal layer (Sqahin-Akyar 2002; Bukte et al. 2004; Ravalji et al. 2006). A thin rim of contrast enhancement limited to the capsule may be detected. Contrast enhancement is not typical since the lesion is usually quiescent. Thin rim of CE, limited to the capsule region, may be detected (usually only one segment) due to focal meningeal adhesions and inflammatory reactions due to previous cyst leakage (Abdel Razek et al. 2009, 2011) (Fig. 11.1).

The CE2 cyst: It appears as a unilocular maternal cyst with peripherally arranged broad daughter vesicles. The presence of smaller daughter cysts within the primary maternal cyst is considered to be pathognomonic of a hydatid cyst. It signifies an attempt at survival by a damaged or dying cyst. Daughter vesicles (broad capsules) are small spheres that carry the protoscoleces. Daughter vesicles are formed from internal budding of the germinal layer. The wall of the daughter cysts appears as low signal intensity (Abdel Razek et al. 2009, 2011). A high-signal-intensity rim may be seen around the maternal cyst on T2-weighted images. This is explained by degenerating larvae releasing metabolic products that disrupt the blood-brain barrier with host inflammatory response (Fig. 11.2).

The CE3 type: It develops from rupture of the primary cyst with endocystic proliferation of the hydatid cyst, and the cyst contents are confined within the pericyst, resulting in maternal cyst with multiple large daughter cysts. The maternal and daughter cysts are isointense on both T1- and T2-weighted images. When the daughter cysts completely fill the maternal cyst, the cysts appear as multiseptated and may produce "grapelike," "wheel-like," "rosette-like," or "honeycomb-like" structures (Abdel Razek et al. 2009, 2011) (Fig. 11.3).

The CE4 type: It appears as a cystic lesion with serpentine bands or floating membranes representing the detached or ruptured membranes. When the viability of the parasite is lost, the intracystic pressure is lowered and the endocystic membranes are detached and float freely. Intracystic wavy or serpentine bands ("water-lily sign") may appear, representing the delaminated germinal layer and rupture of the membranes. The presence of detached membranes with a ball-of-wool appearance is a sign of severe degeneration. Degenerated cysts consist of a heterogeneous, solid-looking pseudotumor that may show a "ball-of-wool sign" as the cystic lesion gradually becomes smaller

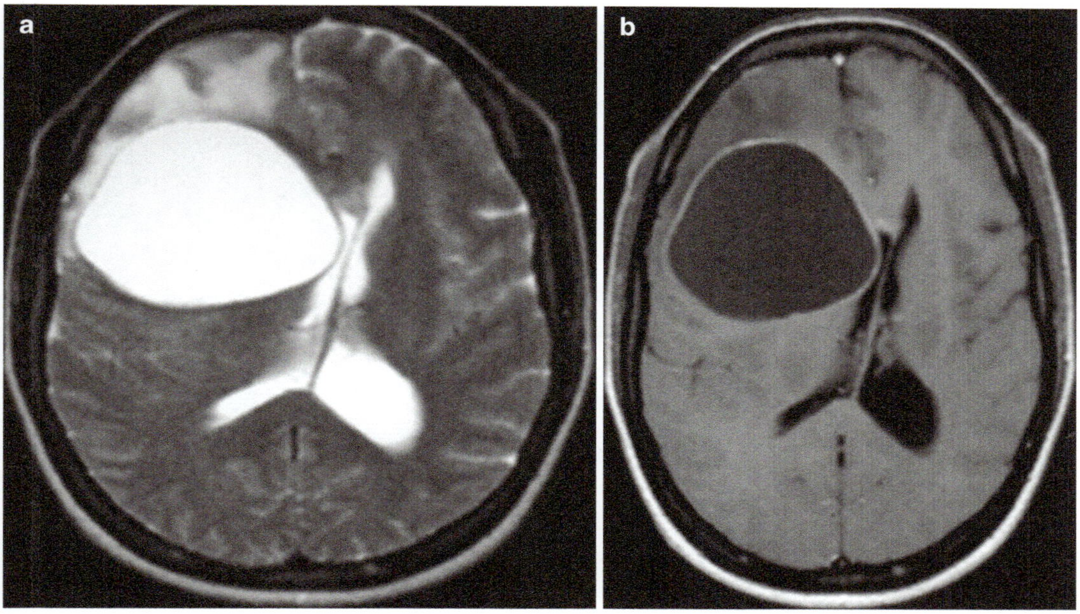

Fig. 11.1 CE1 type of hydatid cyst. (**a**) Axial T2-weighted MRI shows a large well-defined unilocular cystic lesion in the right parietal region with thick hypointense wall and mild marginal edema. (**b**) Post-contrast axial T1-weighted MRI shows homogenous low signal intensity of the cyst with mild marginal contrast enhancement

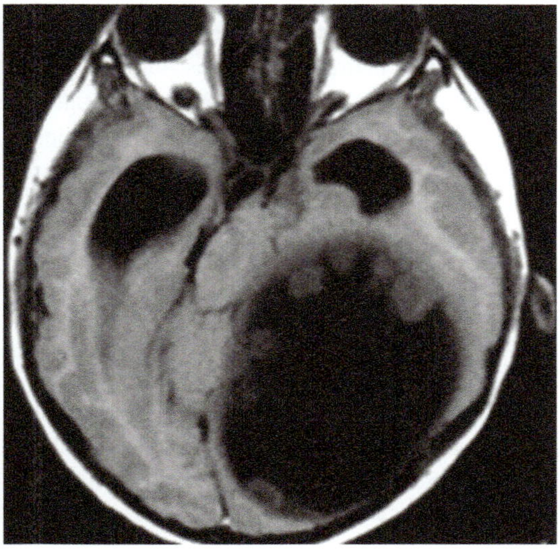

Fig. 11.2 CE2 type of hydatid cyst. Axial T1-weighted MRI shows a large maternal cyst with small peripherally arranged daughter vesicles

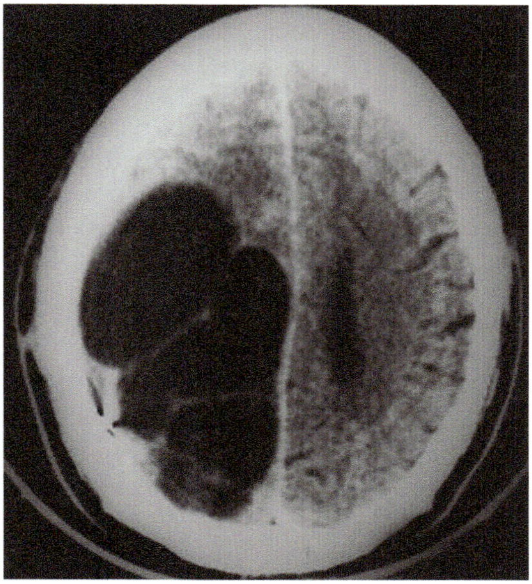

Fig. 11.3 CE3 type of hydatid cyst. Axial CT scan of the brain shows a large cyst with honeycomb appearance after surgery

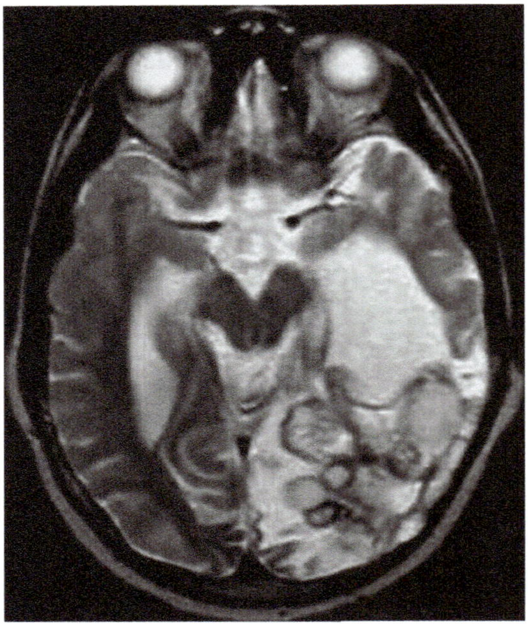

Fig. 11.4 CE4 type of hydatid cyst. Axial T2-weighted MRI shows a large cyst with ball-of-wool appearance in the left occipital region

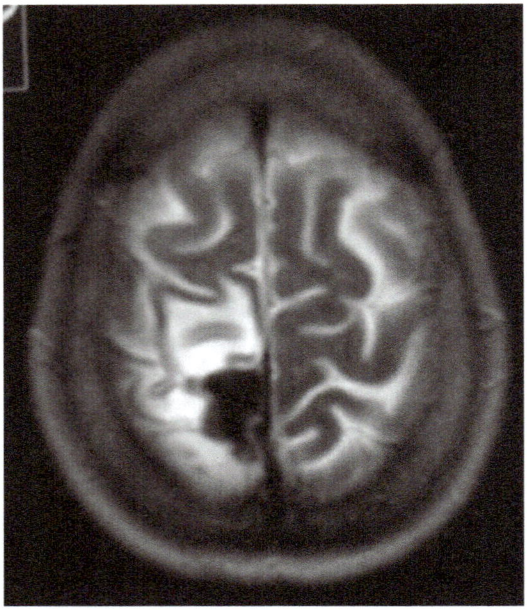

Fig. 11.5 CE5 type of hydatid cyst. Axial T2-weighted MRI shows a hypointense calcified dead cyst in the brain

and solidifies. Degenerating cysts show wavy or serpentine bands or floating membranes representing the detached or ruptured membranes (Abdel Razek et al. 2009, 2011) (Fig. 11.4).

The CE5 type: It is the infertile and dead form of CE. The dead cysts are characterized by a thick calcified wall in 50 % of patients. The degree of calcification varies from partial to complete calcification of the cyst. CT scan is best for detection of calcification. On MRI, the calcified lesion appears as signal void region (Abdel Razek et al. 2009; Basraoui et al. 2010; Bartosch et al. 2011) (Fig. 11.5).

Advanced Magnetic Resonance Imaging

Magnetic Resonance Spectroscopy

MRS may be added to the routine MRI protocol for a more accurate etiological diagnosis of a cystic lesion. MRS of cerebral CE shows dominant resonances of acetate (1.92 ppm), succinate (2.4 ppm), lactate (1.33 ppm), and glycine (3.56 ppm) and small contributions from alanine and isoleucine, leucine, and valine. The most specific metabolite of CE is a peak of succinate (2.4 ppm); however, a succinate peak has also been seen in pyogenic abscesses and neurocysticercosis. Other less-specific metabolites, such as lactate and acetate, are suggestive of infectious diseases. MRS studies ex vivo have found malate (4.3 ppm) and fumarate (6.5 ppm) in fertile cysts (Garg et al. 2002; Chawla et al. 2004; Hosch et al. 2008).

Diffusion Magnetic Resonance Imaging

CE is isointense with cerebrospinal fluid at diffusion-weighted MRI. The apparent diffusion coefficient (ADC) value of CE is $1.33 \pm 0.15 \times 10^{-3}$ s/mm^2 (Kittis et al. 2004).

Special Types

Multiple Hydatid Cysts

Multiple cerebral hydatid cysts, secondary or primary, are rare. Secondary infertile cysts are due to the surgical, spontaneous, or traumatic

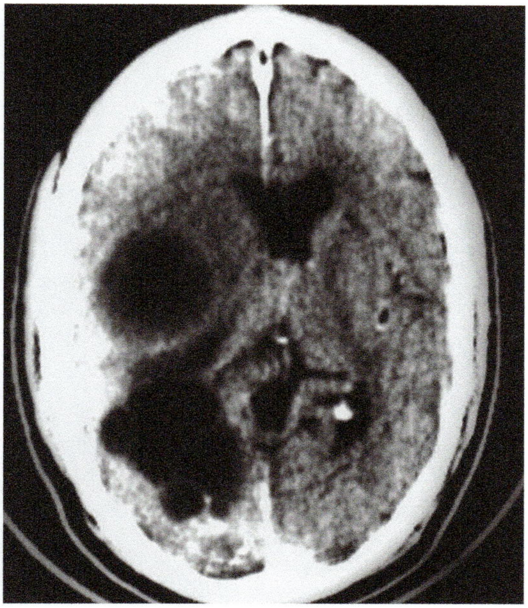

Fig. 11.6 Multiple hydatid cysts. Axial CT scan of the brain shows multiple hydatid cysts are seen in the right cerebral hemisphere

rupture of a viable primary lesion with spilling of the scolices inside the cerebral parenchyma, while multiple primary cysts result from embolization of a ruptured cardiac cyst (Al Zain et al. 2002; Lotfinia et al. 2007; Yurt et al. 2007) (Fig. 11.6).

Extraparenchymal Hydatid Cyst

The reported sites of extraparenchymal hydatid cyst include the subarachnoid space, cisterns, ventricles, pons, cerebellum, aqueduct of Sylvius, extradural space, and diploic space of skull bones (Diren et al. 1993; Tsitouridis et al. 1997; Lakhdar et al. 2010; Wani et al. 2010). Cranial extradural hydatid cyst is extremely rare because the physiologic flow of blood to the brain is mainly through the internal carotid system, so the likelihood of the larvae traveling through the external carotid system is very low (Cemil et al. 2009; Turgut 2010). Primary calvarial hydatid cysts arising from the dipole of the cranial bones with intracranial extension are extremely rare (Erman et al. 2001; Sharma et al. 2011). Different forms of extraparenchymal hydatidosis is discussed in detail in Chap. 21.

Infected Hydatid Cyst

When a secondary process occurs in the cyst, such as infection or rupture, the signal intensity tends to be slightly decreased on T2- and a little higher on T1-weighted images. When rupture, superinfection, or hemorrhage occurs in the cyst, the signal intensity may be slightly decreased on T2-weighted images and slightly increased on T1-weighted images (El-Shamam et al. 2001).

Stroke

Embolic stroke due to rupture of a hydatid cyst in cardiac cavity, a cause of ischemic infarction and multiple metastatic cyst formation, is an extremely rare entity (Martin et al. 1996; Turgut and Bayülkem 1998). Stroke as a complication of cardiac hydatidosis is discussed in detail in Chaps. 21 and 22.

Differential Diagnosis

CE on CT needs to be differentiated from porencephalic cyst, arachnoid cyst, brain abscess, and cystic tumor. Porencephalic and arachnoid cysts are not spherical and are not surrounded entirely by brain parenchyma. Porencephalic cyst shows signs of volume loss and gliosis in adjacent white matter. Arachnoid cyst is extra-axial in location, whereas intra-axial hydatid cyst is surrounded by brain parenchyma all around. Cystic tumor and brain abscess show definite contrast enhancement in the wall and/or mural nodule; perilesional edema is also present in case of abscess (Wani et al. 2010; Bartosch et al. 2011). The presence of multiple daughter cysts and hypointense ring in T2-weighted imaging is characteristic of CE (da Rocha et al. 2005).

Posttreatment

Methods

The treatment of cerebral CE is surgical and the aim of surgery is to excise the cyst completely without rupture to prevent anaphylactic reaction and local recurrence. The most commonly utilized surgical procedure designed to remove the intact cyst completely without rupture is by irrigating saline into the interface between the cyst wall and brain. However, medical treatment with albendazole has been reported with favorable results as an adjunct and, in certain circumstances, as the primary mode of treatment (Wani et al. 2010; Bartosch et al. 2011).

Surgical

The complications of hydatid cyst surgery are various and depend on the location, size, and multiplicity of the cysts. Intraoperative cyst rupture is the most common and serious complication which can lead to widespread dissemination followed by severe inflammatory or anaphylactic response. Subdural effusion occurs due to rapid drop of the intracranial pressure after the removal of the cyst with opening up the subdural space. Porencephalic cysts are abnormal brain cavities resulting from trauma and iatrogenic (postoperative) or perinatal vascular occlusion. These cavities are filled with cerebrospinal fluid and commonly connected with ventricles or subdural spaces (Fig. 11.7). Postoperative hemorrhage has been reported after surgery of hydatid cyst (Duishanbai et al. 2010; Tuzun et al. 2010).

Medical

Chemotherapy could be of great importance in patients with multiple cysts and in those unfit for surgery or suffering from recurrent disease. After medical treatment, the small cysts disappear, while large cysts are reduced in size and appear deformed or collapsed. Disappearance of daughter cysts has also been reported. Small foci of calcification have been seen on CT in the site of prior cysts, 12 ± 18 months after completion of treatment (Kalaitzoglou et al. 1998; Altas et al. 2010) (Fig. 11.7). Recently, MRS has been used for monitoring patient after medical treatment. The change in the levels of the alanine, succinate, acetate, and lactate in the cyst correlated well with the shrinkage and resolution of the cyst (Seckin et al. 2008).

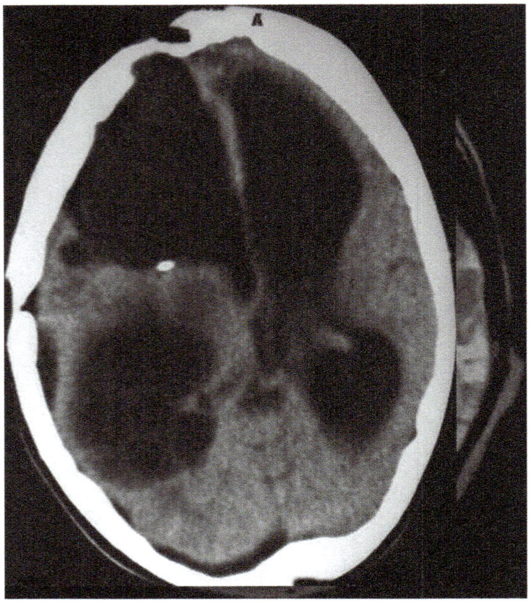

Fig. 11.7 Postoperative hydatid cyst. Axial CT scan shows a well-defined multilocular cyst which is seen in the right temporoparietal region associated with a thin-walled cyst in the right frontoparietal region of encephalomalacia. Note area of calcification is seen along the posterior wall of the cyst

Alveolar Echinococcosis

Alveolar echinococcosis (AE) is an uncommon form of hydatid disease caused by *E. multilocularis*. Cerebral infestation by AE and CE differ: AE occurs in adults who live in rural areas, whereas CE affects mostly children. CE infestation is usually self-limited, whereas AE infestation may appear as an infiltrative lesion in both the liver and brain, which makes total surgical removal difficult (Tunaci et al. 1999; Senturk et al. 2006; Ozdol et al. 2011).

AE features alveolar structures composed of numerous irregular cysts with a diameter between 1 and 20 mm that are not sharply demarcated from surrounding tissue. Central cystic cavities can result from necrosis of the inner part of the cyst. An irregularly thickened and partially calcified wall is present in most cases. This wall lies in the deep gray matter but may be in the posterior fossae. On CT and MRI, the lesions mainly appear as solid or multilocular cystic masses. Calcification and surrounding edema are common findings in these lesions. Peripheral ringlike, heterogeneous, nodular, and cauliflower-like enhancement patterns have all been reported. Perfusion-weighted MRI reveals low regional cerebral blood volume within the lesions because of gliosis and higher values in the periphery because of surrounding inflammation. This infection may mimic malignancy as a result of invasion of adjacent structures and destructive tissue growth (Bensaid et al. 1994; Piotin et al. 1997; Tunaci et al. 1999). On DW-MRI, the lesion is hypointense at b value 1,000 s/mm^2 with ADC value of $2.88 \pm 0.24 \times 10^{-3}$ s/mm^2 (Kittis et al. 2004).

Conclusion

We concluded that imaging is essential to diagnose different forms of intracranial hydatid cyst that represent different developmental and degenerative stages of hydatid cyst. Also, imaging can detect exact location and multiplicity of the lesion. Furthermore, imaging can be used for monitoring patients after surgical or medical treatment. Finally, advanced MRI is helpful for differentiating hydatid cyst from simulating lesions.

References

Abdel Razek A, Shamam O, Abdel wahab N. MR appearance of cerebral cystic echinococcosis: WHO classification. Acta Radiol. 2009;50:549–54.

Abdel Razek A, Watcharakorn A, Castillo M. Parasitic diseases of the central nervous system. Neuroimaging Clin N Am. 2011;21:815–41.

Aiken A. Central nervous system infection. Neuroimaging Clin N Am. 2010;20:557–80.

Al Zain TJ, Al-Witry SH, Khalili HM, Aboud SH, Al Zain Jr FT. Multiple intracranial hydatidosis. Acta Neurochir (Wien). 2002;44:1179–85.

Altas M, Aras M, Serarslan Y, Davran R, Evirgen O, Yilmaz N. A medically treated multiple cerebral hydatid cyst disease. J Neurosurg Sci. 2010;54:79–82.

Bartosch C, Reis C, Castro L. Large solitary cerebral hydatid cyst. Arch Neurol. 2011;68:946–7.

Basraoui D, El Idrissi I, Jalal H, Hiroual M, Essadki O, Ousehal A, Aniba K, Ghannane H, Lmejjati M, Ait Benali S. Intracranial hydatid cysts in children: a report of 9 cases (in French). J Radiol. 2010;91:293–6.

Bensaid A, Dietemann J, Filippe de la Palavesa M, Klinkert A, Kastler B, Gangi A, Jacquet G, Cattin F. Intracerebral alveolar echinococcosis: CT and MRI. Neuroradiology. 1994;36:289–91.

Brunetti E, Kern P, Vuitton DA, Writing Panel for the WHO-IWGE. Expert consensus for the diagnosis and treatment of cystic and alveolar echinococcosis in humans. Acta Trop. 2010;114:1–16.

Bukte Y, Kemanoglu S, Nazaroglu H, Ozkan U, Ceviz A, Simsek M. Cerebral hydatid disease: CT and MRI findings. Swiss Med Wkly. 2004;134:459–67.

Cemil B, Tun K, Gurcay A, Uygur A, Kaptanoglu E. Cranial epidural hydatid cysts: clinical report and review of the literature. Acta Neurochir (Wien). 2009;151:659–62.

Chawla S, Kumar S, Gupta R. Marker of parasitic cysts on in vivo proton magnetic resonance spectroscopy: is it succinate or pyruvate? J Magn Reson Imaging. 2004; 20:1052–3.

da Rocha A, Maia AC, Ferreira NP, do Amaral FL. Granulomatous diseases of the central nervous system. Top Magn Reson Imaging. 2005;16:155–87.

Demir K, Karsli A, Kaya T, Devrimci E, Alkan K. Cerebral hydatid cysts: CT findings. Neuroradiology. 1991;33:22–4.

Diren H, Ozcanli H, Boluk M, Kilic C. Unilocular orbital, cerebral and intraventricular hydatid cysts: CT diagnosis. Neuroradiology. 1993;35:149–50.

Duishanbai S, Jiafu D, Guo H, Liu C, Liu B, Aishalong M, Mijiti M, Wen H. Intracranial hydatid cyst in children: report of 30 cases. Childs Nerv Syst. 2010;26:821–7.

El-Shamam O, Amer T, El-Atta M. Magnetic resonance imaging of simple and infected hydatid cysts of the brain. Magn Reson Imaging. 2001;19:965–74.

Erman T, Tuna M, Göçer I, Ildan F, Zeren M, Cetinalp E. Intracranial intraosseous hydatid cyst. Case report and review of literature. Neurosurg Focus. 2001;11:ECP1.

Foerster B, Thurnher M, Malani P, Petrou M, Carets-Zumelzu F, Sundgren P. Intracranial infections: clinical and imaging characteristics. Acta Radiol. 2007; 48:875–93.

Garg M, Chawla S, Prasad KN, Roy R, Sikora SS, Kumar R, Husain M, Khetrapal CL, Gupta RK. Differentiation of hydatid cyst from cysticercus cyst by proton MR spectroscopy. NMR Biomed. 2002;15:320–6.

Hosch W, Junghanss T, Stojkovic M, Brunetti E, Heye T, Kauffmann GW, Hull WE. Metabolic viability assessment of cystic echinococcosis using high-field 1H MRS of cyst contents. NMR Biomed. 2008;21:734–54.

Kalaitzoglou I, Drevelengas A, Petridis A, Palladas P. Albendazole treatment of cerebral hydatid

disease: evaluation of results with CT and MRI. Neuroradiology. 1998;40:36–9.
Kittis O, Calli C, Yunten N. Report of diffusion-weighted MRI in two cases with different cerebral hydatid disease. Acta Radiol. 2004;45:85–7.
Lakhdar F, Arkha Y, Bougrine M, Derraz S, El Ouahabi A, El Khamlichi A. Posterior fossa extradural and extracranial hydatid cyst. Acta Neurochir (Wien). 2010;56:391–4.
Lotfinia I, Vahedi P, Hadidchi S, Djavadzadegan H. Multiple cerebral hydatid cysts secondary to embolization from intracardiac hydatidosis. Neurosurg Q. 2007;17:134–7.
Martin O, Chimpen R, Reviriego J, Sanchez R. Repeated strokes as a sign of multiple cerebral hydatid cysts (in Spanish). Neurologia. 1996;11:307–9.
Ozdol C, Yildirim AE, Daglioglu E, Divanlioglu D, Erdem E, Belen D. Alveolar hydatid cyst mimicking cerebellar metastatic tumor. Surg Neurol Int. 2011;29:2–13.
Piotin M, Cattin F, Kantelip B, Miralbes S, Godard J, Bonneville J. Disseminated intracerebral alveolar echinococcosis: CT and MRI. Neuroradiology. 1997;39:431–3.
Ravalji M, Kumar S, Shah A, Vaghela D, Makwana G, Singh H. CT and MRI features of the typical and atypical intracranial hydatid cysts: report of five cases. Indian J Radiol Imaging. 2006;16:727–32.
Seckin H, Yagmurlu B, Yigitkanli K, Kars H. Metabolic changes during successful medical therapy for brain hydatid cyst: case report. Surg Neurol. 2008;70:186–9.
Senturk S, Oguz K, Soylemezoglu F, Inci S. Cerebral alveolar echinococcosis mimicking primary brain tumor. AJNR Am J Neuroradiol. 2006;27:420–2.
Sharma AK, Diyora B, Badhe P, Nayak N, Patankar P, Chopra G. Neurological picture. Primary multiple calvarial hydatid cysts–a rare occurrence. J Neurol Neurosurg Psychiatry. 2011;82:349–50.
Sqahin-Akyar G. Computed tomography and magnetic resonance imaging findings in cerebral hydatid disease. Radiography. 2002;8:251–8.
Topal U, Parlak M, Kihc C, Sivri Z, Sadikoglu M, Tuncell E. CT and MRI findings in cerebral hydatid disease. Eur Radiol. 1995;5:244–7.
Tsitouridis J, Dimitriadis AS, Kazana E. MR in cisternal hydatid cysts. AJNR Am J Neuroradiol. 1997;18:1586–7.
Tunaci M, Tunaci A, Engin G, Özkorkmaz B, Ahishali B, Rozanes I. MRI of cerebral alveolar echinococcosis. Neuroradiology. 1999;41:844–6.
Turgut M. Intracranial extradural hydatid cysts: review of the literature. Acta Neurochir (Wien). 2010;152:1805–6.
Turgut M, Bayülkem K. Cerebrovascular occlusive disease: hydatidosis. Childs Nerv Syst. 1998;14:697–9.
Tüzün M, Hekimoglu B. Hydatid disease of the CNS: imaging features. AJR Am J Roentgenol. 1998;171:1497–500.
Tuzun Y, Solmaz I, Sengul G, Izci Y. The complications of cerebral hydatid cyst surgery in children. Childs Nerv Syst. 2010;26:47–51.
Wani N, Kosar T, Khan A, Ahmad S. Multidetector-row computed tomography in cerebral hydatid cyst. J Neurosci Rural Pract. 2010;1:112–4.
Wani NA, Kousar TL, Gojwari T, Robbani I, Singh M, Ramzan A, Khan Q, Kirmani A, Wani A. Computed tomography findings in cerebral hydatid disease. Turk Neurosurg. 2011;21:347–51.
Yurt A, Avci M, Selçuki M, Ozer F, Camlar M, Uçar K, Taşli F, Altinörs N. Multiple cerebral hydatid cysts report of a case with 24 pieces. Clin Neurol Neurosurg. 2007;109:821–6.

Imaging of Spinal Hydatid Disease

12

Alper Dilli, Umit Yaşar Ayaz, Ahmet Tuncay Turgut, and Halil Arslan

Contents

A. Dilli, MD
Department of Radiology, Dışkapı Yıldırım Beyazıt Training and Research Hospital, Ankara, Turkey

U.Y. Ayaz, MD
Department of Radiology, Mersin Women's and Children's Hospital, Mersin, Turkey

A.T. Turgut, MD (✉)
Department of Radiology, Ankara Training and Research Hospital, Angora Park Evleri, Rüyalar Caddesi 31, Mutlukent Mahallesi, TR-06800, Ankara, Turkey
e-mail: ahmettuncayturgut@yahoo.com

H. Arslan, MD
Department of Radiology, Dışkapı Yıldırım Beyazıt Training and Research Hospital, Ankara, Turkey

Introduction

Hydatid disease (echinococcosis) is a parasitic infection caused more frequently by *Echinococcus granulosus* and less frequently by *E. multilocularis* (*E. alveolaris*), the liver and lungs being the most commonly involved organs (Turgut 1997). Involvement of the spine is rare but it is clinically challenging (Fig. 12.1). Alveolar echinococcosis of the spine is much rarer, and imaging findings, such as inhomogeneous osteolysis of vertebral bodies without loss of intervertebral disk height with an associating paravertebral mass, may be nonspecific (Toussaint et al. 2001).

Patients with hydatid disease usually present with symptoms caused by spinal cord or nerve root compression (Akhan et al. 1991; Pandey and Chaudhari 1997; Işlekel et al. 1998; Hilmani et al. 2004; Layadi et al. 2005; Adilay et al. 2007; Gopal et al. 2007; Kaen et al. 2009; Limaiem et al. 2010). Hydatid disease can be seen at any level of the spine (Bouras et al. 1984; Mathuriya et al. 1985; Göçer et al. 1994; von Sinner and Akhtar 1994; Pandey and Chaudhari 1997; Turgut 1997; Singh et al. 1998; Layadi et al. 2005; Adilay et al. 2007; Song et al. 2007; Arif and Zaheer 2009; Senoglu et al. 2009), but thoracic vertebrae are more commonly involved (Polat et al. 2003; Gopal et al. 2007), sometimes misleading to the diagnosis of Pott's disease (Bouras et al. 1984; Turgut 1997; Song et al. 2007) and mimicking tuberculous spondylodiscitis (Tabak et al. 2007). Intradural hydatid at the foramen magnum was reported with all features

M. Turgut (ed.), *Hydatidosis of the Central Nervous System: Diagnosis and Treatment*, DOI 10.1007/978-3-642-54359-3_12, © Springer-Verlag Berlin Heidelberg 2014

of spinomedullary compression including respiratory distress, so hydatid disease should be considered in the differential diagnosis of compressive lesions at the foramen magnum (Mathuriya et al. 1985).

Hydatid cysts were classified according to their relationship with the dura mater, spinal canal, and spinal cord (Pamir et al. 1984; Fahl et al. 1994; von Sinner and Akhtar 1994; Berk et al. 1998; Turgut 2002; Polat et al. 2003; Adilay et al. 2007; Gopal et al. 2007; Arif and Zaheer 2009; Güneş et al. 2009) as intramedullary hydatid cysts, intradural extramedullary hydatid cysts, extradural-intraspinal hydatid cysts (Fig. 12.2), hydatid cysts of the vertebrae (Figs. 12.3, 12.4, 12.5, 12.6, and 12.7), and paravertebral hydatid cysts (Figs. 12.4, 12.8 and 12.9) (Polat et al. 2003). Intradural hydatid cysts are rare (Pamir et al. 1984; Kahilogullari et al. 2005; Arif and Zaheer 2009; Güneş et al. 2009).

Lack of osteoporosis and sclerosis in involved bone, absence of damage to intervertebral disk spaces and vertebral bodies, paraspinal extension, and (in the thoracic spine) involvement of contiguous rib are the most common features of spinal hydatid disease (Polat et al. 2003). Hydatid disease of the spine usually begins in the vertebral body. The cysts show slow growth in the direction of least resistance (Polat et al. 2003; Phatak 2006). With time, the parasite replaces the osseous tissue and destroys the cortex. It then spreads from bone to surrounding tissue such as muscle and the spinal cord (Polat et al. 2003). Extension into the spinal canal results in spinal cord and neural compression (Gopal et al. 2007). Hydatid cysts that lack the typical radiographic appearance may be mistaken for arachnoid cysts (Secer et al. 2008).

Plain X-rays are routinely obtained as a part of initial imaging but radiographic findings of spinal hydatid disease are nonspecific (Fig. 12.3). Plain X-rays may show bone destruction (Fig. 12.4) and sometimes abnormal soft tissue masses in the paravertebral region (Phatak 2006). However, they may show no bony abnormalities (Gopal et al. 2007; Arif and Zaheer 2009). It should be remembered that, radiographically, no sclerosis or periosteal reaction is evident in the early stages of the disease (Farzan et al. 2006).

Computed tomography (CT) and magnetic resonance imaging (MRI) demonstrate cystic cerebral hydatid disease effectively (Bükte et al. 2004) and they also serve for imaging of spinal hydatid disease (Figs. 12.1, 12.2, 12.3, 12.4, 12.5, 12.6, 12.7, and 12.9). After obtaining plain X-rays, CT and MRI should be used for further imaging as diagnostic tools of choice (Göçer et al. 1994; Turgut 1997; Gopal et al. 2007). CT and/or MRI techniques were found to be extremely useful, both for reaching the correct diagnosis and for proper surgical management of hydatid disease (Turgut 2002). CT and MRI have revolutionized neurosurgical practice for the diagnosis of hydatid cysts and allowed early diagnosis of the disease and provided localization of the lesions more accurately than we could do with plain X-ray, and also they could show multiple lesions (Turgut 1997); therefore, they are of value in preoperative planning of the surgical approach to hydatid lesions of the skeleton.

On CT and MRI, the appearance of the cystic fluid resembles that of cerebrospinal fluid (CSF) (Figs. 12.2, 12.3, 12.8, and 12.9) (Polat et al. 2003; Layadi et al. 2005; Gopal et al. 2007; Senoglu et al. 2009). In the past, myelography and CT myelography were used in the diagnosis of spinal hydatid disease (Işlekel et al. 1998), but now MRI has replaced the need for invasive myelography procedures.

Computed Tomography Scan

CT scan is effective in demonstrating the destructive hydatid lesions in vertebrae (Figs. 12.3, 12.4, 12.5, and 12.7), in determining their spread, and in establishing the presence of other hydatid cysts in adjacent soft tissues (Bouras et al. 1984; von Sinner and Akhtar 1994). CT could show multiple hydatid cysts in the ipsilateral psoas (Figs. 12.8) and quadratus lumborum muscles,

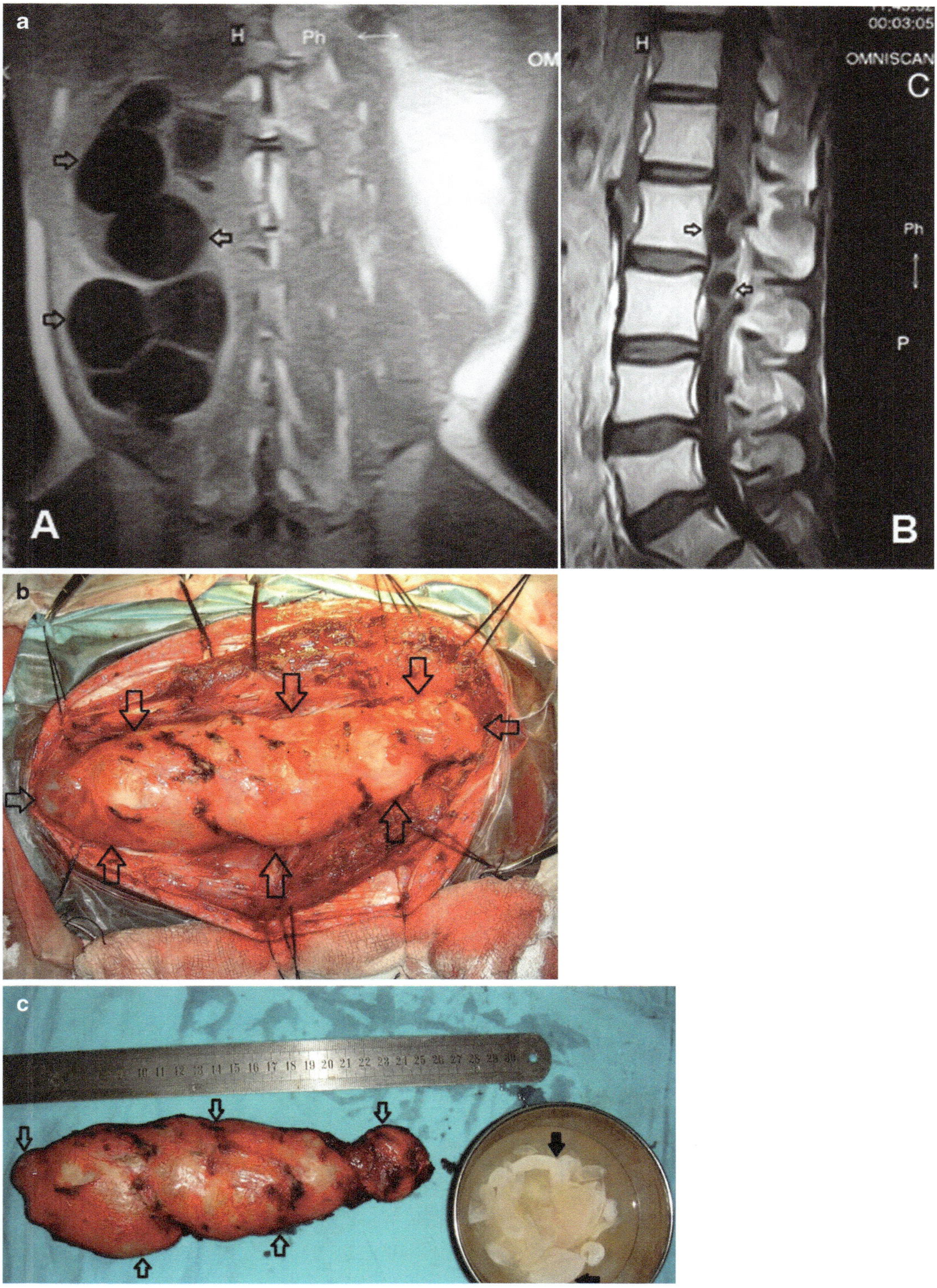

Fig. 12.1 (**a**) Spinal hydatid cysts (*arrows*). (**b**) Spinal hydatid preoperative view (*arrows*). (**c**) Spinal hydatid resected specimen (*arrows*) (Courtesy of D. Chowdhury, MD)

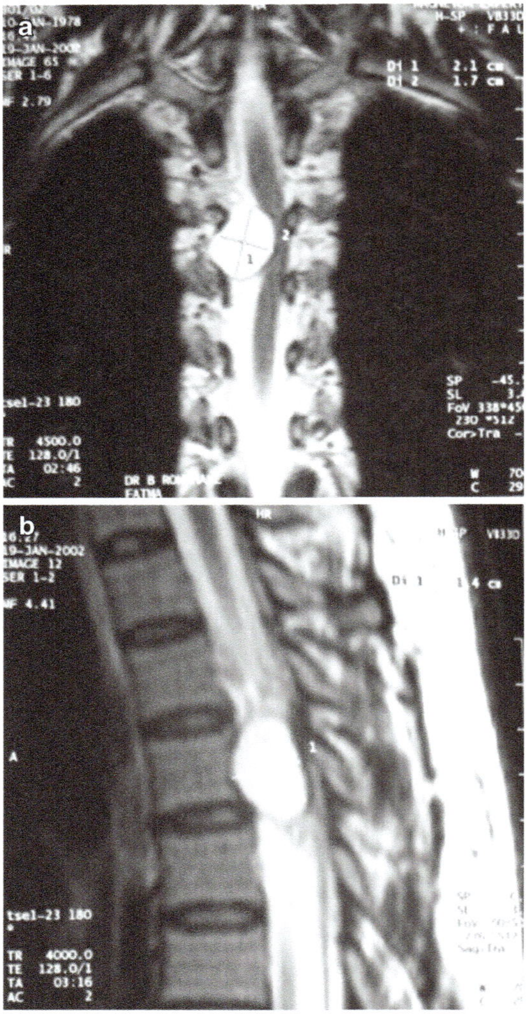

Fig. 12.2 (**a**, **b**) A 24-year-old male patient with extradural hydatid cyst at T4 vertebra corpus level (Courtesy of F. Limaiem, MD)

widening of the neural foramen, and extension of cyst into the neural canal compressing the spinal cord (Phatak 2006).

In a 73-year-old man with sacral/retroperitoneal hydatid disease, CT could demonstrate a large, multiloculated, lytic lesion that expanded anteriorly causing extensive destruction of the sacrum and extending into the sacral canal. CT shows the cystic nature of the lesions which are isodense to CSF (Senoglu et al. 2009), but it is not possible to differentiate an extramedullary hydatid cyst from an arachnoid cyst by using only the CT views (Tuncel 2008).

Usually no rim enhancement is evident after injection of contrast material, but there may be some exceptional cases. CT could show peripheral rim enhancement in a case with an infected intradural hydatid cyst at the foramen magnum (Mathuriya et al. 1985). In a 45-year-old woman with lumbar vertebral hydatid disease, axial contrast-enhanced CT could demonstrate increased contrast enhancement peripheral to the secondary lesions in the erector spinae muscles and spinal canal (Polat et al. 2003).

Contrast enhancement may be seen in alveolar echinococcosis. Contrast-enhanced CT images of an 80-year-old man with primary extrahepatic alveolar echinococcosis showed a multilobulated cystic mass in the right retroperitoneum originating from the psoas muscle, where the cystic components had fluidlike density and thickened septae with mild contrast enhancement. Besides, the lumbar spine presented lytic lesions of the first and second lumbar vertebra with partial cortical destruction (Nell et al. 2011).

Calcification is rare in spinal hydatid disease (Polat et al. 2003). However, on CT scan, the existence of calcification in the cyst wall, appearance of microvesicular polycystic vertebra, or the development of vertebral compression fracture can be observed in the last stage of involvement of the spine (Turgut et al. 2007).

CT was also used for the treatment where CT-guided needle aspiration and hypertonic saline irrigation of a multilocular extradural cervical spinal hydatid cyst causing severe spinal cord compression eliminated the need for emergency surgery and provided complete resolution of the patient's quadriplegia (Spektor et al. 1997).

Magnetic Resonance Imaging

More recently, MRI became the first imaging modality in patients with myelopathy and/or radiculopathy, with multiple daughter cysts within a parent cyst in spinal hydatidosis (Turgut

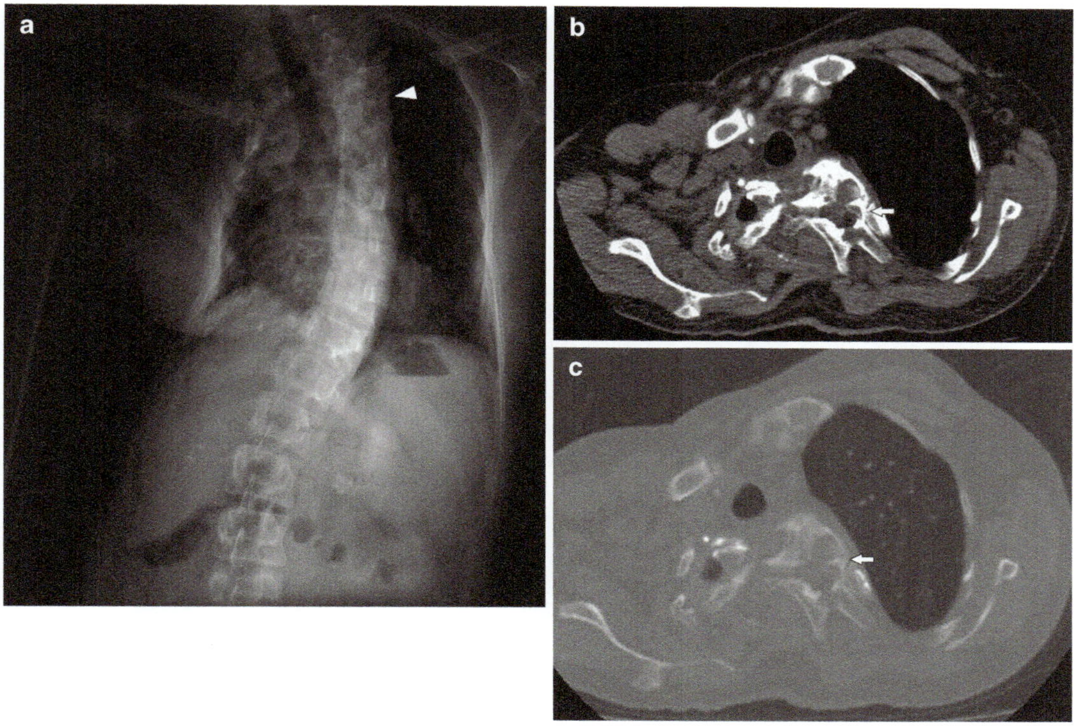

Fig. 12.3 Anteroposterior plain X-ray (**a**) of a 54-year-old male patient with thoracic spinal hydatid disease. There is marked kyphoscoliosis (*arrowhead*). Subtle radiolucent areas can be seen in the upper thoracic vertebrae. Unenhanced axial chest CT images with soft tissue window (**b**) and bone window (**c**) settings demonstrate hypodense cystic lesion in the vertebral corpus, which is isodense to cerebrospinal fluid, causing bone destruction and extending into the upper thoracic spinal canal (*arrow*). Chest deformities and subsequent tracheal deviation are prominent

et al. 2007). Although X-ray or CT images of spinal echinococcosis are similar to tuberculosis, metastases, giant cell tumors, or cysts of the bone, MRI was reported to show distinctive diagnostic features of spinal hydatid disease (Song et al. 2007).

MRI confirms the multicystic/multiloculated/multiseptated nature of the lesion (Figs. 12.1, 12.4, 12.8 and 12.9) (Gopal et al. 2007; Song et al. 2007; Güneş et al. 2009; Kaen et al. 2009; Senoglu et al. 2009; Turan Süslü et al. 2009) and is useful in the demonstration of complications such as spinal cord and/or nerve root compression (Gopal et al. 2007; Kaen et al. 2009).

MRI was stated to be the diagnostic procedure of choice in the face of neurological deficit (Turgut 1997). MRI characteristically shows a lesion resembling a bunch of grapes (Figs. 12.1, 12.8 and 12.9) which can help in distinguishing hydatid infestation from spinal tuberculosis. In spinal hydatid disease, cyst walls are thin and regular (Figs. 12.2 and 12.8); the presence of a markedly hypointense cyst wall on T1-weighted and T2-weighted images and the absence of wall enhancement with gadolinium are characteristic of hydatid disease (Limaiem et al. 2010).

On lumbar MRI of a 36-year-old man with extradural-intraspinal and paravertebral hydatid disease secondary to the spread of vertebral lesions, axial spin-echo T1-weighted image through the L3 vertebra showed multiple hypointense masses in the vertebral body and in the paravertebral and extradural-intraspinal areas, and corresponding axial fast spin-echo T2-weighted image showed multiple areas of increased signal intensity.

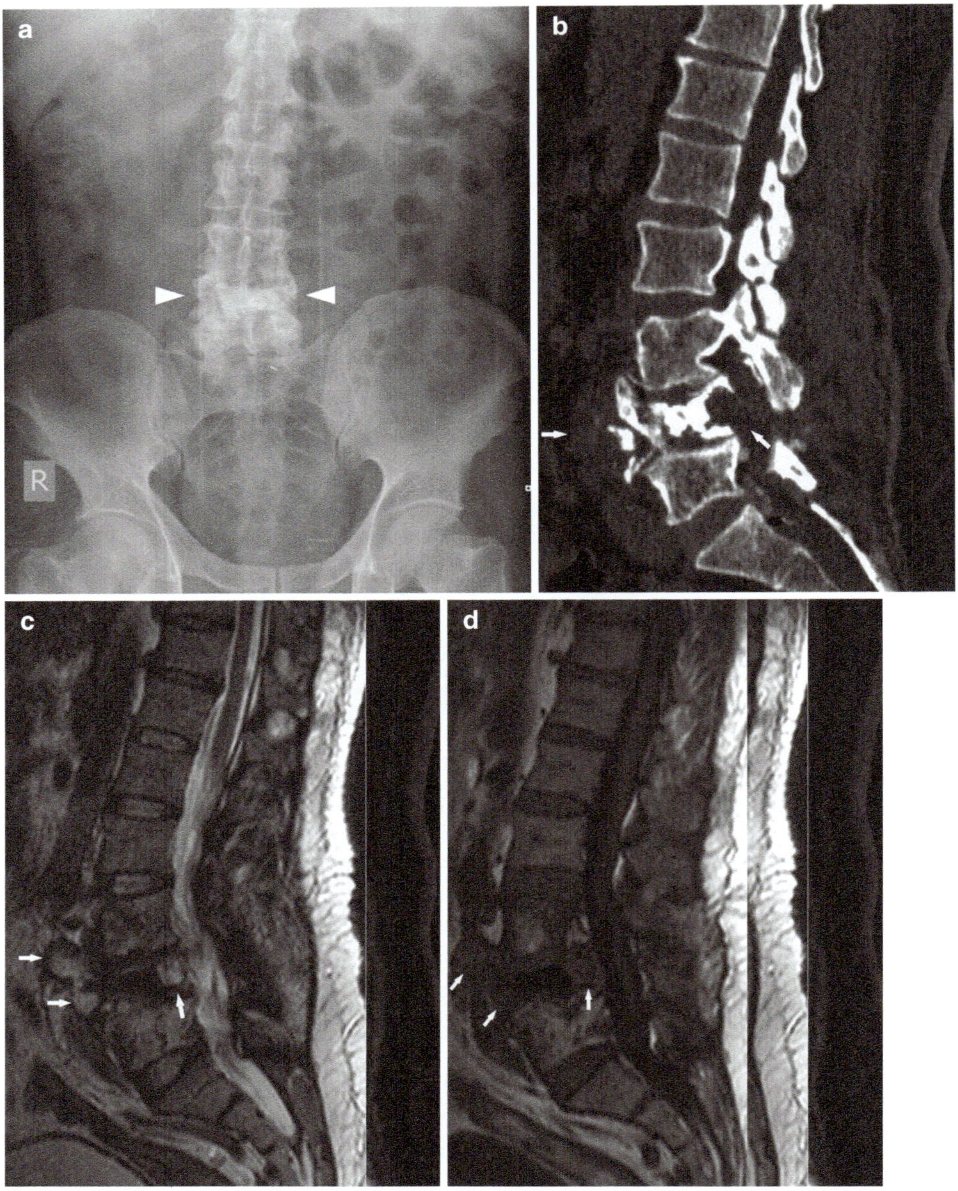

Fig. 12.4 Anteroposterior plain X-ray (**a**) of a 43-year-old male patient with lumbar spinal hydatid disease. Decreased vertebral height and diffuse sclerosis is noticed at L4 vertebra (*arrowheads*). Sagittal reformatted CT image with bone window settings (**b**) demonstrates expansion and destruction at L4 vertebra with both sclerotic and lytic areas (*arrows*). Anterior paravertebral lesions with soft tissue density can also be seen. Sagittal spinal MRI demonstrates loss of height and destructive appearance with associating cystic lesions, hyperintense on T2-weighted image (**c**) and hypointense on T1-weighted image (**d**) (*arrows*), some of which extend into anterior paravertebral areas

Extradural-intraspinal masses had low-signal-intensity rims, and there was also marked destruction of the right anterolateral portion of the vertebral body (Polat et al. 2003). On MRI of another patient, multiple hydatid cysts in ipsilateral psoas and quadratus lumborum

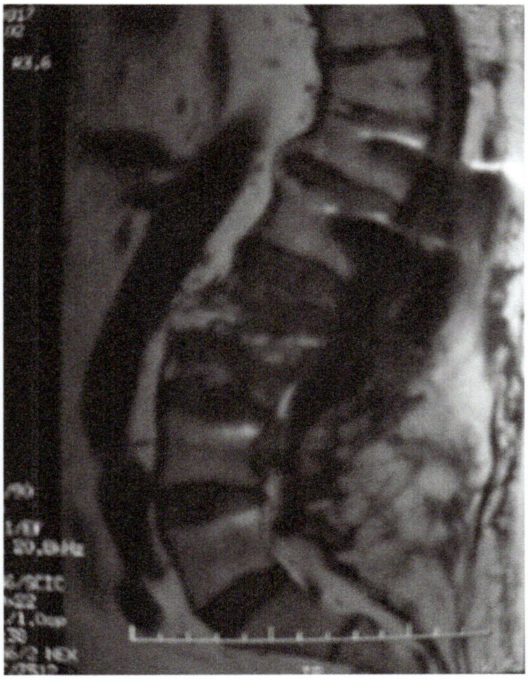

Fig. 12.5 A 59-year-old male patient who was operated 2 years ago had anterior debridement with partial corpectomy and grafting, posterior fusion. Despite the recurrence of disease, chemotherapy was not followed by the patient (Courtesy of A. Herrera, MD, PhD)

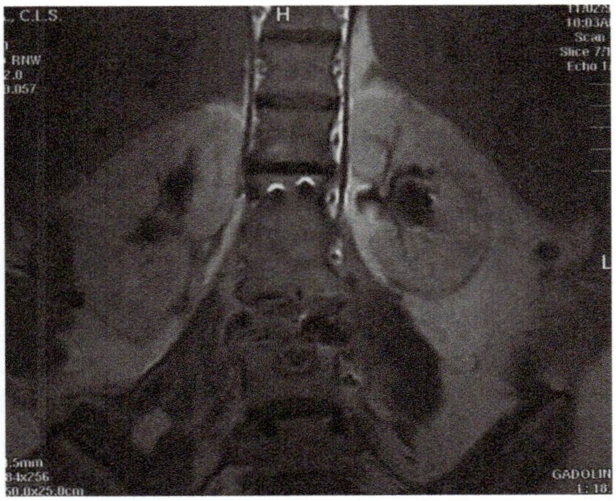

Fig. 12.6 A 46-year-old female patient. MRI lumbar spine hydatid lesions in L3 (Courtesy of A. Herrera, MD, PhD)

muscles were hypointense on T1-weighted images and hyperintense on T2-weighted images (Phatak 2006). In a 73-year-old man with sacral/retroperitoneal hydatid disease, MRI demonstrated a multilobular cystic lesion with thin and regular cyst walls, compressing the nerve roots. The cyst contents were hypointense on T1-weighted images and hyperintense on T2-weighted images, with an intensity similar to that of CSF (Senoglu et al. 2009). In a 25-year-old female, intradural lesions without vertebral involvement at lumbar level demonstrated low-intensity signal on T1-weighted images without enhancement after gadolinium injection and high-intensity signal on T2-weighted images (Hilmani et al. 2004).

In a pediatric case, an intradural, extramedullary cystic lesion which was seen to extend from L1 to L4 spine was hypointense on T1-weighted images and hyperintense on T2-weighted images (Arif and Zaheer 2009). In a 15-year-old male patient with a primary solitary hydatid cyst of the sacral spinal canal, plain X-rays and MRI revealed a widened sacral canal with pressure changes, and MRI confirmed the cystic nature of the lesion which had intensities that were similar to those of CSF (Pandey and Chaudhari 1997).

It should be kept in mind that MRI findings in alveolar echinococcosis of the spine may be nonspecific, unusual, or confusing. In an 80-year-old man with primary extrahepatic alveolar echinococcosis, T2-weighted axial images showed multiple small hyperintense lesions in the right psoas muscle, and corresponding fat-suppressed T1-weighted image after gadolinium administration confirmed the diagnosis of a multicystic mass and delineated the thickened, contrast-enhancing septations around the cystic components. T1-weighted image and T2-weighted STIR image of the lumbar spine in sagittal orientation showed the bone marrow replacement within the first, second, and third lumbar vertebrae (Nell et al. 2011).

MRI has been used postoperatively both to demonstrate recurrent cysts (Fig. 12.5) (Adilay et al. 2007; Arif and Zaheer 2009; Papakonstantinou et al. 2011) and to follow up the patient in order to show no recurrence of spinal cystic lesion (Fig. 12.10) (Arif and Zaheer 2009; Senoglu et al. 2009). On MRI, recurrent

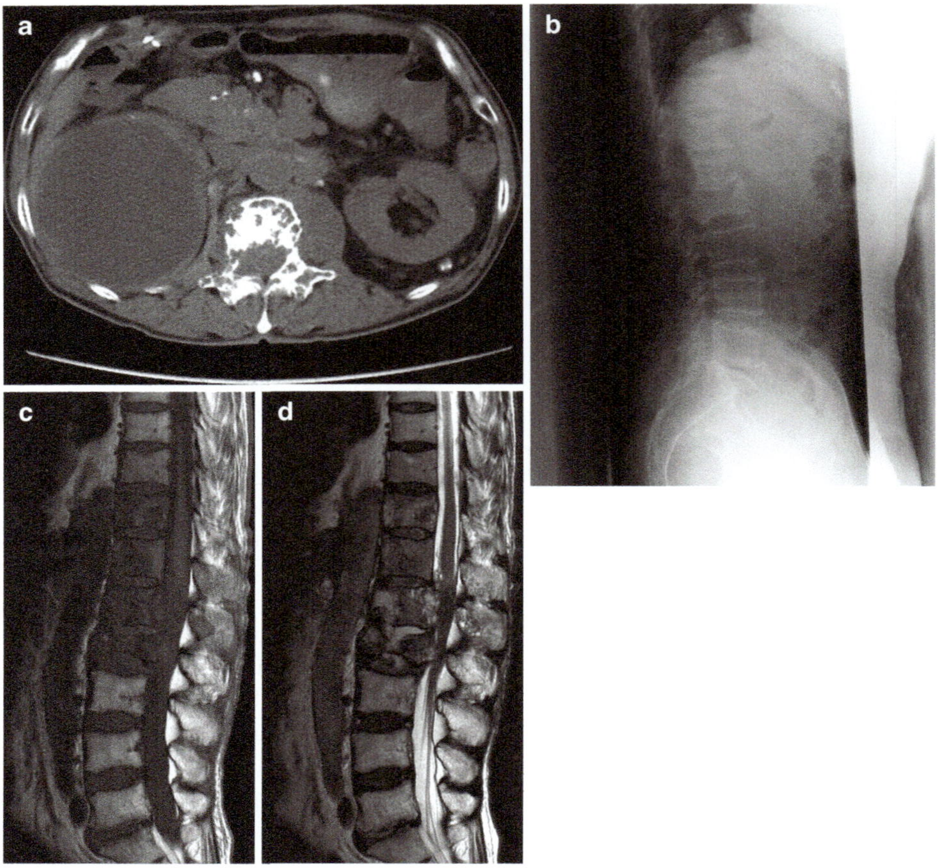

Fig. 12.7 (**a–d**) A 73-year-old male patient. He underwent palliative posterior decompression and instrumentation but died 2 years postoperatively (Courtesy of H. Sudo, MD)

hydatid disease is characterized by extensive involvement of the paravertebral soft tissues, soft tissues of the back at the site of previous laminectomies, and extradural space; extension into the intervertebral disk and iliopsoas muscles and skip lesions in the extradural space are not uncommon (Papakonstantinou et al. 2011).

Diffusion-weighted MRI (DW-MRI) can help differentiate complicated hydatidosis from other cystic lesions (Doganay and Kantarci 2009; Bhake and Agrawal 2010). Conventional MRI and DW-MRI were reported to be useful not only in the diagnosis of intradural extramedullary hydatid disease of the spine but also in determining a treatment protocol. Presence of restricted diffusion shows that the cystic lesions are complicated and infected, which require urgent surgery (Doganay and Kantarci 2009). In a 14-year-old boy, conventional MRI showed cystic multiloculated lesions in the lumbosacral spinal canal which were hypointense on T1 and hyperintense on T2-weighted images. DW-MRI of the boy showed hypointensity in the cystic lesions, and apparent diffusion-coefficient map images showed hyperintensity at the same level, without any evidence of restricted diffusion in the spinal canal (Doganay and Kantarci 2009).

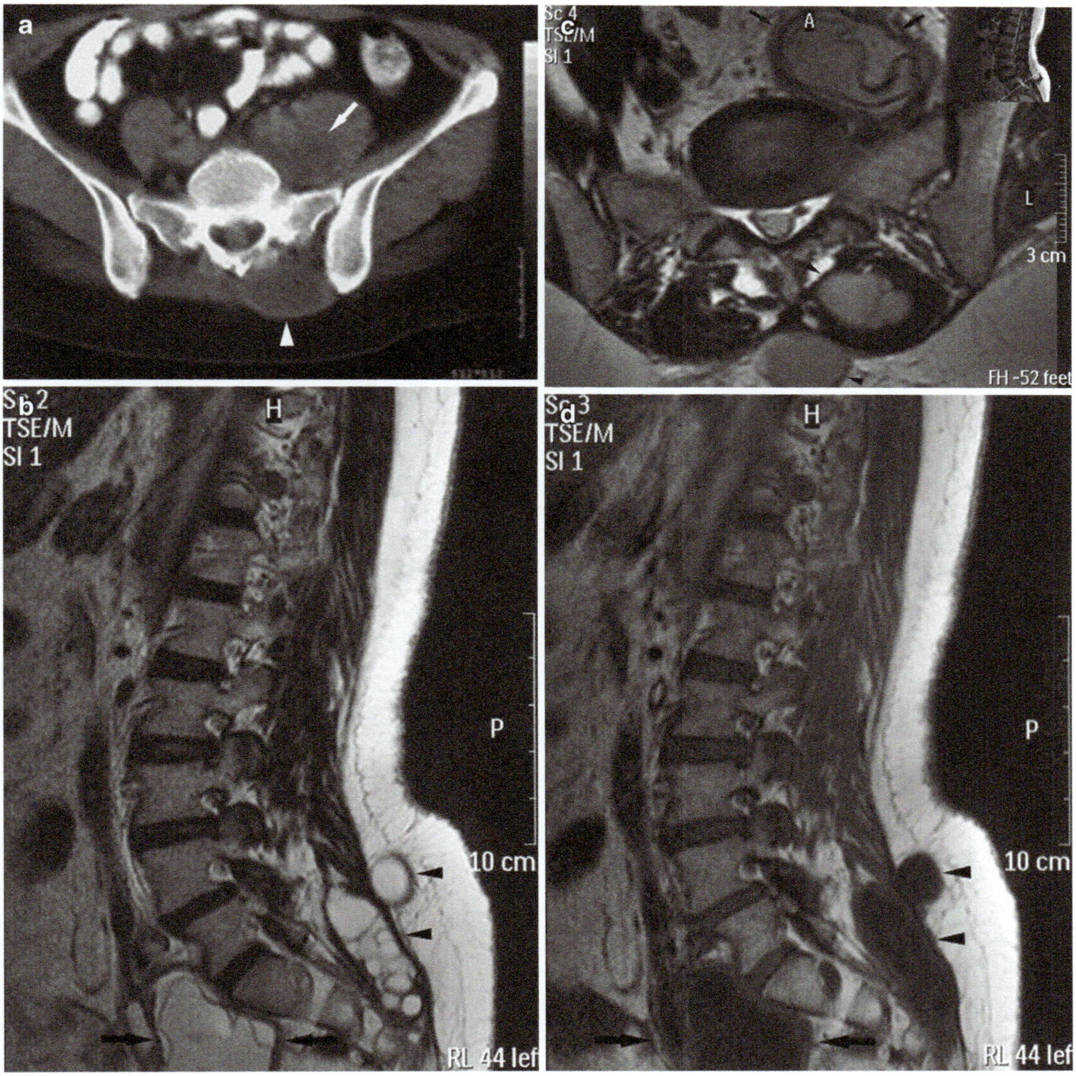

Fig. 12.8 In a 46-year-old female with multiple sacral paraspinal hydatid cysts on the left side, unenhanced axial pelvic CT image (**a**) demonstrates a hypodense hydatid cyst (*white arrow*) in the left psoas muscle which shows a close relation with left sacral neural foramina and nerves. Posterior to the sacrum, another hydatid lesion (*white arrowhead*) is located in the erector spinae muscle. MRI reveals multicystic-multiloculated sacral paraspinal hydatid lesions (*black arrows*: lesion anterior to the sacrum, *black arrowheads*: lesions posterior to the sacrum) as sharply demarcated hyperintense lesions on sagittal T2-weighted (**b**) and axial T2-weighted (**c**) images, which are hypointense on sagittal T1-weighted image (**d**). One of the posteriorly located cysts protrudes into subcutaneous fat (*black arrowhead*). On sagittal (**b**) and axial T2-weighted images (**c**), collapsed germinative membranes inside the cyst in the left psoas muscle were clearly demonstrated (*black arrows*). All the cysts are isointense to cerebrospinal fluid

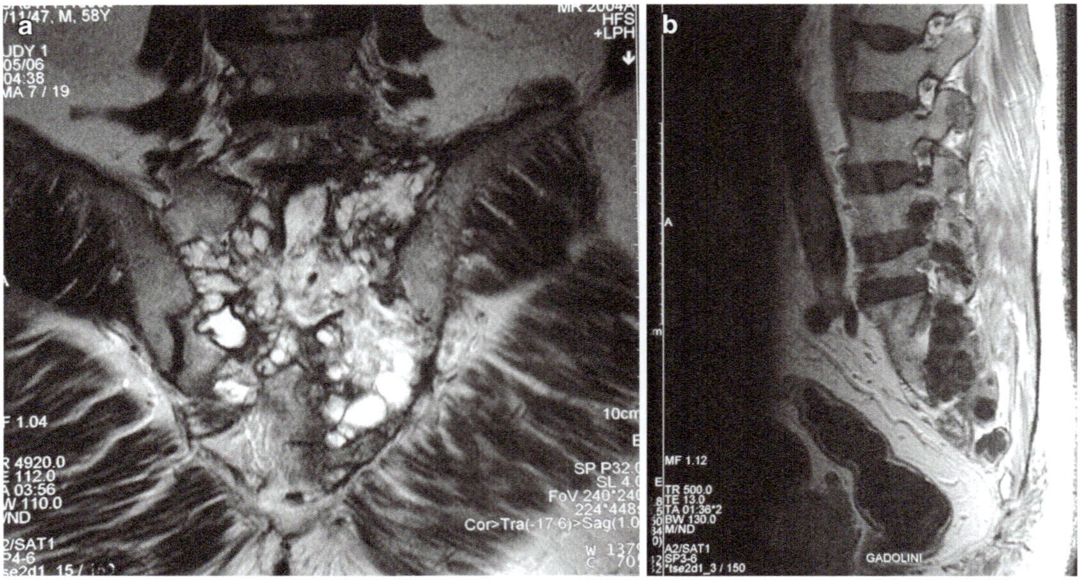

Fig. 12.9 (**a**, **b**) Sacral hydatidosis without accompanying neurological injury in a 61-year-old male patient. The patient with lung and liver hydatid cysts was not treated and transferred to his country of origin, Morocco (Courtesy of A. Herrera, MD, PhD)

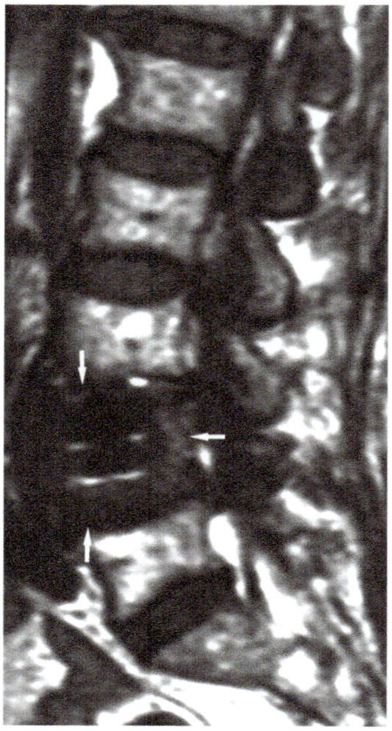

Fig. 12.10 Follow-up imaging of a 56-year-old male patient who was previously operated for lumbar spinal hydatid disease. Sagittal T2-weighted MRI demonstrates loss of height and decreased signal intensity in the operated lumbar vertebra (*arrows*). Neighboring disk spaces are fairly preserved. Despite the unfavorable effects of few metallic artifacts, there is no evidence of recurrent hydatid cyst

Conclusion

In the areas where the disease is endemic, hydatid disease should be considered in the differential diagnosis of a cystic lesion in the spine. In countries where tuberculosis is common, it should be known that spinal hydatidosis simulates tuberculosis spondylitis or chronic osteomyelitis (Turgut et al. 2007). There are ongoing MRI investigations to differentiate alive and fertile cysts from the inactive forms of hydatidosis and to monitor drug therapy (Turgut and Turgut 2010). It seems that MRI is the most efficient imaging modality in diagnosis of spinal hydatid disease and in demonstration of its complications.

Acknowledgments We thank Assistant Professor Ahmet Oguz Hasdemir, MD, Assistant Professor Halil Dönmez, MD, Mehmet Gümüş, MD, and Rukiye Dilli for their assistance.

References

Adilay U, Tuğcu B, Gunes M, Günaldi O, Gunal M, Eseoglu M. Cauda equina syndrome caused by primary lumbosacral and pelvic hydatid cyst: a case report. Minim Invasive Neurosurg. 2007;50:292–5.

Akhan O, Dinçer A, Saatçi I, Gülekon N, Besim A. Spinal intradural hydatid cyst in a child. Br J Radiol. 1991;64:465–6.
Arif SH, Zaheer S. Intradural extramedullary primary hydatid cyst of the spine in a child: a very rare presentation. Eur Spine J. 2009;18 Suppl 2:179–82.
Berk C, Ciftçi E, Erdoğan A. MRI in primary intraspinal extradural hydatid disease: case report. Neuroradiology. 1998;40:390–2.
Bhake A, Agrawal A. Hydatid disease of the spine. J Neurosci Rural Pract. 2010;1:61–2.
Bükte Y, Kemaloglu S, Nazaroglu H, Ozkan U, Ceviz A, Simsek M. Cerebral hydatid disease: CT and MR imaging findings. Swiss Med Wkly. 2004;134:459–67.
Bouras A, Lardé D, Mathieu D, Delépine G, Benameur C, Ferrané J. The value of computed tomography in osseous hydatid disease (echinococcosis). Skeletal Radiol. 1984;12:192–5.
Doganay S, Kantarci M. Role of conventional and diffusion-weighted magnetic resonance imaging of spinal treatment protocol for hydatid disease. J Spinal Cord Med. 2009;32:574–7.
Fahl M, Haddad FS, Huballah M, Kana'an S, Husheimi I, Azizi T. Magnetic resonance imaging in intradural and extradural spinal echinococcosis. Clin Imaging. 1994; 18:179–83.
Farzan M, Mortazavi SMJ, Motamedi M. Hydatid disease of bone. Acta Med Iran. 2006;44:361–4.
Gopal N, Chauhan S, Yogesh N. Primary spinal extradural hydatid cyst causing spinal cord compression. Indian J Orthop. 2007;41:76–8.
Göçer AI, Tuna M, Ildan F, Bağdatoğlu H, Haciyakupoğlu S. Cervical intradural extramedullary hydatid cyst. Turk Neurosurg. 1994;4:169–71.
Güneş M, Akdemir H, Tuğcu B, Günaldi O, Gümüş E, Akpinar A. Multiple intradural spinal hydatid disease: a case report and review of literature. Spine (Phila Pa 1976). 2009;34:E346–50.
Hilmani S, El Malki M, Bertal A, Achouri M, Sami A, Ouboukhlik A, El Kamar A, El Azhari A. Lumbar intradural hydatid cyst. Case report (in French). Neurochirurgie. 2004;50:57–60.
Işlekel S, Erşahin Y, Zileli M, Oktar N, Oner K, Ovül I, Ozdamar N, Tunçbay E. Spinal hydatid disease. Spinal Cord. 1998;36:166–70.
Kaen A, Lagares A, Perez-Nuñez A, Rivas JJ, Ramos A, Lobato RD. Intradural extramedullary spinal hydatidosis: case report. Neurocirugia (Astur). 2009;20: 282–7.
Kahilogullari G, Tuna H, Aydin Z, Colpan E, Egemen N. Primary intradural extramedullary hydatid cyst. Am J Med Sci. 2005;329:202–4.
Layadi F, Boubrik M, Ait El Qadi A, Ait Benali S. Primary sacral epidural hydatid cyst: a case report (in French). J Radiol. 2005;86:1040–2.
Limaiem F, Bellil S, Bellil K, Chelly I, Mekni A, Khaldi M, Haouet S, Zitouna M, Kchir N. Primary hydatidosis of the central nervous system: a retrospective study of 39 Tunisian cases. Clin Neurol Neurosurg. 2010;112:23–8.
Mathuriya SN, Arora OP, Khosla VK, Prabhakar SK, Chopra JS, Kak VK. Infected intradural hydatid cyst at foramen magnum. A case report. Clin Neurol Neurosurg. 1985;87:283–6.
Nell M, Burgkart RH, Gradl G, von Eisenhart-Rothe R, Schaeffeler C, Trappe D, da Costa CP, Gradinger R, Kirchhoff C. Primary extrahepatic alveolar echinococcosis of the lumbar spine and the psoas muscle. Ann Clin Microbiol Antimicrob. 2011;10:13.
Pamir MN, Akalan N, Ozgen T, Erbengi A. Spinal hydatid cysts. Surg Neurol. 1984;21:53–7.
Pandey M, Chaudhari MP. Primary hydatid cyst of sacral spinal canal: case report. Neurosurgery. 1997;40:407–9.
Papakonstantinou O, Athanassopoulou A, Passomenos D, Kalogeropoulos I, Balanika A, Baltas C, Gouliamos A, Guglielmi G. Recurrent vertebral hydatid disease: spectrum of MR imaging features. Singapore Med J. 2011;52:440–5.
Phatak SV. Pictorial essay: spinal echinococcosis. Indian J Radiol Imaging. 2006;16:355–7.
Polat P, Kantarci M, Alper F, Suma S, Koruyucu MB, Okur A. Hydatid disease from head to toe. Radiographics. 2003;23:475–94.
Secer HI, Anik I, Celik E, Daneyemez MK, Gonul E. Spinal hydatid cyst mimicking arachnoid cyst on magnetic resonance imaging. J Spinal Cord Med. 2008;31: 106–8.
Senoglu M, Bulbuloglu E, Demirpolat G, Altun I, Celik M. Combined anterior and posterior approach for sacral/retroperitoneal hydatid cyst disease: case report. Turk Neurosurg. 2009;19:428–32.
Singh S, Korah IP, Gibikote SV, Shyam NK, Nair A, Korula A. Sacral hydatidosis: value of MRI in the diagnosis. Skeletal Radiol. 1998;27:518–21.
Song X, Liu D, Wen H. Diagnostic pitfalls of spinal echinococcosis. J Spinal Disord Tech. 2007;20:180–5.
Spektor S, Gomori JM, Beni-Adani L, Constantini S. Spinal echinococcal cyst: treatment using computerized tomography-guided needle aspiration and hypertonic saline irrigation. Case report. J Neurosurg. 1997;87:464–7.
Tabak O, Yilmaz M, Oz B, Ozaras R, Erdincler P, Mert A, Ozturk R, Tabak F. A vertebral hydatid cyst infection mimicking tuberculous spondylodiscitis. J Infect Chemother. 2007;13:180–2.
Toussaint F, Pere P, Le Chaffotec L, Grandhaye P, Pourel J, Chary-Valckenaere I. Alveolar echinococcosis of the spine. J Clin Rheumatol. 2001;7:248–51.
Turan Süslü H, Ceçen A, Karaaslan A, Börekçi A, Bozbuğa M. Primary spinal hydatid disease. Turk Neurosurg. 2009;19:186–8.
Tuncel E. Clinical radiology (in Turkish). 2nd ed. Bursa: Nobel and Güneş; 2008. p. 944.
Turgut AT, Altin L, Topçu S, Kiliçoğlu B, Altinok T, Kaptanoğlu E, Karademir A, Koşar U. Unusual imaging characteristics of complicated hydatid disease. Eur J Radiol. 2007;63:84–93.
Turgut M. Hydatid disease of the spine: a survey study from Turkey. Infection. 1997;25:221–6.
Turgut M. Hydatidosis of central nervous system and its coverings in the pediatric and adolescent age groups in Turkey during the last century: a critical review of 137 cases. Childs Nerv Syst. 2002;18:670–83.

Turgut M, Turgut AT. Spinal intradural extramedullary hydatidosis: report of 3 cases. Neurosurgery. 2010;67: E1471–2.

von Sinner WN, Akhtar M. Case report 833: primary spinal echinococcosis (Echinococcus granulosus) of lumbosacral spine with destruction of the left pedicles of L3-5 and extension of a large paraspinal cystic mass into the spinal canal. Skeletal Radiol. 1994;23: 220–3.

In Vivo Proton Magnetic Resonance Spectroscopy in Hydatidosis of the Central Nervous System

13

Avinash K. Kanodia

Contents

A.K. Kanodia, MBBS, MD, DM
Department of Radiology, Perth Royal Infirmary, Perth, Scotland, UK

Department of Radiology, Ninewells Hospital, Dundee, Scotland, UK
e-mail: ak_kanodia@rediffmail.com

Introduction

Magnetic resonance spectroscopy (MRS) is a non-invasive technique that is used in clinical and research domains, for detecting various metabolites in normal and abnormal tissues and using them as an important adjunct in making a diagnosis. It has been available for several decades and established itself in a clinical role in various clinical conditions including brain tumours, dysplastic lesions, cystic lesions, epilepsy, etc. and is a powerful research tool in various other conditions (Castillo et al. 1998, 2001; Nelson et al. 2002; Ross et al. 2006). However, it is important to consider the results of MRS in context of the clinical problem and conventional magnetic resonance imaging (MRI), and the potential of being misled exists if the results are considered in isolation. There is also ample evidence in the literature, highlighting the limitations of MRS in certain conditions (Saindane et al. 2002; Szewczyk-Bieda et al. 2011). There is relatively limited literature about the applications of MRS in hydatid cyst and similar cystic lesions that highlights the usefulness and the potential limitations of MRS in the diagnosis of hydatid cyst and its differentiation from other cyst-like conditions of the brain.

Basics of Magnetic Resonance Spectroscopy

MRS utilizes nuclei with an odd number of protons and neutrons, such as ^{1}H, ^{31}P, ^{13}C, ^{19}F and ^{23}Na that have a magnetic moment, the most

M. Turgut (ed.), *Hydatidosis of the Central Nervous System: Diagnosis and Treatment*, DOI 10.1007/978-3-642-54359-3_13, © Springer-Verlag Berlin Heidelberg 2014

common in clinical use being ^1H. When an external magnetic field is applied, the nuclei resonate depending upon the gyromagnetic ratio and the external magnetic field applied (Cousins 1995; Matson et al. 1999). The nuclei in different metabolites resonate at a slightly different frequency compared to a standard, called the chemical shift. Signal acquisition follows a brief excitation of the tissue by the RF pulse, and it is the free induction decay (FID), which is transformed into spectrum by Fourier transformation. The horizontal axis represents the chemical shift, and plotted as parts per million (ppm) of the total resonance frequency, this remains constant for different metabolites. The signal intensity of a spectral peak is indicated by the area under the peak (i.e. the integral of the peak), rather than the height of the peak (Connelly 1996; Castillo et al. 1998). The ^1H MRS technique has the distinct advantage over others in that it can be more easily combined with MRI in the same setting, since it is performed with the same coil and ^1H is naturally more abundant than others.

To determine the volume of tissue from which magnetic resonance spectra are being obtained, two distinct approaches may be employed. First is the single-voxel spectroscopy (SVS) technique in which data is acquired from a single volume of interest (usually a cube of 8 ml or smaller), which can be repeated in other regions of interest. The second technique is chemical shift imaging (CSI) (also called magnetic resonance spectroscopic imaging or MRSI), in which a large region is excited before the signals are spatially encoded. With this technique, data from many voxels can be acquired simultaneously, and the increase in efficiency can be used to obtain smaller voxels (1–2 ml) than is feasible with SVS methods. It has the advantage that prior knowledge of the exact area of abnormality is not necessary (Duncan 1997). Thus maps can be obtained superimposed on the MRI image, where different colours or different shades of a single colour may be used to outline the area having increased concentration of a particular metabolite (Hetherington et al. 1995; Rudkin and Arnold 1999). Two-dimensional CSI is the most common approach; usually the study is done in a transverse plane although it can also be performed in other planes (Hunter and Wang 2001). Even larger volumes can be mapped using 3D CSI. However, the disadvantages over SVS technique are that magnetic field homogeneity is required over a larger area and that signals from individual voxels can contribute to their neighbours along with relatively lesser signal in each voxel (Connelly 1996).

The metabolites that are detectable using ^1H MRS depend on the acquisition conditions used. In SVS technique, the most commonly used localization techniques are point-resolved spectroscopy (PRESS) and stimulated echo method (STEAM). The PRESS technique is able to detect 100 % of all available signals, although only the metabolites with relatively longer or intermediate relaxation times may be seen. PRESS allows for sampling of relatively large volumes of interest (VOI) of tissue (3–27 cm^3). Moreover, to obtain higher signal to noise ratio (SNR), a relatively smaller number of signal averages or number of excitations (NEX) are required (Castillo et al. 1998; Hunter and Wang 2001). STEAM detects 50 % of all available signals, necessitating higher NEX to produce a good SNR. With STEAM, sampling of smaller VOI (1–3 cm^3) can be done, and this technique also allows for visualization of more metabolites with short relaxation times. In both techniques, a water suppression pulse is applied to the suppression of the water signal.

In the normal brain, three metabolites are usually present (Fig. 13.1). *N*-acetyl aspartate (NAA at 2 ppm) is detected mainly by its N-acetyl methyl group. It is a marker of neuronal density and viability, and its concentration decreases with many insults to the brain. In normal spectra, NAA is the largest peak. The choline peak (Cho at 3.2 ppm) contains contributions from glycerophosphocholine, phosphocholine and phosphatidylcholine and reflects total Cho stores. Cho is a constituent of the phospholipid metabolism of the cell membranes and reflects membrane turnover, and it is a precursor of acetylcholine and phosphatidylcholine (Miller 1991). The latter compound is used to build cell membranes, while the former is a critical neurotransmitter. Increased Cho reflects increased membrane synthesis or an increased number of cells (Castillo et al. 1998).

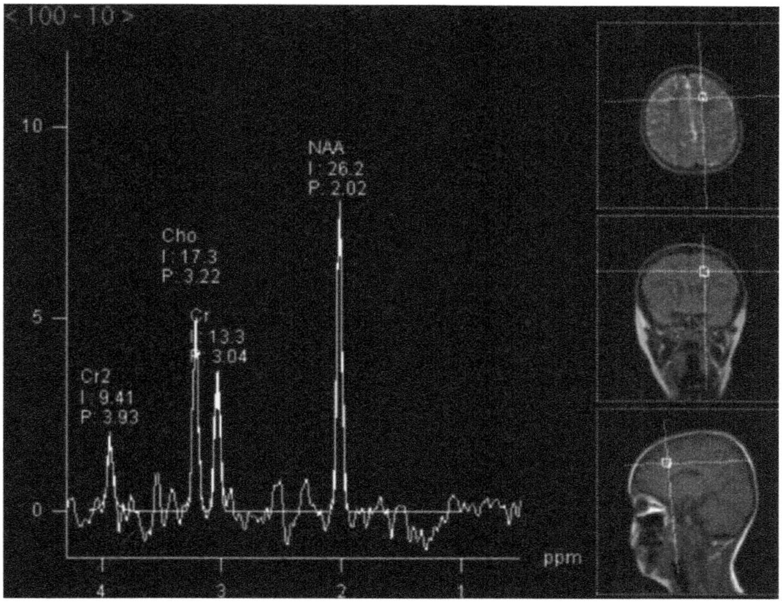

Fig. 13.1 In vivo ^{1}H MRS of the normal brain. Predominantly, three metabolites are seen at TE = 135 ms. These are NAA, Cho and Cr, NAA being the largest, seen at 2 ppm

The creatine peak (Cr at 3 ppm) contains contributions mainly from Cr and Cr phosphate. Cr probably plays a role in maintaining energy-dependent systems in brain cells by serving as a reserve for high-energy phosphates and as a buffer in ATP-ADP reservoir. The overall levels of Cr remain quite stable in most situations, and it is a good internal standard for comparison with other metabolites (Castillo et al. 1998).

Lactate (1.3 ppm) is a nonspecific marker often associated with anaerobic conditions in different situations. The configuration of lactate resonance consists of two distinct, resonant peaks (called a 'doublet') that are due to magnetic field interactions between adjacent protons (J-coupling) (Fig. 13.2). Lactate levels in the brain are normally very low or absent (Fig. 13.1). The presence of lactate indicates that the normal cellular oxidative respiratory mechanism is no longer in effect and that carbohydrate catabolism is taking place. At time to echo, TE = 272 ms, the lactate doublet projects above the baseline, whereas at TE = 136 ms, the lactate doublet is projected below the baseline (Castillo et al. 1998).

The results of MRS are compared and evaluated in various ways. The signal intensities of the metabolites are taken as a ratio against a standard metabolite, which is least likely to change (e.g. Cr in case of ^{1}H MRS). These ratios can be compared by taking the other side as control. Several quantitative methods are also used. The observed signal intensity is multiplied by the 90° pulse voltage, thereby compensating for differences in radiofrequency coil loading, and then comparing the signal intensities between different subjects. Using MRS, the concentration of metabolites can also be measured by determining the effects of T_1 and T_2 relaxation. Another method is that the signal intensity can be calibrated against a standard (phantom) (Gadian et al. 1994; Duncan 1997; Hunter and Wang 2001).

Cysts and Cyst-like Lesions of the Brain

A variety of cysts and cystic lesions can be seen, including arachnoid cysts, porencephalic cysts, neuroglial cysts, epidermoids, large perivascular spaces, cyst or necrosis associated with tumours, abscesses, parasitic cysts such as hydatid and neurocysticercosis (NCC), etc. (Osborn and Preece 2006). While history, clinical features, geographical factors and conventional CT and MRI appearances are often helpful in differentiating these lesions, the appearances are

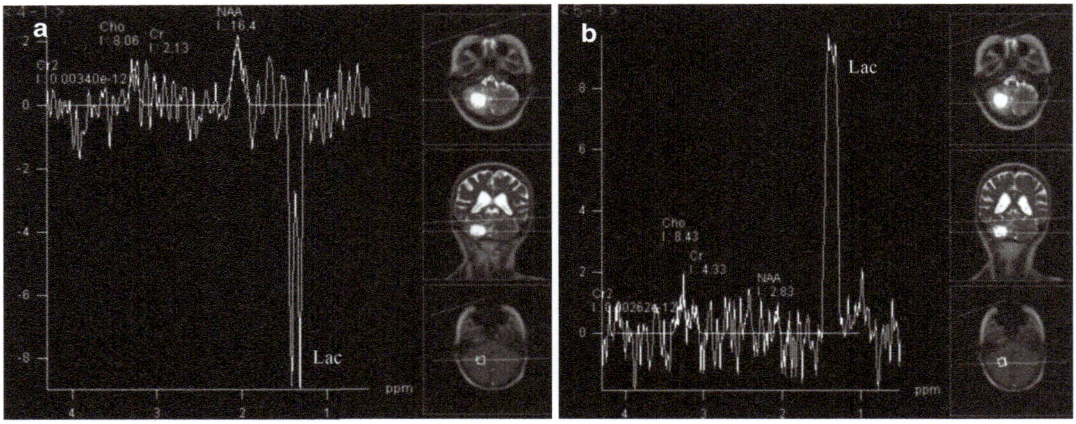

Fig. 13.2 In vivo ^{1}H MRS showing typical lactate peak in a necrotic mass (**a**) shows MRS with TE = 135 ms and (**b**) shows MRS with TE = 270 ms. The typical lactate peak is a doublet, projecting below baseline in (a) and above baseline in (b)

occasionally atypical and can present with diagnostic dilemmas. Since these represent vastly different pathologies requiring different treatment approaches, the importance of accurate diagnosis cannot be overemphasized. ^{1}H MRS utilizes a different, metabolite-based approach and provides a vital clue in several of these difficult situations.

Proton Magnetic Resonance Spectroscopy in Hydatid Cysts

Biochemical Basis of Magnetic Resonance Spectroscopy

In parasitic cysts, some anaerobic metabolism is usually present, even if the aerobic pathway is active to some extent (Garg et al. 2002). As a result, a variety of metabolites involved in anaerobic metabolism are usually found. Of the parasitic cysts, hydatid cyst is a typical example that shares many similarities and some differences with other parasitic cysts. The frequently described metabolites found in hydatid fluid in reasonable amounts are succinate, pyruvate, acetate, lactate and alanine, while a few others such as malate, fumarate, glycine, other amino acids, Cho (and Cho-containing compounds), propionate, etc. are found in smaller amounts or traces (McManus and Smyth 1978; Chang et al. 1998; Garg et al. 2002; Jayakumar et al. 2003). The frequency and success of detection of metabolites depend largely on the technique used.

Pyruvate is a product of glycolysis and reported to be found in abundance in hydatid fluid; investigators have confirmed its presence using mass spectroscopic measurements (Jayakumar et al. 2003). It is also thought to be an indicator of viability as it has not been detectable in cysts that show degeneration on histopathologic examination (Jayakumar et al. 2003). Pyruvate can be metabolized to acetate and lactate which are important and easily detectable metabolites in hydatid fluid, lactate being more prominently seen. Under anaerobic conditions, the partial tricarboxylic acid (TCA) cycle is active, in which phosphoenolpyruvate formed during glycolysis partially converts into oxaloacetate and then further into malate, using malate dehydrogenase (MDH). It further transforms into fumarate and succinate (McManus and Bryant 1995; Garg et al. 2002). In hydatid, the activity of MDH and other related enzymes has been reported as more favourable for succinate production by some of the investigators (Garg et al. 2002), who regard succinate as a very important metabolite present in significant amount in hydatid cysts and have confirmed its presence by specialized techniques (Garg et al. 2002). However, other investigators have given more importance to pyruvate, describing it as a marker of cestodial infestation and have downplayed the importance of succinate by

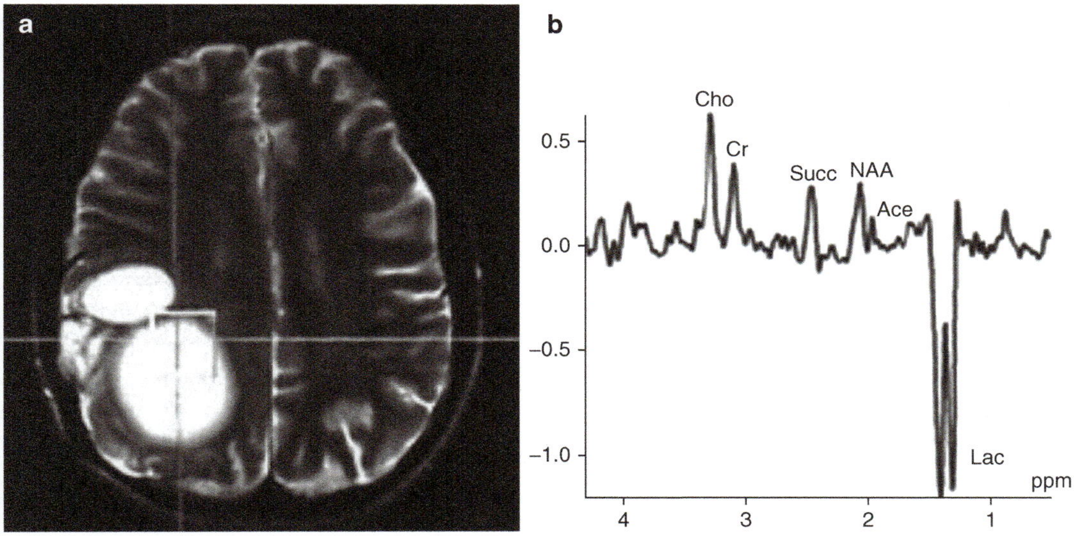

Fig. 13.3 In vivo ^{1}H MRS, showing the voxel over hydatid cyst (**a**) and the spectrum obtained using a TE of 135 ms (**b**). The MRS in (**b**) shows a large inverted lactate peak (*Lac*), a prominent succinate (*Succ*) peak and a smaller acetate peak (*Ace*). Further choline (*Cho*), creatine (*Cr*) and NAA peaks are present due to contamination from the surrounding tissue (From Chand et al. (2005) with permission)

citing low biochemical activity of succinate dehydrogenase (Jayakumar et al. 2003). Therefore, in the literature, there is no consensus on the relative importance of succinate and pyruvate, and as discussed below, it has important ramifications for ^{1}H MRS.

The only significant amino acid found is alanine, which is derived from pyruvate (Kohli et al. 1995; Jayakumar et al. 2003), while others such as leucine, valine and isoleucine are found in small amounts. Fumarate and malate are only detectable in traces but are considered as important metabolites that indicate fertility and can also be useful for differentiation from NCC cysts (Garg et al. 2002).

Technical Factors of In Vivo Proton Magnetic Resonance Spectroscopy

While both PRESS and STEAM techniques have been used, PRESS is more commonly performed. Both SVS and CSI techniques have been successfully used. At 1.5 T, different researchers use (time to repeat) TR of 1,500–3,000 ms with satisfactory results. Usually, a (time to echo) TE of 135–144 ms is used, as the metabolites usually found in hydatids are reasonably detected at these TE values, although some researchers have also used shorter TEs in addition (Chang et al. 1998). A variable NEX can be performed, depending on several factors. It is preferable to obtain the spectrum from the cystic part, avoiding the solid tissue/wall/host tissue as it can result in further metabolites (Fig. 13.3).

Typical Spectrum of In Vivo Proton Magnetic Resonance Spectroscopy in Hydatid Cysts

Of the several metabolites described, only a few are routinely picked up reliably on in vivo ^{1}H MRS due to sensitivity issues. In particular the peak at 2.4 ppm is important as both pyruvate and succinate are detected at 2.4 ppm. These are difficult to differentiate on in vivo ^{1}H MRS, and as discussed above, there is no consensus in the literature as to which of these metabolites are predominantly represented at 2.4 ppm, although their presence has been confirmed in separate studies using different techniques (Garg et al.

2002; Jayakumar et al. 2003, 2004). While this issue is pending, awaiting further investigation, still, a prominent peak at 2.4 ppm (pyruvate/succinate) is one of the most important features in in vivo ^{1}H MRS.

Other important metabolites detected by in vivo technique are lactate (1.3 ppm, seen as a doublet), acetate (1.9 ppm) and alanine (1.5 ppm) (Chang et al. 1998; Garg et al. 2002; Jayakumar et al. 2003). While these could be variable, lactate is usually seen as a significant peak. Acetate is detectable although it is a smaller peak relative to the succinate/pyruvate. As a result, the ratio of succinate/acetate is generally quite high in hydatid cysts and is an important differentiating feature with pyogenic abscesses, where acetate/succinate ratio is high (Poptani et al. 1995; Martinez-Perez et al. 1997; Dev et al. 1998; Chand et al. 2005). It has been further suggested that various metabolites described in hydatid cysts may not be seen in all spectra, due to changes in internal milieu during evolution of the cyst (Jayakumar et al. 2003). Also, various forms of echinococcus may have different consumptions of oxygen and glycogen, thereby producing different concentration of metabolites (Jayakumar et al. 2003). Thus, despite having some uniformity in basic spectra, variations are possible.

Ex vivo ^{1}H MRS detects a larger number of metabolites from hydatid fluid. These include amino acids leucine, valine and isoleucine (0.9–1.2 ppm), glycine (3.56 ppm), Cho (3.2 ppm), malate (4.3 ppm), fumarate (6.5 ppm), glucose and some of the aromatic amino acids (Garg et al. 2002).

In Vivo Proton Magnetic Resonance Spectroscopy in Other Cystic Conditions

Neurocysticercosis

The size and appearance of NCC are usually fairly different from hydatid cysts and rarely present a diagnostic dilemma; however, large and racemose lesions can create difficulty in diagnosis on routine MRI (Jayakumar et al. 2003). The issue becomes important due to the different management of these conditions (medical in NCC versus surgical in hydatid).

Being a parasitic infection, NCC and hydatid have similar metabolic pathways, and ^{1}H MRS in NCC follows closely that of hydatid with minimal differences (Jayakumar et al. 2004). The same metabolites are usually found in vivo, including succinate/pyruvate (2.4 ppm), acetate (1.9 ppm), lactate (1.3 ppm) and alanine (1.5 ppm), although these are generally lower in concentration than hydatid, attributable to a difference in enzyme activity that determines the concentration of these metabolites (Garg et al. 2002; Jayakumar et al. 2004). However, another unidentified peak at 3.3 ppm has been described by Chang et al. 1998, thought to be representing Cho (and Cho-containing compounds) by other authors (Jayakumar et al. 2004), which has not been confirmed but may potentially serve as a differentiating feature.

Ex vivo ^{1}H MRS has additional features helpful in differentiation (Garg et al. 2002). These include the absence of malate and fumarate, which are described in fertile hydatids. Creatine (3 ppm) can also be seen, attributable mainly to diffusion from host tissues (Garg et al. 2002).

Pyogenic Abscess

The in vivo ^{1}H MRS spectrum of pyogenic abscesses is significantly different from hydatid cysts. The presence of an amino acid (AA) peak at 0.9 ppm is usually considered as a sensitive marker, attributed to the presence of proteolytic enzymes, released by neutrophil breakdown (Mishra et al. 2004; Pal et al. 2010). These could sometimes be absent, notably in treated abscesses (Pal et al. 2010). AA peak is not usually encountered as a significant peak in in vivo ^{1}H MRS in hydatid. Lactate (1.3 ppm) is also an important metabolite, sometimes the only metabolite seen such as in treated abscesses (Pal et al. 2010).

Acetate (1.9 ppm) is another very important peak in abscesses caused by anaerobes. It is thought to be a result of enhanced glycolysis, resulting in pyruvate formation that converts into acetate and succinate. Biochemical reactions leading to acetate formation are thought to be more favourable than those leading to succinate formation, leading to prominent acetate peak (Pal et al. 2010). Succinate (2.4 ppm), while usually presenting small amounts, may or may not be detectable by in vivo ^{1}H MRS (Pal et al. 2010). As a result, the ratio of acetate/succinate is quite high as compared to hydatid cysts (Poptani et al. 1995; Martinez-Perez et al. 1997; Dev et al. 1998). Acetate and succinate are not observed in abscesses by aerobic organisms as the pyruvate is metabolized in TCA cycle in the usual manner (Pal et al. 2010).

Cysts/Necrosis Associated with Tumours

A variety of tumours can have cysts, such as pilocytic astrocytomas, or even associated with benign tumours such as meningiomas. High-grade gliomas are more usually associated with necrosis. The ^{1}H MRS spectra limited to the cysts or necrotic parts of tumours usually show a prominent lactate or lactate/lipid peak (1.3 ppm) (Fig. 13.2). Other metabolites are generally absent, unless there is contamination from surrounding solid tissue (Chang et al. 1998).

Epidermoids

Epidermoids usually have typical imaging features on MRI and rarely present a diagnostic difficulty, in relating to hydatid cysts. The in vivo ^{1}H MRS is significantly different from hydatid and shows a relatively small or medium lactate peak (1.3 ppm), while no further metabolites are usually described (Chang et al. 1998).

Other Cysts

A variety of developmental and incidental cysts and cyst-like lesions are encountered, including arachnoid cysts, porencephalic cysts, neuroglial cysts, large perivascular spaces, etc. On in vivo ^{1}H MRS, these are generally devoid of any peaks (Chang et al. 1998), although there is some literature about the presence of excitatory amino acids such as glutamate and aspartate in some of the arachnoid cysts (Hajek et al. 1997). However these are usually seen at much shorter TE values and not at the usual intermediate values used for hydatid cysts.

Conclusion

In vivo ^{1}H MRS can be a useful tool in differentiating cystic lesions of the brain including hydatid cysts especially when used as an adjunct to MRI rather than in isolation. There are significant overlapping features with NCC which are rarely large enough in isolation to present a diagnostic dilemma, while there are sufficient important differentiating features from other cysts lesions. The in vivo ^{1}H MRS features of various cystic conditions have been summarized in Table 13.1.

Table 13.1 Relative importance of different metabolites in cysts/cystic conditions of brain on in vivo ^{1}H MRS

		Succinate/pyruvate (2.4 ppm)	Acetate (1.9 ppm)	Lactate (1.3 ppm)	Alanine (1.5 ppm)	AA peak (0.9 ppm)	Choline[a] (3.3 ppm)
Hydatid cyst		+++	+	+++	+	–	–
Neurocysticercosis		++	+	++	+	–	+
Anaerobic pyogenic abscess	Untreated	+	+++	+++	–	+++	–
	Treated	–	–	++	–	–	–
Tumour cyst and necrosis		–	–	+++	–	–	–
Epidermoids		–	–	+/++	–	–	–
Other cysts		–	–	–	–	–	–

[a]Choline, unconfirmed peak at 3.3 ppm (Chang et al. 1998)

References

Castillo M, Kwock L, Scatliff J, Mukherji SK. Proton MR spectroscopy in neoplastic and non-neoplastic brain disorders. Magn Reson Imaging Clin N Am. 1998;6:1–20.

Castillo M, Smith JK, Kwock L, Proton MR. Spectroscopy in patients with acute temporal lobe seizures. AJNR Am J Neuroradiol. 2001;22:152–7.

Chand K, Kanodia AK, Manpreet G, Neeraj A. In vivo proton magnetic resonance spectroscopy in a known case of intracranial hydatid cyst. Neurol India. 2005;53:337–8.

Chang KH, Song IC, Kim SH, Han MH, Kim HD, Seong SO, Jung HW, Han MC. In vivo single-voxel proton MR spectroscopy in intracranial cystic masses. AJNR Am J Neuroradiol. 1998;19:401–5.

Connelly A. Proton magnetic resonance spectroscopy in epilepsy. In: Casino GD, Jack CR, editors. Neuroimaging in epilepsy: principles and practice. Newton, Mass: Butterworth-Heinemann; 1996.

Cousins JP. Clinical MR, spectroscopy- fundamentals, current applications and future potential. AJR Am J Roentgenol. 1995;164:1337–47.

Dev R, Gupta RK, Poptani H, Roy R, Sharma S, Husain M. Role of in vivo proton magnetic resonance spectroscopy in the diagnosis and management of brain abscesses. Neurosurgery. 1998;42:37–43.

Duncan JS. Magnetic resonance spectroscopy. In: Engel Jr J, Pedley TA, editors. Epilepsy: a comprehensive textbook. Philadelphia: Lippincott-Raven; 1997.

Gadian DG, Connelly A, Duncan JS, Cross JH, Kirkham FJ, Johnson CL, Vargha-Khadem F, Nevile BG, Jackson GD. ^{1}H magnetic resonance spectroscopy in the investigation of intractable epilepsy. Acta Neurol Scand. 1994;152(Suppl):116–21.

Garg M, Chawla S, Prasad KN, Roy R, Sikora SS, Kumar R, Husain M, Khetrapal CL, Gupta RK. Differentiation of hydatid cyst from cysticercus cyst by proton MR spectroscopy. NMR Biomed. 2002;15:320–6.

Hajek M, Do KQ, Duc C, Boesiger P, Wieser HG. Increased excitatory amino acid levels in brain cysts of epileptic patients. Epilepsy Res. 1997;28:245–54.

Hetherington HP, Kuzniecky RI, Pan JW, Vaughan JT, Teeig DB, Pohost GM. Application of high field spectroscopic imaging in the evaluation of temporal lobe epilepsy. Magn Reson Imaging. 1995;13:1175–80.

Hunter JV, Wang ZJ. MR spectroscopy in pediatric neuroradiology. Magn Reson Imaging Clin N Am. 2001;9:165–89.

Jayakumar PN, Srikanth SG, Chandrashekher HS, Kovoor JM, Shankar SK, Anandh B. Pyruvate: an in vivo marker of cestodal infestation of the human brain on proton MR spectroscopy. J Magn Reson Imaging. 2003;18:675–80.

Jayakumar PN, Chandrashekar HS, Srikanth SG, Guruprasad AS, Devi BI, Shankar SK. MRI and in vivo proton MR spectroscopy in a racemose cysticercal cyst of the brain. Neuroradiology. 2004;46:72–4.

Kohli A, Gupta RK, Poptani H, Roy R. In vivo proton magnetic resonance spectroscopy in a case of intracranial hydatid cyst. Neurology. 1995;45:562–4.

Martinez-Perez I, Moreno A, Alonso J, Aguas J, Conesa G, Capdevila A, Arús C. Diagnosis of brain abscess by magnetic resonance spectroscopy. Report of two cases. J Neurosurg. 1997;86:708–13.

Matson GB, Weiner MW, Stark DD, Bradley WG. Spectroscopy in MRI. St. Louis: Mosby; 1999. p. 181–211.

McManus DP, Bryant C. Biochemistry, physiology and molecular biology of Echinococcus. In: Thompson RCA, Lymbery AJ, editors. Echinococcus and hydatid disease. Oxford: CAB International; 1995. p. 135–56.

McManus DP, Smyth JD. Differences in the chemical composition and carbohydrate metabolism of Echinococcus granulosus (horse and sheep strains) and E. multilocularis. Parasitology. 1978;77:103–9.

Miller BL. A review of chemical issues in ^{1}H NMR spectroscopy: N-acetyl-L-aspartate, creatine and choline. NMR Biomed. 1991;4:47–52.

Mishra AM, Gupta RK, Jaggi RS, Reddy JS, Jha DK, Husain N, Prasad KN, Behari S, Husain M. Role of diffusion-weighted imaging and in vivo proton magnetic resonance spectroscopy in the differential diagnosis of ring-enhancing intracranial cystic mass lesions. J Comput Assist Tomogr. 2004;28:540–7.

Nelson SJ, McKnight TR, Henry RG. Characterization of untreated gliomas by magnetic resonance spectroscopic imaging. Neuroimaging Clin N Am. 2002;12:599–613.

Osborn AG, Preece MT. Intracranial cysts: radiologic-pathologic correlation and imaging approach. Radiology. 2006;239:650–64.

Pal D, Bhattacharyya A, Husain M, Prasad KN, Pandey CM, Gupta RK. In vivo proton MR spectroscopy evaluation of pyogenic brain abscesses: a report of 194 cases. AJNR Am J Neuroradiol. 2010;31:360–6.

Poptani H, Gupta RK, Jain VK, Roy R, Pandey R. Cystic intracranial mass lesions: possible role of in vivo MR spectroscopy in its differential diagnosis. Magn Reson Imaging. 1995;13:1019–29.

Ross BD, Colletti P, Lin A. MR spectroscopy of the brain: neurospectroscopy. In: Edelman RR, Hesselink J, Zlatkin M, Crues J, editors. Clinical magnetic resonance imaging. 3rd ed. Philadelphia: Saunders-Elsevier; 2006. p. 1840–910.

Rudkin TM, Arnold DL. Proton magnetic resonance spectroscopy for the diagnosis and management of cerebral disorders. Arch Neurol. 1999;56:919–26.

Saindane AM, Cha S, Law M, Xue X, Knopp EA, Zagzag D. Proton MR spectroscopy of tumefactive demyelinating lesions. AJNR Am J Neuroradiol. 2002;23:1378–86.

Szewczyk-Bieda M, Kanodia AK, Main G, Eljamel MS. ^{1}H MR spectroscopy in gliomatosis: is there a sensitivity issue? Case Rep Radiol. 2011. doi:10.1155/2011/371073.

Surgical Treatment of Spinal Hydatidosis

14

Erdal Kalkan, Fatih Keskin, and Fatih Erdi

Contents

E. Kalkan, MD (✉) • F. Keskin, MD • F. Erdi, MD
Department of Neurosurgery, Meram Faculty of Medicine, Necmettin Erbakan University, Konya, Turkey
e-mail: erdalkalkan62@yahoo.com

Introduction

Spinal hydatid cyst is an important and serious form of hydatid disease which is caused by a cyclophyllid cestode, the echinococcus. *Echinococcus* has four subgroups: *Echinococcus granulosus, E. multilocularis, E. oligoarthus* and *E. vogeli (Pamir et al. 2002). E. granulosus* and *E. multilocularis* are clinically important in humans, and hydatid disease is most commonly caused by the larval stage of *E. granulosus. E. multilocularis* or *E. oligoarthus* are much less important in humans (Pamir et al. 2002; Sengul et al. 2008). The species of *Echinococcus* are discussed in Chap. 3.

Echinococcus has definitive and intermediate hosts. The definitive host is mainly a domestic dog and occasionally other carnivores such as hyenas and jackals. The exact habitat of the adult worm is the jejunum of the definitive host. The parasite has three proglottids: one immature, one mature and one gravid. The gravid proglottid is shed in the excreta of the definitive host and ruptures to release 500–800 ova (Pamir et al. 2002). The intermediate hosts including humans are most commonly sheep, cattle and goats, camel and other herbivores such as deer, kangaroos and wallabies. The intermediate hosts digest the ova in the infected food or water. After digestion of the chitin, outer layer embryos (oncospheres) develop in the intestine to penetrate the duodenal mucosa and disseminate through the portal circulation. The oncospheres which rescue from the immune system of the host develop into cysts in tissues. The cysts consist of an outer fibrous layer

M. Turgut (ed.), *Hydatidosis of the Central Nervous System: Diagnosis and Treatment*, DOI 10.1007/978-3-642-54359-3_14, © Springer-Verlag Berlin Heidelberg 2014

and a cestode-derived inner germinal membrane containing scolices (Pamir et al. 2002).

The hydatid cysts generally occurs (up to 70 %) in the liver and lungs (12–30 %). Bone involvement in hydatid disease has been reported to be only 0.5–4 %, and spinal involvement is found in 50 % of these cases (Ouma 2006). Spinal cyst hydatid can occur by direct extension from pulmonary or pelvic infestation or less commonly begin in the vertebral body (Kalkan et al. 2007; Senoglu et al. 2009). The vertebral body infestation usually begins in the centre of the vertebral corpus and subsequently extends outward into the epidural and paravertebral area (Senoglu et al. 2009).

Vertebral hydatid disease was classified into five groups in 1928 by Dew: intramedullary, intradural extramedullary, extradural, vertebral and paravertebral extending to the spine (Dew 1928). Fiennes and Thomas (1982) reported isolated extradural spinal infestation. Secondary extension from paravertebral tissues or cysts involving the muscles or even the lungs is occasionally seen. In 90 % of cases the disease is confined to the bone and epidural space (Senoglu et al. 2009). Intradural extramedullary involvement is found in only 9 % of the all spinal cases (Figs. 14.1, 14.2, and 14.3); this can be primary (Kalkan et al. 2007) or secondary as a complication of surgery with dural opening or tear (Pamir et al. 2002). Primary intramedullary hydatid cyst is rarely seen (Ley and Marti 1970).

The most common symptoms and signs in vertebral involvement are paraparesis (62 %), increasing back or radicular pain (55 %), sensory loss (36 %), sphincter disturbance (30 %) and paraplegia (26 %). The time period between the onset of the symptoms and medical consultation varies between 6 and 15 months (Thaler et al. 2010).

A full discussion of the clinical findings of spinal hydatidosis is given in Chap. 8.

Pathology

Portovertebral shunts play an important role in most of the genesis of spinal lesions in hydatid cysts. The vertebral body is generally the first target. When echinococcal larvae are carried to a vertebral body, the parasite grows multilocularly along the bony intratrabecular space and infiltrates and destroys the bone like a tumour, because of a lack of defensive reaction of the bony tissue (Işlekel et al. 1998). Pathological fractures occur due to compression or avascular necrosis of the cortical bone. Subsequently the disease usually spreads to the pedicles, laminae or the ribs. The intervertebral discs are spared in the early stages of the disease. Finally the infestation may extend beyond the vertebral body and periosteum with the development of a cyst with space-occupying symptomatology. It was observed that hydrophilic degeneration of the *Echinococcus* embryo without reactive osteitis could develop over a number of years, with damage and erosion

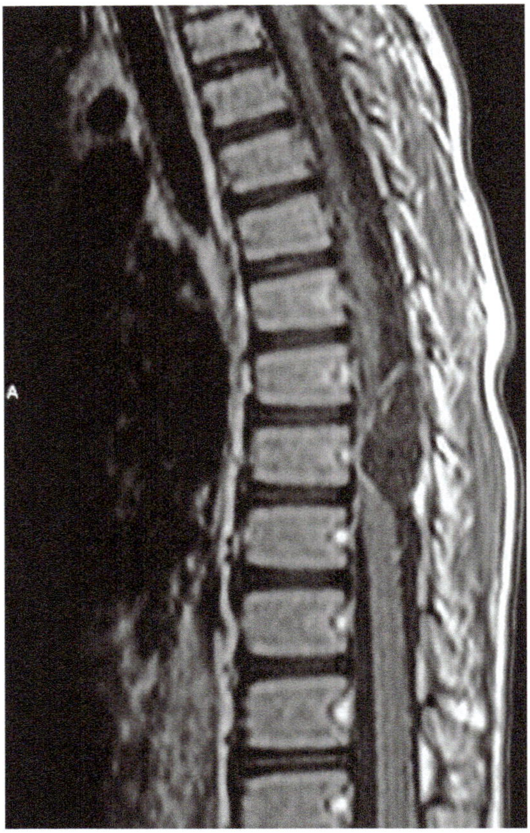

Fig. 14.1 Posteriorly located intradural extramedullary hydatid cyst can be seen on sagittal T1-weighted MRI. The cyst was compressing the spinal cord from the posterior aspect at the T7–8 level

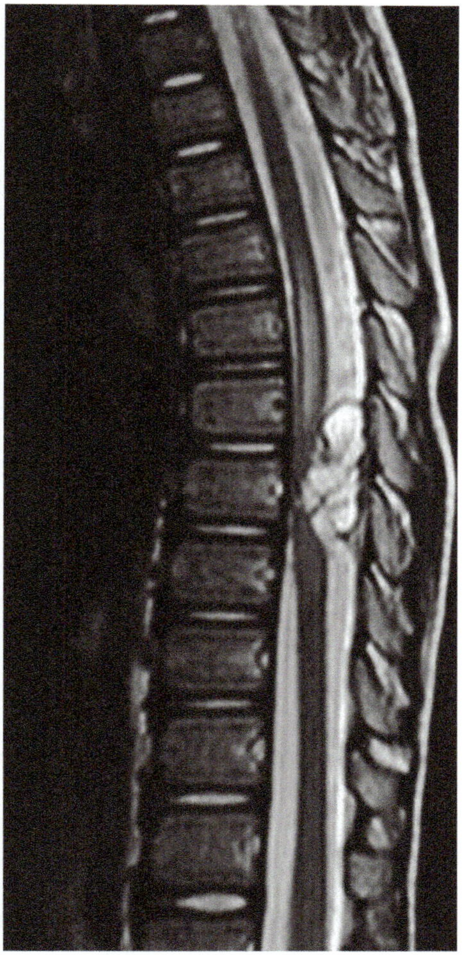

Fig. 14.2 Intradural extramedullary hydatid cyst on T2-weighted sagittal MRI. There was cord oedema

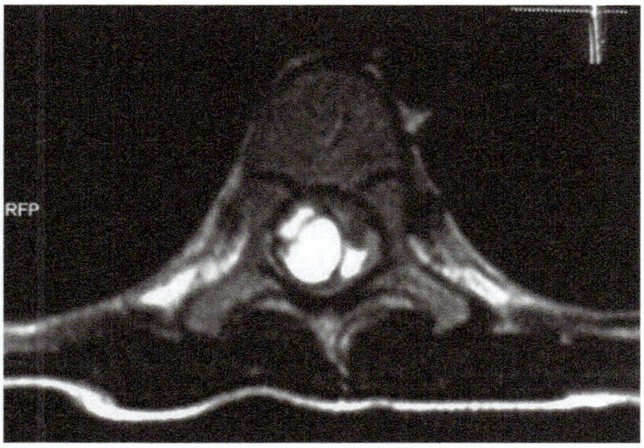

Fig. 14.3 T2-weighted axial MRI shows intradural extramedullary multilocular hydatid cyst. Right-sided lesion was compressing the spinal cord transversely

of the trabecular composition of the bone by the expanding vesicles, with subsequent cystic progression and invasion of all vertebral structures (Tsitouridis and Dimitriadis 1997). When the cyst perforates the cortex, it extends to the paravertebral structures and into the spinal canal or neural foramina (Kalkan et al. 2008). Bone destruction and puslike fluid may be encountered during operation, leading to the name 'ossifluent abscess' (Pamir et al. 2002). Papanikolaou (2008) described three mechanisms for the intraosseous invasion as mechanical, ischaemic and cellular process. The mechanical process affects the surrounding tissues by expansion, compression, dislocation and repression which cause bone and nerve tissue atrophy and osteitis. The ischaemic process affects the nutrient vessels by obstruction and compression which cause bone necrosis and sequestra formation. The cellular process affects the bone tissue by osteoclast proliferation and causes destruction.

The pathology of spinal hydatidosis has been discussed in detail in Chap. 9.

Surgical Treatment of Spinal Hydatidosis

Surgery is currently the mainstay treatment modality for spinal hydatidosis. The first surgical intervention in spinal hydatidosis was reported in 1819 by (Reydellet 1819; Rayport et al. 1964). Most of the cases admitted to surgeons with spinal cord compression syndrome symptomatology are urgent surgeries (Pamir et al. 2002). Patients with spinal hydatid disease usually present with a long history of back pain or other non-specific symptoms of spinal cord compression. Weakness of the limbs occurs in the later stages. Paraplegia or radicular compression is said to occur in 25–84 % of patients (Baysefer et al. 1996). Preoperative diagnosis and the real extent of the disease are very important for operative planning. Preoperative diagnosis of the lesion guides the surgical preference. The correct diagnosis, natural history and serological and radiological studies are essential (Kalkan et al. 2008). Generally, routine laboratory tests do not show specific values. Eosinophilia is mostly limited (15 %) or absent. An intradermal Casoni test result is positive in 95 %, but there are up to 40 % false-positive results. Indirect haemagglutination test and enzyme-linked immunosorbent assay are established methods for the detection of anti-Echinococcus antibodies (immunoglobulin G). Serological tests are 80–100 % sensitive and 88–96 % specific for liver hydatid disease. They have 50–56 % sensitivity for lung disease and only 25–56 % for other organs like spinal cyst hydatid (El-On et al. 2003; Thaler et al. 2010).

Successful treatment of the spinal hydatidosis is challenging because of its invasiveness and its potentially severe complications. Surgical excision is the first and most effective option. The total eradication of the cyst without rupture should be the primary goal of the surgery (Thaler et al. 2010). In clinical practice, however, this is not possible in the spine because there is no one cyst but a multitude of small cysts. Either anterior or posterior approaches can be preferred for the surgical treatment. Pure intradurally or epidurally located lesions at all spinal levels are approached posteriorly. In these cases surgical excision without intraoperative rupture results in cure (Pamir et al. 2002). Bone involvement is very important for defining the recurrence rates. Surgical planning should be made according to this.

Spinal disease most frequently involves the thoracic segments (46–50 %). Lumbar segments (20–29 %) and sacral segments (20–23 %) are also involved frequently. Cervical spine is the least common affected segment (Pamir et al. 2002). Twenty-eight reports of spinal hydatid disease, published during the past five decades, from Turkey, were reviewed, and 71 patients with spinal hydatid disease were collected (Turgut 1997). According to this study, spinal echinococcus involved the thoracic segment of the spine in 35 patients (49 %), the lumbar segment in 28 patients (39 %), the cervical segment in three patients (4 %), the thoracolumbar segment in three patients (4 %) and the sacral segment in one patient (2 %) (Turgut 1997). One patient had non-contagious lesions in the cervical and lumbar segments (Turgut 1997).

Surgical Treatment of Cervical Spinal Hydatidosis

Hydatid disease in the vertebral column is rare in cervical spine. Several procedures can be useful for the spinal hydatid cyst in the cervical region. Cervical laminectomy is the favourite approach for spinal hydatidosis affecting the cervical aspect of the spinal canal. Intradural lesions are also approached posteriorly. The posterior approach to the cervical spine is relatively straightforward and is well known by all neurosurgeons. Avoidance of risk to the anterior vascular and visceral structures is an advantage of this approach. Potentially greater discomfort and longer hospital stays and increased incidence of spinal deformity are the major disadvantages of this surgery. Postlaminectomy kyphosis is common if the laminectomy is performed in an immature spine. Resection of 50 % or more of one facet or its capsule results in a significant risk of subsequent instability (Tandon and Vollmer 2006). The use of lateral mass plating is a significant improvement for the treatment of cervical spine instability. Keller et al. (1997) reported a case of postoperative kyphosis after an anterior corpectomy with simple bony fusion in a spinal hydatid patient. Progressive myelopathy occurred, in this reported patient, and it was successfully treated with a posterior lateral mass plating.

The anterior approach may be utilised for decompression and stabilisation of the cervical spine in a variety of conditions. Anterior approaches including corpectomy with simple bony fusion and corpectomy with anterior plating have been reported for the treatment of cervical spinal hydatidosis (Keller et al. 1997). Anterior instrumentation, in addition to bone grafting, has been generally successful in the cervical spine when treating infection and may obviate the need for posterior instrumentation.

Surgical Treatment of Thoracic Spinal Hydatidosis

Spinal hydatidosis most commonly affects thoracic spinal segment (Figs. 14.4, 14.5, and

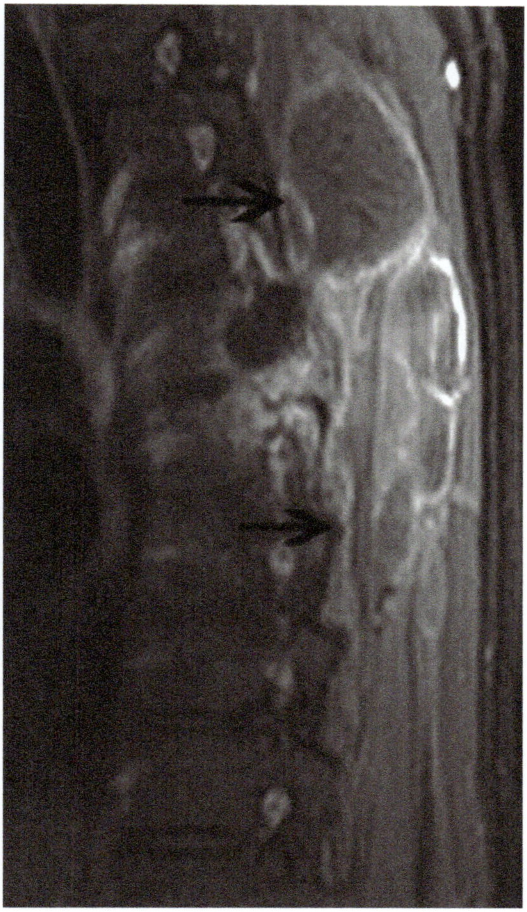

Fig. 14.4 T1-weighted sagittal MRI obtained after contrast administration shows multiloculated cystic lesion at the T4 level. *Black arrows* indicate rim enhancement of the cystic lesion

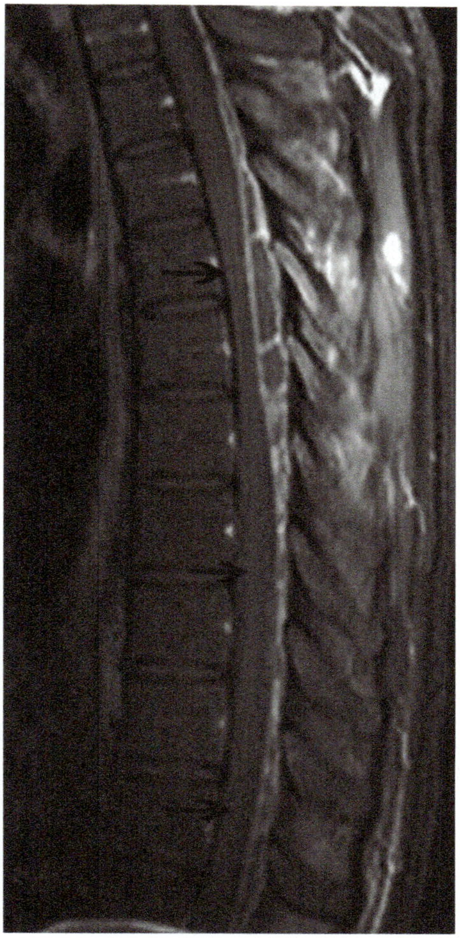

Fig. 14.5 T1-weighted sagittal fat-saturated MRI obtained after administration of intravenous contrast material reveals rim-enhancing loculated cystic lesions through posterior epidural space (*black arrows*)

14.6). The reported approaches in thoracic cases were mainly posterior. The posterior approach via laminectomy is the main choice of treatment (Pamir et al. 2002). Complete surgical removal and most extensive removal of the infected bone must be the goal of the surgery. Decompression of the cord, resection of the cysts, infected bone resection and deformity correction can be done in one approach under direct vision of the cord through a posterior approach (Figs. 14.7 and 14.8). Extradural multiple cysts and cysts located in the bone or in the paravertebral region are the most commonly seen scenario (Figs. 14.9 and 14.10). Daughter cysts may form within the main cyst (Işlekel et al. 1998). Surgical excision without intraoperative cyst rupture results in a cure in pure intradural or pure epidural lesions. In most cases the cysts are multiple and extensive. It is nearly impossible to remove these cysts without rupture. During laminectomy, cysts are almost always ruptured (Işlekel et al. 1998). More extensive lesions with vertebral body involvement can be also approached posteriorly via a transpedicular route (Pamir et al. 2002).

Simple decompression with laminectomy is performed most frequently due to its low morbidity and mortality, but it is not free from risks. Access to the vertebral body through a laminectomy is

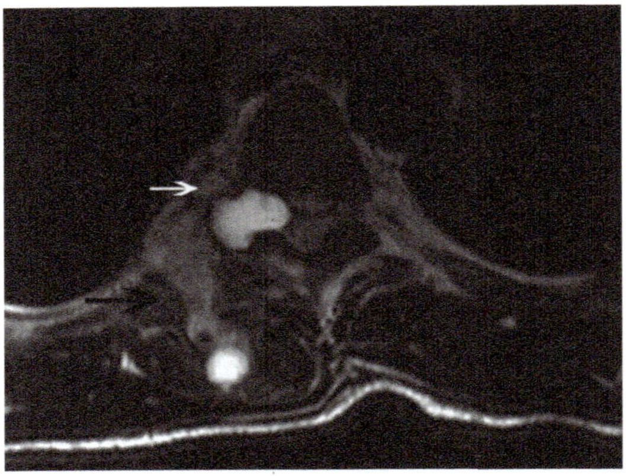

Fig. 14.6 T2-weighted axial MRI reveals heterogeneously hyperintense multiloculated cyst infiltrating paravertebral muscles (*black arrow*) as well as epidural space through neural foramen (*white arrow*)

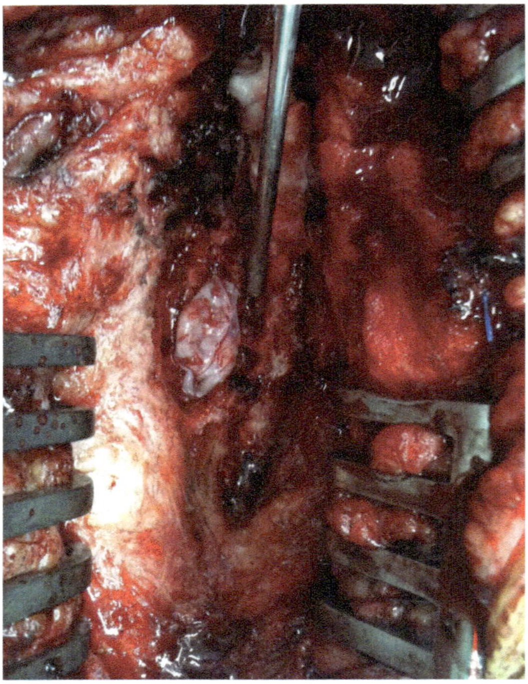

Fig. 14.7 Intraoperative view of a posterior laminectomy site. Extradurally located hydatid cyst can be seen

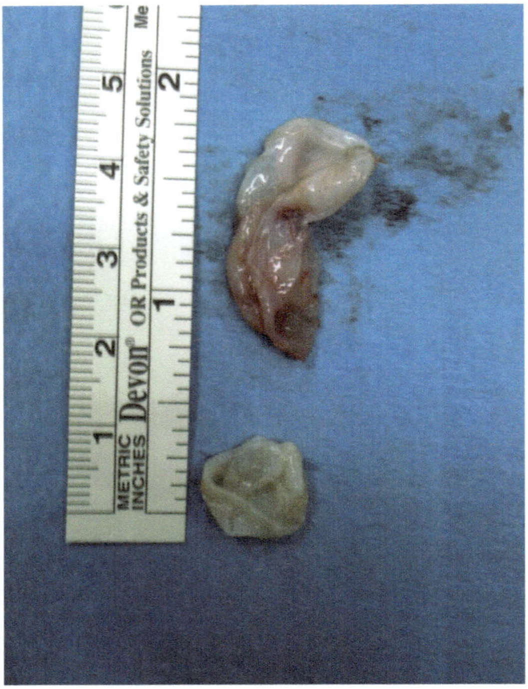

Fig. 14.8 Some of the cysts which were retrieved during surgery

limited, resulting in poor outcomes, especially in recurrent disease. Despite treatment, the disease frequently relapses with progressive destruction of the vertebral column and neurological deterioration (Senoglu et al. 2009). Kaoutzanis et al. (1989) suggested that routine laminectomy for spinal hydatid did not significantly affect the outcome. Turtas et al. (1980) reported a 50 % recurrence rate after posterior decompression alone. Thaler et al. (2010) indicated that partial hydatid cyst resection, inappropriate stabilisation and posterior multilevel laminectomies without posterior stabilisation have led to progressive deformities of the thoracic spine. They concluded that no cases of reoperations due to spinal deformity were found when cyst resection and posterior laminectomy were combined with anterior or posterior stabilisation.

Khazim et al. (2003) reported seven cases of spinal hydatid disease treated with posterior decompression and were followed up for an average of 20 years. They concluded that the long-term results were very poor, with high rates of mortality, localised and extra-vertebral recurrence, significant neurological deficits, spino-cutaneous fistulae, spinal instability and pain. Spinal column deformity often occurs in children after multilevel laminectomies for spinal tumours, and its incidence, in these

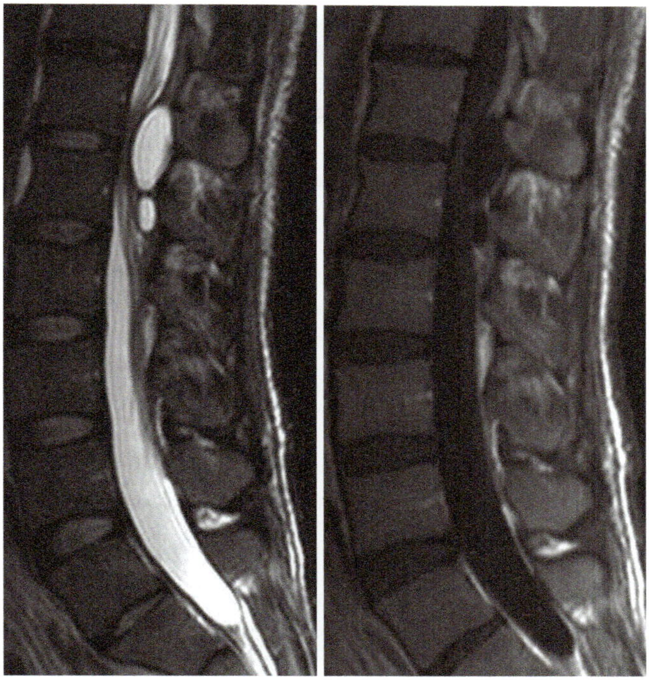

Fig. 14.9 T2- and T1-weighted sagittal contrast-enhanced MRI shows multiloculated hydatid cyst with rim enhancement. The lesion was located in posterior epidural space at the level of T12–L1

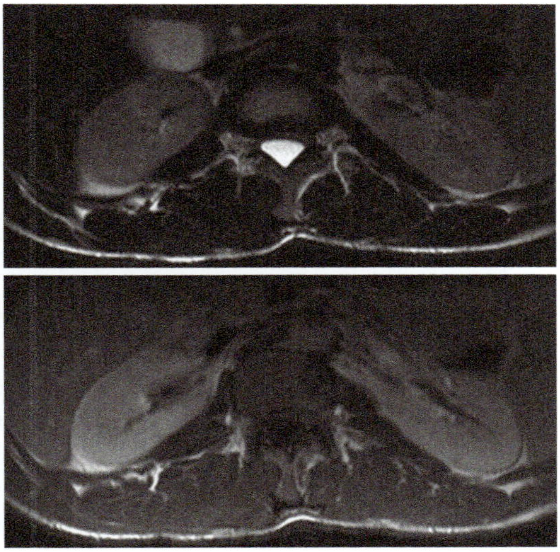

Fig. 14.10 T2- and T1-weighted axial MRI shows cystic lesion which was compressing the dural sac anteriorly

patients, has been reported to be 24–100 % (Papagelopoulos et al. 1997).

Herrera et al. (2005) presented a large series which consisted of 20 spinal hydatid cases. In this series seven thoracic region cases were reported: they exposed the spine posteriorly in all except two patients, and they recommended posterior decompression alone only in cases with isolated neural arch and in extraosseous extradural presentations (Herrera et al. 2005). For the lesions situated in the vertebral body, they recommended an anterior approach to remove the infested bone (Herrera et al. 2005). They also recommended a posterior approach to remove the involved posterior elements and to add a posterior fixation (Herrera et al. 2005). Technically, they used Harrington or Luque spinal instrumentation and pedicle screws for posterior fixation (Herrera et al. 2005).

Khazim (2006) suggested that if stabilisation with pedicle screws is performed, the disease might be iatrogenically seeded into the vertebral body if viable scolices are present at the surgical site. Fusion or stabilisation is not recommended if only partial or complete laminectomy without excessive facet joint excision is performed (Khazim 2006). In our clinical practice we decide to add instrumented fusion depending on whether instability is already present or is created by surgery.

Anterior approach to the thoracic lesions is another alternative for the treatment of thoracic spinal hydatidosis. Transthoracic corpectomy with anterior fusion and anterior approaches with costotransversectomy can also be performed according to the bony involvement of the disease. For lesions situated in the vertebral body, an anterior approach can be used to remove the infected bone (Herrera et al. 2005). Thaler et al. (2010) suggested that anterior compression was falsely treated with posterior laminectomies further destabilising the spine and accelerating the kyphotic deformity. The bony apex due to the kyphotic deformity was continuously causing anterior pressure on the cord causing neurological deterioration with episodes of paraplegia. In a kyphotic deformity, the posterior approach with costotransversectomy gives a perfect view of the operative field especially for the resection of the posterior wall of the bony apex. An anterior approach via thoracotomy would provide a better vessel control in cases of vascular injury; however, it is inappropriate in terms of apical resection and cord control.

Successful anterior approaches, with symptom-free period of 2 or 3 years after surgery, have been reported by some authors (Pamir et al. 2002; Akesen et al. 2011). The cysts which extended into the thoracic cavity via neural foramina can be removed with an anterior approach. Anterior approaches have also been used for complementary treatment strategies for thoracic spinal hydatidosis. Prabhakar et al. (2005) presented a series of four spinal hydatidosis in which they presented two thoracic ones which were treated with combined posterior and anterior approaches. Firstly laminectomy and posterior decompression were performed, and subsequently this surgery was complemented with anterior decompression and fusion. Akesen et al. (2011) presented a case of multilevel thoracic spinal hydatidosis which was treated by a three-level anterior corpectomy after posterior decompression and fusion. They suggested that multilevel spinal involvement should not be a reason to avoid surgical treatment if the lesion can be excised with a three-level corpectomy. Stability of the anterior column must be ascertained to prevent postoperative kyphosis. An extensive resection with stabilisation and grafting is shown to prolong survival in selected cases (Turtas et al. 1980).

After corpectomy a tricortical iliac strut graft or a lyophilised iliac crest allograft or an autologous costal graft can be placed for anterior support. Also a titanium cage packed with autogenous bone graft can be placed in the bone defect formed. Sapkas et al. (1998) reported his concerns about the possible infestation of graft material and advocated the use of acrylic cement for osteosynthesis. Bhojraj and Shetty (1999) have a contrary idea. They suggested that an anterior approach should be avoided to prevent the spread of the disease to the chest and abdominal cavities (Sapkas et al. 1998).

In brief, appropriate surgical treatment would include complete cyst resection without violation of the wall, appropriate decompression of the cord, correction of the deformity and appropriate anterior and posterior instrumented stabilisation techniques (Thaler et al. 2010).

Surgical Treatment of Lumbosacral Spinal Hydatidosis

The lumbar segment is the second most common disease location in spinal hydatidosis (Turgut 1997; Pamir et al. 2002). Simple laminectomy is the most common procedure for surgical treatment (Pamir et al. 2002). This approach allows simple and easy decompression with low morbidity and mortality. But in cases of bone involvement, access to the vertebral body is limited with a laminectomy (Figs. 14.11 and 14.12). In addition spillage of scolices is unavoidable in cases of bone involvement. Laminectomy only may result in rupture of cysts and scolex spillage (Senoglu et al. 2009).

Abdominal retroperitoneal corpectomy with posterior fusion and subsequent surgery for vertebral body was reported in lumbar hydatidosis (Lam et al. 1997). Baysefer et al. (1996) presented a case of L4 vertebral hydatid cyst which was operated through an anterior approach. Anterior spinal decompression by a retroperitoneal abdominal approach was performed. The vertebra was excised and an autologous iliac bone graft was inserted into the defect. Later they performed a posterior fusion for stabilisation.

We have previously reported a case of spinal hydatidosis which eroded the 2nd lumbar vertebral body and pedicle and extended to the paravertebral and abdominal region and neural foramina (Fig. 14.13). The patient was operated through an anterolateral approach, the lesion was removed and L2 partial corpectomy was performed. Interbody fusion was accomplished using an L1–L3 distractable cage, and stabilisation was performed using an L1–L3 bicortical screw-plate system (Fig. 14.14). The patient was symptom-free at his 6-month follow-up, and

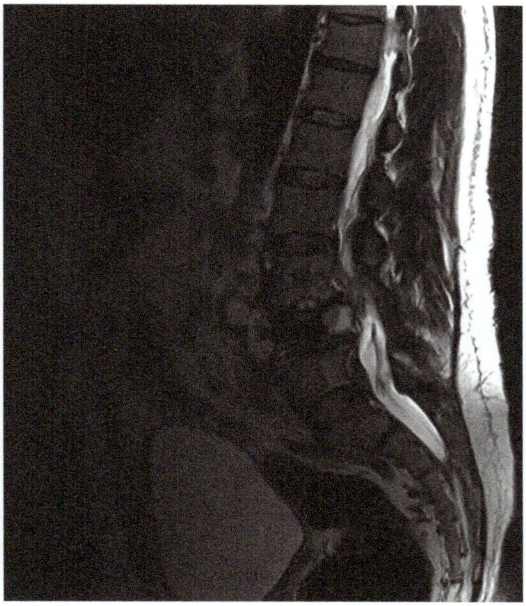

Fig. 14.11 T1-weighted sagittal MRI shows spinal hydatid cyst with L4 corpus involvement. There is bone destruction, partial collapse and retroperitoneal extension

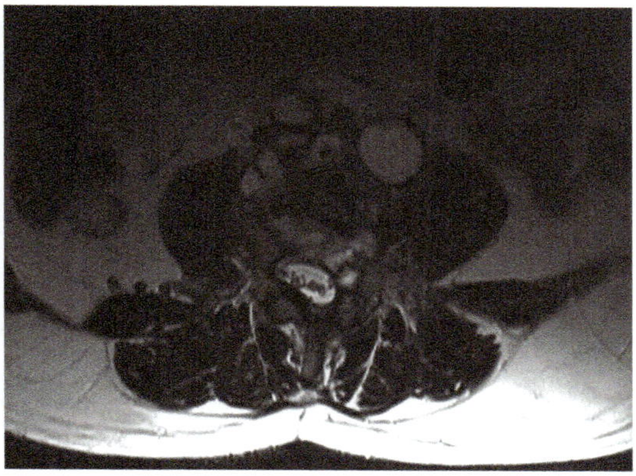

Fig. 14.12 T2-weighted axial MRI sequence through L4 vertebral body. The corpus was almost completely destroyed

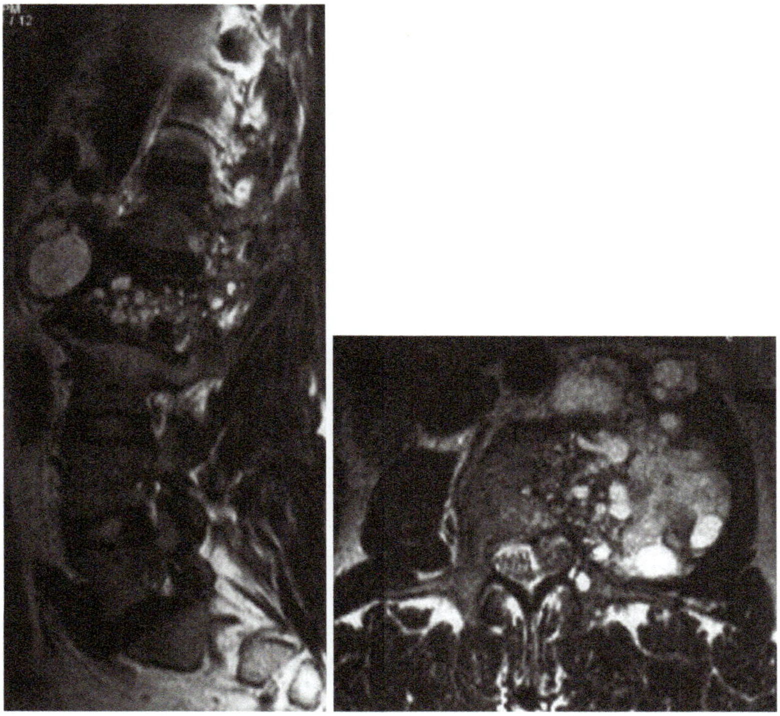

Fig. 14.13 Sagittal T2-weighted (*right*) and axial (*left*) MRI sequences show L2 vertebral body destruction with left psoas expansion. The lesion was extending through the left neural foramen and compressing the root

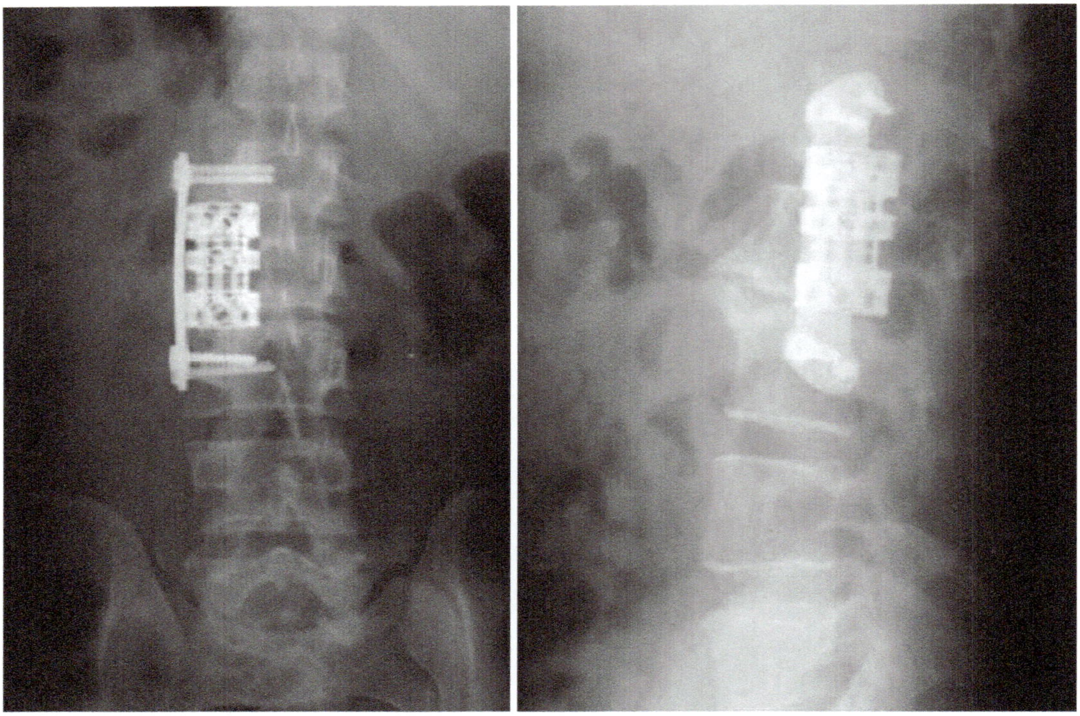

Fig. 14.14 Postoperative plain radiographs of the case shown in Fig. 14.13 show L1–3 distractable cage and L1–3 screw-plate system

magnetic resonance imaging (MRI) revealed total removal of the disease (Kalkan et al. 2008). Senoglu et al. (2009) presented a case of sacral spinal hydatidosis which was treated with combined anterior and posterior approach. Firstly an anterior extraperitoneal approach was performed, and then a posterior approach with bilateral S1 hemilaminectomy was done.

Scolicidal Agents

Although the effectivity is not proven, most surgeons advocate intraoperative scolicidal agents as well as adjuvant pharmacotherapy (Pamir et al. 2002). Scolicidal agents like 3 % hypertonic saline, cetrimide, chlorhexidine, 80 % alcohol, 0.5 % silver nitrate, 10 % formalin, sodium hypochlorite and glycerine phenol are used in abdominal hydatid cyst disease (Pamir et al. 2002; Khazim et al. 2003). The use of povidone iodine as a scolicidal agent is reported in spinal cases, but long-term results are lacking (Pandey and Cahudhari 1997). Hypertonic saline is the most frequently used agent in spinal hydatidosis. Hypertonic saline is a scolicidal agent due to the difference of osmolality between the hypertonic saline and the interior of the cyst. It causes the sclerosis of the cyst (Herrera et al. 2005). Işlekel et al. (1998) reported an operative mortality due to toxic myelitis caused by formalin after a dural tear. Formalin irrigation is also reported to add to the morbidity by increasing tissue necrosis and should be avoided in spinal cases (Pamir et al. 2002).

Chemotherapy for spinal hydatidosis is discussed in detail in Chap. 16.

Minimally Invasive Techniques

Diagnostic or therapeutic fine needle aspiration of hydatid cysts is frequently used in abdominal hydatid disease. Puncture-aspiration-injection-reaspiration (PAIR) refers to an ultrasound-guided technique consisting of puncture and evacuation of the contents of the hydatid cyst, injection of scolicidal agents such as 95 % ethanol and reaspiration of the contents of the cyst. This technique was first developed by Mueller et al. (1985) as an alternative treatment method against surgical excision of the liver hydatid cysts. Spektor et al. (1997) described the successful decompression of an extradural cervical spinal hydatid cyst by computed tomography (CT)-guided fine needle aspiration with complete resolution of quadriplegia. Bilgic et al. (2009) reported a case of primary hydatid cyst of the erector spinae muscle which was treated successfully with PAIR technique. At the final follow-up 26 months after the aspiration, the patient was free of symptoms and ultrasonography revealed solidification of the cyst content and thickening and irregularity of the cyst wall, all of which were considered as signs of cure.

Other minimally invasive techniques such as endoscopic evacuation of cyst material are reported in the literature (Acikgoz et al. 1996). Pamir et al. (2002) suggested that minimally invasive methods may be of value in selected patients with localised spinal disease, in whom surgical therapy is contraindicated. They suggested that these minimally invasive techniques are still experimental and the efficacy and safety has not been established. Potential complications of this technique are anaphylaxis and the risk of iatrogenic spreading (Thaler et al. 2010). In addition, simple drainage of the infested cystic area is reported to result in pyogenic osteomyelitis and is strongly discouraged (Rao et al. 1991). Spector et al. (1997) suggested that with adequate prophylaxis against anaphylaxis and dissemination, CT-guided aspiration of spinal hydatid cysts with hypertonic saline irrigation and subsequent chemotherapy may be an alternative to surgical therapy in selected cases.

Complications

The surgical treatment has some specific and non-specific complications. Cyst rupture is an important complication especially in the pure intradurally or epidurally located hydatid cyst cases without bone involvement. Extreme caution should be taken not to rupture intradural or epidural solitary cysts, as complete removal might potentially result in a cure. If any cyst ruptures into the intradural space, the surgical area should be irrigated with hypertonic saline, but this seems relatively ineffective, and recurrence is unavoidable in these cases (Braithwaite and Lees 1981).

Cyst rupture during surgery has a potentially fatal but rare complication: anaphylactic shock. Turgut (2001) reported 3 deaths from 'anaphylactic shock' out of the 268 reviewed intracranial hydatid cases in the Turkish literature. There is no reported case of anaphylactic shock in spinal hydatid cyst. Recurrence is a major complication of the surgical treatment. The recurrence rate has ranged from 30 to 100 %. The average number of procedures per patient has been reported as 2.6–4.6 (Khazim et al. 2003).

Infection, deep venous thrombosis, pulmonary embolism, cerebrospinal fluid leakage, postoperative mortality and increased neurological deficit are some important non-specific complications of surgical treatment. A mortality rate of 0–3 % is reported which progressively increases to 15 % in reoperations (Pamir et al. 2002). Işlekel et al. (1998) reported on the death of a case due to formalin irrigation, the formalin having seeped into the CSF through an intraoperative tear of the dura.

Complications of spinal hydatidosis are discussed in detail in Chap. 18.

Surgical Results

The prognosis of vertebral hydatidosis is very poor, especially if neurological deficits are present. Even with extensive surgery results are far from being curative and recurrences are almost universal (Pamir et al. 2002). Up to 40 % of patients are reported to have recurrent symptomatology within 2 years from the initial operation. In recurrent lesions the major goal is restoration of neurological status and preservation of spinal stability. The presence of disease involving the paravertebral tissues further warrants the use of adjuvant therapy. Nevertheless, most patients experience a downhill course with worsening neurological status and progressive destruction of the vertebral column with multiple recurrences. The incidence of paraplegia in recurrent disease is reported to be as high as 45 %. Recurrence is considered a bad prognostic factor in spinal hydatid disease. Operative mortalities up to 14.4 % were reported in recurrent cases. Most patients having such treatment have had several operations for recurrence.

Keller et al. (1997) reported a cervical case operated on six times with preservation of spinal stability and neurological status. They concluded that despite multiple recurrences, spinal stability could be achieved and should be the goal. Recurrences occur 2–28 months (mean, 25.2 months) after the initial operation. The recurrence rate for intradural extramedullary disease is reported to be low. The high recurrence rate is primarily responsible for the poor survival rate in only 5 years after the onset of symptoms. Lam et al. (1997) reported that the average age at death is 41 years. Operative mortality rates up to 15 % are reported in the literature and are known to increase with subsequent operations. Paraplegia due to recurrent disease is reported to be as high as 45 % (Pamir et al. 2002). Overall mortality rates were reported as 14–58 % for groups of patients with or without paraplegia (Khazim et al. 2003).

Khazim et al. (2003) suggested that the poor results of surgical treatment can be partially explained by the fact that the diagnosis was not suspected until the lesion was encountered intraoperatively. They concluded that a high level of suspicion is paramount in making the diagnosis. This is more important in countries where the disease is not endemic.

Işlekel et al. (1998) reported a case which was operated in a western country where the hydatid disease is not endemic. The pre- and postoperative diagnoses were a dermoid cyst. Opening of the dura during the first operation presumably led to the intradural invasion and recurrences. This patient was operated upon eight times and died of renal complications.

Conclusion

Spinal hydatidosis should be considered as a locally aggressive tumour, the treatment of which ideally should be radical excision of all affected tissues with a margin of healthy tissue. Technically, this is very unlikely to be achieved because of the absence of distinct anatomic planes, containment within small spaces having bony boundaries and the existence of neural structures in close vicinity. Nevertheless, marginal or intralesional excision of the hydatid lesions is possible through combined anterior and posterior approaches.

References

Acikgoz B, Sungur C, Ozgen T, Camurdanoglu M, Berker M. Endoscopic evacuation of sacral hydatid cysts: case report. Spinal Cord. 1996;34:361–4.

Akesen B, Ermutlu C, Aydinli U. Spinal hydatidosis. Report of a case treated by three level corpectomy, anterior and posterior instrumentation. J Turk Spinal Surg. 2011;22:45–50.

Baysefer A, Gonül E, Canakci Z, Erdogan E, Aydogan N, Kayali H. Hydatid disease of the spine. Spinal Cord. 1996;34:297–300.

Bhojraj SY, Shetty N. Primary hydatid disease of the spine: an unusual cause of progressive paraplegia. Case report and review of the literature. J Neurosurg. 1999;91:216–8.

Bilgic S, Kose O, Sehirlioglu A, Safaz I, Ozkan H. Primary paraspinal hydatid cyst treated with puncture, aspiration, injection and re-aspiration (PAIR) technique: a case report. Eur Spine J. 2009;18 Suppl 2:165–7.

Braithwaite PA, Lees RF. Vertebral hydatid disease: radiological assessment. Radiology. 1981;140:763–6.

Dew HR. Hydatid disease. Its pathology, diagnosis and treatment. Sydney: Australasian Medical Publishing Co Ltd; 1928. p. 429.

El-On J, Ben-Noun L, Galitza Z, Ohana N. Case report: clinical and serological evaluation echinococcosis of the spine. Trans R Soc Trop Med Hyg. 2003;97:567–9.

Fiennes AG, Thomas DG. Combined medical and surgical treatment of spinal hydatid disease: a case report. J Neurol Neurosurg Psychiatry. 1982;45:927–30.

Herrera A, Martínez AA, Rodríguez J. Spinal hydatidosis. Spine (Phila Pa 1976). 2005;30:2439–44.

Işlekel S, Erşahin Y, Zileli M, Oktar N, Oner K, Ovül I, Ozdamar N, Tuncbay F. Spinal hydatid disease. Spinal Cord. 1998;36:166–70.

Kalkan E, Cengiz SL, Ciçek O, Erdi F, Baysefer A. Primary spinal intradural extramedullary hydatid cyst in a child. J Spinal Cord Med. 2007;30:297–300.

Kalkan E, Torun F, Erdi F, Baysefer A. Primary lumbar vertebral hydatid cyst. J Clin Neurosci. 2008;15:472–3.

Kaoutzanis M, Anagnostopoulos D, Apostolou A. Hydatid disease affecting the vertebrae. Acta Neurochir (Wien). 1989;98:60–5.

Keller TM, Schweitzer JS, Helfend LK, Chappel T. Treatment of progressive cervical spinal instability secondary to hydatid disease. A case report. Spine (Phila Pa 1976). 1997;22:915–9.

Khazim RM. Spinal hydatid disease. South Med J. 2006;99:114.

Khazim R, Fares Y, Heras-Palou C, Ruiz Barnes P. Posterior decompression of spinal hydatidosis: long term results: Fundacion Jimenez Diaz, Madrid, Spain. Clin Neurol Neurosurg. 2003;105:209–14.

Lam KS, Faraj A, Mulholland RC, Finch RG. Medical decompression of vertebral hydatidosis. Spine (Phila Pa 1976). 1997;22:2050–5.

Ley A, Marti A. Intramedullary hydatid cyst. Case report. J Neurosurg. 1970;33:257–9.

Mueller PR, Dawson SL, Ferrucci Jr JT, Nardi GL. Hepatic echinococcal cyst: successful percutaneous drainage. Radiology. 1985;155:627–8.

Ouma JR. Echinococcosis-a rare spinal disorder. S Afr Med J. 2006;96:680–2.

Pamir MN, Ozduman K, Elmaci I. Spinal hydatid disease. Spinal Cord. 2002;40:153–60.

Pandey M, Cahudhari MP. Primary hydatid cyst of sacral spinal canal: case report. Neurosurgery. 1997;40:407–9.

Papagelopoulos PJ, Peterson HA, Ebersold MJ, Emmanuel PR, Choudhury SN, Quast LM. Spinal column deformity and instability after lumbar or thoracolumbar laminectomy for intraspinal tumors in children and young adults. Spine (Phila Pa 1976). 1997;22: 442–51.

Papanikolaou A. Osseous hydatid disease. Trans R Soc Trop Med Hyg. 2008;102:233–8.

Prabhakar MM, Acharya AJ, Modi DR, Jadav B. Spinal hydatid disease: a case series. J Spinal Cord Med. 2005;28:426–31.

Rao S, Parikh S, Kerr R. Echinococcal infestation of the spine in North America. Clin Orthop Relat Res. 1991;271:164–9.

Reydellet. Moelle epiniere, medulla spinalis ou dorsalis. In: Dictionaire des medicales, par une societede medecins et des chirurgiens, vol. 33. Paris: C.I.F. Panckoucke; 1819:538–68 in (Rayport M, Wisoff HS, Zaiman H. Vertebral echinococcosis: report of case of surgical and biological therapy with review of the literature. J Neurosurg. 1964; 21: 647–59.)

Sapkas GS, Stathakopulos DP, Babis GC, Tsarouchas JK. Hydatid disease of bones and joints. 8 cases followed for 4–16 years. Acta Orthop Scand. 1998;69:89–94.

Sengul G, Kadioglu HH, Kayaoglu CR, Aktas S, Akar A, Aydin IH. Treatment of spinal hydatid disease: a single center experience. J Clin Neurosci. 2008;15:507–10.

Senoglu M, Bulbuloglu E, Demirpolat G, Altun I, Celik M. Combined anterior and posterior approach for sacral/retroperitoneal hydatid cyst disease: case report. Turk Neurosurg. 2009;19:428–32.

Spektor S, Gomori JM, Beni-Adani L, Constantini S. Spinal echinococcal cyst: treatment using computerized tomography guided needle aspiration and hypertonic saline irrigation. Case report. J Neurosurg. 1997;87:464–7.

Tandon N, Vollmer DG. Posterior approaches to the cervical spine. In: Fesler GR, Sekhar L, editors. Atlas of neurosurgical techniques, spine and peripheral nerves. New York: Thieme; 2006.

Thaler M, Gabl M, Lechner R, Gstöttner M, Bach CM. Severe kyphoscoliosis after primary Echinococcus granulosus infection of the spine. Eur Spine J. 2010;19:1415–22.

Tsitouridis I, Dimitriadis AS. CT and MRI in vertebral hydatid disease. Eur Radiol. 1997;7:1207–10.

Turgut M. Hydatid disease of the spine: a survey study from Turkey. Infection. 1997;25:221–6.

Turgut M. Intracranial hydatidosis in Turkey: its clinical presentation, diagnostic studies, surgical management and out-come, a review of 276 cases. Neurosurg Rev. 2001;24:200–8.

Turtas S, Viale ES, Pau A. Long term results of surgery for hydatid disease of the spine. Surg Neurol. 1980;13:468–70.

Surgical Treatment of Cerebral Hydatidosis

15

Sailike Duishanbai and Hao Wen

Contents

S. Duishanbai, MD, PhD
Department of Neurosurgery,
First Teaching Hospital of Xinjiang Medical University,
Xinjiang, China
e-mail: serickd@yahoo.com

H. Wen, MD, PhD (✉)
Department of General Surgery,
First Teaching Hospital of Xinjiang Medical University,
No1 Liyusha, Urumqi, Xinjiang 830054, China
e-mail: dr.wenhao@163.com

Surgical Indications

There are no clear-cut surgical indications for intracranial hydatid cysts in the existing medical literature. Unlike other intracranial lesions, an intracranial hydatid cyst has its own characteristic, biological behavior, and clinical manifestations, such as benign growth, relatively mild neurological deficit, and large size at presentation (Turgut 1997; Duishanbai et al. 2011). Owing to such distinct characteristics, almost all patients with intracranial hydatid cysts need to undergo one or more surgical interventions for the rapid relief of intracranial pressure or decompression of surrounding neural, vascular, and parenchymal brain tissues. Increased intracranial pressure and progressive neurological deficit are the main surgical indications. Surgical treatment is mandatory for all patients once the correct diagnosis is made, except for patients with multiple organ involvement in poor general conditions and deep-located cysts in which surgery may produce additional neurological deficit or even death. Recurrent hydatid cysts, multiple hydatid cysts, and hydatid cysts which are resistant to chemotherapy still need surgical treatment (Yurt et al. 2007).

Preoperative Care

Preoperative chemotherapy, albendazole, is not indicated for primary intracranial solitary hydatid cysts, while intracranial hydatid cyst with

M. Turgut (ed.), *Hydatidosis of the Central Nervous System: Diagnosis and Treatment*,
DOI 10.1007/978-3-642-54359-3_15, © Springer-Verlag Berlin Heidelberg 2014

extraneuronal involvement still needs preoperative chemotherapy (Turgut 2001; Duishanbai et al. 2010). Epilepsy is one of the common symptoms of supratentorial intraparenchymal hydatid cyst; thus, antiepileptic drugs are recommended for such a subgroup of patients. Intermittent usage of dehydrating agents such as 20 % mannitol is recommended for patients with increased intracranial pressure who are at risk of developing brain herniation or impending loss of vision. Good nutritional status and absence of other associated infections are important for a successful surgical treatment. Intraoperative antibiotics are also recommended for all surgical cases. Usually, blood preparation is not mandatory except for infants or children with big cyst which needs large craniotomies.

Surgery

Anesthesia

Patients with an intracranial hydatid cyst receive general anesthesia. General anesthesia should be deep enough to prevent brain bulging and inadvertent movement of the patient.

Positioning

The positioning of the patient depends on the location of the given cyst. Supine and lateral positions are used for supratentorial hydatid cysts, and prone and sitting positions are used for infratentorial ones. To facilitate the delivery process of a hydatid cyst by gravity, head positioning is very important. At the time of delivery, the surgeon should be able to rotate or lower the head at will to facilitate the delivery. So, the patient's head should not be securely fastened to the operating table (Turgut 2001, 2002; Duishanbai et al. 2011).

Craniotomy

Craniotomies for the removal of cerebral hydatid cysts are always larger in size than the standard neurosurgical craniotomies for other space-occupying lesions, as well as large skin flaps (Duishanbai et al. 2010). Commonly used approaches may include temporo-frontal, temporo-fronto-parietal, and temporo-parieto-occipital approaches. On rare occasions, cysts are found in the orbit, pons, intra- or parasellar regions, cerebellopontine angle, thalamus and petroclivus, aqueduct of Sylvius, and jugular foramen; and those may need more sophisticated surgical approaches (Gökalp and Erdoğan 1988; Kayaoglu 2008; Kamath et al. 2009). Multiple cerebral hydatid cysts may need multiple craniotomies (Akdemir et al. 2007; Yurt et al. 2007).

Surgical Procedures

Surgery is the method of choice for the treatment of cerebral hydatid cysts whenever possible, but alone it may not cure hydatid cyst in some conditions such as multiple hydatid cysts in deep locations and multiple organ involvement (Turgut 2001). Although the Dowling-Orlando technique has long been used as a golden surgical technique for the treatment of cerebral hydatid cysts, it is not always applicable to the hydatid cyst in extraneural spaces and atypical areas such as the orbit, epidural spaces, brain stem, periventricular regions, cavernous sinus, and basal cisterns (Rivierez et al. 1992; Yüceer and Gökalp 1998; Yilmazlar and Aksoy 1999; Khaldi et al. 2000; Rumboldt et al. 2003; Beskonakli et al. 2005; Boudawara et al. 1975). Although the removal of a solitary cerebral hydatid cyst can easily and safely be achieved by a modified Dowling's technique in uncomplicated cases, complete removal of multiple cysts or those located in atypical areas is usually difficult, and radical extirpation of the cyst is not possible without rupture. In these cases, techniques other than Dowling's technique, such as puncture-aspiration-injection-reaspiration (PAIR) of the cyst, may be used. The materials used in irrigation are devitalizing solutions like 0.1–1 % cetrimide, chlorhexidine, 80 % alcohol, 0.5 % silver nitrate, 10 % formalin, sodium hypochlorite, glycerin-phenol, and hypertonic saline. Up until now, the main surgical choice for the removal of intracranial hydatid cysts may include (a) the modified Dowling-Orlando technique, (b) the percutaneous

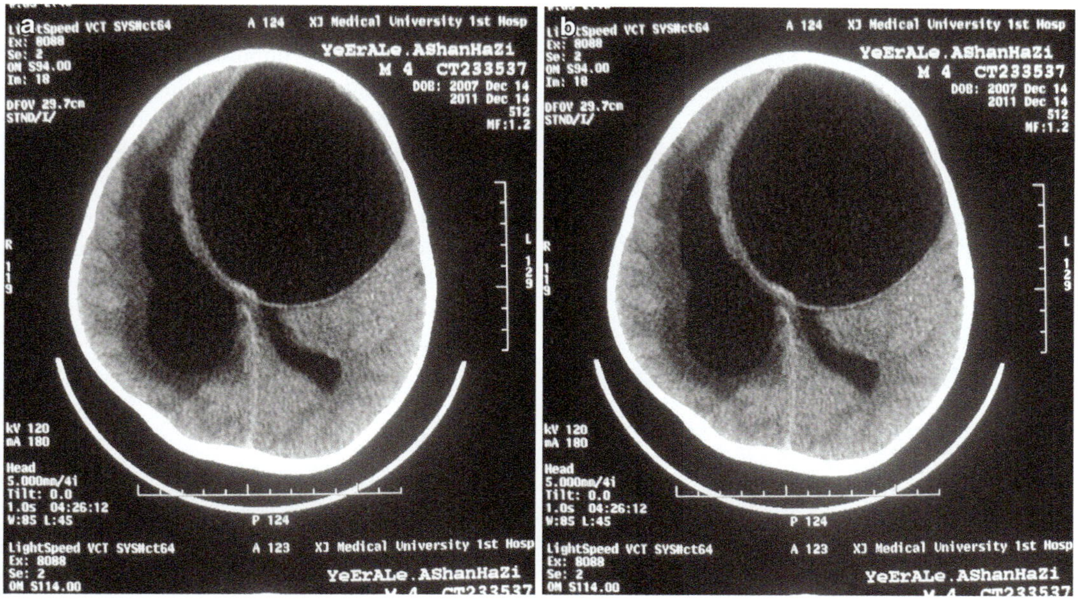

Fig. 15.1 A plain CT showing a giant frontal hydatid cyst in a 4-year-old Kazakh boy (**a**) and an intubated patient and a large skin incision marked in supine position with the head turned a little toward the opposite side of the lesion (**b**)

or intraoperative PAIR method, (c) microsurgery, or (d) a combination of the above three methods. Surgical strategy should be tailored according to the type of cyst for a favorable outcome with minimal mortality and morbidity (Turgut 2001). Hydatid cysts which are located in extradural spaces and in the orbit can be removed with microsurgical techniques (Gazzaz et al. 2000; Erman et al. 2001; Turgut 2001). Akdemir et al. (2007) and Cemil et al. (2009) reported that hydatid cysts of the internal acoustic canal and jugular foramen have been removed via retrosigmoid suboccipital craniotomy.

Modified Dowling-Orlando Technique

After the correct diagnosis, patients with cerebral hydatid cyst may be treated on an emergency basis or as elective surgery according to the neurological symptoms and signs (Fig. 15.1a). Herniated cases or cases that are at risk of herniation should be treated urgently. The timing of surgery is based on the neurological and neuroimaging findings. Early cyst extirpation (within 3 days) is reserved for giant hydatid cysts that cause severe neurological deficits, and late extirpation (more than 3 days) is performed in patients who have relatively small cysts and those which need to undergo further evaluation for the differential diagnosis or to improve their general condition (Turgut 2001, 2002).

Positioning

The patient should be positioned in the correct operating position according to the location and size of the given cyst, and the head should not be fastened securely to the operating table for the possible changes in its position intraoperatively (Haddad and Haddad 2003) (Fig. 15.1b).

Craniotomy

The craniotomy should be planned to be larger than craniotomies utilized in usual space-occupying lesions, and the excess should be planed toward the inferior edge of the cyst (Fig. 15.2). It is preferable to use clamps rather than Raney scalp clips to secure hemostasis of the scalp. The sharp edges of the Raney scalp clips may injure the falling cyst. It is preferable to use a manual burr hole handle and a Gigli saw than an electric or air-powered drill because the vibrations of the later may rupture

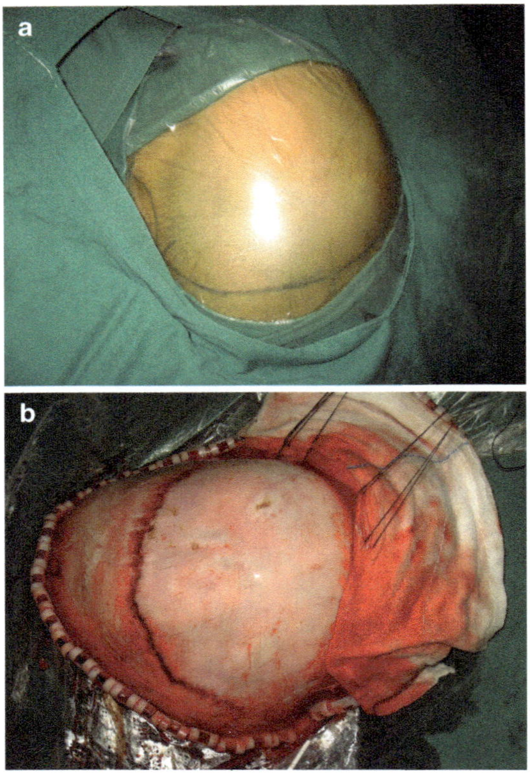

Fig. 15.2 A plain CT showing the operating filed sterilized and draped (**a**) and a large skin flap reflected (**b**)

a cyst in its proximity. The bone flap is then carefully lifted and separated from the underlying dura matter and removed as a free flap (Fig. 15.3a). One must be sure not to leave sharp bony edges in the field. These should be carefully trimmed and smoothened to prevent and inadvertent rupture of the cyst (Haddad and Haddad 2003).

The dura is carefully opened starting away from the expected position of the cyst, and any adhesions to the underlying brain or ectocyst should be released carefully (Fig. 15.3b). Tucking of the dura is strongly recommended after the opening of the dura, not before, to prevent possible injury of superficially lying cysts. On illumination, through the thinned dura, cyst fluid may be observed in some patients once the cranium has been opened (Fig. 15.3c). Usually there is a very thin cortical tissue, if any, under the dura mater (Fig. 15.3c).

Operative Field Draping

This is of paramount importance. It may prevent cyst rupture, and in case of such inadvertent rupture, this draping will minimize the damage. Fine gauze imbibed with 0.1 % Cetrimide is placed around the bone edges of the craniotomy, as well as over the normal brain tissue. The same type of gauze covers all clamps and/or Raney scalp clips and fishhooks if in use. Rolls of wet gauze are tucked between the edges of the dura and the cortex to prevent the seepage of fluid into the base of the brain, in case of rupture.

The Delivery

Usually a small surface of the cyst appears through the cortex. This area is not large enough to permit the safe delivery of the cyst. The arachnoid is carefully opened. As seen in Fig. 15.3d, "episiotomies" are performed in silent areas. While carrying these episiotomies, no cautery, uni- or bipolar, should be used. Any significant blood vessel should be clipped and not coagulated. These vascular clips could be removed at the end of surgery and the blood vessels coagulated then. The episiotomies are carried though the depth of the cortex until the cyst wall is seen (Fig. 15.3e). At this stage the "membranes" should be ruptured to allow a normal delivery. The membrane in these cases is the pericyst. In the brain, there is a very fine pericyst which at times may rupture spontaneously. If it remains intact, it will hamper delivery. One can tear it with a blunt instrument. Once the apparent portion of the pericyst is resected, the head of the patient is readjusted in a way to have the cyst in the most dependent position (Fig. 15.3f). A band of soft gauze, soaked in cetrimide, is laid on the cortex from the interphase between the cyst and cortex, in its most dependent position and extending to the receptacle which will receive the specimen. This receptacle should contain some cetrimide to prevent the direct fall of the cyst against the container's solid bottom. A fine pliable rubber tube is inserted in the space between the pericyst and ectocyst, and a 0.1 % Cetrimide solution is gently injected to break the adhesive effect between the peri- and ectocyst and to float the cyst (Fig. 15.3g). At this moment Credé's maneuver by pressing on the cortex

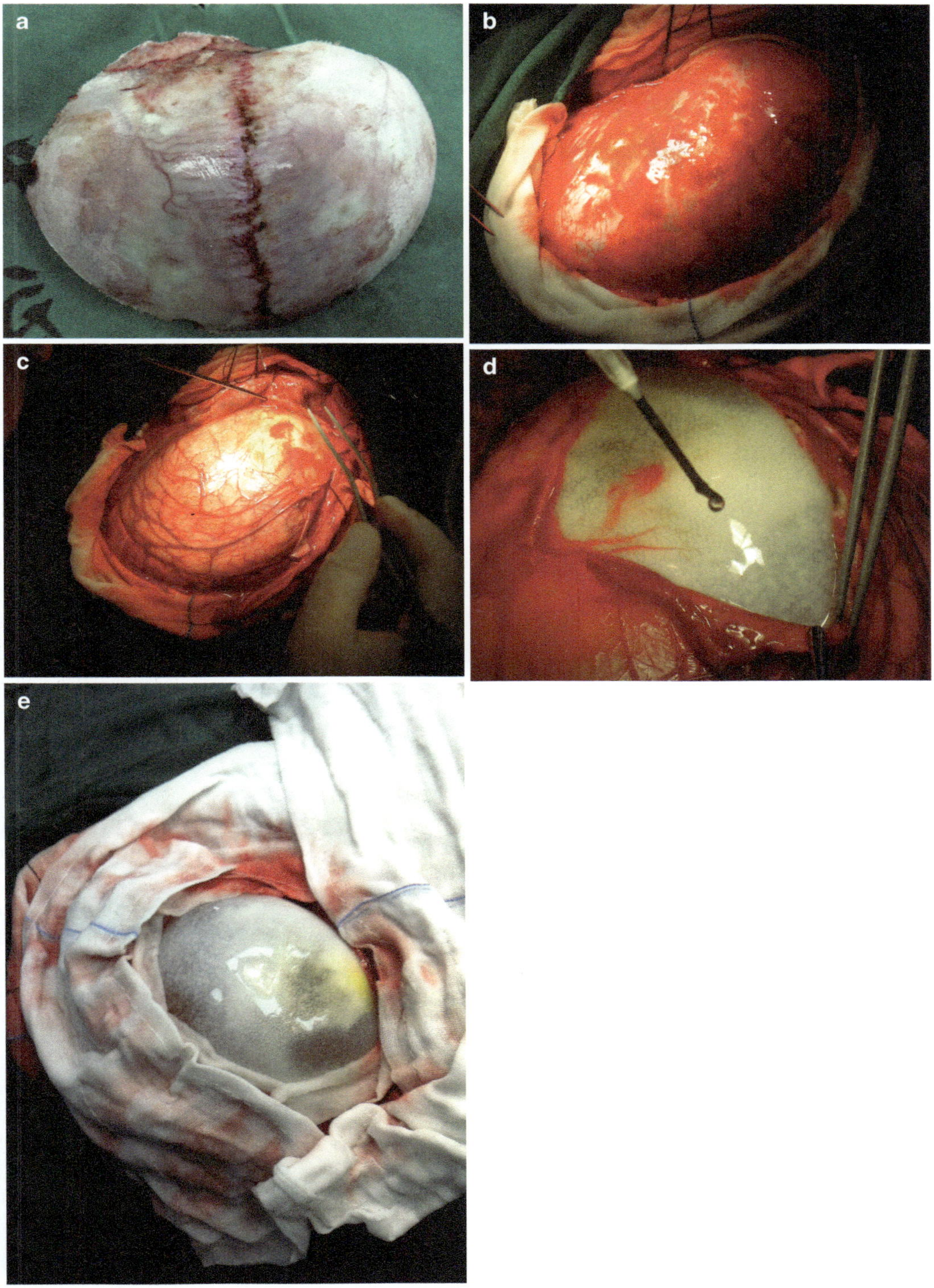

Fig. 15.3 A plain CT showing a large free bone flap removed (**a**), a tense dura (**b**), a thin layer of cortical tissue overlying the hydatid cyst (**c**), a meticulous cortical dissection performed to expose the cystic wall (**d**), the entire cystic wall exposed (**e**), the operating table tilted toward the lesion side and the head of the patients lowered and a fine plastic tube inserted between the cystic wall and brain tissue (**f**), floating of hydatid cyst after injecting saline with the syringe (**g**), intactly removed hydatid cyst in a bowel with water (**h**), and the irrigation procedure after the removal of the hydatid cyst (**i**)

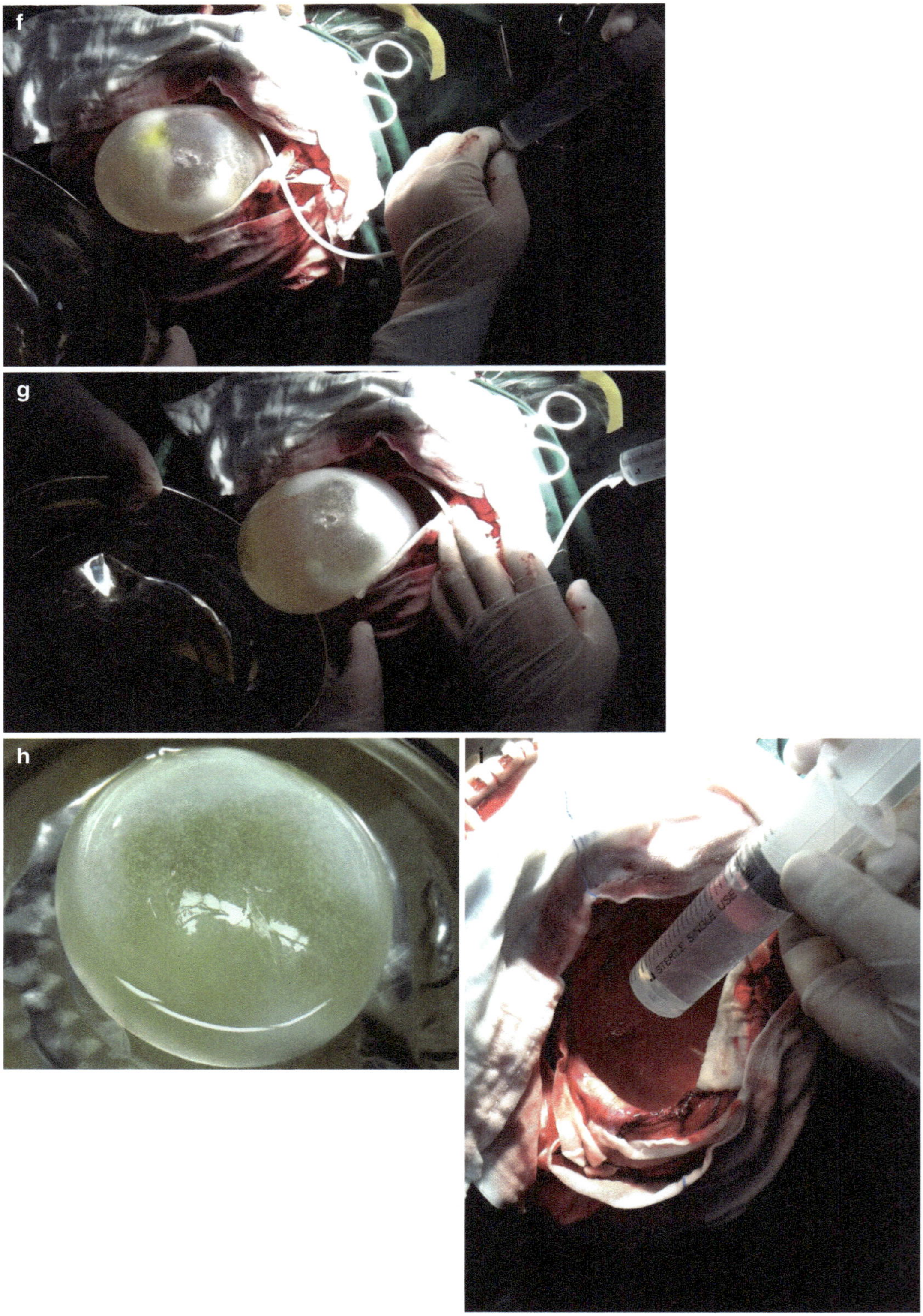

Fig. 15.3 (continued)

superior to the cyst and asking the anesthesiologist to compress both jugular veins in the neck in an effort to increase the intracranial pressure and gradually expulsing the cyst. In case the cyst does not come out, the head is further lowered until the cyst flows out of its cavity in the brain into the prepared receptacle (Fig. 15.3h). It is extremely important to maintain a blunt wide brain retractor in the upper portion of the cavity to prevent the brain from collapsing, which may tear crossing the veins, and to simultaneously fill the cavity with cetrimide while the cyst is being delivered (Fig. 15.3i). Once the cyst is delivered, hemostasis is completed and all the gauze is retrieved. The closure of the craniotomy is then performed in the usual manner (Turgut 2001; Haddad and Haddad 2003; Izci et al. 2008; Duishanbai et al. 2011).

Delivery of Deep Lesions

In case the cyst does not present on the surface of the cortex, the latter should be cut with a fine blunted tip pair of scissors in a silent area overlying the cyst. The opening is enlarged and deepened, with blunt dissection, until the pericyst appears. This procedure, which was called by one of the authors a "cesarean section," should be performed with extreme care lest the cyst rupture. We have used the cortical ultrasound to detect the remaining distance between the cyst and our instrument. In case the cyst is large, its delivery is similar to the cortical cyst. However, more frequently, one is dealing with small cyst, and we found that an appropriate size kitchen spoon is very helpful in raising the cyst into the receptacle.

Puncture-Aspiration-Injection-Reaspiration (PAIR) Technique

This technique should only be used in case the previously described delivery technique is impossible to use. This, as its name indicates, involves the puncture of the cyst with a fine needle and aspirating its content and partially and carefully injecting a scolicidal solution which should be left in place for a minimum of 10 min. Then the remaining fluid is reaspirated, and the collapsed chitinous membrane is removed with a forceps. The problem in this procedure is that there is always spillage around the needle puncture, and if the cyst is rapidly and completely emptied, it collapses and cannot be refilled properly. Although the area of spillage is irrigated with a scolicidal solution to prevent anaphylactic complications and recurrences, each puncture invariably leads to some spillage of the contents into the operative field, and cyst recurrences are frequent. For example, total removal of a pontine hydatid cyst is practically impossible with Dowling's technique, which requires forcing saline beneath the cyst in order to displace it outward.

The PAIR technique was introduced in the mid-1980s for treating liver hydatid cyst (Filice and Brunetti 1997). It is usually used for cerebral hydatid cyst in deep location or eloquent areas where removal of the hydatid cyst without rupturing is impossible or may cause additional neurological deficit (Muthusubramanian et al. 2009). Non-intentional burr hole draining was reported, but it is a very risky procedure (Anvari et al. 2009). The PAIR technique should always be performed by skilled and experienced physicians well prepared to deal with complications. According to expert recommendations, the PAIR should be accompanied by chemotherapeutic coverage to minimize the potential risk of secondary echinococcosis. In this indication, albendazole is given in daily oral doses of 10 mg/kg of body weight 24–4 h before and 15–30 days after the intervention (World Health Organization Informal Working Group of Echinococcosis 2001). There are several case reports which speak of a successful outcome in removing pontine, basal ganglion and in the interpeduncular cistern hydatid cysts (Boudawara et al. 1999; Erşahin et al. 1995; Yilmazlar and Aksoy 1999; Beskonakli et al. 2005).

Microsurgery

Hemispheric hydatid cysts usually do not need a surgical microscope, but hydatid cysts in deep locations, eloquent areas, and around vital structures need good illumination and magnification for fine dissections on the approach to the cyst or around the cyst wall. We recommend that microsurgery be applied in deep-seated lesions. The use of the magnification during the early part of the surgery of a hydatid cyst is extremely helpful because, at a crucial stage of the procedure, it prevents inadvertent damage to the very thin cyst wall and allows development of the critical surgical plane (Kurtsoy et al. 1999; Balak et al. 2006). Gamma knife treatment has been tested in only a limited number of cases (Schnider 1999).

Postoperative Care

It is recommended that the patients should stay in a neurosurgical intensive care unit overnight until the anesthesia wears off. Antiepileptic drugs may be administered and patients' activities restricted to limit fluctuations in intracranial pressure during the early postoperative period. Albendazole is administered at a dose of 10 mg/kg for 3 months in case of cyst rupture (Duishanbai et al. 2010). Postoperative neuroimaging, computed tomography (CT) or magnetic resonance imaging (MRI), is recommended in the first postoperative day to excluding complications.

Surgical Results and Complications

The results of surgical treatment depend on several factors, including the location, size, and multiplicity of the cysts (Uzun et al. 2010). Giant cysts with a thick wall are no more difficult to remove than smaller ones, which are prone to rupture (Turgut 2001, 2002). Furthermore, it is considered that patients with multiple cysts have high morbidity and mortality rates owing to the number of surgical interventions needed to remove them all, but these patients frequently tolerate multiple surgical procedures. The ratio of cysts to patients was 2.2, and the recurrence and mortality rates for intracranial hydatid cysts were 14 and 10 %, respectively (Turgut 2002). Although it is rarely possible to expel a cyst intact from an extradural localization in the central nervous system without rupturing it, its rupture into this space, fortunately, does not inevitably lead to a severe anaphylactic response, in contrast to widespread subarachnoid dissemination. Cysts in deep locations have posed surgical problems, and some cysts have inadvertently ruptured during surgery. In the postoperative period, subdural effusions and porencephalic cysts can occur as a complication in children and adolescents (Sandhu et al. 2000; Tuzun et al. 2010).

Brain abscess has also been reported to be a rare complication (Kabatas et al. 2009). The shunting procedure is a technique used when postoperative CT/MRI shows ventricular dilatation, subdural effusion, and/or porencephalic cyst. Complications of surgical intervention depend on several factors including the location, size, and multiplicity of the cysts, as well as the presence of contamination (Ozek 1994). Recently, Ciurea et al. (2006) reported that the dimensions of the lesions had a strong influence on the possibility of total removal and on the rates of recurrence and postoperative complications. The most common complication is a rupture of the cyst into the subarachnoid space, which leads to widespread dissemination into the subarachnoid space, followed by severe anaphylactic reaction. If the cyst membrane is torn intraoperatively, the area of spillage is irrigated with hypertonic saline solution or cetrimide to prevent recurrences. However, while doing PAIR, each puncture invariably leads to some spillage of the contents into the operative field, and cyst recurrences are extremely dangerous. Advances in diagnostic and surgical techniques have greatly improved the prognosis of patients with intracranial hydatidosis. Unfortunately, however, delivery of the cyst with extradural localization is rarely possible without rupture, in contrast to parenchymal cystic lesions. Disseminated, multiple intracranial cystic lesions, development of systemic implantations, and failure to remove the primary focus are the main causes of poor outcome.

These complications are discussed in Chap. 17.

Long-Term Surgical Outcome

The treatment of choice for the intracranial hydatid cyst is surgical, but the long-term results of the surgical treatment differ according to the location, size, and multiplicity or extraneuronal involvement. In general, primary solitary cerebral hydatid cyst which has been removed unruptured will have excellent outcome with or without postoperative albendazole treatment, while intraoperative ruptured hydatid cysts, multiple hydatid cysts, and hydatid cysts with extraneuronal involvement have a poor outcome and would need postoperative long-term albendazole treatment (Altinörs et al. 2000; Onal et al. 2001; Turgut 2001, 2002; Tuzun et al. 2004; Ciurea et al. 2006). Disseminated, multiple intracranial cystic lesions, development of systemic implantations, and failure to remove the primary focus are the main causes of poor outcome.

Conclusion

Intact surgical removal of the cyst with its contents is the method of choice of treatment in the majority of intracranial hydatid cyst using the modified Dowling's technique whenever feasible. Hydatid cysts in deep and critical areas of the brain, multiple intracranial hydatid cysts, hydatid cysts with multiple organ involvement, and ruptured cysts at surgery would need chemotherapy, albendazole. Based on the literature review, optimal management strategy for a patient with intracranial hydatidosis is given in Fig. 15.4 (Turgut 2001, 2002).

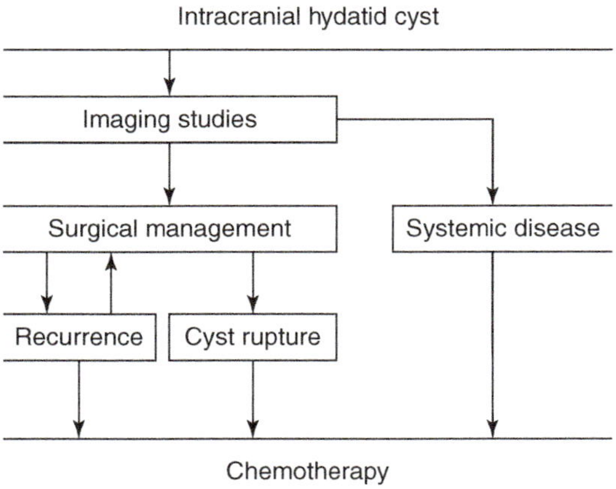

Fig. 15.4 Algorithm depicting the imaging and treatment management pathways for central nervous system hydatidosis in pediatric and adolescent patient groups (Adapted from Turgut (2001) p. 296)

Acknowledgments We would like to thank Fuad Sami Haddad, MD, for his supervision, invaluable inputs, and final correction of the manuscript in English.

References

Akdemir G, Dağlioğlu E, Seçer M, Ergüngör MF. Hydatid cysts of the internal acoustic canal and jugular foramen. J Clin Neurosci. 2007;14:394–6.

Altinörs N, Bavbek M, Caner HH, Erdogan B. Central nervous system hydatidosis in Turkey: a cooperative study and literature survey analysis of 458 cases. J Neurosurg. 2000;93:1–8.

Anvari M, Amirjamshidi A, Abbassioun K. Gradual and complete delivery of a hydatid cyst of the brain through a single burr hole, a wrong happening! Childs Nerv Syst. 2009;25:1639–42.

Balak N, Cavumirza C, Yildirim H, Ozdemir S, Kinay D. Microsurgery in the removal of a large cerebral hydatid cyst: technical case report. Neurosurgery. 2006;59:485–6.

Beskonakli E, Solaroglu I, Tun K, Albayrak L. Primary intracranial hydatid cyst in the interpeduncular cistern. Acta Neurochir (Wien). 2005;147:781–3.

Boudawara MZ, Jemel Jr H, Guevera A. Surgical treatment of hydatid cysts of the central nervous system in the pediatric age (Dowling's technique). Childs Brain. 1975;1:4–213.

Boudawara MZ, Jemel H, Ghorbel M, Triki C, Soussi R, Ben Ali H, Mhiri C, Ben Mansour H. Hydatid cysts of the brain stem. Two cases (in French). Neurochirurgie. 1999;45:321–4.

Cemil B, Tun K, Gurcay AG, Uygur A, Kaptanoglu E. Cranial epidural hydatid cysts: clinical report and review of the literature. Acta Neurochir (Wien). 2009;151:659–62.

Ciurea AV, Fountas KN, Coman TC, Machinis TG, Kapsalaki EZ, Fezoulidis NI, Robinson JS. Long-term surgical outcome in patients with intracranial hydatid cyst. Acta Neurochir (Wien). 2006;148:421–6.

Duishanbai S, Jiafu D, Guo H, Liu C, Liu B, Aishalong M, Mijiti M, Wen H. Intracranial hydatid cyst in children: report of 30 cases. Childs Nerv Syst. 2010;26:821–7.

Duishanbai S, Geng D, Liu C, Guo HR, Hao YJ, Liu B, Wang YX, Luo K, Zhou K, Wen H. Treatment of intracranial hydatid cysts. Chin Med J (Engl). 2011;124:2954–8.

Erman T, Tuna M, Göçer I, Ildan F, Zeren M, Cetinalp E. Intracranial intraosseous hydatid cyst: case report and review of literature. Neurosurg Focus. 2001;11:ECP1.

Erşahin Y, Mutluer S, Dermirtaş E, Yurtseven T. A case of thalamic hydatid cyst. Clin Neurol Neurosurg. 1995;97:321–3.

Filice C, Brunetti E. Use of PAIR in human cystic echinococcosis. Acta Trop. 1997;64:95–107.

Gazzaz M, Bouyaakoub FA, Akhaddar A, Derraz S, Elkhamlichi A. Epidural hydatid cyst of the posterior fossa (in French). Neurochirurgie. 2000;46:387–90.

Gökalp HZ, Erdoğan A. Hydatid cyst of the aqueduct of Sylvius. Case report. Clin Neurol Neurosurg. 1988;90: 83–5.

Haddad FS, Haddad GF. Overview of brain hydatid and its surgical management. Personal experience with cyst delivery. Pan Arab J Neurosurg. 2003;7:33–41.

Izci Y, Tüzün Y, Seçer HI. Cerebral hydatid cysts: technique and pitfalls of surgical management. Neurosurg Focus. 2008;24:E15.

Kabatas S, Yilmaz C, Cansever T, Gulsen S, Sonmez E, Altinors MN. The management of a complicated brain hydatid cyst: case report. Neurol Neurochir Pol. 2009; 43:575–8.

Kamath SM, Mysorekar VV, Rao SG, Varma RG. Intraventricular hydatid cyst in a child. Indian J Pathol Microbiol. 2009;52:571–2.

Kayaoglu CR. Giant hydatid cyst in the posterior fossa of a child: a case report. J Int Med Res. 2008;36:198–202.

Khaldi M, Mohamed S, Kallel J, Khouja N. Brain hydatidosis: report on 117 cases. Childs Nerv Syst. 2000;16:765–9.

Kurtsoy A, Oktem IS, Koç RK, Akdemir H, Menkü A, Tucer B. Successful surgical treatment of a thalamic hydatid cyst with contralateral transcallosal approach. Case report and review of the literature. Pediatr Neurosurg. 1999;31:96–9.

Muthusubramanian V, Pande A, Vasudevan MC, Ravi R. Surgical management of brainstem hydatid cyst -an unusual site. Surg Neurol. 2009;71:103–6.

Onal C, Unal F, Barlas O, Izgi N, Hepgul K, Turantan MI, Canbolat A, Turker K, Bayindir C, Gokay HK, Kaya U. Long-term follow-up and results of thirty pediatric intracranial hydatid cysts: half a century of experience in the Department of Neurosurgery of the School of Medicine at the University of Istanbul (1952–2001). Pediatr Neurosurg. 2001;35:72–81.

Ozek MM. Complications of central nervous system hydatid disease. Pediatr Neurosurg. 1994;20:84–91.

Rivierez M, el-Azhari A, el Tantaoui M, Alaoui M. Hydatid cyst of the cavernous sinus. A case (in French). Neurochirurgie. 1992;38:46–9.

Rumboldt Z, Jednacak H, Talan-Hranilović J, Rumboldt T, Kalousek M. Unusual appearance of a cisternal hydatid cyst. AJNR Am J Neuroradiol. 2003;24: 112–4.

Sandhu P, Saggar K, Sodhi KS. Neurological picture. Multiple hydatid cysts of the brain after surgery. J Neurol Neurosurg Psychiatry. 2000;68:97.

Schnider P. Gamma knife radiosurgery in cerebral echinococcosis. Clin Infect Dis. 1999;28:409.

Turgut M. Primary intracranial extradural hydatid cyst extending above and below the tentorium. Br J Neurosurg. 1997;11:587.

Turgut M. Intracranial hydatidosis in Turkey: its clinical presentation, diagnostic studies, surgical management, and outcome. A review of 276 cases. Neurosurg Rev. 2001;24:200–8.

Turgut M. Hydatidosis of central nervous system and its coverings in the pediatric and adolescent age groups in Turkey during the last century: a critical review of 137 cases. Childs Nerv Syst. 2002;18:670–83.

Tuzun Y, Kadioglu HH, Izci Y, Suma S, Keles M, Aydin IH. The clinical, radiological and surgical aspects of cerebral hydatid cysts in children. Pediatr Neurosurg. 2004;40:155–60.

Tuzun Y, Solmaz I, Sengul G, Izci Y. The complications of cerebral hydatid cyst surgery in children. Childs Nerv Syst. 2010;26:47–51.

Uzun MA, Koksal N, Ozkan OF, Kayahan M, Tilki M, Gunes P, Ozkan P. Gastric duplication cyst in an adult. J Coll Physicians Surg Pak. 2010;20:335–6.

World Health Organization Informal Working Group of Echinococcosis. Puncture, aspiration, injection, reaspiration. An option for the treatment of cystic echinococcosis. Document WHO/CDS/CSR/APH/2001.6. Geneva: World Health Organization; 2001. p. 1–40.

Yilmazlar S, Aksoy K. Approach via the floor of the fourth ventricle for hydatid cyst of the pons. Pediatr Neurosurg. 1999;31:326–9.

Yüceer N, Gökalp HZ. Periventricular hydatid cyst. J Neurosurg Sci. 1998;42:173–5.

Yurt A, Avci M, Selçuki M, Ozer F, Camlar M, Uçar K, Taşli F, Altinörs N. Multiple cerebral hydatid cysts. Report of a case with 24 pieces. Clin Neurol Neurosurg. 2007;109:821–6.

Chemotherapy for Central Nervous System Hydatidosis

16

Sipho K. Dlamini and Ntobeko B.A. Ntusi

Contents

S.K. Dlamini, MBChB, FCP(SA)
Department of Medicine, Groote Schuur Hospital, University of Cape Town, Cape Town, South Africa

N.B.A. Ntusi, MB, ChB, FCP(SA) (✉)
Department of Cardiovascular Medicine, John Radcliffe Hospital, Oxford, OX3 9DU, UK

Department of Medicine, Groote Shuur Hospital, Cape Town, South Africa
e-mail: ntobekon@yahoo.com

Introduction

A larval form of the parasite *Echinococcus* (family Taeniidae) causes hydatidosis, of which four species result in human disease: *Echinococcus granulosus* (cystic hydatid disease), *E. multilocularis* (alveolar hydatid disease), *E. vogeli* (polycystic type), and *E. oligarthus*. Consequent to the ubiquitous nature of *E. granulosus*, cystic echinococcosis is an important public health concern, with a global disease burden of 1,009,662 people and 3.6 million disability-adjusted life years (DALYs) (Budke et al. 2006). The species of *Echinococcus* is discussed in Chap. 3.

Central nervous system (CNS) hydatidosis is uncommon, occurring only in 2–3 % of cases of hydatidosis (Altinörs et al. 2000; McManus et al. 2003), and is usually caused by cystic echinococcosis and very rarely by alveolar echinococcosis (Turgut 2001; McManus et al. 2003). CNS hydatidosis may be classified into two forms according to the location of a given cyst, (a) intracranial and (b) spinal hydatid disease, which have different clinical manifestations and management approaches. CNS hydatid disease is diagnosed with neuroimaging such as computed tomography (CT) and magnetic resonance imaging (MRI) complemented by immunodiagnostic techniques (Figs. 16.1, 16.2, and 16.3).

The historical management of patients with CNS hydatidosis has been surgery, as it was the only modality of treatment available. Current treatment options include surgery, percutaneous

M. Turgut (ed.), *Hydatidosis of the Central Nervous System: Diagnosis and Treatment*,
DOI 10.1007/978-3-642-54359-3_16, © Springer-Verlag Berlin Heidelberg 2014

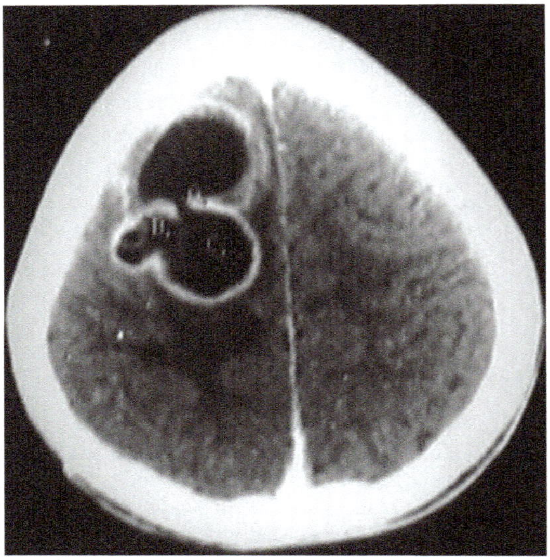

Fig. 16.1 CT scan of a 10-year-old male patient showing a hydatid cyst in the frontoparietal region (Courtesy of F. Limaiem, MD)

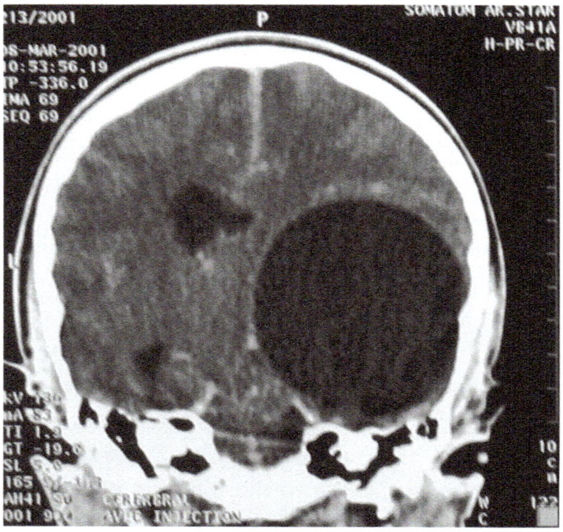

Fig. 16.2 CT scan of a 12-year-old male patient showing hydatid cyst in the right temporoparietal region (Courtesy of F. Limaiem, MD)

evacuation, chemotherapy with benzimidazoles, and the watch and wait approach. The decision on which the treatment strategy is approached must be individualized for each patient, and combination therapy is often employed. Indications for treatment are complex and based on the

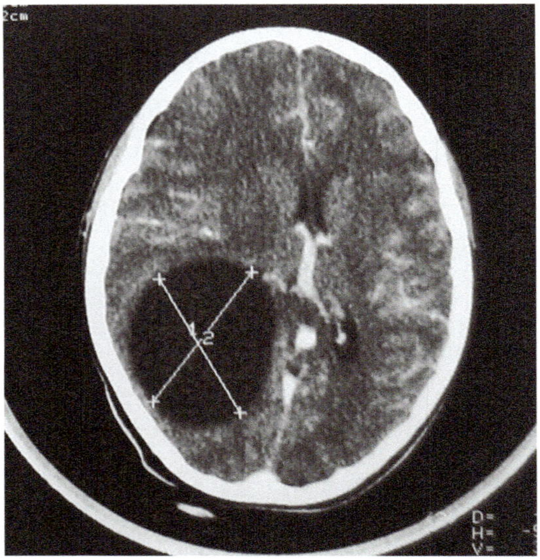

Fig. 16.3 CT scan of a 15-year-old female patient showing hydatid cyst in the right occipital region (Courtesy of F. Limaiem, MD)

characteristics of the cyst and other factors such as available medical/surgical expertise, equipment, and the ability of the patient to adhere to long-term monitoring (Brunetti et al. 2010). Spinal hydatid disease and alveolar CNS echinococcosis are treated primarily surgically and often with adjuvant chemotherapy.

Cystic Central Nervous System Hydatidosis

Cystic CNS hydatidosis is managed with surgery as the initial mode of therapy. Either surgery is combined with chemotherapy or, in some instances, chemotherapy is used singularly. Surgical therapy results in the complete resolution of lesions in the majority of cases. The response to albendazole (ABZ) is reported to be 64–100 % (Todorov et al. 1992a, b; Kalaitzoglou et al. 1998), and there have been a few case reports that have reported complete resolution of lesions following ABZ therapy. Both surgery and chemotherapy, alone or in combination, may result in complete eradication of cystic CNS hydatidosis.

Alveolar Central Nervous System Hydatidosis

Alveolar CNS hydatidosis is managed primarily with surgery where complete resection of the lesion is mandatory. This should be followed by chemotherapy for a limited period thereafter (2 years is recommended). Where surgery is not feasible, then chemotherapy, ABZ, or mebendazole (MBZ) as the only mode of therapy is acceptable, and this is usually administered long term or even lifelong. Since the introduction of chemotherapy after 1976, the 10-year survival has increased from less than 10 to 85–90 % in the chemotherapy era (Ammann and Eckert 1996).

Indications for Chemotherapy for Hydatidosis of the Central Nervous System

Surgery remains the first line of therapy for CNS hydatidosis and is the most effective form of therapy. Chemotherapy for CNS hydatidosis became a reality with the introduction of the two benzimidazoles, MBZ and ABZ, respectively, in 1976 and in 1982. Flubendazole (FBZ) was also shown to be effective for treatment of cystic echinococcosis (Ceballos et al. 2011) but is less efficacious than ABZ and is not used for the management of CNS hydatidosis. ABZ is most widely utilized, owing to its higher absorption in the gut and better gastrointestinal tolerability. Over the last 30 years, the use of chemotherapy in hydatidosis has evolved with a consensus now established on the indications, dosage, and follow-up of patients following initiation of therapy with benzimidazoles (World Health Organization [WHO] Informal Working Group on Echinococcosis 1996).

Traditional indications for chemotherapy for CNS hydatidosis include multiple or multiseptate cysts, large cysts (>10 cm), and cysts that are difficult to reach surgically or where the surgery would be clearly hazardous (El-On 2003; Ntusi and Horsfall 2008) (Table 16.1). Furthermore, patients with recurrence of CNS hydatid cysts are treated medically (Stojkovic et al. 2009), as are those for whom surgery would be contraindicated. There have been few case reports of the use of ABZ as the sole treatment of CNS hydatidosis with complete resolution of lesions on imaging (Kalaitzoglou et al. 1998; Ntusi and Horsfall 2008) in instances in which surgery was not feasible. However, there is no clinical trial evidence for the superiority of ABZ versus surgery for CNS hydatidosis.

Table 16.1 Indications for chemotherapy for central nervous system hydatidosis

1. Multiple/multiseptate cysts
2. Large cysts (>10 cm)
3. Cysts difficult to reach via surgery
4. Recurrent CNS hydatid cysts
5. Surgery is contraindicated
6. Cases where surgery is clearly hazardous

The adjunctive use of benzimidazoles before or after invasive procedures is now commonly practiced. The rationale for this indication is that perioperative administration may be important for cyst volume reduction and in minimizing the risk of rupture during the procedure (Morris 1987; Horton 1989).

In alveolar CNS hydatidosis, adjunctive chemotherapy with ABZ or MBZ following surgery is always indicated. In this instance, chemotherapy must be administered for a minimum of 2 years, and patients should be monitored for 10 years thereafter (Hemphill and Müller 2009). In instances where surgery is not feasible for alveolar hydatidosis, it is recommended that chemotherapy be used long term or lifelong. Currently, no evidence or guidelines are available for the perioperative use of benzimidazoles for alveolar CNS echinococcosis.

Indications for Surgical Treatment of Hydatidosis of the Central Nervous System

Surgery remains the cornerstone of management for uncomplicated cysts in CNS hydatidosis. The aim of surgical therapy is radical removal of the cyst without spillage of its content. Single lesions are more amenable to surgical removal compared to multiple lesions. All forms of spinal hydatid disease and alveolar CNS echinococcosis are treated surgically (Turgut 1997; Bresson-Hadni et al. 2000; Turgut 2001), as are lesions with bone involvement. Furthermore, patients who remain refractory to medical therapy or show progressive neurological decline despite chemotherapy should be considered for surgical treatment (Stojkovic et al. 2009).

Medical Chemotherapy for Hydatidosis

Benzimidazoles

Mechanism of Action

The action of benzimidazoles is their inhibitory effect on the uptake of glucose by the parasite, thus leading to the depletion of glycogen stores (Sheth 1975). The drug inhibits glucose uptake by the cestode, but does not affect serum glucose concentration in humans (Fierlafijn 1971). The benzimidazoles also result in degenerative alterations in the germinal layer of the cyst, leading to cellular autolysis (Schantz et al. 1982). In vitro studies have demonstrated disruption of microtubule structure and function in metacestodes treated with ABZ (Lacey 1988). Furthermore, benzimidazoles have been shown to have a higher affinity for parasite tubulin compared to that of the human host (Friedman and Platzer 1980; Gottschall et al. 1990), explaining their selective capacity for parasite immobilization and death.

Evidence of Efficacy

Benzimidazoles form the mainstay of medical chemotherapy for CNS hydatidosis. The efficacy of MBZ has been reported variably, with no consensus regarding the effective dose or optimal duration of therapy (El-On 2003). ABZ is more effective in the treatment of hydatidosis, most likely related to its superior intestinal absorption and particularly the higher penetration of its metabolite, ABZ sulfoxide, into the cyst cavity (Davis et al. 1989; Casado et al. 1996). ABZ is most efficacious in young cysts and in cysts less than 8 cm in size (Todorov et al. 1992a, b; Teggi et al. 1993).

There are limited data from randomized clinical trials, demonstrating efficacy of the benzimidazoles in the management of hydatidosis. FBZ has been shown to be inferior to ABZ and MBZ (Davis et al. 1986). Several trials have demonstrated the superiority of ABZ to MBZ, with a response rate of 75–85 % versus 50–60 %, respectively (Saimot et al. 1983; Todorov et al. 1992a, b; Teggi et al. 1993; Liu and Weller 1996; Luchi et al. 1997). The results of chemotherapy are affected by cyst characteristics such as size, age, and location, as well as by host characteristics (El-On 2003). ABZ is associated with evidence of radiological improvement in hydatid cysts in 68–82 % of patients (Falagas and Bliziotis 2007; Stojkovic et al. 2009). Prolonged courses of ABZ have been shown to be effective in the management of CNS hydatidosis (Teggi et al. 1993; Ntusi and Horsfall 2008).

Administration and Dosing

MBZ is given orally. About 2–10 % of the drug is absorbed intestinally and converted to its active metabolites, ABZ sulfoxide and ABZ sulfone, by the liver (El-On 2003). MBZ is excreted in the bile as glucuronide or a sulfate conjugate (Gottschall 1993). The usual dose in adults is 40–50 mg/kg/day, given in three equally divided doses after meals. Treatment is usually given for 3–6 months (Table 16.2).

ABZ is also given orally. Its absorption in the gastrointestinal tract is better than for MBZ. It is metabolized by the liver to ABZ sulfoxide. The standard dose is 10–15 mg/kg/day, usually 800 mg/day, given in two equally divided doses. Absorption is improved by a fatty meal. Therapy is given for 3–6 months. Previously, ABZ was given for 4 week courses, followed by two drug-free intervals, due to safety concerns. Nevertheless, continuous therapy does not increase side effects (Teggi et al. 1993).

Pharmacokinetics

MBZ is minimally absorbed in the gut, with 95 % of the drug being bound to proteins. Metabolism

Table 16.2 Administration and dosing of chemotherapy for central nervous system hydatidosis

Chemotherapy	Mechanism of action	Dose	Duration	Side effects
Mebendazole	Inhibition of glucose uptake by parasite Disruption of microtubules by inhibition of the polymerization of tubulin into microtubules	40–50 mg/kg/day in three divided doses	3–6 months	Nausea, vomiting, diarrhea, and abdominal pain
Albendazole	Inhibition of glucose uptake by parasite Disruption of microtubules by inhibition of the polymerization of tubulin into microtubules	10–15 mg/kg/day in two divided doses	3–6 months	Gastrointestinal disturbances, abnormalities in liver function, leukopenia, and hematuria
Praziquantel	Increases the cell permeability to calcium in cestodes	25 mg/kg/day (in combination with albendazole)	No clear data	Dizziness, headache, malaise, abdominal pain, and nausea

is extensively hepatic. The time from ingestion to peak serum concentration is 2–4 h, with a half-life of elimination of 1–12 h. Excretion is primarily in feces, with very little in the urine.

ABZ has a good volume of distribution within the hydatid cysts and the cerebrospinal fluid, with protein-binding capacity of 70 %. Metabolism primarily takes place in the liver mainly through sulfoxidation (and less through hydrolysis and oxidation), with extensive first-pass effect. The time from ingestion to peak serum concentration is 2–5 h. The half-life of elimination is 8–12 h. The drug is excreted in the urine and feces (de Silva et al. 1997).

Adverse Effects

The adverse effects of the benzimidazoles may be related to the drug itself or its metabolites, but, for the most part, both drugs are well tolerated. Because of its poor absorption, MBZ has a better side effect profile than ABZ. Common adverse reactions include abdominal pain, diarrhea, and vomiting. CNS reactions include dizziness, drowsiness, headaches, and seizures. Reversible hepatotoxicity is well documented, with increase in liver enzymes. Dermatologic reactions may include angioedema, exanthema, itching, urticaria, toxic epidermal necrolysis, and Steven-Johnson syndrome. Less commonly, the benzimidazoles may be associated with hypersensitivity, hematuria, or bone marrow suppression (neutropenia or agranulocytosis).

Contraindications

Benzimidazoles should not be used in patients with liver disease or bone marrow suppression. ABZ and MBZ are relative contraindications in pregnancy, as they have been shown to induce embryotoxicity and teratogenicity in rats. However, they have been shown not to cause harm in human pregnancy (Bradley and Horton 2001).

Praziquantel

Mechanism of Action

Praziquantel (PZQ) is a heterocyclic pyrazinoisoquinoline that is effective against protoscoleces and therefore active against early cysts having no activity against mature cysts. PZQ increases the cell permeability to calcium in cestodes, causing contractions, increased motility, and paralysis of the worm musculature leading to detachment of their suckers. The in vivo consequence of PZQ is dislocation of the worm in the intestines and loss of sensitivity of the skin to proteolytic enzyme activity (Doenhoff et al. 2008).

Evidence of Efficacy

PZQ, in combination with ABZ, has been shown to be better than ABZ alone (Cobo et al. 1998; Mohamed et al. 1998). However, the role of PZQ as single therapy for CNS hydatidosis has not been defined (Wen et al. 1993). Furthermore, there is evidence for improved outcomes when

PZQ is combined with ABZ for management of cyst spillage pre- and post-intervention (Cobo et al. 1998) compared to either drug alone.

Administration and Dosing

PZQ is administered orally and given at a dose of 25 mg/kg/day alone or in combination with ABZ.

Pharmacokinetics

Over 80 % of the orally administered PZQ is absorbed via the intestines. Metabolism is hepatic, with extensive first-pass effect and 80 % protein-binding capacity. PZQ increases the serum concentration of ABZ fourfold. The time from ingestion to peak serum concentration is 1–3 h. The half-life of elimination is 0.8–1.5 h for the drug and 4.5 h for the metabolites. Excretion is mostly in the urine.

Adverse Effects

PZQ is usually well tolerated. It may cause abdominal discomfort and nausea. Dizziness, fever, headache, seizures, and malaise have been described. Less commonly, the drug may cause hepatotoxicity, ventricular fibrillation, atrioventricular block, ventricular ectopy, and hypersensitivity.

Contraindications

PZQ should be used with caution in patients with cardiovascular disease, hepatic impairment, and history of seizures. There are no adequate studies in human pregnancy.

Monitoring Response to Treatment

Monitoring of patients treated for CNS hydatidosis, known as pharmacovigilance, is important for evaluating the success of chemotherapy and presence of adverse reactions and complications. Cysts can grow at a rate of 1–50 mm per year, persist for years without change, rupture or collapse, or disappear completely following treatment. The optimal approach to monitoring must be individualized for each patient.

The ideal monitoring strategy involves repeat imaging at 3–6-month intervals until the CNS findings are stable and thereafter followed by monitoring every 12–24 months. In the first 3 months of treatment, evaluation every 2–4 weeks of leukocytes and liver enzymes is recommended. The use of serological markers to assess response or relapse of hydatid disease is currently not recommended as serological tests may be elevated despite complete removal of cysts with surgery.

Watch and Wait Approach

The "watch and wait" approach is one of the recognized strategies which have evolved over the decades in the management of hydatidosis, even though there is still no clear-cut data evaluating its role as a treatment strategy. In cases where patients have inactive or degenerating cysts, it may be appropriate to observe these without any medical therapy (Junghanss et al. 2008; Brunetti and Junghanss 2009). CNS hydatid disease requires close follow-up with neuroimaging.

Prevention of Hydatidosis

Prevention of cystic hydatid disease can be achieved by avoidance of dogs, in particular stray dogs. Prohibiting home slaughter of domestic animals (e.g., sheep) will avoid dogs consuming infected viscera. Careful rinsing of vegetables and contaminated fresh produce may reduce infection. Prevention of alveolar echinococcosis requires avoidance of foxes and other infected canid hosts.

In theory it is possible to prevent echinococcosis through vaccination of the intermediate host (sheep) and the definitive host (dog). However, at present there is no vaccine against cystic echinococcosis available for dogs. Important strategies in prevention of human hydatidosis and elimination of the parasite in the hosts include regular deworming of dogs and the controlled slaughtering of infected sheep. Such efforts have led to disease eradication in the first world, and it is estimated that in places where the disease is endemic, it could take 20 years to achieve this (WHO Informal Working Group on Echinococcosis 1996).

Conclusion

CNS hydatidosis remains an uncommon complication of human echinococcal infestation. Surgery is the first line and most effective form of therapy for cystic and alveolar CNS disease. Chemotherapy is usually administered in combination with surgical management. Chemotherapy with ABZ (with or without PZQ) is effective in the management of patients not amenable to surgery or in those with pre- and post-intervention cyst spillage.

References

Altinörs N, Bavbek M, Caner HH, Erdogan B. Central nervous system hydatidosis in Turkey: a cooperative study and literature survey analysis of 458 cases. J Neurosurg. 2000;93:1–8.

Ammann RW, Eckert J. Cestodes: Echinococcus. Gastroenterol Clin North Am. 1996;25:655–89.

Bradley M, Horton J. Assessing the risk of benzimidazole therapy during pregnancy. Trans R Soc Trop Med Hyg. 2001;95:72–3.

Bresson-Hadni S, Vuitton DA, Bartholomot B, Heyd B, Godart D, Meyer JP, Hrusovsky S, Becker MC, Mantion G, Lenys D, Miguet JP. A twenty year history of alveolar echinococcosis: analysis of a series of 117 patients from Eastern France. Eur J Gastroenterol Hepatol. 2000;12:327–36.

Brunetti E, Junghanss T. Update on cystic hydatid disease. Curr Opin Infect Dis. 2009;22:497–502.

Brunetti E, Kern P, Vuitton DA. Expert consensus for the diagnosis and treatment of cystic and alveolar echinococcosis in humans. Acta Trop. 2010;114:1–16.

Budke CM, Deplazes P, Torgerson PR. Global socioeconomic impact of cystic echinococcosis. Emerg Infect Dis. 2006;12:296–303.

Casado N, Pérez-Serrano J, Denegri G, Rodríguez-Caabeiro F. Development of a chemotherapeutic model for the in vitro screening of drugs against *Echinococcus granulosus* cysts: the effects of albendazole- albendazole sulfoxide combination. Int J Parasitol. 1996;26:59–65.

Ceballos L, Elissondo C, Sánchez Bruni S, Denegri G, Lanusse C, Alvarez L. Comparative performance of flubendazole and albendazole in cystic echinococcosis: ex vivo activity, plasma/cyst disposition, and efficacy in infected mice. Antimicrob Agents Chemother. 2011;55:5861–7.

Cobo F, Yarnoz C, Sesma B, Fraile P, Aizcorbe M, Trujillo R, Diaz-de-Liaño A, Ciga MA. Albendazole plus praziquantel versus albendazole alone as a pre-operative treatment in intra-abdominal hydatidosis caused by *Echinococcus granulosus*. Trop Med Int Health. 1998;3:462–6.

Davis A, Pawlowski ZS, Dixon H. Multicentre clinical trials of benzimidazolecarbamates in human echinococcosis. Bull World Health Organ. 1986;64:383–8.

Davis A, Dixon H, Pawlowski ZS. Multicentre clinical trials of benzimidazole-carbamates in human cystic echinococcosis (phase 2). Bull World Health Organ. 1989;67:503–8.

de Silva N, Guyatt H, Bundy D. Anthelmintics. A comparative review of their clinical pharmacology. Drugs. 1997;53:769–88.

Doenhoff MJ, Cioli D, Utzinger J. Praziquantel: mechanisms of action, resistance and new derivatives for schistosomiasis. Curr Pin Infect Dis. 2008;21:659–67.

El-On J. Benzimidazole treatment for cystic echinococcosis. Acta Trop. 2003;85:243–52.

Falagas ME, Bliziotis IA. Albendazole for the treatment of human echinococcosis: a review of comparative clinical trials. Am J Med Sci. 2007;334:171–9.

Fierlafijn E. Mebendazole in enterobiasis. JAMA. 1971;218:1051.

Friedman PA, Platzer EG. Interaction of anthelmintic benzimidazoles with Ascaris suum embryonic tubulin. Biochem Biophys Acta. 1980;630:271–8.

Gottschall PE. Infectious disease, interleukin-1 and central nervous system. J Fla Med Assoc. 1993;80:127–9.

Gottschall DW, Theodorides VJ, Wang R. The metabolism of benzimidazole anthelmintics. Parasitol Today. 1990;6:115–24.

Hemphill A, Müller J. Alveolar and cystic echinococcosis: towards novel chemotherapeutic treatment options. J Helminthol. 2009;83:99–111.

Horton RJ. Chemotherapy of Echinococcus infections in man with albendazole. Trans R Soc Trop Med. 1989;83:97–102.

Junghanss T, da Silva AM, Horton J, Chiodini PL, Brunetti E. Clinical management of cystic echinococcosis: state of the art, problems, and perspectives. Am J Trop Med Hyg. 2008;79:301–11.

Kalaitzoglou I, Drevelengas A, Petridis A, Palladas P. Albendazole treatment of cerebral hydatid disease: evaluation of results with CT and MRI. Neuroradiology. 1998;40:36–9.

Lacey E. The role of the cytoskeletal protein, tubulin, in the mode of action and mechanisms of drug resistance to benzimidazoles. Int J Parasitol. 1988;18:885–936.

Liu LX, Weller PF. Antiparasitic drugs. N Eng J Med. 1996;334:1178–84.

Luchi S, Vincenti A, Messina F, Parenti M, Scasso A, Campatelli A. Albendazole treatment of human hydatid tissue. Scand J Infect Dis. 1997;29:165–7.

McManus DP, Zhang W, Li J, Bartley PB. Echinococcosis. Lancet. 2003;362:1295–304.

Mohamed AE, Yasawy MI, Karawi MA. Combined albendazole and praziquantel versus albendazole alone in the treatment of hydatid disease. Hepatogastroenterology. 1998;45:1690–4.

Morris L. Pre-operative albendazole therapy for hydatid cysts. Br J Surg. 1987;74:805–6.
Ntusi NBA, Horsfall C. Severe disseminated hydatid disease successfully treated medically with prolonged administration of albendazole. Q J Med. 2008;101:745–6.
Saimot AG, Meulemans A, Cremieux AC, Giovanangeli MD, Hay JM, Delaitre B, Coulaud JP. Albendazole as a potential treatment for human hydatidosis. Lancet. 1983;2:652–6.
Schantz PM, van den Bossche H, Eckert J. Chemotherapy for larval Echinococcus in animals and humans: report of a workshop. Z Parasitenkd. 1982;67:5–26.
Sheth UK. Mechanisms of anthelmintic action. Prog Drug Res. 1975;19:147–57.
Stojkovic M, Zwahlen M, Teggi A, Vutova K, Cretu CM, Virdone R, Nicolaidou P, Cobanoglu N, Junghanss T. Treatment response of cystic echinococcosis to benzimidazoles: a systematic review. PLoS Negl Trop Dis. 2009;3:e524.
Teggi A, Lastilla MG, De Rosa F. Therapy of human hydatid disease with mebendazole and albendazole. Antimicrob Agents Chemother. 1993;37:1679–84.
Todorov T, Mechkov G, Vutova K, Georgiev P, Lazarova I, Tonchev Z, Nedelkov G. Factors influencing the response to chemotherapy in human cystic echinococcosis. Bull World Health Organ. 1992a;70:347–58.
Todorov T, Vutova K, Mechkov G, Georgiev P, Petkov D, Tonchev Z, Nedelkov G. Chemotherapy of human cystic echinococcosis: comparative efficacy of mebendazole and albendazole. Ann Trop Med Parasitol. 1992b;86:59–66.
Turgut M. Hydatid disease of the spine: a survey from Turkey. Infection. 1997;25:221–6.
Turgut M. Intracranial hydatidosis in Turkey: its clinical presentation, diagnostic studies, surgical management, and outcome. A review of 276 cases. Neurosurg Rev. 2001;24:200–8.
Wen H, New RR, Craig PS. Diagnosis and treatment of human hydatidosis. Br J Clin Pharmacol. 1993;35:565–74.
WHO Informal Working Group on Echinococcosis. Guidelines for the treatment of cystic and alveolar echinococcosis in humans. Bull World Health Organ. 1996;74:231–42.

Complications of Cerebral Hydatidosis

17

Fuad Sami Haddad

Contents

F.S. Haddad, BA, MD, FRCS(C), FACS, ABNS
Department of Surgery,
American University of Beirut Medical Center,
Beirut, Lebanon
e-mail: fshaddad@aub.edu.lb

Introduction

The frequency and the seriousness of the complications in hydatid disease brought us to compare its course to a malignant condition as early as 1963 (Haddad FS et al. 1963). These complications of cerebral hydatidosis are studied in three time frames, the preoperative, operative, and postoperative periods. In the preoperative period, these complications are blindness, calcification of the cyst, infected and complicated cysts, caseation, formation of "chitinoma," hydrocephalus, leakage of cyst fluid in the surrounding brain, spontaneous intracranial rupture of the cyst, bulging and thinning of the skull in the vicinity of the cyst, perforation of the skull and or dura by the intact cyst, cerebral stroke and hydatid embolization from disease in the heart, infertility due to cyst pressure on the hypothalamo-pituitary axis, and nephrotic syndrome. In the treatment period, these complications are inadvertent rupture or intentional cyst puncture, cystoperitoneal shunt, cysto-atrial shunt, anaphylactic shock, and complications of medicinal treatment. During the posttreatment period, these complications are recurrences; porencephalic cyst; subdural effusion; pneumo- or hydrocephalus; bleeding in the epidural, subdural, or intraparenchymal spaces; wound infection; meningitis and abscess formation; cerebrospinal fluid leaks; pulmonary embolism; calcifications; glioma; choreiform movements; mental retardation; seizures; and death.

M. Turgut (ed.), *Hydatidosis of the Central Nervous System: Diagnosis and Treatment*,
DOI 10.1007/978-3-642-54359-3_17, © Springer-Verlag Berlin Heidelberg 2014

Complications During the Pretreatment Period

Blindness

It is one of the worst complications. It is due to the delay in the institution of treatment in a patient who suffers from marked increase in intracranial pressure accompanied by papilledema. In hydatid of the brain, the patient is often a child, and the separation of the sutures as well as the slow progression of increased intracranial pressure is not accompanied by the usual drowsiness, nausea, and vomiting seen in other brain expanding lesions. Thus, severe papilledema is often seen in conjunction with a relatively well-conserved physical and mental condition and may be overlooked. Blindness usually affects both eyes simultaneously and is irreversible. Decreased visual acuity, which may be the only symptom, sets in gradually and might not be of the same intensity in both eyes. This decreased acuity is an important warning and if taken seriously should lead to an early intervention which might reverse the process either partially or totally.

Calcification

This is a very rare condition (Legrè and Massad 1957; Alvarez et al. 1982). Robinson (1961) evaluated it at 1 % and Abderrahmen et al. (2007) at less than 1 % of all cerebral hydatid cysts. Ouboukhlik et al. (1994) report 4 calcified cysts out of 48 cases. The author of this chapter has seen only one such case out of 39 operated cases. Kooy (1940) was the first to describe a linear calcification in the wall of a cerebral hydatid cyst, and Roger (1944) was the first to describe a circular and globular calcification. Since then a number of cases have been reported (Legrè and Massad 1957; Samiy and Zadey 1965; Gomori et al. 1988; Rudwan and Khaffaji 1988; Nurchi et al. 1992; Peter et al. 1994; Choukri et al. 2001; Bouaziz 2005; Turgut et al. 2007). These calcifications were observed in different time frames. They have been noticed as early as 6 months after the onset of symptoms (Samiy and Zadey 1965) and as late as 20 years (Choukri et al. 2001). On plain x-ray, the calcification appears as a linear (Kooy 1940), curvilinear (Roger 1944), or nonhomogeneous mass (Abderrahmen et al. 2007). It involves the pericyst and may rarely extend into the ectocyst (Acquaviva et al. 1966; Alvarez et al. 1982). Intracystic calcifications are rare and may represent calcifications in the wall of the enclosed daughter cysts (Aksungur et al. 1994). Rudwan and Khaffaji (1988) believed this intracystic calcification "most likely represented a calcified collapsed cyst membrane."

These calcifications are best demonstrated on computed tomography (CT) scans. In calcified cysts, the pericyst may enhance on gadopentate magnetic resonance imaging (MRI) (Aksungur et al. 1994). On histopathologic examination, the surrounding brain reveals the presence of gliosis and macrophages (Alvarez et al. 1982). It is usually assumed that calcified cysts are dead cysts (Aksungur et al. 1994). However, it has been shown that some of these calcified cysts contain viable brood capsules and are still fertile (Samiy and Zadey 1965; Choukri et al. 2001).

The pathogenesis of such calcifications is not well known but is attributed by Radwan and Khaffaji (1988) to "degeneration" of the cyst. Robinson (1961) sees it as a sign of healing. Often the calcified pericyst is adherent to the ectocyst either by strands of tissue or over a variable surface area. These adhesions are more severe when the cyst is in contact with the dura or the falx. It is important to realize, prior to surgery, that the cyst is calcified, as it might change the plan of the intervention. In this case, surgery is usually difficult and may result in further complications (Rudwan and Khaffaji 1988; Peter et al. 1994). Some have removed the calcified pericyst with the cyst as it is sometimes impossible to separate them from each other. What follows is a personal case which illustrates the previous two subdivisions on blindness and calcification.

Case 1

NM, a 13-year-old girl, was admitted to hospital on November 28, 1965, complaining of bouts of headache of 4-year duration, worse on the right side, and accompanied by vomiting. In the past

2 years, her vision had gradually decreased until she became completely blind. In the past 6 months, she complained of weakness on the left side, especially in the upper extremity. Examination revealed a fully conscious, well-oriented, totally blind patient with bilateral optic atrophy. There was loss of position sense and astereognosia in the left hand with a bilateral Babinski sign. The patient brought with her plain x-rays showing separation of the sutures and a thin rim of calcification in the right posterior parietal region. A right carotid arteriogram revealed an anterosuperior shift of the terminal branches of the anterior cerebral as well as those of the middle cerebral arteries by an avascular mass within the rim of calcification. At operation, the dura was adherent to the underlying brain by multiple thin strands of fibrous tissue. These were released. In the occipital region, where the bone was extremely thin, the brain had been spliced open by the calcified shell which was partially adherent to the dura. The entire area was freed, and the shell of calcium was carefully removed over an area of 3.5 cm in diameter to uncover the ectocyst. Clearly the calcium lay in a thickened pericyst and did not involve the ectocyst. Attempts at delivering the cyst were not successful because of adhesions between the ectocyst and the calcified pericyst. The opening was enlarged by carrying three episiotomies in the brain, especially toward the occipital lobe which, in the present case, was safe in view of the blindness, and the ectocyst was further uncovered over an area 5 cm in diameter. In two areas, the cyst wall was very thin, and great care was taken not to rupture it. The head of the patient was tilted, and the jugular veins were compressed in an attempt at raising the intracranial pressure and expulsing the cyst. Fluid was injected in the bed of the cyst. What we have called the Credé maneuver – pressure on the brain to help deliver the cyst (Haddad and Haddad 2000; Haddad and Haddad 2003) – was possible in this case in spite of the calcified shell surrounding the cyst. The cyst was beginning to deliver (Fig. 17.1a). As it was dropping into the basin, it tore because of some unnoticed adhesions of the ectocyst to the calcified pericyst in its medial region. A most interesting finding was observed. No fluid was present in the mother cyst which, in turn, was filled with daughter

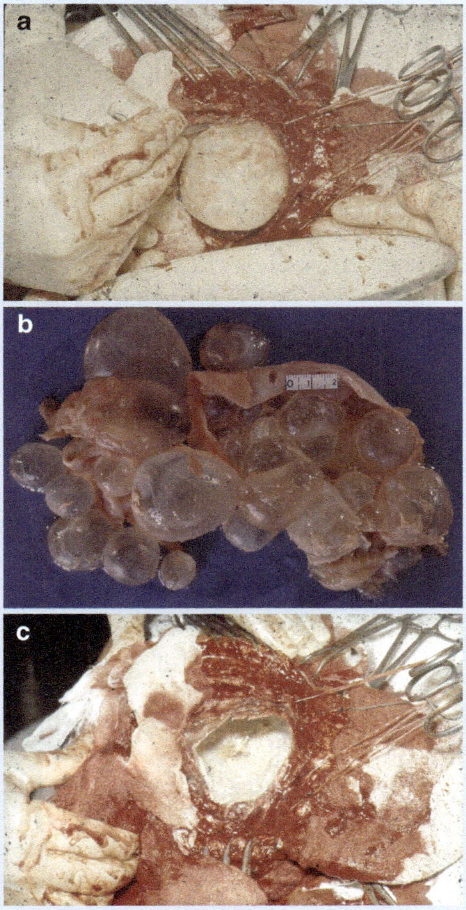

Fig. 17.1 (**a**) Delivering the cyst by applying the Credé maneuver. (**b**) Opened cyst showing the multitude of daughter cysts. (**c**) The cavity left by the cyst, note the uncollapsed cyst bed because of the calcification

cysts, some of which were attached to the endocyst (Fig. 17.1b). The cavity, left by the cyst, did not collapse due to the calcification of the pericyst (Fig. 17.1c). This cavity was thoroughly irrigated with saline, and the wound was closed. Seen 13 months later, on December 28, 1966, the patient was perfectly normal except for blindness.

Infected or Complicated Cysts

Although most authors use the term "infected," some use the term "infected or complicated" cyst (El-Shamam et al. 2001). The term complicated is more appropriate as, in spite of an extensive search in the literature, nothing has been found concerning the pathogenesis nor the pathogens in these cases. The cultures of the pus in the cases of Ersahin et al. (1993) and Turgut et al. (1997) did not yield any growth. In these cases, rim enhancement and paracystic edema are seen on computed tomography (CT) scan (Krawjewski and Stelmasiak 1991). The best method of diagnosis is by magnetic resonance imaging (MRI) which reveals "varying degrees of perifocal edema and contrast enhancement" (El-Shamam et al. 2001), and Nourbakh et al. (2010) report on T2 imaging a "hyperintense area of perifocal edema, complete and incomplete (segment) rim of contrast enhancement." These cysts become so adherent to the surrounding brain that their delivery intact becomes next to impossible (Rudwan and Khaffaji 1988). Mathuriya et al. (1985) described a case of infected intradural extramedullary hydatid cyst at the foramen magnum.

In 1948 Obrador and Urquiza reported a 9-year-old girl who harbored a "large" infected cyst in the left frontoparietal region. This was excised, and the culture of the pus did not yield any growth. This case is interesting because the abscess had formed around a shrunken hydatid vesicle measuring 7 cm in length. It is not clear whether the abscess was primarily pericystic or intracystic, and, with the rupture of the cyst in situ (see section "Spontaneous intracerebral rupture of the cyst"), the pus poured to the outside. Zahed et al. (2010) reported a case of infected hydatid cyst occurring prior to surgical intervention in a 20-year-old female suffering from a tender cystic swelling over the right temporal region associated with proptosis of the eye on the same side. The histopathology of the excised specimen was reported as an infected hydatid. The frequency of these infected cysts is extremely low, yet El-Shamam et al. (2001) found 4 out of 16 cases, and Kocaman et al. (1999) reported it in 3 out of 23 cases. An interesting case is that of Erongun et al. (1994) where an infected cyst was removed from the left occipital lobe of a 12-year-old boy with multiple adjacent cysts which were not infected. Twenty days after surgery, a cyst was found on CT scan in the left temporoparietal region. The family refused surgery. Fifty days later the child went into deep coma and died in spite of a rapid decompression by needle aspiration. The author does not mention the consistency of the fluid obtained.

Could it be possible that the cyst, which was found in the left temporoparietal region, had been missed at the time of surgery and, relieved from the surrounding pressure, rapidly expanded, in a matter of 70 days? This lapse of time is too short for a new cyst to produce symptoms.

Another interesting case is that of Goinard and Descuns (1952) where a thin blade of sterile pus was localized in the space between the ectocyst and a markedly thickened pericyst.

Other single cases have been reported in the literature (Obrador and Urquiza 1948; Arana-Iniguez and San Julian 1955; Boixados 1973; Mathuriya et al. 1985; Turgut et al. 1997; Turgut and Turgut 2002; Polat et al. 2003).

Although the content of these complicated cysts were considered as sterile, from the point of view of hydatid recurrence, the case of Yuceer et al. (1998), proved the opposite. They reported on a case 12-year-old child. A year earlier, the patient harbored "a large hydatid cyst with rim enhancement and calcification of the cyst wall." At operation the cyst ruptured and "purulent material" was drained. The patient presented a year later with multiple recurrent cysts in the bed of the previously removed infected and calcified cyst. This is why these cysts have to be as carefully delivered as are regular hydatid cysts.

Caseation

Caseation of the cyst content was described by Kooy (1940) in two cases. Both cases had peripheral calcifications. In one of these cases, the caseous material contained hooklets, and in the second there was a conglomeration of daughter cysts. It is not known whether these hydatid particles were active or dead. Radwan and Khaffaji (1988) reports on a patient whose cyst was filled with "mucoid gelatinous material," and there were adhesions between the dura, arachnoid, and overlying cortex. This case too showed, on plain skull films, a "fairly round, calcified lesion. When the cyst capsule was incised, mucoid gelatinous material was evacuated." No other reference related to caseation was found in the literature.

Chitinoma

Nanassis et al. (1999) resected from the frontal lobe of a 35-year-old woman a solid, partially cystic tumor, with focal calcifications, which on pathologic examination revealed an "acellular eosinophilic material with focal necrosis that surrounded typical protoscolices of Echinococcus granulosus." This acellular material was identified as chitin, hence the nomination of this mass "chitinoma." This term has been refuted by Turgut and Turgut (2002). It is interesting to note that there is a great deal of resemblance between this present case and those reported under "caseation," which leads one to believe that this might be a more advanced case of caseation.

Hydrocephalus

Although hydrocephalus is not expected to be associated with such large cerebral supratentorial cysts, it does occur. El-Shamam et al. (2001) detected, on MRI, 4 preoperative hydrocephalics out of 16 patients and in only one was the cyst in the posterior fossa. Abbassioun et al. (1978) described two cases of hydrocephalus out of two posterior fossa cysts discovered on CT scan. Villarejo et al. (1983) reported such a case that required a ventriculoperitoneal shunt preoperatively later removed together with the cyst.

Leakage

Leakage of hydatid fluid in the surrounding tissues was reported to occur through a "thick porous" cyst wall (Griponissiotis 1957). This leakage produces a chronic type of inflammation with adhesions of the cyst wall to the surrounding tissues and its invasion with leucocytes. On CT scan and MRI, edema is observed in the surrounding brain. The description of the case of Gonzalez-Ruiz et al. (1990) is reminiscent of such a condition, although the authors believed it was an intracerebral rupture of the cyst. There was a hyperdense cyst wall visible on CT scan; the cyst was tightly adherent to the dura "producing inflammation and subsequent gliosis of the surrounding brain." Could this leakage be the precipitating factor for the calcification in the pericyst? Nothing is found in the literature to refute or confirm this presumption. This condition makes the "delivery" of the cyst much more hazardous.

Spontaneous Intracerebral Rupture of the Cyst

This is an exceptionally rare condition and is accompanied by severe pericystic edema (Ozek 1994). It is usually ushered by an abrupt and important deterioration in the clinical status of the patient and may lead to dissemination of the disease. No reason for the spontaneous rupture of such cysts has been advanced except for that given by Griponissiotis (1957). He suggested that head injury may cause a cyst, adherent to the parietal dura, to rupture in the extradural space giving rise to numerous extradural cysts. He gave such an example. One of the causes of multiplicity of hydatid cysts in the brain may be due to the advent of a single cyst rupturing spontaneously in situ, as suggested by Nurchi et al. (1992). These authors removed approximately 30 cysts, measuring between few millimeters and 8 cm, from a single location (the right occipital lobe).

Bulging and Thinning of the Skull

The continued pressure and constant pulsations of those cysts lying adjacent to the peripheral dura, against the skull, produce, with time, bulging of the skull which may be extreme (Samiy and Zadey 1965). The skull in this area may become excessively thin. This thinning of the skull, described as early as 1888 by Vergo in the right frontal region in a 10-year-old child (quoted by Simpson and Verco 1976), may render the bone paper thin, a finding called "the parchment skull sign." Dew described this aspect of hydatid disease as early as 1934. Phillips (1948) describes a case where "the bone was so thin that the flap could be cut with a strong scissors" (see Case 8).

Cysts Perforating the Skull and/or Dura

Phillips (1948) states that the "cyst had eroded the calvarium and was presenting beneath the scalp." The skull is more at risk than the dura because the latter is more elastic. Should the pressure persist, the already thinned and necrotic skull disintegrates. This perforation was very well shown on a lateral MRI view in the article of Polat et al. (2003), where the brain, containing a cyst, passed through the skull to rest under the galea. Tizniti et al. (2000) describe a similar case. Goinard and Descuns (1952) made note of a case where the cyst had perforated the dura. It has also been described in intracranial extradural cysts (Samiy and Zadey 1965; Sharma et al. 2010; Zahed et al. 2010). Griponissiotis (1957) believed the pathogenesis of such a condition is due to an injury to the skull in the presence of an intracranial hydatid cyst attached to the dura. The latter ruptures and the cyst is forced outside the dura.

Stroke and Embolism of Cerebral Arteries

Stroke as a complication of cardiac hydatidosis is described in Chap. 22. Suffice it to say that this type of embolism is seen with ruptured cysts within the left cardiac chambers or wall as well as post excision of such cysts (Vaquero et al. 1982). It may produce multiple secondary brain cysts (Turgut et al. 1997; Ugur et al. 1998; Ait Ben Ali et al. 1999), a stroke (Martín Oterino et al. 1996; Yaliniz et al. 2004; Acarturk et al. 2004) which might be fatal (Byard and Bourne 1991; Ulgen et al. 2000), or both (Abbassioun et al. 1978; El Khamlichi 1993; Benomar et al. 1994; el Quessar et al. 1996; Kocaman et al. 1999).

Infertility

Tiberin et al. (1984) report a case of galactorrhea, amenorrhea, secondary sterility, and gain of weight of 2-year duration in a 29-year-old woman in whom no endocrinologic or gynecologic cause could be found and who recovered with restoration of fertility following the removal of an intact left frontal lobe cyst. Mazor et al. (1986) report on a similar case of a patient aged 31 who got pregnant less than 2 months following the excision of a left frontal lobe hydatid cyst, after 13 years of sterility. Both believe that this condition could be due to pressure exerted by the cyst on the hypothalamic-pituitary axis.

It would be interesting to include under this section the case of an 18-year-old male reported by Ozgen et al. (1984) who had an intrasellar cyst operated through a transsphenoidal approach. The hormonal profile which was on the low side preoperatively returned to normal within 10 months.

Nephrotic Syndrome

Sharma et al. (2010) report on a patient suffering from an extradural intracranial hydatid cyst associated with a nephrotic syndrome. This condition did not respond to the usual medical treatment but subsided when the cyst was removed. They believe that there must be cause-to-effect relationship between these two conditions. This syndrome was also reported, in the same article, secondary to pulmonary and hepatic hydatidosis.

Complications During the Treatment Period

There are two types of treatment: surgical and medical. These may be used simultaneously or separately, and each has its own set of complications.

Complications Related to the Surgical Act

These complications are many. In a review of 25 cases, Tuzun et al. (2010) reported 20 complications related to the surgical act.

Inadvertent Cyst Punctures During Ventriculography

Puncture of the cyst during ventriculography used to be one of the major complications when that test was about the only one available for diagnosis and localization of brain masses. This brought Brailsford (1931) to condemn its use when hydatid was suspected. When the cyst is punctured, the risk of spillage of hydatid fluid in the brain is very substantial, and recurrences may ensue. Philips (1948) warned against this complication and so did Griponissiotis (1957). Accidental cystography used not to be infrequent (Dew 1934). Fortunately, with the advent of the newer imagery techniques, including CT and MRI, this complication is only of historical importance. This complication is well represented in the following case.

Case 2

NT, a 10-year-old girl, was seen in June 1957 suffering from headache of 7-month duration accompanied by progressive right-sided weakness of 6.5-month duration. On examination, she had tremors in the right hand and crackpot resonance. Plain skull x-ray revealed separation of sutures. Ventriculography was carried out, and the cyst was inadvertently punctured. The films revealed a cyst in the left parietal region (Fig. 17.2). A small craniotomy was performed, and, through the intact dura, the cyst was twice filled with 1 % formalin which was left in the cyst cavity for 5 min each time and then irrigated profusely with normal saline solutions. The dura was then opened and the cyst removed through a small cortical incision. A severe postoperative reaction occurred, accompanied by fever, subsiding on the 13th postoperative day. A month after surgery, the patient was well. No further follow-up was possible.

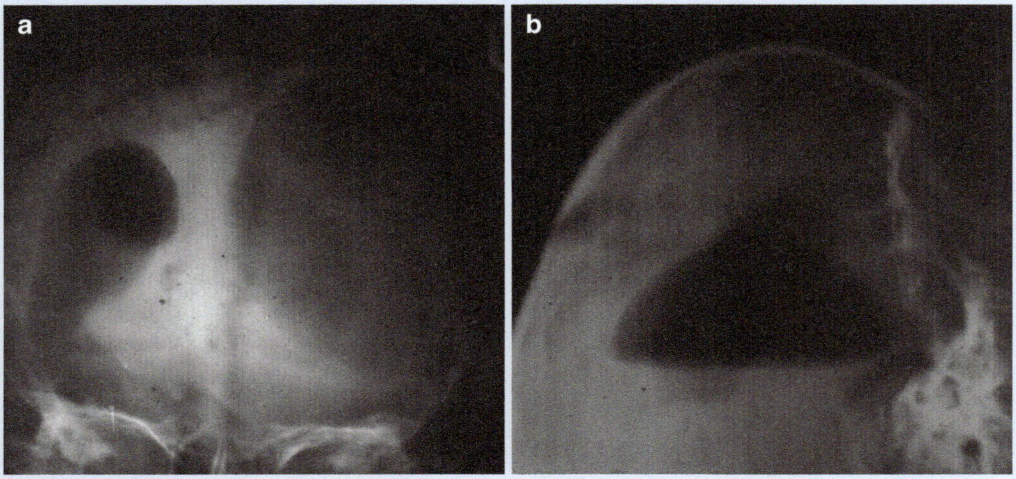

Fig. 17.2 (a) Ventriculography showing the injected cyst in AP projection. (b) Brow up lateral projection

Intentional Cyst Puncture

Cyst puncture is only indicated in extremis. It should never be carried out to decompress the brain before or at surgery. This is a most dangerous procedure as shown in the following case.

Case 3

RM, an 11-year-old boy, was seen for the first time on January 19, 1980, for headache of 3-year duration diagnosed as migraine. A month prior to his consultation, the headache became very severe, and a plain skull x-ray revealed separation of the sutures, with a decreased uptake in the left frontal area on isotope scanning. On examination there was no papilledema, but a crackpot resonance was obtained. Because of the above and his relatively good general condition, he was suspected of harboring a cerebral hydatid cyst. His family preferred him to be operated in France. His brother, a medical student who was accompanying him, was told that this was most probably a hydatid cyst and was asked to warn his surgeon in Paris not to puncture the lesion and that he, the surgeon, should be aware of that diagnosis and should do his best to deliver the cyst intact. The surgeon did not heed the advice and thought he was dealing with a cystic astrocytoma. When the dura was opened, the brain bulged, and the surgeon introduced a needle in the brain to reduce the pressure. Clear fluid spurted out and the brain relaxed; the surgeon carried out an incision in the cortex and pulled the chitinous membrane, closed the wound, and discharged the child in perfect health. This child was well until 8 months later, August 1980, when he suffered from headaches. CT scan of the brain became available in Lebanon; it was performed and revealed a cyst in the operative field. He was advised surgery but was lost to follow-up until March 28, 1981, at which time he suffered from severe weakness in the upper extremities with bilateral Babinski sign, absent knee and ankle jerks, saddle anesthesia, and urinary retention. He was being treated for a Guillain-Barré syndrome. A cisternal myelogram (CT myelography was not yet in use) revealed a complete block at C6. Following that test, the patient became completely paralyzed from C6 down with a flicker of movement in the left lower extremity. An emergency lumbar myelogram was performed with a puncture at L5–S1 to delineate the lower extent of the lesion. It revealed multiple subarachnoid space-occupying lesions extending from S2 to L2. The contrast medium did not flow beyond L2. The findings were suggestive of multiple subdural spinal hydatid cysts. An emergency surgery was performed on March 31, 1981, first on the cervical spine, from where a 3 cm cyst was removed intact from the spinal subarachnoid space at the C6 level. Then a laminectomy from S2 to L2 was performed, and four cysts were removed, two intact and two ruptured; the latter two had been punctured at the time of myelography (the needle punctures were clearly seen). The cervical and lumbar areas were thoroughly irrigated with 0.1 % cetrimide solution and the wounds closed. The patient gradually recovered his movements and sensations in the upper and lower extremities. Two weeks later, a myelogram, using the residual dye left in the spinal canal, revealed the presence of more cysts in the dorsal region (Fig. 17.3a). On April 16, a third laminectomy, joining the previous cervical and lumbar laminectomies, was performed, and the remaining six subarachnoid cysts were delivered intact from the dorsal region (Fig. 17.3b). The patient made a perfect recovery except for some urgency on urination and was discharged on May 1, 1981. On November 30, 1981, about 7 months after his discharge from hospital, he was readmitted because of bouts of headache and vomiting of 3-week

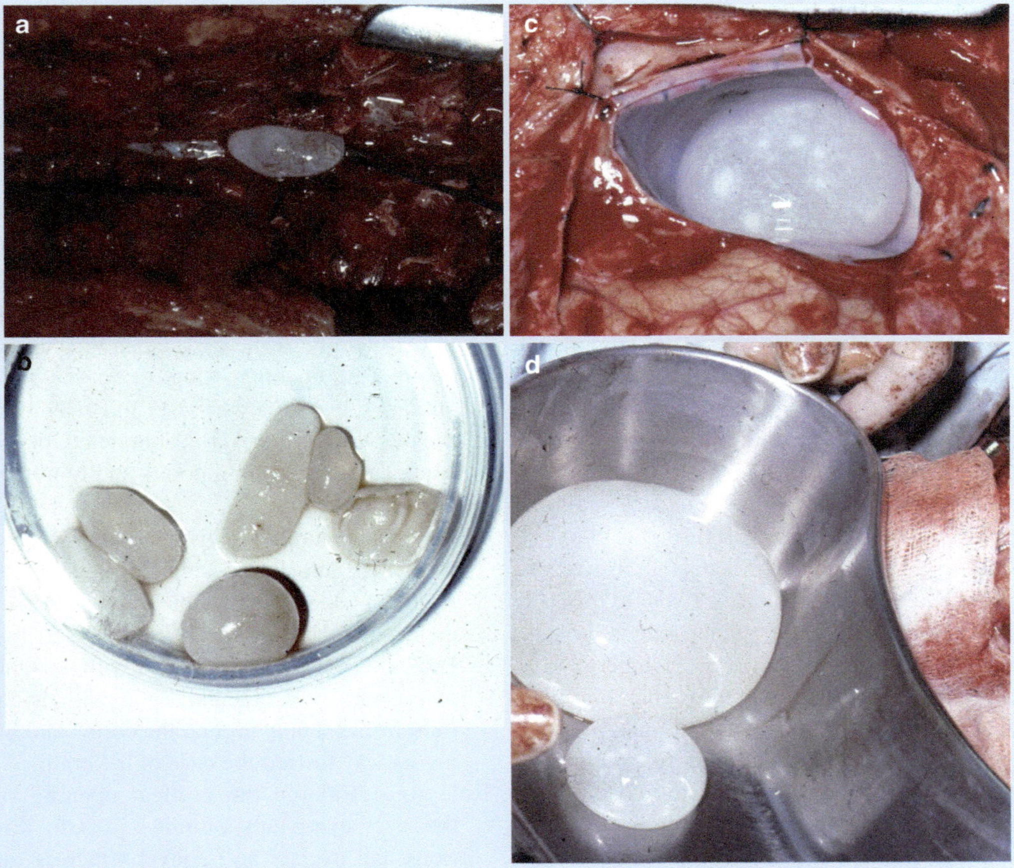

Fig. 17.3 (a) Delivery of cyst from the subdural space. (b) Cysts lying in a petri dish delivered from the dorsal space. (c) Cyst in situ in the cavity left by the previous surgery (note the thickened glistening pericyst). (d) Two recurring delivered cerebral cysts in a basin and the cavity left behind

duration. About 23 months from the initial surgery, on December 1, 1981, the left frontal craniotomy was reopened, and two recurrent frontal cysts were removed intact from the bed of the original cyst (Fig. 17.3c, d). Since then he has done well.

Cyst Rupture

The most important and most catastrophic complication in surgery of brain hydatid is the inadvertent or intentional rupture of the cyst in situ at the time of surgery. It is generally estimated that 25 % of all operated cases rupture. Do these cysts have a topographic predilection for rupture during surgery? Deep-seated cysts tend to rupture more often than superficial ones, and cysts around the brain stem are more difficult to deliver intact. Onal et al. (2001) found that cysts in the frontal location were more prone to rupture and seven out of his eight cases, in this location, did rupture.

Most of these cysts are fertile, and, upon rupturing, the brain is flooded with hydatid fluid, disseminating the hydatid sand over a large area. However, only few cysts develop, rarely exceeding a dozen in number. The question which has not yet been answered is why, while such a large number of scolices (it is estimated that one cubic centimeter of hydatid fluid contains 400,000 scolices) soak the brain, only a few, if any, hatch and only a relatively small number of cysts develop (Case 3). Is it due to the host or to the parasite? Is it that when a scolex hatches, it produces some kind of an enzyme that inhibits the hatching of other scolices? Or is it that the brain develops a certain immunity against the parasite? In some cases, the seeding may reach the spinal subdural space. Case 3 is such an example.

What is the percentage of recurrences following cyst rupture? Griponissiotis (1957) reports on four cysts ruptures out of a total of eight cases, and out of the four there was only one recurrence. He attributes this low incidence of recurrence in ruptured cysts to the fact that he did sterilize the cyst by injecting in it formalin and by washing the cavity left by the cyst with formalin.

It takes an average of 6 months for these recurrent cysts to become fertile and 1 year to produce symptoms. Therefore, the golden rule is: in case a cyst ruptures intraoperatively, it is imperative to investigate the patient within 6 months, even though the patient may be asymptomatic. A negative investigation does not entirely exclude the possibility of a recurrence at a later date. This is why, if the investigations at 6 months are negative, the search should be repeated every 4–6 months for 4 years, as a 4-year period was found to be the maximum time for a recurrence to occur. In case recurrent cysts are found, it is indicated to operate on them before they become fertile, i.e., before 6 months elapse especially that these recurrent cysts usually lie deeper in the brain and their delivery, intact, becomes more difficult. They may at times be found within the lateral ventricle (Case 4) or even in the spinal subarachnoid space (Case 3). In case the cyst recurs in the same place occupied by the original one, often the pericyst is much thicker than usual and is adherent to the adjoining brain and may mimic the appearance of the ectocyst. There may also be fluid between the thickened pericyst and the ectocyst as in our Case 3 (Fig. 17.3c).

To prevent such complications, in case of rupture, it is advisable to adapt surgery in a way to reduced damages to a minimum. As Benjamin Franklin once said "an ounce of prevention is worth a pound of cure." What kind of prevention should be applied? If one adopts the following five rules, one is prone not only to prevent rupture but, in case of rupture, to minimize the damage:

Rule one: Do not allow any sharp instrument or material to be found in or near the surgical field. Cover with wet gauze all Raney clips, and cover all sharp objects in the vicinity of the cyst, like clamps, hooks, bony edges, etc., with a wet gauze.

Rule two: Do not use the cautery (uni- or bipolar) in the vicinity of the cyst. Open the cortex or enlarge the opening using a pair of scissors and applying clips whenever indicated. After the delivery of the cyst is completed, one can coagulate the bleeding points and remove the clips if necessary.

Rule three: Cover all the visible cortex with soft, wet gauze and place a long strip of soft gauze from the edge of the visible cyst to the receptacle which is supposed to receive it intact. Pack the cortex-dura interface with wet gauze to prevent an accidental flood with hydatid fluid from seeping around the cortex and finding its way toward the base of the brain.

Rule four: Enlarge the cortical opening over the cyst using episiotomies in safe directions and excise the pericyst which is quite thin but may impair the normal delivery of the cyst. The pericyst is always present but is translucent and may be difficult to see. It often ruptures spontaneously. The unaware surgeon may believe the ectocyst is starting to rupture.

Rule five: Imbibe all the surrounding gauze with 0.1 % cetrimide solution and in case of rupture irrigate the entire field with the cetrimide solution before and after removing the surrounding gauze. Cetrimide in this concentration is innocuous to the brain but is a powerful scolicidal solution (Frayha et al. 1981; Frayha et al. 1997). Do not use hypertonic saline and certainly not formalin. The use of formalin may be fatal (Kocaman et al. 1999).

If these five rules are followed, the possibility of intact delivery of the cyst is enhanced, and, in case of rupture, recurrences are reduced to a very low percentage.

Cystoperitoneal Shunt

Peter et al. (1994) mention the insertion of a "cystoperitoneal" shunt as an emergency "by a resident." The cyst was removed a year later together with the shunt and the patient developed abdominal cysts.

Cysto-Atrial Shunt

El-Khamlichi et al. (1980) report a case, erroneously diagnosed as an intra-axial tumor, who underwent a cysto-atrial shunt and who developed an infection and meningitis followed by death, and it was on autopsy that the real nature of the disease was discovered.

Anaphylactic Shock

Much has been said and written about anaphylactic shock, especially in case of cyst rupture during surgery; yet there are very few case reports relating to this condition. De Durana et al. (1997) report on a male who was seen in the emergency department with urticaria, angioedema, syncope, and severe hypotension with positive hydatid serological tests, a year prior to the appearance of a cerebral cyst on computed tomography of the brain. It is difficult to accept any cause and effect of these reactions to the cerebral cyst. Kaya et al. (1975) report on a case that died 1 day after surgery, where "the hydatid fluid spilled into the subarachnoid space during the removal of the parapontine cyst; hyperthermia and severe allergic reactions were noted and death was probably due to anaphylactic shock." The authors of the article themselves are in doubt about anaphylactic shock and use the term "probably." Turgut (2001), who reviewed 47 articles in the Turkish literature, collected three deaths from "anaphylactic shock" out of 268 cases but does not describe the facts.

Complications Related to Nonsurgical Treatment

Albendazole and Mebendazole Treatment

If given for a long period of time, they may produce mild to moderate rise in the level of liver enzymes, alopecia, and bone marrow suppression. All these complications are reversible upon the cessation of treatment (Nourbakhsh et al. 2010).

Praziquantel Treatment

I have no experience with this drug and could not find except one reference related to the complications of this drug in humans by Zhang and Zhang (2011) who report on a case of recrudescence of fever following the treatment with this drug. I refer here to Chap. 16 of this book where the authors Dlamini and Ntusi state that "Praziquantel is usually well-tolerated." It may cause abdominal discomfort and nausea. Dizziness, fever, headache, seizures, and malaise have been described. Less commonly, the drug may cause hepatotoxicity, ventricular fibrillation, atrioventricular block, ventricular ectopy, and hypersensitivity.

Complications During the Postoperative Period

Some of these complications are specific to hydatid disease, and others are common to all other craniotomies.

Specific Complications

Recurrence

Recurrence is about the most common complication. It should be differentiated from a de novo cyst. Recurrence comes as the consequence of the spillage of fertile hydatid fluid in or over the brain due to puncture or rupture of the cyst preoperatively or during surgery. Preoperatively, the cyst puncture may be accidental as in ventriculography or for diagnostic purposes or it may be intentional as for preoperative decompression. Intraoperatively its rupture may again be intentional or inadvertent.

Not all cysts that rupture at surgery recur. In the series of Krawjewski and Stelmasiak (1991), only two recurred out of six ruptured cysts; Tuzun et al. (2010) reports one of three cases that recurred. All six ruptured cases of El-Shamam et al. (2001)

recurred, and only two cases recurred out of seven in the series of Ersahin et al. (1993). The major reason why not all ruptured cysts recurred is that those cysts may have been sterile at the time of surgery. Another reason may be that the surgeon sterilizes the cyst before he tackles it using different solutions like hypertonic salt solution, cetrimide, absolute alcohol, silver nitrate solution, or formaldehyde. The latter three solutions are not safe for use, as disability or death may ensue.

The rate of recurrence following cyst rupture is hard to evaluate because most authors report only one or a small number of cases and follow-ups are scarce and inadequate. Statistics in this respect are erroneous because, especially in the Mediterranean regions, if the disease recurs the patient seeks the opinion of another neurosurgeon and the original one may not know of the recurrence. Therefore, these statistics tend to underestimate the true recurrence rate which have been evaluated in a wide range. Ciurea et al. (1995) reported a recurrence rate of 40.7 % in a series of 27 patients, Onal et al. (2001) reported 4 out of 30 (14 %), and Tuzun et al. (2010) reported one recurrence out of 25 operated patients (4 %).

It is interesting to note that the rupture of these cysts was used by many surgeons, to determine the growth rate of hydatid cysts in the brain. They would measure the size of the recurrent cyst at the time of the redo surgery and divide it by the time elapsed between the insemination and delivery thus obtaining the so-called growth factor. None took into consideration that this growth is not a linear one but depends greatly on the intracranial pressure as well as the location of the cyst. Obviously cysts would grow in a virgin relaxed brain quicker that it would in a tense brain.

Case 4

MG, an 8-year-old boy, was admitted to hospital on October 6, 1953, for headache and vomiting accompanied by blurred vision of 4-month duration. Twenty days prior to admission, he gradually developed spasticity on the left side of the body. On physical examination, he was mentally clear and well oriented with crackpot resonance of the skull and a convergent squint. Bilateral papilledema was present. There was spastic paresis of the left side of the body with a left Babinski sign and clonus of the left foot. Plain skull x-rays revealed widening of the sutures. Casoni, Weinberg, and purified protein derivative tests were negative. A ventriculography revealed the presence of a large mass in the left frontal region. As there were no neurosurgeons in the country, a general surgeon drilled a burr hole in the left frontal region, and a cyst appeared under the dura. It was aspirated. The chitinous membrane was pulled out and the reconstructed cyst measured 5.5 cm in diameter. The patient made a good recovery. He was readmitted about a year later to another hospital where we are told another brain cyst was removed. The details of this admission are not available. On October 10, 1955, he was readmitted because of severe bouts of headaches, vomiting, and a left-sided spasticity. The right frontal craniotomy was reopened, and more than 30 cysts were removed, measuring from 1 to 7 cm in diameter. Unfortunately two small cysts ruptured. The area was thoroughly washed with hypertonic saline solution. The lateral ventricle was then opened, and a large intact cyst was removed from within it using a sterile teaspoon. Following this surgery, he was seen at different time intervals for seizures. He was seen about a year ago and is still doing well.

Porencephalic Cyst

Usually the brain reshapes postoperatively and fills the cavity left behind by the cyst so that it may be difficult to tell where the cyst was. However, in a substantial number of cases, especially when the cyst is large (estimated size at 5 cm or more), a porencephalic cavity remains in the field. Tuzun et al. (2004) recorded 4 such cavities out of 25 operated patients and Ersahin et al. (1993) 2 out of 19. These porencephalic cavities are most usually asymptomatic and need no further attention. However, this was not the case in the second patient of De Villiers Hamman and Joubert (1957) who presented a year later with a right hemiparesis and aphasia (the latter symptom is extremely rare in hydatid disease) and was operated for a possible recurrence. At surgery a large porencephalic cyst was found, and no recurrence was observed. This is the problem we faced with our radiologist who insisted that there was a recurrence and forced our hand to reoperate the following patient.

Case 5

RJ, a 21-year-old female, was operated on March 18, 1994, by a colleague for a right parietal hydatid cyst. The patient reported that her previous surgeon had told her family that "some spillage of the cyst content occurred during delivery." She received albendazole for 3 months after surgery. She was readmitted in our service on November 2, 1994, at which time an MRI revealed "a 2 cm well circumscribed cystic lesion in the right parietal lobe compatible with local recurrence of previously excised hydatid cyst" (Fig. 17.4). The patient was operated, and only gliosis surrounding a cystic area was found. Last seen on July 1, 1998, she was doing well.

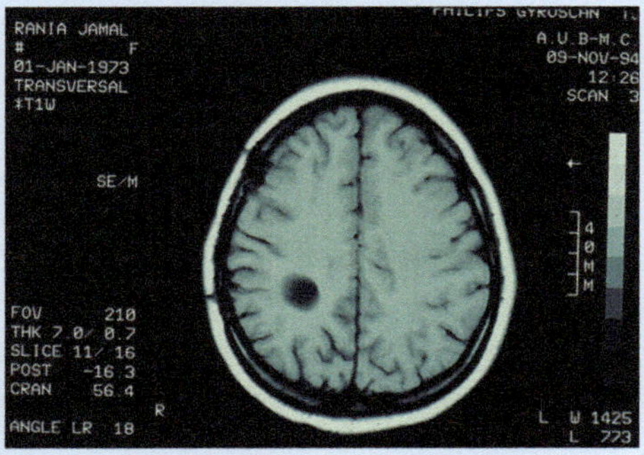

Fig. 17.4 Porencephalic cyst seen on MRI in the right parietal white matter mistaken for a recurrence

Kocaman et al. (1999) reported on two patients who needed a porencephalic cystoperitoneal shunt. These porencephalic cysts may be associated with a subdural effusion. They often last for a very long period of time.

Case 6

HI, a 10-year-old boy, was admitted to the American University Medical Center of Beirut on December 19, 1994, suffering from dizziness and headache of 1 month duration. On examination he had a left hemianopsia, papilledema, and a right Babinski sign. He brought with him an MRI revealing a 10.5 × 9.5 cm cyst in the right parietotemporal region (Fig. 17.5a). The cyst was delivered but leaked through

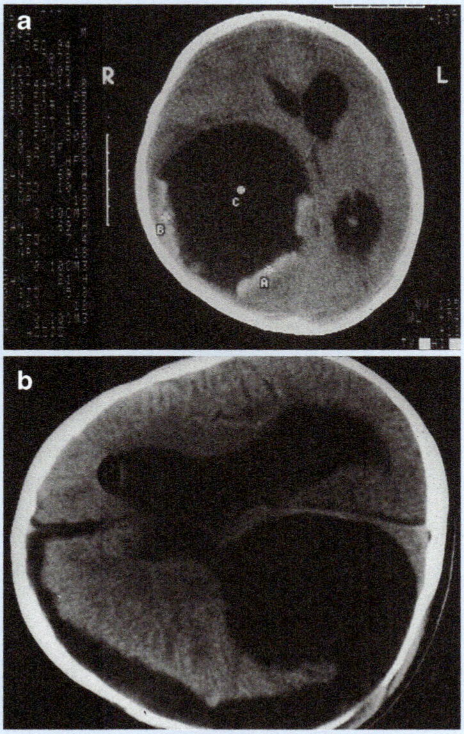

Fig. 17.5 (**a**) Pre-op MRI revealing a 10.5 × 9.5 cm hydatid cyst with multiple overgrowth of the germinative membrane. (**b**) Post-op MRI showing a large porencephalic cyst in continuity with a subdural hygroma

a pinhole. The entire field was thoroughly irrigated with 1 in 1,000 cetrimide. Readmitted 13 months later on January 17, 1996, because of headache, a large porencephalic cyst was discovered, and a cystoperitoneal shunt was planned. A needle was introduced into the cyst, and the fluid did not flow out; it had to be aspirated. In view of the low pressure in the cyst, it was decided against a shunt. Patient was seen 10 months later, on November 20, 1996; he was still asymptomatic, and his immunohemagglutination was negative.

Subdural Effusion

This is not an uncommon complication (Tuzun et al. 2004; Yuceer et al. 1998). In one report it occurred in three out of five operated patients (Abbassioun et al. 1978) and in another in 7 out of 25 operated cases (Tuzun et al. 2010). It may be connected to a porencephalic cyst as is seen in the case of HI (Fig. 17.5b). Immediately after surgery, this represents the fluid which was injected in the cyst bed just before the final dural closure to eject all the air that had filled the surrounding spaces. This fluid is later replaced by cerebrospinal fluid. Very often this condition does not need any intervention, and the fluid is gradually and spontaneously absorbed within 2–3 months (Abbassioun et al. 1978). The subdural fluid should not be aspirated with a syringe or evacuated by drainage. It is not a helpful procedure because the space will quickly refill with fluid or air. Subdural effusion very rarely produces increased intracranial pressure. In such very exceptional cases, a subdural-peritoneal shunt is of help (Tuzun et al. 2010).

Pneumocephalus

Pneumocephalus has been reported in 12 % of cases in the postoperative period (Tuzun et al. 2004). It is of no consequence and disappears within few days without any specific treatment.

Hydrocephalus

This complication is quite rare. It has been described by Ersahin et al. (1993) who report on one case who needed a ventriculoperitoneal shunt after surgery and so did Kocaman et al. (1999).

Intracerebral Bleed

Intracerebral bleed has been occasionally reported (Tuzun et al. 2004). Griponissiotis (1957) lost a patient from hemorrhage "resulting from an attempt to remove a very thick capsule." Radwan and Khaffaji (1988) reported on a patient who developed an intracerebral, intraventricular, and extracerebral hematoma which was evacuated; but the patient deteriorated progressively, developed hydrocephalus, and died 7 months later.

The etiology of such bleeds is legion, but most frequently bleeds occur after the delivery of a cyst which had leaked, ruptured, or was infected in situ prior to surgery. These three conditions often produce adhesions of the cyst to the adjoining brain tissue through the pericyst rendering delivery difficult and hazardous. Tuzun et al. (2004) lists the following causes of postoperative bleed: uncontrolled bleed from a hidden area, difficult dissection, retraction, vessel injury by needle, bleeding from a residual lesion, local hemodynamic changes, and hypertension during surgery and during recovery from anesthesia.

Postoperative Calcification

St. George et al. (2003) reported a complicated case in whom postoperative calcification occurred. A 9-year-old boy was harboring a 5 cm hydatid cyst diagnosed as a "porencephalic" cyst of the parietal lobe. This was treated with aspiration. The cyst got infected with "mixed organisms," and an Ommaya reservoir was inserted for repeated aspiration and local instillation of gentamicin. The patient also received parenteral antibiotics until the returns from aspiration became culture negative. It is interesting to note that, 6 years later (1981), a multiloculated cyst was found at the site of the original one from which sterile "thick purulent fluid" was aspirated and patient was started on mebendazole. A left parietal craniotomy was performed, and multiple cysts containing scolices and brood capsules were delivered with calcifications in the walls of the larger ones. In 1984, 3 years after the excision of the cysts, a calcification was observed on CT scan at the site of surgery. Twelve years later the patient developed a malignant glioma at the site of the previously removed hydatid cyst. In this case it is not clear whether this calcification had a direct relation to the cyst or whether it was a consequence of the infection or whether it was part of the glioma.

A real postoperative calcification was seen in the bed of the delivered cyst in one of our patients.

Case 7

HQ, a 23-year-old male, was seen for the first time on October 14, 1981, suffering from generalized headache of 1-month duration. Examination was negative, and he was managed conservatively. The headache persisted, and on December 17, 1981, he had developed papilledema. A CT was performed and revealed a very large cystic mass, in the left parietal region which was considered an abscess or a hydatid cyst. He was urgently admitted to hospital where he was operated, and the mass proved to be a hydatid cyst (Fig. 17.6a) which was delivered intact. On April 14, 1993, i.e., 12 years after surgery, the patient returned complaining of some headache in the left side

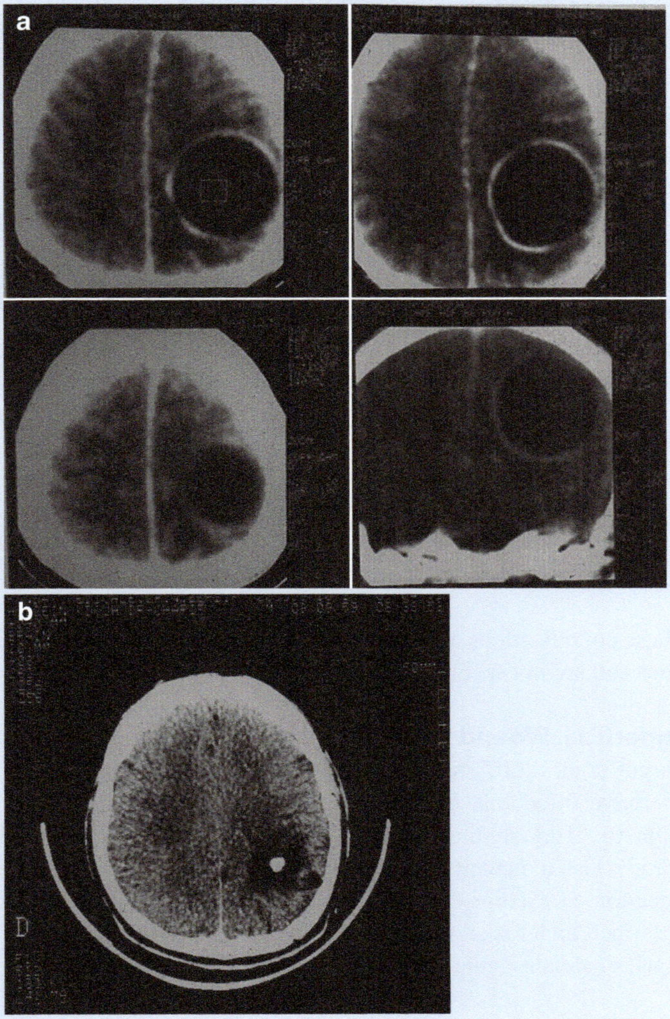

Fig. 17.6 (**a**) Preoperative CT showing the left parietal hydatid cyst. (**b**) Gliosis with central calcification at the site of the hydatid cyst removed 12 years earlier

of the head, and a CT revealed an area of gliosis with a central calcification at the site of the previous hydatid cyst. This calcification is most probably in the pericyst left behind (Fig. 17.6b).

Glioma

St George et al. (2003) report on a case described in the previous section ("Postoperative calcification") of a man who developed a malignant glioma, in the same location from which 22 years earlier a hydatid cyst was removed, and ponder whether it is "possible that the glioma arose as a result of chronic changes induced by previous hydatid?" No other reference for such a transformation has been found in the literature.

Choreiform Movements

These movements were described in the postoperative period in one case in which the cyst was delivered from the basal ganglia area. That patient was free from these symptoms prior to surgery (Turgut 2001).

Delayed Mental Development

It is interesting to note that 3 out of 12 operated children (ages not recorded) reported by Krajewski and Stelmasiak (1991) "showed retardation of mental development." All three children had a persistent porencephalic cyst.

Nonspecific Complications

These complications are common to all craniotomies and are not specific to hydatidosis.

Superficial Wound Infection

Turgut et al. (2007) reported four cases of postoperative infections out of 268 cases retrieved from the Turkish literature, and Griponissiotis (1957) lost a patient because of postoperative infection. St. George et al. (2003) reported a case, described under section "Postoperative calcification", of an iatrogenic infection.

Meningitis and Abscess

Meningitis was reported by Turgut et al. (2007) in 1 case out of 268. Krajewski and Stelmasiak (1991) reported 2 cases of nonbacterial meningitis occurring immediately after surgery, out of 12 operated patients, as well as one case of meningitis appearing a year after the third operation for recurrent hydatid disease. Mircevski et al. (1985) reported on three deaths from a series of nine intraventricular cysts, one of whom, a 5-year-old girl harboring a fourth ventricular cyst, died from purulent meningitis. Samiy and Zadeh (1965) reported a 9-year-old girl who developed meningitis due to a cerebrospinal fluid fistula and died 3 months after surgery. Botteau et al. (2003) describe a case of eosinophilic meningitis which occured following excision of a cerebral hydatid cyst and resolved under chorticosteroid therapy. Ouboukhlik et al. (1994) reported on a case in which an abscess developed in the cavity left by the cyst needing a second operation.

Deep Venous Thrombosis

Turgut et al. (2007) reported 2 out of 268 cases.

Pulmonary Embolism

The case of Tiberin et al. (1984) developed "a delayed massive pulmonary embolism (which) responded well to anticoagulation therapy."

Cerebrospinal Fluid Leak

Turgut et al. (2007) reported 1 out of 268 cases, and Samiy and Zadeh (1965) described one case which led to meningitis (see section "Meningitis and abscess").

The above three subsections are not all inclusive. Although little was found in the literature about these three types of complications, obviously they must have occurred more frequently but have not been reported.

Subdural Hematoma

Subdural hematoma has been described on the opposite side of surgery and proved to be fatal (Garcia-Uria et al. 1980). This is probably due to the decompression that occurred following the evacuation of the cyst. The positioning of the head during surgery is of paramount importance; were the patient lying on the normal side of the head, the weight of the brain would have avoided this complication. Turgut (2001) reports on 4 cases out of 268 but does not mention the side relative to surgery nor the outcome.

Epidural Hematoma

This complication was reported in one out of 25 operated cases (Tuzun et al. 2010). The extreme decompression within the skull may be inductive to such a complication. This is why it is advisable to place retention sutures from the dura to the pericranium at the start of surgery, which will obliterate the extradural space and will not allow the dura to peel off.

Seizures

Focal cerebral seizures occur in approximately one-third of patients before surgery (Arseni and Marinescu 1974) and show a wide range of frequency from 7 to 48.5 % depending on different authors (Goinard and Descuns 1952; Arseni and Marinescu 1974; Ersahin et al. 1993). The electroencephalography is not pathognomonic of hydatid disease and often shows delta wave activity (Arseni and Marinescu 1974). These seizures frequently improve following surgery. However, de novo seizures do occur postoperatively; 4 out of 59 operated patients were reported by Arseni and Marinescu (1974), 4 out of 30 by Onal et al. (2001), 4 out of 23 by Kocaman et al. (1999), and 10 out of 48 by Ouboukhlik et al. (1994). These patients do require long-term antiepileptic therapy.

Postoperative Mortality

In hydatid disease, like all major intracranial surgery, mortality depends a great deal on the preoperative condition of the patient (our Case 8) and the localization of the cyst(s) (Barjhoux et al. 1970) as well as on the expertise and dexterity of the surgeon. It ranges from zero percent in some series (Tuzun et al. 2010) up to 25 % or 26.6 % in other series (Kaya et al. (1975).

Case 8

FM, a 2-year-old boy, was admitted to hospital for seizures, headaches, vomiting, and right hemiplegia. He was diagnosed as harboring a brain space-occupying lesion. He developed chicken pox, and the pediatrician insisted on discharging him, to be readmitted for surgery in 3 weeks' time. He was lost to follow up until he reappeared, on February 1958, at the age of 5 years, with a right hemiplegia, diplopia, and vomiting. On examination he was drowsy and had fits of unconsciousness accompanied by generalized spasticity with head turning to the right side. He had an enlarged head mainly in the left parietal region with crackpot resonance. He had bilateral papilledema and a bilateral Babinski sign. An emergency right carotid angiogram was performed revealing a large avascular, rounded space-occupying lesion in the left hemisphere mainly in the parietotemporal region. Chest x-ray was negative, and blood examinations revealed zero eosinophils, a negative indirect hemagglutination test, and a 1/4 Weinberg test. By the time the patient was taken to the operating room, his pupils had become dilated and nonreactive to light. A scalp flap was rapidly turned, and the skull was cut with a pair of scissors. When the dura was opened, a large cyst appeared (Fig. 17.7a). It was delivered intact and weighed 1.7 kg (probably the largest cerebral cyst on record) (Fig. 17.7b). Postoperatively the patient started to recover very gradually, his pupils came down, and he began to respond to painful stimuli but passed away on the fourth postoperative day from aspiration pneumonia.

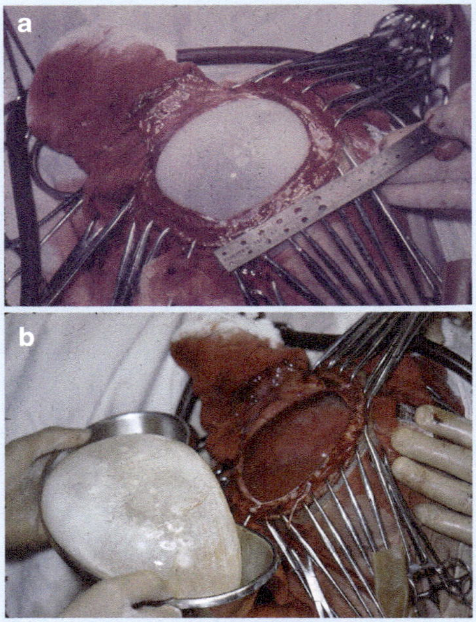

Fig. 17.7 (**a**) Cyst as it appeared upon the reflection of the dura. (**b**) Cyst delivered intact into a basin

Conclusion

Complications of cerebral hydatid disease are multiple. Most of them are avoidable if the nature and progression of this disease is well understood. Although some are of a minor nature, others may be very serious and even lethal.

Acknowledgments I am indebted to Miss Aida Farha and her staff, at the Saab Medical Library at the American University of Beirut, for their help in obtaining valuable references. To Dr. Sherreen Khayrallah go my thanks for going over the English of this chapter and to Drs. Georges F. Haddad and Souheil F. Haddad for reviewing the text and suggesting many important corrections.

References

Abbassioun K, Rahmat H, Amelie NO, Tafazoli M. Computerized tomography in hydatid cyst of the brain. J Neurosurg. 1978;49:408–11.

Abderrahmen K, Aouidj ML, Kallel J, Khaldi MM. Calcified cerebral hydatid cyst (in French). Neurochirurgie. 2007;53:371–4.

Acarturk E, Zeren A, Koc M, Yaliniz H, Bicakci S, Demir M. Left ventricular hydatid cyst presenting with acute ischemic stroke: case report. J Am Soc Echocardiogr. 2004;17:1009–10.

Acquaviva R, Tamic PM, Bau P, Lebascle J, Kendoudi H. Les formes involuées des kystes hydatiques cérébraux. L Med Maroc. 1966;2:317–22.

Ait Ben Ali S, Hilmani S, Choukri M, Sami A, El Azhari A, Achouri M, Ouboukhlik A, El Kamar A, Boucetta M. Multiple cerebral hydatid cysts of cardiac origin. A case report (in French). Neurochirurgie. 1999;45:426–9.

Aksungur EH, Oguz M, Bicakci K, Altay M. Cerebral hydatid lesion with daughter cysts: MR and CT findings. AJR Am J Roentgenol. 1994;163:1269–70.

Alvarez F, Garcia-Blanquez M, Oliver B, Manrique M. Calcified cerebral hydatid cyst. Surg Neurol. 1982;17:163–4.

Arana-Iniguez R, San Julian J. Hydatid cysts of the brain. J Neurosurg. 1955;12:323–35.

Arseni C, Marinescu V. Epilepsy in cerebral hydatidosis. Epilepsia. 1974;15:45–54.

Barjhoux P, Avocat L, Gilbertas A, Girona GC, Rochet M. Localisation cérébrale terminale d'une échinococcose alvéolaire hépatique et pulmonaire. A propos d'une observation. Arch Fr Mal App Dig. 1970;59:709–20.

Benomar A, Yahyaoui M, Birouk N, Vidailhet M, Chkili T. Middle cerebral artery occlusion due to hydatid cysts of myocardial and intraventricular cavity cardiac origin. Two cases. Stroke. 1994;25:886–8.

Boixados JR. Hidatidosis del sistema nervioso central. Madrid: Publicaciones Controladas; 1973. 144 p.

Bottieau E, David P, Dewitte O, Jacobs F. Eosinophilic meningitis, following incomplete resection of a meningeal hydatid cyst. Scand J Infect Dis. 2003;35:898–901.

Bouaziz M. Calcified cerebral hydatid cyst: a case report. Sante. 2005;15:129–32.

Brailford JF. Hydatid disease in England. Br Med J. 1931;1:133–6.

Byard RW, Bourne AJ. Cardiac echinococcosis with fatal intracerebral embolism. Arch Dis Child. 1991;66:155–6.

Choukri M, Bertal A, Lakhdar A, Achouri M, Ouboukhlik A, el Kamar A, el Azhari A. Calcified cerebral hydatid cyst. Report of a case. J Neuroradiol. 2001;28:261–3.

Ciurea AV, Vasilescu G, Nuteanu L, Carp N. Cerebral hydatid cyst in children. Experience of 27 cases. Childs Nerv Syst. 1995;11:679–85.

De Villiers HH, Joubert MJ. A review of hydatid disease of the brain. S Afr Med J. 1957;31:1163–7.

Dew HR. Hydatid disease of the brain. Surg Gynec Obst. 1934;59:321–9.

Dew HR. Hydatid disease of the brain. Arch Int Hidatid. 1967;13:132–44.

Diaz de Durana MD, Lopez A, Fraj J. Anaphylaxis and cerebral hydatid disease. Ann Intern Med. 1997;126:745.

El Khamlichi A, El Ouarzazi A, Chkili T, Medejel A, Alaoui MF. Les formes ataxiques du kyste hydatique de l'encéphale. Maroc Med. 1980;11:85–90.

El Khamlichi A. Kyste hydatique de la loge caverneuse. Une observation. Neurochirurgie. 1993;39:55–7.

El Quessar A, Benabdejlil M, Mansouri A, el Hassani MR, Chakir N, Jiddane M, Benomar A, Yahyaoui M, Chkili T, Boukhrissi N. Cerebral vascular accidents due to hydatid embolisms. Apropos of 2 cases. J Neuroradiol. 1996;23:74–8.

El-Shamam O, Amer T, Abo El-Atta M. Magnetic resonance imaging of simple and infected hydatid cyst of the brain. Magn Reson Imaging. 2001;19:965–74.

Erongun U, Ozkal E, Acar O, Kocaogullar Y. Multiple and infected cerebral hydatid cysts. Case report. Neurosurg Rev. 1994;17:77–81.

Ersahin Y, Mutluer S, Guzelbag E. Intracranial hydatid cysts in children. Neurosurgery. 1993;33:219–25.

Frayha GJ, Bikhazi KJ, Kachachi TA. Treatment if hydatid cysts (Echinococcus granulosus) by Cetrimide. Trans R Soc Trop Med Hyg. 1981;75(3):447–50.

Frayha GJ, Smyth JD, Gobert JG, Savel J. The mechanisms of action of antiprotozoal and anthelmintic drugs in man. Gen Pharmacol. 1997;28:273–99.

Garcia-Uria J, Cabezudo J, Nombela L. Subdural hematoma as a complication in the surgical removal of intracranial hydatidosis. Acta Neurochir (Wien). 1980; 52:51–4.

Goinard P, Descuns P. Les kystes hydatiques du nevraxe. Rev Neurol. 1952;86:369–415.

Gomori JM, Cohen D, Eyd A, Pomeranz S. Water lily sign in CT of cerebral hydatid disease: a case report. Neuroradiology. 1988;30:358.

Gonzalez-Ruiz CA, Isia A, Perez-Higueras A, Blazquez MG. Unusual CT image of a cerebral hydatid cyst. Pediatr Radiol. 1990;20:283–4.

Griponissiotis B. Hydatid cyst of the brain and its treatment. Neurology. 1957;7:789–92.

Haddad FS, Haddad FS, Haddad SI. La malignité de l'échinococcose. Rev Med Moyen Orient. 1963;20: 270–5.

Haddad FS, Haddad GF. Overview of brain hydatid and its surgical management: personal experience with cyst delivery. Pan Arab J Neurosurgery. 2003;7:33–41.

Haddad GF, Haddad FS. Management of hydatid cyst of the brain. Contemp Neurosurg. 2000;22:1–6.

Kaya U, Ozden B, Turker K, Tarcan B. Intracranial hydatid cysts: study of 17 cases. J Neurosurg. 1975;42: 580–4.

Kocaman S, Ersahin Y, Mutluer S. Cerebral hydatid cysts in children. J Neurosci Nurs. 1999;31:270–7.

Kooy FM. Two cases of old caseous hydatid cysts. S Afr Med J. 1940;14:47–9.

Krawjewski R, Stelmasiak Z. Cerebral hydatid cysts in children. Childs Nerv Syst. 1991;7:154–5.

Legrè J, Massad A. Etudes radiologiques des calcifications intra-craniennes. J Radiol Electrol. 1957;38:645–62.

Martín Oterino JA, Chimpén Ruiz VA, Reviriego Jaén G, Sánchez Rodríguez A. Repeated strokes as a sign of multiple cerebral hydatid cysts. Neurologia. 1996;11:307–9.

Mathuriya SN, Arora OP, Khosla VK, Prabhakar SK, Chopra JS, Kak VK. Infected intradural hydatid cyst at foramen magnum. A case report. Clin Neurol Neurosurg. 1985;87:283–6.

Mazor M, Picard R, Tauber E, Hagay ZJ, Leiberman JR. Restoration of fertility following excision of an intracranial hydatid cyst (in French). J Gynecol Obstet Biol Reprod (Paris). 1986;15:909–11.

Mircevski M, Mircevska D, Boyadziev I, Basevska R. Voluminous intraventricular hydatid cysts in children (in French). Neurochirurgie. 1985;31:425–8.

Nanassis K, Alexiadou-Rudolf C, Tsitsopoulos P, Tzioufa V, Pestas G, Grigoriou K. Solid cerebral echinococcosis mimicking a primary brain tumor. Neurosurg Rev. 1999;22:58–61.

Nourbakhsh A, Vannemreddy P, Minagar A, Toledo EG, Palacios E, Nanda A. Hydatid disease of the central nervous system: a review of literature with an emphasis on Latin American countries. Neurol Res. 2010;32:245–51.

Nurchi G, Floris F, Montaldo C, Mastio F, Peltz T, Coraddu M. Multiple cerebral hydatid disease: case report with magnetic resonance imaging study. Neurosurgery. 1992;30:436–8.

Obrador S, Urquiza P. Two cases of cerebral abscess of unusual nature: tuberculous abscess and suppurated hydatid cyst. J Neurosurg. 1948;5:572–8.

Onal C, Unal F, Barlas O, Izgi N, Hepgul K, Turantan MI, Canbolat A, Turker K, Bayindir C, Gokay HK, Kaya U. Long-term follow-up and results of thirty pediatric intracranial hydatid cysts: half a century of experience in the department of neurosurgery of the School of Medicine at the University of Istanbul (1952–2001). Pediatr Neurosurg. 2001;35:72–81.

Ouboukhlik A, Choukri M, Elazhari A, Elkamar A, Boucetta M. Cerebral hydatid cyst. Apropos of 48 cases (in French). Neurochirurgie. 1994;40:242–6.

Ozek MM. Complications of central nervous system hydatid disease. Pediatr Neurosurg. 1994;20:84–91.

Ozgen T, Bertan V, Kansu T, Akalin S. Intrasellar hydatid cyst. Case report. J Neurosurg. 1984;60:647–8.

Peter JC, Domingo Z, Sinclair-Smith C, de Villiers JC. Hydatid infestation of the brain: difficulties with computed tomography diagnosis and surgical treatment. Pediatr Neurosurg. 1994;20:78–83.

Phillips G. Primary cerebral hydatid cysts. J Neurol Neurosurg Psychiatry. 1948;11:44–52.

Polat P, Kantarci M, Alper F, Suma S, Koruyucu MB, Okur A. Hydatid disease from head to toe. Radiographics. 2003;23:475–94.

Robinson RG. Complications neurologiques de la maladie hydatique. World Neurol. 1961;2:426–32.

Roger H. Les kystes hydatiques du cerveau. Med Trop. 1944;4:89–110.

Rudwan MA, Khaffaji S. CT of cerebral hydatid disease. Neuroradiology. 1988;30:496–9.

Samiy E, Zadey FA. Cranial and intracranial hydatidosis with special reference to roentgen ray diagnosis. J Neurosurg. 1965;22:425–33.

Sharma T, Khosla VK, Brar R. Primary extradural hydatid cyst associated with nephrotic syndrome in a pediatric patient. Childs Nerv Syst. 2010;26:1247–9.

Simpson DA, Verco PW. Cerebral hydatid cysts in Colonial Australia. Surg Neurol. 1976;6:377–80.

St George EJ, Hillier CEM, Hatfield R. Glioma after cerebral hydatid disease. Childs Nerv Syst. 2003;19: 837–40.

Tiberin P, Heilbronn YD, Hirsch M, Barmeir E. Giant cerebral Echinococcus cyst with galactorrhea and amenorrhea. Surg Neurol. 1984;21:505–6.

Tizniti S, Allali N, El Quessar A, Chakir N, El Hassani MR, Jiddane M. An unusual cerebral hydatid cyst. J Neuroradiol. 2000;27:200–2.

Turgut M. Intracranial hydatidosis in Turkey: its clinical presentation, diagnostic studies, surgical management and out-come, a review of 276 cases. Neurosurg Rev. 2001;24:200–8.

Turgut AT, Turgut M. Infected or complicated hydatid cyst case mimicking a primary brain tumor (letter). Neurosurg Rev. 2002;25:191.

Turgut AT, Altin L, Topçu S, Kiliçoğlu B, Altinok T, Kaptanoğlu E, Karademir A, Koşar U. Unusual imaging characteristics of complicated hydatid disease. Eur J Radiol. 2007;63:84–93.

Turgut M, Benli K, Eryilmaz M. Secondary multiple intracranial hydatid cysts caused by intracerebral embolism of cardiac echinococcosis: an exceptional case of hydatidosis. Case report. J Neurosurg. 1997;86:714–8.

Tuzun Y, Kadioglu HH, Izci Y, Suma S, Keles M, Aydin IH. The clinical, radiological and surgical aspects of cerebral hydatid cysts in children. Pediatr Neurosurg. 2004;40:155–60.

Tuzun Y, Solmaz I, Sengul G, Izci Y. The complications of cerebral hydatid cyst surgery in children. Childs Nerv Syst. 2010;26:47–51.

Ugur HÇ, Attar A, Bagdatoglu C, Erdogan A, Egemen N. Secondary multiple intracranial hydatid cysts caused by intracerebral embolism of cardiac echinococcosis. Acta Neurochir (Wien). 1998;140:833–4.

Ulgen MS, Alan S, Karadede A, Aydinalp O, Toprak N. Cardiac hydatid cysts located in both the left ventricular apex and the intraventricular septum: case report. Heart Vessels. 2000;15:243–4.

Vaquero J, Jimenez C, Martinez R. Growth of hydatid cysts evaluated by CT scanning after presumed cerebral hydatid embolism: case report. J Neurosurg. 1982;57:837–8.

Villarejo F, Blazquez MG, Arcas J, Pascual-Castroviejo I, Esteban F. Hydatid cyst of the posterior fossa: case report. Neurosurgery. 1983;12:228–9.

Yaliniz H, Tokcan A, Ulus T, Kisacikoglu B, Salih OK, Topcuoglu MS, Poyrazoglu H, Alhan C. A rare presentation of cardiac hydatid cyst: stroke and acute aortic occlusion. Heart Surg Forum. 2004;7E:364–6.

Yuceer N, Guven MB, Yilmaz H. Multiple hydatid cysts of the brain: a case report and review of the literature. Neurosurg Rev. 1998;21:181–4.

Zahed HM, Mizanur RM, Mohammad BS. Cranial hydatid abscess. Trop Doct. 2010;40:255–6.

Zhang SX, Zhang TY. Temperature recrudescence caused by praziquantel treatment after falling to normal automatically in acute schistosomiasis patients: a report of 19 cases. Zhongguo Xue Xi Chong Bing Fang Zhi Za Zhi. 2011;23:411–27.

Complications of Spinal Hydatidosis

18

Hideki Sudo

Contents

H. Sudo, MD, PhD
Department of Advanced Medicine
for Spine and Spinal Cord Disorders,
Hokkaido University Graduate School of Medicine,
North-15, West-7, Kita-ku,
Sapporo, Hokkaido 060-8638, Japan
e-mail: hidekisudo@yahoo.co.jp

Introduction

It has been reported that hydatid disease involving the vertebral body and paraspinal muscles is rare, even in rural areas where echinococcosis is endemic. The treatment of choice for spinal hydatidosis is surgical resection of the affected vertebrae combined with stabilization, followed by postoperative adjuvant chemotherapy. Nevertheless, the recurrence rate is extremely high, and radical resection is often impossible to achieve in cases of extradural lesions involving the spine due to rupture of the hydatid cyst during surgery.

Complicated Hydatid Cysts of the Spine

Epidemiology

Spinal hydatid cysts account for 1 % of all cases of hydatid disease and 50 % of cases of hydatid disease of the bone (Szypryt et al. 1987; Schnepper and Johnson 2004; Herrera et al. 2005). Cysts can be located in the thoracic spine (50 %), lumbar spine (20 %), sacral spine (20 %), or cervical spine (10 %) (Turgut et al. 2007). It has been reported that hydatid disease involving the vertebral body and paraspinal muscles is rare even in rural areas where echinococcosis is endemic (Szypryt et al. 1987; Sudo and Minami 2010).

Epidemiology of hydatidosis is discussed in detail in Chaps. 2, 3, 4, and 8.

M. Turgut (ed.), *Hydatidosis of the Central Nervous System: Diagnosis and Treatment*,
DOI 10.1007/978-3-642-54359-3_18, © Springer-Verlag Berlin Heidelberg 2014

Characteristics of Cystic Lesions

In contrast to the infestation of other body tissues, infestation of the bones including the vertebral column provides an appropriate microenvironment for viable parasites (Turgut et al. 2007). In vertebral hydatidosis, the parasites spread along the intratrabecular spaces, destroying the bone, although intervertebral discs are usually preserved because the disease tends to propagate beneath the periosteum and ligaments (Herrera et al. 2005). In addition, spinal hydatid cysts have thinner walls because of decreased inflammatory response against them and reduced fibrotic reaction (Tali 2004; Turgut et al. 2007). Clinically, unilocular type I cysts, unilocular type II cysts with daughter vesicles or detached membranes, and unilocular type III calcified cysts are frequently observed (Polat et al. 2003; Turgut et al. 2007).

Vertebral Involvement and Pathological Fracture

Hydatid cysts in the vertebral column are usually asymptomatic until a pathological fracture develops. Herrera et al. (2005) reported that only 5 patients showed back or sacral pain out of the 20 operated patients. In a review of 14 cases of spinal hydatidosis, Haddad and Bitar (1997) reported that pain was the most common symptom (13 out of 14 cases). Other symptoms were incontinence of urine, weakness, and sciatica. Signs include weakness and spasticity. The findings on spinal radiography are mostly nonspecific, though they have a characteristic imaging appearance on computed tomography (CT) or magnetic resonance imaging (MRI). Plain spinal radiography sometimes shows an "absent pedicle sign"-like spinal tumor. On CT, a spinal hydatid cyst has a typical appearance of a large non-enhancing cyst of cerebrospinal fluid density, with no pericystic edema and no enhancement after injection of the contrast medium (Turgut et al. 2007). Frequently, they have a honeycomb appearance due to a multiplicity of small cysts within the bone marrow. Large unicystic lesion is very rare; it may be found in the paraspinal area. Absence of osteoporosis and sclerosis in the host vertebrae as well as lack of damage in the adjacent intervertebral disc space also indicates this disease (Turgut et al. 2007).

MRI is the preferred imaging modality for the diagnosis of spinal hydatidosis. On MRI, the involved vertebra has a heterogeneous medium to low signal intensity on T1-weighted images and high signal intensity on T2-weighted images. The daughter cysts are more hypointense than the parent cyst on T1-weighted images, whereas they are of slightly higher signal intensity in comparison with the parent cyst on T2-weighted images (von Sinner et al. 1991; Turgut et al. 2007).

In advanced cases, mild kyphotic deformity of the spine is observed due to compression fracture or collapse of the affected vertebra. Persistent pain and deformity is caused by either collapse of the spine or extension of the process beyond the skeletal confines (Tabak et al. 2007).

This material is discussed in detail in Chap. 8.

Spinal Canal Compromise

Although it is not specific to spinal hydatidosis, radicular pain and myelopathic pain with back pain are the most typical symptoms. Neurological deterioration will result in paraplegia in 25–50 % of cases (Normelli et al. 1998; Schnepper and Johnson 2004). Spinal hydatid cysts can be extradural, subdural, subarachnoidal, or intramedullary (Akhan and Ozmen 1999; Turgut et al 2007) and are usually situated in the dorsal region. They may generate medullary or radicular symptoms according to their location (Karadereler et al. 2002). A primary spinal intradural extramedullary hydatid cyst is extremely rare. Kalkan et al. (2007) reported this lesion in a child as follows: an 8-year-old boy presented with back pain, left leg pain, and difficulty in walking. The patient had no other signs of systemic hydatid cyst disease. An intradural extramedullary cystic lesion was identified with MRI and shown to be a hydatid cyst by histopathological examination after surgical removal. In MRI examination, an intradural extramedullary hydatid cyst has two dome-shaped ends but no debris in its lumen and has sausage-like appearance. Cyst walls are extremely thin and regular and have no septation (Kalkan et al. 2007).

Hydatid cysts that lack the typical radiographic appearance may be mistaken for arachnoid cysts. Secer et al. (2008) documented these cysts as follows: arachnoid cysts occur as single or multiple cysts. Because they have long T1 and T2 relaxation times, they demonstrate a homogeneous signal pattern similar to that of cerebrospinal fluid: hypointense on T1-weighted and hyperintense on T2-weighted images. One of the differential diagnoses of a spinal arachnoid cyst is a unilocular type 1 hydatid cyst. Unilocular type 1 hydatid cysts usually have thinner walls than their counterparts. However, arachnoid cysts are an exception because of the existence of a decreased inflammatory response.

Paraspinal Extension

When vertebral body destruction and paravertebral soft tissue involvement are observed, tuberculous spondylodiscitis can be confused with hydatid cysts. Tabak et al. (2007) documented a vertebral hydatid cyst mimicking tuberculous spondylodiscitis. They reported that the macroscopic destruction of the vertebrae observed during the surgery was typical of spinal tuberculosis; therefore, antituberculous therapy was initiated before the histopathological reports verifying the presence of *Echinococcus* was obtained. Other differential diagnoses should be established for pyogenic brucellosis, other granulomatous infections affecting the vertebral bodies causing paravertebral abscesses, and tumors (Tabak et al. 2007).

Infection of Cystic Lesion

Turgut et al. (2007) reported that superimposed pyogenic infections involving the spine may develop in some cases, particularly those cases in which cyst rupture occurs spontaneously. In complicated cases, osseous structures, such as vertebrae, constitute a friendly microenvironment for the development of a chronic infection resistant to treatment. On CT or MRI, there may be atypical features such as irregularity of the cyst wall contour, enhancement of the surrounding rim, isodensity, or heterogeneity of the cyst content.

Complications Related to Surgery

Surgical Indications for Spinal Hydatidosis

The treatment goals of spinal hydatidosis are to resect the infested lesion, alleviate pain, prevent neurological deficit, and establish spinal stability. Although the appropriate treatment varies with patient condition and cyst characteristics, including size and location, surgical intervention is mostly indicated in patients with spinal hydatidosis. Patients should be operated as soon as diagnosed unless there is a contraindication for surgery. The earlier the surgery is carried out, the better is the prognosis. One should not wait until surgery becomes a palliative treatment. Conversely, there is no clear consensus regarding which patient should undergo surgical treatment in cases of diffuse spread of the infection within multiple vertebrae and paraspinal muscles (Figs. 18.1, 18.2, 18.3, 18.4, 18.5, and 18.6). Possible indications for palliative surgery in such cases may include vertebral collapse causing intractable pain, spinal cord compression causing progressive neurological compromise, and a life expectancy of at least 3 months, in line with the recommendations regarding palliative surgery for metastatic spinal tumors (Oda et al. 2006).

Surgical Procedures

Laminectomy with complete resection of the cysts is the most frequently performed procedure. A posterior approach should be used to resect the involved posterior element and add

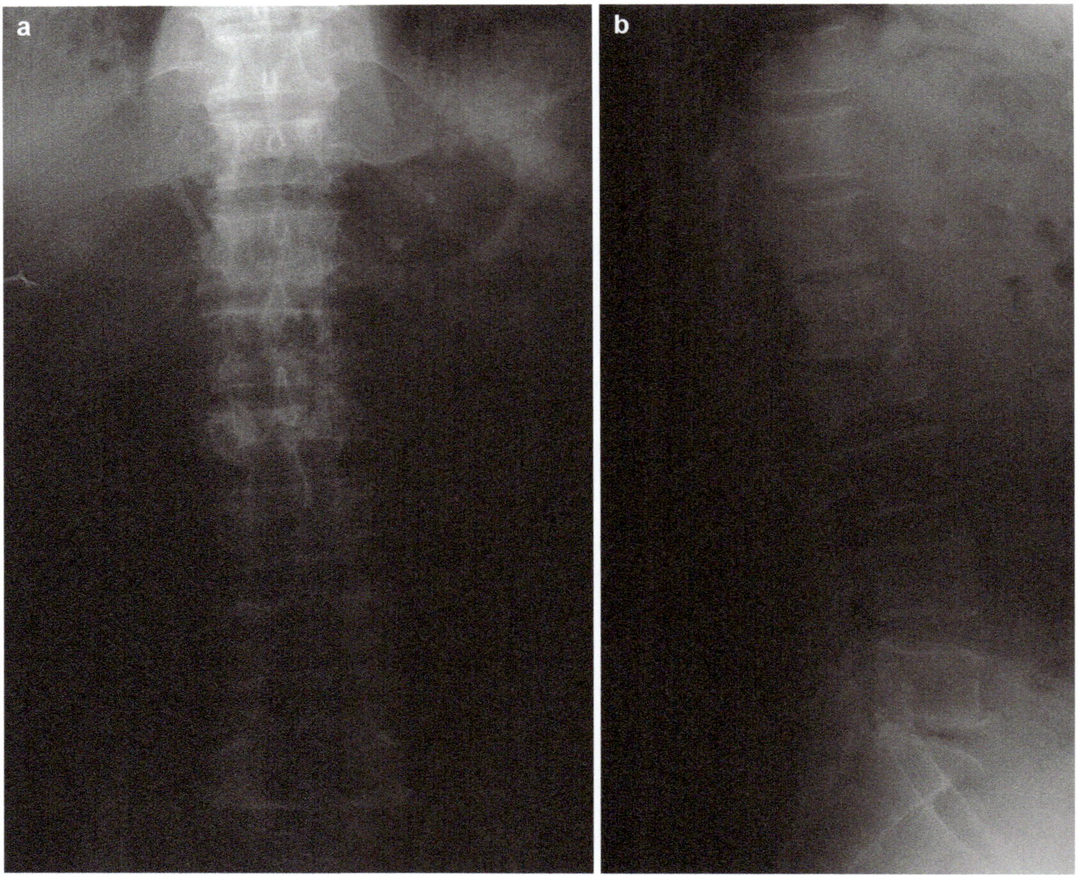

Fig. 18.1 A 73-year-old man presented with increasing low back and leg pain. Plain lumbar spinal radiography showed a compression fracture within the L2 vertebra as well as the "absent pedicle sign" at both L1 and L2. (**a**) Anteroposterior view. (**b**) Lateral view. In this patient, a hydatid cyst of the liver caused by *Echinococcus multilocularis* was surgically resected 30 years before the time of presentation

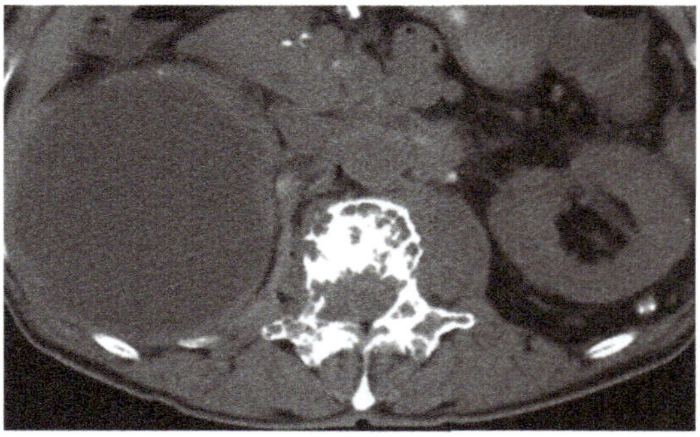

Fig. 18.2 CT shows the presence of multiloculated osteolytic lesions in the vertebral body and posterior elements. Periosteal reactions were observed

posterior fixation. Care should be taken to avoid implant protrusion into the dorsal skin, decubitus ulcer formation, and vertebral fractures in the adjacent segments after posterior spinal reconstruction. An anterior approach to perform total corpectomy and bone grafting with a cage may be used when most of the disease is located in the vertebral body (Charles et al. 1988; Herrera et al. 2005). The anterior approach is useful for curative resection of infected vertebrae; however, care must be taken to avoid spread of the disease to the chest and abdominal cavities (Bhojraj and Shetty 1999). Surgical procedures used in spinal hydatidosis are discussed in detail in Chap. 14.

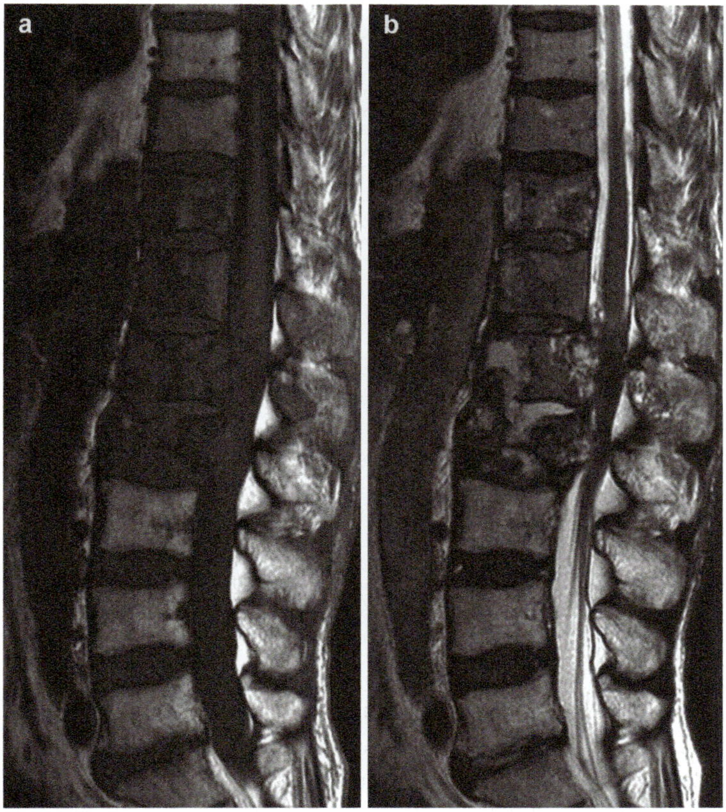

Fig. 18.3 Sagittal MRI views show multiseptated and multicystic lesions. Epidural extension of soft tissue with cord compression is also seen. T1-weighted (**a**) and T2-weighted (**b**) image

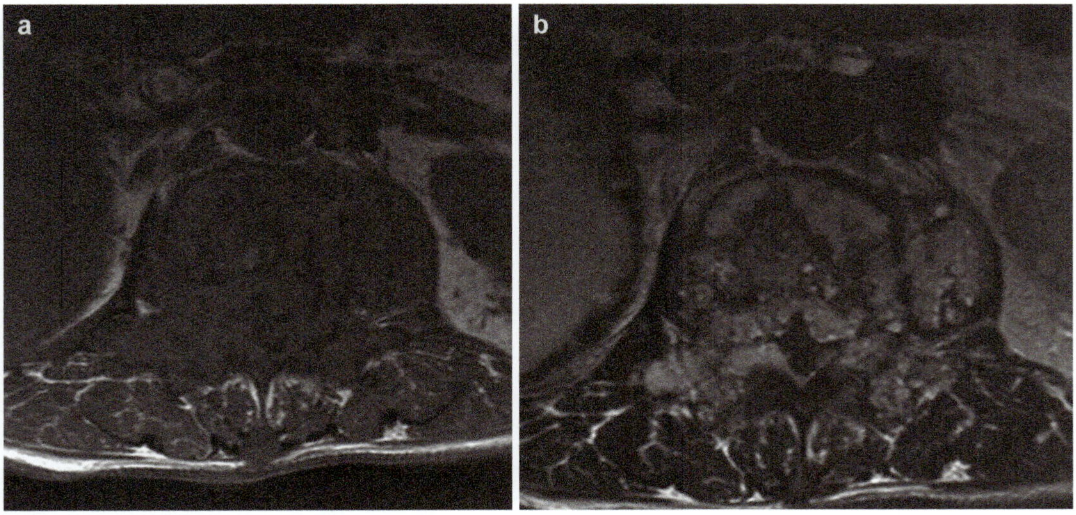

Fig. 18.4 Axial T1 (**a**) and T2 (**b**) MRI demonstrate involvement of neural structures, paraspinal muscles, and the liver

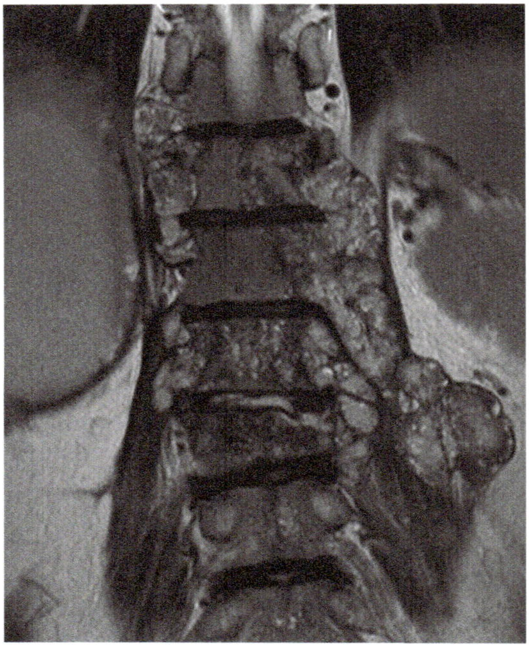

Fig. 18.5 Coronal T2-weighted MRI shows the presence of a complex T2 hyperintense mass in the paravertebral region with multiple septa

Surgery-Related Complications

Surgical Site Infection

In hydatid of the spine, there is not one cyst around which dissection can be carried out. The bone is infiltrated with a great number of minute cysts. In cases where leaked fluid containing parasites is left behind at the surgical site, concerns are raised about delay of skin closure, leading to deep pyogenic infection. It is particularly a cause of concern when surgical intervention is complicated by cerebrospinal fluid leakage. In this case, lumbar drainage may be required. Intensive muscle closure is also required during surgery to avoid fluid leakage. A plastic surgical procedure, such as musculocutaneous flap transfer, is often required for chronic infection. Although there have been few reports about larger series of spinal hydatidosis, Herrera et al. (2005) reported that 50 % of recurrence cases also have chronic wound infection with chronic productive sinuses that required several surgical debridements. Because surgery for spinal hydatidosis is extensive and

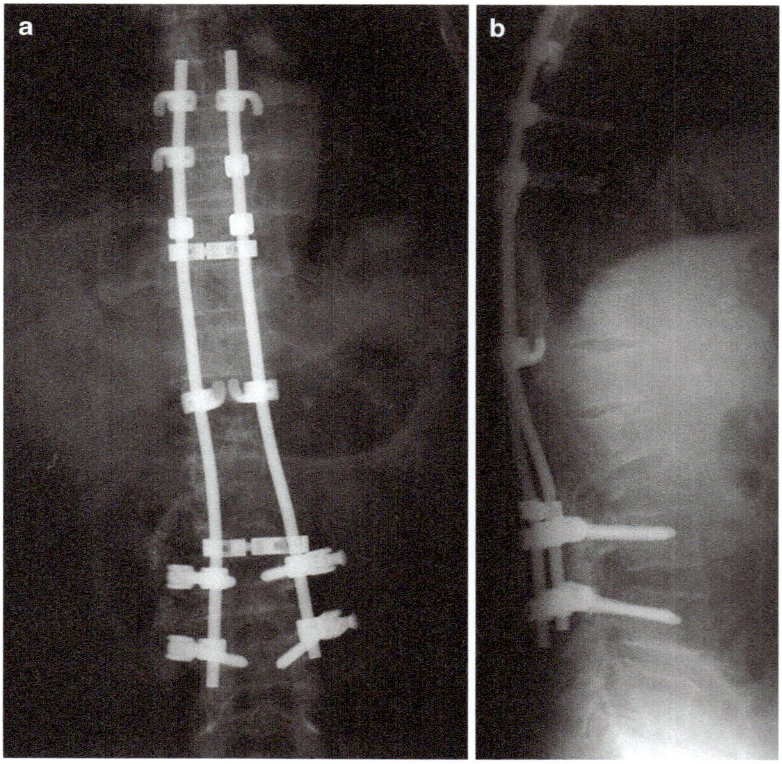

Fig. 18.6 Palliative surgery was performed with posterior decompression and instrumentation for persistent leg pain. Leg pain was significantly reduced. Spinal stability was maintained until the patient died (2 years after the surgery) (Courtesy of S. Satoh, MD) (**a**) Anteroposterior view. (**b**) Lateral view

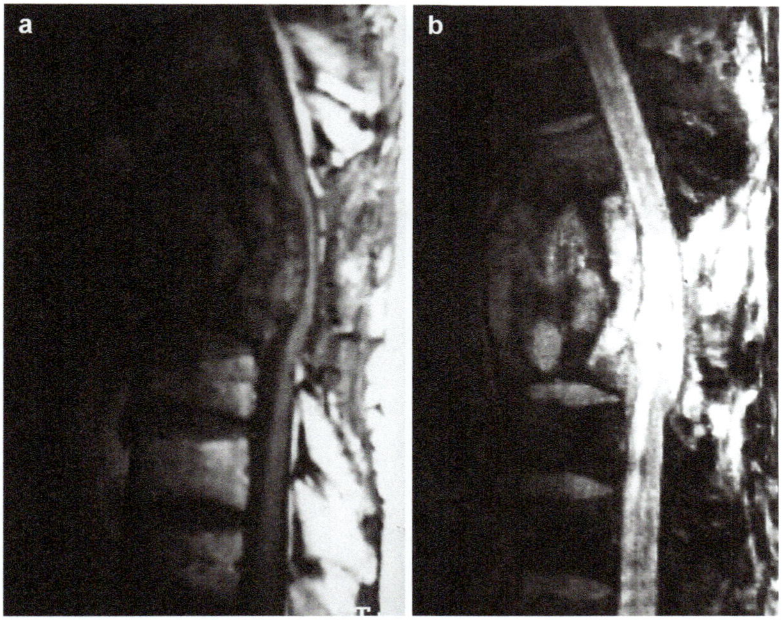

Fig. 18.7 Recurrence of spinal hydatidosis. A 52-year-old man presented with intractable leg pain and motor paralysis. Two years before the time of presentation, anterior mass resection and autologous fibular grafting had been performed, followed by posterior decompression and fusion using an iliac bone graft at T6–T9. MRI shows cysts extending into the canal and compressing the spinal cord. T1-weighted (**a**) and T2-weighted (**b**) image

the reappearance of postoperative surgical wound infection is frequent, perioperative antibiotic therapy is important.

Rupture of Cysts and Allergic Reactions

Another surgery-related complication is allergic reaction caused by rupture of the cyst. This reaction ranges from mild hypersensitivity to fatal anaphylaxis (Kök et al. 1993; Wellhoener et al. 2000; Laifer et al. 2002). Because spinal hydatidosis is usually advanced, rupture of the cyst into the surrounding tissue will already have occurred and the possibility of serious allergy manifesting during surgery is regarded as extremely low. However, this possibility makes close monitoring mandatory during surgery, with facilities available for treating potential complications, particularly anaphylactic shock and laryngeal edema (Khuroo et al. 1997).

Complications After Surgery

Recurrence

Recurrence remains a major problem in spinal hydatidosis (Figs. 18.7, 18.8, 18.9, and 18.10); the literature cites a rate of 30–100 % (Schnepper and Johnson 2004). The thin wall may easily rupture, either spontaneously or due to surgery, resulting in recurrence of multiple cysts (Schnepper and Johnson 2004). It is extremely difficult to resect the extradural lesions involving the spine without rupturing the hydatid cyst because the cysts are contained in narrow spaces within bone boundaries (Schnepper and Johnson 2004; Tabak et al. 2007). Therefore, the management of echinococcal cysts usually involves a combination of surgical resection and antihelminthic therapy.

Adjunctive Chemotherapy

Adjunctive chemotherapy before and after surgery appears to reduce the risk of recurrence by inactivating protoscolices and lessening the tension of cysts for easier cyst resection (Tabak et al. 2007). Administration of either albendazole or mebendazole is recommended to reduce the risk of secondary hydatidosis (Erzurumlu et al. 2000). Chemotherapy for spinal hydatidosis is discussed in detail in Chap. 16.

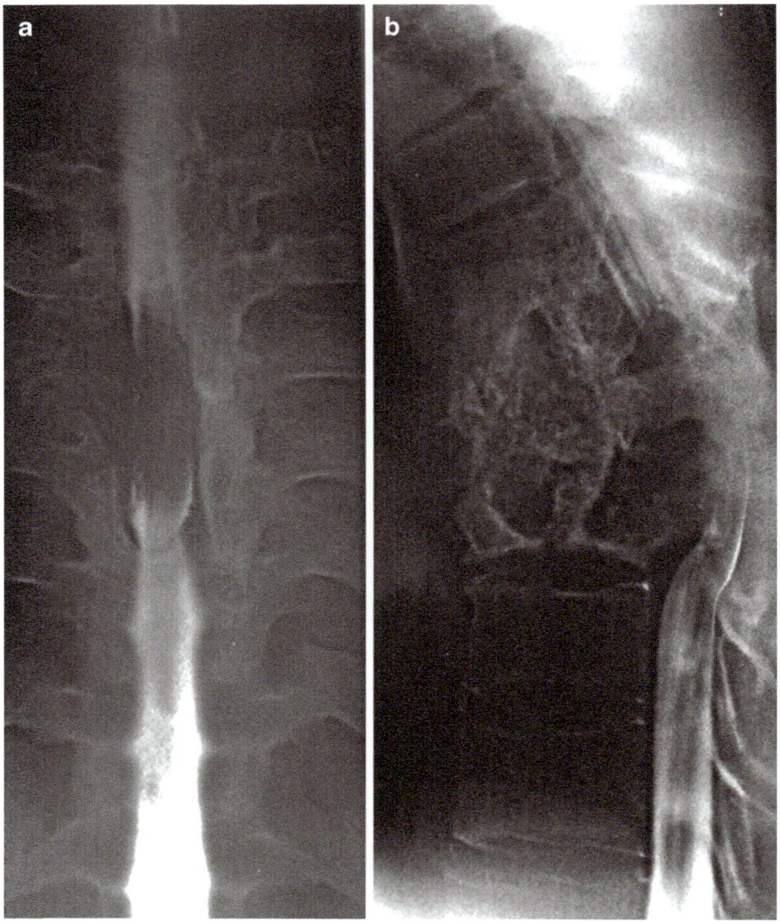

Fig. 18.8 Myelo-tomogram. Note that even after the spinal fusion was completed, the grafted bone was destroyed by recurrent cysts (**a**) Anteroposterior view. (**b**) Lateral view

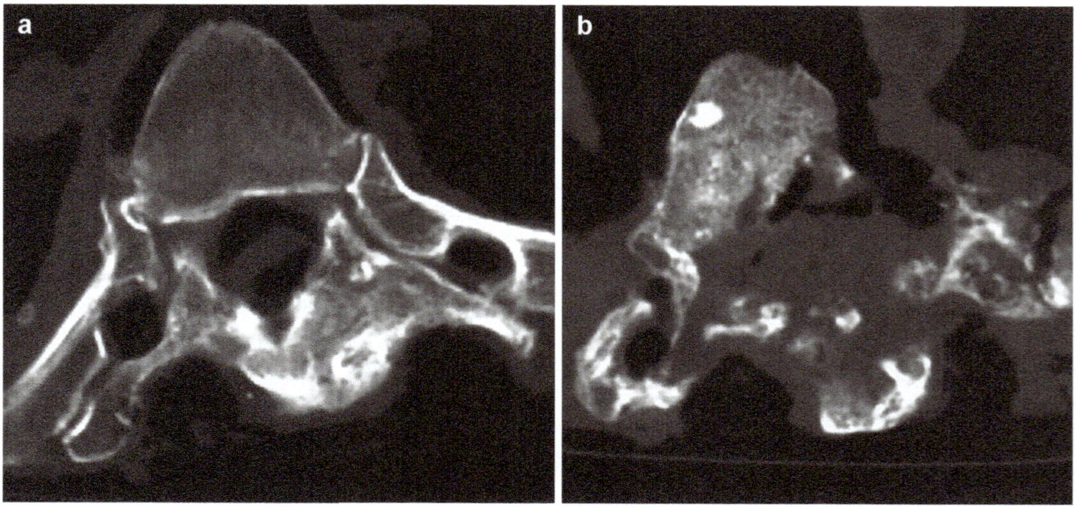

Fig. 18.9 CT showing the completed spinal fusion after the previous surgery (**a**), but recurrence of spinal hydatidosis destroyed the fusion mass (**b**)

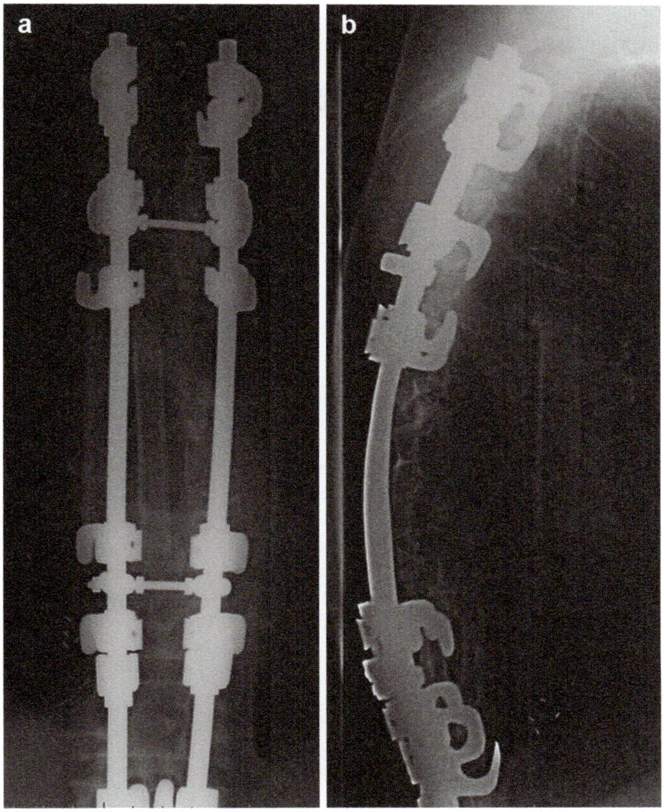

Fig. 18.10 Following posterior decompression and fusion, anterior mass resection and vascularized fibular grafting was performed in a second operation (**a**) Anteroposterior view. (**b**) Lateral view

Other Preventive Measures

Intracystic injections of 10 % formalin, 0.5 % silver nitrate, hydrogen peroxide, 1 % aqueous iodine, and hypertonic saline solutions have been used to destroy the residual larvae (Erşahin et al. 1993), although these remain unproven. Irrigation of the surgical site with hypertonic saline or diluted betadine solution after the cyst resection may help destroy and disrupt the parasite (Schnepper and Johnson 2004; Herrera et al. 2005). Hypertonic saline is a scolicidal agent because the difference of osmolality between the hypertonic saline and the interior of the cyst causes sclerosis of the cyst. Bavbek et al. (1992) documented that the operation area was soaked with 3 % NaCl-wetted patties for a few minutes, which were then removed, and the area was washed with normal 0.09 % NaCl.

Prognosis

Due to the high rate of recurrence, spinal hydatidosis has poor prognosis and has been compared to spinal malignancy. Reported mortality rates range from 3 to >50 % (Bettaieb et al. 1978; Karray et al. 1990; Schnepper and Johnson 2004). Radical resection is sometimes impossible to achieve in cases of extradural lesions involving the spine. Comprehensive evaluation of the patient is important during treatment. Assessment factors should include general complications, other hydatid lesions, prognosis, lifestyle, pain, and the absence or presence of paralysis.

Conclusion

The treatment goals of spinal hydatidosis are to resect the infested lesion, to alleviate pain, to prevent neurological deficit, and to establish spinal stability. Nevertheless, it is extremely difficult to resect the extradural lesions involving the spine without rupturing the hydatid cyst. Therefore, the management of echinococcal cysts usually involves a combination of surgical resection and antihelminthic therapy. Comprehensive evaluation of the patient is also important to prevent complications of spinal hydatidosis.

References

Akhan O, Ozmen M. Percutaneous treatment of liver hydatid cysts. Eur J Radiol. 1999;32:76–85.
Bavbek M, Inci S, Tahta K, Bertan V. Primary multiple spinal extradural hydatid cysts. Case report and review of the literature. Paraplegia. 1992;30:517–9.
Bettaieb A, Khaldi M, Ben Rhouma T, Touibi S. Spinal echinococcosis; clinical study of 32 cases (in French). Neurochirurgie. 1978;24:205–10.
Bhojraj SY, Shetty NR. Primary hydatid disease of the spine: an unusual cause of progressive paraplegia. Case report and review of the literature. J Neurosurg. 1999;91:216–8.
Charles RW, Govender S, Naidoo KS. Echinococcal infection of the spine with neural involvement. Spine (Phila Pa 1976). 1988;13:47–9.
Erşahin Y, Mutluer S, Güzelbağ E. Intracranial hydatid cysts in children. Neurosurgery. 1993;33:219–24.
Erzurumlu K, Hökelek M, Gönlüsen L, Tas K, Amanvermez R. The effect of albendazole on the prevention of secondary hydatidosis. Hepatogastroenterology. 2000;47:247–50.
Haddad FS, Bitar E. Primary hydatid disease of the spine: report of 14 cases and review of the literature. Pan Arab J Neurosurg. 1997;1:46–52.
Herrera A, Martínez AA, Rodríguez J. Spinal hydatidosis. Spine (Phila Pa 1976). 2005;30:2439–44.
Kalkan E, Cengiz SL, Ciçek O, Erdi F, Baysefer A. Primary spinal intradural extramedullary hydatid cyst in a child. J Spinal Cord Med. 2007;30:297–300.
Karadereler S, Orakdögen M, Kiliç K, Ozdogan C. Primary spinal extradural hydatid cyst in a child: case report and review of the literature. Eur Spine J. 2002;11:500–3.
Karray S, Zlitni M, Fowles JV, Zouari O, Slimane N, Kassab MT, Rosset P. Vertebral hydatidosis and paraplegia. J Bone Joint Surg Br. 1990;72:84–8.
Khuroo MS, Wani NA, Javid G, Khan BA, Yattoo GN, Shah AH, Jeelani SG. Percutaneous drainage compared with surgery for hepatic hydatid cysts. N Engl J Med. 1997;337:881–7.
Kök AN, Yurtman T, Aydin NE. Sudden death due to ruptured hydatid cyst of the liver. J Forensic Sci. 1993;38:978–80.
Laifer G, Marti W, Wiesner W, Fluckiger U. Balancing on the edge. Lancet. 2002;360:1746.
Normelli HC, Aaro SI, Follin PH. Vertebral hydatid cyst infection (Echinococcus granulosus): a case report. Eur Spine J. 1998;7:158–61.
Oda I, Abumi K, Ito M, Kotani Y, Oya T, Hasegawa K, Minami A. Palliative spinal reconstruction using cervical pedicle screws for metastatic lesions of the spine: a retrospective analysis of 32 cases. Spine (Phila Pa 1976). 2006;31:1439–44.
Polat P, Kantarci M, Alper F, Suma S, Koruyucu MB, Okur A. Hydatid disease from head to toe. Radiographics. 2003;23:475–94.
Schnepper GD, Johnson WD. Recurrent spinal hydatidosis in North America. Case report and review of the literature. Neurosurg Focus. 2004;17:E8.
Secer HI, Anik I, Celik E, Daneyemez MK, Gonul E. Spinal hydatid cyst mimicking arachnoid cyst on magnetic resonance imaging. J Spinal Cord Med. 2008;31:106–8.
Sudo H, Minami A. Neurological picture: a widespread echinococcosis of the spine. J Neurol Neurosurg Psychiatry. 2010;81:892.
Szypryt EP, Morris DL, Mulholland RC. Combined chemotherapy and surgery for hydatid bone disease. J Bone Joint Surg Br. 1987;69:141–4.
Tabak O, Yilmaz M, Oz B, Ozaras R, Erdincler P, Mert A, Ozturk R, Tabak F. A vertebral hydatid cyst infection mimicking tuberculous spondylodiscitis. J Infect Chemother. 2007;13:180–2.
Tali ET. Spinal infections. Eur J Radiol. 2004;50:120–33.
Turgut AT, Altin L, Topçu S, Kiliçoğlu B, Aliinok T, Kaptanoğlu E, Karademir A, Koşar U. Unusual imaging characteristics of complicated hydatid disease. Eur J Radiol. 2007;63:84–9.
von Sinner W, te Strake L, Clark D, Sharif H. MR imaging in hydatid disease. AJR Am J Roentgenol. 1991;157:741–5.
Wellhoener P, Weitz G, Bechstein W, Djonlagic H, Dodt C. Severe anaphylactic shock in a patient with a cystic liver lesion. Intensive Care Med. 2000;26:1578.

Outcome and Follow-up of Patients with Cerebral Hydatidosis

19

Deme Raja Reddy

Contents

D.R. Reddy, MD, MBBS, FRCS (E), FRACS, FICS
Department of Neurosurgery,
Nizam's Institute of Medical Sciences,
Hyderabad, India

Department of Neurosurgery,
Apollo Hospital, Room No. 39, Jubilee Hills,
Hyderabad 500096, India
e-mail: palvashareddy@gmail.com

Introduction

The ideal and generally accepted treatment of hydatid disease involving the central nervous system (CNS) is surgical and that medical treatment should be restricted to nonoperable patients. The outcome of treatment depends on many factors such as the species of echinococcal infestation, whether it is primary or secondary, single or multiple; the anatomical location and dimension of the lesion; the result of surgical intervention; the presence and extent of the disease in other parts of the body; and the type and the duration of drug therapy in cases with rupture of a cyst or of cysts during surgery (Saidi 1976; Altinors et al. 2000; Khaldi et al. 2000; Turgut 2002; McManus et al. 2003; Sayek et al. 2001; Izci et al. 2008; Duishanbai et al. 2010). Prognosis is also different for osseous echinococcal lesions of the cranial bones (or the vertebral column), which secondarily involve the neural elements (Reddy et al. 1972, 1979). The cranial hydatidosis and the vertebral hydatidosis are types of bony hydatid disease which produces few pericystic formations and such lesions confined inside bony tissue enlarge by the formation of a large number of daughter cysts with attendant risk of spillage during their removal and inevitable recurrence of the disease at a later stage. Bony hydatidosis causes few tissue reactions by the host, and the value of drug treatment in such cases is questionable. The outcome also varies with the anatomical location of the lesion, depending upon whether it is epidural,

M. Turgut (ed.), *Hydatidosis of the Central Nervous System: Diagnosis and Treatment*,
DOI 10.1007/978-3-642-54359-3_19, © Springer-Verlag Berlin Heidelberg 2014

subdural, or subarachnoid or it involves the brain or spinal cord parenchyma. Certain locations of hydatid cysts such as cavernous sinus, interpeduncular region, intraventricular region, and brainstem make a total intact excision difficult (Copley et al. 1992; Kiresi et al. 2003; Hamamci et al. 2004; Beskonakli et al. 1996; Gana et al. 2008; Muthusubrahmanian et al. 2009; Guzel et al. 2008; Furtado et al. 2009). The result also depends upon whether calcification is present or not as well as whether an infection is involved (Turkoglu et al. 2005; Abderrahmen et al. 2007).

Species of Echinococcal Infestation

The outcome of therapy mostly depends upon the type of species of the cestode infestation. There are four main species of the larval stage of tape worm, namely, *E. granulosus*, *E. multilocularis* (*alveolaris*), *E. vogeli*, and *E. oligarthus*. *E. granulosus* is the most common infestation worldwide, whereas *E. multilocularis* is prevalent in the northern hemisphere including Alaska, Canada, Siberia, and Central Europe but has recently been increasingly reported in more temperate regions of Eastern France, Nebraska, Illinois, and Turkey (Aydin et al. 1986; Algros et al. 2003). Dog is the host for *E. granulosus* infection; livestock and humans are intermediate hosts. Infection with the remaining types of echinococcosis is rather rare since wild animals such as fox and rodents are the hosts in such types of echinococcal infection (Romig 2003). The presence of fertile scolices and whether they are single or multiple differentiates the first two species of echinococcus infestation. The alveolar echinococcosis is an aggressive disease and eventually invades contiguous structures with tumorlike progression. Usually found in the liver, it can metastatize to the lungs and brain (Kappagoda et al. 2011). Lesions of *Echinococcus multilocularis* in the brain are of firm consistency with a jellylike material, and they mimic brain tumors (Senturk et al. 2006). Infection with *E. alveolaris* has a relatively poor prognosis compared to *E. granulosus* infestations, and in untreated cases it has a mortality of 90–100 % after 10 years (Ehrhardt et al. 2007). In some countries the clinical picture of the hydatid disease may be due to both an *E. granulosus* and an *E. alveolaris* infection. There are reports that there could be infestation by cystic as well as alveolaris types in a single individual (Meade and Barnett 1941). The last two are Neotropic species of echinococcosis which are prevalent in certain parts of Central and South America. Only three cases of *E. oligarthus* and 200 cases of *E. vogeli* cases have been reported from 12 countries in Central and South America (D'Alessandro and Rausch 2008). No cases of cerebral involvement by these species of echinococcal infection have been reported so far, but in other organs they produce invasive lesions like multilocularis, and hence their prognosis should be poor. Single large cysts associated with *E. granulosus* infection can be extirpated without spillage in the majority of cases, and usually the surgical results are better in such cases. For example, in the series of Ciurea et al. (2006), there were only 3 multiple cysts out of 76, and of the single cysts, 56 (73.7 %) could be excised without rupture. There was only one death due to an anaphylactic shock in those 56 cases where as all three patients with multiple cysts died. In contrast cystic lesions which are located in deeper areas or in eloquent regions may not be amenable for complete excision. All cerebral alveolar lesions are secondary, and all patients do have hepatic lesions, and some may have pulmonary lesions too. Sometimes alveolar cerebral lesions had been excised completely, but the patients had succumbed to irreversible liver disease (Wang et al. 2009). In general it may be admitted that all types of cerebral echinococcosis are serious, but the alveolar echinococcosis is worse.

Primary or Secondary

A hydatid lesion in the CNS is classified as primary lesion, when there are no recognizable lesions in other parts of the body (Dew 1928, 1955). Such a hydatid lesion of the brain arises from an onchosphere which is initially deposited in the brain by the blood stream after a successful passage through the hepatic and pulmonary filtering systems. In contrast the secondary hydatid cysts of the brain are those which originate from scolices or brood capsules belonging to a primary hydatid disease elsewhere. They have landed secondarily in the brain. Obviously management of primary lesions is better than those with secondary lesions affecting other organs. Primary cerebral lesions are usually single, but multiple lesions are reported very rarely. It is supposed that multiple cerebral lesions will develop, if the content of the ruptured cyst gets directly in the arterial circulation (Mancuso et al. 1997; Karadag et al. 2004). Some primary lesions could be in different hemispheres. Some primary lesions especially those involving the spine may develop by spreading through the venous or lymphatic route. Primary lesions are mainly in the cerebral hemispheres in the middle cerebral artery territory, but they have also been reported to occur in the intracranial epidural space (Beskonakli et al. 1996), spinal epidural, vertebral, and rarely in spinal intradural and extramedullary locations. Management of primary lesion in any location results in good surgical outcomes (Pasaoglu et al. 1989; Arif and Zaheer 2009). Favorable long-term outcome has been reported for the excision of primary solitary cerebral lesions in children, and this supports the assumption that these lesions in the pediatric age group are mainly primary (Lunardi et al. 1991). They reported on 12 children, of which one patient suffered from a secondary brain cyst. Eight of the 12 patients who had a mean follow-up of 28 years were still living and enjoying good health at the time of the report. In contrast to primary lesions, the secondary lesions are infertile since they lack brood capsules and scolices (Mancuso et al. 1997).

Solitary or Multiple

Cerebral hydatid cysts are nearly always solitary, and in one series of 135 cerebral lesions, only 2 were multiple (Iplikcioglu et al. 1989). But in a large study which was performed by Turgut (2002), there were 92 (77 %) solitary cases out of 119 and the rest were multiple in 27 (23 %). There were 20 cases with involvement of spine 1 in this series. After surgery there was recurrence in 22 % of cases, in which 6 solitary and 12 multiple lesions occurred. Al-Zain et al. (2002) reviewed all the cases of multiple intracranial hydatidosis and collected 77 cases from the literature. These cases often have serious neurological deficits, and frequently the outcome of surgery was not satisfactory, and in only 46.4 % of cases, a good outcome could be achieved. Overall the mortality in multiple cases was 17.6 %. Five of the patients had more than one recurrence which had appeared from 3 months to 3 years after surgery. Recurrent disease is defined as the appearance of new active cysts after therapy, and a rising titer is of value regarding the diagnosis of recurrence (Sielaff et al. 2001). The chance of recurrence is higher in multiple cases with multiple lesions after surgery. Multiple secondary hydatid cysts can develop by embolism from cardiac echincoccosis and echinococcosis of great arterial vessels (Mancuso et al. 1997; Turgut et al. 1997).

Unusual Locations

Hydatid disease is endemic in many parts of the world, and it can develop in any part of the body. The location is mostly hepatic (75 %) and pulmonary (15 %), and only 10 % other parts of the body are affected (Kiresi et al. 2003). There are some rare sites in the brain where hydatid lesions can occur: cavernous sinus, interpeduncular region, sella, brainstem and cerebellopontine angle, lateral ventricles, and cerebellar hemispheres. Occasionally hydatid could exist along with primary brain tumor (Ozgen et al. 1984; Copley et al. 1992; Beskonakli et al. 1996; Hamamci et al. 2004; Evliyaoglu and Keskil 2005; Gana et al. 2008; Guzel et al. 2008; Furtado et al. 2009; Muthusubrahmanian et al. 2009; Siddiqui et al 2010). The prognoses in cases of hydatid disease involving rare sites especially those in deeper locations are poor.

Laboratory Diagnosis of Echinococcosis

Casoni's test is not very helpful in the diagnosis of hydatid disease involving the CNS (Fairley and Kellaway 1933). However, a positive result with complement fixation test before the first operation on any cyst provides definite evidence of hydatid disease. In the diagnosis of recurrent disease, the skin tests are not helpful. Assessment of the extent of the skin response in such tests is no method for monitoring the disease or adapting the medication. Hence a great number of immunological assays have been developed for the detection of antibodies to anti-hydatid cyst antibodies. Detection of circulating antibodies may be more useful for the immune diagnosis of hydatid disease (Sadjjadi et al. 2009). Tests which are available for the diagnosis of the hydatid disease are enzyme-linked immunosorbent assay, indirect hemagglutination or immunofluorescent assay, radioallergosorbent testing, and latex fixation tests. All of these tests are sensitive but are compromised by nonspecific cross-reactivity with *Helminthes* other than echinococcosis. A positive result of one of these tests should be confirmed by the use of a more specific test. The results of standard serological tests are positive in over 90 % of patients with hepatic cysts but only in about 50 % of those with pulmonary disease and only in 25–36 % in other organs (Karadereler et al. 2002). In a series of 25 cerebral hydatid cysts, the serological tests were positive in only 3 cases (Tuzun et al. 2010). The problems with the laboratory diagnosis of the hydatid disease very often lead to difficulties in the preoperative diagnosis and planning of treatment of the hydatid disease involving the brain in non-endemic areas.

Treatment

The management strategies available for the treatment of echinococcosis depend on the cyst stage and include puncture-aspiration-injection-reaspiration (PAIR), surgery, antiparasitic chemotherapy, and expectant management (Tirnaksiz and Dogan 2004). Positron emission tomography scan and contrast-enhanced ultrasound of the liver involvement might help in guiding the treatment of hepatic lesions by the visualization of metabolic activity and vascularization pattern of echinococcal lesions. Surgical excision and alternative techniques to surgery such as fine needle aspiration and injection of scolicidal drugs and puncture of the cyst, aspiration of the fluid followed by introducing a protoscolicidal agent, and then reaspiration (PAIR procedure) are reported (von Sinner et al. 1995) for abdominal lesions. However, the ideal treatment of intracranial and cerebral lesions is their total surgical excision. PAIR procedure may be necessary in cases of deep-seated or difficult cerebral cystic lesions. Medical treatment is indicated when a cyst ruptures or the disease involves the other organs. Intracranial hydatid cysts grow very rapidly, and some may grow as much as 10 cm per year, and hence their excision is preferred as a mode of therapy (Kirimlioglu et al. 2001). The rate of growth of cerebral hydatid cysts is variable; it can be 1–10 cm per year according to various reports (Vaquero et al. 1982; Sierra et al. 1985).

Surgical Treatment

Surgical treatment remains the preferred management for active hydatid disease, and the aim of the surgery is to excise the cyst or cysts in toto without soiling and complete obliteration of the resulting dead space (Dowling and Orlando 1929; Normelli et al. 1998; Kirimlioglu et al. 2001; Abdel Razek et al. 2009; Tuzun et al. 2010; Mohindra et al. 2011) (Figs. 19.1, 19.2, 19.3, 19.4, and 19.5).

Sometimes successful excision of the alveolar lesions which are in an accessible location followed by a piecemeal of those in difficult locations resulted in good neurological recovery (Wang et al. 2009). Alveolar type of hydatid disease may sometimes mimic a brain tumor, and its total excision may be difficult (Senturk et al. 2006; Ma et al. 2009). Rarely granulosus lesions could be multiple and may be present in different hemispheres, and such cases need planned excision in one or more stages (Yuceer et al. 1998). Liver and lung disease may be responsible for delayed deaths later on in spite of chemotherapy. In a Chinese study, two of the six surgically treated cases of cerebral hydatid disease of the alveolar type died due to end-stage liver disease (Wang et al. 2009). In a recent study, injection of 0.04 % chlorhexidine into the cysts (hepatic) for 5 min had been shown to kill all the live scolices and there was no recurrence over a follow-up period of 2 years (Topcu et al. 2009). However, this method is yet to be tried in cerebral and cranial hydatid disease. One has to study the deleterious effects of 0.04 % chlorhexidine to the brain, if that were to get spilled over accidentally during the operation. Effective scolicidal agent is useful especially while removing the cysts containing fertile scolices. Viability and fertility of the protoscolices and viable germinal layer determine the recurrence of the disease at a later date (Manterola et al. 2006). Orbital location of hydatid disease is a rare type of infestation, and total extirpation of the cysts without rupture may be difficult, and in such cases recurrence is the result (Fig. 19.6; Ghosh et al. 2008). Endoscopic approaches are available in the management of orbital hydatid disease. Cranial and vertebral hydatid disease invariably recurs because of spillage of large numbers of daughter cysts. Long-term chemotherapy preferably a combination of albendazole and praziquantel is recommended in such cases. Recurrence of spinal disease even with chemotherapy may benefit

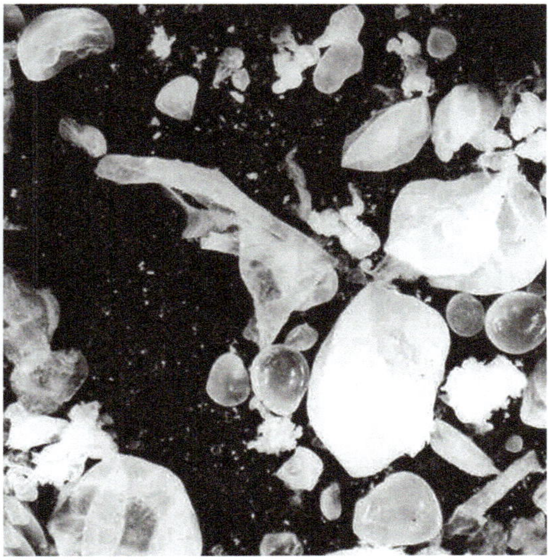

Fig. 19.1 Enormous numbers of cysts of different sizes in a case of cranial hydatid disease in frontal region involving orbit with spread into the intracranial epidural space. Recurrence of the lesion occurred 1 year later in spite of prolonged chemotherapy

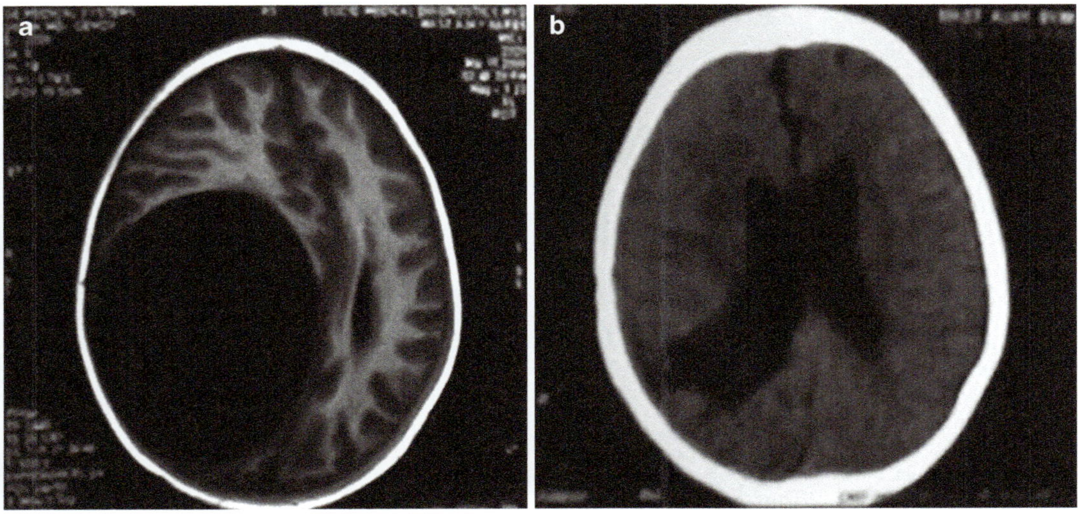

Fig. 19.2 (**a**, **b**) Single primary cystic lesions of the type depicted above, even if large reaching on to the surface in accessible areas are amenable for complete excision with a cure. Preop scan on the left and post-op scan on the right side

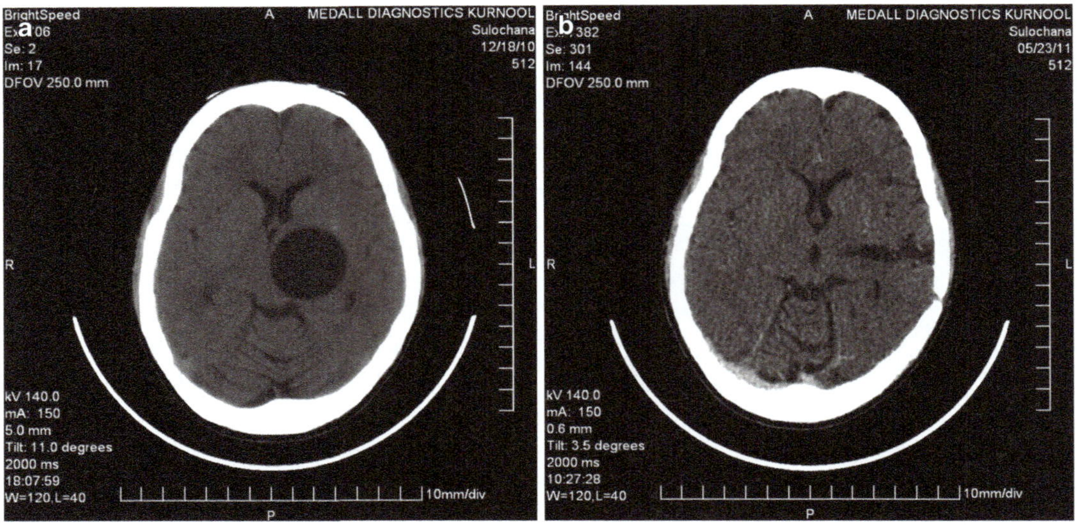

Fig. 19.3 (**a**, **b**) The best surgical outcomes are recorded also in cases of hydatid disease of the central nervous system when the lesion is primary solitary and even if it is located in deeper areas of the brain as shown above. This kind of lesion needs planning and requires microsurgical methods for excision without spillage. Same is true for rare primary spinal epidural and intradural and extramedullary lesions. Scans shown in this figure belong to a 24-year-old lady from an endemic area of hydatid disease. Picture on the left is before surgery, and the scan on the right side is after the total excision of solitary primary lesion. Microscopic excision is helpful in these cases which provide good illumination and careful dissection. Adults seek treatment earlier, and the lesions tend to be smaller in size as compared to those of children where the cysts grow to a large size and their excision without breaking of the cyst may sometimes be difficult due its sheer size with thin walls especially towards the ventricle

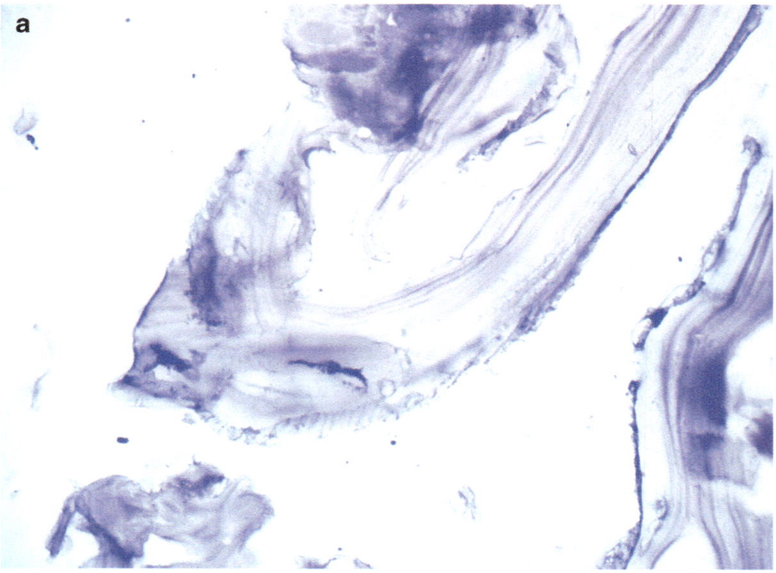

Fig. 19.4 (**a**, **b**) Laminated membrane of the hydatid cyst wall with an inner germinal layer. Hematoxylin and eosin magnification 110× on left (**a**) and 200× (**b**) on the right side, respectively

Fig. 19.4 (continued)

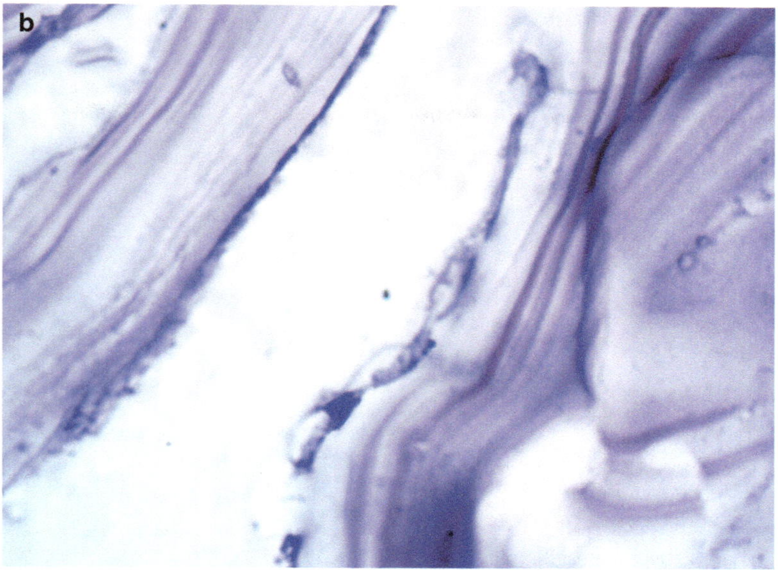

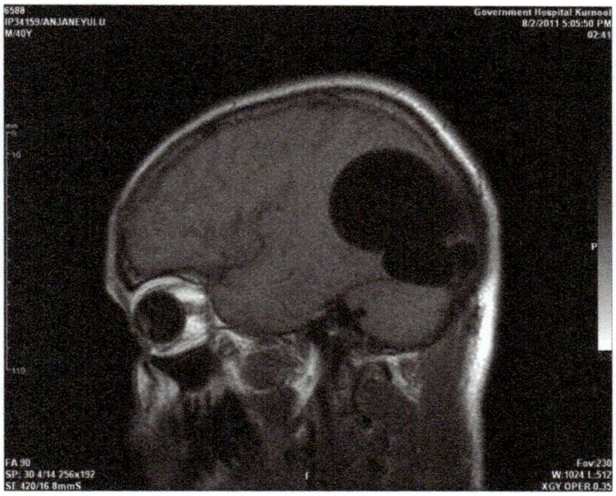

Fig. 19.5 A 40-year-old male with right parieto-occipital primary multiple hydatid cysts in close proximity

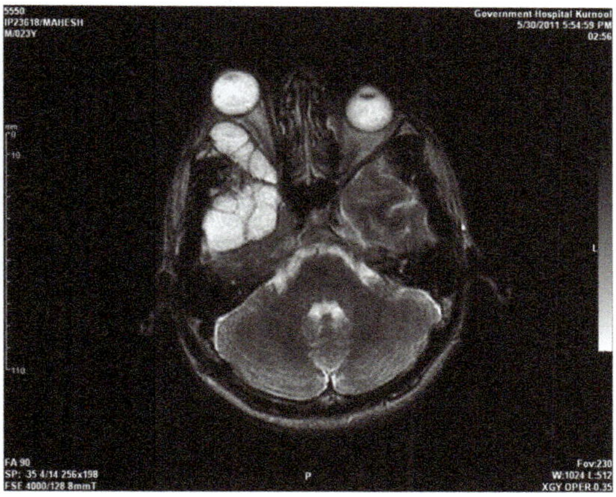

Fig. 19.6 A 23-year-old male with recurrent hydatid cysts involving the orbit, frontal, and temporal regions

from reoperative surgery since the recurrent cysts may be without a brood capsule and hence they may not recur again. Intact excision was possible in 119 cases out of 137 cases of cerebral hydatid disease (Turgut 2002). In 22 % of cases, recurrence was noted and surprisingly recurrence occurred in 7 of the cases which were removed intact. Recurrence was expected in such of those cases which ruptured during surgery, and these were 7 out of 31 (Turgut 2002). Recurrence in those cases depends upon the presence of live protoscolices, and these can be estimated per field, and it is also known that fertile cysts contain malate fumarate along with other resonances. Greatest number of viable protoscolices was observed in multiple cysts in comparison to single cysts (Manterola et al. 2006). Preoperative studies will help in planning the surgery as well

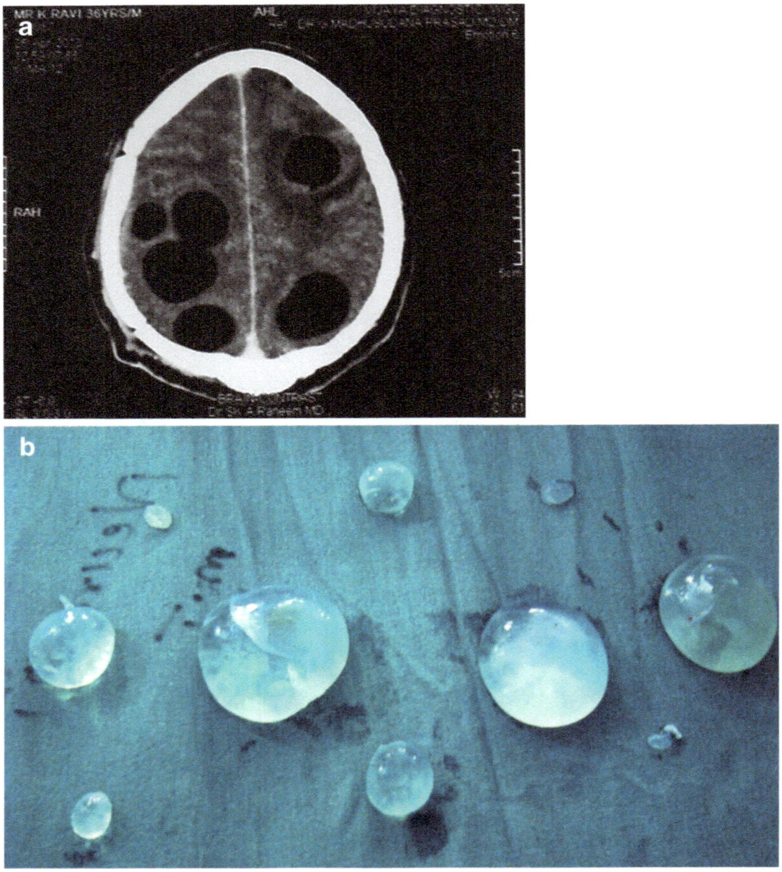

Fig. 19.7 (**a**, **b**) A 34-year-old male with recurrence after rupture during first operation. There were six large lesions and a few smaller lesions which were all removed with good outcome

as the precautions that should be taken to avoid risks of surgery. Microscopic surgery gives good illumination and helps in proper dissection of the cysts. Cyst rupture during surgery is always critical, and the recurrence depends upon whether the lesion is primary or secondary. In one study with long-term follow-up, out of 29 cases operated, 18 were removed intact and 8 cases ruptured, of which 5 are dead (63 %) and they were all primary. In contrast 3 cases also ruptured and they were secondary and they are alive proving that secondary lesions are not fertile. Recurrence after rupture is a problem, and even if there are many lesions, they should be removed and the results can be gratifying (Fig. 19.7). The complications of cerebral hydatid cyst surgery are not uncommon which require prompt diagnosis and treatment (Tuzun et al. 2010). Subdural effusion and porencephaly are the delayed complications, whereas hemorrhage in the operated site and extradural hematomas are immediate problems. Rarely there could be infected hydatid cysts which need antibiotic coverage (Obrador and Urquiza 1948; Arana-Iniguez and Julian 1954).

Medical Treatment

Medical treatment may be chosen if patients are not eligible for surgery or the cysts are present in many organs. Albendazole, mebendazole, and praziquantel are the main drugs used as antiparasitic medication for the treatment of echinococcal infection (Davis et al. 1989; Gil-Grande et al. 1993). Albendazole is a broad-spectrum benzimidazole which is preferred over mebendazole because it is better absorbed and achieves higher blood, cyst wall, and fluid concentrations. Both act by inhibition of tubulin polymerization resulting in the loss of cytoplasmic microtubule formation inhibition and the inhibition of the glucose uptake of the parasites leading to cell autolysis (Silva et al. 2004; Kappagoda et al. 2011). Albendazole sulfoxide, the active metabolite, reaches predictable levels in serum after an oral dose; cyst fluid levels are slowly reaching therapeutic levels and are less predictable; thus a prolonged duration of treatment is required. It is effective against the larval forms of echinococcal infection. Albendazole results in disappearance of up to 48 % of cysts and a substantial reduction in size of the cysts in another 28 %. It is another drug for the treatment of hydatid disease, but it does not produce adequate serum levels which are able to kill the germinal membrane alone and can be used along with albendazole. It increases serum concentrations of albendazole to the fourfold and can be used in combination, which is advisable (Sihota and Sharma 2000; Jamshidi et al. 2008). The duration of anthelmintic treatment could be up to 5 months or longer. Anthelmintic therapy is beneficial and indicated in patients with spillage or in those patients with disease in other parts of the body, like the liver and lungs. Severe disease in organs other than the CNS may be responsible for delayed deaths. The response to albendazole treatment for cerebral hydatid disease can be monitored with CT and MRI imaging (Kalaitzoglou et al. 1998). There are reports that a viable residual spinal hydatid cyst disappeared with albendazole therapy (Baykaner et al. 2000). Preoperative combination chemotherapy is more effective for post-spillage prophylaxis than albendazole or praziquantel alone (Morris 1987). There are also reports claiming that albendazole is not effective in the treatment of hepatic hydatid cysts (Kapan et al. 2008).

Hydatid Disease in Other Parts of the Body

Presence of hydatid lesions in other parts of the body also determines the outcome of treatment (Fig. 19.8). In a recent study, six cases of intracranial hydatid cysts were operated, but two of these subsequently died from severe forms of liver involvement sometime later (Wang et al. 2009). These cases had no recurrence of cerebral lesions even though they were removed piecemeal. Liver transplantation is now possible in cases with hepatic hydatid disease. Same may also happen in the cases with involvement in other parts of the body such as the lungs. Turgut (1997) reviewed the hydatid disease of the spine in Turkey and reported that 14 out of 18 cases of hydatid disease had pulmonary involvement. Naturally, disease in other parts of the body dictates the outcome of hydatid involving the CNS.

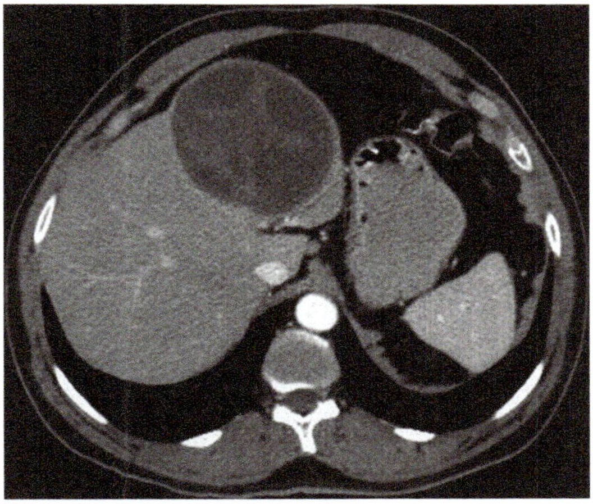

Fig. 19.8 Central nervous system hydatid disease with involvement of liver that determines the ultimate outcome of the patient. Echinococcosis of the alveolaris type invariably has the liver involvement, and their survival depends upon the liver status

Delayed Complications

Sometimes hydatid cyst could be associated with other primary lesions of the brain such as acoustic neurinoma and glioma. Prognosis depends upon the other associated disease (Cohen et al. 1997). Delayed development of glioma at the same site of previous hydatid cyst raises the doubt whether constant irritation may be responsible for its development (George et al. 2003). But glioma development in this case could have been incidental also.

Outcome and Prognosis of Hydatid Disease Involving the Central Nervous System

Hydatid disease causes considerable mortality and morbidity, and a large population around the world is affected by the disease (McManus et al. 2003). Surgical removal of the clinically symptomatic primary cysts is curative, and treatment with anthelmintics in nonoperable cases is only palliative. Long-term experience of the treatment of alveolar types of hydatid disease is not rewarding (Pau et al. 1987; Reuter et al. 2001; Buttenschoen and Buttenschoen 2003; Buttenschoen et al. 2009). Forty-two percent of cases were cured, and in the remaining 58 %, palliative treatment alone was possible.

The Australian Hydatid Registry contained 1,802 cases by the end of 31 March in 1945, and only 16 of the cases showed a brain involvement. The registry estimated the deaths from hydatid disease as 16.6 %, but they cautioned that this number was fallacious since this was the number of patients with hydatid disease who died in hospitals (Barnett 1936). In a survey the number of hydatid deaths till then were given as 276, but the actual number of dead was 534 because more deaths occurred in the homes of the diseased. Probably the best strategy of any public health policy should be prevention and control of the hydatid disease. Each country needs to find the echinococcal species causing the disease and the definitive and intermediate hosts responsible in the life cycle of the parasite (Palmer et al. 1996). In some countries both forms of the disease, *E. granulosus* and *E. alveolaris*, may be prevalent. For India the definitive host is the domestic dog and the intermediate hosts are sheep, goat, and cattle. In a study on the incidence of hydatid infestation in intermediate hosts in Kurnool of Andhra Pradesh, India infection rates of goats, sheep, and cattle were 16.96, 21.75, and 60.94 %, respectively. 33.3 % of dogs were positive in Kurnool region (Reddy et al. 1968; Reddy and Murthy 1986). These facts emphasize the importance to control the disease in intermediate hosts and definitive hosts to contain the hydatid disease (Reddy 2009).

Conclusion

Long-term outcome of cerebral hydatidosis can be summarized as follows: (1) Surgical treatment remains the preferred management of active hydatid disease involving the brain; (2) the best surgical outcomes are recorded in cases of cystic hydatid disease where the lesion is primary solitary and is located in an accessible area which can be excised without rupture; (3) the excision of alveolar type of echinococcosis is only palliative in nature; and (4) the presence of hydatid disease in other parts of the body besides the brain determines the long-term outcome of cerebral echinococcosis.

References

Abdel Razek AA, El-Shamam O, Abdel Wahab N. Magnetic resonance appearance of cerebral cystic echinococcosis. World Health Organization (WHO) classification. Acta Radiol. 2009;5:549–54.

Abderrahmen K, Aoudi ML, Kallel J, Khaldi MM. Calcified cerebral hydatid cyst (in French). Neurochirurgie. 2007;53:371–4.

Al Zain TJ, Al-Witry SH, Khalili HM, Aboud SH, Al Zain Jr FT. Multiple intracranial hydatidosis. Acta Neurochir (Wien). 2002;144:1179–85.

Algros MP, Majo F, Bresson S, Hadni S, Koch IJ, Goddard J, Cattin B, Delbosc B, Kantelip B. Intracerebral alveolar echinococcosis. Infection. 2003;31:63–5.

Altinors N, Bavbek M, Caner H, Erdogan B. Central nervous system hydatidosis in Turkey: a cooperative study and literature survey analysis of 458 cases. J Neurosurg. 2000;93:1–8.

Arana-iniguez R, Julian JS. Hydatid cysts of the brain. J Neurosurg. 1954;3:232–5.

Arif SH, Zaheer S. Intradural extramedullary primary hydatid of the spine in a child: a very rare presentation. Eur Spine J. 2009;18:179–82.

Aydin Y, Barlas O, Yolas C, Aydin IH, Ceviz A, Aladag A, Oren D, Akdemir D. Alveolar hydatid disease of the brain. Report of four cases. J Neurosurg. 1986;65:115–9.

Barnett L. Deaths from hydatid disease. Aust N Z J Surg. 1936;5:237–43.

Baykaner MK, Dogulu F, Ozturk G, Edali N, Tall T. A viable residual spinal hydatid cyst cured with albendazole. J Neurosurg. 2000;93:142–4.

Beskonakli E, Cayli S, Yalcinlar Y. Primary intracranial extradural hydatid cyst extending above and below the tentorium. Br J Neurosurg. 1996;10:315–6.

Buttenschoen K, Buttenschoen DC. Echinococcus granulosus infection: the challenge of surgical treatment. Langenbecks Arch Surg. 2003;388:218–30.
Buttenschoen K, Buttenschoen DC, Gruener B, Kern P, Beger HG, Henne-Bruns D, Reuters S. Long term experience of alveolar echinococcosis. Langenbecks Arch Surg. 2009;394:689–98.
Ciurea AV, Fontas KN, Coman TC, Machinis TG, Kapsalaki EZ, Fezoulidis NI, Robinson JSW. Long -term surgical outcome in patients with intracranial hydatid cyst. Acta Neurochir (Wien). 2006;148:421–6.
Cohen JE, Ginsberg HJ, Tsai EC, Schwartz ML, Petrocelli S. Hydatid cyst and brain tumor in the same location. Case illustration. J Neurosurg. 1997;86:312.
Copley IB, Fripp PJ, Albert M, Erasmus M, Otto DDV. Unusual presentations of cerebral hydatid disease in children. Br J Neurosurg. 1992;6:203–10.
D'Alessandro A, Rausch RL. New aspects of Neotropical polycystic (Echinococcus vogeli) and unicystic (Echinococcus oligarthus) Echinococcosis. Clin Microbiol Rev. 2008;21:380–401.
Davis A, Pawloski ZS, Dixon H. Multicentre clinical trials of benzimidazole carbamates in human echinococcosis. Bull World Health Organ. 1989;67:503–8.
Dew HR. Hydatid disease. Sydney: The Australian Medical Publishing Company Ltd; 1928.
Dew HR. Primary cerebral hydatid disease. Aust N Z J Surg. 1955;24:161–71.
Dowling E, Orlando RG. Quite hidatico del lobulo frontal derecho. Rev Assoc Med Argent. 1929;4:209–17.
Duishanbai S, Jiafu D, Guo H, Liu C, Liu B, Aishalong M, Mijiti M, Wen H. Intracranial hydatid cyst in children: report of 30 cases. Childs Nerv Syst. 2010;26:821–7.
Ehrhardt AR, Reuter S, Buck AK, Haenle MM, Mason RA, Gabelmann A, Kern P, Kratzer W. Assessment of disease activity in alveolar echinococcosis: a comparison of contrast enhanced ultrasound, three-phase helical CT and [(18)F] fluorodeoxyglucose positron emission tomography. Abdom Imaging. 2007;32:730–6.
Evliyaoglu C, Keskil S. Possible spontaneous "birth" of a hydatid cyst in to the lateral ventricle. Childs Nerv Syst. 2005;21:425–8.
Fairley KD, Kellaway CH. The value of laboratory investigations in the diagnosis of hydatid infestation. Aust N Z J Surg. 1933;2:236–43.
Furtado SV, Vishvanathan K, Nandita G, Reddy K, Hegde AS. Multiple fourth ventricular hydatidosis. J Clin Neurosci. 2009;16:110–2.
Gana R, Skhissi M, Maagili R, Bellakhadar F. Multiple infected cerebral hydatid cysts. J Clin Neurosci. 2008;15:591–3.
George EJ, Hillier CEM, Hatfield R. Glioma after cerebral hydatid disease. Childs Nerv Syst. 2003;19:837–40.
Ghosh A, Saha S, Jha A, Chandra S. Orbital hydatid cyst-a rare case report. Indian J Otolaryngol Head Neck Surg. 2008;60:191–3.
Gil-Grande LA, Prieto JG, Brasa C, Casado N. Randomized control trial of efficacy of albendazole in intra-abdominal hydatid disease. Lancet. 1993;342:1269–72.
Guzel A, Tatli M, Maciaczyk J, Altinors M. Primary cerebral intraventricular hydatid cyst: a case report and review of the literature. J Child Neurol. 2008; 23:585–8.
Hamamci EO, Besim H, Korkmaz A. Unusual locations of hydatid disease and surgical approach. ANZ J Surg. 2004;74:356–60.
Iplikcioglu AC, Ozer AF, Benli K, Isik N, Erbengi A. Multiple cerebral hydatid cysts: report of two cases. Br J Neurosurg. 1989;3:217–20.
Izci Y, Tuzun Y, Secer HI, Gonul E. Cerebral hydatid cysts: technique and pitfalls of surgical management. Neurosurg Focus. 2008;24:E15.
Jamshidi M, Mohraz M, Zangench M, Jamshidi A. The effect of combination therapy with albendazole and praziquantel on hydatid cyst treatment. Parasitol Res. 2008;103:195–9.
Kalaitzoglou I, Drevelengas A, Petridis A, Palladas P. Albendazole treatment of cerebral hydatid disease: evaluation of results with CT and MRI. Neuroradiology. 1998;40:36–9.
Kapan S, Turhan AN, Kalayci V, Alis H, Aygun E. Albendazole is not effective for primary treatment of hepatic hydatid cysts. J Gastrointest Surg. 2008;12:867–71.
Kappagoda S, Singh U, Blackburn BG. Antiparasitic therapy. Mayo Clin Proc. 2011;86:561–83.
Karadag O, Gurelik M, Ozum U, Goksel HM. Primary multiple cerebral hydatid cysts with unusual features. Acta Neurochir (Wien). 2004;146:73–7.
Karadereler S, Orakdogen M, Kilic K, Ozdogan C. Primary spinal extradural hydatid cyst in a child: case report and review of the literature. Eur Spine J. 2002;11:500–3.
Khaldi M, Mohamed S, Kallel J, Khouja N. Brain hydatidosis: report on 117 cases. Childs Nerv Syst. 2000;16:765–9.
Kiresi DA, Karabacakoglu A, Odev K, Karakose S. Uncommon locations of hydatid. Acta Radiol. 2003;44:622–36.
Kirimlioglu V, Akoglu M, Oner K, Pekcan M. Hypertonic saline in hydatid disease. World J Surg. 2001;25:975–9.
Lunardi P, Missori P, Lorenzo ND, Fortuna A. Cerebral hydatidosis in childhood: a retrospective survey with emphasis on long-term follow-up. Neurosurgery. 1991;29:515–8.
Ma L, Liu WK, Mao BY, Zhang YK. An Echinococcosis multilocularis presenting as a giant anterior cranial basilar tumor. Neurol Sci. 2009;30:247–9.
Mancuso P, Noubari BA, Gurusinghe NT. Multiple primary cerebral cysts: case report. Br J Neurosurg. 1997;11:248–9.
Manterola C, Vial M, Melo A, Oberg TM, Fonseca F. Viability and fertility of human hepatic hydatid cysts. World J Surg. 2006;30:227–32.
McManus DP, Zhang W, Li J, Bartley PB. Echinococcosis. Lancet. 2003;362:1295–304.
Meade JA, Barnett L. Echinococcosis alveolaris (alveolar hydatid disease), associated with ordinary hydatid cysts of the liver. Aust N Z J Surg. 1941;10:317–27.

Mohindra S, Savardekar A, Gupta R, Tripathi M, Rane S. Varied types of intracranial hydatid cysts: radiological features and management techniques. Acta Neurochir (Wien). 2011;154:165–72.

Morris DL. Preoperative albendazole therapy for hydatid cyst. Br J Surg. 1987;74:805–6.

Muthusubrahmanian V, Pande A, Vasudevan MC, Ravi R. Surgical management of brainstem hydatid cyst- an unusual site. Surg Neurol. 2009;71:103–6.

Normelli HCM, Aaro SI, Follin PH. Vertebral hydatid cyst infection (Echinococcus granulosus)- a case report. Eur Spine J. 1998;7:158–61.

Obrador S, Urquiza P. Two cases of cerebral abscess of unusual nature- tuberculous abscess and suppurated hydatid cyst. J Neurosurg. 1948;5:572–6.

Ozgen T, Bertan V, Kansu T, Akalin S. Intrasellar hydatid cyst- case report. J Neurosurg. 1984;60:647–8.

Palmer SR, Biffin AH, Craig PS, Walters TM. Control of hydatid disease in Wales. Br Med J. 1996;312:614–5.

Pasaoglu A, Orhon C, Adkemir H. Multiple primary hydatid cysts of the brain. Turk J Pediatr. 1989;31:57–61.

Pau A, Brambilla M, Cossu M, Sehrbundt Viale E, Turtas S. Long term follow-up of the surgical treatment of the intracranial hydatid disease. Acta Neurochir (Wien). 1987;88:116–8.

Reddy DR. Managing cerebral and cranial hydatid disease. Neurol India. 2009;57:116–8.

Reddy DR, Murthy JMK. Parasitic intracranial space occupying lesions in children in India. Childs Nerv Syst. 1986;2:244–7.

Reddy CR, Narasiah IL, Parvathi G, Rao MS. Epidemiology of hydatid disease in Kurnool. Indian J Med Res. 1968;56:1205–20.

Reddy DR, Rao BD, Subrahmanian MV. Hydatid disease of the central nervous system. Indian J Surg. 1972;34:191–5.

Reddy DR, Muralidhar B, Rajyalakshmi K, Reddy VV, Rammohan S, Verma JR. Intradiploic hydatid cyst of the occipital bone in a child-a case report. Indian Pediatr. 1979;16:647–50.

Reuter S, Nussle K, Kolokythas O, Haug V, Rieber A, Kern P, Krawtzer W. Alveolar liver echinococcosis: a comparative study of three imaging techniques. Infection. 2001;29:119–25.

Romig T. Epidemiology of echinococcosis. Langenbecks Arch Surg. 2003;388:209–17.

Sadjjadi SM, Sadaghat F, Hosseini SV, Sarkari B. Serum antigen and antibody detection in echinococcosis: application in sero-diagnosis of human hydatidosis. Korean J Parasitol. 2009;47:153–7.

Saidi F. Hydatid cysts of the central nervous system. In: Farrokh S, editor. Surgery of hydatid disease. London: W. B. Saunders Company Ltd; 1976. p. 352–76.

Sayek I, Onal C, Unal F, Barla SO, Izgi N, Hepgul K, Turantan MI, Canbolat A, Turker K, Bayindir C, Gokay HK, Kaya U. Long-term follow-up and results of thirty pediatric intracranial hydatid cysts: half a century of experience in the department of neurosurgery of the school of medicine at the University of Istanbul (1952–2001). Pediatr Neurosurg. 2001;35:72–81.

Senturk S, Oguz KK, Soylemezoglu F, Inci S. Cerebral alveolar echinococcosis mimicking primary brain tumor. AJNR Am J Neuroradiol. 2006;27:420–2.

Siddiqui MA, Rizvi SW, Rizvi SA, Ahmad I, Ullah E. Atypical multifocal hydatid disease of the cranial vault. Simultaneous orbital and extradural meningeal involvement. Emerg Radiol. 2010;17:427–30.

Sielaff TD, Taylor B, Langer B. Recurrence of hydatid disease. World J Surg. 2001;25:83–6.

Sierra J, Oviedo J, Berthier M, Leiguarda R. Growth rate of secondary hydatid cysts of the brain- case report. J Neurosurg. 1985;62:781–2.

Sihota R, Sharma T. Albendazole therapy for a recurrent orbital hydatid cyst. Indian J Opthalmol. 2000;48:142–3.

Silva MA, Mirza DF, Bramhall SR, Mayer AD, McMaster P. Treatment of hydatid disease of the liver. Evaluation of a UK experience. Dig Surg. 2004;21:227–33.

Tirnaksiz MB, Dogan R. Cystic hydatid disease: current trends in diagnosis and management. Surg Today. 2004;34:987–96.

Topcu O, Sumer Z, Tuncer E, Aydin C, Koyuncu A. Efficacy of chlorhexidine gluconate during surgery for hydatid cyst. World J Surg. 2009;33:1274–80.

Turgut M. Hydatid disease of the spine: a survey of study from Turkey. Infection. 1997;25:221–6.

Turgut M. Hydatidosis of the central nervous system and its coverings in the pediatric and adolescent age groups in Turkey during the last century: a critical review of 137 cases. Childs Nerv Syst. 2002;18:670–83.

Turgut M, Benli K, Eryilmaz M. Secondary multiple intracranial hydatid cysts caused by intracerebral embolism of cardiac echinococcosis: an exceptional case of hydatidosis. J Neurosurg. 1997;86:714–8.

Turkoglu OF, Solaroglu I, Tun K, Beskonakli E, Taskin Y. Secondary infection of intracranial hydatid cyst with clostridium ramosum. Childs Nerv Syst. 2005;21:1004–7.

Tuzun Y, Solmaz I, Sengul G, Izci Y. The complications of cerebral hydatid cyst surgery in children. Childs Nerv Syst. 2010;26:47–51.

Vaquero J, Jimenez C, Martinez R. Growth rate of hydatid cysts evaluated by CT scanning after presumed cerebral hydatid embolism. Case report. J Neurosurg. 1982;57:837–8.

Von Sinner WN, Nyman R, Lanzawi T, Ali AM. Fine needle aspiration biopsy of hydatid cysts. Acta Radiol. 1995;36:168–72.

Wang J, Cai B, You C. Surgical treatment options for cerebral alveolar echinococcosis: experience in six patients. Neurol India. 2009;57:157–61.

Yuceer N, Guven MB, Yilmez H. Multiple hydatid cysts of the brain-a case report and review of the literature. Neurosurg Rev. 1998;21:181–4.

Outcome and Follow-up of Patients with Spinal Hydatidosis

20

Lukas K. Postl and Chlodwig Kirchhoff

Contents

L.K. Postl, cand. Med • C. Kirchhoff, MD (✉)
Klinik und Poliklinik für Unfallchirurgie,
Klinikum Rechts der Isar,
Technische Universitaet Muenchen,
Ismaningerstrasse 22, Muenchen 81675, Germany
e-mail: chlodwig.kirchhoff@mri.tum.de

Introduction

The following chapter focuses on outcome and follow-up of patients suffering from spinal hydatidosis, i.e., the cystic as well as the alveolar form. In general, intraspinal hydatidosis differs from the intracranial form not only regarding the primary manifestation and treatment but also regarding follow-up and recurrence. Although several characteristics apply to the cystic as well as the alveolar form, detailed information is provided separately in each specific section.

The intraosseous growth of hydatid disease progresses relatively slowly and asymptomatically, developing diverticulated cysts along the intratrabecular spaces. Usually hydatid disease becomes clinically symptomatic in the extraosseous stage, when cysts excavate into the extradural and paraspinal regions, compromising nerve roots and the spinal cord causing objective sensory and motor disturbances at the level of the involved vertebrae (Herrera et al. 2005; Sengul et al. 2008; Belhassen-Garcia et al. 2011). However, local recurrence of hydatid disease does not typically begin in the vertebral body. But it also can relapse in the paravertebral, paraspinal, or intraspinal portion and therefore become clinically apparent early after negative restaging. Several authors describe a "malignancy" or "white cancer" when reporting on hydatid disease (Haddad et al. 1963; Turgut 1997; Viljoen and Crane 2008).

According to our opinion every patient suffering from hydatid disease needs a clearly structured aftercare and follow-up calendar including

M. Turgut (ed.), *Hydatidosis of the Central Nervous System: Diagnosis and Treatment*,
DOI 10.1007/978-3-642-54359-3_20, © Springer-Verlag Berlin Heidelberg 2014

physical examination, imaging, as well as serologic tests. This follow-up should also be individualized and consider the surgical progress, i.e., in case surgical spreading of the echinococcosis is likely, the follow-up needs to be adapted. Regarding the best follow-up imaging modality, it can be stated that hydatid extension into the extradural space or para-osseous soft tissues may not be detected by spine radiographs (Bron et al. 2007; Celik et al. 2010).

The imaging features of intraspinal hydatid cyst usually comprise multiple spherical lesions with clearly defined borders, containing fluid that is similar to cerebrospinal fluid (CSF) in intensity on both computed tomography (CT) scan and magnetic resonance imaging (MRI). Due to the need for repetitive scanning on a regular basis, for several reasons, we regard MRI as the imaging technique, since it allows for an early diagnosis of spinal cord compression and for a more accurate localization of intra- and paraspinal manifestation if multiplanar images are acquired (Pamir et al. 2002; Limaiem et al. 2010). On MRI it is possible to detect both the exact anatomical location of the lesion and the viability of the hydatid cysts. On T2-weighted images, a cystic lesion has a high intensity, whereas a decrease in signal indicates a necrotic cyst. Thus, a decreased signal in this sequence is a characteristic indicator for a necrotic cyst. Furthermore, the layers of the cyst can only be demonstrated by MRI, and the pericyst may show enhancement after contrast material administration due to its rich vascularization. Figures 20.1 and 20.2 demonstrate MRI findings.

Localization

The outcome of hydatid disease significantly depends on the location of the lesions. In this context the classification of Braithwaite and Lees provides an initial reference for the expected outcome (Braithwaite and Lees 1981). According to their anatomic location, cysts can be divided into intramedullary, intradural-extramedullary, extradural, spinal (vertebral), and paraspinal lesions extending into spinal structures. Besides these anatomic references, especially the spinal level influences the neurologic outcome. There is a remarkable difference regarding the outcome between cervical, thoracic, lumbar, and sacral manifestations of the spinal hydatid disease, especially in advanced stages when irreversible nerve tissue damage exists.

Aftercare

Surgical decompression and chemotherapy are the principal forms of treatment in pediatric and adolescent cases of spinal hydatidosis. Unfortunately even with extensive surgery, results are far from being curative. The recurrence and mortality rates for intraspinal hydatid disease range up to 50 and 15 %, respectively (Taratuto and Venturiello 1997; Toussaint et al. 2001; Wang et al. 2009). Up to 40 % of patients are reported to have recurrent symptomatology within 2 years after the initial operation (Spies et al. 2008; Takci et al. 2008; Taghipoor and Razmkon 2009). As the recurrence rate is high, adjuvant anthelmintic agents are recommended following surgery. Anthelmintic drugs are strongly recommended in case of recurrence, systemic disease, intraoperative rupture or puncture, poor suitability for surgery, and prophylaxis (Papagelopoulos et al. 1997; Schnepper and Johnson 2004; Romig 2009; Sharma et al. 2011). However, a clearly structured aftercare and follow-up calendar including physical examination, imaging, as well as serologic testing is mandatory. In parallel to the aftercare of soft tissue sarcoma, we recommend restaging every 3 months for the first 2 years. This should include CT scans of the abdomen and MRI of the spine. In the following the intervals can be reduced to twice a year up to year 5 and once a year until year 10 after onset of the disease.

The imaging features of intraspinal hydatid cyst usually comprise multiple spherical lesions with clearly defined borders, containing fluid with similar CSF intensity on both CT and MRIs. Though, due to the need for repetitive scanning on a regular basis, we regard MRI for several reasons as the best imaging technique, since it allows early diagnosis of spinal cord compression and

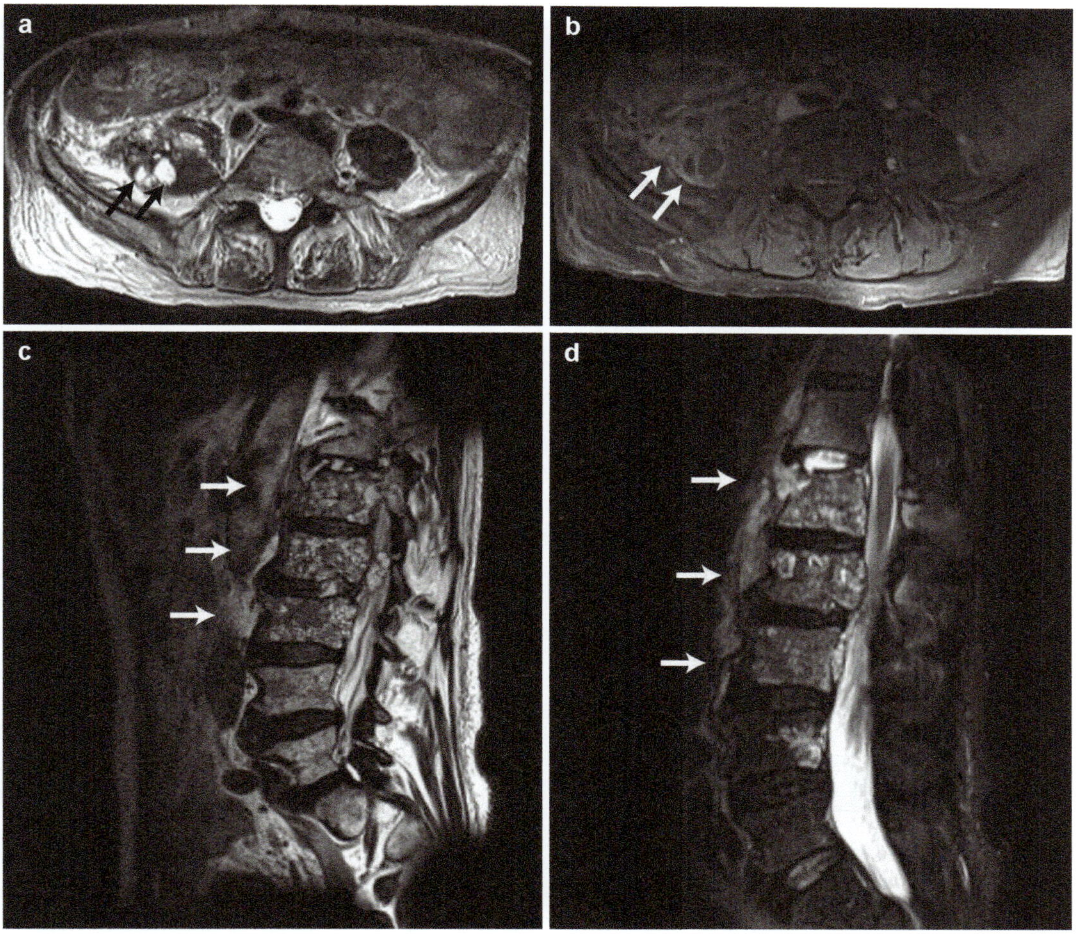

Fig. 20.1 The figure demonstrates the MRI findings of an 80-year-old male patient, initially presenting with recurrent abdominal pain and pain in the upper lumbar spine from lumbar vertebrae L1 to L3 without neurological deficit. (**a**) The T2-weighted axial MRI shows multiple small hyperintense lesions in the right psoas muscle (*arrows*). The corresponding fat-suppressed T1-weighted image after gadolinium administration (**b**) confirmed the diagnosis of a multicystic mass and delineated the thickened, contrast-enhancing septations around the cystic components (*arrow*). T1-weighted image (**c**) and T2-weighted STIR image (**d**) of the lumbar spine show the bone marrow replacement within the first, second, and third lumbar vertebrae (*arrows*). The lesions comprise of cystic and solid components

more accurate localization of intra- and paraspinal manifestation if multiplanar images are acquired. On MRI it is possible to detect the exact anatomical location of the lesion and to show the viability of the hydatid cysts. On T2-weighted images, a cystic lesion has a high intensity, and a decrease in signal indicates a necrotic cyst. Thus, a decreased signal in this sequence is a characteristic indicator of a necrotic cyst. Furthermore, the layers of the cyst can only be demonstrated by MRI, and the pericyst may show enhancement after contrast material administration due to its rich vascularization. In particular positron emission tomography scanning in combination with CT scan or MRI might show active lesions at a time when clinical symptoms are absent or unspecific and recurrence of parasitic tissue is not detectable by conventional imaging (Brunetti et al. 2010). Imaging of spinal hydatid disease is discussed in Chap. 12.

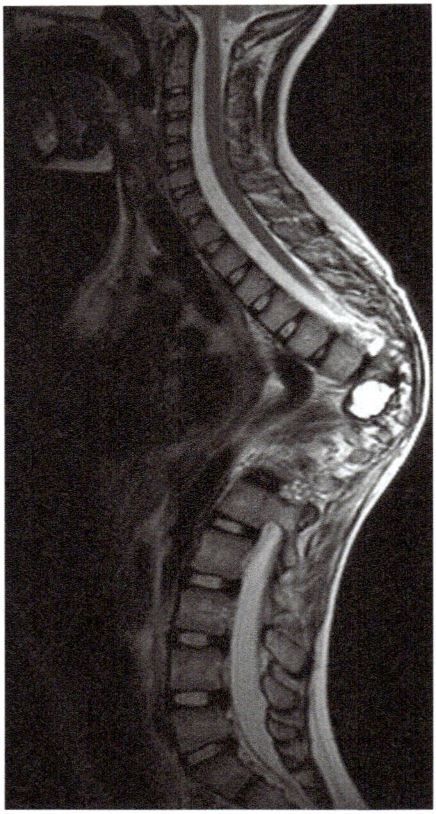

Fig. 20.2 The figure presents the MRI of a 6-year-old girl with primary *Echinococcus granulosus* infection of the spine being treated with various interventions. Now presenting recurrence of infection due to incomplete cyst resection and inappropriate surgical measures causing progressive kyphoscoliotic deformity, spinal stenosis, cord compression, and neurologic injury. At the presentation at our institution, she was wheelchair bound. The clinical investigation revealed gibbus in the middle thoracic spine with a Cobb angle of 110°, cord compression at the apex, and paraplegia with Frankel Grade C

Blood tests should include benzimidazole blood levels as well as serological tests (Nell et al. 2011). Determination of benzimidazole blood levels, 4 h after the morning dose, is recommended 1, 4, and 12 weeks after initiating drug therapy. Detection of antibody directed to echinococcal polypeptide antigens has the highest degree of specificity. Enzyme-linked immunosorbent assay (ELISA), indirect hemagglutination, and complement fixation tests are reported to be 80–100 % sensitive and 88–96 % specific in abdominal disease. However, the sensitivity decreases abruptly to 25–56 % in extrahepatic disease which limits their use in the diagnosis or follow-up for primary bone disease. Second-line tests like immunoblotting (antigen 5 precipitation: arc-5 test) may be used for confirmation after ELISA and hemagglutination. Laboratory findings of patients with spinal hydatidosis are discussed in Chap. 10.

Benzimidazole Treatment

Albendazole should be administered orally at a dose rate of 10–15 mg/kg/day divided into two doses (WHO 1996). In practice a daily dose of 800 mg is applicable to adults. Intermittent or cyclic treatment is no longer necessary, since albendazole treatment is well tolerated and it has been reported that a dose rate of 20 mg/kg/day is tolerated for up to 5 years. Alternatively if albendazole is not enough tolerated or available, mebendazole could be administered at a daily dose rate of 40–50 mg/kg/day. Benzimidazoles are generally well tolerated. Adverse reactions include hepatotoxicity, alopecia, gastrointestinal disturbances, and leucopenia (Vuitton 2009). Moreover the only contraindication for benzimidazoles is pregnancy. Albendazole is the most widely used benzimidazole worldwide. Benefits of albendazole are a better bioavailability to achieve higher plasma levels, an easy administration, and an overall better efficacy. However, benzimidazoles in general are only parasitostatic and do not erase *E. multilocularis* metacestodes.

Cystic Echinococcosis

Neurological Deficit

The neurological and orthopedic symptoms can often be reduced or eliminated by surgery and/or anthelmintic treatment for a certain time, but very often only a short follow-up is reported, and it remains doubtful if the patient was cured (Arif and Zaheer 2009; Kotil et al. 2010; Thaler et al. 2010; Scarlata et al. 2011). In recurrent cases multiple interventions can be reasonable to preserve or even improve the spinal stability and the neurological status, but cure of disease is usually not possible (Keller et al. 1997).

Treatment Characteristics

Benzimidazole treatment is recommended for a period of at least 3 months. Although these drugs are well tolerated, Pamir et al. (1984) do state that there is no clear evidence that further administration is lowering the recurrence rate. Nevertheless, Turgut (1997) report that the drugs could effectively keep the disease asymptomatic for a prolonged time.

Several authors stress that imaging should not be the only means for diagnosing a recurrent disease, because a residual cavity is very hard to differentiate. In this regard symptoms seem to have a certain impact. Lawn et al. (2004) found that during post-surgical follow-up, the immunoglobulin G subclass IgG2 antibody response provides a reasonable correlate of disease activity, and Nouir et al. (2008) found that immunoblotting can be a useful approach for monitoring post-treatment follow-up.

Recurrence Rate

Recurrence During Anthelmintic Therapy

Conservative treatment seems to be effective and the recurrence rate of conservatively treated patients is significantly lower than the rate of surgically treated patients without chemotherapy. Nevertheless, very often patients present with neurological symptoms that urgently require surgical decompression.

Recurrence After Surgery

Total excision of the cysts should be the aim of treatment, but in the majority of cases, this cannot be obtained and recurrence is reported. Therefore up to 40 % of cases show recurrence within 2 years of initial operation (Turtas et al. 1980). Nevertheless, the excision of intradural and extradural lesions without osseous involvement could theoretically be curative when the cysts remain intact (Bettaieb et al. 1978; Pamir et al. 1984). But in most cases a complete removal of cyst cannot be performed without damaging the nerve roots (Turgut and Turgut 2010). Osseous involvement causes a multivesicular and diffuse infiltration of the vertebrae (Ozek 1994). Due to this fact the surgery at the vertebrae will lead to spillage of the scolices (Baysefer et al. 1996; Islekel et al. 1998). In this context Turgut (1997) were able to show that the recurrence rate of spinal lesions is significantly higher (33 %, $n=41$) than the rate of intraspinal lesions without or minor bone involvement (<6 %, $n=27$). Both surgery and anthelmintic therapy should be considered. Some authors recommend administering lifelong chemotherapy. Most patients suffer from multiple recurrences, worsening of disease, and very often restoration of the spine to improve and preserve neurological status and spine stability.

Prognosis

The recurrence rate is reported in up to 40 % of all cases, but the recurrence probability for a single case depends very much on the localization of the lesion and in case of a surgery on the progress of the intervention. The literature does provide case reports and reviews, but larger studies on echinococcosis of the spine are scarce. Most publications only report on a period of a few years post operation, and reliable data on, e.g., the survival time for cases with spine affection, is missing.

Alveolar Echinococcosis

Treatment Characteristics

Although postoperative benzimidazole therapy is obligatory in all cases, generally accepted guidelines concerning presurgical anthelmintic treatment and the duration of treatment after surgery are not available. Brunetti et al. (2010) recommended temporary treatment after complete resection. Reuter et al. (2000a, b) require a benzimidazole treatment for a period of at least 2 years post surgery, since residual echinococcosis might remain undetected and follow-up of patients should be at least 10 years. In cases of a subtotal surgery or in inoperable cases, long-term or even lifelong benzimidazole therapy is necessary. Ammann and Eckert (1996) provided evidence that long-term benzimidazole therapy in subtotal resected lesions causes a significant improvement of the 10-year survival rate. According to the authors the 10-year survival rate in an untreated historical control group was found to be 6–25 % and could be increased to 80–83 % in patients receiving long-term benzimidazole therapy. Further long-term anthelmintic treatment also lowers the recurrence rate (Torgerson et al. 2008).

Serological tests in the follow-up seem to be predicative. Scheuring et al. (2003) reported that anti-Em2 and anti-Em18 antibodies rapidly decreased after total resection of lesions and became undetectable. Serological analysis in the follow-up provides reliable information about clinical status and efficiency of treatment of patients with alveolar echinococcosis; thus there is a close relationship between clinical regression and specific serology (Tappe et al. 2009). But unfortunately in patients with subtotal resections and under benzimidazole treatment, the interpretation of serological test is more complex.

Recurrence Rate and Prognosis

Reliable data on recurrence prognosis of the spinal alveolar echinococcosis is even scarcer than data on the prognosis of the cystic echinococcosis. Only a few cases have been published so far (Claudon et al. 1987; Duewell et al. 1990; Merkle et al. 1997; Reuter et al. 2000a, b; Sudo and Minami 2010). For alveolar echinococcosis in general (for all lesions and not only for lesions of the spine), it has been stated that treatment had improved average life expectancy at time of diagnosis—while it had been 3 years in the 1970s, it has reached 20 years in 2005 (Nouir et al. 2008). The recurrence rate seems to be lower under benzimidazole treatment.

Conclusion

Based on our experience and literature data on spinal hydatidosis, the following points are concluded:

1. The outcome will differ for cases of cystic echinococcosis and alveolar echinococcosis.
2. The location of the lesions will strongly influence the outcome and should be considered regarding follow-up.
3. Structured aftercare and follow-up calendar including physical examination, imaging, as well as serologic tests are crucial.
4. Surgical decompression and chemotherapy are the principal forms of treatment in cases of spinal hydatidosis. Unfortunately, even with extensive surgery, results are far from being curative.

References

Ammann RW, Eckert J. Cestodes. Echinococcus. Gastroenterol Clin North Am. 1996;25:655–89.

Arif SH, Zaheer S. Intradural extramedullary primary hydatid cyst of the spine in a child: a very rare presentation. Eur Spine J. 2009;18:179–82.

Baysefer A, Gonul E, Canakci Z, Erdogan E, Aydogan N, Kayali H. Hydatid disease of the spine. Spinal Cord. 1996;34:297–300.

Belhassen-Garcia M, Carpio-Perez A, Blanco JF, Velasco-Tirado V, Pardo-Lledias J. Recurrent spinal echinococcosis. Int J Infect Dis. 2011;15:e435–6.

Bettaieb A, Khaldi M, Ben Rhouma T, Touibi S. Spinal echinococcosis; clinical study of 32 cases (in French). Neurochirurgie. 1978;24:205–10.

Braithwaite PA, Lees RF. Vertebral hydatid disease: radiological assessment. Radiology. 1981;140:763–6.

Bron JL, van Kemenade FJ, Verhoof OJ, Wuisman PI. Long term follow-up of a patient with disseminated spinal hydatidosis. Acta Orthop Belg. 2007;73:678–82.

Brunetti E, Kern P, Vuitton DA. Expert consensus for the diagnosis and treatment of cystic and alveolar echinococcosis in humans. Acta Trop. 2010;114:1–16.

Celik C, Sasmaz MF, Oktay F, Ucan H, Kaptanoglu E. Paraplegia associated with spinal hydatid cyst: a case report. Spine (Phila Pa 1976). 2010;35:E356–8.

Claudon M, Bracard S, Plenat F, Regent D, Bernadac P, Picard L. Spinal involvement in alveolar echinococcosis: assessment of two cases. Radiology. 1987;162:571–2.

Duewell S, Marincek B, von Schulthess GK, Ammann R. MRT and CT in alveolar echinococcosis of the liver (in German). Rofo. 1990;152:441–5.

Haddad FS, Haddad FS, Haddad SI. La malignité de l'échinococcose. Rev Med Moyen Orient. 1963;20: 270–5.
Herrera A, Martinez AA, Rodriguez J. Spinal hydatidosis. Spine (Phila Pa 1976). 2005;30:2439–44.
Islekel S, Ersahin Y, Zileli M, Oktar N, Oner K, Ovül I, Ozdamar N, Tuncbay E. Spinal hydatid disease. Spinal Cord. 1998;36:166–70.
Keller TM, Schweitzer JS, Helfend LK, Chappell T. Treatment of progressive cervical spinal instability secondary to hydatid disease. A case report. Spine (Phila Pa 1976). 1997;22:915–9.
Kotil K, Tari R, Savas Y. Medical treatment of primary extradural solitary lumbar hydatid disease. J Clin Neurosci. 2010;17:793–5.
Lawn SD, Bligh J, Craig PS, Chiodini PL. Human cystic echinococcosis: evaluation of post-treatment serologic follow-up by IgG subclass antibody detection. Am J Trop Med Hyg. 2004;70:329–35.
Limaiem F, Bellil S, Bellil K, Chelly I, Mekni A, Khaldi M, Haouet S, Zitouna M, Kchir N. Primary hydatidosis of the central nervous system: a retrospective study of 39 Tunisian cases. Clin Neurol Neurosurg. 2010; 112:23–8.
Merkle EM, Kramme E, Vogel J, Krämer S, Schulte M, Usadel S, Kern P, Brambs HJ. Bone and soft tissue manifestations of alveolar echinococcosis. Skeletal Radiol. 1997;26:289–92.
Nell M, Burgkart RH, Gradl G, von Eisenhart-Rothe R, Schaeffeler C, Trappe D, da Costa CP, Gradinger R, Kirchhoff C. Primary extrahepatic alveolar echinococcosis of the lumbar spine and the psoas muscle. Ann Clin Microbiol Antimicrob. 2011;10:13.
Nouir NB, Nuñez S, Frei E, Gorcii M, Müller N, Gianinazzi C, Mekki M, Nouri A, Babba H, Gottstein B. Post-surgical follow-up (by ELISA and immunoblotting) of cured versus non-cured cystic echinococcosis in young patients. Parasitology. 2008;135: 105–14.
Ozek MM. Complications of central nervous system hydatid disease. Pediatr Neurosurg. 1994;20:84–91.
Pamir MN, Akalan N, Ozgen T, Erbengi A. Spinal hydatid cysts. Surg Neurol. 1984;21:53–7.
Pamir MN, Ozduman K, Elmaci I. Spinal hydatid disease. Spinal Cord. 2002;40:153–60.
Papagelopoulos PJ, Peterson HA, Ebersold MJ, Emmanuel PR, Choudhury SN, Quast LM. Spinal column deformity and instability after lumbar or thoracolumbar laminectomy for intraspinal tumors in children and young adults. Spine (Phila Pa 1976). 1997;22: 442–51.
Reuter S, Jensen B, Buttenschoen K, Kratzer W, Kern P. Benzimidazoles in the treatment of alveolar echinococcosis: a comparative study and review of the literature. J Antimicrob Chemother. 2000a;46:451–6.
Reuter S, Seitz HM, Kern P, Junghanss T. Extrahepatic alveolar echinococcosis without liver involvement: a rare manifestation. Infection. 2000b;28:187–92.
Romig T. Echinococcus multilocularis in Europe-state of the art. Vet Res Commun. 2009;33:31–4.
Scarlata F, Giordano S, Saporito L, Marasa L, Li Pani G, Odierna A, Scaglione V, Di Carlo P, Romano A. Cystic hydatidosis: a rare case of spine localization. Infez Med. 2011;19:39–41.
Scheuring UJ, Seitz HM, Wellmann A, Hartlapp JH, Tappe D, Brehm K, Spengler U, Sauerbruch T, Rockstroh JK. Long-term benzimidazole treatment of alveolar echinococcosis with hematogenic subcutaneous and bone dissemination. Med Microbiol Immunol. 2003;192:193–5.
Schnepper GD, Johnson WD. Recurrent spinal hydatidosis in North America. Case report and review of the literature. Neurosurg Focus. 2004;17:E8.
Sengul G, Kadioglu HH, Kayaoglu CR, Aktas S, Akar A, Aydin IH. Treatment of spinal hydatid disease: a single center experience. J Clin Neurosci. 2008;15: 507–10.
Sharma AK, Diyora B, Badhe P, Nayak N, Patankar P, Chopra G. Neurological picture. Primary multiple calvarial hydatid cysts-a rare occurrence. J Neurol Neurosurg Psychiatry. 2011;82:349–50.
Spies C, Weisskopf M, Ohnsorge JA. Intraspinal echinococcosis within the lumbar spine of an 18-year-old male patient (in German). Z Orthop Unfall. 2008;146:463–7.
Sudo H, Minami A. Neurological picture. A widespread echinococcosis of the spine. J Neurol Neurosurg Psychiatry. 2010;81:892.
Taghipoor M, Razmkon A. Neurological picture. Huge primary intracranial hydatid cysts. J Neurol Neurosurg Psychiatry. 2009;80:1149.
Takci E, Sengul G, Akar A, Uslu H, Alper F, Erdogan F, Aydin IH. Alveolar echinococcosis of the brain in five patients. J Clin Neurosci. 2008;15:1105–9.
Tappe D, Frosch M, Sako Y, Itoh S, Grüner B, Reuter S, Nakao M, Ito A, Kern P. Close relationship between clinical regression and specific serology in the follow-up of patients with alveolar echinococcosis in different clinical stages. Am J Trop Med Hyg. 2009; 80:792–7.
Taratuto AL, Venturiello SM. Echinococcosis. Brain Pathol. 1997;7:673–9.
Thaler M, Gabl M, Lechner R, Gstottner M, Bach CM. Severe kyphoscoliosis after primary Echinococcus granulosus infection of the spine. Eur Spine J. 2010; 19:1415–22.
Torgerson PR, Schweiger A, Deplazes P, Pohar M, Reichen J, Ammann RW, Tarr PE, Halkik N, Müllhaupt B. Alveolar echinococcosis: from a deadly disease to a well-controlled infection. Relative survival and economic analysis in Switzerland over the last 35 years. J Hepatol. 2008;49:72–7.
Toussaint F, Pere P, Le Chaffotec L, Grandhaye P, Pourel J, Chary-Valckenaere I. Alveolar echinococcosis of the spine. J Clin Rheumatol. 2001;7:248–51.
Turgut M. Hydatid disease of the spine: a survey study from Turkey. Infection. 1997;25:221–6.
Turgut M, Turgut AT. Spinal intradural extramedullary hydatidosis: report of 3 cases. Neurosurgery. 2010;67: E1471–2.

Turtas S, Viale ES, Pau A. Long-term results of surgery for hydatid disease of the spine. Surg Neurol. 1980; 13:468–70.

Viljoen H, Crane J. Hydatid disease of the spine. Spine (Phila Pa 1976). 2008;33:2479–80.

Vuitton DA. Benzimidazoles for the treatment of cystic and alveolar echinococcosis: what is the consensus? Expert Rev Anti Infect Ther. 2009;7:145–9.

Wang J, Cai B, You C. Surgical treatment options for cerebral alveolar echinococcosis: experience in six patients. Neurol India. 2009;57:157–61.

WHO. Guidelines for treatment of cystic and alveolar echinococcosis in humans. WHO Informal Working Group on Echinococcosis. Bull World Health Organ. 1996;74:231–42.

Unusual Presentations of Hydatidosis of the Central Nervous System

21

Alexandru-Vlad Ciurea, Horatiu-Alexandru Moisa, and Dan Aurel Nica

Contents

A.-V. Ciurea, MD, PhD, MSc, Dr. h.c. Mult. (✉)
H.-A. Moisa, MD
Department of Neurosurgery, Sanador Medical Center Hospital, 9 Sevastopol Street, Sector 1, Bucharest 010991, Romania

Department of Neurosurgery, "Carol Davila" University School of Medicine, 8 Eroii Sanitari Boulevard, Bucharest 050474, Romania
e-mail: rsn@bagdasar-arseni.ro, prof.avciurea@gmail.com

D.A. Nica, MD, PhD
Department of Neurosurgery, St. Pantelimon Emergency University Hospital, 340-342 Soseaua Pantelimon Hwy, Sector 2, Bucharest, Romania

Introduction and General Data

Hydatid disease is an anthropozoonosis caused by the larval cysts of *Echinococcus granulosus*, a small, cosmopolite, cyclophyllid cestode (tape worm) currently found throughout the world.

History of hydatidosis is given in detail in Chap. 1 of the book.

Morphology and Classification

Currently, the *Echinococcus* genus (of the *Taenoides* family) is represented by four subspecies which were found in human beings: (1) *E. granulosus*, (2) *E. multilocularis*, (3) *E. oligarthus*, and (4) *E. vogeli* (Eckert et al. 2001).

The subspecies of hydatidosis in the world are discussed in Chaps. 2, 3, and 4.

Unusual Manifestations of Craniocerebral Hydatid Disease

By unusual presentations of hydatid disease, we understand the extremely rare situations that some clinicians might never actually see in their practice. The cases mentioned here come as a result of personal experiences of the authors and a review of the world literature.

Hydatid disease can theoretically be positioned anywhere within the skull, thanks to its hematogenous dissemination. From the known data in the literature, we mention hydatid disease

M. Turgut (ed.), *Hydatidosis of the Central Nervous System: Diagnosis and Treatment*, DOI 10.1007/978-3-642-54359-3_21, © Springer-Verlag Berlin Heidelberg 2014

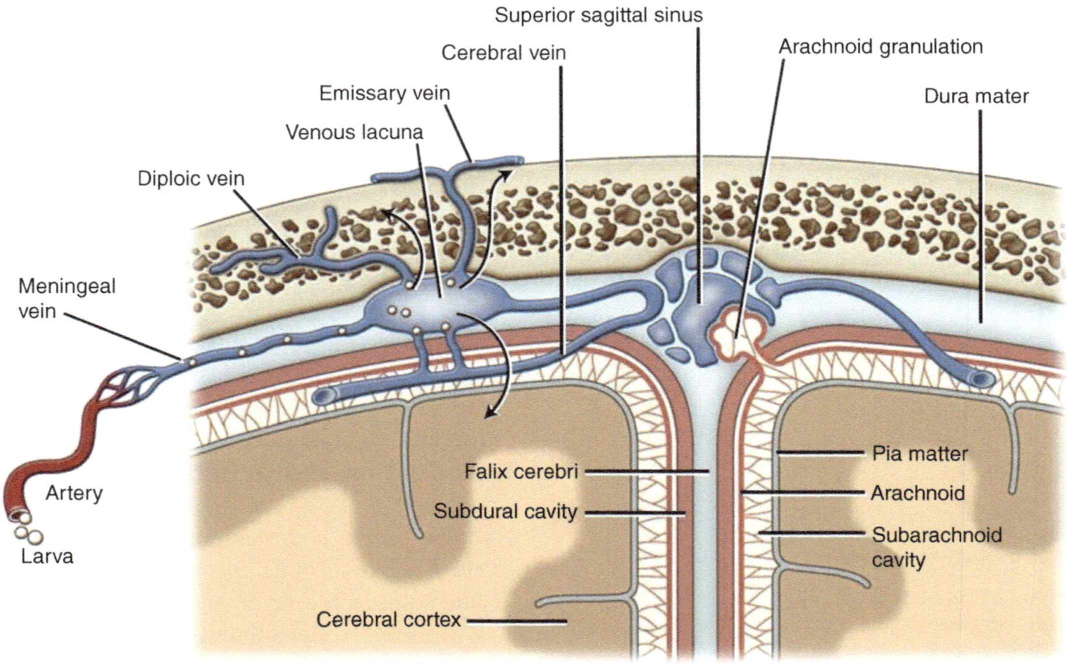

Fig. 21.1 The vascular dissemination of hydatidosis

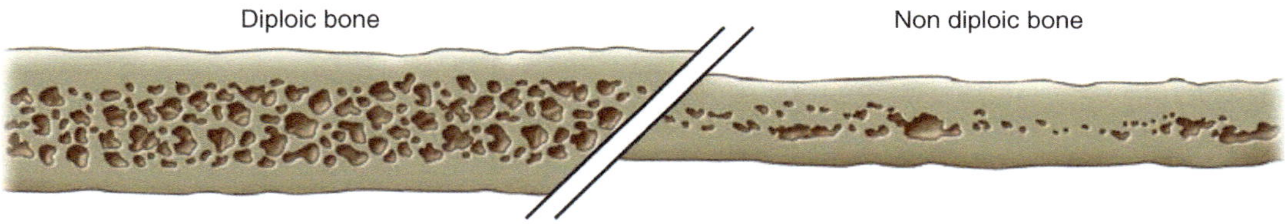

Fig. 21.2 Diploic vs. nondiploic sagittal bone section

positioned in the epidural space, within the meninges (intradural), subdural, subarachnoid, intracerebral, intraventricular, periventricular, cisternal, intrasinusal (vascular), in the brainstem, in the thalamus, and in the bony skull. All these manifestations are considered to be completely unusual. Among these, the most frequent are those located within the tissue of the central nervous system (CNS) due to the intense vascularization of the brain and better conditions for the larvae of *E. granulosus* (Fig. 21.1).

Calvarium

Hydatid disease in the calvarium is usually the rarest in the CNS. Anatomically, the bones of the calvarium, which has a protective function toward the brain, are made of one layer of spongious bony tissue flanked on the outside and on the inside by two other layers of compact laminar bone tissue such is the case of diploic bones (Figs. 21.2 and 21.3).

The bones of the base of the skull are nondiploic and the core spongious bony tissue may be very little represented or absent. While bones of the calvarium are more prone to destruction by hydatid cysts, the bones of the skull base can also be involved, although this situation is much rarer (Fig. 21.4). The first one to describe bone destruction as a consequence of hydatid cysts in the skull was Monro in 1811 (Arseni et al. 1981). There were other scarce presentations in the literature of hydatid disease in the diploe (in 1872 by

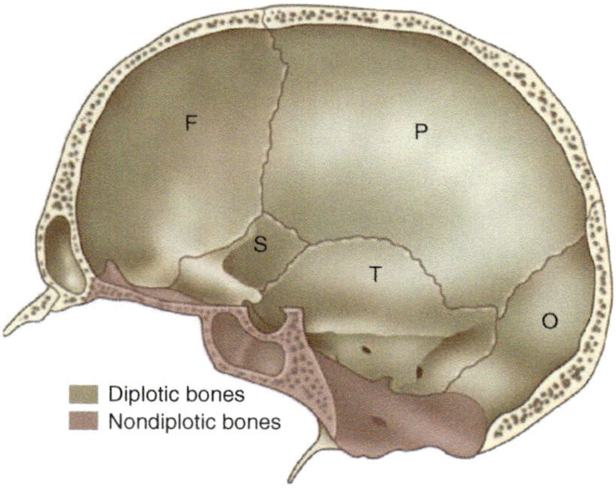

Fig. 21.3 Sagittal cut-through section of the skull showing the distribution of the diploic and nondiploic bones. *F* Frontal bone, *P* parietal bone, *T* temporal bone, *S* sphenoid bone, *O* occipital bone

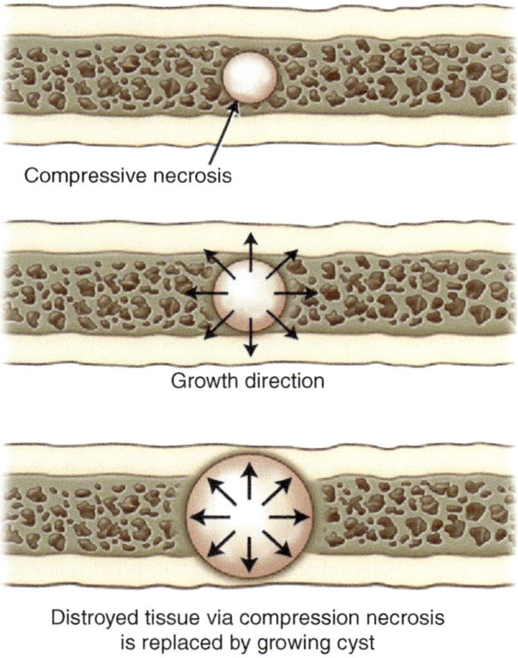

Fig. 21.4 Hydatid cyst growing in the diploe. The inner and outer tables are gradually spread apart by the eccentrical growth of the cyst

Verdale, in 1901 by Herrera and Cranwell, in 1909 by Goyanes). Felix Deve himself managed in 1949 to gather 637 cases of hydatid disease in the skeleton, of which 22 cases were positioned at the level of the calvarium (quoted from Arseni et al. 1981). Another peculiar manifestation of hydatidosis is in the petrous part of the temporal bone. Three such cases were presented in the literature by Schroeder et al. 1953 (quoted from Arseni et al. 1981).

The pathogenic mechanism of hydatid disease in the calvarium is quite difficult to explain. Arseni and Samitca mention in 1957 in their monograph regarding hydatidosis a single case of hydatid disease in the cranial vault. As to the bones of the skull base, researchers such as Arana Iniguez showed that 7.6 % out of 145 cases of cerebral hydatid disease attacked the bony structures, especially the petrous portion of the temporal bone (quoted from Arseni et al. 1981). Recently, a case in which an *E. granulosus* cyst produced a brain abscess in a 28-year-old patient has been reported (Llanes et al. 2008). In this case, the evacuation of the brain abscess was performed with a combined otolaryngologic and neurosurgical procedure (canal wall down mastoidectomy and temporal craniotomy) (Llanes et al. 2008). Another rarity we found in skull vault-related unusual presentations of hydatidosis is the presence of the disease in the viscerocranium – especially the sinuses. The maxillary sinus (Goldsher et al. 1983) and maxillary antrum (Copley et al. 1992) are two of the rarest locations for hydatidosis in the skull even in the endemic areas across the world.

The surgical approach for hydatid cysts in the skull vault doesn't present too many surgical difficulties. Many authors recommend an oval incision in the skin, in the form of a horseshoe to provide an intact removal of the hydatid cyst penetrating the calvarium. In endemic areas, the diagnosis must be clearly made, absolutely without biopsy and without compromising the integrity of the cyst in the subjacent structures including the bone and meninges. In non-endemic areas, a case of multifocal hydatidosis, metastasized or polycystic, has to be correctly diagnosed. In this respect, all the investigative data has to be correlated so that the diagnosis and surgical approach are not carried out inappropriately (Fig. 21.5). One case stands out. It is the case of a 14-year-old boy which after birth started showing a particular progressive deformity of the calvarium. Despite what looked like hydrocephalus or scaphocephalus, the child showed satisfactory results in school. The child started suffering from latero-cervical

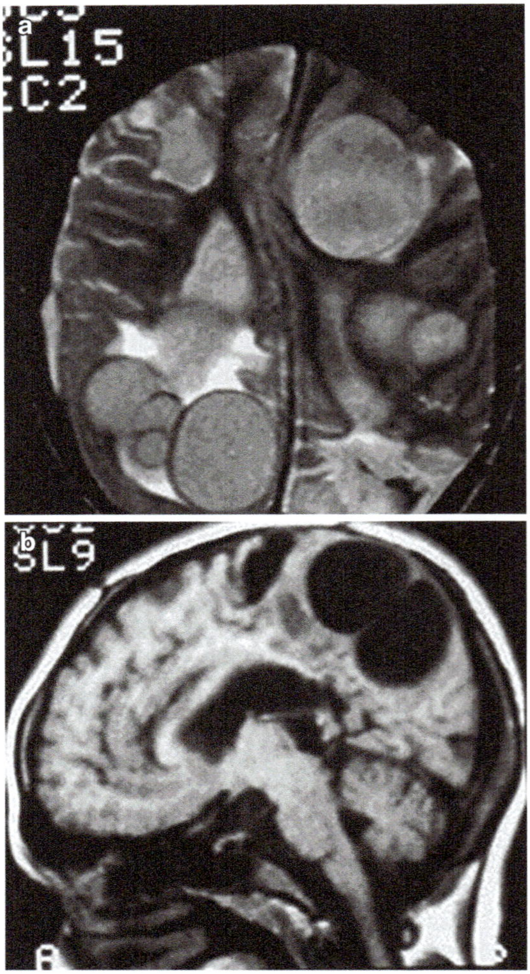

Fig. 21.5 Axial (**a**) and sagittal (**b**) MRIs of multiple hydatid cysts in the brain

pain which irradiated to the back of the head and associated with nausea and lately with intermittent vomiting. The radiograph showed a characteristic cyst-like formation 12 cm in length and 5 cm thick. Once opened, the calvarium contained more than 80 microcysts ranging from 3 mm to 5 cm. At the periphery of the cyst, the calvarium measured 1.5 cm in thickness. The depressed inner sheath of the bone was also removed (thus complete craniectomy was achieved) with a minimal blood loss and well-tolerated surgery. A few hours after surgery, shock installed; however, the patient managed to withstand due to glucose serum and blood perfusions. Twelve hours postoperative the patient started showing right-sided hemiplegia with cerebral edema. Gradually the patient recovered and left the hospital with a minimal deficit which was completely resolved 4 months after surgery (Fig. 21.6).

The hydatidosis of the skull is discussed in Chap. 5 in detail.

Craniocerebral Extradural

Extradural hydatid disease occurs at the moment when one or more *E. granulosus* oncospheres end up via the bloodstream in the epidural space of the cerebrospinal axis; this includes the skull and spine. The space we are referring to consists of the space enclosed between the outer surface of the dura mater and the internal surface of the skull which continues through the foramen magnum downward with the internal surface of the spinal canal, lined by the tectorial membrane, posterior longitudinal ligament, and yellow ligament and is filled with the peridural adipose tissue (Figs. 21.7, 21.8, and 21.9).

After the larva has penetrated the inner bone layer, it will grow outside of the dura mater, developing into a substantial cyst of viscous consistency. The cyst will then compress the brain matter leading to the characteristic symptoms. The clinical features of this manifestation are dominated by the slow evolution of the cyst which is translated into a raised intracranial pressure syndrome and diminished visual acuity. Patients usually end up at the hospital when the cyst has exaggerated dimensions (Arseni et al. 1981). Sporadic manifestations of extradural hydatidosis in the literature have also been found more recently (Sharma et al. 2010). The extradural meningeal space is generally affected during a multifocal hydatid disease (Siddiqui et al. 2010).

Interesting enough is the fact that more and more unusual manifestations of extradural hydatid disease appear in the literature. We mention only for historical purpose six cases (Arseni et al. 1981).

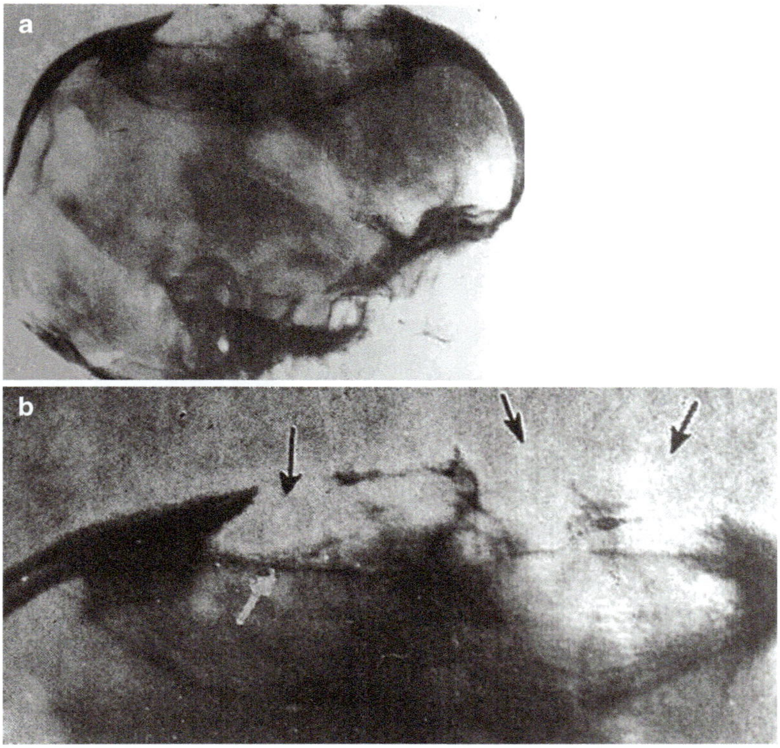

Fig. 21.6 (**a**) Lateral radiograph showing the cyst. Note the length and the width of the displacement of the inner and outer sheath of the calvarium. (**b**) Radiograph centered on the cyst. *Arrows* represent areas where the hydatid cyst has destroyed the outer sheath of the calvarium

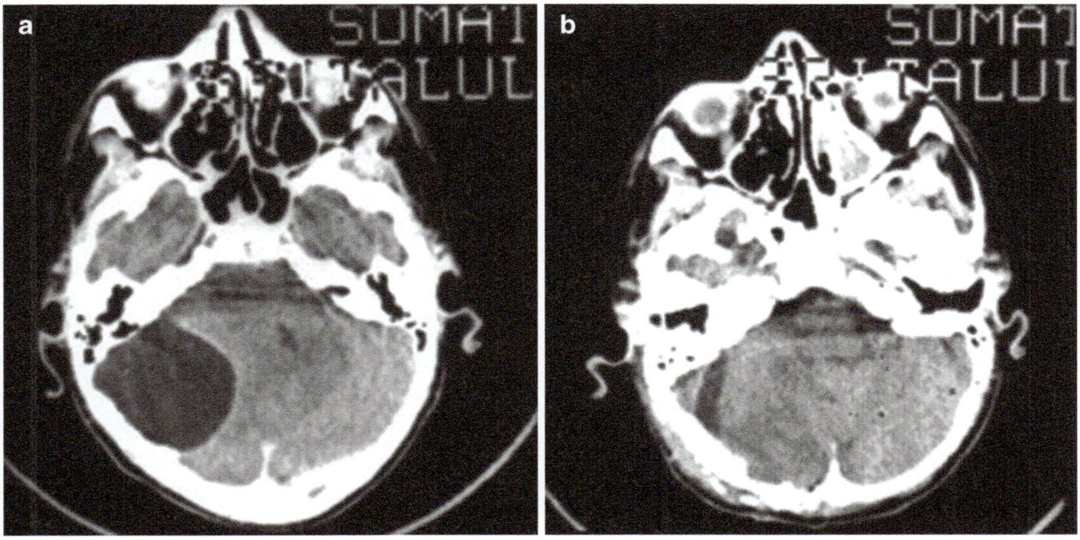

Fig. 21.7 Preoperative (**a**) and postoperative (**b**) aspects of an extradural hydatid cyst in the posterior fossa

We describe two such cases: one is mentioned in the literature in 1949 (Arseni et al. 1981). Here, the patient, a young child, had a large destruction of bony substance associated with an enormous cyst 425 cm^3 in volume that contained nine daughter cysts which varied in size. The child died 4 days after surgery as a result of violent epileptic seizures triggered by 100,000 units

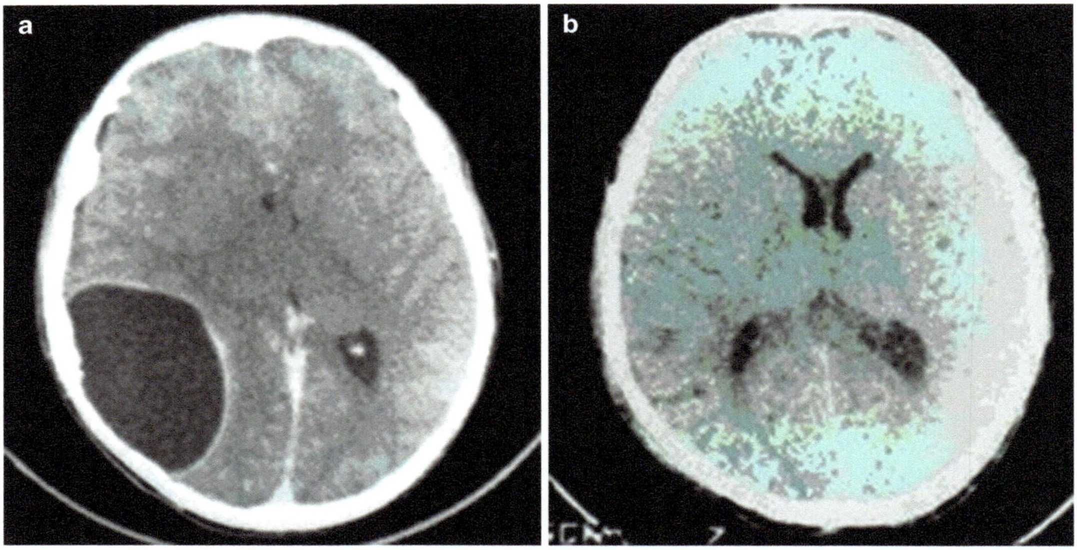

Fig. 21.8 Preoperative (**a**) and postoperative (**b**) aspects of an extradural hydatid cyst in the parietooccipital region of the brain

of penicillin administered at the site of the cyst. The second case was published in 1959 (Arseni et al. 1981). The patient showed a left frontal pulsatile tumefaction. The cyst had drilled through the walls of the left frontal sinus, and the secondary sinusitis masked the presence of the cyst. Three such cases are presented by Arseni et al. (1981) as part of their personal list of cases.

Craniocerebral Extradural Sellar

An extremely interesting case was signaled in the Maghreb where a young Bedouin woman became fertile again 13 years after a hydatid cyst that was pushing against her pituitary stalk was removed. The removal of the cyst returned full hormonal functions (Mazor et al. 1986) (Fig. 21.10).

We are familiar with one other case of such nature, taken from the literature, in which a 38-year-old woman manifesting hypothalamic stupor and absolute mutism presented a hydatid cyst in the area between the diencephalon and pituitary gland. The patient unfortunately died and the cyst was found at autopsy, lying behind the optic chiasmus and in front of the pons. The cyst was herniating between the hemispheres and was the size of a pigeon egg (Arseni et al. 1981). The cyst developed in the tissue of the pituitary gland, the ceiling of which got atrophic and resorbed through a slow process of compression which was doubled by a flattening of the neural portion as well as the whole infundibulo-tuberian area. One such case was also depicted by Arseni et al. (1981) as part of their personal experience in Fig. 21.11.

Craniocerebral Extradural Parasellar

Another case of multiple hydatid cysts was spotted in a patient from an endemic area, a 21-year-old man presenting with multiple cranial nerve palsy, impaired eyesight, raised intracranial pressure, and a computed tomography (CT) image showing a hypodense mass with septations and a hyperdense rim. The case pointed out the presence of a parasellar hydatid cyst (Behari et al. 1997).

The recommended surgical approach in such situations is the pterional basal one or the fronto-temporo-orbito-zygomatic one, which can be extended to the needs of the surgeon. The approach is executed in such a way that it will allow the widest exposure of the cyst to permit a complete intact cyst removal. Under no circumstance should the integrity of the cyst be disrupted (Fig. 21.12).

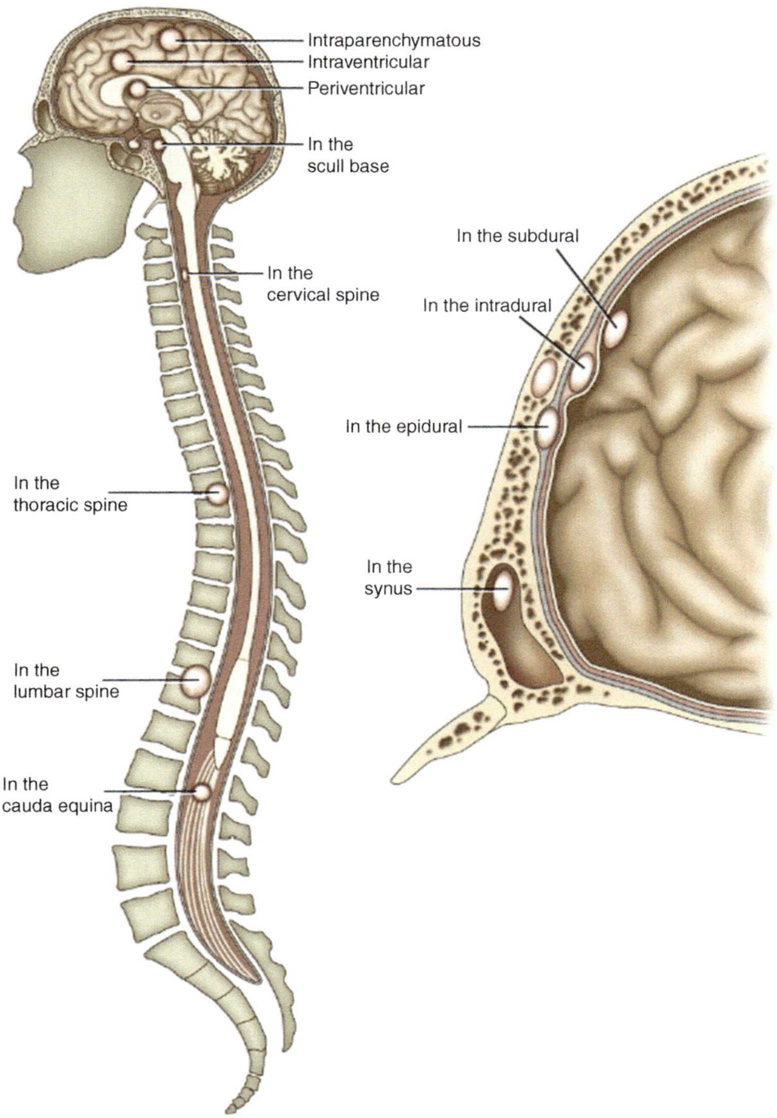

Fig. 21.9 Distribution of the dura mater and the development of various hydatid cysts

Craniocerebral Intradural and Subdural

Unlike neurocisticercosis, literature data shows extremely few cases of intradural manifestations of hydatidosis. Not even data from endemic areas is significant. We describe the case of a 6-year-old child, in which an *E. granulosus* cyst developed between the dura mater and the arachnoid membrane. The cyst had destroyed the frontoparietal skull as it had grown in all directions unhindered (Arseni et al. 1981) (Fig. 21.13).

One other interesting case we found is that of a hydatid cyst which laid both extradurally and subdurally. The larva which traveled via the middle meningeal artery positioned itself in the dura mater. Given the particularities of the dural blood network, the parasite most likely stopped in the deepest layer, which is very similar to the lymphatic capillaries. From here on, the parasite starts to grow and develop more or less as in the case we invoked, in the tissue underneath the dura mater, separated from the cortex by the leptomeninges (Arseni et al. 1981). It is most likely that after the larva perforated the dura mater, it was able to grow both subdurally and epidurally. We feel forced to mention that usually hydatid cysts remain attached to the inner surface of the dura mater.

The surgical approach in such situations is conducted via a wide skin incision that will encircle the whole surface of the cyst. The craniotomy/craniectomy should resect a surface of the skull wider than the cyst. These rare situations cannot be handled through a minimally invasive approach as the purpose of the procedure is to expose the cyst and the adjacent and subjacent structures. The removal of the cyst will be made via the intact enucleation of Arana Iniguez. It consists of delivering the cyst by introduction of a flexible catheter between the cyst and the receiving cavity while injecting hypertonic fluid (Kalangu et al. 2011). A general rule for the

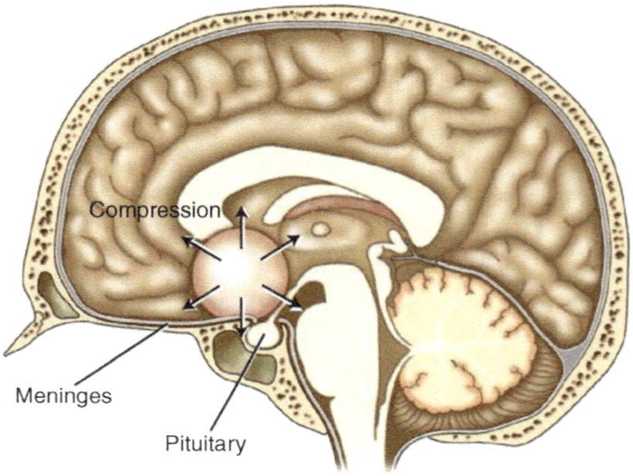

Fig. 21.10 Example of hydatid cyst compressing against the pituitary stalk

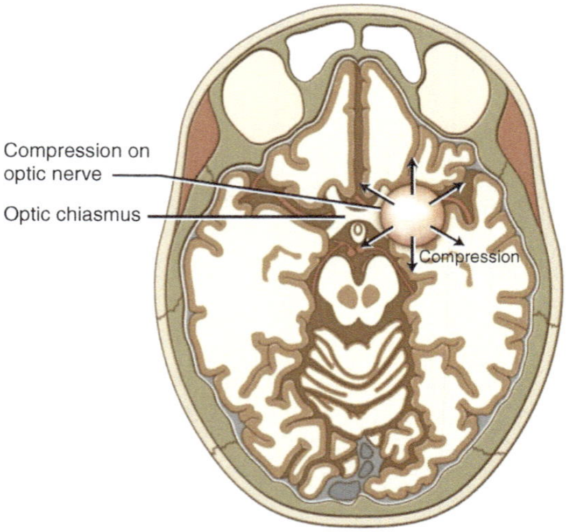

Fig. 21.12 An artistic illustration showing a hydatid cyst in the right parasellar area

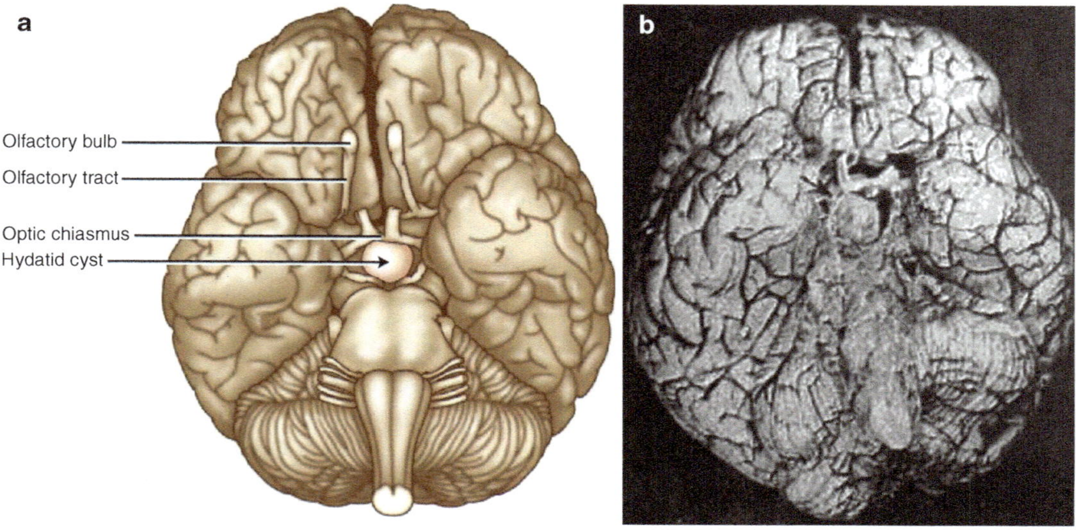

Fig. 21.11 (**a**) Pathology finding of a hydatid cyst behind the optic chiasmus and in front of the pons. Courtesy of the C. Arseni pathology museum. (**b**) Pathology finding of a hydatid cyst behind the optic chiasmus and in front of the pons (Courtesy of the C. Arseni pathology museum)

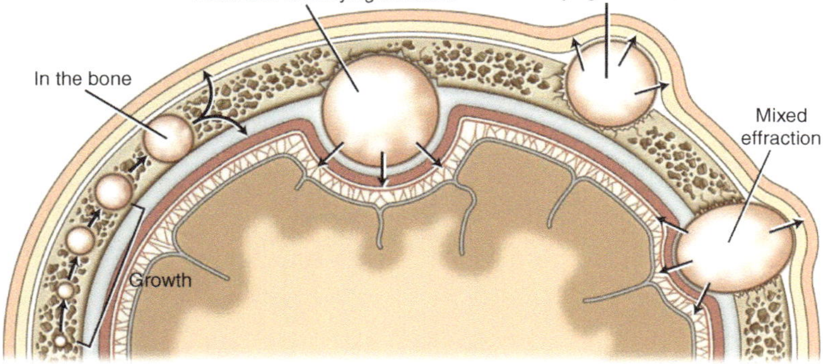

Fig. 21.13 Possibilities of evolution for a hydatid cyst

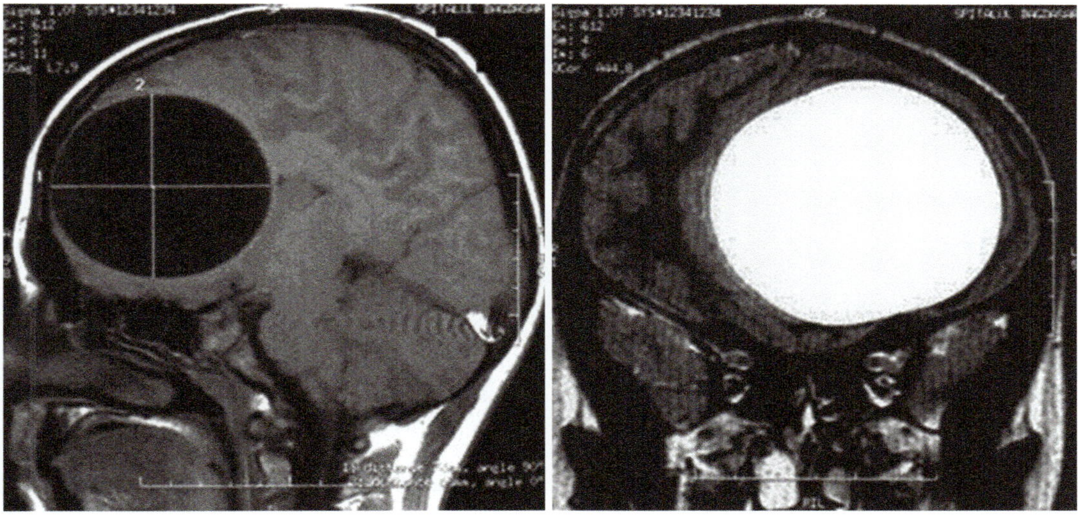

Fig. 21.14 A gigantic frontal cyst

removal of the cysts: preserve the integrity of the cyst at all costs.

The case of subdural hydatid disease is the same as intradural hydatidosis. These are very rare manifestations (Arseni et al. 1981). In the series reported by C. Arseni and V. Marinescu, there are no cases of such nature (Arseni et al. 1981).

Intraencephalic

All the literature data mention the prevalence of hydatidosis in the cerebral hemispheres. Most of the cases of intracerebral hydatidosis are present in the left hemisphere. These cysts can reach tremendous dimensions and volumes, for example, 770 g, as described by Bahloul et al. (2009) (Figs. 21.14 and 21.15).

Cerebral

There is a series of articles worth mentioning in this chapter, as hydatid cysts can take various forms and can come in a wide array of presentations. In one case the hydatid cyst had the unusual appearance of a hemorrhagic infarct (Kanj et al. 2010).

Another strange appearance of a hydatid cyst brought into discussion a strange area of edema resembling a cystic astrocytoma involving a cerebral hemisphere (Bahloul et al. 2009).

The most extreme situation we ever came across was that of a 7-year-old girl. The first manifestation of hydatid disease was raised

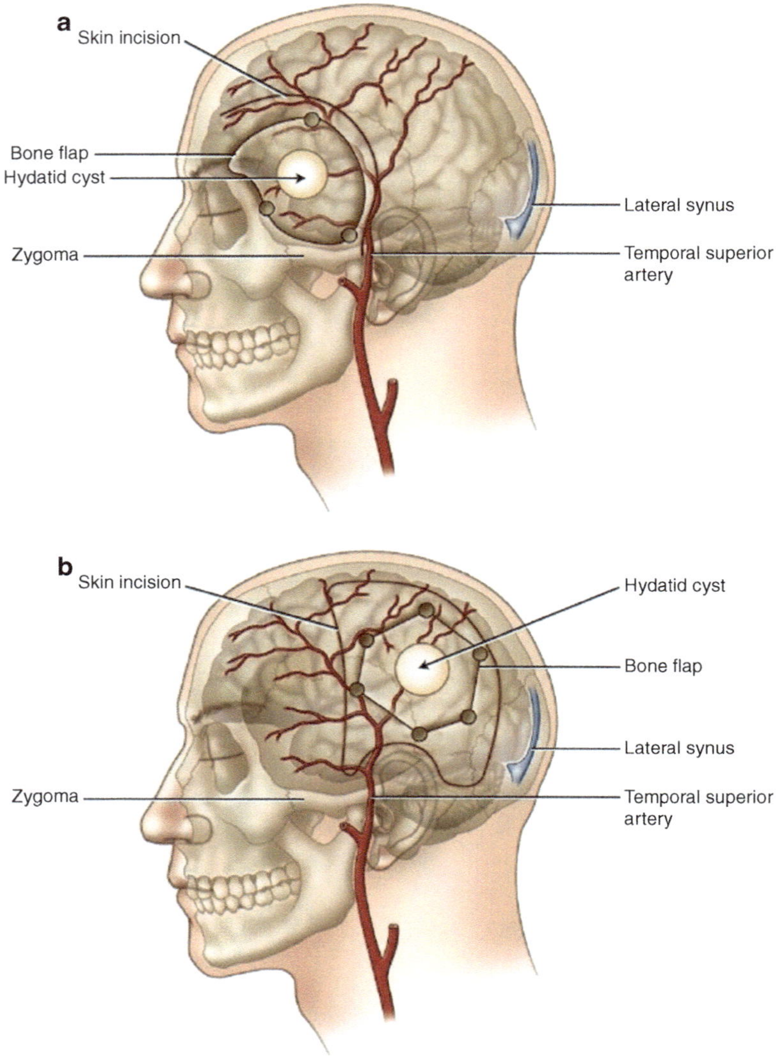

Fig. 21.15 The surgical approach for the craniotomy. (**a**) Frontotemporal hydatid cyst. (**b**) Parietal hydatid cyst. Note: Remember the necessity for large bone flaps

intracranial pressure syndrome. Unfortunately, before the primary ruptured *E. granulosus* cyst was detected in the myocardium of the left ventricle, the patient underwent nine operations over an 8-year period for hydatid embolism affecting the brain among other clinical manifestations. The case was reported by Turgut et al. (1997). The multiple hydatid cysts were the result of a hydatid embolus coming from the heart. Such a possibility must always be taken into account when multiple hydatid cysts are present. Cardiac hydatid disease can generate emboli which in turn can determine reinfections of the brain (Turgut et al. 1997). Stroke as a complication of cardiac hydatidosis is discussed in Chap. 22 in detail.

Cerebral alveolar echinococcosis is a rare but possible manifestation that has a poor prognosis. We report having found in the literature an unusual case presenting with disseminated intracranial lesions secondary to primary hepatic infection (Piotin et al. 1997).

Cerebellar

All the literature data that presents wide series of cases show hydatid cysts in the cerebellum,

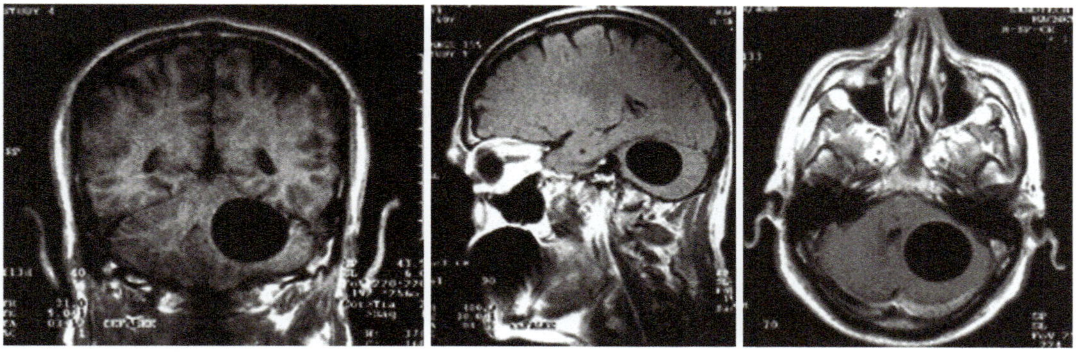

Fig. 21.16 Different views showing a unique cerebellar hydatid cyst

occurring mostly in children. Arseni et al. (1981) collected all the cases in the literature reporting only one case of unique primary cerebellar manifestation of hydatid disease.

In such cases neuroimaging is conclusive just as in cerebral manifestations of hydatid disease (Fig. 21.16). We have personally come across hydatid cysts in the cerebellum. One of our patients was a 9-year-old boy presenting with ataxia and cerebellar syndrome. The investigations showed a large dimension hydatid cyst which was completely excised without incident. Given the young age of the patient, no loss of function occurred and the overall recovery was favorable (Figs. 21.16 and 21.17).

We also report here having found in the modern literature one case involving the cerebellum and the maxillary antrum, a case first described by Copley et al. in 1992.

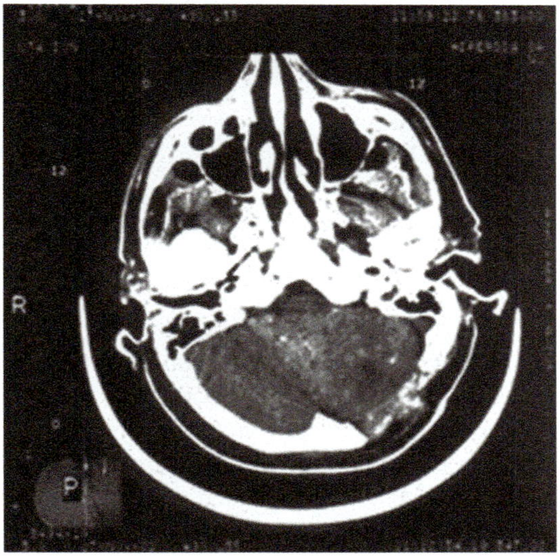

Fig. 21.17 Postoperative aspect of the intervention

Ventricular and Periventricular

Hydatid cysts in the ventricles are reported in all the literature. Of course, this situation is much rarer than in neurocisticercosis (Arseni et al. 1981). In the personal series presented by Arseni et al. in 1981, we noticed five cases of hydatid disease in the lateral ventricles – one in the third ventricle and four cases in the fourth ventricle with a total of ten. This stands for 8.4 % of all intracranial hydatid cysts in Romania at the time.

We present two cases involving the ventricles. The first one is that of a 45-year-old female patient with two primary cerebral hydatid cysts, each one of them being positioned in a separate hemisphere. Imaging studies revealed no evidence of hydatid disease elsewhere in the body. The cysts were removed during two separate interventions. Though the cyst in the right posterior parietal lobe was delivered unruptured, 7 months later, a new cyst was detected in the same cavity, which seems to show relatively rapid growth in a year. The latter was also delivered intact. This case is presented here for its unusual features such as having two primary cerebral hydatid cysts simultaneously in separate hemispheres, one of which partly localized intraventricular, and the occurrence of a new cyst in the

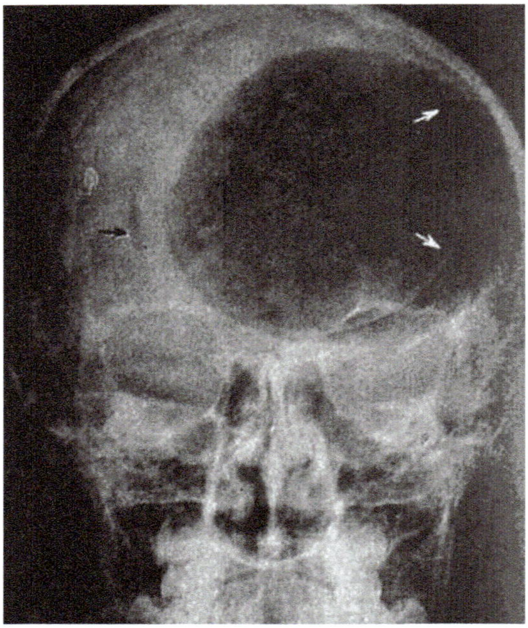

Fig. 21.18 Ventriculography showing a gigantic hydatid cyst in the left ventricle. The right lateral ventricle (*black arrow*) and the contour of the cyst (*white arrows*)

same cavity following intact removal of the previous cyst (Karadağ et al. 2004).

Another reported case shows that hydatid disease can manifest through hemichorea. The discovered cyst was situated periventricular (Iplikçioğlu et al. 1992).

The last article we quoted for this topic shows three children with hydatid disease of the central nervous system. In two patients the lateral ventricles were involved, while one case involved the cerebellar hemisphere. In addition, one child presented with a deposit in the maxillary antrum (Copley et al. 1992) (Fig. 21.18).

The intraventricular hydatidosis is discussed in Chap. 7 in detail.

Brainstem and Basal Ganglia

Such a location is exceptional, even regarding hydatid disease. Even wide series of cases such as those of Paillas and Bonnal or Arseni and Marinescu contain no such cases (Arseni et al. 1981).

In the last years reports from endemic areas have shown sporadic manifestations of such difficulty. Without regard to all difficulties concerning diagnosis and surgical treatment, total removal and good global outcome were achieved.

We present three such cases in which the brainstem and basal ganglia were involved. The first case presents an extremely rare case of a thalamic cyst with a successful total removal via contralateral transcallosal approach (Kurtsoy et al. 1999). The second case (Muthusubramanian et al. 2009) shows a hydatid cyst in the brainstem of a 40-year-old female. She presented with headache, progressive right-sided weakness, double vision, and unsteadiness of gait of 1-month duration. On examination, she had a left one-and-a-half syndrome, right hemiparesis, and left cerebellar signs. CT and MRI scans of the brain revealed a solitary, cystic lesion in the brainstem more toward the left side with features suggestive of hydatid cyst. A left retromastoid craniectomy was performed, followed by a left middle cerebellar peduncle approach. Aspiration of the cyst and total excision of the cyst followed. Postoperatively, the patient improved progressively and was asymptomatic with minimal left cerebellar signs at 1-year follow-up. Last but not least, the third case comes with a completely exceptional manifestation: pontine hydatid cyst in association with an acoustic neurinoma (Mascalchi et al. 1991).

Unusual Positions in the Venous Sinuses

During a multifocal infection with *E. granulosus*, there is an extremely low chance that the larva will position itself in the cavernous sinus generating all the associated symptoms. Such a situation is more than exceptional, but we found a case in the literature coming from Turkey (Kireşi et al. 2003).

Cisternal

The existence of hydatidosis in the cisternal spaces must not be neglected given the capacity of *E. granulosus* larvae to disseminate via the cerebrospinal fluid (CSF) (Andronikou et al. 2002).

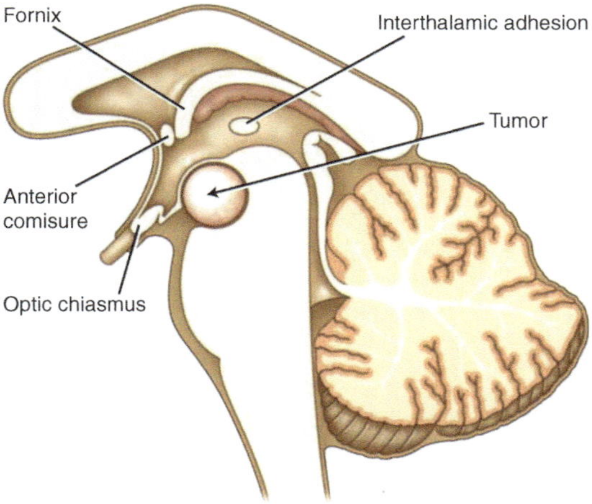

Fig. 21.19 A hydatid cyst in the interpeduncular cistern

Generally any case of multiple hydatid cysts must be carefully investigated for any overlooked hydatid cysts in the skull. This includes the cisternal spaces as well.

We present two cases. The first one is the case of an isolated multilocular hydatid cyst occurring in the basilar cisterns, with nondependent levels of different signal intensities shown on MRIs. Three portions were visualized on T1-weighted images: the hyperintense inferior aspect, the isointense central part, and the superior aspect of lower signal intensity. The inferior portion was hypointense on T2-weighted images. This unusual appearance was caused by layering of hydatid sand and may represent a characteristic feature of hydatid disease (Rumboldt et al. 2003). The second one is the first case in the literature of a hydatid cyst in the interpeduncular cistern (Beskonakli et al. 2005) (Fig. 21.19).

Orbital

Orbital hydatid cysts are known in the entire world as rare manifestations of *E. granulosus* infection. There are various references in the literature regarding the primary orbital manifestations of hydatidosis or orbital manifestations of hydatidosis during multiple dissemination. We will not insist upon these due to their description in Chap. 23 (Figs. 21.20 and 21.21).

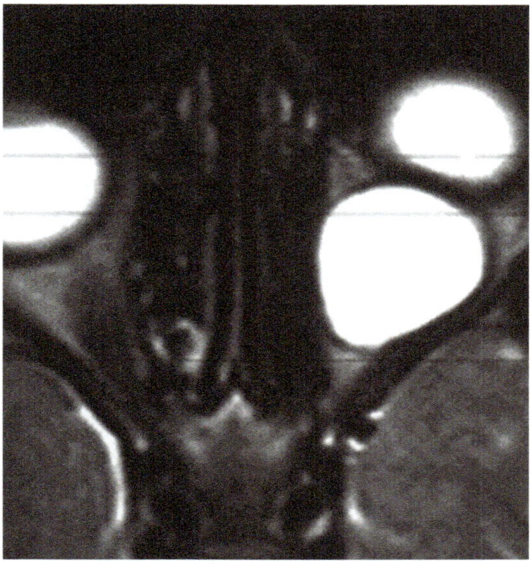

Fig. 21.20 A hydatid cyst in the orbit

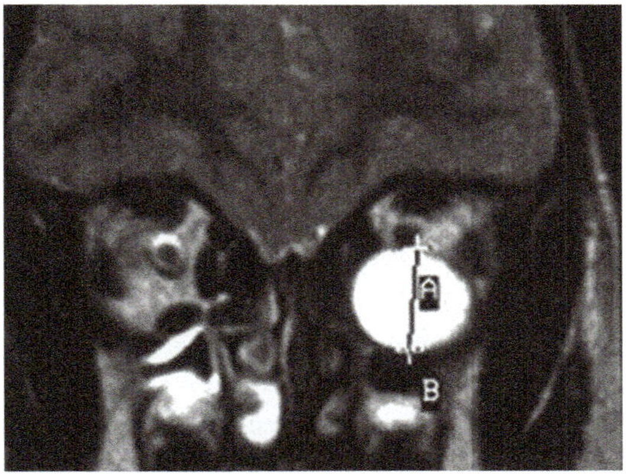

Fig. 21.21 A hydatid cyst in the orbit. *A* represents the coronal diameter of the presented cyst, *B* represents the cyst itself

Unusual Manifestations of Vertebromedullary Hydatid Disease

Although it accounts for 0.5–2 % of all the cases in the literature involving bone dissemination (Papakonstantinou et al. 2011), spinal hydatid disease is much more frequently met than that of the skull given the capacity of the protoscoleces to disseminate via blood and CSF. A second fac-

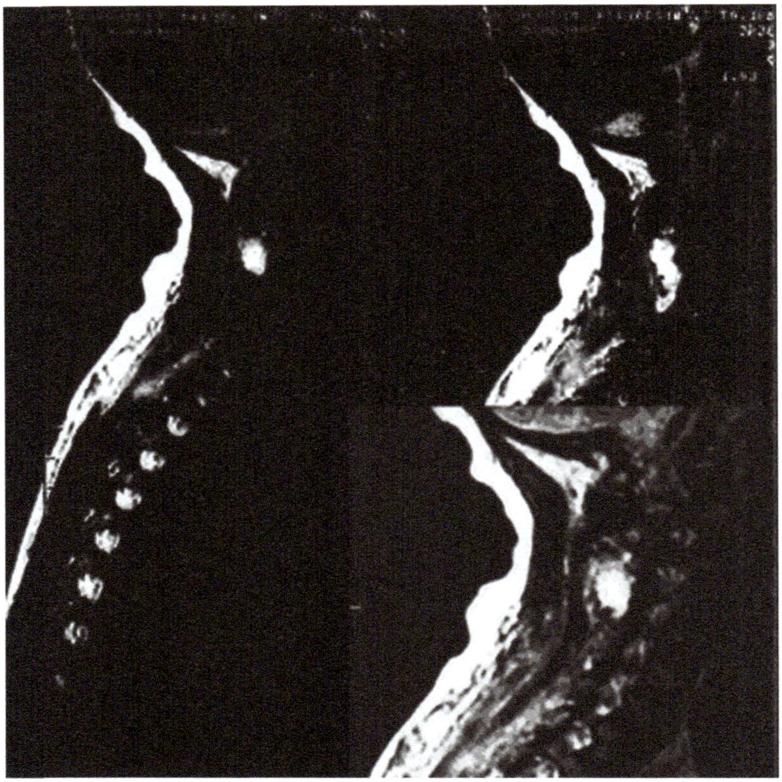

Fig. 21.22 An extreme hydatid cyst in the spine

tor facilitating this migration is the intense vascularization of the spine which often proves to be a dissemination pathway for several pathologies including cancer and polio.

In Deve's series from 1949 there are 281 cases of hydatid disease in the spine – including the sacrum (quoted from Arseni et al. 1981). This stands for 44.2 % of all the manifestations of hydatidosis in the skeleton. Research data advocates for the preponderant disposition of hydatid disease in the thoracic vertebrae.

All the classic authors – Arana Iniguez, Acquaviva, Arseni, and Marinescu – describe multiple cases of hydatid disease in the spine, with a maximum of incidence at patients well past their third decade of life and of male gender. In all these situations multiple hydatid cysts were present in all the patients.

It is Deve who suggested two possible pathways of spinal infestation (quoted from Arseni et al. 1981). One pathway is the pathogenic dissemination of the parasitic embolus from the lung, for example, to the spine via the blood and the other via effraction from the pleura to the extraosseous space.

In the actual literature spinal hydatid disease is widely mentioned. A noticeable aspect is the danger posed by infections with alveolar hydatid disease which has a more severe prognosis. The hydatidosis of the spine and spinal cord is discussed in detail in Chaps. 8, 9, 12, 14, and 20.

Vertebral (Bone Involvement)

Although vertebral hydatid disease has been mentioned in all the studies regarding parasitoses, in the western European countries and in the United States, cases like these are now considered true curiosities. Hydatid disease in the spine attacks all levels – including the cervical spine and lumbar spine – and if untreated can lead up to multilevel vertebral instability as a result of progressive bone destruction. We personally came across one case of hydatid disease manifesting itself in the cervical spine (Fig. 21.22).

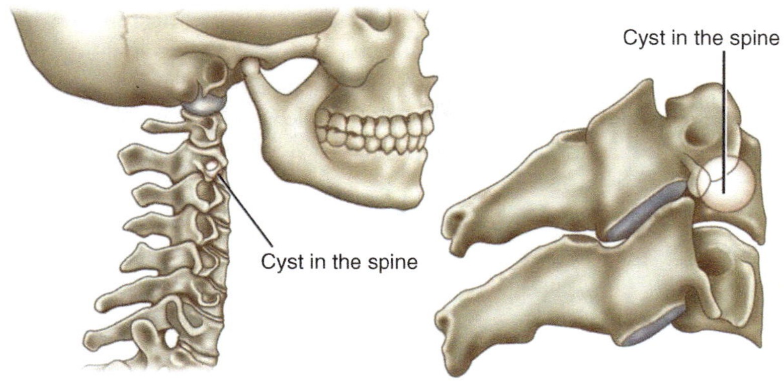

Fig. 21.23 Artistic illustration of the cyst we describe based on the image above

The case we present is old. At the time of the surgery, the true nature of the cystic lesion was only suspected. The diagnosis was confirmed intraoperatively (Fig. 21.23).

Spinal Extradural

Ever since the papers of Deve 1926 mentioning only two cases (quoted by Arseni et al. in 1981), extradural manifestations of hydatidosis were mentioned despite its very low frequency; these cases are reported in the endemic areas. In 1946, two Romanians (Cosacescu and Vereanu) reported a cyst, the size of a chicken egg, which had eroded the spinous processes and the laminae of the S1 and S2 vertebrae (quoted from Arseni et al. 1981). Benhamou and Goinard (1929) mention seven such cases (quoted from Arseni et al. 1981). Chitkara and Colab mention a 17-year-old male with a hydatid cyst positioned at the level of the T1-T2 vertebrae, extradural, on the left side (quoted from Arseni et al. 1981). The cyst formed a cavity at the level of the intervertebral foramen and had an unfortunate evolution which left the patient paraplegic. The pathology findings showed a 3.81 cm cyst. Lagrot and Colab found in an 8-year-old female patient a hydatid cyst the size of a walnut at the level of the L1 vertebral body (quoted from Arseni et al. 1981). The literature of the twentieth century contains sporadic cases of extradural hydatid cysts; however, we feel that we need to present twenty-first-century cases.

In this respect we came up with a series of cases we found in the literature which are perfect for the illustration of extradural space involvement with hydatid disease of the spine. The first case we present is a study on four patients. Out of those four, hydatid disease involved the lumbar spine in two patients, the thoracolumbar spine in one patient, and the lumbosacral in the last patient. All four patients had extensive involvement of the extradural space (Papakonstantinou et al. 2011).

The youngest patient ever met was a 4-year-old boy. He manifested a primary spinal extradural hydatid cyst in the thoracic spine (Eloqayli et al. 2010). For didactic purposes we mention the fact that primitive manifestations of hydatid disease in the spine are referred to as "Hydatid Pott Disease."

According to Arseni et al. (1981) the vertebral body implications manifest as follows: 45 % of all parasitic involvement is placed in the vertebral body, 19 % attacks the posterior arch of the vertebra, and 36 % of all parasitic disseminations at this level attack both the body and the arch. A modern study however shows that hydatid cysts can attack the vertebral laminae, the spinous processes, the pedicles, the articular processes, and the transverse processes as well.

Spinal Intradural and Subdural

The medical literature contains sporadic cases of intradural hydatid disease of the spine. These cases are considered to be exceptional. Most of the cases reported to present intradural manifestations of hydatidosis in the spine have their authenticity discussed. A multivesicular hydatid disease could easily be mistaken for a neurocisticercosis case. In 1932 Deve presented only three cases (quoted from Arseni et al. 1981). Goinard and Descuns (1952) presented another three (quoted from Arseni et al. 1981). Grossiord et al. (1955) noted in a female patient in Ethiopia several crowded hydatid vesicles in a tight web made out of arachnoid fibers (quoted from Arseni et al. 1981). The roots of the cauda equina were stuck together. The postoperative evolution of the patient was positive in spite of anal sensitivity impairment and paraplegia. The pronounced adhesive arachnoiditis explained the absence of the parasite in the cephalic subarachnoid spaces. A more recent case describing an intradural cyst was reported by Fahl et al., in 1994.

Spinal Intramedullary

Intramedullary hydatidosis is known and reported by all the classic authors including Acquaviva, Arseni, and Colab. Research data is consistent showing affections mostly at thoracic levels. In the Arseni-Marinescu-Ciurea statistics, out of 35 cases of hydatidosis in the spinal cord, 20 are at the thoracic level (Arseni et al. 1981). In the number of reported hydatid disease manifestations in the spine, there are some unusual cases worth mentioning.

Arseni et al. (1981) reported a single such case of spinal manifestation. The patient was a 41-year-old female previously operated for a pulmonary hydatid cyst 1 year earlier. The patient was admitted for motor deficit of the legs, trophic disturbances, sphincteric disturbances, and impaired sensitivity. She manifested flask paraplegia, abolished osteotendinous reflexes, urinary incontinence, and xantochromic CSF.

A wide T_6-T_{12} laminectomy was performed. The dural sack was incised widely. A series of yellowish, fragile membranes that had been wrapped around the medulla were removed. Having proceeded lower, toward the inferior pole of T_{12}, the surgeon was able to identify a white milky membrane that had developed caudally for 12 cm in the shape of a cyst and another one of 10 cm which was side by side with the first one. The medulla had holes in it, and after the surgery, the patient did not improve.

The existence of two cysts in the spine comes as a hint toward the idea that a first cyst had ruptured and disseminated either in the spinal or cephalic CSF. In the current data available, intramedullar hydatid cysts behave exactly like a perfectly delimited medullar compression. In this respect the differential diagnosis must be made with any kind of cystic tumor at this level.

The perfect targets for this affection are young people coming from the rural parts of countries in endemic areas. Multiple disseminations and perfectly delimited cystic lesions indicate the diagnosis and the treatment. The cyst's integrity must be preserved. The surgical treatment imposes a gentle delimitation with cottonoid and the delivery of the cyst via hypertonic fluid injection in the receiving cavity with a flexible catheter.

Conclusion

The following is concluded: (1) Hydatid disease classically involves the liver, lungs, and brain but can involve almost any organ and numerous organs simultaneously. (2) Whether hydatid disease is discovered incidentally or by intentional imaging, extended imaging is recommended to identify multifocal disease. (3) All patients with one known cyst should undergo a minimum CT scan of the abdomen, chest, and brain. The combination of clinical history, imaging findings, and serologic test results usually helps the diagnosis. (4) Imagistic findings are pathognomonic for hydatid disease. (5) Hydatid cysts represent a delayed emergency due to their compression on the central nervous system. (6) Any kind of hydatid cyst – single or multiple – must be immediately removed surgically. (7) There is no temporization and the treatment must not be delayed. Through anthelmintic medication the cysts die but they remain as physical compressive elements. (8) The treatment of hydatid disease is prophylactic – targeted on disrupting the vicious circle taking place between dogs and men. A good sanitary education and hygiene will lead rapidly to the lowering of the number of people infested.

References

Andronikou S, Welman CJ, Kader E. Classic and unusual appearances of hydatid disease in children. Pediatr Radiol. 2002;32:817–28.

Arseni C, Ciurea AV, Cristescu A, Horvath L, Marinescu V. Parasitoses of the central nervous system. Bucharest: The Scientific and Encyclopedic Publishing House; 1981.

Bahloul K, Ouerchefani N, Kammoun B, Boudouara MZ. Unusual brain edema caused by an intracranial hydatid cyst: case report and literature review. Neurochirurgie. 2009;55:53–6.

Behari S, Banerji D, Phadke RV, Shukla S, Krishnani N, Chhabra DK. Multiple infected extradural parasellar hydatid cysts. Surg Neurol. 1997;48:53–7.

Benhamou ED, Goinard P. L'echinococcose intra-rachidienne. Rev Neurol. 1929;2:657–97.

Beskonakli E, Solaroglu I, Tun K, Albayrak L. Primary intracranial hydatid cyst in the interpeduncular cistern. Acta Neurochir (Wien). 2005;147:781–3.

Copley IB, Fripp PJ, Erasmus AM, Otto DD. Unusual presentations of cerebral hydatid disease in children. Br J Neurosurg. 1992;6:203–10.

Deve F. CR Soc Biol (Paris). 1926;94:440

Eckert J, Gemmell MA, Meslin FX, Pawłowski ZS. WHO/OIE manual on echinococcosis in humans and animals: a public health problem of global concern. Paris: World Organization for Animal Health (Office International des Epizooties)/World Health Organization; 2001.

Eloqayli H, Matalka I, Daoud S. Primary spinal extradural hydatid cyst in a 4-year-old child. Br J Neurosurg. 2010;24:602–3.

Fahl M, Haddad FS, Hubballah M, Kan'an S, Husheimi I, Azizi T. Magnetic resonance imaging in Intradural and extradural spinal echinococcosis. Clin Imaging. 1994; 18:179–83.

Goinard P, Descuns P. Les kystes hydatiques du névraxe. Rev Neurol. 1952;86:369–415.

Goldsher M, Eliachar I, Joachims Z, Golz A. Primary hydatid cyst of the maxillary sinus. J Laryngol Otol. 1983;97:869–70.

Grossiord A, Pecker J, Bitry-Boely C. Vesicular echinococcosis of the cauda equina. Bull Mem Soc Med Hop Paris. 1955;71:289–94.

Iplikçioğlu AC, Ozek MM, Ozer AF, Ozgen T. Periventricular hydatid cyst presenting with hemichorea. Childs Nerv Syst. 1992;8:292–3.

Kalangu K, Kato Y, Dechambenoit G. Essential practice of neurosurgery. Nagoya: Access Publishing; 2011.

Kanj AH, Fares YH, Yehya RR, Hamzeh FF. Unusual appearance of a cerebral hydatid cyst as a hemorrhagic infarct. Neurosciences (Riyadh). 2010;15:275–6.

Karadağ O, Gürelik M, Ozüm U, Göksel HM. Primary multiple cerebral hydatid cysts with unusual features. Acta Neurochir (Wien). 2004;146:73–7.

Kireşi DA, Karabacakoğlu A, Odev K, Karaköse S. Uncommon locations of hydatid cysts. Acta Radiol. 2003;44:622–36.

Kurtsoy A, Oktem IS, Koç RK, Akdemir H, Menkü A, Tucer B. Successful surgical treatment of a thalamic hydatid cyst with contralateral transcallosal approach. Case report and review of the literature. Pediatr Neurosurg. 1999;31:96–9.

Llanes EG, Stibal A, Mühlethaler K, Vajtai I, Häusler R, Caversaccio M. Echinococcosis presenting as an otogenic brain abscess: an unusual lesion of the middle ear cleft and temporal lobe. Auris Nasus Larynx. 2008;35:115–20.

Mascalchi M, Ragazzoni A, Dal Pozzo G. Pontine hydatid cyst in association with an acoustic neurinoma: MR appearance in an unusual case. AJNR Am J Neuroradiol. 1991;12:78–9.

Mazor M, Picard R, Tauber E, Hagay ZJ, Leiberman JR. Restoration of fertility following excision of an intracranial hydatid cyst. J Gynecol Obstet Biol Reprod (Paris). 1986;15:909–11.

Muthusubramanian V, Pande A, Vasudevan MC, Ravi R. Surgical management of brainstem hydatid cyst -an unusual site. Surg Neurol. 2009;71:103–6.

Papakonstantinou O, Athanassopoulou A, Passomenos D, Kalogeropoulos I, Balanika A, Baltas C, Gouliamos A, Guglielmi G. Recurrent vertebral hydatid disease: spectrum of MR imaging features. Singapore Med J. 2011;52:440–5.

Piotin M, Cattin F, Kantelip B, Miralbès S, Godard J, Bonneville JF. Disseminated intracerebral alveolar echinococcosis: CT and MRI. Neuroradiology. 1997; 39:431–3.

Rumboldt Z, Jednacak H, Talan-Hranilović J, Rumboldt T, Kalousek M. Unusual appearance of a cisternal hydatid cyst. AJNR Am J Neuroradiol. 2003;24:112–4.

Schroeder AH, Medoc J. Quiste hidático de cerebro. Archivos de pediatría del Uruguay. 1953;24:559–580.

Sharma T, Khosla VK, Brar R. Primary extradural hydatid cyst associated with nephrotic syndrome in a pediatric patient. Childs Nerv Syst. 2010;26:1247–9.

Siddiqui MA, Rizvi SW, Rizvi SA, Ahmad I, Ullah E. Atypical multifocal hydatid disease of cranial vault: simultaneous orbital and extradural meningeal involvement. Emerg Radiol. 2010;17:427–30.

Turgut M, Benli K, Eryilmaz M. Secondary multiple intracranial hydatid cysts caused by intracerebral embolism of cardiac echinococcosis: an exceptional case of hydatidosis. Case report. J Neurosurg. 1997;86:714–8.

Stroke as a Complication of Cardiac Hydatidosis

22

Mehmet Turgut, Ahmet Tuncay Turgut, and Vikram S. Dogra

Contents

M. Turgut, MD, PhD
Department of Neurosurgery, Adnan Menderes University School of Medicine, Aydin, Turkey
e-mail: drmturgut@yahoo.com

A.T. Turgut, MD
Department of Radiology, Ankara Training and Research Hospital, Ankara, Turkey

V.S. Dogra, MD (✉)
Department of Imaging Sciences, University of Rochester School of Medicine, Rochester, NY 14642, USA
e-mail: vikram_dogra@urmc.rochester.edu

Introduction

Hydatid disease is still a serious disease in some regions of the world such as Australia, New Zealand, North Africa, Europe, Asia Minor, the Middle East, and South America, while it is not a major public health problem in most Western countries (Byard and Bourne 1991; Turgut and Bayülkem 1998; Turgut 2001, 2002). The epidemiology of *Echinococcus* in the world is discussed in Chaps. 2, 3, and 4.

Hydatidosis is commonly caused by *Echinococcus granulosus*. The normal life cycle of the tapeworm *E. granulosus* involves passage from definitive carnivore hosts, with transmission of eggs to an accidental intermediate host. Infection of humans with the cestode is usually caused by inadvertent contamination with eggs from infected dogs as follows: (1) by eating contaminated vegetables, (2) by soiling their mouth after patting infested dogs, or (3) by inhaling dust carrying dried ova (Haddad and Haddad 2005). The ova hatch in the intestine, and the larvae reach the liver, through the portal system, where a hydatid cyst may be formed, but the ova may bypass the liver and settle in the lung (Haddad and Haddad 2005). Routes of infestation and site of primary echinococcal cysts in man are the intestine (very rare), liver (75 %), lungs (8.5 %), and heart (0.5 %), and then muscles (5.5 %), spleen (2.5 %), kidney (2.0 %), brain (1.5 %), bone (1.5 %), and miscellaneous parts (3.5 %) via systemic circulation (Peters et al. 1945). Thus, it is obvious that the heart and brain are quite infrequently affected

M. Turgut (ed.), *Hydatidosis of the Central Nervous System: Diagnosis and Treatment*, DOI 10.1007/978-3-642-54359-3_22,

organs, although multiorgan involvement is common in hydatid disease.

Cardiac Hydatidosis

Cardiac involvement by *E. granulosus* is rare and has a reported incidence of 0.5 % of cases in the literature (Peters et al. 1945), because contraction of the heart provides natural resistance to the maintenance of viable hydatid cysts. The first report of hydatidosis of the heart dates from 1836, and the first successful surgical operation for hydatid disease in the left ventricular wall of the heart was performed in 1932 (quoted from Peters et al. 1945).

At present, it is commonly accepted that the oncosphere reaches the cavities of the heart through the coronary arteries by traveling through the myocardium or through pulmonary veins. In cases of cardiac hydatidosis, the most common location is the left ventricle (60 %), followed by the right ventricle (17 %), interventricular septum (9 %), right atrium (8 %), left atrium (4 %), interatrial septum (2 %), and pericardium (very rarely) (Fig. 22.1) (Aleksic-Shihabi and Vidolin 2008; Byard 2009). Amongst these anatomical chambers of the heart, a high frequency of left ventricular hydatidosis is possibly due to various factors including dominance of the left coronary artery, the presence of a big myocardial mass in the left ventricle, and different pressure gradients (Thameur et al. 2001). It has been suggested that hydatid cysts in the pericardium generally occur as a result of rupture of a primitive cardiac cyst (Deve 1946).

As a rule, left-sided cysts tend to grow subepicardially, while right-sided cysts have a tendency to expand subendocardially (Dursun et al. 2008). There are five patterns of hydatid disease of the heart: (1) dead calcified cysts, (2) living intact cysts, (3) ruptured pericardial cysts, (4) pediculated intracavitary cysts, and (5) ruptured intracavitary cysts (Peters et al. 1945). A ruptured cyst is a serious complication of cardiac hydatidosis. It is important to know that right ventricular cyst rupture leads to pulmonary embolus, severe anaphylactic shock, or sudden death (Dursun et al. 2008). The ruptured hydatid cyst results in systemic emboli in organs supplied by the aortic circulation such as the (1) brain (64 %), kidney (17.5 %), spleen (17.5 %), and liver (1 %) (Peters et al. 1945).

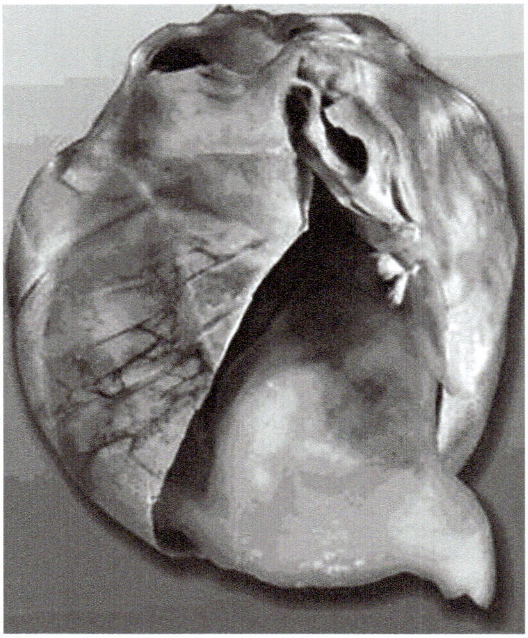

Fig. 22.1 Macroscopic photo of the heart at autopsy demonstrates hydatid cyst filling the left ventricle as a cause of sudden death (From Byard (2009), with permission)

Clinically, the following sequential stages of the hydatid disease develop after direct rupture of a primitive cyst of the heart:

1. Onset stage, characterized by general malaise with signs of anaphylaxis ranging from only a rash to an allergic shock
2. Asymptomatic stage, characterized by embolic dissemination of the parasite into various organs in the body through the pulmonary or systemic aortic circulation
3. Metastatic stage, characterized by development of pulmonary or visceral secondary hydatidosis within the host
4. Complication stage, characterized by development of various complications such as bacterial infection of the pericyst cavity, related to the secondary localization of the hydatidosis (Deve 1946)

Importantly, it has been noted that the aforementioned four stages are independent of the location of the rupture (intracavitary, intramyocardial, or intrapericardial) (Thameur et al. 2001). It has been reported that the intrapericardial location occurs as a result of rupture of a primitive hydatid lesion (Dursun et al. 2008). The early diagnosis and treatment of cases with cardiac hydatidosis during the initial phase of rupture characterized by the history of allergic reactions is very important to prevent possible fatal risk of rupture. As expected, the diagnosis of cardiac hydatid cyst is easy when the secondary location is symptomatic (Thameur et al. 2001).

In the cases of cardiac hydatidosis, chest pain and cough are the most common initial signs, followed by fever, arrhythmias, cardiac syncope, acute myocardial infarction, pulmonary hypertension, pericarditis, pulmonary embolism, anaphylactic shock, or unexpected death (Aleksic-Shihabi and Vidolin 2008). The sudden death in cases with cardiac hydatidosis results from "obstruction" of the chambers of the heart or "embolism" of pulmonary or carotid arteries by migrated cyst fragments, following intracavitary rupture of the cyst in the right or left heart (Thameur et al. 2001).

The symptoms and signs depend on the anatomical location of the hydatid embolus, including the cerebral arteries, the abdominal aorta, or its branches including the extremity arteries. Imaging studies such as plain radiography, computed tomography (CT), magnetic resonance imaging (MRI), and ultrasonography (US) provide very useful information for the diagnosis of cardiac hydatid disease, although echocardiography (EC) remains the most efficient diagnostic method (Aleksic-Shihabi and Vidolin 2008). In clinical practice, hydatid cyst of the heart is generally sterilized before removal with 30 % hypertonic saline solution or other scolicidal agents including 0.1–1 % cetrimide, 2 % formalin, 1 % iodine, or 0.5 % silver nitrate (Maroto et al. 1998).

Cerebral Hydatidosis

Cerebral hydatid cyst can be single fertile "primary" containing hydatid sand or multiple metastatic "secondary," which is sterile and does not have a germinative layer, due to spontaneous, surgical, or traumatic rupture of a primary cyst (Fig. 22.2) (Turgut and Bayülkem 1998; Turgut 2001, 2002; Byard 2009). It is well known that the sterile cysts do not form secondary cysts in case of rupture, if no sand is present in the cyst (Haddad and Haddad 2005). Nevertheless, there is no consensus as to the route the larvae take from the gut to the brain for primary hydatidosis: the larvae

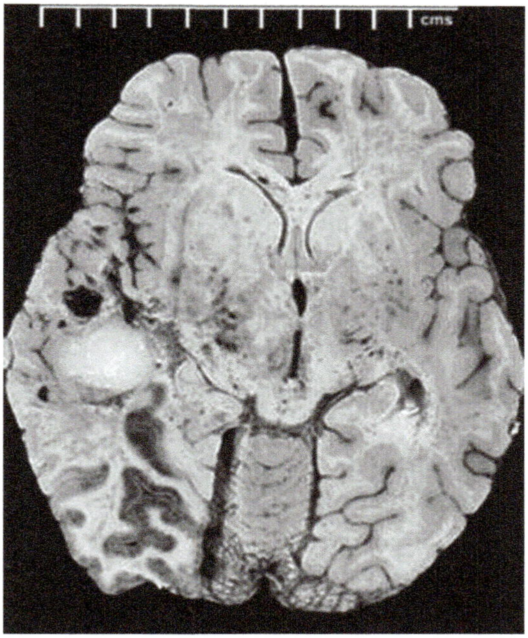

Fig. 22.2 Macroscopic photo of the brain at autopsy reveals a large hydatid cyst in the left temporal lobe (From Byard (2009), with permission)

reach the right heart through the inferior vena cava and the brain in case of a patent septal cardiac foramen or arteriovenous channels in the lung (Haddad and Haddad 2005). On the other hand, as described above, secondary cysts in the brain result from the rupture of the primary cysts localized in the left compartments of the heart.

In general, the clinical picture is dominated by the symptoms of increased intracranial pressure (IICP) with or without hydrocephalus in children, while in adults, the focal neurological signs related to infarcts or cysts located in the watershed of the abovementioned cerebral arteries, such as hemiparesis, epileptic seizures, and aphasia, are usually the first to appear (Abada et al. 1977; Turgut and Bayülkem 1998; Turgut 2001, 2002). It has also been reported that children with multiple hydatid may present with focal neurological signs (Turgut and Bayülkem 1998; Turgut 2001, 2002).

Neuroimaging modalities, such as CT and MRI, are the most valuable diagnostic tools for diagnosing cerebral hydatid disease. Typically, hydatid cyst has a density similar to that of cerebrospinal fluid on CT scans and MRI (Haddad and Haddad 2005). It is important to know that multiple cysts are more often seen in cases secondary to cardiac embolization

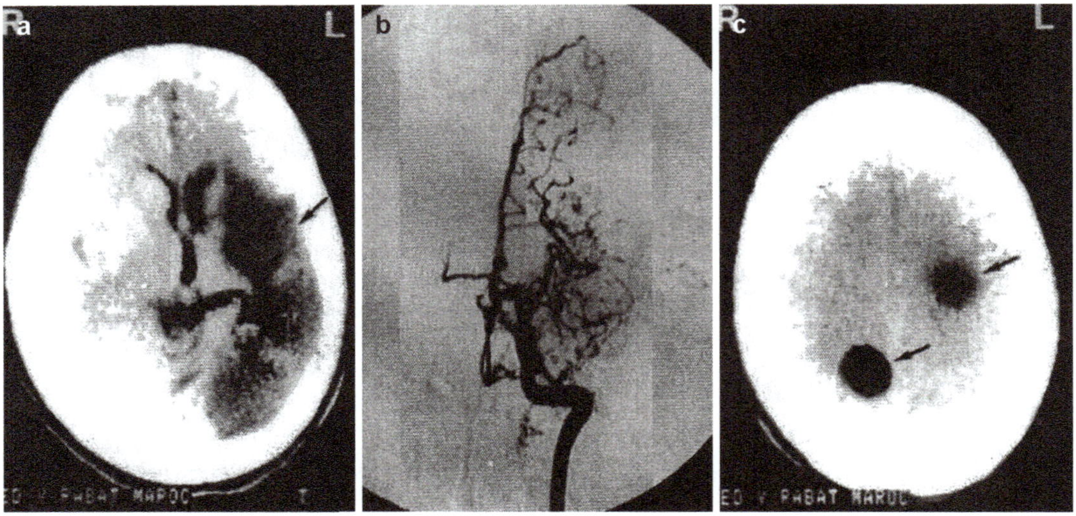

Fig. 22.3 Development of cyst in a previously infarcted region of the brain following hydatid occlusion of the cerebral artery. (**a**) CT shows infarct (*arrow*) of the left middle cerebral artery (MCA). (**b**) Angiogram demonstrates occlusion of the left MCA. (**c**) CT displays cystic lesions (*arrows*) in the infarcted region of the brain (From Benomar et al. (1994), with permission)

through the vascular system (Turgut et al. 1997). In some cases with hydatidosis, the pericyst layer may be calcified owing to the calcium deposition, and there is no peripheral enhancement of the cyst. Recently, it has been suggested that the differentiation of fertile and sterile cysts may be possible with proton MR spectroscopy (Garg et al. 2002).

Today, the treatment of choice is surgical removal of the cysts if possible. In complicated cases, various techniques including tapping of the cyst and injection of a devitalizing solution such as formalin or hypertonic saline other than the Dowling-Orlando technique may be useful before removal of the cyst (Turgut 2001). Rupture of the cyst into the subarachnoid space as complication of surgery may result in severe anaphylactic response (Buris et al. 1987).

Anthelmintics are recommended in patients with multiple cysts and in those unfit for surgery or suffering from recurrent disease (Turgut and Bayülkem 1998; Turgut 2001, 2002). In such instances, anthelmintics such as mebendazole, liposomal and tablet albendazole, or praziquantel should be administered during the perioperative period, although the efficacy of medical treatment is questionable in hydatidosis. Nonetheless, large and symptomatic cysts should be surgically treated first, and the patient should be closely followed up for the need for reoperation in the future.

In addition to different chemotherapeutical agents, clinical and imaging findings of cerebral hydatidosis are discussed in detail in Chaps. 6, 11, and 16.

Stroke as a Complication of Cardiac Hydatidosis

"Stroke" as a complication of cardiac hydatidosis, a cause of ischemic or hemorrhagic infarction and multiple metastatic cyst formations, is an extremely rare entity (Byard and Bourne 1991; Turgut et al. 1997; Turgut and Bayülkem 1998). It results from spontaneous, traumatic, or surgical rupture of a fertile cardiac cyst and embolization of the germinative membrane, scolices, or portions of endocyst. Basically, there are two pathological types of "stroke" from cardiac embolization: (1) acute obstruction of a cerebral artery, partial or complete, with a piece of embolized cyst membrane and (2) development of multiple cyst formations in the infarcted area following embolism of scolices during the course of several months. In young patients with the diagnosis of stroke, subsequent development of "cerebral cyst" within the necrotic area of the brain tissue, called "cerebral infarct," strongly suggests embolism of ruptured cardiac hydatid

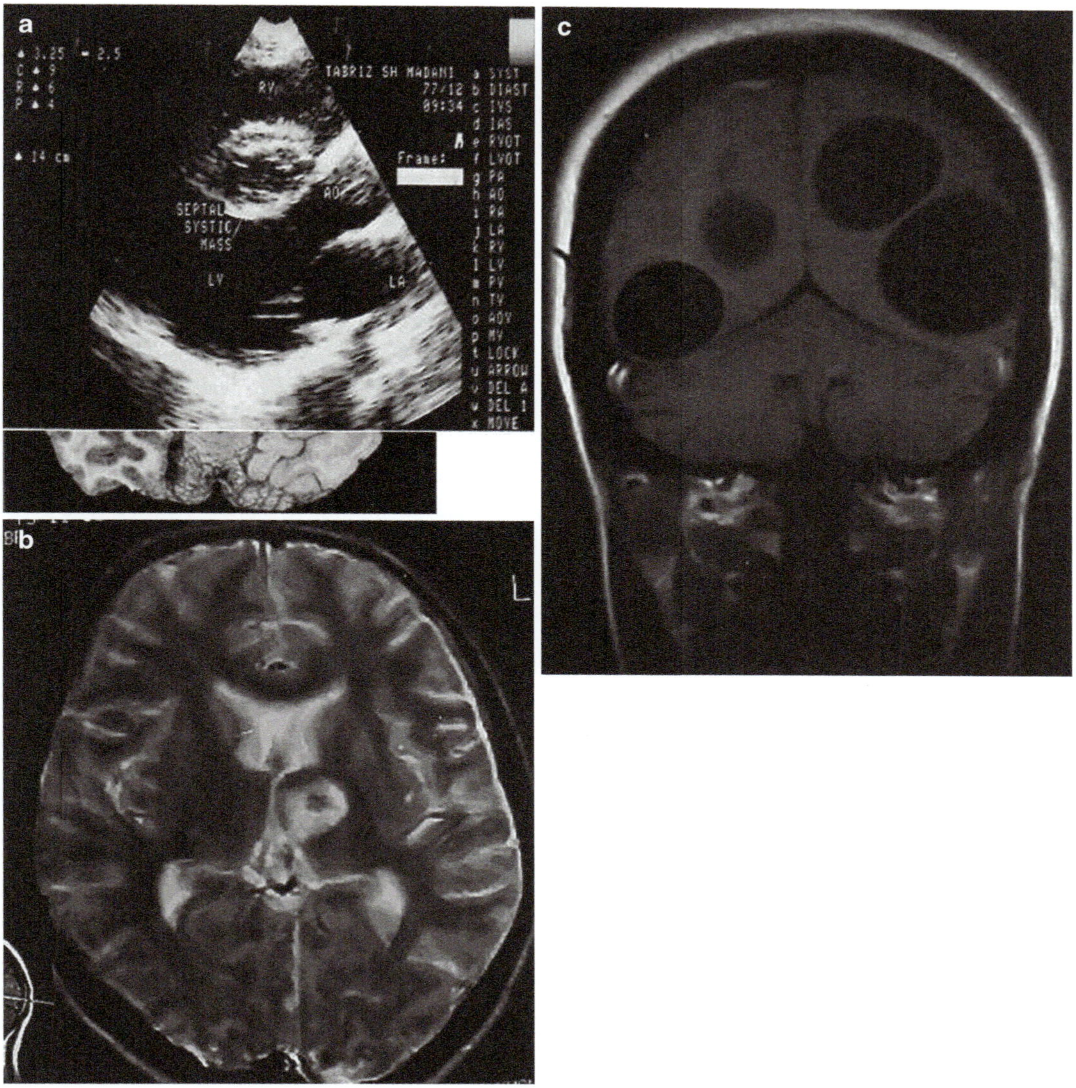

Fig. 22.4 Stroke as a complication of cardiac hydatidosis with an interval of 2 years between infarction and cyst formation. (**a**) Echocardiography shows a cystic mass in the ventricular septum of the heart. (**b**) Axial T2-weighted MRI demonstrates hyperintense cystic foci in the left basal ganglia. (**c**) Axial T2-weighted MRI shows multiple cystic cerebral lesions in both hemispheres (From Lotfinia et al. (2007), with permission)

cysts (Figs. 22.3 and 22.4) (Benomar et al. 1994; Lotfinia et al. 2007). As a rule, the cerebral embolism called "stroke" usually occurs when portions of a ruptured hydatid cyst travel from the left side of the heart to the brain (Turgut et al. 1997). For this reason, a routine investigation for cardiac hydatidosis as a possible source of a cerebral embolus should be undertaken, if patient has hydatid disease in other organs.

We reviewed the scientific literature for all published articles containing cases of "stroke" as a complication of cardiac hydatidosis with/without multiple metastatic hydatid cysts of the brain published to date. In this review, all published case reports, case series, and abstracts found in congress abstract books on stroke as a complication of cardiac hydatidosis were included. If a case appeared in more than one paper on this subject, the earlier report was omitted. Also, dubious cases with no data available to the authors were excluded (Gessini and Giammusso 1957; Preda et al. 1963; Thameur et al. 2001; Díaz and Maillo 2002).

Altogether, 41 articles were selected, containing 41 cases of "stroke" as a complication of cardiac hydatidosis with/without multiple metastatic hydatid cysts of the brain (Peters et al. 1945; Paillas et al. 1962; Chin et al. 1981; Vaquero et al. 1982; Petrov 1987; Borisenko et al. 1990; Byard and Bourne 1991; Benomar et al. 1994; Talaslioglu et al. 1994; el Quessar et al. 1996; Turgut et al. 1997; Evliyaoglu et al. 1998; Kabbaj et al. 1998; Marcì et al. 1998; Ugur et al. 1998; Maffeis et al 2000; Ulgen et al. 2000; Kemaloğlu et al. 2001; Cakir et al. 2002; Trehan et al. 2002; Singh et al 2003; Acarturk et al. 2004; Bükte et al. 2004; Karabay et al. 2004; Pillai et al. 2004; Yaliniz et al. 2004; Itumur et al. 2006; Yaliniz et al. 2006; Lotfinia et al. 2007; Aleksic-Shihabi and Vidolin 2008; Ašanin et al. 2008; Goz et al. 2008; Kumar and Hasan 2008; Byard 2009; Kanj et al. 2010; Kojundzic et al. 2010; Sabouni et al. 2010; Cansu et al. 2011; Ekici et al. 2011; Fabijanić et al. 2011; Potapov et al. 2011). Nevertheless, the cases cited in this chapter do not constitute all of those in the literature because of the unsuitability of some of the reports for proper analysis and the inaccessibility of certain papers. The details of the 41 cases of "stroke" as a complication of cardiac hydatidosis with/without multiple metastatic hydatid cysts of the brain are listed in Tables 22.1 and 22.2.

In this meta-analysis, only 7 (17 %) of the 41 patients of "stroke" as a complication of cardiac hydatidosis in the literature were reported in the period of 1945–1987 and the remaining 34 (83 %) cases in the period of 1990–2011. Importantly, 33 (80 %) of the 41 cases reported were from the Middle East, Mediterranean, or Eastern Europe countries. In all these patients the cerebrovascular condition was caused by rupture of an intracardiac hydatid cyst. There were 24 (59 %) male and 17 (41 %) female patients. Their ages ranged from 4 to 70 years, and 30 (73 %) of the 41 patients reported were clustered in the age between the first and third decades inclusively (Table 22.1).

Locations of Cyst(s)

In all but only two cases, detailed information for the cardiac anatomical location of the hydatid cyst(s) was available. In the cases of cardiac hydatidosis complicated with "stroke" in the literature, there was more than one cyst in the heart, and the most common location of the cyst(s) was the left ventricle (57 %), followed by the septum (13 %), left atrium (13 %), pericardium (11 %), and right atrium (4 %). With the exclusion of only one case without any information, the condition was caused by spontaneous rupture of a primary intracardiac hydatid cyst in 36 (90 %) patients and by surgical rupture of a primary intracardiac hydatid cyst in four (Table 22.1).

Out of 41 cases of "stroke" as a complication of cardiac hydatidosis, 24 (59 %) have single/multiple ischemic/hemorrhagic infarct(s), while 27 (66 %) have single/multiple hydatid cysts. In a total of 10 patients, however, single/multiple hydatid cyst(s) developed within the infarcted cerebral tissue with an interval ranging from a few months to 5 years (Table 22.2). Anatomically, cerebral hydatid embolism from the rupture of a fertile intracardiac hydatid cyst affected the regions of middle cerebral artery, the internal carotid artery, the basilar artery, or peripheral arterial branches (Table 22.2).

Other organs involved by hydatidosis as a result of systemic embolization from the ruptured cyst were the liver in 14 cases, kidney in 8 cases, spleen in 5 cases, lung in 3 cases, eyeball in 2 cases, and thyroid and cecum in 1 case each, in addition to obstruction of the distal branches of the aorta including the renal artery, splenic artery, and femoral artery (Table 22.1).

Clinical Features

Clinical, neuroimaging, and surgical findings are summarized in Table 22.2. Motor weakness, hypoesthesia, IICP, epileptic seizure, and unconsciousness were the most common presenting symptoms in patients with single/multiple infarct(s) and/or metastatic hydatid cysts of the brain. The presenting symptoms were related to (1) embolization from heart with cerebral ischemia and infarction or (2) the mechanical effects of growth and compression of adjacent parenchyma by intracranial hydatid cysts, although they were nonspecific.

Table 22.1 Summary of the 41 reported cases with stroke as a complication of cardiac hydatidosis published in the world literature to date: demographic data and cardiac findings

Author(s)	Country	Year of publication	Patient age (years), sex	Systolic murmur	EC	Location of cyst(s) in the heart	Other organ involvement	Result of serological study	Type of rupture
Peters et al.	USA	1945	5, F	NS	NS	LV[e]	Liver	NS	Spontan
			24, M	NS	NS	LA[e]	NS	NS	Spontan
			45, F	NS	NS	LA, P, IVS, LV[e]	Kidney, spleen, thyroid, ICA, MCA, superior mesenteric artery, renal artery, splenic artery	NS	Spontan
Paillas et al.	France	1962	17, M	(–)	NS	LV[e]	ICA, eyeball, foramen ovale	NS	Spontan
Chin et al.	Australia	1981	37, M	NS	(–)	P	(–)	(+)	Spontan
Vaquero et al.	Spain	1982	37, M	NS	(–)	P, LV	NS	NS	Surgical
Petrov	Bulgaria	1987	32, M	NS	(–)	LV[e]	(–)	NS	Spontan
Borisenko et al.	USSR	1990	11, F	(+)	(+)	LV	(–)	(+)	Spontan
Byard and Bourne	Australia	1991	7, M	NS	(–)	LV	Liver	NS	Spontan
Talaslıoglu et al.	Turkey	1994	19, F	NS	(+)	NS	NS	NS	Spontan
Benomar et al.	Morocco	1994	21, F	NS	(–)	P, LA, LV	Kidney, liver, spleen	NS	Spontan
			40, F	NS	(+)	LV	Kidney, liver, spleen	(+)	Spontan
el Quessar et al.	Morocco	1996	21, F	NS	(–)	P, LV	Kidney, liver, spleen	NS	Spontan
			40, F	NS	(+)	LV	Kidney, liver, spleen	(+)	Spontan
Turgut e al.	Turkey	1997	7, F	(+)	(+)	LV	Femoral artery	NS	Spontan
Ugur et al.	Turkey	1998	18, F	NS	(–)	IVS	NS	NS	Spontan
Kabbaj et al.	Morocco	1998	28, M	NS	(+)	LV	Kidney, liver	(+)	Spontan
Evliyaoglu et al.	Turkey	1998	24, M	NS	(+)	LV	NS	NS	Spontan
Marci et al.	Italy	1998	26, F	(+)	(+)	LV	(–)	(+)	Spontan
Ulgen et al.	Turkey	2000	70, M	NS	(+)	IVS, LV	Liver	(+)	Spontan
Maffeis et al.	Brazil	2000	57, M	NS	(+)	LV	NS	NS	Spontan
Kemaloglu et al.	Turkey	2001	7, F	NS	(+)	LV	NS	NS	Spontan
Cakir et al.	Turkey	2002	6, F	(–)	(+)	LV	(–)	(+)	Spontan
Trehan et al.	India	2002	13, M	(+)	(+)	RA, LA, IAS	Liver	(–)	Spontan

(continued)

Table 22.1 (continued)

Author(s)	Country	Year of publication	Patient age (years), sex	Systolic murmur	EC	Location of cyst(s) in the heart	Other organ involvement	Result of serological study	Type of rupture
Singh et al.[a]	India	2003	13, M	(+)	(+)	RA, LA, IAS	Liver	(+)	Spontan
Acarturk et al.	Turkey	2004	15, M	NS	(+)	LV	Liver, abdominal aorta	NS	Spontan
Pillai et al.	UAE	2004	36, F	NS	(+)	LV	Eyeball	NS	Spontan
Karabay et al.	Turkey	2004	19, M	NS	(+)	IAS, RA, LA	Liver	NS	Spontan
Yaliniz et al.	Turkey	2004	16, M	NS	(+)	LV	Liver	(+)	Surgical
Bükte et al.[b]	Turkey	2004	7, F	NS	(+)	LV	NS	NS	Spontan
Itumur et al.	Turkey	2006	24, M	(+)	(+)	LV	(–)	NS	Spontan
Yaliniz et al.[c]	Turkey	2006	16, M	NS	(+)	LV	Liver	(+)	Surgical
Lotfinia et al.	Iran	2007	17, F	(+)	(+)	S	(–)	NS	Spontan
Aleksic-Shihabi and Vidolin	Croatia	2008	27, M	(+)	(+)	LV, P	(–)	(+)	Surgical
Kumar and Hasan	India	2008	4, M	NS	(–)	LV, P	Lung	(+)	Surgical
Goz et al.	Turkey	2008	24, M	NS	(+)	LV	NS	(–)	Spontan
Ašanin et al.	ME	2008	22, M	NS	(+)	LA	Liver, mediastinum	(+)	Spontan
Byard[d]	Australia	2009	12, M	NS	(–)	LV	Liver	NS	Spontan
Kanj et al.	Lebanon	2010	32, F	NS	(–)	NS	NS	NS	NS
Sabouni et al.	Iran	2010	12, M	NS	(+)	IVS	Kidney, cecum	(+)	Spontan
Kojundzic et al.	Croatia	2010	34, M	(+)	(–)	LV	Lung	(+)	Spontan
Cansu et al.	Turkey	2011	7, M	(–)	(+)	LV	Liver	(+)	Spontan
Potapov et al.	Russia	2011	21, M	NS	(+)	LV	Kidney	(+)	Spontan
Ekici et al.	Turkey	2011	12, M	NS	(+)	LA	(–)	(–)	Spontan
Fabijanić et al.	Croatia	2011	24, F	(–)	(+)	LV	Lung	(–)	Spontan

Abbreviations: *NS* not stated, *USSR* Union of Soviet Socialist Republics, *UAE* United Arab Emirates, *USA* United States of America, *ME* Montenegro, *F* female, *M* male, *LV* left ventricle, *LA* left atrium, *P* pericardium, *S* septum, *IVS* interventricular septum, *IAS* interatrial septum, *RA* right atrium, *ICA* internal carotid artery, *MCA* middle cerebral artery, *EC* echocardiography, *Spontan* spontaneous

[a]The case reported by the authors had already been described by Trehan et al. earlier

[b]The case reported by the authors had already been described by Kemaloglu et al. earlier

[c]The case reported by the authors had already been described by same authors earlier

[d]The case reported by the author had already been described by Byard & Bourne earlier

[e]In these cases, location of the cyst(s) in the heart was determined at autopsy

Table 22.2 Summary of the 41 reported cases with stroke as a complication of cardiac hydatidosis published in the world literature to date: cerebral findings, treatment, and outcome

Author(s)	Presenting symptoms	Imaging study	Kind of cerebral lesion(s)			Location of cerebral lesion(s) (No. of cysts)[e]	Anthel treatment	No. of surgery (cardiac/cerebral)[g]	Outcome
			Infarct	Cyst	Interval				
Peters et al.	NS	NS	(–)	(+)	(–)	Cerebral (1)	NS	0/1	Died
	IICP, right hemiparesis, aphasia	NS	(–)	(+)	(–)	Left T, right O, left P (6)	NS	0/3	Died
	Seizure, coma	NS	(+)	(–)	(–)	Right MCA and ICA	NS	0/0	Died
Paillas et al.	Vertigo, IICP, left hemihypoesthesia and hemiparesis, visual loss and proptosis on right side, seizure	Angio, EEG	NS	(+)	(–)	Right FT (3)	NS	0/1[h]	Died
Chin et al.	IICP, fever, neck stiffness, right hemiparesis	CT	(+)	(–)	(–)	Right cerebellum, both MCA	MEB	1/0[i]	No follow-up
Vaquero et al.	Left hemiparesis	CT	(+)	(+)	5 years	Right MCA, right P, left P, left O (3)	NS	1/2	No follow-up
Petrov	Seizure, coma	Angio	(+)	(–)	(–)	Right MCA[f]	(–)	0/0	Died
Borisenko et al.	Right hemiparesis, loss of speech	CT, MRI, US, Scint	(+)	(+)	9 months	Left MCA, left O (3)	(–)	NS	NS
Byard and Bourne	Unconsciousness, seizure	(–)	(+)	(–)	(–)	Both MCA	NS	0/0	Died
Talaslıoglu et al.	IICP	MRI	(–)	(+)	(–)	NS	NS	0/9	No recur at 2 years
Benomar et al.	Left hemiparesis, IICP, left hemihypoesthesia, fever	CT, Angio	(+)	(+)	9 months	Right MCA, brainstem	NS	0/1	Died
	Right hemiparesis, aphasia	CT, Angio	(+)	(+)	1 year	Left MCA	MEB	0/0	No change at 1 year
el Quessar et al.	Fever, urticaria, left hemiparesis, IICP	CT, MRI, Angio	(+)	(+)	A few months	Right MCA	NS	1/1[j]	Died
	Right hemiplegia, aphasia	CT, Angio	(+)	(+)	A few months	Left MCA	MEB	0/0	No follow-up
Turgut e al.	Left hemiparesis, IICP, cyanosis, double vision	CT, MRI, Angio	(–)	(+)	(–)	Both F (17), both PO (3), both P (8), right O (1)	MEB+ALB	1/8[j]	No recur at 2 years

(continued)

Table 22.2 (continued)

Author(s)	Presenting symptoms	Imaging study	Kind of cerebral lesion(s)			Location of cerebral lesion(s) (No. of cysts)[e]	Anthel treatment	No. of surgery (cardiac/cerebral)[g]	Outcome
			Infarct	Cyst	Interval				
Ugur et al.	Left hemiparesis, IICP	CT	(–)	(+)	(–)	Right F, P and both PO (7)	ALB	0/1	No follow-up
Kabbaj et al.	Left hemiplegia, facial paralysis, aphasia	CT	(+)	(–)	(–)	Right MCA	NS	1/0	No follow-up
Evliyaoglu et al.	Right hemiparesis, aphasia	CT, US	(+)	(+)	6 months	Left MCA, left F (3) right T (mult)	NS	0/2	Died
Marci et al.	Right hemiplegia	CT, MRI, US	(+)	(–)	(–)	Left MCA	ALB	1/0	No follow-up
Ulgen et al.	Vertigo, syncope, cardiac arrest	MRI	(+)	(–)	(–)	MCA	(–)	0/0[j]	Died
Maffeis et al.	Right hemiparesis	CT, MRI, Angio	(+)	(–)	(–)	Left ICA, right cerebellum	ALB	1/0	Well at 6 weeks
Kemaloglu et al.	Right hemiparesis, dysphasia, seizure, facial paresis	CT, MRI, US	(+)	(+)	6 months	Both PO (2)	MEB	1/1	Partial recovery at 3 months
Cakir et al.	Hemiparesis, speech disturbance	CT, US	(–)	(+)	(–)	Left PO (1)	MEB	1/1	No recur at 2 months
Trehan et al.	Right hemiparesis	CT, Angio, US	(+)	(–)	(–)	Left basal ganglia	ALB	1/0	Complete recovery at 1 month
Singh et al.[a]	Right hemiparesis	CT, Angio, US	(+)	(–)	(–)	Left basal ganglia	NS	NS	NS
Acarturk et al.	Right hemiparesis, seizure, aphasia	MRI, US	(+)	(–)	(–)	Left capsulostriatum	ALB	1/0[j]	Partial recovery and no recur at 6 months
Pillai et al.	Left proptosis, diplopia	CT, US	(–)	(+)	(–)	Both P (mult)	NS	0/0[j]	No follow-up
Karabay et al.	IICP	CT, MRI	(–)	(+)	(–)	Left F (1)	ALB	1/0	Well at 6 months

Yaliniz et al.	Right hemiparesis, aphasia	CT, MRI, US	(+)	(–)	(–)	Left MCA	ALB	1/0[j]	Complete recovery at 5 months
Bükte et al.[b]	Right hemiparesis, dysphasia, seizure, facial paresis	CT, MRI, US	(+)	(+)	6 months	Both PO (2)	MEB	1/1	Partial recovery at 3 months
Itumur et al.	Right hemiparesis, IICP, dysphasia	MRI	(–)	(+)	(–)	Left cerebrum (18)	ALB	1/2	No recur at 6 months
Yaliniz et al.[c]	Right hemiparesis, aphasia	CT, MRI, US	(+)	(–)	(–)	Left MCA	ALB	1/0[j]	Complete recovery at 5 months
Lotfinia et al.	IICP, coma, left hemiparesis, visual loss	CT, MRI	(+)	(+)	2 years	Left basal ganglia, left PO, right TP, right O (5)	ALB	2/2	No recur at 2 years
Aleksic-Shihabi and Vidolin	Left hemiparesis, IICP, facial paresis	CT	(–)	(+)	(–)	Right PO (1)	ALB	2/1	No follow-up
Kumar and Hasan	Right hemiplegia, fever	CT, MRI	(+)	(–)	(–)	Left basal ganglia	ALB	1/0	No follow-up
Goz et al.	Right hemiparesis	CT, MRI US	(–)	(+)	(–)	Left P, O, F and cerebellum (NS)	ALB	1/2	No recur at 15 months
Asanin et al.	Right hemiparesis, aphasia, TIA	CT, MRI	(+)	(–)	(–)	Left MCA	NS	0/0[j]	NS
Byard[d]	Unconsciousness	(–)	(+)	(–)	(–)	Both MCA	NS	0/0	Died
Kanj et al.	Right hemiparesis, IICP	CT, MRI	(+)	(+)	11 months	Left MCA, left FP (2)	NS	0/1	No follow-up
Sabouni et al.	Left hemiparesis, IICP, facial paresis	CT, US	(–)	(+)	(–)	Right T, both centrum semiovale (5)	ALB+PRAZ	1/1[j]	No follow-up
Kojundzic et al.	Left hemiparesis, IICP, facial paresis, left hemihypoesthesia	CT, MRI, US	(–)	(+)	(–)	Right T, P, O (3)	ALB	1/2[j]	No follow-up
Cansu et al.	Bilateral hemiparesis, unconsciousness, fever, seizure, ulcer of limb	CT, MRI US	(+)	(–)	(–)	Left FPO	ALB	1/0[j]	No follow-up

(continued)

Table 22.2 (continued)

Author(s)	Presenting symptoms	Imaging study	Kind of cerebral lesion(s)			Location of cerebral lesion(s) (No. of cysts)[e]	Anthel treatment	No. of surgery (cardiac/cerebral)[g]	Outcome
			Infarct	Cyst	Interval				
Potapov et al.	Left hemiparesis, IICP, right hemianopsia	CT, MRI, MR tracto	(–)	(+)	(–)	Right P, left PO (6)	NS	0/1[k]	Complete recovery at 4 months
Ekici et al.	Left hemiparesis, IICP, seizure	CT, MRI US	(–)	(+)	(–)	Right PO (3)	ALB	0/(mult)[k]	No follow-up
Fabijanić et al.	Syncope	US	NS	(+)	NS	NS (NS)	ALB+PRAZ	1/1[j]	No recur at 1 year

Abbreviations: *NS* not stated, *CT* computed tomography, *MRI* magnetic resonance imaging, *IICP* increased intracranial pressure, *TIA* transient ischemic attack, *Angio* angiography, *Scint* scintigraphy, *ICA* internal carotid artery, *MCA* middle cerebral artery, *F* frontal, *T* temporal, *P* parietal, *O* occipital, *FP* frontoparietal, *PO* parieto-occipital, *FPO* fronto-parieto-occipital, *anthel* anthelmintic, *MEB* mebendazole, *ALB* albendazole, *PRAZ*, praziquantel, *recur* recurrence, *MR tracto* MR tractography, *mult* multiple

[a]The case reported by the authors had already been described by Trehan et al. earlier

[b]The case reported by the authors had already been described by Kemaloglu et al. earlier

[c]The case reported by the authors had already been described by same authors earlier

[d]The case reported by the author had already been described by Byard & Bourne earlier

[e]No. of cysts within the brain tissue

[f]In this case, two hydatid cysts were removed from the right MCA at autopsy

[g]No. of operations include cardiac (first) and brain (second) operations

[h]In this patient, carotid sympathectomy and cervical ganglion resection were also done for occlusion of ICA

[i]In this patient, only pericardial puncture was done as a diagnostic procedure

[j]An additional surgery was done for involvement of other organs such as the lung, liver, intestine, eyeball, abdominal aorta, or femoral artery by hydatid cysts

[k]The patient was treated surgically with the aid of a neuronavigation system

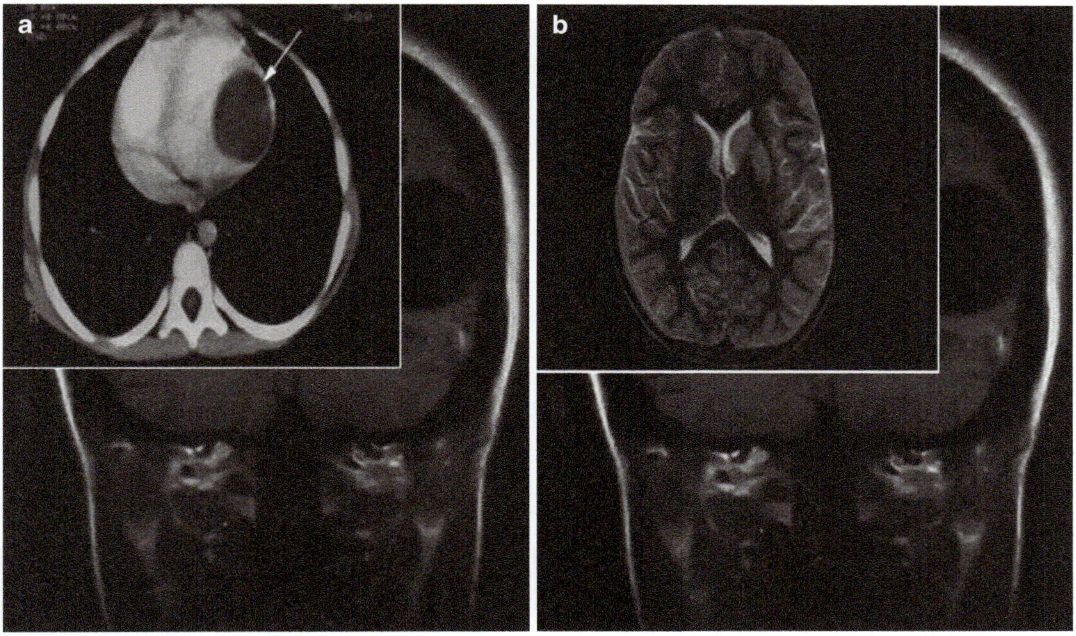

Fig. 22.5 Stroke as a complication of cardiac hydatidosis. (**a**) Axial contrast-enhanced CT of thorax shows a well-defined cystic mass (*arrow*) in the left ventricle of the heart. (**b**) Axial T2-weighted MRI shows hyperintense lesions in the left basal ganglia (From Kumar and Hasan (2008), with permission)

Interestingly, there were no EC signs of cystic formation in the heart in 10 (27 %) of 37 patients with detailed information. In addition, physical examination revealed a systolic murmur in only 8 cases with cardiac hydatidosis complicated with single/multiple hydatid cysts. Similarly, results of serologic tests for hydatid disease were negative in 4 (25 %) of 20 patients with detailed information (Table 22.1).

Imaging Findings

Radiological information for three patients was not available and data for these patients are not included. Thus, all but one were investigated by neuroimaging studies including CT, MRI, angiography, US, or MR tractography and at autopsy in five (Figs. 22.3, 22.4, 22.5, and 22.6) (Benomar et al. 1994; Turgut et al. 1997; Lotfinia et al. 2007; Kumar and Hasan 2008). In these cases, characteristic findings of cerebral hydatidosis were well-defined, smooth, thin-walled, spherical, homogeneous cystic lesions with no contrast enhancement, no calcification, and no surrounding edema. On the other hand, the diagnosis of intracardiac hydatidosis was confirmed by EC in 27 of 41 patients (Table 22.2).

Treatment

Excluding the eight cases without cardiac or intracranial surgery, 32 reported patients with detailed information had surgery ranging from one to nine operations. In cases of "stroke" with/without multiple metastatic hydatid cysts of the brain as a complication of cardiac hydatidosis, the number of cerebral cysts ranged from 1 to 29. Technically, complete removal of multiple cysts or those with atypical localization was usually difficult and radical extirpation of the cyst was not possible without rupture, although removal of a single cerebral hydatid cyst was achieved by the Dowling-Orlando technique without any difficulty. Anthelmintics such as mebendazole, albendazole, and praziquantel were administered in all but only three cases reported in the literature (Table 22.2).

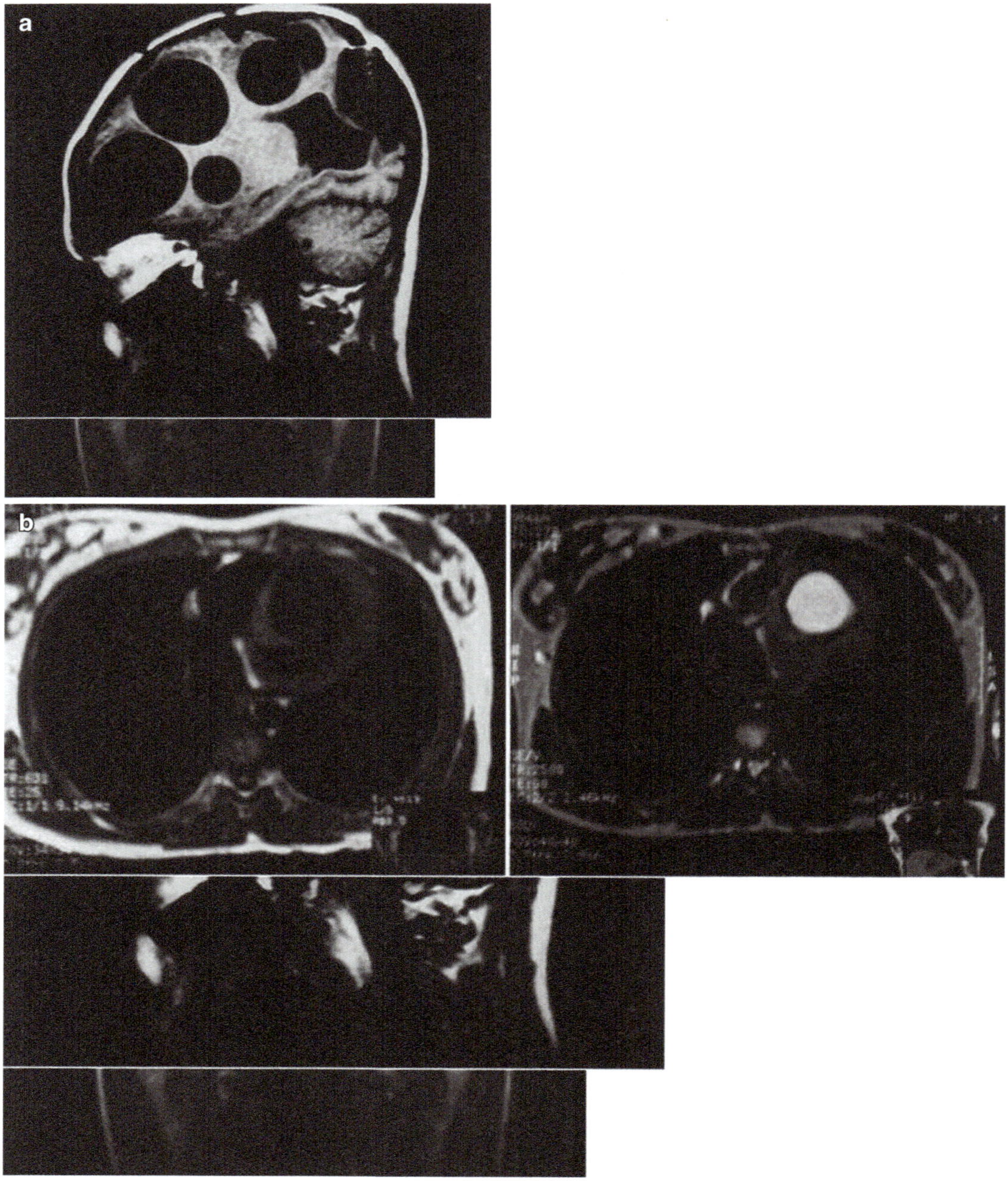

Fig. 22.6 Stroke as a complication of cardiac hydatidosis. Axial T1 (**a**) and T2 (**b**) -weighted MRI shows a giant hydatid cyst in the interventricular septum of the heart (Reproduced, with permission, from Turgut et al.: J Neurosurg 1997;86:716)

Prognosis

Some patients died preoperatively of cerebral infarction caused by embolized fragments from a ruptured cardiac hydatid cyst that was found at autopsy (Peters et al. 1945; Petrov 1987; Byard and Bourne 1991; Ulgen et al. 2000), but almost all the other patients underwent surgical intervention. We found that, in a review of the literature, outcome information for 14 patients was not available and there were a total of 10 (24 %) deaths (Table 22.2).

Conclusion

The following conclusions may be gleaned from the present chapter and the review of the series of cardiac hydatidosis as a source of cerebral embolism from the published literature:

1. In most cases, the diagnosis is difficult in cardiac hydatidosis, owing to the presence of long latency period and nonspecific findings, but early diagnosis and treatment are important.
2. As a rule, the hydatid cyst embolism is an infrequent but serious complication of cardiac hydatidosis in geographic locations where the disease is endemic, because it remains a possible cause of sudden death.
3. In cases with cerebral hydatidosis presenting as "stroke," a persistent investigation is required to detect new hydatid cyst formation in the heart as a source of embolism, as demonstrated by some authors (Turgut et al. 1997; Evliyaoglu et al. 1998; Itumur et al. 2006; Goz et al. 2008; Kojundzic et al. 2010; Ekici et al. 2011).
4. Importantly, the neurosurgeon must always remember that all of multiple secondary cerebral cysts can seldom be removed without rupture, but there is no risk of rupture in the infertile secondary cerebral cysts.
5. Finally, as a rule, especially in pediatric and young patients with otherwise unexplained cerebral embolism, a careful search for the possibility of cardiac cyst as a source of embolism should be undertaken in patients with multiple intracranial hydatid cysts because the combined therapy with surgical treatment and chemotherapy would not be successful without removal of the intracardiac hydatid cyst.

Acknowledgments Thanks to Dimitar Vuchev and Stefan Sivkov, who translated some texts from Bulgarian and Russian to English, and Bülent Bozdoğan for having translated some texts from French and Spanish to English. We especially would like to thank Fuad Sami Haddad for having reviewed the text in English.

References

Abada M, Galli I, Bousallah A, Lehmann G. Hydatid cysts of the brain. Diagnostic and therapeutic problems apropos of 100 cases (in French). Neurochirurgie. 1977;23:195–204.

Acarturk E, Ozeren A, Koc M, Yaliniz H, Bicakci S, Demir M. Left ventricular hydatid cyst presenting with acute ischemic stroke: case report. J Am Soc Echocardiogr. 2004;17:1009–10.

Aleksic-Shihabi A, Vidolin EP. Cystic echinococcosis of the heart and brain: a case report. Acta Med Okayama. 2008;62:341–4.

Ašanin B, Milić I, Milović Z. Echinococcosis cerebri: report of two less common cases. Facta Univ Ser Med Biol. 2008;15:64–7.

Benomar A, Yahyaoui M, Birouk N, Vidailhet M, Chkili T. Middle cerebral artery occlusion due to hydatid cysts of myocardial and intraventricular cavity cardiac origin. Two cases Stroke. 1994;25:886–8.

Borisenko VV, Shukin ID, Kugoev AI. Ischemic infarction in a patient with echinococcosis of the heart and brain (in Russian). Klin Med (Mosk). 1990;68: 122–4.

Bükte Y, Kemaloglu S, Nazaroglu H, Ozkan U, Ceviz A, Simsek M. Cerebral hydatid disease: CT and MR imaging findings. Swiss Med Wkly. 2004;134:459–67.

Buris L, Takacs P, Varga M. Sudden death caused by hydatid embolism. Z Rechtsmed. 1987;98:125–8.

Byard RW. An analysis of possible mechanisms of unexpected death occurring in hydatid disease (echinococcosis). J Forensic Sci. 2009;54:919–22.

Byard RW, Bourne AJ. Cardiac echinococcosis with fatal intracerebral embolism. Arch Dis Child. 1991;66: 155–6.

Cakir O, Eren N, Kilinc N. Cardiac hydatic cyst causing cerebral emboli in a child. Pediatr Cardiol. 2002;23: 555–6.

Cansu A, Cakir M, Dilber E, Gedikli O, Cansu A, Kul S, Erduran E. Cardiac echinococcosis associated with cerebrovascular occlusive disease and subcutaneous bullous eruptions and ulcers. Ann Trop Paediatr. 2011; 31:251–4.

Chin DD, Rice JP, Lequesne DM. Hydatid cyst of the heart presenting as cerebral and cerebellar infarction. Med J Aust. 1981;2:556–7.

Deve F. Echinococcose Secondarie. Paris: Mason Edit; 1946. p. 17–8.

Díaz P, Maillo A. Middle cerebral artery occlusion after cerebral hydatic embolism in a pediatric patient: case report (in Spanish). Neurocirugia (Astur). 2002;13: 216–8.

Dursun M, Terzibasıoglu E, Yilmaz R, Cekrezi B, Olgar S, Nisli K, Tunaci A. Cardiac hydatid disease: CT and MRI findings. AJR Am J Roentgenol. 2008;190: 226–32.

Ekici MA, Ekici A, Per H, Tucer B, Kumandas S, Kurtsoy A. Concomitant heart and brain hydatid cyst without other organ involvement: a case report. Düşünen Adam J Psychiatry Neurol Sci. 2011;24:155–9.

el Quessar A, Benabdejlil M, Mansouri A, el Hassani MR, Chakir N, Jiddane M, Benomar A, Yahyaoui M, Chkili T, Boukhrissi N. Cerebral vascular accidents due to hydatid embolisms. Apropos of 2 cases (in French). J Neuroradiol. 1996;23:74–8.

Evliyaoglu C, Yuksel M, Gul B, Kaptanoglu E, Yaman M. Growth rate of multiple intracranial hydatid cysts assessed by CT from the time of embolisation. Neuroradiology. 1998;40:387–9.

Fabijanić D, Bulat C, Letica D, Nenadić D, Pešutić-Pisac V, Carević V. Echocardiographic appearance of a hydatid cyst of the papillary muscle and chordae tendineae. J Clin Ultrasound. 2011;39:431–3.

Garg M, Gupta RK, Prasad KN, Sikora SS, Pal L, Chawla S, Kumar R, Husain M, Saxena S, Husain N, Roy R. Fertility assessment of hydatid cyst by proton MR spectroscopy. J Surg Res. 2002;106:196–201.

Gessini L, Giammusso V. An exceptional cause of internal carotid thrombosis: echinococcal cyst of carotid bifurcation; angiographic demonstration of a collateral circle of the external carotid through the ophthalmic artery (in Italian). Minerva Neurochir. 1957;1:23–6.

Goz M, Cakir O, Kilinc N, Eren MN. A case of multivesicular cardiac hydatid cyst with cerebral involvement. Turk J Thorac Cardiovasc Surg. 2008;16:186–8.

Haddad FS, Haddad GF. Hydatid disease of the central nervous system. Personal experience: its appearance, management, and outcome in the brain and the spine. Neurosurg Q. 2005;15:33–41.

Itumur K, Tamam Y, Karabulut A, Guzel A, Kilic N. Co-occurrence of cardiac and cerebral hydatid cysts: a case report. Scott Med J. 2006;51:50.

Kabbaj N, Chat L, Dafiri R, Imani F. Rare cause of ischemic cerebrovascular infarct in a young patient: cardiac hydatic cyst (in French). J Radiol. 1998;79:53–6.

Kanj AH, Fares YH, Yehya RR, Hamzeh FF. Unusual appearance of a cerebral hydatid cyst as a hemorrhagic infarct. Neurosciences (Riyadh). 2010;15:275–6.

Karabay O, Onen A, Yildiz F, Yilmaz E, Erdal CA, Sanli A, Kilci G, Algin I, Itil O, Açikel U. The case of a cyst hydatid localized within the interatrial septum. Jpn Heart J. 2004;45:703–7.

Kemaloğlu S, Ozkan U, Bükte Y, Acar M, Ceviz A. Growth rate of cerebral hydatid cyst, with a review of the literature. Childs Nerv Syst. 2001;17:743–5.

Kojundzic SL, Dolic K, Buca A, Jankovic S, Besenski N. Hydatid disease with multiple organ involvement: a case report. Macedonian J Med Sci. 2010;3:154–8.

Kumar S, Hasan R. Recurrent cardiac hydatidosis in a child presenting as acute stroke. Ind J Thorac Cardiovasc Surg. 2008;24:24–7.

Lotfinia I, Vahedi P, Hadidchi S, Djavadzadegan H. Multiple cerebral hydatid cysts secondary to embolization from intracardiac hydatidosis. Neurosurg Q. 2007;17:134–7.

Maffeis GR, Petrucci O, Carandina R, Leme Jr CA, Truffa M, Vieira R, Schelini F, Metze K, Nogueira EA. Cardiac echinococcosis. Circulation. 2000;101:1352–4.

Marcì M, Ponari A, Finazzo F, Battaglia A. Echocardiographically diagnosed cardiac echinococcus complicated by embolic intraventricular thrombus. J Am Soc Echocardiogr. 1998;11:1158–60.

Maroto LC, Carrascal Y, Lopez MJ, Forteza A, Perez A, Zavanella C. Hydatid cyst of the interventricular septum in a 3.5-year-old child. Ann Thorac Surg. 1998; 66:2110–1.

Paillas J, Bonnal J, Payan H, Berard-Badier M. Thrombosis of the internal carotid artery revealing ruptured cardiac echinococcosis and followed by intracranioorbital hydatidosis (in French). Sem Hop (Paris). 1962;38:1200–3.

Peters J, Dexter L, Weiss S. Clinical and theoretical considerations of involvement of the left side of the heart with echinococcal cysts. A review of the literature with a report of five new cases including one observed by the authors. Am Heart J. 1945;29:143–7.

Petrov S. Echinococcosis of the heart and parasitic embolism of a cerebral artery (in Bulgarian). Vutr Boles. 1987;26:86–8.

Pillai AK, Pillai MV, Vohra S, Oommen EB. Multiple central nervous system hydatidosis secondary to cardiac echinococcosis. Indian J Radiol Imaging. 2004;14:81–3.

Potapov AA, Goriaĭnov SA, Okhlopkov VA, Kravchuk AD, Zakharova NE, Podoprigora AE, Kurnosov AB, Khit' MA, Panina TN, Eliseeva NM. Multiple echinococcosis of brain, heart and kidneys (in Russian). Zh Vopr Neirokhir Im N N Burdenko. 2011;75:57–65.

Preda I, Moraru I, Manolescu A. Rapid posttraumatic death from cerebral embolism in the case of a myocardial hydatid cyst with secondary echinococcosis (in French). Ann Med Leg Criminol Police Sci Toxicol. 1963;43:481–2.

Sabouni F, Ferdosian F, Mamishi S, Nejat F, Monnajemzadeh M, Rezaei N. Multiple organ involvement with hydatid cysts. Iran J Parasitol. 2010;5:65–70.

Singh NP, Arora SK, Gupta A, Anuradha S, Sridhara G, Agarwal SK, Gulati P. Stroke: a rare presentation of cardiac hydatidosis. Neurol India. 2003;51:120–1.

Talaslioglu A, Ersoy AO, Soyuer A, Koksal E, Tomar A. A case of cerebral emboli due to cardiac hydatid cyst (in Turkish). Proceedings of the 30th National Neurology Congress. Adana, Turkey. 1994; p. 87.

Thameur H, Abdelmoula S, Chenik S, Bey M, Ziadi M, Mestiri T, Mechmeche R, Chaouch H. Cardiopericardial hydatid cysts. World J Surg. 2001;25:58–67.

Trehan V, Shah P, Yusuf J, Mukhopadhyay S, Nair GM, Arora R. Thromboembolism: a rare complication of cardiac hydatidosis. Indian Heart J. 2002;54:199–201.

Turgut M. Intracranial hydatidosis in Turkey: its clinical presentation, diagnostic studies, surgical management, and outcome. A review of 276 cases. Neurosurg Rev. 2001;24:200–8.

Turgut M. Hydatidosis of central nervous system and its coverings in the pediatric and adolescent age groups in

Turkey during the last century: a critical review of 137 cases. Childs Nerv Syst. 2002;18:670–83.
Turgut M, Bayülkem K. Cerebrovascular occlusive disease: hydatidosis. Childs Nerv Syst. 1998;14:697–9.
Turgut M, Benli K, Eryılmaz M. Secondary multiple intracranial hydatid cysts caused by intracerebral embolism of cardiac echinococcosis: an exceptional case of hydatidosis. Case report. J Neurosurg. 1997;86:714–8.
Ugur HC, Attar A, Bagdatoglu C, Erdogan A, Egemen N. Secondary multiple intracranial hydatid cysts caused by intracerebral embolism of cardiac echinococcosis. Acta Neurochir (Wien). 1998;140:833–4.
Ulgen MS, Alan S, Karadede A, Aydinalp O, Toprak N. Cardiac hydatid cysts located in both the left ventricular apex and the intraventricular septum: case report. Heart Vessels. 2000;15:243–4.
Vaquero J, Jimenez C, Martinez R. Growth of hydatid cysts evaluated by CT scanning after presumed cerebral hydatid embolism. Case report. J Neurosurg. 1982; 57:837–8.
Yaliniz H, Tokcan A, Ulus T, Kisacikoglu B, Salih OK, Topcuoglu MS, Poyrazoglu H, Alhan C. A rare presentation of cardiac hydatid cyst: stroke and acute aortic occlusion. Heart Surg Forum. 2004;7:E364–6.
Yaliniz H, Tokcan A, Salih OK, Ulus T. Surgical treatment of cardiac hydatid disease: a report of 7 cases. Tex Heart Inst J. 2006;33:333–9.

Hydatidosis of the Orbit

23

Subrahmanyam Mallajosyula, Syeed Mehbub Ul Kadir, Fuad Sami Haddad, and Sucharitha Ramavath

Contents

S. Mallajosyula, MS, DO, FUBC, FUW (✉)
Orbit and Ophthalmic Plastic Services,
Sankar Foundation Eye Hospital,
Vishakhapatnam, India
e-mail: subrahms@yahoo.com

S.M. Ul Kadir, MS, FSIO
Department of Oculoplasty, National Institute of Ophthalmology & Hospital, Dhaka, Bangladesh

F.S. Haddad, BA, MD, FRCS(C), FACS, ABNS
Department of Surgery, American University of Beirut Medical Center, Beirut, Lebanon

S. Ramavath, MBBS, MS, FSIO
Department of Oculoplasty,
Vasan Eye Care, Bangalore, India

Introduction

Hydatidosis of the orbit is of rare occurrence, and very few, if any, have a wide experience of this disease in this location. We shall endeavor to use the experience of many other authors to present an as accurate as possible picture of this clinical presentation and its management.

Incidence

Hydatid disease of the orbit is rare, even in endemic areas, and accounts for less than 1 % of all hydatid cysts (Gomez Morales et al. 1988; Betharia et al. 2002). To our knowledge orbital hydatid cyst has never been described bilaterally. It commonly occurs as a primary cyst or may be associated with cysts in other locations (Sami et al. 1995; Jimenenez-Mejias et al. 2000). An orbital cyst is located in the retrobulbar space either within the muscle cone or outside, especially in the superolateral or superomedial aspect of the orbit (Alparslan et al. 1990; Guerinel et al. 1991; Gomez Morales et al. 1988). In an exceptional case the cyst was located in the medial rectus muscle (Kiratli et al. 2003). Hydatid cyst is the second most common parasitic cystic lesion in the orbit, after cysticercosis. Hydatid cysts account for 0.3–5 % of all orbital diseases (Xiao and Xueyi 1999; Subrahmanyam et al. 2008). In our series of 1,700 cases of proptosis, in only seven patients was it due to a hydatid cyst.

M. Turgut (ed.), *Hydatidosis of the Central Nervous System: Diagnosis and Treatment*,
DOI 10.1007/978-3-642-54359-3_23,

Hydatidosis usually affects children and young adults. In a review article of 35 cases by Gomez Morales et al. (1988) the age range was 2–57 years, with a mean age of 16 years (Gomez Morales et al. 1988). Most of the patients are in the second decade of life below the age of 16 years. Elders are rarely affected. Xiao and Xueyi (1999) reviewed their hospital records and issues of Chinese medical journals between 1956 and 1994 and found 18 cases of orbital hydatid cyst, including ten cases from their hospital. Among the 18 cases, 7 were males and 11 were females, with an age range of 3–55 years; 15 cases were below the age of 16. However, orbital hydatidosis can occur in older people and was reported in five patients between the ages of 70 and 74 years (Sangawe et al. 1982; Lerner et al. 1991; Abbassi et al. 2007; Jeblaoui et al. 2008; Limaiem et al. 2010) (see Table 23.1).

Clinical Features

Unilateral, progressive, axial or non-axial, non-tender, non-pulsatile proptosis is the most common presentation of orbital hydatidosis and was present in almost all reported cases (Turgut et al. 2004; Garrity and Henderson 2007; Subrahmanyam et al. 2008). This proptosis is irreducible. Usually, the proptosis is of a few months' duration up to 2 years and may be associated with mild pain or discomfort. In our experience, hydatid cysts are the most common intraconal cystic lesions that occur in young patients. As the mass increases in size, it can cause relative afferent pupillary defect, choroidal folds, edema of the optic disc, limitation in ocular motility, and visual impairment (Turgut et al. 2004; Garrity and Henderson 2007; Subrahmanyam et al. 2008). In a meta-analysis, conducted in Turkey (Turgut et al. 2004), slow progressive unilateral proptosis, with or without pain, was the most frequent clinical manifestation (80 %). The other presenting symptoms were visual loss (48 %), periorbital pain (24 %), chemosis (16 %), and headache (12 %). Refractive errors, corneal complications due to exposure, decrease vision due to keratitis and optic nerve compression. Diplopia due to ocular motility restriction can be a rare symptom (Crompton et al. 1985; Kiratli et al. 2003). If they are non-axial, they may be palpable and may even present under the conjunctiva (Mehta et al. 2010). It may be associated with chemosis of the conjunctiva (Talib 1972b; Hanioglu et al. 1997; Betharia et al. 2002).

In long-standing cases, the cyst can grow to a very large size, deforming the globe (Akhan et al. 1998; Subrahmanyam et al. 2008). In a child, the course can be more rapid and may suggest an orbital sarcoma. Orbital hydatid cysts associated with exudative retinal detachment which settled after a total excision of the cyst were reported (Gelisken et al. 1994). Other unusual presentations would include spontaneous rupture of the mother cyst as in the case reported by Ozek et al (1993). A 52-year-old female presented with a 6-month history of painless proptosis of the right eye and a 4-day history of total visual loss associated with severe orbital pain. She had very gross proptosis (28 mm). Intraoperatively a ruptured mother cyst was found with 3 daughter cysts which were removed. The patient was managed successfully with irrigation of the orbital cavity with 3 % sodium chloride solution and oral mebendazole.

Orbital cysts are most often isolated but can be associated with hydatidosis elsewhere in the body, like the lung, liver, and brain (Betharia et al. 2002; Papathanassiou et al. 2008; Siddiqui et al. 2010). Hence, in orbital hydatid disease cases, a whole-body computed tomography (CT) scan and a head magnetic resonance imaging (MRI) scan are mandatory to insure that no other dissemination exists.

Diagnostic Procedures

The plain X-ray, a long forgotten diagnostic procedure, shows thinning and at times erosion of one of the walls of the orbit, the nearest to the cyst. In western countries MRI scan of the orbit is the gold standard imaging technique. However, in endemic countries, the more economic CT scans show a well-encapsulated cys-

Table 23.1 Summary of the 234 reported cases with orbital hydatidosis published in the world literature to date

Author(s)	Country	Year of publication	No. of cases and sex	Age (in years) and side	Proptosis	Visual loss	Location[a]	Surgery[a]	Cyst rupture[a]	Remarks[a]
Wood	South Africa	1925	2F, 1NS	16L, 25R, 3L	3+	2+	Intracon (3)	Operated (3)	Ruptured (3)	Pain in orbit (2)
Seale	South Africa	1926	1F	8R	+	+	Sup-med	Curetting	+	
Handousa	Egypt	1951	2F, 1M	12, 12R, 1L	3+	NS	Intracon (2)	NS (2), 1+	1=0;1=; NS (1)	Palpable (3)
Mazhar	Aden	1954	2F	35L, 35R	2+	2+	Sup-lat	Ant approach	Ruptured (2)	Both were palpable
Lidgett	Australia	1955	1M	55L	NS	NS	Upper med	Orbitonasal	NS	Hypophoria
Tonjum	Sweden	1963	1F	55R	+	+	Sup-lat	Krönlein	+	No systemic HC found
Van Selm	South Africa	1964	5	5<10	5+		Muscle cone (4)	Lat (4), sup (1) orbito	Aspirated	Review of patients below 13
Mehra et al.	India	1965	1M	30R	+	+	Sup-med	Trans-sup lid	Ruptured	
Reddy et al.	India	1970	1M	13L	+	+	Intraorbital	Lat orbito	Ruptured	5×5 cm
Baghdassarian and Zakharia	Lebanon	1971	2M, 1F	31M, 6M, 7F	3+	3+	Med (3), sup (2), inf (1)	Krönlein (1), lid incision (2)	3+	Negative follow-up at 6 months, 18 yrs, and 13 yrs
Talib	Iraq	1972a, b	11M, 11F	11<20 L/R=2/1	18+	NS	Sup-lat or sup-med	Dickson Wrght	NS	Ten years experience left/right=2/1
Zakharia et al.	Lebanon	1972	3	2<15						Unilateral exophthal (85)
Sevel and Sapeika	South Africa	1977	6M, 5F	11 below 17	11+	7+	Retrobulb (11)	Transcutaneous (5), lat orbito (6)	Ruptured (11)	
Amaya et al.	Bolivia	1980	3							
Apple et al.	Cameroun	1980	1NS	6R	+	–	NS	Orbital exploration	–	Pallor of fundus
Danziger and Price	South Africa	1980	1F	9L	+		Med	Done	Biopsy	Papilledema
Okelo et al.	Kenya	1980	1M	17R	+	+	Floor of orbit	NS	NS	
Toledo and Szelagowski	Argentina	1980	1M	18R	+	+	Muscle cone	Operated	NS	
Agarwal et al.	India	1982	1M	38	+	None	Left orbit	Mebendazole	None	HC in spleen
Hamza et al.	Tunisia	1982	9	NS	+	NS	NS	NS	NS	Study of 55 cases
Kars et al.	Turkey	1982	1M, 1F	7L, 11R	2+	+, +	Retrobulb	Cranio (2)		1st case reoperated

(continued)

Table 23.1 (continued)

Author(s)	Country	Year of publication	No. of cases and sex	Age (in years) and side	Proptosis	Visual loss	Location[a]	Surgery[a]	Cyst rupture[a]	Remarks[a]
Sangawe et al.	India	1982	1M	70R	+	+	Intraorbital	Enucl	Aspirated	Chemosis
Klaus and Chana	Kenya	1983	2M, 7F	6–25	9+					Average age 18.8
Lamba et al.	India	1983	1M	Young R	+	+	Upper med	Ant orbito	None	Restriction all eye mov
Bassiri and Jabi	Lebanon	1984	1F	56	+	NS	Intraorbital	Cranio	NS	Chest cyst, ptosis
Crompton et al.	Australia	1985	1M	59	NS	NS	Infraorbital	Sinusecto	NS	Diplopia
Staindl and Krenkel	Germany	1985	1F	5	NS	NS	Orbit	NS	NS	Liver cyst
Chana et al.	Kenya	1986	5F, 2M	5 < 15, 5L–2R	7+	7+	Intraorbital (7)	NS	3	
Khalili	Iraq	1987	5M, 10F	10–50	15+	11+	NS	Done	NS	
Gomez et al.	Argentina	1988	35	26 < 16	25+	7+	Orbital	Orbito (28)	NS	41 yrs experience
Lopera et al.	Venezuela	1989	1F	61L	+	NS	Sup nasal	Cranio	+	*E. oligarthrus*
Alparslan et al.	Turkey	1990	1M, 1F	11L, 6R	2+	+, +	Upper med	Orbito	None, +	
Lerner et al.	Argentina	1991	1F	73L	+	+	Inf lat orbit	Krönlein	+	
Nahri	Egypt	1991	1M, 1F	6L, 4L	2+	0	Intarcon (1)	Orbito (2)	Aspirated (2)	No recurrence in 24 and 18 months
Turgut et al.	Turkey	1992	1M	5L	+	+	Muscle cone	Cranio	Ruptured	Chest HC
Diren et al.	Turkey	1993	1F	10R	+	NS	Retrobulb	Cysts removed in one stage (3)	NS	HC in right frontal lobe and left ventricle
Malde et al.	USA	1993	1M	33L	+		Sup orbital	Orbito	None	
Ozek et al.	Turkey	1993	1F	52R	+	+	Sup orbital	Kronlein	Ruptured	
Mohammad et al.	Egypt	1994	1F	15R	+	None	Intracon	Anteromedial	Ruptured	Neck and liver cysts
Sperryn and Corr	South Africa	1994	10	Mean age 16 (3–41)	10+	4+	Intracon (5)	NS	NS	Ten-year review
Fink et al.	Canada	1995	1M	4 1/2 R	+	NS	Lat upper	NS	NS	Liver HC
Saenz-Santamaria et al.	Spain	1995	1M	8	NS	NS	NS	Aspiration	Aspirated	1 of 15 cases
Sami et al.	Morocco	1995	5M, 5F	Mean 25	10+	7+	Intraorbital	Cranio (9)	None	Frontotemporal (1)
Sharma et al.	India	1995	1M, 1F	18L–25L	2+	+, +	Orbito, NS	Rupture, NS	+, NS	
Sodhani et al.	India	1996	1F	25R	+	None	Intraorbital	Lat orbito	Aspirated	
D'Alessandro	Columbia	1997	NS	NS	NS	NS	Intraorbital	NS	NS	*E. oligarthrus* (2)
Ergün et al.	Turkey	1997	1F, 3M	3 < 15	+	2+	Intraorbital	Cranio (4)	4, PAIR	
Gokcek et al.	Turkey	1997	1F	60L	+	+			+	
Hanioglu et al.	Turkey	1997	1M	4L	+	+	Inf-med	Exploration	Aspirated	Infiltrated maxillary sinus

Karakas et al.	Turkey	1997	2M	54R–6L	+	+	Intraorbital	Cranio		Papilledema
Saygi et al.	Turkey	1997	1M	4L	+	+	Med orbital	NS	Aspirated	Partial removal of cyst
Akhan et al.	Turkey	1998	1M	21R	+	NS	Retrobulb	PAIR	Aspirated	Diplopia
Basset et al.	Suriname	1998	1M	6L	+	+	Intraorbital	Cranio	Ruptured	*E. oligarthrus*
Rastogi et al.	India	1998	1M	25R	+	+	Retrobulb	Enucl	Ruptured	Multiple daughter cysts
Belmekki et al.	Morocco	1999	8	1–15	NS	NS	NS	NS		Out of 54 children
Chaabouni et al.	Tunis	1999	1M	5L	+	None	Inf lat orbit	Cranio	None	No systemic disease
Xiao and Xueyi	China	1999	7M, 11F	15 < 16	14+	6+	Intracon (11)	Orbito (13)	PAIR	38-year review. 8116 cases of HC
Zahawi et al.	Iraq	1999	1M, 3F	Mean 21.3						4 out of 92 HC cases
Zaidi	Libya	1999	1M	19		+		+		
Zaidi	Austria	1999	1		+	+			None	Systemic hydatidosis
Jimenenez -Mejias et al.	Spain	2000	1M	22L	+	+	Sup-lat	Lat orbito	+	No recurrence in 7 yrs
Kargi and Kargi	Egypt	2000	1M	4L	+	+	Inf-med	Subtotal excision	Aspirated	No recurrence in 3 yrs
Sihota and Sharma	India	2000	1M	14L	+	+	Entire orbit	Albendazole	None	2 previous surgeries
Aksoy et al.	Turkey	2001	1M	4R	+	NS	Intracon	Lat orbito	None	Cysts in liver and lungs
Gokcek et al.	Turkey	2001	1M	4	+	+	Intraorbital	Lat orbito	Intact	Papilledema
Betharia et al.	India	2002	1F	35L	+	+	Sup-med	Cryoextract	Aspirated	Systemic disease
Kaymaz et al.	Turkey	2002	1F	8R	+	NS	Intraorbital	Lat orbito	None	
Betharia et al.	India	2003	9	NS	NS	NS	NS	Surgery (9)	NS	Double wall sign
Kiratli et al.	Turkish	2003	1F	20R	NS	None	Med rectus	+		Pain on eye mov
Souhail et al.	Morocco	2003	2	NS	2+	NS	NS	NS	NS	
Cooney et al.	Kenya	2004	NS	NS	NS	NS	Retro-orbital	NS	NS	710 cases reviewed
Turgut et al.	Turkey	2004	25	18 < 20; 11R, 13L	20+	11+	Intracon (9)	Enucl (4); orbito (10)	9	Review of 30 yrs
Diatchuk et al.	Israel	2005	1M	14R	+	NS	Extraconal	PAIR	1	
Murthy et al.	India	2005	1F	14R	+	+	30 cysts	Enucl		*E. oligarthrus*
Ciurea et al.	Hungary	2006	1M, 1F	15L, 4L	2+	2+	Intracon	Cranio (2)	1	
Ryou et al.	Korea	2002	1F	33R	+	+	Intracon	Lat orbito	+	Pain in affected eye

(continued)

Table 23.1 (continued)

Author(s)	Country	Year of publication	No. of cases and sex	Age (in years) and side	Proptosis	Visual loss	Location[a]	Surgery[a]	Cyst rupture[a]	Remarks[a]
Abbassi et al.	Morocco	2007	1M	70L	NS	+	Multiple	Medical	None	Headache and neck mass
Sanli et al.	Turkey	2007	1F	22R	+	+	NS	Cranio	None	
Ali et al.	Pakistan	2008	2	NS	NS	NS	NS	Lat orbito (2)	NS	Over a period of 7 yrs
Jeblaoui et al.	Tunisia	2008	1M	72L	+	+	Postero-lat	Lat orbito	None	
Papathanassiou et al.	Greece	2008	1	Child				Albendazole	None	Lung and liver
Groves et al.	Kenya	2009	1F	25R	+	None	Postero-med	Aspiration	+	Into nose and fronto-ethmoid sinus
Bagheri et al.	Iran	2010	1M, 1F	11L, 8R	2+	1+, 1−	Intracon (2)	Lat orbito (2)	1+ and 1−	A case had 2 previous surgeries and one *E. alveolaris*
Benazzou et al.	Morocco	2010	6M, 4F	7 below 12	10+	8+	Retrobulb (10)	Cranioto (10)	Ruptured (9)	CNS HC 135 cases
Limaiem et al.	Tunisia	2010	1M	74L	+	+	Retrobulb	Cranioto	Rupture	
Mehta et al.	Turkey	2010	1F	35L	+	+		Trans conjunctiva	+	Double wall sign
Siddiqui et al.	India	2010	1M	7L	+	+	Thru roof	Aspirat	Punctured	Extension of epidural
Yazdani et al.	Iran	2010	1F	14R	+	+	Subtemporal	Caldwell-Luc	None	Multiple brain HC
Bhaduri et al.	India	2011	1F	40L	+	+	Intracon	Enucl	NS	
Menghi and Gatta	Argentina	2011	1F	41R	+	NS	Orbit	Surgery	Ruptured	
Sharma et al.	India	2011	1M	6L	+	+	Outside muscle cone	Extended lat orbito	Aspirated	Eye pushdown and lat. bilobed cyst
Yurt et al.	Turkey	2011	1M	3L	+		Retro-orbital	Lat orbito	None	Adherent to lat rectus
Holland	India	2012	8		8+	6+	Upper med	Conjunctiva	Aspirated (8)	Formalin injection
Kahveci	Turkey	2012	1F	6L	+	+	Inf lat orbit	Cranioto	PAIR	
Somay et al.	Turkey	2012	1M	10	NS	NS	Intracon	Cranio	None	

Abbreviations: *NS* not stated, *ant* anterior, *lat* lateral, *med* medial, *sup* superior, *inf* inferior, *F* female, *M* male, *R* right, *L* left, *CNS* central nervous system, *exophthal* exophthalmos, *HC* hydatid cyst, *intracon* intraconal, *mov* movement, *cranio* craniotomy, *cryoextrat* cryoextraction, *Enucl* enucleation, *orbito* orbitotomy, *PAIR* puncture-aspiration-injection of scolicidal fluid-reaspiration, *retrobulb* retrobulbar, *sinusecto* sinusectomy, *yr(s)* year(s)

[a]Numbers within the brackets show no. of cases for each entity

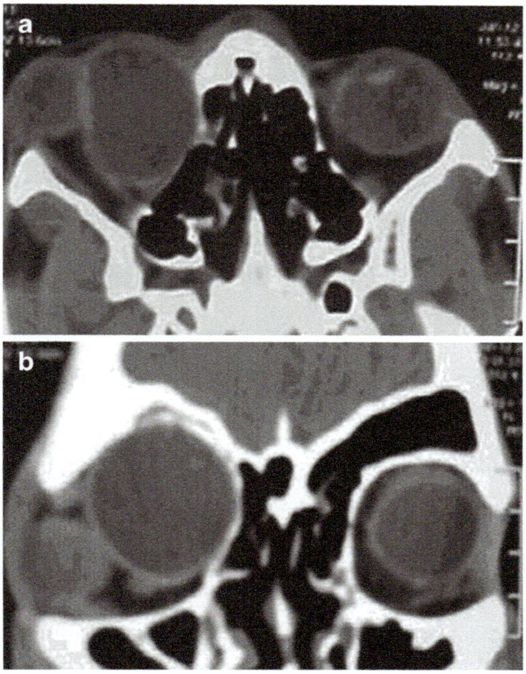

Fig. 23.1 (**a**) Axial section of CT scan of orbit showing a very large, thin-walled hydatid cyst displacing the globe laterally. The size of the cyst is larger than the eyeball. Look at the bony "excavation" with very smooth margins of the medial wall which denotes a "chronic course" of a "benign lesion." (**b**) Coronal section of CT scan of the orbit showing a very large, isodense cystic lesion displacing the globe inferolaterally and it dwarfs the globe

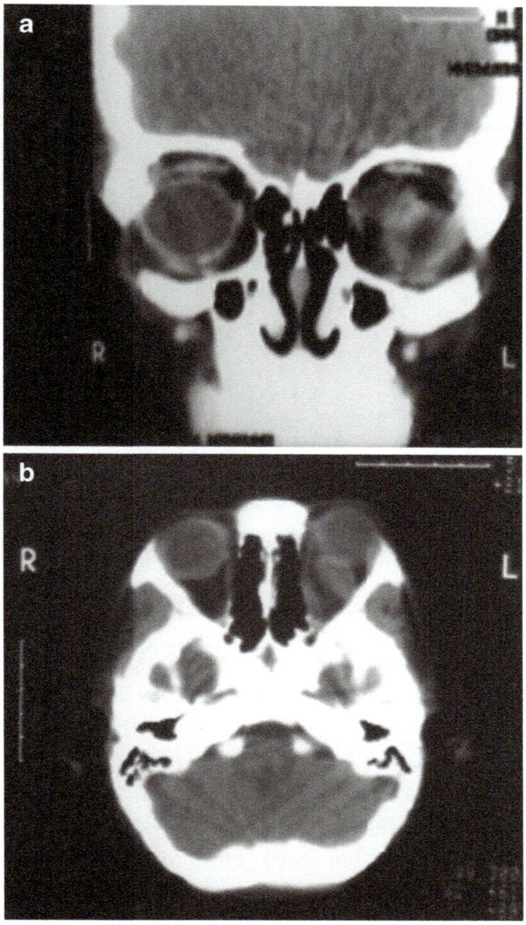

Fig. 23.2 (**a**) Coronal view and (**b**) axial view. A 28-year-old male patient; CT scan of the orbit shows hydatidosis of the orbit (Courtesy of F. Limaiem)

tic mass with cyst fluid showing attenuation values of 3–30 HU (Figs. 23.1, 23.2, and 23.3). The mass can indent and deform the globe. Calcification of the internal septa may be seen. MRI is the alternative choice of imaging diagnostic techniques. MRI shows a low-intensity signal on T_1-weighted images and a high-intensity signal on T_2-weighted images (Diren et al. 1993; Gokcek et al. 1997).

B-scan ultrasound of the orbit shows confirmatory diagnostic double wall sign; spoke wheel pattern and water lily sign are seen with cyst calcification (Malde et al. 1993). The double wall sign described by Betharia et al. (2002) was considered diagnostic of hydatid disease of the orbit. However, this double wall sign was described by Kashyap et al. (2009) in a case of an orbital schwannoma with cystic degeneration.

Other investigations are as follows:

- Hemogram is usually normal.
- Stool examination does not show eggs or cysts.
- Casoni's intradermal test is positive in 75 % of the people (Subrahmanyam et al. 2008).
- Counter immunoelectrophoresis (Kiratli et al. 2003).
- Fine-needle aspiration biopsy: microscopic analysis of the cyst fluid shows scolices and hooklets (Saenz-Santamaria et al. 1995). However, this test is strongly contraindicated.
- Enzyme-linked immunosorbent assay (ELISA) and the indirect hemagglutination test are highly sensitive procedures for serum screening; sensitivity rates vary from 60 to 90 %.

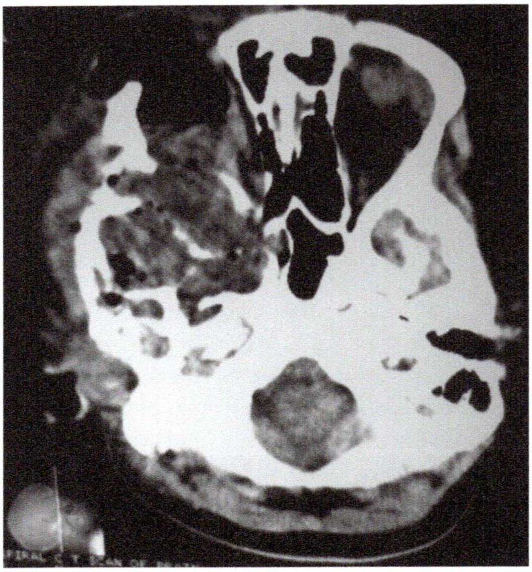

Fig. 23.3 A hydatid abscess entering into the right orbit from the surrounding anatomic structures (Courtesy of M.Z. Hossain)

Pathology

The cyst is pearly white and has a wall consisting of three layers. Unlike in brain cysts, where the pericyst is so thin that it may go unnoticed, the pericyst in retro-orbital cysts may be well formed. This is due to the proximity of fibrous tissue in the orbit. The ectocyst is a structureless, acellular, laminated, homogeneously basophilic material. The ectocyst cyst is laminated and has the characteristic "coats of an onion" appearance (Garrity and Henderson 2007). The endocyst may show overgrowth and is the germinative layer. The clear fluid filling the cyst may show hooklets and scolecesif the cyst is intact and productive. In long-standing cysts, specks of calcium may be present. Some may contain daughter cysts.

Management

Surgery

The aim of surgery is to deliver the entire cyst intact and not to spill any of its content in the orbit or the adjoining tissues. We feel it is best achieved through a subfrontal approach. We believe surgery of orbital hydatid cysts is a neurosurgical procedure and not an ophthalmological one. The essence is to deliver the cyst intact, without rupturing it, a result which is seldom achieved through an ophthalmological approach especially in those cysts located in the medial aspect of the orbit.

The eyelids should be closed with a scotch tape or a tarsorrhaphy to protect the cornea. The draping is an essential part of this procedure. The drapes should be laid loose over the affected eye to allow an eventual Credè procedure. The incision is a regular bifrontal incision, behind the hair line, if possible going way down to below the zygoma on the affected side sparing the seventh nerve on that side. The soft tissues are reflected over the eyes. They should be held high up away from the forehead and eyes, to allow for the surgeon's hand to reach the affected eye from over the drapes during surgery. A frontal free bone flap is raised as close to the supracillary ridge as possible, possibly including it. In case the frontal sinus is in the way, it should be opened, exenterated, and its inner wall completely removed. The basal frontal dura is peeled off the base of the skull until the anterior clinoid process, covered with a 0.1 % cetrimide-wetted gauze, and retracted up and back with a self-retaining retractor. The orbital roof is nibbled away carefully with a small bone rongeur and the entire roof as well as part of its lateral orbital wall is removed. The bony edges are smoothened all around the bony resection and covered with gauze imbibed in cetrimide. A thick thread or fine tape is passed under the levator palpebrae superioris, the rectus oculi superioris, and the superior oblique muscles. These are retracted in a direction not to hinder the delivery of the cyst and would depend on the position of the cyst. The periorbita is opened and the orbital fat dissected with care with a blunt instrument. Once the cyst is seen, it should be carefully uncovered from fat until the pericyst is seen. The pericyst should be dissected carefully and excised over as large an area as possible. There is no need to resect the entire pericyst. When the cyst comes clearly into view and is uncovered as far and as well as possible, the surgeon places two fingers over the drape covering the closed eyelids and presses on the eyeball, through the drapes, using the Credè method to deliver the cyst. In case it does not come out easily, a blunt instrument is passed under the cyst and cetrimide solution is injected behind the cyst through a fine flexible rubber catheter. This maneuver is repeated until the cyst is delivered in the field; it is then scooped with a small tablespoon and placed in a basin.

In case the cyst is inadvertently ruptured, the fluid should be immediately aspirated and the entire operative area washed thoroughly with cetrimide. Then the gauze in the field should be carefully removed after sucking the excess fluid to avoid any fluid dripping from it and the field is again washed with cetrimide. The wound is then closed in the usual manner.

The wall of the cyst is very thin and may rupture very easily during surgery. To prevent rupture of the cyst, after exposing it, its contents are aspirated to shrink it in size (Fig. 23.4). Then, it can be easily removed with the help of cryo (Subrahmanyam et al. 2008) (Fig. 23.5). These two procedures should be reserved for cases which cannot be removed otherwise and only in extreme need.

Previously, the aspiration of the cyst, establishment of the diagnosis, reinflation of the mass with some agent (e.g., hypertonic saline, alcohol, formalin) to detach the scolices from the inner germinal wall, a second aspiration to empty the cyst, and followed by extirpation of the endocyst with or without the overlying ectocyst were done by many surgeons, the so-called PAIR procedure (Chana et al. 1986).

Nahri (1991) first used the cataract cryoprobe in two cases. An initial aspiration helps the cyst to collapse so that the outer fibrous wall is easily tented and grasped with nontoothed forceps and the needle puncture site is snipped open. The endocyst is attached to the cryoprobe and completely extracted. There were no recurrences during 18–24 months of follow-up, but we prefer the delivery of the intact cyst as described above.

Gokcek et al. (1997) recommends total removal of the cyst by means of a microdissection technique. Afterwards, Akhan et al. (1998) proposed a percutaneous treatment as an alternative approach to conventional surgery. Under ultrasonographic guidance, the cyst was aspirated with 15 % hypertonic saline and then reaspirated without complication. Twenty-one months later,

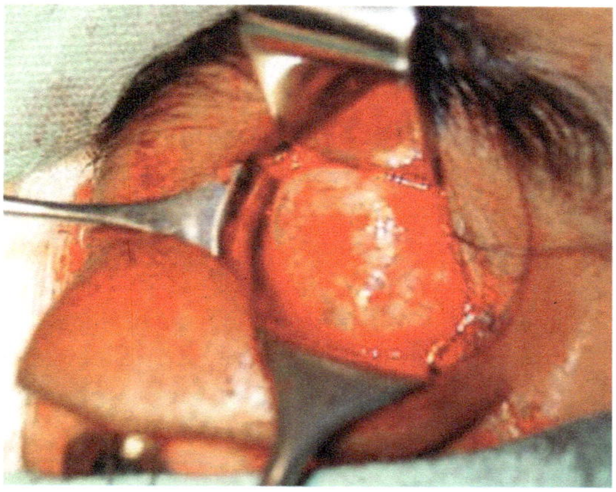

Fig. 23.4 After exposing the cyst, the contents are aspirated to shrink the cyst and facilitate its removal without rupturing the cyst wall

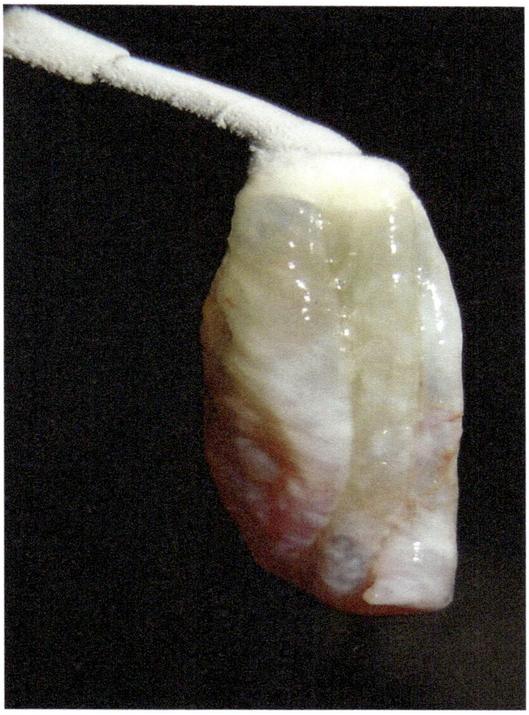

Fig. 23.5 The shrunken cyst was removed with the help of a cryo

imaging of the shrunken mass showed a volume of only 0.5 ml, and the patient was asymptomatic. Recently, Jimenenez-Mejias et al. (2000) described a case wherein the cyst ruptured during surgical removal. The surgical field was irrigated with hypertonic saline solution, and the remnants of the cyst were excised.

Anaphylaxis is a complication that the surgeon is worried about which can occur due to the rupture of the cyst during surgery. The incidence was about 2.25 % and no mortality was reported due to anaphylactic shock (Li et al. 2011).

Medical

Medical management with oral albendazole at a dose of 400 mg/day for 3 months in combination with praziquantel at a dose of 1,200 mg, every 8 hours, has been tried for primary as well as for recurrent cases of orbital hydatidosis with some success (Chana et al. 1986; Sihota and Sharma 2000). Oral albendazole is continued for 3 months after surgery. In another comparative study on hydatidosis of the liver, it was found that in the patients who received preoperative albendazole for 12 weeks prior to surgery, there were no viable cysts at the time of surgery compared to 95% of those who did not receive albendazole prior to surgery. There was no recurrence in the first group, whereas in the second group, the recurrence rate was about 17 % (Chana et al. 1986). Hence, there is a definite role for pharmaceutical management and all the patients in whom the cyst ruptures during surgery should receive oral albendazole. It would also be recommended that, whenever possible, this drug should be used preoperatively.

Conclusion

This rare condition, orbital hydatid cyst, is an important part of the study of human echinococcosis. It can be the sole body cyst or it may be associated with cyst elsewhere in the body such as the liver, spleen, etc. Its surgical delivery is the treatment of choice. It is recommended that the patient receive medicinal treatment preoperatively and that this treatment be continued in case of cyst puncture or rupture for a period of at least 3 months. A combination of albendazole and praziquantel is recommended.

References

Abbassi R, Kacemi L, Bricha M, El Quessar A, El Hassani MR, Chakir N, et al. Cervico-facial hydatid disease: a case report. J Radiol. 2007;88(Pt I):1725–7.

Agarwal MB, Kamdar MS, Tilve GH, Bapat RD, Vakil NB, Desai MB. Splenic and orbital hydatid cysts and treatment with mebendazole (a case report). J Postgrad Med. 1982;28:115–7.

Akhan O, Bilgic S, Akata D, Kiratli H, Ozmen MN. Percutaneous treatment of an orbital hydatid cyst: a new therapeutic approach. Am J Ophthalmol. 1998;125:877–9.

Aksoy FG, Tanrikulu S, Kosar U. Inferiorly located retrobulbar hydatid cyst: CT and MRI features. Comput Med Imaging Graph. 2001;25:535–40.

Ali M, Khan H, Khan KH, Khwanzada K, Ayub S, Rahman S. Cranioorbital hydatidosis. J Pediatr Neurol. 2008;6:125–8.

Alparslan L, Kanberoglu K, Peksayar G, Cokyüksel O. Orbital hydatid cyst: assessment of two cases. Neuroradiology. 1990;32:163–5.

Amaya C, Villarejo F, Izquierdo JM, Perez-Higueras A, Blazquez MG. Hydatid cyst: unusual cause of unilateral exophthalmos. Surg Neurol. 1980;14:351–4.

Apple DJ, Fajoni ML, Garland PE, Kuhr L, Moel SA. Orbital hydatid cyst. J Pediatr Ophthalmol Strabismus. 1980;17:380–3.

Baghdassarian SA, Zakharia H. Report of three cases of hydatid cyst of the orbit. Am J Ophthalmol. 1971;71:1081–4.

Bagheri A, Fallahi MR, Yazdani S, Rezaee Kanavi M. Two different presentations of orbital echinococcosis: a report of two cases and review of the literature. Orbit. 2010;29:51–6.

Bassiri A, Jabi A. Computerised tomography in orbital echinococcosis. Br J Radiol. 1984;57:270–2.

Basset D, Girou C, Nozais IP, D'Hermies F, Hoang C, Gordon R, et al. Neotropical echinococcosis in Suriname: Echinococcus oligarthrus in the orbit and Echinococcus vogeli in the abdomen. Am J Trop Med Hyg. 1998;59:787–90.

Belmekki M, El Bakkali M, Abdellah H, Benchrifa F, Berraho A. Epidemiology of orbital processes in children. 54 cases (in French). J Fr Ophthalmol. 1999;22:394–8.

Benazzou S, Arkha Y, Derraz S, El Ouahabi A, El Khamlichi A. Orbital hydatid cyst: review of 10 cases. J Craniomaxillofac Surg. 2010;38:274–8.

Betharia SM, Pushker N, Sharma V, Avinash M, Kashyap S. Disseminated hydatid disease involving orbit, spleen, lung and liver. Ophthalmologica. 2002;216:300–4.

Betharia SM, Sharma V, Pushker N. Ultrasound findings in orbital hydatid cysts. Am J Ophthalmol. 2003; 135:568–70.

Bhaduri G, Chatterjee SS, Gayen S, Goswami S. Hydatid cyst of orbit. J Indian Med Assoc. 2011;109:681–2.

Chaabouni M, Ben Zina Z, Ben Ayez H, Tounsi R, Trigui A, Ben Mansour H. Kyste hydatique de l'orbite: localisation intra-orbitaire unique. A propos d'une observation. J Fr Ophthalmol. 1999;22:329–34.

Chana HS, Klauss V, Shah A. Orbital hydatid disease in Kenya. Am J Trop Med Hyg. 1986;35:991–4.

Ciurea AV, Giuseppe G, Machinis TG, Coman TC, Fountas KN. Orbital hydatid cyst in childhood: a report of two cases. South Med J. 2006;99:620–4.

Cooney RM, Flanagan KP, Zehyle E. Review of surgical management of cystic hydatid disease in a resource limited setting: Turkana, Kenya. Eur J Gastroenterol Hepatol. 2004;16:1233–6.

Crompton JL, Iyer PV, Merry DJ, Tomich J, Perrett LV. Hydatid cyst: an unusual cause of diplopia. Aust N Z J Ophthalmol. 1985;13:195–203.

D'Alessandro A. Polycystic echinococcosis in tropical America: Echinococcus vogeli and E. oligarthrus. Acta Trop. 1997;67:43–65.

Danziger A, Price H. Computed tomographic findings in orbital echinococciasis; case report. J Comput Assist Tomogr. 1980;4:128–9.

Diatchuk V, Rumelt S, Rehany U. Orbital hydatid cyst manifested as expanding exophthalmos following blunt orbital trauma. J Pediatr Ophthalmol Strabismus. 2005;42:369–71.

Diren HB, Ozcanli H, Boluk M, Kilic C. Unicellular orbital, cerebral and intraventricular hydatid cysts. Neuroradiology. 1993;35:149–50.

Ergün R, Ökten AI, Yüksel M, Gül B, Evliyaoðlu C, Ergüngör F, et al. Orbital hydatid cysts: report of four cases. Neurosurg Rev. 1997;20:33–7.

Fink AM, Newman DE, Stringer DA. Pediatric case of the day. Radiographics. 1995;15:731–4.

Garrity JA, Henderson JW. Cyst and cele. In: Hendersons orbital tumor. 4th ed. Philadelphia: Lippincott Williams & Wilkins; 2007. p. 34–61.

Gelisken F, Erda S, Kreissig I. Exudative retinal detachment in intraorbital echinococcal cyst (in German). Klin Monbl Augenheilkd. 1994;205:109–11.

Gokcek C, Gökçek A, Akif Bayar M, Tanrikulu S, Buharali Z. Orbital hydatid cyst: CT and MRI. Neuroradiology. 1997;39:512–5.

Gokcek C, Bayar N, Buharai Z. Total removal of an unruptured orbital hydatid cyst. Can J Ophthalmol. 2001;36:218–20.

Gomez Morales A, Croxatto JO, Crovetto L, Ebner R. Hydatid cysts of the orbit. A review of 35 cases. Ophthalmology. 1988;95:1027–32.

Groves MW, Muller S, Gathere S, Gachii A, 3rd Johns MM. Pathology quiz case 1. Sino-orbital cystic echinococcosis (CE). Arch Otolaryngol Head Neck Surg. 2009;135:1056, 1058–9.

Guerinel CL, Roux FX, Bonin A, Lucerna S, Lariche B. Intra-orbital hydatid cyst. An uncommon site of hydatidosis. Discussion apropos of a recent case (in French). Neurochirurgie. 1991;37:200–5.

Hamza R, Touibi S, Jamoussi M, Bardi-Bellagha I, Chtioui R. Intracranial and orbital hydatid cysts. Neuroradiology. 1982;22:211–4.

Handousa AB. Proptosis caused by hydatid disease. Br J Ophthalmol. 1951;35:607–13.

Hanioglu S, Saygi S, Yazar Z, Saltik G, Gürsel E. Orbital hydatid cyst. Can J Ophthalmol. 1997;32:334–7.

Holland H. Hydatid of the orbit. Br J Ophthalmol. 2012;32:395–6.

Jeblaoui Y, Bouguila J, Yacoub K, Bouguila H, Ben Neji N, Besbes G. Orbital hydatid cyst. Rev Stomatol Chir Maxillofac. 2008;109:117–9.

Jimenenez-Mejias ME, Alarcon-Cruz JC, Marquez-Rivas FJ, Palomino-Nicas J, Montero JM, Pachón J. Orbital hydatid cyst: treatment and prevention of recurrences with albendazole plus praziquantel. J Infect. 2000;41:105–7.

Kahveci R, Sanli AM, Gurer B, Sekerci Z. Orbital hydatid cyst. J Neurosurg Pediatr. 2012;9:42–4.

Karakaş HM, Tokoglu F, Kacar M, Boyacigil S. Retrobulbar hydatid cyst: assessment of two cases. Australas Radiol. 1997;41:179–80.

Kargi SH, Kargi E. An unusual case of orbital hydatid cyst: a surgical emergency. Ann Plast Surg. 2000;44:574.

Kars Z, Kansu T, Ozcan OE, Erbengi A. Orbital echinococcosis. Report of two cases studied by computerized tomography. J Clin Neuroophthalmol. 1982;2:197–9.

Kashyap S, Pushker N, Meel R, Sen S, Bajaj MS, Khuriajam N, et al. Orbital schwannoma with cystic degeneration. Clin Exp Ophthalmol. 2009;37:293–8.

Kaymaz M, Dogulu F, Kurt G, Kardes O, Baykaner MK. Orbital hydatid cyst. Case illustration. J Neurosurg. 2002;97:724.

Khalili AH. CT values in orbital hydatid cyst. Comput Radiol. 1987;11:193–7.

Kiratli H, Bilgic S, Oztürkmen C, Aydin O. Intramuscular hydatid cyst of the medial rectus muscle. Am J Ophthalmol. 2003;135:98–9.

Klauss V, Chana HS. Ocular tumors in Africa. Soc Sci Med. 1983;17:1743–50.

Lamba PA, Bhatia PC, Jain M, Baweja U. Hydatid cyst of orbit. Indian J Ophthalmol. 1983;31:23–5.

Lerner SF, Gomez Morales A, Croxatto JO. Hydatid cyst of the orbit. Arch Ophthalmol. 1991;109:285.

Li Y, Zheng H, Cao X, Liu Z, Chen L. Demographic and clinical characteristics of patients with anaphylactic shock after surgery for cystic echinococcosis. Am J Trop Med Hyg. 2011;85:452–5.

Lidgett K. Hydatid cyst of the orbit: report of a case. Med J Aust. 1955;42:796.

Limaiem F, Bellil S, Bellil K, Chelly I, Mekni A, Khaldi M, et al. Primary orbital hydatid cyst in an elderly patient. Surg Infect. 2010;11:393–5.

Lopera RD, Meléndez RD, Fernandez I, Sirit J, Perera MP. Orbital hydatid cyst of Echinococcus oligarthrus in a human in Venezuela. J Parasitol. 1989;75: 467–70.

Malde HM, Gadkari SS, Chadha D, Gondhalekar N. Water lily sign in an orbital hydatid cyst. Spontaneous

rupture of an intraorbital hydatid cyst. A rare cause of acute visual loss. J Clin Ultrasound. 1993;21:458–9.
Mazhar M. Hydatid cyst of the orbit. Br J Ophthalmol. 1954;38:753.
Mehra KS, Banerjee C, Somani PN, Rajyashree K. Hydatid cyst in orbit. Acta Ophthalmol (Copenh). 1965;43:761–3.
Mehta M, Sen S, Sethi S, Pushker N, Bajaj MS, Chandra M. Large orbital hydatid cyst presenting as subconjunctival mass. Ann Trop Med Parasitol. 2010;104:601–4.
Menghi CI, Gatta CL. Unusual localization of an hydatid cyst: first reported case in Buenos Aires, Argentina. Braz J Infect Dis. 2011;15:81–2.
Mohammad Ael-N A, Ray CJ, Karcioglu ZA. Echinococcus cysts of the orbit and substernum. Am J Ophthalmol. 1994;118:676–8.
Murthy R, Honavar SG, Vemuganti GK, Naik M, Burman S. Polycystic echinococcosis of the orbit. Am J Ophthalmol. 2005;140:561–3.
Nahri GE. A simplified technique for removal of orbital hydatid cysts. Br J Ophthalmol. 1991;75:743–5.
Okelo GB, Kyobe J, Shah AK, Musyoki JJ. Retro-orbital hydatid: case report. East Afr Med J. 1980;57:285–8.
Ozek MM, Pamir MN, Sav A. Spontaneous rupture of an intraorbital hydatid cyst: a rare cause of acute visual loss. J Clin Neuroophthalmol. 1993;13:135–7.
Papathanassiou M, Petrou P, Zampeli E, Vergados I, Paikos P. Disseminated hydatid disease in a child: albendazole treatment of orbital cyst. Eur J Ophthalmol. 2008;18:1034–6.
Rastogi A, Arora R, Chaturvedi K. Orbital hydatid cyst: an unusual presentation. Orbit. 1998;17:107–11.
Reddy MV, Satyndran OM, Krishna KS. Orbital hydatid cyst. J Indian Med Assoc. 1970;55:203–4.
Ryou JY, Kim KH, Kim SY. Hydatid cyst of the orbit (in Korean). J Korean Ophthalmol Soc. 2002;47:484–8.
Saenz-Santamaria J, Moreno-Casado J, Nunez C. Role of fine-needle biopsy in the diagnosis of hydatid cyst. Diagn Cytopathol. 1995;13:229–32.
Sami A, Achouri M, Harouch M, Choukry M, Ouboukhlik A, Elkamar A, et al. Intra-orbital hydatid cysts. 10 cases (in French). Neurochirurgie. 1995;41:398–402.
Sangawe JL, Chitra NV, Venkataramaiah NR, Van Raalte JA. Hydatid cyst of the orbit. J Trop Med Hyg. 1982; 85:149–51.
Sanli M, Sabuncuoğlu H, Keskin T. Primary intraorbital hydatid cyst: an unusual location, case report and review of the literature. Minim Invasive Neurosurg. 2007;50:367–9.
Saygi HS, Yazar Z, Saltik G, Gürsel E. Orbital hydatid cyst. Can J Ophthalmol. 1997;32:334–7.
Seale EA. A case of Hydatid cyst of the orbit: Removal of cyst with preservation of eye and vision. Br Med J. 1926;1(3412):910–1.
Sevel D, Sapeika RJ. Hydatid cyst of the orbit. Surv Ophthalmol. 1977;22:101–5.
Sharma R, Vashisht S, Berry M. Orbital hydatid cysts: sonographic and CT appearance. Australas Radiol. 1995;39:246–8.
Sharma RL, Thakur RC, Sud C, Sareen A. Extended lateral orbitotomy, an effective procedure to excise large orbital hydatid cyst: a rare case. Ann Trop Med Public Health. 2011;4:45–7.
Siddiqui MA, Rizvi SW, Rizvi SA, Ahmad I, Ullah E. Atypical multifocal hydatid disease of cranial vault: simultaneous orbital and extradural meningeal involvement. Emerg Radiol. 2010;17:427–30.
Sihota R, Sharma T. Albendazole therapy for a recurrent orbital hydatid cyst. Indian J Ophthalmol. 2000; 48:142–3.
Sodhani P, Das DK, Natarajan R, Khan IU. Cytological diagnosis of orbital echinococcosis. Diagn Cytopathol. 1996;15:52–3.
Somay H, Emon ST, Orakdogen M, Berkman MZ. A primary orbital hydatid cyst. J Clin Neurosci. 2012;19: 898–900.
Souhail H, Mahi M, Akjouj S, Elhassani MR, Chakir N, Jiddane M. A rare cause of exophthalmos, hydatid cyst of the orbit. Presse Med. 2003;32:457–9.
Sperryn CW, Corr PD. CT evaluation of orbital hydatid disease: a review of 10 cases. Clin Radiol. 1994;49: 703–4.
Staindl O, Krenkel C. Echinococcosis of the orbit (in German). HNO. 1985;33:404–8.
Subrahmanyam M, Ather M, Madini P. Parasitic cysts of orbit. In: Subrahmanyam M, editor. Surgical atlas of orbital diseases. 1st ed. New Delhi: Jaypee Brothers; 2008. p. 206–18.
Talib H. Orbital tumours in Iraq. Ann R Coll Surg Engl. 1972a;51:31–40.
Talib H. Orbital hydatid disease in Iraq. Br J Surg. 1972b;59:391–4.
Toledo EC, Szelagowski JC. Unilateral exophthalmos in orbital echinococciasis. J Comput Assist Tomogr. 1980; 4:127.
Tonjum AM. Hydatid cyst of the orbit. Acta Ophthalmol (Copenh). 1963;41:445–8.
Turgut M, Saglam S, Ozcan OE. Orbital hydatid cyst. Report of a case followed by serial computed tomography. J Clin Neuroophthalmol. 1992;12:43–6.
Turgut AT, Turgut M, Kosar U. Hydatidosis of the orbit in Turkey: results from review of the literature 1963-2001. Int Ophthalmol. 2004;25:193–200.
Van Selm J. Some orbital swelling in children. S Afr Med J. 1964;38:590–2.
Wood DJ. Hydatid cysts of the orbit. Br J Ophthalmol. 1925;9:4–6.
Xiao A, Xueyi C. Hydatid cysts of the orbit in Xinjiang: a review of 18 cases. Orbit. 1999;18:151–5.
Yazdani N, Basam A, Heidarali M, Sharif Kashani S, Hasibi M, Mokhtari Z. Infratemporal hydatid cyst: a case presenting with blindness. J Laryngol Otol. 2010; 124:456–9.
Yurt A, Secer M, Selcuki M. Large primary intraorbital hydatid cyst. Childs Nerv Syst. 2011;27:693–5.
Zahawi HM, Hameed OK, Abalkhail AA. The possible role of the age of the human host in determining the localization of hydatid cysts. Ann Trop Med Parasitol. 1999;93:621–7.
Zaidi M. An unusual case of orbital hydatid cyst: a surgical emergency. Ann Plast Surg. 1999;42:327–9.
Zakharia HS, Asdourian K, Matta CS. Unilateral exophthalmos. Aetiological study of 85 cases. Br J Ophthalmol. 1972;56:678–86.

Alveolar Hydatidosis of the Central Nervous System

24

Sikó Barabási Sándor

Contents

S.B. Sándor, DVM, Dr. Univ., MSc, PhD
Department of Ecological and Biotechnological Systems, Faculty of Environmental Science, Babeş-Bolyai University Cluj-Napoca, Extension of Sfântu Gheorghe, Stadionului Str. 14., Sfântu Gheorghe RO-520064, Romania
e-mail: siko.b.sandor@gmail.com

Introduction

Alveolar echinococcosis (AE) is caused by the larval stage of the fox tapeworm *Echinococcus multilocularis*. This cestode has a sylvatic life cycle in foxes (as the definitive hosts) and in arvicolid rodents (voles), which represent the larval metacestode stage (as intermediate hosts). Foci of human AE also occur where foxes or domestic dogs are fed on infected rodents and where there is accidental ingestion of *E. multilocularis* eggs from canine fecal matter (McManus et al. 2011; Sikó 2011a).

Alveolar hydatid disease (AHD) occurs in at least 42 countries of the Northern Hemisphere. Recent studies in Europe and Asia have shown that the endemic area of *E. multilocularis* is larger than previously known, and the parasite has regionally expanded from rural to urban areas. In addition, increasing fox populations may be associated with higher infection risk in humans with a phase lag of 10–20 years in Europe.

AHD is an aggressive and a highly lethal parasitic infection caused by the larval stage of *E. multilocularis*. It is characterized by the appearance of a tumor with extensive character, primarily in the liver of intermediate hosts including humans. The tumor has a pronounced pseudomalignant growth and can induce metastasis to different organs (Sikó 2011b). The diagnosis and the treatment are difficult. AHD is a life-threatening parasitosis. Mortality rate is 94–100 % in patients diagnosed late or undiagnosed and untreated. Long incubation period (10–15 years), considerable hospital costs

M. Turgut (ed.), *Hydatidosis of the Central Nervous System: Diagnosis and Treatment*,
DOI 10.1007/978-3-642-54359-3_24, © Springer-Verlag Berlin Heidelberg 2014

(17,800 USD/patient/year), low survival rate, expansive character of the area of distribution, increase in human cases from year to year, and persistence of the parasite in nature are sufficient arguments for AHD caused by the larval form of *E. multilocularis* to be considered as a first emergency parasitic disease in Europe.

Cerebral hydatid disease is very rare, representing only 2 % of all cerebral space-occupying lesions even in the countries where the disease is endemic (Bükte et al. 2004). Alveolar hydatid cysts constitute 3 % of cerebral hydatid cyst cases (Senturk et al. 2006; Ozdol et al. 2011). Intracranial AE accounts for about 1 % of all cases of AE and is generally considered to be fatal (Yang et al. 2005).

The first AE lesion in the brain was reported in 1884 (Devé 1946). A European study of 600 cases of AE collected up to the year 1932 showed that in only 31 cases was the brain involved (WHO 1996). Altinors et al. (2000) found a total of 219 cases of intracranial echinococcosis in the 5-year period 1994–1999 in Turkey. Of these 16 were AE. Two of them were AE with no extra central nervous system (CNS) involvement. The proportion of CE:AE cases in various studies from Turkey was 1,109:169 (Torgerson et al. 2010). A large study in China suggested that 4 % of AE cases had neurological involvement (Jiang et al. 2005). Likewise, a large European study found 17 of 559 (3 %) cases of AE had brain involvement (Kern et al. 2003).

Table 24.1 Cases of the *Echinococcus multilocularis* infection in definitive hosts, in intermediate hosts, or in humans reported in central and eastern parts of Europe and in Turkey

Country	Year	Host
Poland	1995–2006	Fox
	1955–2007	Human
Slovenia	2006–2007	Human
Hungary	1988	Human
	2003, 2008–2009	Fox
Slovakia	1999, 2001	Fox
	2009	Dog
	2000–2008	Human
Bulgaria	1980	Rodents
Turkey	1934, 1939	Human
	1965	Fox
Greece	1978	Human
Moldavia	1961	House mouse
	1971	Fox, raccoon dog, human
Ukraine	1957, 2006–2008	Fox
Romania	2009, 2011	Fox, voles, human
Armenia	1958	Human
Belarus	1957, 1958	Rodents
	2001, 2003	Fox
Lithuania	2003, 2009	Beaver
	2005–2006	Dog, pig
	1997–2006	Human
	2001–2004	Fox
Latvia	2008	Fox
Estonia	2005	Fox
Russia	1957	Fox
	1966	Wild cat
	1970, 1972, 1998	Fox, human
Kyrgyzstan	2010	Fox

Adapted from Sikó (2011a)

Epidemiology

In 1980 in Europe the *E. multilocularis* was known and described in only four countries (Austria, France, Germany, and Switzerland). In 1996 the number of these countries has reached 9. The presence of the parasite is reported more frequently in Eastern Europe (Slovakia, Hungary, Ukraine, Bulgaria, and Romania), Turkey, Asia (Russia, Kazakhstan, and China), North America (Dakota), and Japan (Table 24.1). In most countries AE has already an endemic character and is still expanding with alarming rapidity. Epidemiology of alveolar hydatidosis is discussed in Chap. 4.

The main source of infection and life cycle in Europe is forestry including mainly the European red fox (*Vulpes vulpes*) and several species of rodents as intermediate hosts: water mouse (*Arvicola terrestris*), field mouse (*Microtus arvalis*), forest mouse (*Clethrionomys glareolus*), and other species. Foxes can spread oncospheres of tapeworm in an area over 18 ha and at distances over 15–16 km. Also, from a single stool containing oncospheres, in 10 days they can disperse distances of over 80 m from the excrement in question. Increasing fox populations and extending their life by urban territories is an increased risk factor for humans, and this is all the more so as these animals, the definitive hosts, show no clinical signs to a massive 100,000 tapeworm infection.

The *E. multilocularis* oncospheres are viable outdoors 3–8 months during summer and autumn and in cold temperatures in winter up to 8 months.

Foxes and small rodents represent the natural hosts of parasite. Naturally the parasite transmits between foxes or dogs and small mammals, while humans are aberrant intermediate hosts. Transmission of AE to humans is by consumption of parasite eggs which are excreted in the feces of the definitive hosts: foxes and, increasingly, dogs (Sikó 2011a). Human infection can be through direct contact with the definitive host or indirectly through contamination of food and contaminated green vegetables and fruits or possibly water with parasite eggs.

The incubation period is long (5–15 years); the parasitic tissue grows slowly and is of the infiltrating type. The liver is the organ primarily involved. Metastasis may occur and can involve virtually any organ. In systematic surveys, metastasis to the brain was reported in only 1–3 % of patients with AE (Bresson-Hadni et al. 2000; Kern et al. 2003). Among possible metastases of hepatic AE, locations to the brain are rare, usually fatal, and they have especially been assigned to concomitant immune suppression (Yang et al. 2005; Tappe et al. 2008). Brain metastasis is considered a sign of the terminal phase of the disease (Barjhoux et al. 1970; Bresson-Hadni et al. 2000). Few reports on the rare primary infections of the brain have been published (Aydin et al. 1986; Qiu et al. 1986). Pregnancy has been proposed to play a role as a predisposing factor for cerebral metastasis in AE (Yang et al. 2005).

Pathophysiology and Pathogenesis

AHD is very aggressive. Lesions develop rapidly in the liver where an invasive pseudomalignant (paraneoplastic) mass may be produced. This may spread locally to adjacent organs such as the lung or metastasize to distant structures (Sikó 2011b).

According to the results of animal experiment in Japan, the mechanism of metastasis was due to the detached proliferated bud, even very small or only a few nuclei entering the blood vessels (Matsuhisa et al. 1996). Nevertheless, it was incapable of causing metastasis if protoscoleces were injected into the vessels.

In the European registry 34 % of patients who have metacestode lesions in the liver have simultaneously a lesion in one or more extrahepatic organs, at the time when the patients reach medical attention (Kern et al. 2003).

The metacestode was characterized by internally protrusive hyperplasia from the mother alveolar wall into the alveolar cavity and then proliferation extending continuously to reach the opposite wall of the cavity. So, septum-like budding was formed. Sometimes two or more proliferative sites on the alveolar wall propagated simultaneously into the cavity in opposite directions and mingled with each other to form a septum dividing the mother cyst to form two or more small alveoli (Jiang et al. 2005).

After ingestion of contaminated foods and/or water, embryos of *E. multilocularis* migrate through the portal system to the liver where vesicular masses are formed. The disease may extend gradually to adjacent organs or spread via the bloodstream (hematogenous metastasis) to distant areas such as the brain. Primary affected is usually the liver, and then the secondary localization by metastasis is in the lung. Bensaid et al. (1994) report a patient with right frontal lobe and palpebral lesions secondary to a primary hepatic focus with secondary lesion in the lung. The intracerebral, frontal lobe, palpebral lobe, disseminated, or other CNS localizations appeared usually after the lung metastasis due to an immunosuppressive effect of parasite.

Sato et al. (1998) made an experimental infection of larval *E. multilocularis* in the rodent brain attempting to establish a murine model for cerebral AE. Mice and jirds (*Meriones* genus) were injected intracranially with 10 % of a homogenated hydatid cyst mass. Small cystic larvae were observed macroscopically in the cranial cavity 1, 2, and 5 months post infection in both mice and jirds. Some larval cysts from both rodents contained mature or immature protoscoleces. In mice, the laminated layer was found in the lateral ventricle 2 months post infection but without protoscoleces. At 5 months post infection, larger larval cysts were found in the cranial cavity of a mouse, which also demonstrated partial palsy of the legs. A laminated layer with mature protoscoleces was observed in the third ventricle, and the mouse also harbored, in the left lung, a larval cyst containing protoscoleces surrounded by lymphocytes. Jirds were also found to be infected with metacestodes in the cranial cavity, but neither unusual behavior nor establishment of cysts inside the brain was observed in jirds during the course of infection.

Clinical Features

In the cerebral AE the lesions may remain asymptomatic until they are quite large. The clinical presentation usually includes symptoms of increased intracranial pressure, progressive and severe headaches (vomiting, motor weakness, etc.), seizures, cranial nerve findings, and visual disturbances (Takci et al. 2008). Ozdol et al. (2011) present a case of a 23-year-old man with nausea, imbalance, occasional urinary and fecal incontinence, and a severe headache for 1 month. These symptoms were caused by multiple calcified mass lesions in the right upper lobe of the lung and right liver and another solid tumor between the right kidney and liver. Other symptoms such as hemiparesis, seizures, visual field alteration, and gait disorders may vary with the location of the metacestode. Cerebral AHD can also cause intracranial hypertension, seizures, and focal neurological deficits. However, the clinical course is usually more rapid and more severe than in cystic hydatid disease. AE cases are usually present in adults. The average age of patients with cerebral AE is significantly higher than the age of those with cystic echinococcosis (Ammann and Eckert 1996).

Types of Lesions

The infiltrating growth of *E. multilocularis* metacestode is particularly significant because it may resemble a neoplasm, the so-called malignant hydatid disease. It is especially serious when the *E. multilocularis* lesions involve the brain, termed a "fatal disease" (Qiu et al. 1986). Cerebral metastasis of primary hepatic AE is often multifocal (Tappe et al. 2008). The cerebral AE is present like multiple intracranial masses which show cauliflower-like contrast enhancement pattern on magnetic resonance imaging (MRI) (Tunaci et al. 1999).

Based on imaging characteristics the AE lesions are divided into three types: (1) solid type (a solid lesion without liquid necrosis or only small patches of necrosis), (2) mixed type (solid component surrounding large and/or irregular liquid necrosis area), and (3) pseudocystic type (large cyst without visible solid component).

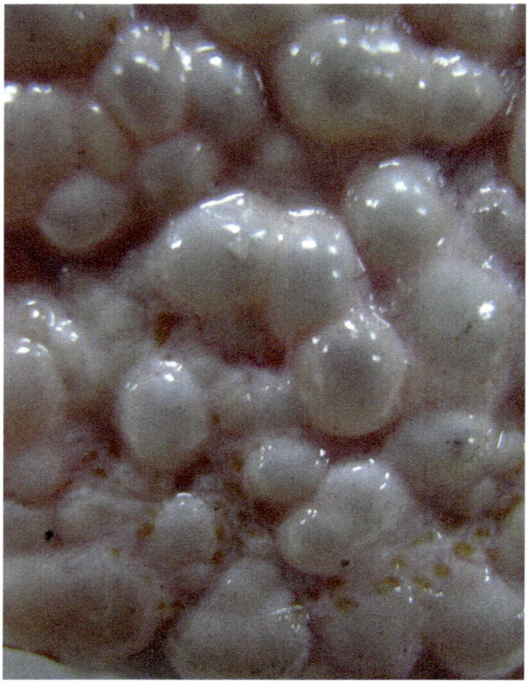

Fig. 24.1 Alveolar echinococcosis an expansive tumoral formation

Calcification in alveolar echinococcosis may be categorized into three patterns: (1) mild calcification (inconspicuous calcification or punctuate scattered calcification), (2) moderate calcification (coastline calcification located at the periphery of the lesion, with or without the central dot-calcification), and (3) abundant calcification (large calcified deposits) (Wang et al. 2011).

According to the Chinese records, intracranial AE can be subdivided into three types: (a) monomassive type, (b) multifocal type, and (c) extracerebral type (Qiu et al. 1986). The volumes of the lesions are variable, between $6.0 \times 4.5 \times 3.5$ cm^3 and $9.0 \times 6.5 \times 8.5$ cm^3 (Qiu et al. 1986).

The most frequent morphological profile of AE is represented by a heterogeneous, infiltrative, and destructive mass (Fig. 24.1), with irregular outlines and a nonvascular and necrotic center. The cyst it appears as a spongy structure, resembling a crumb

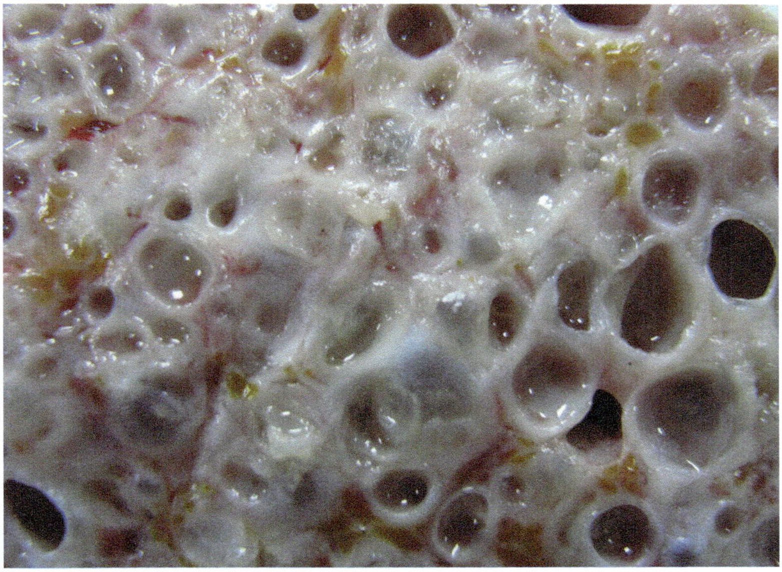

Fig. 24.2 The internal spongy structure of the tumoral formation

of cheese, with empty cavities or with a gray jelly content (Fig. 24.2). Most of the cavities do not have a well-defined content. In other samples, the formation had mainly a cystic structure, without a divided multivesicular character. In the intracerebellar tissues the metacestode showed a pale yellow mass. Calcification and perilesional edema are prominent (Algros et al. 2003).

In contrast with *E. granulosus*, the *E. multilocularis* cysts are small, group in clusters, elicit a severe inflammatory reaction from the host, and tend to metastasize both locally and distantly. Within the CNS, they usually are located within the brain parenchyma. Intracranial AE is thought to be rare with CNS involvement usually a manifestation of metastases from a primary lesion.

AHD is a biologically aggressive infestation mimicking a malignant neoplasm as assessed radiologically and macroscopically (Ozdol et al. 2011). AE develops within the liver as a rapid invasive pseudomalignant growth and may metastasize to different organs. AE involvement of the brain and liver is similar to an infiltrative tumor (Sikó 2011a, b).

Cerebral cystic echinococcosis lesions are usually single. The cerebral alveolar echinococcosis lesions may be single (and multiseptated) or multiple (Tunaci et al. 1999). Piotin et al. (1997) reported a disseminated intracerebral AE case, secondary to primary hepatic infection. Oktar et al. (1999) described a brain computed tomography (CT) which showed multiple intracranial lesions with remarkable peritumoral cerebral edema. Hakan and Aker (2001) describe a 53-year-old man who presented with headache and right-sided seizures, and on MRI multiple cranial lesions were seen (Figs. 24.3 and 24.4). There were three multiloculated cystic lesions, in the left cerebellum, in the right occipital and left frontal lobes, and two solitary lesions, in the left frontal and left parietal lobes. CT showed multiple masses in the liver and lung. Aydinli et al. (2008) reported a 62-year-old man who had liver AHD with simultaneous lung and brain metastases. Other intracranial localizations were reported in the right frontal lobe and palpebral lesions secondary to a primary hepatic focus with secondary lesion in the lung (Bensaid et al. 1994).

The histopathological examination reveals a diffuse growth composed of compartments that are filled with a gelatinous matrix and many brood capsules and protoscoleces filled with necrotic tissue (Sikó 2011a, b). The larval cestodes of *E. multilocularis* produce a typical infiltration and induce destruction of the organ. The human organism responds with a granulomatous inflammatory reaction and peripheral formation of granulation tissue. In centripetal direction, the adventitial layer's components are formed by the fibroconjunctive reaction; inflammatory cells are

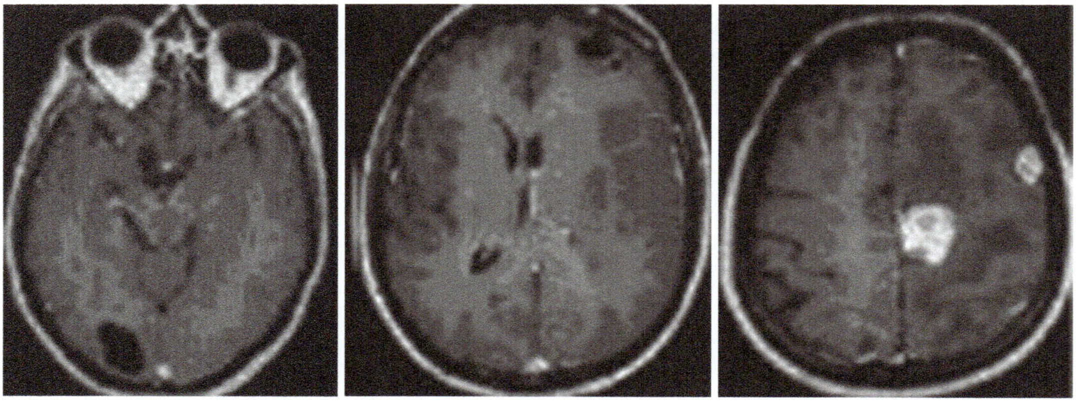

Fig. 24.3 Sagittal T1-weighted MRIs with a subcortical, solitary multilocular cystic lesion (From Hakan and Aker (2001), with permission)

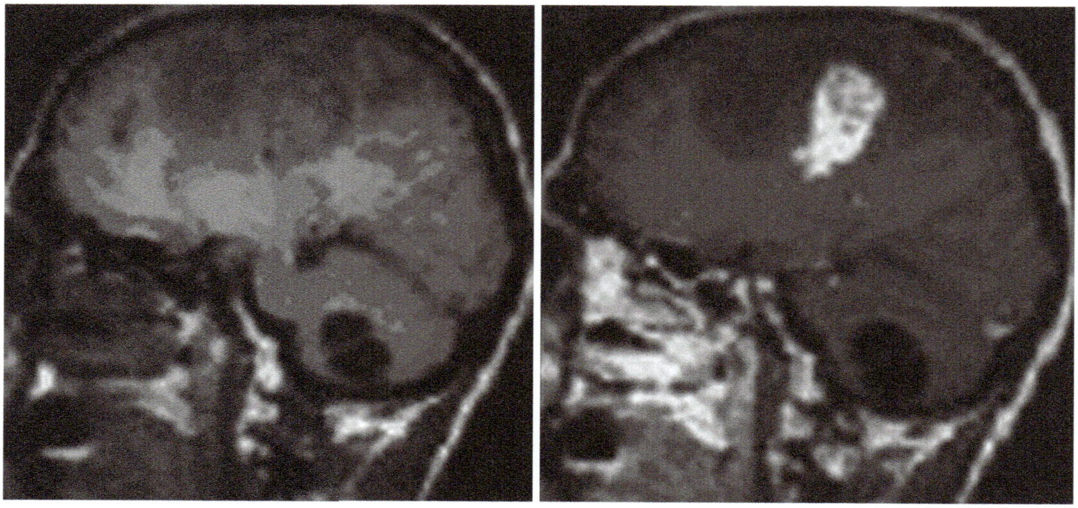

Fig. 24.4 Axial CT of the head after contrast administration. The multiloculated cystic lesions in right occipital, in left frontal lobe, and solitary lesions, one in left frontal and the other one in left parietal lobe (From Hakan and Aker (2001), with permission)

present. In the peripheral areas lymphocytes and monocytes dominate. They are followed by a rich infiltration of the giant cells and a decrease of the inflammatory local reaction (Fig. 24.5). These structures were gradually replaced by a fibroconjunctive reaction. The surrounding brain tissues show edema, degeneration of neurons, proliferation of gliocytes, and an increase in the number of vessels with distension of lumen by engorgement and complicated by focal necrosis (Qiu et al. 1986; Sikó 2011a, b).

Poorly hyalinized cuticle and more cellular reaction, especially with multinucleated giant cells, could be seen in the dense fibrous tissue infiltrated by an inflammatory cell layer. The cuticular layer is mono- or multistratified, formed by concentric conjunctival tissue layers, which penetrate in the cystic cavity and develop many anastomoses conferring it a multivesicular aspect. In the spaces between these blade cells similar to giant cells, we could also notice rare histiocytes and eosinophils. Due to the multitude of anasto-

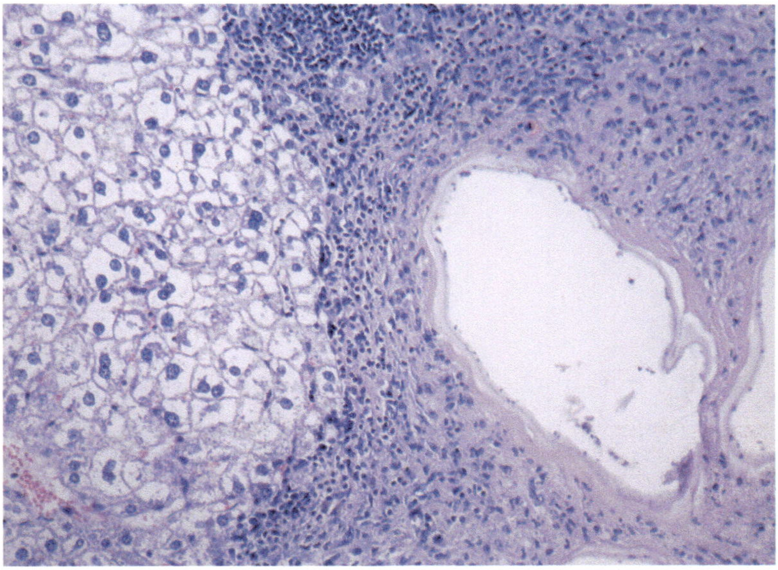

Fig. 24.5 Inflammatory local reaction with multinucleate giant cells, lymphocytes, plasmocytes, and macrophages. Hematoxylin-eosin stain, ×200

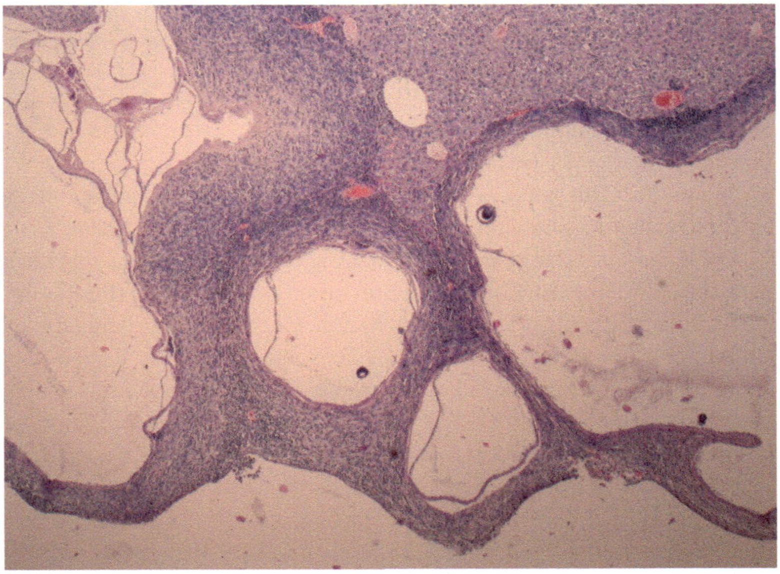

Fig. 24.6 Anastomosis with an invasive character. Pappenheim's stain, ×40

moses, the cyst is a structure with an invasive character (Fig. 24.6). In most cases there were collapsed cysts characterized by a fragmented or folded laminar layer and massive necrosis.

The germinative layer which lines the new formed cavities has a plasmatic structure with rare multinucleate cells. This layer has many young cells and gives a rhizoid aspect characteristic of malignant tissues. Some cysts contained remnants of a single germinative layer.

Studies aiming at the histological aspects have suggested that *E. multilocularis* produces multilocular alveolar cysts (1–10 mm in diameter) that resemble alveoli. They grow by means of exogenous proliferation with cysts that progressively invade the tissue by means of peripheral extension

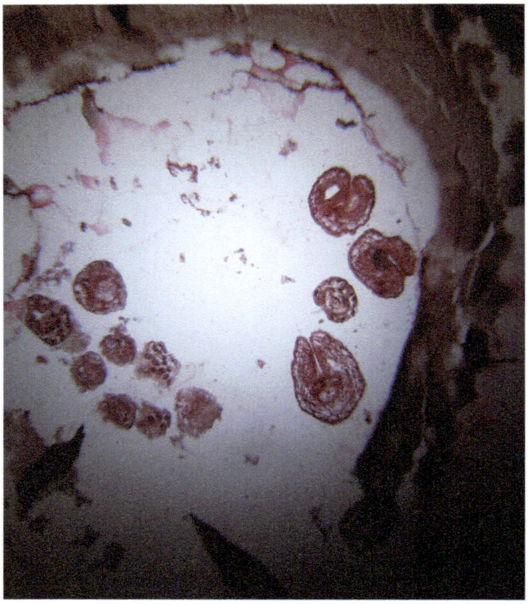

Fig. 24.7 Protoscoleces in the cyst of alveolar echinococcosis. Hematoxylin-eosin stain, ×40

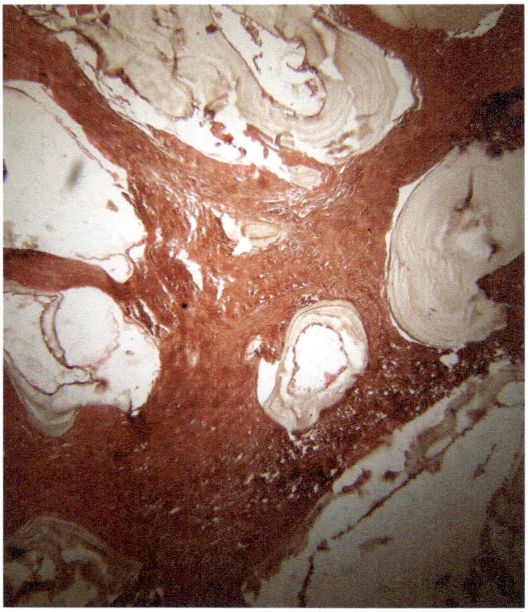

Fig. 24.8 Infiltrative and invadant character of alveolar echinococcosis. Hematoxylin-eosin stain, ×40

of the processes originating in the germinal layer. The larvae cause invasive and destructive changes in the tissue. This area is separated from the parenchyma by inflammatory cells.

The lesions are characterized by many alveoli with different sizes and shapes. Observation of the alveolar wall shows that the thick, noncellular, laminated outer layer looks bank-like, sometimes folding within the alveolar cavity. The thin, germinal inner membrane lined by a single layer cell is usually deficient due to detachment. Brood capsule or protoscoleces were occasionally seen (Fig. 24.7). The lesion may be complicated by central necrosis, producing a cavity or pseudocyst after liquefaction. In the periphery of alveoli group, there is hyperplasia of fibroconnective tissue and cellular infiltration of eosinocytes, lymphocytes, plasma cells, and giant cells, forming a typical alveococcus nodule (Fig. 24.8).

Histopathological examination reveals a periodic acid-Schiff (+) cuticular membrane with wide areas of necrosis and inflammation which are typical for AE. They are usually supratentorial and within the watershed zone of the middle cerebral artery; however, infratentorial AE is extremely rare.

Diagnosis

The diagnosis of AE is based on case history, clinical findings, morphological lesions identified by imaging techniques, the polymerase chain reaction (PCR), or immunofluorescence/immunohistochemistry and immunodiagnosis.

Early diagnosis of AE can result in significant improvements in the quality of the management and treatment. In most cases, the early stages of infection are asymptomatic, so that methods that are inexpensive and relatively easy to use are required for large-scale screening of populations at high risk (Zhang et al. 2003; Zhang and McManus 2006).

The diagnosis of AE has improved due to the use of new or more optimal methods for purification of *Echinococcus* antigens from somatic materials, by the application of molecular tools for parasite identification and the synthesis of recombinant diagnostic antigens and immunogenic peptides (Zhang et al. 2003).

Any person with the following findings might be diagnosed with alveolar echinococcosis: a slowly growing tumor – signs and symptoms vary with tumor location, size, and type (solid, partly multivesicular, centrally necrotic), visualized by imaging techniques (Kern 2010).

A case is verified if at least two of the following four parameters are fulfilled: (1) typical organ lesions detected by imaging techniques such as abdominal ultrasound, CT, and MRI; (2) detection of *Echinococcus* sp.-specific serum antibodies by tests of high sensitivity and confirmed by assays with high specificity; (3) histopathology compatible with a metacestode of *E. multilocularis*; and (4) detection of *E. multilocularis* nucleic acid in a clinical specimen.

AHD causes different neuroimaging findings, on the CT scan or MRI, because the lesions are multiple and surrounded by edema and show ringlike enhancement. The CT and MRI appearances of cerebral alveolar echinococcosis have rarely been reported. On CT and MRI, cerebral AE lesion appears as a solid, semisolid, or multilocular cystic mass with definite margins and surrounding contrast enhancement. Calcification and surrounding edema are common (Algros et al. 2003). Contrast enhancement occurs within the region of inflammatory reaction around the cysts (Bensaid et al. 1994; Reittner et al. 1996). Bükte et al. (2004) described a case where the CT and MRI showed a well-defined, multicystic appearance with a central solid component and calcifications. In the cerebral AE, CT showed a well-defined, multiseptated mass consisting of hyperdense solid and hypodense cystic components and hyperdense calcifications (Bükte et al. 2004).

On MRI the metacestode mass showed a multicystic appearance with a central solid component and punctate calcifications with contrast enhancement of the wall, and solid components. The solid components were iso-/hyperintense. The cystic components were hypointense. The lesion presented as an intracranial mass which is slightly hyperdense on CT scans and very hypointense with central hyperintensity on T2-weighted MRIs. The hypointensity on T2-weighted MRIs appears to be characteristic of lesions of cerebral alveolar echinococcosis. The lesion exhibited marked contrast enhancement on both CT and MRIs and is accompanied by extensive white matter edema (Wada et al. 1996).

The alveolar hydatidosis of the spinal canal may be visualized by MRI, although the findings are nonspecific. Usually the CT scan is better than MRI to demonstrate bone erosion in vertebral bodies. The CT is a superior method in detecting calcification of the cyst wall or septa. The MRI method is the better method in detecting multiplicity and defining the anatomic relationship of the lesion with the adjacent structures and helps in surgical planning (Bükte et al. 2004).

Asanuma et al. (2003) had intracranially injected 36 female Wistar rats (6–8 weeks old) with a 10 % homogenate of echinococcal larval tissues. They observe a neoplastic fine structure of the rat brain. The T2-weighted MRIs revealed a hyperintense region in the cerebral cortex at 2 weeks after injection. At 3 weeks after injection, this region was found to have cysts on the basis of results of histological examination. Unmarked areas corresponding to hyperplasia and the subsequent calcification of the cuticular layer, at 6 and 13 weeks after injection, respectively, were observed in T2-weighted and proton density MRIs. Using this secondary cerebral AE animal model, it was concluded that the MRI method was suitable for early detection of secondary cerebral AE (Sato et al. 1998).

Immunodiagnosis provides such an approach and can also confirm clinical findings. The immunologic diagnosis is not accurate due to cross-reaction with other parasitic diseases or false-negative results in patients with intact cystic hydatid lesions. Immunofluorescence, indirect hemagglutination tests, enzyme-linked immunosorbent assay (ELISA), and immunoelectrophoresis with antigenic extracts of *E. multilocularis* are usually supportive laboratory tests for a diagnostic accuracy. However, the serological cross-reactions between various cestodes and between cestodes and the phylogenetically related trematodes may occur.

The serodiagnosis of AE provides a complementary role to other procedures in early detection of the infection. The methods are similar to those used for CE, but serological tests for antibody detection are generally more reliable. The Em2, a species-specific native antigen isolated from the metacestode of *E. multilocularis*, has been used for immunodiagnosis of human AE with encouraging results. The sensitivities of Em2 in ELISA varied depending on the geographic origin of the patient. They ranged between 77 and 92 %. The Em2^{plus} ELISA, a combination of Em2 with a recombinant protein designated II/3–10, increased the sensitivity to 97 % (Zhang et al. 2003; Zhang and McManus 2006; Brunetti et al. 2010).

DNA probes and PCR may be applied to differentiate between *Echinococcus* spp. In order to confirm the assumed echinococcal etiology of these lesions, Georges et al. (2004) and Tappe et al. (2008) used a specialized PCR with primers directed against the spliced leader RNA gene in chromosomal echinococcal DNA on a cerebrospinal fluid sample of the patient. PCR has been used to confirm the echinococcal etiology of lesions in unusual locations. Diverse protocols have been developed to detect echinococcal nucleic acids in biological samples, and PCR is increasingly being accepted as a complementary diagnostic tool for echinococcosis.

Differential Diagnosis

The differential diagnosis of cerebral AE includes the following: cystic echinococcosis, tuberculosis, bacterial abscesses, fungal infections, glial tumor, invasive brain tumors, and metastases (Isik et al. 2007). The differential diagnosis encompasses coenurosis (a single, large grapelike mass in the brain without other organ involvement), cysticercosis (small cysts in multiple brain locations and in the muscles, the grapelike racemose type in the cisternae), brain paragonimiasis, toxoplasmosis, glioma, and cerebral metastasis of malignant neoplasias. In the case presented, the cerebral lesions were not biopsied due to their location (Tappe et al. 2008).

McManus et al. (2011) described a case in China, when in a patient the primary diagnosis was of undifferentiated metastatic cancer in the liver and brain, with current pulmonary bacterial infection. After a systematic review of her clinical records, it was suspected that the patient had hepatic AE which had metastasized to the brain and lungs. This case demonstrated that differential diagnosis for AE should generally include assessment for the presence of tumors and other lesions such as abscesses caused by tuberculosis, which may require specific pathological examination or molecular analysis of biopsy material to provide a definitive diagnosis.

Epidemiologically, the infection of *E. multilocularis* is endemic in high-altitude zones and areas of cold climate; *E. granulosus* infection is mostly seen in areas of moderate climate. Both may however be seen outside endemic areas due to migration from endemic areas or due to tourism. Infestation with *E. multilocularis* is a more malignant disease, referred to as AE. In AE the latter lacks limiting membrane thus can grow aggressively.

Radiological differentiation from brain tumor is difficult. The diagnosis should be suggested by evidence of a primary hepatic focus, appropriate clinical history, high prevalence of the infection in the host's geographic location, and laboratory findings (Reittner et al. 1996; Piotin et al. 1997; Tunaci et al. 1999). The clinical manifestations of alveolar hydatidosis are nonspecific and similar to those caused by primary or metastatic brain tumors. The cyst of AE differs from that of cystic echinococcosis in that it grows by external budding of the germinal membrane with progressive infiltration of the surrounding tissue (Kammerer 1993; Bükte et al. 2004).

Histopathological examination is necessary for a definite and certain diagnosis.

Immunofluorescence, passive hemagglutination tests, ELISA, and immunoelectrophoresis with antigenic extracts of *E. multilocularis* may provide a diagnosis. Serological testing can be positive, but this does not always help make a definite differentiation between the infections of *E. granulosus* or *E. multilocularis*.

Imaging techniques may be more sensitive than serodiagnosis.

Basically, in an immunodiagnostic process, an 18-kDa antigen (Em18) from PSC of AE was reported as being a highly species-specific (96.8 %) and sensitive (97 %) antigen with potential not only for differentiation of AE from either CE or other helminth infections but also for differentiation of active from inactive AE. Subsequently, Em18 was shown to be a fragment of the C-terminal of Em10, and the recombinant protein was recognized by 87.1 and 90.3 % of 31 serum samples from AE patients in ELISA and immunoblotting, respectively. Recombinant Em18-ELISA and Em18-immunoblot assays have proved invaluable for differentiating AE from CE infection, the former also being useful for evaluating the efficacy of treatment in patients with AE (Zhang et al. 2003; Zhang and McManus 2006; Brunetti et al. 2010).

Prognosis

The cerebral AE has a poor prognosis. Locations to the brain are usually fatal (Yang et al. 2005)

Treatment

AHD is a life-threatening parasitosis (Wang et al. 2009). The first attempt of medical treatment of AE was by Hanstein (1957). The initial start of chemotherapy dates to 1974 when benzimidazole compounds were demonstrated to be effective against larval *Echinococcus*. The first agents used were mebendazole and its fluorine analogue flubendazole. Doses of mebendazole ranging from 15 to 60 mg/kg/day have been administered to human subjects. Duration of therapy is not exactly known; it may be continued for months or in some cases for years. Another benzimidazole compound, albendazole, is better absorbed and diffusion of its metabolites into tissues and cysts is far higher than with mebendazole. Dosage of albendazole is 10–15 mg/kg/day.

Mebendazole and albendazole are the drugs of choice for the long-term treatment of AE. The mebendazole or albendazole treatment followed up for an average of 42 months had a success rate in 80–97 % and was defined as non-progression for more than 1 year (Reuter et al. 1998).

Radical resection is generally considered as the only method of surgical treatment. The standard treatment of cerebral AHD consists of open brain surgery and systemic albendazole therapy postoperatively (Wang et al. 2009). Surgical excision of solitary lesions of *E. multilocularis* has been described. However, cyst rupture during removal may lead to dissemination and/or chemical meningitis. Fatal anaphylactic shock has also been described (Hakan and Aker 2001). Radical excision should be performed for all accessible surgical lesions. The surgical treatment for multiple cerebral lesions is usually palliative with alternative chemotherapeutics for at least 2 years.

Several cycles of postoperative albendazole chemotherapy are almost always required (Ozdol et al. 2011). Gamma knife radiosurgery may be an alternative to surgery for patients with inoperable alveolar hydatid cysts or with a high risk of surgery and anesthesia (Schmid et al. 1998; Yamamoto 1999).

The decision making to choose between the surgery and medical treatment with albendazole or mebendazole must take into account the surgical mortality (≥2 %), postoperative complications (8–25 %), recurrence rate after surgery (2–25 %), and cure rate with medical treatment (30–40 %). Definitive treatment still consists of surgical removal. Takci et al. (2008) showed that radical surgery combined with antihelmintic therapy of sufficient duration is mandatory to prevent the progression of symptoms, but the disease continues to be difficult to cure. Surgical removal of alveolar cysts usually requires resection of adjacent tissue, and this may cause neurological deficits if the lesion is located in an eloquent cerebral area.

In the encephalic localizations, Weber et al. (1988) suggest the treatment with flubendazole, with a 4-year follow-up. Albendazole administration should follow or even precede the surgical procedure or may be used as primary therapy for patients with inoperable alveolar hydatid disease. The drug is given 10 mg/kg body weight per day for lifetime. Using this approach, 90 % of lesions regress or remain static, and only 10 % continue to grow. Isik et al. (2007) suggested a postoperative treatment started on albendazole at a daily dosage of 800 mg for 3 months. The patient has remained free of any mass lesion for 5 years. Albendazole (800 mg, 3 × 28-day treatment cycle, followed by a 14-day albendazole-free interval) and cefotaxime were prescribed for postoperative treatment (Ozdol et al. 2011). A further operation was performed to resect the lesion in the lung a month after intracranial surgery. Postoperative early CT examination and MRI performed 6 months after surgery showed no recurrence. However, Li et al. (2010) reviewed by a follow-up of 1–7 years 17 cases of complicated AE in multiorgans (liver, lung, and brain). They concluded when more than two organs are involved by AE lesion, it was rather difficult to diagnose and cure. Thus the life quality and long-term survival of patients were seriously endangered.

It is concluded that cerebral *E. multilocularis* lesions are amenable to surgery and that their removal provides useful prolongation of life despite the presence of hepatic or pulmonary disease. In any case long-term chemotherapy may be indicated as a life-saving measure for patients with severe liver dysfunction but is associated with a relatively high risk of proliferation of intraoperatively undetected parasite remnants.

For AE, early diagnosis and radical (tumor-like) surgery followed by anti-infective prophylaxis with albendazole remain the key elements. However, most patients with AE are diagnosed at a later stage, when radical surgery (distance of larval to liver tissue of >2 cm) cannot be achieved. The backbone of AE treatment remains the continuous medical treatment with albendazole and, if necessary, individualized interventional measures (Brunetti et al. 2010).

Prevention

AHD may be prevented by reducing human contact with definitive host feces. Any person who lives in an area where *E. multilocularis* is found in rodents and wild canines should take the following precautions to avoid infection:

- Do not touch a fox or other wild canines, dead or alive, unless you are wearing gloves. Hunters and trappers should use plastic gloves to avoid exposure.
- Do not keep wild animals, especially wild canines, as pets or encourage them to come close to your home.
- Do not allow your dogs and cats to wander freely or to capture and eat rodents.
- If you think that your pet may have eaten rodents, consult your veterinarian about the possible need for preventive treatments.
- Wash your hands with soap and warm water after handling dogs or cats and before handling food.
- Teach children the importance of washing hands to prevent infection.
- Do not collect or eat wild fruits or vegetables picked directly from the ground. All wild-picked foods should be washed carefully or cooked before eating.
- AE can be effectively controlled and prevented when care is taken to avoid exposure and contact with wild animals such as foxes, coyotes, and dogs and by limiting the interactions between dogs and rodent populations.
- Do not allow dogs to feed on rodents and other wild animals.

Conclusion

Hepatic failure, local extension, or metastases to the vital organs lead to mortality. In untreated patients the mortality may reach 90 %. In the present case, there were multifocal brain lesions, hepatic failure, and superimposed secondary infection. In patients with multiple cerebral lesions who live in or have visited an endemic area and especially if there has been contact with foxes, dogs, or rodents, *E. multilocularis* should be remembered in the differential diagnosis. AE remains today a very lethal disease. The cerebral lesions may be multiloculated, solid, solitary, or multiple and may involve the infra- or supratentorial areas.

References

Algros MP, Majo F, Bresson-Hadni S, Koch S, Godard J, Cattin F. Intracerebral alveolar echinococcosis. Infection. 2003;31:63–5.

Altinors N, Bavbek M, Caner HH, Erdogan B. Central nervous system hydatidosis in Turkey: a cooperative study and literature survey analysis of 458 cases. J Neurosurg. 2000;93:1–8.

Ammann RW, Eckert J. Cestodes. Echinococcus. Gastroenterol Clin North Am. 1996;25:655–89.

Asanuma T, Matsumoto Y, Takiguchi M, Inanami O, Nakao M, Nakaya K, Ito A, Hashimoto A, Kuwabara M. Magnetic resonance imaging and immunoblot analyses in rats with experimentally induced cerebral alveolar echinococcosis. Comp Med. 2003;53: 649–56.

Aydin Y, Barlas O, Yolaş C, Aydin IH, Ceviz A, Aladağ A, Ören D, Akdemir D. Alveolar hydatid disease of the brain. Report of four cases. J Neurosurg. 1986;65: 115–9.

Aydinli B, Aydin U, Yazici P, Oztürk G, Onbaş O, Polat KY. Alveolar echinococcosis of liver presenting with neurological symptoms due to brain metastases with simultaneous lung metastasis: a case report. Turkiye Parazitol Derg. 2008;32:371–4.

Barjhoux P, Gilbertas A, Girona GC, Rochet M. Terminal cerebral localization of hepatic alveolar and pulmonary echinococcosis. Apropos of a case. Arch Fr Mal App Dig. 1970;59:263–4.

Bensaid AH, Dietemann JL, Filippi de la Palavesa MM, Klinkert A, Kastler B, Gangi A. Intracranial alveolar echinococcosis: CT and MRI. Neuroradiology. 1994;36:289–91.

Bresson-Hadni S, Vuitton DA, Bartholomot B, Heyd B, Godart D, Meyer JP, Hrusovsky S, Becker MC, Mantion G. A twenty-year history of alveolar echinococcosis: analysis of a series of 117 patients from eastern France. Eur J Gastroenterol Hepatol. 2000;12: 327–36.

Brunetti E, Kern P, Vuitton DA. Expert consensus for the diagnosis and treatment of cystic and alveolar echinococcosis in humans. Acta Trop. 2010;114:1–16.

Bükte Y, Kemanoğlu S, Nazaroğlu H, Özkan Ü, Ceviz A, Şimşek M. Cerebral hydatid disease: CT and MR imaging findings. Swiss Med Wkly. 2004;134: 459–67.

Devé F. L'echinococcose alvéolaire secondaire. Paris: Masson; 1946.

Georges S, Villard O, Filisetti D, Mathis A, Marcellin L, Hansmann Y, Candolfi E. Usefulness of PCR analysis for diagnosis of alveolar echinococcosis with unusual localizations: two case studies. J Clin Microbiol. 2004;42:5954–6.

Hakan T, Aker FV. A case report of fatal echinococcosis. Ann Neurosurg. 2001;1:14–9.

Hanstein H. Medical therapy of multilocular echinococcosis. Dtsch Med Wochenschr. 1957;82:316–7.

Isik N, Silav G, Cerçi A, Karabagli P, Elmaci I, Kalelioglu M. Cerebral alveolar echinococcosis. A case report with MRI and review of the literature. Neurosurg Sci. 2007;51:145–51.

Jiang P, McManus DP, Jones M. Liver alveolar echinococcosis in China: clinical aspect with relative basic research. World J Gastroenterol. 2005;11:4611–7.

Kammerer WS. Echinococcosis affecting the central nervous system. Semin Neurol. 1993;13:144–7.

Kern P. Clinical features and treatment of alveolar echinococcosis. Curr Opin Infect Dis. 2010;23:505–12.

Kern P, Bardonnet K, Renner E, Auer H, Pawlowski Z, Ammann RW, Vuitton DA, Kern P. European echinococcosis registry: human alveolar echinococcosis, Europe, 1982–2000. Emerg Infect Dis. 2003;9:343–9.

Li HT, Tuerganaili H, Ayifuhanahan, Shao YM, Zhao JM, Ran B, Wen H. Clinical experiences in the treatment of human multi-organ alveolar echinococcosis by surgery and drugs. Zhonghua Yi Xue Za Zhi. 2010;90: 2839–42.

Matsuhisa T, Uchino J, Sato N, Furuya K, Fujioka Y. Which component makes distant metastasis of alveolar echinococcosis, germinal cells or protoscolices? In: Uchino J, Sato N, editors. Strategy for eradication of alveolar echinococcosis of the liver. Sapporo: Fuji Shoin Publishers; 1996. p. 233–7.

McManus DP, Li Z, Yang S, Gray DJ, Yang YR. Case studies emphasising the difficulties in the diagnosis and management of alveolar echinococcosis in rural China. Parasit Vectors. 2011;4:196.

Oktar N, Karabiyikoğlu M, Demirtaş E, Altintaş N, Korkmaz M, Özdamar N. Cerebral alveolar echinococcosis. Review of the literature and report of a case. Norol Bil D Turkish J Neurological Sci. 1999;16:1.

Ozdol C, Yildirim AE, Daglioglu E, Divanlioglu D, Erdem E, Belen D. Alveolar hydatid cyst mimicking cerebellar metastatic tumor. Surg Neurol Int. 2011; 2:13.

Piotin M, Cattin F, Kantelip B, Miralbes S, Godard J, Bonneville JF. Disseminated intracerebral alveolar echinococcosis: CT and MRI. Neuroradiology. 1997;39: 431–3.

Qiu M, Hun ZS, Liu SC, Wen Li C, Wang S, Bao LS. Intracranial alveolar echinococcosis in China: discussion of surgical treatment. Acta Neurochir (Wien). 1986;82:123–7.

Reittner P, Szolar DH, Schmid M. Case report. Systemic manifestation of Echinococcus alveolaris infection. J Comput Assist Tomogr. 1996;20:1030–2.

Reuter S, Kratzer W, Kurz S, Wellinghausen N, Kern P. Chemotherapy of alveolar echinococcosis with benzimidazoles. A prospective long-term study. Med Klin (Munich). 1998;93:463–7.

Sato Y, Nakao M, Nakaya K, Ito A. Experimental infection of larval Echinococcus multilocularis in the rodent brain as a model for cerebral alveolar echinococcosis. J Helminthol. 1998;72:59–64.

Schmid M, Pendl G, Samonigg H, Ranner G, Eustacchio S, Reisinger EC. Gamma knife radiosurgery and albendazole for cerebral alveolar hydatid disease. Clin Infect Dis. 1998;26:1379–82.

Senturk S, Oguz KK, Soylemezoglu F, Inci S. Cerebral alveolar echinoccosis mimicking primary brain tumor. AJNR Am J Neuroradiol. 2006;27:420–2.

Sikó BS. Echinococcosis with E. multilocularis in Romania. Aetiology, epidemiology, diagnosis and control of the disease. PhD thesis, USAMV Cluj Napoca; 2011a.

Sikó BS. Alveolar echinococcosis. A paraneoplasic zoonosis recent confirmed in Romania. Internat. Congress of Oncology, Neptun, Romania, Workshop 2; 2011b.

Takci E, Sengul G, Akar A, Uslu H, Alper F, Erdogan F. Alveolar echinococcosis of the brain in five patients. J Clin Neurosci. 2008;15:1105–9.

Tappe D, Weise D, Ziegler U, Müller A, Müllges W, Stich A. Brain and lung metastasis of alveolar echinococcosis in a refugee from a hyperendemic area. J Med Microbiol. 2008;57:1420–3.

Torgerson PR, Keller K, Magnotta M, Ragland N. The global burden of alveolar echinococcosis. PLoS Negl Trop Dis. 2010;4:e722.

Tunaci M, Tunaci A, Engin G, Ozkorkmaz B, Ahishali B, Rozanes I. MRI of cerebral alveolar echinococcosis. Neuroradiology. 1999;41:844–6.

Wada H, Takahashi S, Higano S, Tominaga T, Sakamoto K. CT and MR imaging findings in a case of cerebral alveolar echinococcosis masquerading as brain tumor. Nippon Igaku Hoshasen Gakkai Zasshi. 1996;56: 608–9.

Wang J, Cai B, You C. Surgical treatment for cerebral alveolar echinococcosis: experience in six patients. Neurol India. 2009;57:157–61.

Wang J, Xing Y, Ren B, Xie W, Wen H, Liu W. Alveolar echinococcosis: correlation of imaging type with PNM stage and diameter of lesions. Chin Med J. 2011;124:2824–8.

Weber M, Vespignani H, Jacquier P, Gérard A, Claudon P, Bracard S, Floquet J. Neurological manifestations of alveolar echinococcosis. Rev Neurol (Paris). 1988;144: 104–12.

WHO Informal Working Group on Echinococcosis. Guidelines for treatment of cystic and alveolar echinococcosis in humans. Bull World Health Organ. 1996; 74:231–42.

Yamamoto M. Gamma knife radiosurgery: technology, applications, and future directions. Neurosurg Clin N Am. 1999;10:181–202.

Yang YR, Vuitton DA, Jones MK, Craig PS, McManus DP. Brain metastasis of alveolar echinococcosis in a hyperendemic focus of Echinococcus multilocularis infection. Trans R Soc Trop Med Hyg. 2005;99:937–41.

Zhang W, McManus DP. Recent advances in the immunology and diagnosis of echinococcosis. FEMS Immunol Med Microbiol. 2006;47:24–41.

Zhang W, Li J, McManus DP. Review concepts in immunology and diagnosis of hydatid disease. Clin Microbiol Rev. 2003;16:18–36.

Control and Prevention of Hydatidosis

25

Jorge A. Guisantes

Contents

J.A. Guisantes, MD, PhD
Department of Immunology, Microbiology and Parasitology, Faculty of Pharmacy, University of the Basque Country, Paseo de la Universidad No. 7, Vitoria 01006, Spain
e-mail: jorgegdb@telefonica.net

Introduction

The control of the parasitic zoonoses is encompassed by a complex group of actions because of its existence in the life cycle of animal hosts (domestic and wild) as well as humans. This complexity is the reason why – despite knowing thoroughly the life cycle of *Echinococcus granulosus* and their mechanisms of transmission – hydatidosis continues to be an important zoonosis in many regions of the world.

This chapter aims at describing the main methods recommended and employed to control cystic hydatidosis or cystic echinococcosis (CE) in control programs in several countries. Additionally, standards and recommendations for prevention are also described.

Biology and Life Cycle

Cystic hydatid disease in man is a parasitic zoonosis; men can be infected during the metacestode stage of the tapeworm *E. granulosus*. The adult worm lives in the small intestine of dogs and other canids; the parasite eggs are excreted in the feces of these animals, which may thus contaminate soil, grass, and water. The transmission of *E. granulosus* usually occurs through domestic livestock and dogs and other canids (Fig. 25.1). Man is an aberrant intermediate host of *E. granulosus* because the parasite cannot complete its development in humans. Ten strains or genotypes are described in *E. granulosus* using mitochondrial gene analysis and are numbered

M. Turgut (ed.), *Hydatidosis of the Central Nervous System: Diagnosis and Treatment*, DOI 10.1007/978-3-642-54359-3_25,

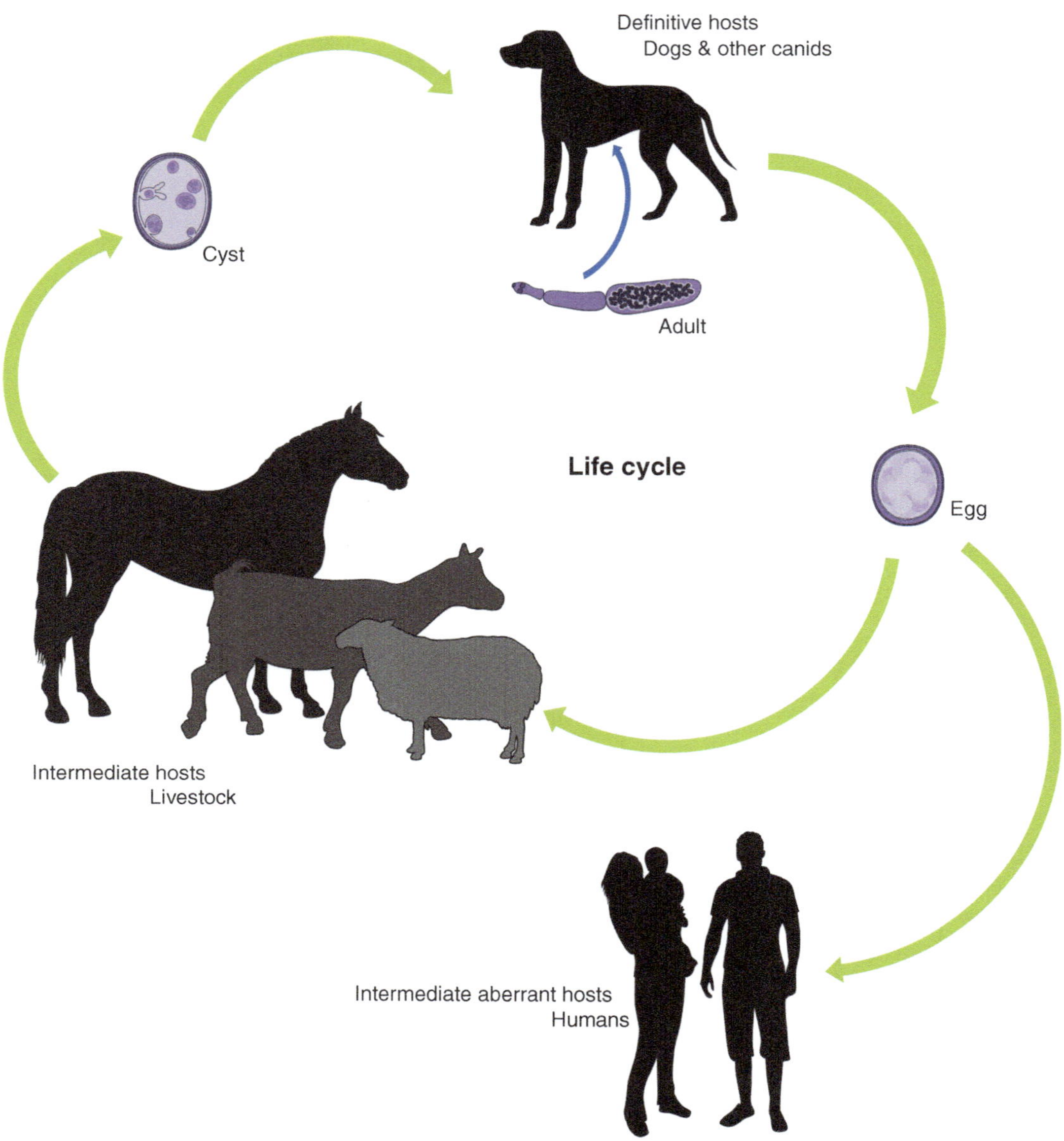

Fig. 25.1 Life cycle of *Echinococcus granulosus*

G1 to G10 (Kamenetzky et al. 2002; Lavikainen et al. 2006; McManus and Thompson 2003). The preponderant strain is the sheep-dog strain or G1 genotype, but other genotypes include horses, cattle, camels, pigs, and cervids as intermediate hosts. The existence of these strains currently leads to consider the existence of an *E. granulosus* complex or new species in relation to these strains. In this regard, have been elevated to species *E. granulosus sensu stricto* (G1, G2 and G3), *E. equinus* (G4), *E. ortleppi* (G5) and *E. canadensis* (G6, G7,G8, G9, G10) have been elevated to species *E. granulosus* sensu stricto (G1, G2, and G3). Recently the lion strain has been proposed as a new species: *E. felidis* (McManus 2011). The knowledge about the predominant strain in a particular country or region is important for the design of more efficient control programs (Pearson et al. 2002).

The eggs passed in the feces of dogs are the infective stage for the intermediate host like domestic livestock, wild intermediate hosts, and humans, where the oncospheres develop into hydatid cysts (Fig. 25.1). The number of eggs produced varies between 100 and 1,500 per proglottid (Thompson 1995), and a dog may have hundreds of adult cestodes. Therefore, an infected dog can spread thousands of fertile eggs of *Echinococcus* that may remain viable for months in the environment.

Each hydatid cyst may have thousands of protoscolices in brood capsules. When dogs ingest raw offal containing hydatid cysts from intermediate hosts, each evaginated protoscolex attaches between the villi of the small intestine and, in about 40 days, develops a mature adult tapeworm. An interesting fact is that the protoscolices of *E. granulosus* have a double biotic potential: if ingested by dogs, they result in adult worms, but if they fall into serous cavities (e.g., pleural or peritoneal cavities) of an intermediate host, including man, they can redevelop into a new cyst (secondary hydatidosis).

Control

Approaches and Options

According to Gemmell and Schantz (1997), control may be defined as an active implementation of a program to limit the prevalence of a specific disease by a recognized authority on an instruction from the legislature. It is different from eradication that Gemmell and Schantz (1997) defined as the purposeful reduction of specific disease prevalence to the point of continued absence of transmission within a specific area by means of a time-limited campaign.

The preventive and control programs require interrupting the life cycle of the parasite acting on the epidemiological chain. For this it is necessary to act on the following: (a) the definitive hosts (dogs and other canids); (b) the herbivorous intermediate hosts such as sheep, cattle, and goats and a rather large number of other suitable hosts such as camels, pigs, horses, etc.; (c) the human population; and (d) other stages of the life cycle.

Since 1863 several programs of control have been employed in many countries. Several of them have been employed in islands such as Iceland (1863–1960), New Zealand (1938–2002), Tasmania (1964–1996), Falkland Islands (1965–1997), Cyprus (1971–1985), and Sardinia (1960–1997), with different efficacy reviewed by Craig and Larrieu (2007).

From the analysis of the control programs developed in continental and insular countries, it is apparent that two main approaches were employed (Gemmell and Schantz 1997; Gemmell 2001): (a) a "horizontal" approach based on health education, sanitation improvement, meat inspection and slaughterhouses facilities, and developing safe water supplies and (b) "vertical" approach that targets the parasite by testing dogs, regular dosing of dogs with praziquantel, and massive reduction of dog populations, including baseline surveys and continuing surveillance of livestock and human infections. These approaches are not mutually exclusive (Gemmell and Schantz 1997; Gemmell et al. 2001). Certainly, the "horizontal approach" is cheaper than the "vertical" approach.

According to Gemmell and Schantz (1997) and Gemmell et al. (2001) and based on previous experiences, the control programs can be divided into four phases: (a) planning phase, (b) attack phase, (c) consolidation phase, and (d) maintenance of eradication phase. During the planning phase, the support of the control authority must be obtained, and the plan should establish methods of control, cost-benefit ratios, and the extent and duration of the program.

In the attack phase, the control measures to be applied must be targeted to the parasite and its definitive hosts; this includes dog-dosing campaigns with praziquantel, massive reduction of dog populations, regulation on dog feeding practice, ruling the keeping of dogs, and introducing an obligatory dog license fee that allows to create a record of rural and urban dogs. This is a costly phase.

In the consolidation phase, the campaign must be focused on at-risk areas as farms are identified using trace-back of the livestock through slaughterhouses surveillance. A trace-forward of the livestock of these farms must be also implemented. During this phase the quarantine of infected farms is important and the dog registration should continue.

The maintenance of eradication phase can begin once the parasite has been potentially eliminated. During this phase, specific activities of previous phases cease, and vigilance activities are employed (e.g., trace-back from slaughterhouses). It is important that the dog registration still takes place during this phase (Gemmell and Schantz 1997; Gemmell et al. 2001). During the planning or preparatory phase taking into account the cost-benefit ratios, five options can be discerned (Gemmell and Schantz 1997; Gemmell et al. 2001):

Option 1: No control, for a variety of reasons such as lack of resources.

Option 2: Implement a horizontal approach.

Option 3: A slow attack option oriented toward preventing the dog's infection from raw offals by testing dogs and creating legislation for quarantining farms still harboring infected animals. This slow attack option may last for more than 30 years.

Option 4: A fast attack option A, which includes an educational approach, legislation, and surveillance of the human and animal population, as in option 3, but in addition the dog population must be drastically reduced. This attack phase can last more than 30 years.

Option 5: A fast attack option B, where all dogs are treated with praziquantel at predetermined intervals. The duration of this attack phase may be as short as 10–15 years. According to Gemmell and Schantz (1997), options 3, 4, and 5 are "vertical" approaches.

Craig and Larrieu (2007) summarize and simplify the approaches to control in slow track and fast track. The slow-track relies on specific health education, meat inspection, and upgrading of slaughterhouses. This approach was the only one employed in the Iceland program for many years and was successful (Craig and Larrieu 2007); however, most authors consider that the use of slow track as the sole tool of control does not lead to a significant reduction in transmission (Gemmell and Schantz 1997; Lloyd et al. 1998; Craig and Larrieu 2007). On the other hand, Wales' experience showed that although the unique use of education failed to reduce the transmission of echinococcosis, it had a positive effect on the praziquantel dosing of dogs by the farmers (Lloyd et al. 1998). The fast-track option leads to a shorter time to control the transmission of echinococcosis.

Based on the proposal of Gemmell et al. (2001), Craig and Larrieu (2007) described better the options for control of echinococcosis, which are as follows:

Option 1: Decision not to proceed because CE is not a public health problem, funding is not available, socio-economics features, and other reasons.

Option 2: Implementation of a long-term (slow-track) approach. Experience in some countries indicates that it would require 30–100 years to be fully implemented.

Option 3: Vertical slow-track approach incorporating at least annual testing of dogs together with on-site education of owners and quarantine of positive dogs.

Option 4: Vertical fast-track approach with elimination of stray dogs and euthanasia of positive dogs. Employed in Cyprus, this approach was effective after 10–15 years.

Option 5: Vertical fast-track approach including regular treatment of all registered dogs with praziquantel. Employed in New Zealand after 1990, it was effective after 10–15 years.

Health Education

Health education, as mentioned, is one of the tools for the control and prevention of echinococcosis, both in slow-track and fast-track approaches. Even in some control programs, such as Iceland (1863–1960), it was the only action taken during many years, and it recorded good results. Health education is a multidisciplinary activity, which requires knowledge of medical sciences, teaching, and communication methods. For the purposes of this paper, health education is defined as a specialty that uses educational principles to promote changes in behavior with regard to health in the individual and the community.

According to Parodi et al. (2001), health education includes three types of activities that tend to be dependent on one another:

1. Information: It involves the transfer of expert knowledge to the group targeted. This activity aims to highlight certain points to get the community to actively participate in preventive actions.
2. Health education sensu strictu: It is aimed to target groups who are not professionally concerned about the problem, such as schoolchildren or the public at large.
3. Occupational training: It targets those who must implement health standards in their professional activities (e.g., farmers and butchers).

The objectives of health education are for the community to support the programs and to be able to influence the importance of health priorities (Parodi et al. 2001). Therefore, health education must be included in all control programs previously defined. It is necessary to enhance the use of new technologies of communication and the spread of knowledge.

Costs and Benefits

The cost-effectiveness analysis and cost-benefit analysis are important tools to compare alternative echinococcosis control programs. For an economic evaluation it will be necessary to estimate the costs of the control program and losses produced by the disease (Nonnemaker and Schantz 1997). There are three types of costs to evaluate: (a) costs of CE in humans, (b) costs of the disease in animals, and (c) costs of the control program.

The cost of control programs must be evaluated realistically, taking into account that there are programs that will be necessary to implement over many years, supported by government budgets. Per Nonnemaker and Schantz (1997), the cost-benefit analysis is more comprehensive than cost-effectiveness analysis, and it determines if the net benefits of a control program outweigh the net cost to society. Whenever possible, the interruption of a control program for lack of funds should be avoided; sufficient funding from the legislature to complete this period of the program should always be in place. Loss of confidence by the government, resulting from inadequate data about evidence of success in the program, may result in a premature withdrawal of funding (Gemmell et al. 2001). To obtain sufficient funds in the budget, it is necessary to make a good analysis of the costs and benefits of the program because an economic evaluation of the effect of the disease should be an integral part of any control program. Therefore, it is necessary to sustain with data that CE has an important economic impact on human health and livestock production (Torgerson 2003a). Human health costs include human morbidity and mortality cost. Morbidity costs should include costs of diagnosis, surgical and medical treatments, nursing care, and paid sick leaves. It must also be considered that hydatidosis is a long-term disease that affects the quality of life both in undiagnosed individuals and in surgically treated individuals (Torgerson and Dowling 2001). The burden of CE may be also estimated using nonfinancial metrics such as the disability-adjusted life year (DALY) defined as a measure of overall disease burden and expressed as the number of years lost due to ill-health, disability, or early death, as proposed by Torgerson (2011). As Torgerson (2003b) said, the mortality costs are difficult to calculate because the value of life is a controversial subject and has been calculated in a number of ways. Because of these difficulties many economists prefer to use the concept of DALYs. It should be noted that the costs of human health are very different in poor countries as compared to the rich developed countries.

The cost estimates for livestock production are based on prevalence of CE in livestock, the value of livestock-related products, and an evaluation of likely production losses. It is accepted that infected animals have a reduction in the growth, milk production, and fecundity. Moreover, after inspection at slaughterhouses, the infected viscera (mainly the liver and lungs) are confiscated and destroyed. Because of all these factors, CE has important costs in livestock.

In a study made in Jordan, a country of lower-middle income with a population of 5,100,981,

Torgerson et al. (2001) estimates annual economic loss attributable to hydatidosis in animals and humans from US$ 2,602,215 to 6,533,661 with a median of US$ 3,874,070. In another study made in Wales, an endemic region of the United Kingdom, a wealthy and industrialized economy, Torgerson and Dowling (2001) estimate an annual human cost of hydatidosis of US$ 1million and perhaps as much as US$ 7.9 million. In Spain, a European country with 47,021,031 inhabitants, a study made by Benner et al. (2010) estimates the overall economic loss attributable to CE in animals and humans in 2005 at 148,964,534 euros. In China, in the province of Sichuan, with 84 million inhabitants, a study made by Budke et al. (2005) quantified the annual combined human and animal economic losses by CE at US$ 218,676 if only liver-related losses in sheep, goats, and yaks are taken into account. However, total annual losses can be nearly US$ 1 million if additional livestock production losses are assumed. Data such as those presented above serve as examples of arguments that must be handled with the government authorities to justify the cost of control programs.

Pharmacological Treatment of Dogs

The antihelminthic treatment of dogs is included in all programs of control. The drug of choice is praziquantel (5 mg/kg/bw) administered orally at intervals of 6 weeks. This interval was based on the prepatent period of infection with *E. granulosus* and has proven to be effective in preventing transmission Cabrera PA et al. (2002). Depending on the program of different countries, the praziquantel dosing is done by the owners of the dogs or by technicians in charge of the program, and the drug may be free or payable by owners.

Reduction of Dog Population

The reduction of dog population was implemented in some programs. A massive reduction of dog population was employed in the control program of Cyprus between 1970 and 1985. The drastic measure taken was the elimination of stray and unattended dogs. During the first year of the campaign, more than 18,000 stray and unattended dogs were killed. All dogs that tested positive for *E. granulosus* were also killed, and a dog registration fee was introduced (Craig and Larrieu 2007). This massive killing of dogs is not currently accepted.

In the current Control Program of Echinococcosis in Uruguay, since 2007, they have introduced a voluntary and free surgical castration of owned dogs. The spaying of stray dogs is also performed. The spaying is performed in dogs of both sexes by veterinarians in mobile units throughout the country. From January 2007 to October 2011, 100,440 dogs have been spayed. This action has the approval of the Society for the Protection of Animals of Uruguay and is made together with a campaign on responsible dog ownership (Ferreira and Irabedra 2007; Guisantes 2009; Purpura 2011).

Controlled Slaughter of Cattle

Measures must be taken to prevent that raw offal is eaten by dogs. Safe slaughtering includes veterinary inspection and improving facilities of abattoirs. The adoption of laws that forbid illegal killing is very important. The measures on home slaughter should be based on health education, especially in rural areas.

Vaccination

The vaccination against CE in livestock may be an important tool of control. The preparation of a vaccine (EG95) to protect sheep, goats, and bovines against hydatidosis is an important advance in this field (Lightowlers et al. 1996; Heath et al. 2003; Zhang and McManus 2008; Jensen and Thevenet 2011). The large-scale trials made in China and Argentina confirmed the efficacy of the dog vaccine developed by Lightowlers et al. (1996), and leads to their incorporation into future control options. The vaccine is a recombinant protein cloned from the oncosphere, which is injected together with Quil A subcutaneously on two occasions 1 month or more apart and induces protection against *E. granulosus* which lasts for at least 12 months. A trial of vaccination of bovines with EG95 (5 doses) was also successful (Heath et al. 2011). However, operational difficulties and problems in field applications may limit the application in some countries (Mujica et al. 2011).

Surveillance

Epidemiological surveillance is defined as the ongoing and systematic collection, analysis, and interpretation of health data in the process of describing and monitoring a health event. This information is used for planning, implementing, and evaluating public health interventions and programs. Surveillance data are used both to determine the need for public health action and to assess the effectiveness of programs.

As recommended by Schantz (1997), the epidemiological surveillance applied to CE requires the measurement of infection in dogs and intermediate hosts (including humans) and the description of those factors relating to the hosts, the agent, and the environment pattern of distribution and transmission. Therefore, there is a significant relationship between surveillance and control because surveillance provides the baseline data necessary for any control program.

The surveys enable establishing the importance of CE in a country or region, obtaining baseline data and an insight into the process of transmission, and providing baseline information for formulating effective control policies for some or all the affected areas and information against which to monitor the progress of control (Gemmell et al. 2001). All this information should be obtained in the planning phase of the control program. The surveillance surveys must include data on human hydatidosis, data on canine echinococcosis, and data on prevalence of CE in livestock.

Data on Human Hydatidosis

These data are very important and may be obtained from different sources described in the following sections as annual surgical and treatment incidence, ultrasonographic (US) surveys, and serologic surveys.

Annual Surgical and Treatment Incidence

This data is the gold standard (Craig and Larrieu 2007). It must be expressed in total patients per 100,000 rural and/or total/rural population. These rates should be classified by age, sex, ethnic group, residence, occupation, etc. The incidence in children is important because it gives data on recent transmission. This data is of great value for monitoring the success of the control program.

Ultrasonographic Surveys

US is an excellent screening technique which has been employed in several control programs (Schantz 1997; Cohen et al. 1998; Larrieu et al. 2000; Frider et al. 2001; Wen et al. 2002; Macpherson et al. 2003; Guisantes 2009). US is a technique with good sensitivity, specificity, and clinical correlation. Its use in surveys has high acceptability to the population, and it can explore the abdominal organs, provide immediate results, has low cost, and can be used under field conditions (Gemmell 2001).

Serologic Surveys

Immunodiagnostic tests may be employed to evaluate the prevalence of hydatidosis. To be applied in seroepidemiologic studies, these tests must have good sensitivity, specificity, and predictive values. As part of this approach, a screening test of high sensitivity as the enzyme-linked immunosorbent assay must be employed, as well as a confirmatory test with high specificity as immunoblot. However, the immunodiagnostic tests have certain limitations: a) a variable proportion of persons with CE do not have detectable antibodies; b) the presence of antibodies not give information on the location, size and other data of the cyst; and c) the existence of cross-reactivity with other parasitic diseases (Gemmell et al. 2001). Currently it is accepted that a mass screening by US with confirmatory serologic testing is a good approach to surveillance of hydatidosis (Cohen et al. 1998).

Data on Canine Echinococcosis

The detection of *E. granulosus* in the definitive host plays a pivotal role in the transmission dynamics of CE. It represents a crucial milestone in the development of epidemiological studies and implementation of control programs in endemic areas (WHO/OIE 2001). Therefore, it is crucial to determine the prevalence of this zoonosis to have reliable methods of diagnosis in dogs and to develop appropriate control programs (Guisantes 2011). The methods in the following sections have been employed for the premortem and postmortem (necropsy) diagnosis in dogs.

Postmortem Diagnosis: Necropsy

The study of the small intestine during necropsy is the most reliable indicator of the prevalence and changes in patterns of infection of dogs with *E. granulosus* (WHO/OIE 2001). The parasitological examination by necropsy was the recommended method for the diagnosis in feral and unwanted dogs (Gemmell et al. 2001). Given its diagnostic accuracy, it is critical to include in all programs for the control of echinococcosis and other parasitic zoonoses, at least, a study based on necropsy. Nevertheless, this is a laborious and ethically questionable procedure, which is not suitable for mass screening.

Premortem Diagnosis in Dogs

This diagnosis includes the following: arecoline purging method, serologic diagnosis, coproantigen detection, and detection of copro-DNA.

Arecoline Purging Method

Identifying *E. granulosus* in feces after treatment with arecoline hydrobromide was discontinued in many control programs due to the many drawbacks.

Serologic Diagnosis

Since its proposal by Gasser et al. (1988), the detection of parasite-specific antibodies in serum has been used in several studies like Benito et al. (2006) in many countries and continents. However, this method has several drawbacks, which include the following: (a) variable informed diagnostic sensitivity (35–90 %), depending on the antigens, countries, and regions studied; (b) false-positives because some studies in endemic areas have found high positivity in noninfected dogs (diagnosed by arecoline); (c) it does not always indicate current infection; and (d) there is no correlation between the number of parasites and the serologic response.

Coproantigen Detection

Since the reports of Allan et al. (1992) and Deplazes et al. (1992), the method has been used worldwide in many studies (Jenkins et al. 2000; Benito et al. 2006) and control programs (Craig and Larrieu 2007; Ferreira and Irabedra 2007; Guisantes 2009). At present, the main advantages may be summarized (Guisantes 2011) as follows: (a) it is positive in the prepatent period; (b) it is an indicator of current infection; (c) it has a good sensitivity and specificity with some antigens and methods; (d) improves the results obtained by arecoline; (e) it can be applied to the analysis of individual cases or in larger studies; and (f) a properly treated sample can be stored and shipped at room temperature. The advantages of this method are the reason why the study of *Echinococcus* coproantigens is the recommended procedure by most authors nowadays. Presently, it is the most suitable method for the diagnosis of *E. granulosus* in dogs applicable to control programs, and its use in many countries has given good results.

Detection of Copro-DNA

The introduction of molecular methods based on polymerase chain reaction (PCR) should provide the required specificity and sensitivity for the detection of *E. granulosus* in dogs. This methodology is reported in many interesting papers, such as Cabrera M et al. (2002a), Abbasi et al. (2003), Dinkel et al. (2004), Stefanic et al. (2004), Varcasia et al. (2006), Naidich et al. (2006), Boufana et al. (2008), and Armua-Fernandez et al. (2011). Copro-PCR methods could be used for confirmation of coproantigen-positive stool samples. Naidich et al. (2006) propose that in areas where control programs and surveillance for canine echinococcosis are undertaken, the copro-PCR could be used to verify that dogs are not longer infected with *E. granulosus* due to its high sensitivity and specificity. Whenever technological and economic conditions allow it, the detection of copro-DNA in feces is another good option for diagnosis in dogs. Its application in control programs worldwide will lead to a better large-scale evaluation of this methodology.

Data on Prevalence of Cystic Echinococcosis in Livestock

These data are very important to know the prevalence in a country or region before beginning a control program and to track its success. A proper inspection of meat in slaughterhouses is essential for a good surveillance. The prevalence data on livestock is usually supplied by the control authorities from slaughterhouses data. It is also important to trace back infected animals arriving to abattoirs to identify the infected farms and regions. In summary, an adequate surveillance system is very important to develop an efficient control program with a good cost-benefit relation.

Prevention

All control measures discussed above are directed toward prevention of infection. In relation to such measures, the prevention of human infection by *E. granulosus* eggs is based primarily on health education. It is important to determine the personal, socioeconomic, and environmental risk factors involved in the transmission of human hydatidosis in each country or region (Carmona et al. 1998; WHO/OIE 2001; Larrieu et al. 2000). One risk is the lack of potable water and the use of rural water tanks that collect rainwater from the ground surface and roofs (Carmona et al. 1998). All personnel handling dogs in endemic areas should be aware of the health risk of acquiring hydatidosis and must take safety precautions.

At a personal level, the prevention is mainly based on simple rules of personal hygiene, such as avoiding contact with unknown dogs that may be infected, washing hands before eating, and washing vegetables before eating them raw. Dog owners should treat the dogs regularly with praziquantel and avoid feeding them with raw offal potentially infected with cysts. The analysis of dog feces through the study of coproantigens is also a measure of safety at the household level.

Conclusion

The following concepts may be gleaned from this chapter:

1. Despite knowing thoroughly the life cycle of *E. granulosus* and their mechanisms of transmission, CE continues to be an important zoonosis in many regions of the world.
2. The control of CE includes a complex group of actions, due to the existence of human and animal hosts in the life cycle of *E. granulosus*.
3. A varied number of approaches and options to control CE have been employed in several countries, with different results.
4. The approaches to control CE have been well summarized by Craig and Larrieu (2007), both for slow-track and fast-track implementations. The slow-track is a long-term implementation that relies on specific health education, meat inspection, and upgrading of slaughterhouses. The slow-track implementation includes a vertical slow-track approach, which incorporates at least annual testing of dogs together with on-site education of owners and quarantine of positive dogs. The vertical fast-track approach also includes elimination of stray dogs and euthanasia of positive dogs and may add a regular treatment of all registered dogs with praziquantel.
5. Health education is a key tool for the control and prevention of CE, both in slow-track and fast-track approaches.
6. The cost-effectiveness analysis and cost-benefit analysis are important tools to compare alternative echinococcosis control programs.
7. The control measures of CE include pharmacological treatment of dogs, reduction of dog population, controlled slaughter of cattle, and vaccination.

8. The surveillance data is crucial to determine the need for public health action and to assess the effectiveness of the programs. The surveillance surveys must include data on human hydatidosis, data on canine echinococcosis, and data on prevalence of CE in livestock.
9. The control measures described are aimed to prevent CE in animals and in men, but of all these control measures, the prevention of human infection by *E. granulosus* eggs is based primarily on health education. Additionally, prior to taking any preventative measures, it is important to determine the personal, socioeconomic, and environmental risk factors involved in the transmission of human hydatidosis in each country or region.

Acknowledgments The author thanks his daughters Marina E. Guisantes, B.A., for drawing the life cycle of *E. granulosus* (Fig. 25.1), and Isabel P. Guisantes, B.B.A., M.P.M., for reviewing and editing the English version of the paper.

References

Abbasi I, Branzenburg A, Campos-Ponce M, Abdel Hafez SK, Raoul F, Craig PS, Hambuger J. Copro-diagnosis of Echinococcus granulosus infection in dogs by amplification of a newly identified repeated DNA sequence. Am J Trop Med Hyg. 2003;69:324–30.

Allan JC, Craig PS, Garcia Noval J, Mencos F, Liu D, Wang Y, Wen H, Zhou P, Stringer R, Rogan M, et al. Coproantigen detection for immunodiagnosis of echinococcosis and taeniasis in dogs and humans. Parasitology. 1992;104(Pt 2):347–56.

Armua-Fernandez MT, Nonaka N, Sakurai T, Nakamura S, Gottstein B, Deplazes P, Phiri IG, Katakura K, Oku Y. Development of PCR/Dot blot assay for specific detection and differentiation of taeniid cestode eggs in canids. Parasitol Int. 2011;60:84–9.

Benito A, Carmena D, Joseph L, Martínez J, Guisantes JA. Dog echinococcosis in northern Spain: comparison of coproantigen and serum antibody assays with coprological exam. Vet Parasitol. 2006;142:102–11.

Benner C, Carabin H, Sanchez-Serrano LP, Budke CM, Carmena D. Analysis of the economic impact of cystic echinococcosis in Spain. Bull World Health Organ. 2010;88:49–57.

Boufana BS, Campos-Ponce M, Naidich A, Buishi I, Lahmar S, Zeyhle E, Jenkins DJ, Combes B, Wen H, Xiao N, Nakao M, Ito A, Qiu J, Craig PS. Evaluation of three PCR assays for the identification of the sheep strain (Genotype 1) of Echinococcus granulosus in canid feces and parasite tissues. Am J Trop Med Hyg. 2008;78:777–83.

Budke CM, Jiamin Q, Qian W, Torgerson PR. Economic effects of echinococcosis in a disease-endemic region of the Tibetan Plateau. Am J Trop Med Hyg. 2005;73:2–10.

Cabrera M, Canova S, Rosenzvit M, Guarnera E. Identification of Echinococcus granulosus eggs. Diagn Microbiol Infect Dis. 2002a;44:29–34.

Cabrera PA, Lloyd S, Haran G, Pineyro L, Parietti S, Gemmell MA, Correa O, Morana A, Valledor S. Control of Echinococcus granulosus in Uruguay: evaluation of different treatment intervals for dogs. Vet Parasitol. 2002b;103:333–40.

Carmona C, Perdomo R, Carbo A, Alvarez C, Monti J, Grauert R, Stern D, Perera G, Lloyd S, Bazini R, Gemmell MA, Yarzabal L. Risk factors associated with human cystic echinococcosis in Florida, Uruguay: results of a mass screening study using ultrasound and serology. Am J Trop Med Hyg. 1998;58:599–605.

Cohen H, Paolillo E, Bonifacino R, Botta B, Parada L, Cabrera P, Snowden K, Gasser R, Tessier R, Dibarboure L, Wen H, Allan JC, Soto de Alfaro H, Rogan MT, Craig PS. Human cystic echinococcosis in a Uruguayan community: a sonographic, serologic and epidemiologic study. Am J Trop Med Hyg. 1998;59:620–7.

Craig PS, Larrieu E. Control of cystic echinococcosis/hydatidosis. In: Molyneux HD, editor. Control of human parasitic diseases. Amsterdam: Academic; 2007. p. 443–508.

Deplazes P, Gottstein B, Eckert J, Jenkins DJ, Ewald D, Jimenez-Palacios S. Detection of Echinococcus coproantigens by enzyme-linked immunosorbent assay in dogs, dingoes and foxes. Parasitol Res. 1992;78: 303–8.

Dinkel A, Njoroge EM, Zimmermann A, Wälz M, Zeyhle E, Elmahdi IE, Mackenstedt U, Romig T. A PCR system for detection of species and genotypes of the Echinococcus granulosus-complex, with reference to the epidemiological situation in eastern Africa. Int J Parasitol. 2004;34:645–53.

Ferreira C, Irabedra P. Cystic echinococcosis as a public health problem in Latin America and new approaches to its control. Neotrop Helminthol. 2007;1:55–7.

Frider B, Moguilensky J, Salvitti J, Odriozola M, Cantoni G, Larrieu E. Epidemiological surveillance of human hydatidosis by means of ultrasonography: its contribution to the evaluation of control programs. Acta Trop. 2001;79:219–23.

Gasser RB, Lightowlers MW, Obendorf DJ, Jenkins D, Rickard MD. Evaluation of a serological test system for the diagnosis of natural Echinococcus granulosus infection in dogs using E. granulosus protoscolex and oncosphere antigens. Aust Vet J. 1988;65:369–73.

Gemmell MA, Schantz PM. Formulating policies for control of Echinococcus granulosus: an overview of planning, implementation and evaluation. In: Andersen EL, Ouhelli H, Kachani M, editors. Compendium on cystic echinococcosis. Provo: Brigham Young University Press Services; 1997. p. 329–45.

Gemmell MA, Roberts TC, Beard S, Campano Diaz JR, Lawson JR, Nonnemaker JM. Control of Echinococcus granulosus. In: Eckert J, Gemmell MA, Meslin F-X, Pawlowski ZS editors. WHO/OIE Manual on echinococcosis in humans and animals. Paris: World Health Organization for Animal Health; 2001, p. 195–204.

Guisantes JA. [The control of echinococcosis/hydatidosis in Uruguay.] (in Spanish). Zoonosis; 2009;1:42–4.

Guisantes JA. The diagnosis of Echinococcus granulosus infections in dogs. Abstracts book of the XXIV World Congress of Hydatidology. Urumqi; 14–18 Sept 2011. p. 68.

Heath DD, Jensen O, Lightowlers MW. Progress in control of hydatidosis using vaccination – a review of formulation and delivery of the vaccine and recommendations for practical use in control programmes. Acta Trop. 2003;85:133–43.

Heath D, Robinson C, Shakes T, Lightowlers MW. Vaccination of bovines against Echinococcus granulosus (CE). Abstracts book of the XXIV World Congress of Hydatidology. Urumqi; 14–18 Sept 2011. p. 203.

Jenkins DJ, Fraser A, Bradshaw H, Craig PS. Detection of Echinococcus granulosus coproantigens in Australian canids with natural or experimental infection. J Parasitol. 2000;86:140–5.

Jensen O, Sanchez-Thevenet P. Hydatidosis by Echinococcus granulosus: update and description of the situation in Patagonia (Argentina). In: Esteves A, editor. Research in Helminths. Kerala: Transworld Research Network; 2011. p. 21–40.

Kamenetzky I, Gutierrez AM, Canova SG, Haag KL, Guarnera EA, Parra A, Garcia GE, Rosenzvit MC. Several strains of Echinococcus granulosus infect livestock and humans in Argentina. Infect Genet Evol. 2002;2:129–36.

Larrieu E, Costa MT, Cantoni G, Labanchi JL, Bigatti R, Pérez A, Araya D, Mancini S, Herrero E, Talmon G, Romeo S, Thakur A. Control program of hydatid disease in the Province of Rio Negro, Argentina, 1980–1997. Bol Chil Parasitol. 2000;55:49–53.

Lavikainen A, Lehtinen MJ, Laaksonen S, Agren E, Oksanen A, Meri S. Molecular characterization of Echinococcus isolates of cervid origin from Finland and Sweden. Parasitology. 2006;133:565–70.

Lightowlers MW, Lawrence SB, Gauci CG, Young J, Ralston MJ, Maas D, Heath DD. Vaccination against hydatidosis using a defined recombinant antigen. Parasite Immunol. 1996;18:457–62.

Lloyd S, Walters TMH, Craig PS. The use of sentinel lambs to survey the effect of an education programme on control on transmission of Echinococcus granulosus in South Powys, Wales. Bull World Health Organ. 1998;76:469–73.

Macpherson CNL, Bartholomot B, Frider B. Application of ultrasound in diagnosis, treatment, epidemiology, public health and control of Echinococcus granulosus and E. multilocularis. Parasitology. 2003;127:S21–35.

McManus DP. Current status of the genetics of Echinococcus species. Abstracts book of the XXIV World Congress of Hydatidology. Urumqi; 14–18 Sept 2011. p. 133.

McManus DP, Thompson RCA. Molecular epidemiology of cystic echinococcosis. Parasitology. 2003;127: S37–51.

Mujica G, Herrero E, Chioso C, Labanchi JL, Perez A, Gatti A, et al. A field study evaluation of the EG95 vaccine against ovine hidatidosis: first communication. Abstracts book of the XXIV World Congress of Hydatidology. Urumqi; 14–18 Sep 2011. p. 202.

Naidich A, McManus DP, Canova SG, Gutierrez AM, Zhang W, Guarnera E, Rosenzvit MC. Patent and prepatent detection of Echinococcus granulosus genotypes in the definitive host. Mol Cell Probes. 2006;20: 5–10.

Nonnemaker JM, Schantz PM. Economic evaluation techniques as tools for the planning and evaluation of echinococcosis control programs. In: Andersen EL, Ouhelli H, Kachani M, editors. Compendium on cystic echinococcosis. Provo: Bringham Young University Press Services; 1997. p. 319–28.

Parodi P, Mantovani A, Seimenis A. Public health education in control programmes. In: Eckert J, Gemmell MA, Meslin F-X, Pawlowski ZS, editors. WHO/OIE manual on echinococcosis in humans and animals. Paris: World Health Organization for Animal Health; 2001. p. 219–24.

Pearson M, Le TH, Zhang LH, Blair D, Dai THN, McManus DP. Molecular taxonomy and strain analysis in Echinococcus. In: Craig P, Pawlowski ZS, editors. Cestode zoonoses: echinococcosis and cysticercosis. Amsterdam: Ios Press; 2002. p. 205–19.

Purpura R. Zoonotic control and animal protection (in Spanish). Zoonosis (Montevideo). 2011;1:8–10.

Schantz PM. Sources and uses of surveillance data for cystic echinococcosis. In: Andersen EL, Ouhelli H, Kachani M, editors. Compendium on cystic echinococcosis. Provo: Brigham Young University Press Services; 1997. p. 72–84.

Stefanic S, Shaikenov BS, Deplazes P, Dinkel A, Torgerson PR, Mathis A. Polymerase chain reaction for detection of patent infections of Echinococcus granulosus ("sheep strain") in naturally infected dogs. Parasitol Res. 2004;92:347–51.

Thompson RCA. Biology and systematics of Echinococcus. In: Thompson RCA, Lymberi AJ, editors. Echinococcus and hydatid disease. Wallingford: CAB International; 1995. p. 1–50.

Torgerson PR. Economic effects of echinococcosis. Acta Trop. 2003a;85:113–8.

Torgerson PR. Transmission dynamics and control options for Echinococcus granulosus. Parasitology. 2003b; 127(suppl):S143–58.

Torgerson PR. How to assess the socio-economic burden of Echinococcosis? Methods and pitfalls. Abstracts book of the XXIV World Congress of Hydatidology. Urumqi; 14–18 Sept 2011. p. 164.

Torgerson PR, Dowling PM. Estimating the economic effects of cystic echinococcosis. Part 2: an endemic

region in the United Kingdom, a wealthy industrialized economy. Ann Trop Med Parasitol. 2001;95:177–85.
Torgerson RP, Dowling PM, Abo-Shehada MN. Estimating the economic effects of cystic echinococcosis. Part 3: Jordan, a developing country with lower-middle income. Ann Trop Med Parasitol. 2001;95:595–603.
Varcasia A, Canu S, Lightowlers MW, Scala A, Garippa G. Molecular characterization of Echinococcus granulosus strains in Sardinia. Parasitol Res. 2006;98:273–7.
Wen H, Chai J-J, Wang JC, Wang S-H, Wang X-Y, Feng X-H, Zhou H-X. Hydatid control within a continental system in P. R. China. In: Craig P, Pawlowski ZS, editors. Cestode zoonosis: echinococcus and cysticercosis. Amsterdam: Ios Press; 2002. p. 355–66.
WHO/OIE. In: Eckert J, Gemmell MA, Meslin F-X, Pawlowski ZS, editors. Control of echinococcosis. Chapter 6. Paris: WHO for Animal Health; 2001.
Zhang W, McManus DP. Vaccination of dogs against Echinococcus granulosus: a means to control hydatid disease? Trends Parasitol. 2008;24:419–24.

Index

M. Turgut (ed.), *Hydatidosis of the Central Nervous System: Diagnosis and Treatment*,
DOI 10.1007/978-3-642-54359-3, © Springer-Verlag Berlin Heidelberg 2014

Batch number: 10705706

Printed by Printforce, the Netherlands

JOHANNES KAUFMANN

Parasitic Infections of Domestic Animals

A Diagnostic Manual

Springer Basel AG

Author

Dr. J. Kaufmann
Bundesamt für Veterinärwesen
Sektion Tierversuche und
Alternativmethoden
Schwarzenburgstr. 161
CH-3097 Liebefeld/Bern
Switzerland

This publication was sponsored by
the Ciba-Geigy Foundation for Cooperation with Developing Countries, Basel, Switzerland,
the Ciba-Geigy Ltd., Animal Health Division, Basel, Switzerland and
the Swiss Development Cooperation, Berne, Switzerland

A CIP catalogue record for this book is available from the Library of Congress, Washington, D.C., USA

Deutsche Bibliothek Cataloging-in-Publication Data

Kaufmann, Johannes:
Parasitic infections of domestic animals : a diagnostic manual/
Johannes Kaufmann. - Basel ; Boston ; Berlin : Birkhäuser, 1996
ISBN 978-3-0348-7668-1

The publisher and editor can give no guarantee for the information on drug dosage and administration contained in this publication. The respective user must check its accuracy by consulting other sources of reference in each individual case.

Originally published by Birkhäuser Verlag in 1996
Softcover reprint of the hardcover 1st edition 1996

Printed on acid-free paper produced from chlorine-free pulp. TCF ∞
Typography and book design: Markus Etterich, Basel

ISBN 978-3-0348-7668-1 ISBN 978-3-0348-7666-7 (eBook)
DOI 10.1007/978-3-0348-7666-7
9 8 7 6 5 4 3 2 1

The author would like to dedicate this manual to his teacher and friend

Prof. Bernd Hörning

Bernd Hörning was Professor of Parasitology at the Veterinary Faculty of Berne, Switzerland. He retired in 1992. His extensive knowledge and commitment to Veterinary Parasitology and his amicable attitude towards students and colleagues should be honored with the present manual.

Contents

II Parasites of Cattle

1 Stages in the gut and faeces

2 Stages in the blood and circulatory system

3 Stages in the urogenital system

4 Stages in internal organs

III Parasites of Sheep and Goats

Foreword

It is a great pleasure for me to introduce this manual for the diagnosis of parasites of domestic animals. It is a unique publication in many respects. Books concerning parasitic animal diseases – comprehensive textbooks, but also field manuals – abound. These generally deal with aetiology, clinical signs and pathology, as well as control and treatment. However, while methods for diagnosis are often mentioned, these are rarely sufficiently practical and specific to allow the personnel in field laboratories to reach a concise, rapid diagnosis of the parasite species involved in any particular case. *Parasitic Infections of Domestic Animals* succeeds in redressing these shortcomings.

That such a work ever came to fruition at all is to the credit of its principal author Dr. Johannes Kaufmann, head of the Diagnostic Section of the Institute of Parasitology at the University of Berne, Switzerland. In the late 1980s Dr. Kaufmann worked in a field laboratory of the International Trypanotolerance Centre in Gambia. While there he became acutely aware of the need for practical literature on parasite diagnosis. After returning to Switzerland he took on the gargantuan task of compiling such a work himself. Supplementing the material gleaned from his field work, Dr. Kaufmann has brought together a great deal of information from various institutes and universities.

The result is an impressively comprehensive, beautifully illustrated and, above all highly serviceable manual. It is easy to consult. Its systematic and colour-coded layout allows the user to steer swiftly and surely through a vast amount of information. Clinical pictures and figures show the parasite stage of diagnostic interest, facilitating a rapid and accurate diagnosis. The book has been designed to be used by veterinarians and technicians, by teachers and students – in fact, by anyone dealing with the diagnosis of diseases in domestic animals. On another practical level, it will enable meat inspectors and other public health officials to identify parasites of animals which may infect humans. While originally meant for use primarily in Africa, the book's relevance is by no means limited to this continent, since most of the economically important parasites considered in detail (e.g. coccidia of poultry, gastrointestinal nematodes of ruminants, strongyles of horses, *Ascaris* and trichinellosis of swine etc.) occur world-wide.

But what good is a well-conceived manual, intelligently and copiously illustrated if it fails to reach those workers in need of it most? The expense of publishing a work of this type, accompanied as it is by approximately 320 color and 400 black and white illustrations is close to prohibitive. That the price has nonetheless been set at a very reasonable level is only possible thanks to generous financial aid from *ciba* Basle, Switzerland, the Swiss Development Cooperation, Berne, Switzerland and the University of Berne, Switzerland. This is the final factor to assuring that *Parasitic Infections of Domestic Animals* will become a well-thumbed bench book in many laboratories world-wide.

Gerrit Uilenberg
Cargese, September 1995

Introduction

The present manual is intended as a tool for the identification of cosmopolitan parasites affecting domestic animals. Special attention has been paid to imported or autochthonous parasitic infections occurring in African livestock, including dromedaries. In the course of compiling this work, a summary was made of the activities of some 300 institutions (national veterinary health departments, research institutes, universities, private enterprises etc.) dealing with the research, diagnosis and control of parasitic diseases in Africa. Both francophone and anglophone literature has been considered.

Laboratories dealing with the diagnosis of parasitic diseases need to rely on well-furnished libraries in order to cover the vast spectrum of parasites causing disease. Nevertheless, many laboratories, especially those in developing countries, do not have access to such resources.

It is for such situations – when technical information is needed but no library is available – that this manual was designed. It contains, in condensed form, all the information, necessary for a rapid and accurate diagnosis of parasitic infections of domestic animals.

Disease may be initiated either by *adult parasites* or by their *immature stages* and very often the identification of a particular parasite is based on *morphological details,* to which special attention has been paid in this manual. Histopathological sections have been included where pathological alterations need to be elucidated. Indirect diagnosis by immunological techniques is indicated where it plays a practical role. These techniques are described in the initial chapter, METHODS.

Molecular biological techniques have gained an increased significance in the detection of parasitic infections even under field conditions because of their high diagnostic specificity and sensitivity. Furthermore, samples may be collected in the field (e.g. squash blots on to filter papers) and transported easily (often without refrigeration) over long distances to laboratories, where the analysis can be carried out. A special section in the METHODS chapter has been devoted to this highly important and fascinating technology.

Sometimes the species diagnosis is relevant for the control, but very often a genus diagnosis is sufficient. This manual is not intended to serve as a textbook. It is meant to be a technical tool and located on the laboratory bench. The Standard Nomenclature of Animal Parasitic Diseases (SNOAPAD) taxonomy is used in order to allow access to specific literature, some of which is mentioned under the section FURTHER READING. Latin names of parasites which are no longer standard in the current scientific literature but still widely in use in certain publications and geographic areas are mentioned as synonyms in brackets.

In order to meet the requirements of laboratories operating under field conditions, a procedure for achieving a rapid and pragmatic diagnostic decision was established. Parasites of cattle, small ruminants, equine, swine, dromedaries and poultry are described in 6 chapters. Each chapter is divided into the 5 stages in which parasites may occur: stages found in the gut and faeces (■ 1), stages found in the blood and circulatory system (■ 2), stages found in the urogenital system (■ 3), stages found in internal organs (■ 4) and stages found on the body surface (■ 5). Under each of these stages parasites are dealt with in a stereotypic manner: protozoa, helminths (trematodes, cestodes and nematodes) and arthropoda (arachnids and insects). Information relevant to each parasite is presented in the following order: scientific name of the parasite (taxon), synonyms, common name of the parasite or the disease caused by the parasite, species description containing biological data, host spectrum, geographic distribution, symptoms, significance of the parasite, diagnosis, therapy and prophylaxis. A numeric key of the source of each illustration is indicated in brackets [ ] at the end of each legend and refers to the BIBLIOGRAPHY. Parasites which are not species-specific are described in the chapter of that particular livestock species in which they play the most important role and a cross-reference (☞) is made to other animal species or organ systems in which they may also occur.

If a genus is described as a group (e.g. *Trichostrongylus* spp.) essential information is provided under "• General features". If several parasite species or genera can be controlled in a similar manner, therapy and prophylaxis may then be indicated for these species or genera collectively. If infections are arthropod-borne, information will be given on the biology of the respective vector.

Rickettsiaceae (*Ehrlichia* spp., *Anaplasma* spp., *Cowdria ruminantium*, *Eperythrozoon* spp. and others) form an important group of "parasite-like" pathogens and are often found in blood or tissue smears made for the detection of blood parasites. Some important species of Rickettsia are described in the present manual for differential diagnosis.

This manual is presented in the hope that it may assist all those colleagues struggling in their daily work with the diagnosis and control of livestock diseases all over the world. The manual wells from a great sympathy for those people "fighting at the front" under difficult field conditions, in regions where human survival is linked to the health of livestock often perilously endangered by a variety of deleterious conditions, among which parasitic infestation may be highly significant.

I

Methods

CONTENTS

1.1 Detection of helminth eggs, larvae, oocysts and sporocysts of protozoa in faeces

Table 1 Methods for the detection of parasite stages in faeces

Method	Detection
Sedimentation	
• in water	Eggs of *Fasciola* spp.; *Paramphistomum* spp.; *Dicrocoelium* spp.; oocysts of *Eimeria leuckarti* (equines)
• in 0.85% saline	Eggs of *Schistosoma* spp.
Flotation	
• with $ZnCl_2$ solution	Eggs of cestodes and nematodes; $ZnSo_4$, (*SG=1.30) oocysts and sporocysts of protozoa except *Eimeria leuckarti* (equines)
• with NaCl solution	Eggs of *Strongyloides* spp.; strongyles, (*SG=1.20) Ascaris spp., *Toxocara* spp., *Oxyuris* spp., *Anoplocephala* spp., *Moniezia* spp., oocysts of protozoa, *Trichuris* spp. and *Capillaria* spp.
Baermann apparatus	Larvae of lungworms, hatched larvae of strongyles and Strongyloides (in older samples)

*SG = specific gravity; concentrations of $ZnCl_2$- and NaCl solutions ☞ Table 2

General rule for the selection of solution for concentrating parasite stages

- saturated NaCl for floating strongyle eggs
- sedimentation in H_2O for trematode eggs
- saturated NaCl (SG=1.204) is a general purpose solution

Table 2: Flotation solutions

Chemical	g to be disolved in 1000 ml of water	SG* at 20°C
NaCl	360	1.2
$NaNO_3$	350	1.2
$ZnCl_2$	436	1.3
$ZnSO_4$ 7 x H_2O	703	1.3
Sugar	550	1.3

*SG= specific gravity

1.2 Collection and examination of faeces

Faeces intended for parasitological examination should be collected from the rectum, using disposable plastic gloves. The sample is collected into the hand of the glove which is turned inside out, air is expressed and the glove is tied at the wrist. Freshly expelled faeces can also be used for examination as long as it is not contaminated with soil and dirt. This is especially important since many free living nematode larvae may occur in the environment, making a proper diagnosis difficult or impossible. Eggs may develop rapidly to a stage in which it is difficult to identify them.

The detection of parasite stages in faeces from animals suffering from diarrhoea may be markedly impaired. The diagnosis of parasitism by microscopic techniques is more reliable when repeated examinations are made. For example, negative results are sometimes obtained from faecal examinations if the parasites are not mature enough to deposit eggs. This might also occur during the encysted stage of certain parasites, such as strongyles or oesophagostomes. Tapeworm segments often leave the digestive tract without disintegrating, and negative results may be obtained unless segments are detected.

1.3 Direct smear method

It is possible to demonstrate the presence of parasite stages (eggs or larvae of helminths, oocysts of coccidia) by the examination of a thin smear of emulsified faeces. A small quantity of faeces is placed on a slide, mixed with some droplets of water and a cover slip is placed on the fluid. The slide is investigated using a magnification of 50 and 250×. This method, however, suffers from the drawbacks that (a) it is effective only where the concentration of parasite stages is high, (b) it is frequently difficult to identify them since they are partially covered by detritus and (c) quantitative results cannot be obtained.

Parasites found with the direct smear method:

- coccidia species and helminth eggs (only when high numbers of oocysts or eggs are present);
- cestode and trematode eggs (mainly in birds)

1.4 Flotation method

Separating the eggs from faecal debris by floating them on a variety of solutions. When faeces are emulsified in liquids of high specific gravity and either centrifuged or allowed to stand, the worm eggs and many protozoan cysts float to the top while the heavy coarse debris settles to the bottom. The top film can then be removed and examined. Nematode and cestode eggs float in a liquid with a specific gravity of between 1.10 and 1.20. Trematode eggs, which are much heavier, require a specific gravity of 1.30–1.35.

Procedure

1. Place a lump of faeces about the size of a walnut (5–10 g or a few faecal pellets of sheep or goats) in a shell vial, cup or glass.

2. Add approximately 50–100 ml of tap water and mix thoroughly with a spatula until all the faecal material is broken down.

3. The mixture is poured through a wire mesh screen with an aperture of 500–800 µm to remove large lumps. The strained fluid is caught in a bowl. The screen is rinsed with water and the debris left on the screen is discarded.

4. Transfer the suspension to a conical measure and fill with tap water to the top allow to settle for 30 min.

5. Discard the supernatant carefully to a remaining sediment of approx. 10 ml.

6. The sediment is stirred and a sample of 2 ml is poured into a centrifuge tube.

7. The tube is placed in the centrifuge. With a pipette, saturated NaCl is added until a convex meniscus stands above the top of the tube.

8. A thick 19 x 19 mm square cover glass is placed on the tube, ensuring that no bubble is trapped under it. The cover glass may additionally be coated with a solution of egg white / glycerol (1: 1) to improve adherence of the eggs.

9. The tube is centrifuged at 2000 rpm for 2–3 min. (In the absence of a centrifuge let the sample stand for 30 to 60 min.)

10. Pick off the cover glass and place the sample on a slide and examine under a microscope by using a magnification of 32–100×.

Parasite stages found with the flotation method: eggs of cestodes and nematodes; larvae of lungworms; oocysts of coccidia (except *Eimeria leuckarti*). Trematode eggs are not satisfactorily detected with the flotation method (☞ Sedimentation method).

1.5 Sedimentation method

Heavy parasite eggs sink to the bottom of solutions used in the flotation techniques.

Procedure

1.–5.: ☞ Flotation method (1.4)

6. Add water to a point a little below the top of the measure and allow to settle again for 3 min.

7. After sedimentation the supernatant is again drawn off, a few drops of methylene blue (5%) added and the sediment screened in aliquots of 5 ml, using a low power stereomicroscope. Any trematode eggs are readily visible (brown or yellow colored) against the pale blue background.

Parasite stages detected with the sedimentation method:

- eggs of *Fasciola* spp., *Dicrocoelium* spp., *Paramphistomum* spp., *Schistosoma* spp., *Gastrodiscus* sp.;
- larvae of lungworms;
- oocysts of *Eimeria leuckarti* (equines)

1.6 McMaster method

This technique is used where the number of eggs or larvae per gram of faeces should be counted.

Procedure

1. Weigh 3 g of faeces and add 42 ml tap water.

2. Homogenize and pour suspension through a 250 μm aperture sieve, collecting the filtrate.

3. Collect the filtrate, agitate and fill a test tube of 15 ml volume.

4. Centrifuge at 2000 rpm for 2 min.

5. Pour off the supernatant, agitate sediment and fill tube to previous level with flotation solution.

6. Invert tube 6 times and remove fluid with pipette to fill both chambers of McMaster slide quickly.

7. Examine one chamber and multiply number of eggs or larvae under one etched area by 100, or two chambers and multiply by 50 to arrive at the number of eggs per gram (epg) of faeces.

Remark: It is impossible to calculate from the epg the actual worm population of the host. Nevertheless, egg counts in excess of 1000 are generally considered indicative of heavy infections. However, a low epg is not necessarily indicative of very low infections, since one part of the worm population may just have started to reach patency but may already cause disease. Alternatively, the epg may be affected by developing immunity. The eggs of some species, such as certain ascarids, *Strongyloides, Oxyuris, Trichuris* and *Capillaria*, can be easily recognized morphologically. However, with the exception of *Nematodirus* spp., the common trichostrongyle eggs require more detailed analysis (measurements) for differentiation. The diagnosis "strongyle egg" is usually sufficient for practical purposes. (Figure 1)

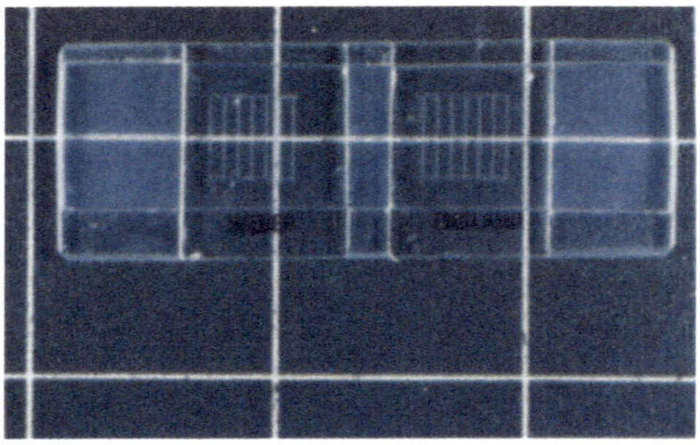

Fig. 1
McMaster chamber for the quantification of parasite eggs in faeces

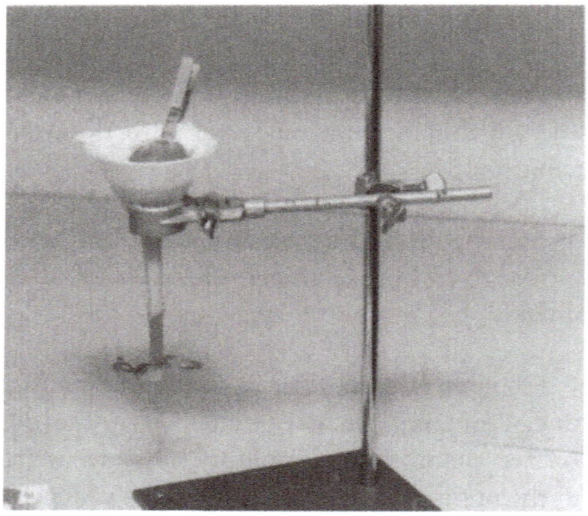

Fig. 2
The Baermann apparatus consists of a funnel held in a retort stand. A rubber tube attached to the bottom of the funnel is constricted by a clip. Faeces are wrapped in gauze and attached with a clothes-peg to the funnel. The larvae leave the faeces, migrate through the gauze to the sediment

1.7 Baermann method

Larvae of lungworms (third-stage larvae of gastrointestinal nematodes) migrate actively into the aqueous phase of the Baermann apparatus. This consists of a glass or plastic funnel held in a retort stand. A rubber tube attached to the bottom of the funnel is constricted by a clip. A sieve (aperture 250 µm) is placed on top of the funnel, which has been partially filled with water. A double layer of gauze is placed on top of the sieve. Faeces are placed on the gauze, and the funnel is slowly filled with water until the faeces are immersed. The apparatus is placed over night at room temperature, during which the larvae migrate out of the faeces and through the sieve to sediment in the neck of the funnel. The clip on the rubber is then opened and the water in the neck of the funnel collected in a small beaker for microscopic examination in a Petri dish. (Figure 2)

A simple adaptation of the above method is to suspend the faeces enclosed in gauze in a urine glass filled with water and leave over night. The larvae will leave the faeces, migrate through the gauze and settle at the bottom of the glass. The sediment is examined under the low power microscope as above.

Parasite stages detected with the Baermann method:

- Larvae of lungworms (*Dictyocaulus* spp., *Muellerius* spp., *Cystocaulus* spp., *Protostrongylus* sp., *Metastrongylus* spp., *Crenosoma* spp.)
- larvae of strongyles

Cave: When faecal samples were collected from the ground, masses of free living nematodes may leave the faeces and appear in the sediment of the Baermann funnel.

1.8 Culture and recovery of third-stage larvae

Faecal culture provides an environment suitable for the hatching of helminth eggs and for their development to the infective stage. The general method described below is suitable for the culture of trichostrongylid or strongylid eggs in the faeces of ruminants, pigs and horses.

Procedure
The faeces should be moist and crumbly but not really wet. Very dry faeces should not be used for culture. If the faeces are very wet, then charcoal, peat moss or vermiculite should be added until the correct consistency is obtained.

1. Faeces are broken up finely using a spatula.

2. Wide-mouthed glass or plastic jars are filled with the mixture, closed with the lid and incubated at 27°C for 7 or at 20°C for 10–20 days. Fungi are sometimes troublesome but indicate that the conditions in the culture are ideal. The growth of fungi can be reduced by stirring the culture each day.

3. Larvae are best recovered using the Baermann apparatus. The culture is removed from the incubator and the faeces are tipped out of the culture dish onto the double layer of gauze of the Baermann apparatus (+ above), distributing it as evenly as possible over the whole area.

4. The culture vessel (lid, jar, dish, etc.) is washed with a small quantity of water. The water is then tipped into the Baermann apparatus.

5. The Baermann apparatus is allowed to stand for 24 hours, or at least over night, during which time the larvae will have migrated through the screen into the bottom of the funnel from where they may be drawn for examination.

1.9 Identification of third-stage larvae of nematodes

Procedure

1. Larvae are killed by the addition of Lugol's iodine to the larval suspension on a microscope slide. Iodine kills the larvae and stains the free-living nematodes yellow while parasitic third-stage larvae remain unstained. A coverslip is placed on the prepared suspension before examination.

2. Microscopic examination at a magnification of 60–80 ×. Some details may only be seen at a magnification of 250 ×.

3. Parasitic larvae appear translucent and almost colourless while free-living nematodes are stained yellow with the iodine. Parasitic larvae show a well defined cuticular sheath (with few exceptions). Characteristics which permit differentiation of the different larvae are shape and internal structure of the head region, number and shape of the intestinal cells, relative size of the sheath tail and shape of the larvae's tail. Lungworm larvae, especially *Dictyocaulus viviparus*, are usually coiled.

1.10 Staining *Cryptosporidia* spp. in faecal smears

Procedure

1. Air-dry thin faecal smears and pass quickly through a flame.

2. Stain with Ziehl-Neelsen's carbol-fuchsin solution (Merck Diagnostica no. 9215) for 2 min.

3. Rinse with tap water.

4. Rinse for a few seconds with acid alcohol (3% hydrochloric acid in 70% ethanol).

5. Rinse again with tap water.

6. Counter stain with Brilliant Green (0.5%; Sigma no. B-6756) for 2 min.

7. Rinse again with tap water.

8. Air-dry the slide. Microscopic examination at 1000×, using immersion oil. Cryptosporidia appear as bright red granules on a blue-green background (☞ CATTLE, ■ 1).

Alternative method

3 µl diarrhoeic faeces and 3 µl carbol-fuchsine (Merck no. 9215) are mixed, and a thin smear is made. After air-drying, the slide is examined at a magnification of 1000 ×, using immersion oil. The oocysts measure 4–5 µm in diameter and appear as thick-walled, red granules.

1.11 Scotch tape method

Procedure

1. A transparent scotch tape, approximately 4 cm in length is pressed onto the skin of the anus and then placed on a microscopic slide.

2. Microscopic examination at a magnification of 32–100 ×.

Remark: This method is widely used to detect eggs of oxyurids (*Enterobius vermicularis, Oxyuris equi* etc.) in animals and man.

1.12 Sodium Acetate Formaldehyde (SAF) method

Procedure

1. Fixation of 2–5 g faeces in SAF solution (15 g sodiumacetate, 20 ml of a 100% acetic acid, 40 ml of a 40% formaldehyde and 925 ml water).

2. Mix thoroughly and pass suspension through a gauze (placed in a funnel) into a tube.

3. Centrifuge at 2000 rpm for 1 min.

4. Discard supernatant to a remaining sediment of 1 ml.

5. Resuspend the sediment with 7 ml of NaCl phys.

6. Add 2 ml of ether, cover the tube with a rubber and mix the contents vigorously.

7. Centrifuge at 2000 rpm for 3 min.

8. Discard the supernatant carefully and transfer some droplets of the sediment onto a microscopic slide. Place a coverslip onto the sample.

9. Microscopic examination at a magnification of 400 ×.

Remark: This method is widely used to detect protozoan parasites (*Entamoeba* spp., *Giardia* spp., *Balantidium* spp., *Eimeria spp.*) in the faeces.

2 Examination of material for *Trichinella spiralis*

2.1 Demonstration of encysted larvae of *T. spiralis* in muscle fibre (Compressorium method)

Procedure

0.5–1.0 g muscle, usually pillars of the diaphragm, are subdivided into small pieces approximately 3 × 10 mm and crushed firmly between pieces of plate glass. For this purpose a product called "compressorium" is available on the marked. The samples are compressed heavily with thumb screws. The samples should be almost transparent for the examination at a magnification of 50 × with a dissecting microscope. Larvae of *T. spiralis* are infective to man. Great care must be taken in handling infected or suspect material.
(Figure 3)

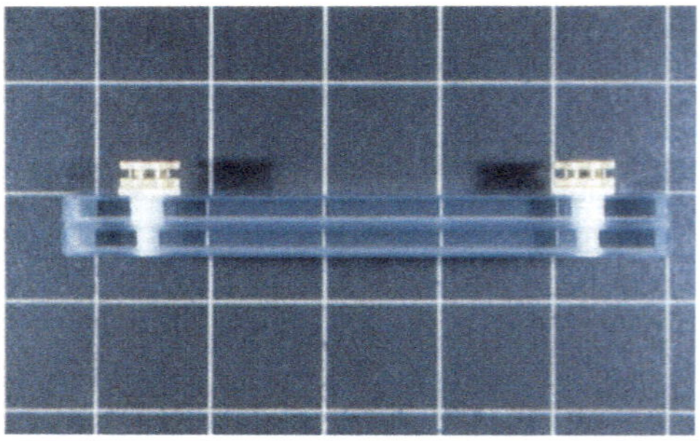

Fig. 3
Compressorium method: Samples of muscles are cut into small pieces and crushed between two glass plates. The samples are compressed heavily with thumb screws until they are almost transparent

2.2 Digestion of muscle for the release of encysted larvae of *T. spiralis*

Procedure

1. The 100 g sample is finely chopped in a chopper/blender or cut manually into small pieces.

2. Transfer the chopped material to a 3 l beaker. Add 10 g of pepsin, dissolved in 2 l of tap water, to give an activity of 2000 FIP (= Fédération Internationale Pharmacie); 30,000 units FB (British Pharmacopoeia) or 10,000 NF (US Nat. Formula).

3. Add 16 ml hydrochloric acid (25%) and place a magnetic stirrer rod in the beaker.

4. Place the beaker on a heated magnetic stirrer which has been pre-set to maintain a temperature of the solution at 44–46°C.

5. After 30 min digestion transfer the contents of the beaker through a mesh screen (aperture of 180 µm) into a 2-l separating funnel. The debris in the screen is gently washed with a fine spray of water in order to remove larvae which may have been trapped on the screen.

6. Sediment for 30 min and run off 40 ml of the sediment into a 50 ml measuring cylinder. Allow to settle for 10 min, then siphon off 30 ml of the supernatant fluid. The sediment is resuspended with a further 30 ml of water and allowed to sediment for 10 min before 30 ml of the supernatant fluid is siphoned off.

7. Pour the remaining 10 ml into a ruled Petri dish (parallel lines 5 mm apart). Dilute the suspension with tap water if it contains a lot of undigested particles.

8. Examine the sediment using a dissecting microscope at a magnification of 20–50 ×.

Remar: Predilection sites are tongue, masseter, intercostal and diaphragm muscles. 10 g samples of each animal are collected and digested. When many animals need to be examined, it is recommended to take 10 g sample of diaphragm pillar tissue from each animal and bulk these to form composite samples with a maximum of 100 g.

Alternative method (for digestion if there is no heatable magnetic stirrer available):

The digested fluid and the tissue are placed in a 3l Erlenmeyer (conical) flask which is maintained at 37°C in a water bath or in an incubator. In this case the flask is shaken every 30 min for 4–5 h.

Remark: The use of pre-prepared and preheated pepsin-HCl solution may be easier and reduce the digestion period markedly.

3 Haematology

3.1 Bloodsmear and Giemsa-stain

Procedure

1. Apply a small drop of blood from a microhaematocrit capillary tube or a pipette to the slide approximately 20 mm from one end.

2. Place a spreader on the slide at an angle of 20–30°C. Draw it back to make contact with the blood.

3. Allow the blood to run to each end of the spreader. Spread the blood along the slide in a fairly rapid but smooth motion.

4. Quickly air-dry the slide and label it with a pencil or a diamond tipped pencil.

5. Fix the thin smear for 1 min in methyl alcohol.

6. Place it in an inverted position in Giemsa-stain (1.5 ml in 15 ml distilled water buffered to pH 7.2) for 30 min.

7. Wash the slide with water and drain in an upright position to dryness.

8. Examine with a microscope at a magnification of 100 and 1000 ×, using immersion oil. (Figure 4)

3.2 Diff-Quick®

This is a rapid staining method for blood smears.

The Diff-Quick® (Baxter Dade AG, 3186 Dü-

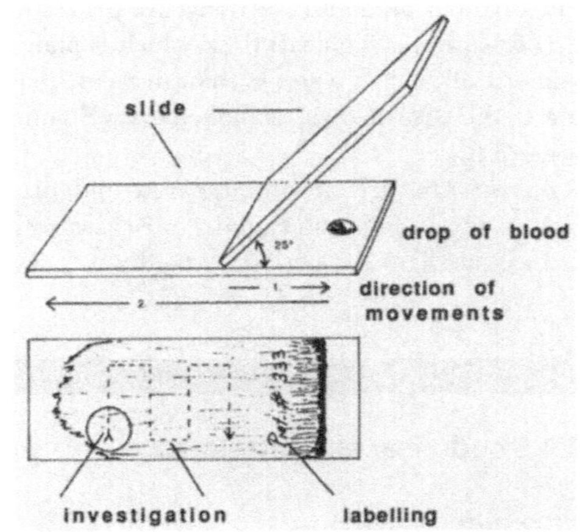

Fig. 4
Preparation of a bloodsmear. A small drop of blood is applied to the slide approximately 20 mm from one end. A spreader (or another clean slide) is placed on the slide at an angle of 20-30° and drawn back to make contact with the blood. The blood is allowed to run to each end of the spreader. The blood is spread along the slide in a fairly rapid but smooth motion [57].

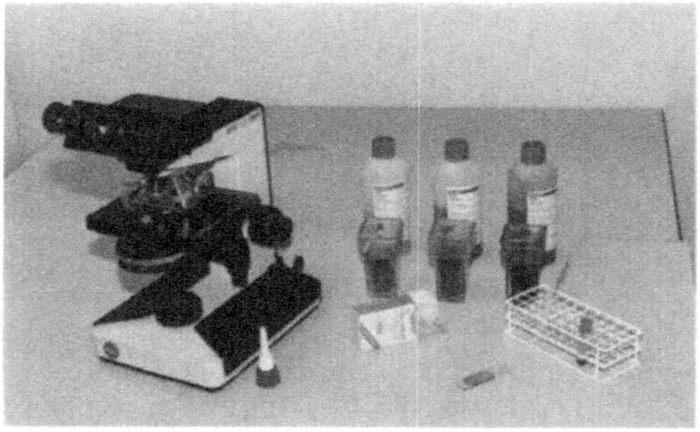

Fig. 5
A good quality high power microscope is an important tool in every diagnostic laboratory. A standard equipment should contain the following magnifications: 32 × 100 ×, 400 × and for the investigation of blood smears 1000 × with oil immersion.
Rapid staining methods for bloodsmears are of great practical use in the routine diagnostic laboratory. The previously air-dried smears are fixed and stained in only 15 s by three consecutive brief immersions in the pre-prepared staining solutions.

dingen, Switzerland) staining set contains solutions for rapid staining of blood smears, yielding results comparable to the Pappenheim technique (Giemsa-May-Grünwald). By consecutive brief immersions in the Dade Diff-Quick Solutions, the previously air-dried smears are fixed and stained in only 15 s. As samples, freshly collected EDTA blood, but also smears from biopsies and other material may easily and quickly be stained with this method.
(Figure 5)

3.3 QBC®

A screening method for rapid detection of blood parasites (*Babesia* spp., *Trypanosoma spp.*, microfilariae etc.)
Originally developed for the diagnosis of malaria, the QBC® (Becton Dickinson, One Becton Drive, Franklin Lakes, N.J. 07417) is also a highly sensitive and rapid method for the diagnosis of blood parasites in animals. The QBC method concentrates the parasitized cells into a narrow zone of the micro blood tube that is examined under a fluorescence microscope. The test capillaries are internally coated with acridine orange and anticoagulants. Expansion of the centrifugally separated cell layers is achieved with a plastic float. With the QBC method, blood parasites may be detected and identified within a few minutes. The method is dependent on a micro capillary centrifuge and a fluorescence microscope.

3.4 Dark ground / phase contrast buffy coat method

Procedure

1. Determine the PCV by the microhaematocrit method.

2. Cut the microhaematocrit tube with a diamond tipped pencil one mm below the buffy coat to include the top layer of red cells.

3. Express the contents of the capillary tube onto a clean slide, mix and cover with a coverslip.

4. Examine the preparation using phase contrast or darkground microscopy at a magnification of 100–400×.

Remark: A number of 10–20 fields should be examined. *Trypanosoma* spp. species may be identified using characteristics listed in Table 7. Giemsa-stained smears can be prepared from buffy coat. Microfilariae are commonly found with the dark ground buffy coat method.

4 Entomology

4.1 Skin scraping

Procedure

1. Scrapings are taken from the affected area by means of a scalpel or a "sharp-edged spoon". The area selected for scraping should be at the edge of a visible lesion and the hair over this area should be clipped away. It is useful to moisten the skin with liquid paraffin so that scrapings adhere to the scalpel. Scraping should be continued until a slight amount blood oozes from the surface.

2. The material is transferred to a slide and a drop of oil is added.

3. A coverslip should then be applied and the sample examined under a low magnification (100 ×).

Remark: If during this initial examination no mites are detected a further sample may be heated on a slide with a drop of 10% KOH. After allowing this preparation to clear for 5–10 min it should be re-examined.

5 Immunological methods

5.1 Introduction

Many parasites of veterinary importance stimulate the production of antibodies in the blood of the host which can be detected, using appropriate serological techniques. The sero-diagnosis is dependent on a specific antigen-antibody response.

A number of serological techniques are available for diagnosis of parasitic infections for routine diagnosis. The indirect fluorescent antibody test (IFAT) is among the most important and most simple techniques for the indirect detection of *Babesia equi*, *B. caballi*, *B. divergens*, *B. bovis*, *Toxoplasma gondii* and *Neospora* spp. infections. The IFAT will be described in detail below.

5.2 Indirect Fluorescent Antibody Test (IFAT)

The test depends upon a reaction between a particulate antigen and immune serum. The globulins of the latter are made visible under ultra-violet light after reaction with fluorescein-labelled anti-species serum (conjugate). The test may be carried out on sera from a variety of hosts for which suitable conjugates are available. (Figure 6)

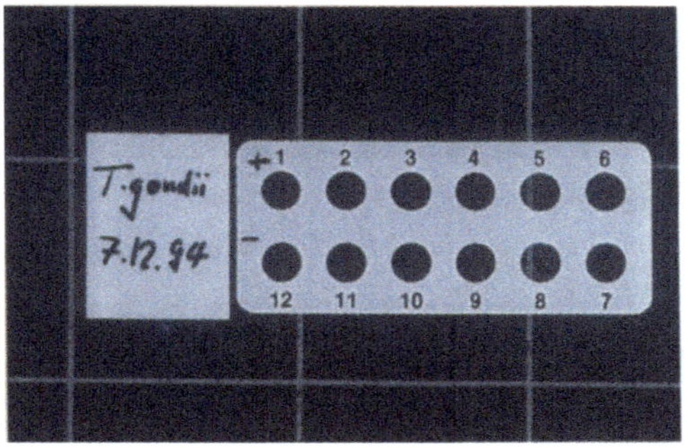

Fig. 6
Antigen is fixed onto defined areas of commercially available IFAT slides. For each individual test a positive and a negative control should be included. In addition, a PBS control may be used to indicate reaction of the conjugate with the antigen directly. Diluted test sera are applied in 10 µl spots onto the slide.

***Preparation of antigen slides for Babesia* spp.:**

1. Blood from a highly parasitaemic animal (between 5–20% of the erythrocytes should be infected) is collected into heparinised tubes.

2. The blood is washed 3 times in phosphate buffered saline solution* (PBS; pH 7.2), centrifuging for 10 min at 1000 rpm between each wash. The supernatant and white cell layer are removed.

3. Two volumes of PBS are added to the packed red cells; the mixture is agitated.

4. If special IFAT slides are available 10 µl of erythrocyte suspension is applied to each hole. If normal slides are used smears are to be made which evenly cover the whole slide.

5. The smears are air-dried** and then wrapped carefully in aluminum foil, sealed in an airtight plastic bag and stored at –20°C (storage up to 1 year) or –80°C (storage for 2–3 years).

* *Phosphate buffered saline solution (PBS) pH 7.2: 87.8 g NaCl, 10.91 g Na_2HPO_4 anhydrous, 2.77 g NaH_2PO_4. Make this up to 1 l with distilled water. Dilute 1/10 with distilled water before use.*

** *Some antigens such as* Toxoplasma gondii *and* Neospora *spp. tachyzoites should be fixed in acetone for 5 min before freezing.*

Procedure (IFAT)
1. Allow antigen slides to reach room temperature.

2. Mark out the slides (if necessary), using a diamond pencil.

3. Prepare serum dilutions (1/20 up to 1/2560) in PBS (pH 7.2).

4. Apply 10 µl spots to the slide, including a positive, a negative and a PBS control.

5. Incubate in a moist chamber at 37°C for 30 min.

6. Rinse with PBS and wash twice with PBS, 5 min each. Allow to dry.

7. Apply fluorescein-labelled conjugate at correct dilution* (1/100 –1/1000). Incubate (in dark) in a moist chamber at 37°C for 30 min.

8. Rinse with PBS and wash twice with PBS, 5 min each. Allow to dry.

9. Mount in 90% glycerol in PBS.

10. Examine under UV illumination at a magnification of 400 ×. Sera dilutes at 1/80 (depending on the particular antigen) and above showing strong fluorescence of the parasites are usually considered to be positive. Special attention should be paid to the pattern of fluorescence in the test sera compared with the controls. This demands experience of the observer!

The following conjugates should be used according to the host species:

- Horse: anti-horse immunoglobulin
- Cattle: anti-bovine immunoglobulin

Individual batches of antigen and conjugate should be titrated against each other using control sera to optimise the conjugate dilution.

5.3 Enzyme linked immunosorbent assay (ELISA)

The antigen is attached to the plastic wells. The antibodies in the test serum when present attach to the antigen. The retained antibody is detected by an anti-species serum conjugated to an enzyme (mostly alkaline phosphatase) which in the presence of a suitable substrate produces a colour reaction, the intensity of which is proportional to the antibody titer. The ELISA is one of the most commonly used serological tests today. The test is dependent on well defined antigens and controls. For the precise reading of the intensity of the colour reaction may be assessed by a spectrophotometric determination (ELISA reader). In veterinary parasitology the ELISA technique is used for *Trichinella spiralis, Hypoderma bovis* and *Toxoplasma gondii.*

5.4 Immunoblotting (Western blot)

Antigen samples are separated in an analytical gel, for example an SDS polyacrylamid gel. The resolved molecules are transferred electrophoretically to a nitrocellulose membrane in a blotting tank. The blot is then treated sequentially with an antibody to the specific antigen, and washed, and then a radiolabelled conjugate to detect antibodies is bound to the blot. The principle is similar to that of ELISA. After washing again, the blot is placed in contact with an X-ray film in a cassette. The autoradiograph is developed and the antigen bands which have bound the antibody are visible. The technique can be modified for use with an enzyme coupled conjugate, and the bound material can be detected by treatment with a chromogen which deposits an insoluble reagent directly onto the blot. (Figure 7)

5.5 Complement Fixation Test (CFT)

Complement is fixed during the reaction between some antigens and antibodies. By conducting this reaction in the presence of measured amounts of complement and then detecting the remaining unfixed amount with a separate antigen-antibody reaction, a quantification

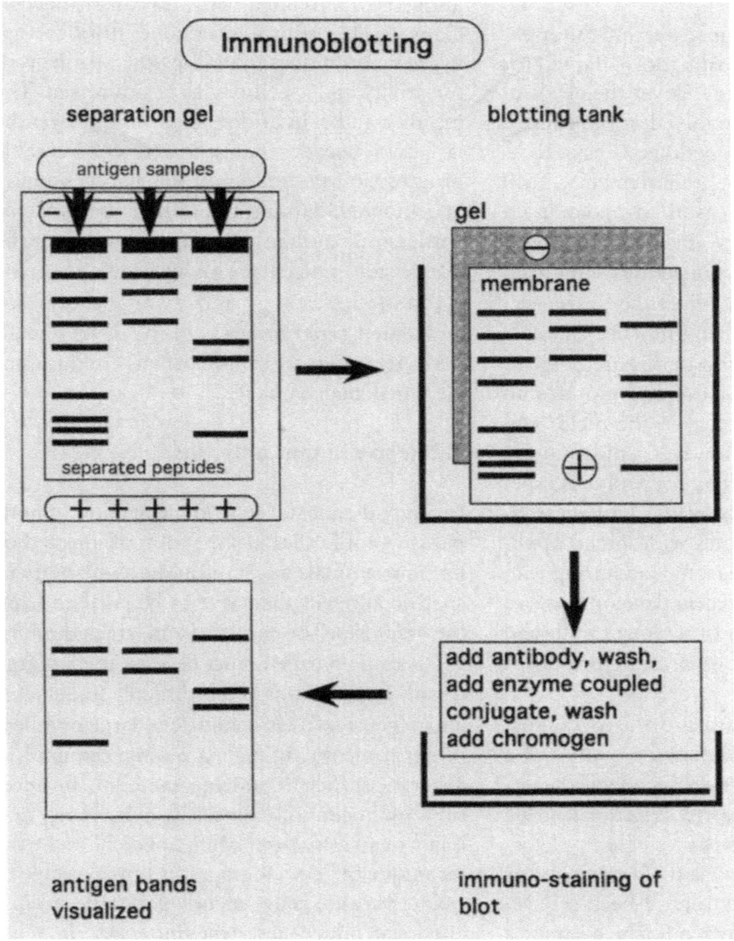

Fig. 7
Immunoblotting:
schematic procedure

of the complement fixing activity of the original serum is obtained. The CFT is required by many national authorities as an import control of horses with regard to *Babesia equi*, *Babesia caballi* and *Trypanosoma equiperdum*, although it is less sensitive than the IFAT. More and more, the CFT is replaced by IFAT and ELISA.

6 Molecular biological techniques

By Dirk Dobbelaere* and Isabel Roditi**
**Institute of Animal Pathology and **Institute of General Microbiology, University of Berne, Switzerland*

6.1 Introduction

A microscope, a well-trained eye and the application of immunodiagnostic tools adapted for the field will, by and large, cover the needs of the person in the field involved in the routine diagnosis of parasitic infections. If easy techniques fulfill diagnostic requirements, then there is indeed every reason to avoid more sophisticated technology. Fieldworkers have established valuable connections to local authorities and animal owners and are well aware of the factors that influence parasite infection and transmission in this area. In this capacity, they function more and more as an important interface between the field and research laboratories. However, epidemiological studies are often called for and it is especially in this area that molecular biology techniques have started to find widespread applications. For this reason, acquiring an elementary insight into recent developments in molecular diagnostics is of interest to all who deal with the diagnosis of parasitic infections.

Sensitivity and specificity are the two most important criteria that define the quality of a diagnostic technique. We are faced with several situations where parasite detection can be very difficult. The parasite often eludes detection by microscopy because the organisms, or the cells infected by them, have been sequestered to parts of the body from which samples cannot easily be taken without invasive manipulations; the number of parasites in circulation can therefore be extremely low. In eradication programs or epidemiology studies, it is important to monitor carrier-status, the presence of reservoirs and the infection rates of transmitting vectors. This requires the direct demonstration of parasites, since the presence of antibodies does not allow a distinction between past and current infections. New DNA technologies now provide valuable tools for solving these problems since they can both detect and identify parasites.
Specificity becomes crucial whenever a distinction needs to be made between pathogenic and non-pathogenic parasites that are closely related. Cross-reactivity in diagnostic tests with antigens of unrelated parasites can also occur. Considerable efforts have gone into developing new techniques that allow the problems of sensitivity and specificity to be addressed. The rapid spread of hybridoma technology over the last two decades has allowed considerable progress in fine-tuning serological techniques and monoclonal antibodies have become the cornerstone of many diagnostic kits. Over the last decade, molecular biology has also become a routine technology and its application has stimulated rapid progress in the development of reagents that are capable of identifying a single unicellular parasite.

6.2 Recombinant antigens

In many diagnostic tests, the detection of antiparasite antibodies in the serum of infected or immune animals depends on the availability of specific antigens that have to be purified from the organism. The parasite from which the antigen is to be purified must be available in large quantities, which is often difficult to achieve, and expensive in vitro culture or large numbers of experimental animals are often required to generate sufficient starting material. In addition, significant differences in yield, purity and quality can arise from batch to batch. Using the technique of gene cloning, it is now possible to isolate parasite genes encoding a single antigen and to introduce these genes into bacteria, yeast or mammalian cells, where they can be expressed in large quantities as a recombinant antigen. It is also possible to "engineer" these antigens and remove those parts that are responsible for cross-reactivity with other organisms. This way, a continuous and reliable source of diagnostic antigens is guaranteed and increased specificity can also be achieved. Importantly, this technique also applies for antigens of parasites which can never be maintained in vitro or collected in large enough quantities for antigen production.

6.3 Detection and identification of parasites using nucleic acid probes

The use of immunodiagnostic methods for the detection of parasites has certain limitations. Demonstrating antibodies against a parasite provides little information on whether the parasite is still present in the animal's body and in primary infections, disease will mostly develop well before antibodies become detectable. For this reason there is a need to be able to detect parasites directly. Several highly sensitive and specific techniques have been developed that rely on the demonstration of parasite nucleic acid sequences. These techniques depend either on the use of DNA probes or on the polymerase chain reaction (PCR). Both will be discussed below.

6.3.1 Techniques based on DNA probes

The genetic material (genome) of parasites that are considered distinct species show significant differences, which one could call their "genomic signature", allowing them to be distinguished from each other. Technologies now exist that enable the isolation and identification of such specific sequences, resulting in the generation of DNA probes which can be used in a variety of assays. DNA probes can be long, consisting of several thousands of nucleotides or be limited to as little as 20 or 30 nucleotides, also called oligonucleotides.

A deciding factor contributing to sensitivity is the number of times that the target sequence occurs in the genome. Ribosomal genes are usually present in large numbers and for this reason the development of DNA probes and investigations on phylogenetic relationship between parasites have often relied heavily on finding species-specific differences in the ribosomal genes. Repetitive sequences which are not derived from the ribosomal genes, however, are equally useful and have also been used for species identification.

In order to allow detection, parasite DNA needs to be immobilised on a nitrocellulose or nylon membrane. Alkaline denaturation causes the separation of the DNA strands, making the sequences accessible and allowing the DNA probe to bind to the target sequence by a process called hybridisation. Binding of the probe to parasite sequences can be demonstrated by labelling it prior to hybridisation.

In past years, the detection of nucleic acids used to depend almost entirely on the use of radioactively labelled probes. More recent developments, however, have led to the appearance of a wide range of labelling kits in which colour reactions or chemiluminescence are used to demonstrate specific hybridisation. This new technology offers many advantages. The expensive laboratory set-up required for the safe handling, storage and disposal of radioactive substances has become unnecessary. Importantly, the problem of radioactive decay of probes is now eliminated and specific reagents can be stored and used over a long period of time in a standardised way. Indeed, with a minimum of equipment and imagination, DNA probes could be used under the most primitive field-laboratory conditions.

There are several easy ways in which parasite nucleic acids can be transferred to membranes. Droplets of fluid to be tested for the presence of parasites (such as blood, lymph, spinal fluid or stool samples) can simply be applied to membranes and left to dry in a process called "dot-blot". In many cases, drying is sufficient to expose the DNA. Parasites that are surrounded by a strong cyst wall, however, will require processing prior to application to a membrane. Parasite-containing vectors, such as infected tsetse flies, ticks, snails etc., can also be squashed onto membranes ("squash-blots"). "Touch-blots" made from lesions have also been used for the diagnosis of *Leishmania* infection, where parasite strain-identification is important for deciding on the strategy of treatment which is often associated with severe side-effects. Using recombinant DNA technology, probes have now been developed which also allow different *Leishmania* strains or geographical isolates to be distinguished from each other.

Membranes on which material has been blotted can be dried and stored for a long time before analysis. This makes it possible to collect many samples during separate field trips and then to process them all together upon return to the laboratory. Figure 8 shows a squash blot prepared from snails in which different larval stages of *Fasciola hepatica* could be detected using a DNA probe which hybridises to repetitive DNA fragments present in the genome of *F. hepatica*. This example illustrates another advantage of using techniques that depend on detecting genomic sequences. Whereas the morphology and the antigenic repertoire of the different life-cycle stages of a parasite can vary extensively, the parasite genome is very stable. Morphological identification, especially when mixed infections occur or when many samples need to be examined,

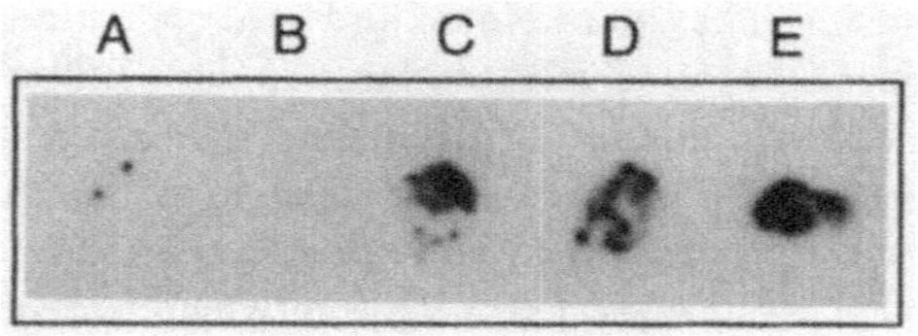

Fig. 8
Detection of isolated larvae of *Fasciola hepatica* and of larval stages in snail 'squash blots'. In position A, two *F. hepatica* rediae, collected from an infected snail, were deposited onto the filter; in position B, an uninfected snail was squashed onto the filter (no signal detectable) and in C to E, whole snails infected with *F. hepatica* were crushed onto the filter. The filter was hybridised with a ^{32}P-labelled DNA probe (Fhr-IV) which hybridises to repetitive DNA fragments present in the genome of *F. hepatica*. The filter was exposed overnight to X-ray film.

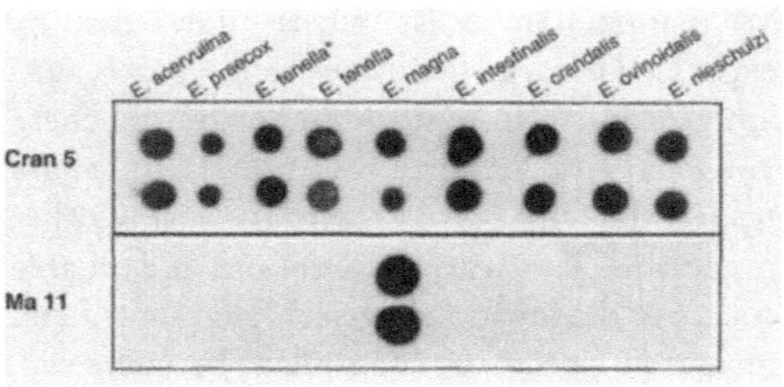

Fig. 9
Specific detection of *Eimeria magna* DNA by 'dot blot analysis'. DNA was isolated from different *Eimeria* species and spotted in duplicate onto two filters. Each dot contains approximately 10 nanograms of genomic DNA. One filter was hybridised with the 32P-labelled DNA probe, Cran 5, which detects repetitive sequences of all *Eimeria* species. The second filter was hybridised with the probe, Ma11, which hybridises exclusively with *E. magna*. The *E. tenella* isolate labelled with (*) also contained *E. acervulina*.

can be difficult and time-consuming and may require expertise which is not always available. Species-specific probes can thus often help to circumvent problems associated with the identification of parasites by light microscopy. An example for the use of a species-specific DNA probe which is capable of distinguishing *Eimeria magna* from several other *Eimeria* species by 'dot blot' analysis is shown in Figure 9.

When treated with a minimum of care, parasite nucleic acids are more stable than most antigens on which immunodiagnostic techniques depend. For a more detailed analysis of field samples and the characterisation of new strains, especially within the context of epidemiological surveys, it is often necessary to collect and store parasites. Most samples can be stored indefinitely in 70% ethanol/1mM EDTA and intact DNA can easily be analysed at a later point. Such analysis involves the extraction of DNA from samples, digestion with a number of empirically chosen restriction enzymes, separation of the DNA fragments by electrophoresis, transfer by capillary blotting to a membrane and hybridisation with specific probes (-called southern blot hybridisation). Figure 10 summarizes this procedure and Figure 11 demonstrates how a specific probe is capable of dis-

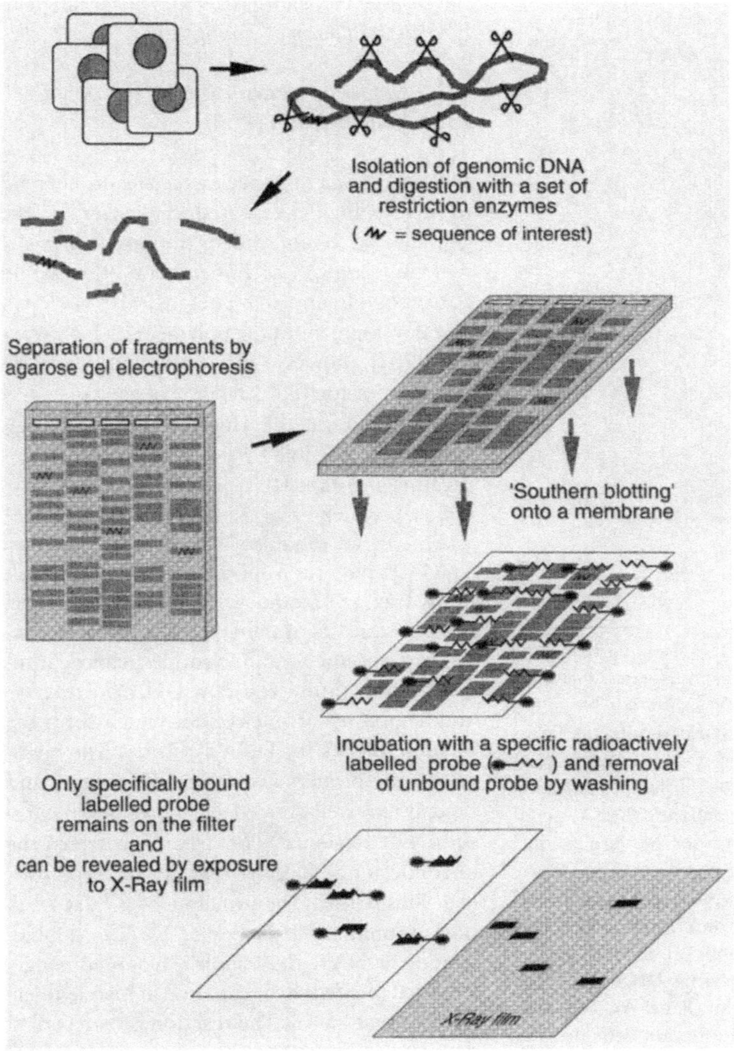

Fig. 10
The principle of Southern blot analysis. Genomic DNA is extracted from an organism (here shown as a collection of cells) and digested with a restriction enzyme that cuts the genomic DNA into many fragments of different sizes. These DNA fragments can be separated, based on their different sizes, by electrophoresis in an agarose gel. The separated fragments are then blotted onto a nylon or nitrocellulose filter by a procedure called southern blotting. The DNA is fixed onto the filter by baking the filter or by UV-cross-linking. The filter is subsequently incubated with a radioactively labelled DNA probe, specific for the sequence of interest, which will hybridise to homologous sequences present on the filter. Unbound probe is washed away and only specifically bound probe remains on the filter. Specific hybridisation of the radioactive probe can be visualised by exposing an X-ray film to the filter (autoradiography). Black bands will appear where the probe hybridised to the filter.
Remark: Probes can now also be labelled enzymatically; incubation with the enzyme's substrate then results in the generation of either a colour reaction on the filter or chemiluminescence, which can be detected by X-ray film.

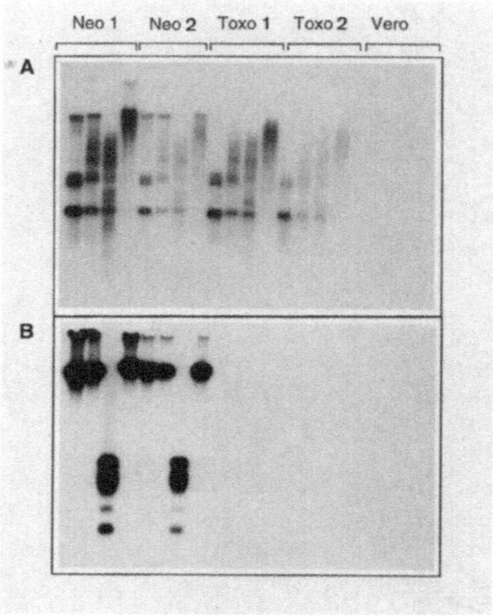

Fig. 11
Southern blot analysis of DNA isolated from two Neospora and two Toxoplasma isolates. Genomic DNA was extracted from two different Neospora isolates (Neo 1 and Neo 2) and two different Toxoplasma strains (Toxo 1 and Toxo 2). Each DNA sample was digested with four different restriction enzymes, BamHI, HindIII, HaeIII and PstI. As a control, DNA was also isolated from the Vero cell line in which the parasites were propagated in culture. The DNA fragments were separated by agarose gel electrophoresis and blotted onto a filter. The filter was hybridised first with a DNA probe which detects both Neospora and Toxoplasma DNA sequences and exposed to an X-ray film (Panel A). The similarity in the pattern of hybridisation demonstrates the close relationship between the two organisms. The probe was then removed from the filter by process called 'stripping' and the filter subsequently rehybridised with a Neospora-specific probe (Panel B). The specificity of this probe is demonstrated by the fact that no hybridisation can be observed where the Toxoplasma DNA was blotted onto the filter. Note that none of the probes hybridises to the DNA isolated from the Vero cells.

tinguishing *Neospora* from the morphologically virtually identical *Toxoplasma*.

6.3.2 Detection of parasites by the polymerase chain reaction (PCR)

Despite the fact that species-specific probes tend to detect highly repeated sequences in the genome, the limits of detection are still in the nanogram range (for *Eimeria* spp., this would correspond to approximately 10^3-10^4 oocysts). The development of the polymerase chain reaction (PCR), however, has opened up extensive possibilities for the detection of parasites and pathogens in general. This technique was originally made possible by the discovery of a temperature-resistant DNA polymerase (Taq polymerase) which was isolated from *Thermus aquaticus*, an organism found in hot springs. The PCR requires a special piece of equipment known as a "thermocycler". A PCR reaction mixture consists of the DNA sample to be tested, two specific oligonucleotides, called primers, a temperature resistant DNA polymerase and a mixture of nucleotides which form the building blocks for DNA synthesis. The oligonucleotide primers are designed to match and bind at two well-defined sites of a known parasite DNA sequence. The distance between the oligonucleotide binding sites is exactly known (e.g. 800 bases), The principle of a PCR reaction is summarised in Figure 12. The double-stranded DNA in the sample is first made single stranded (melted) by incubation at high temperature (about 95°C). The reaction is then cooled down to a lower temperature (e.g. 55°C) at which the primers can bind to the specific target sequences in the DNA sample. The temperature is then raised again to 72°C at which the polymerase synthesizes two new strands of DNA using the specific primers as the starting point and the specific target DNA fragment as a template. These three events, melting, primer annealing and DNA synthesis constitute one cycle. By continuously repeating this cycle, the polymerase synthesizes increasing numbers of copies of the target sequence and the fragment is thus "amplified" so that it can easily be detected by agarose gel electrophoresis. Starting with

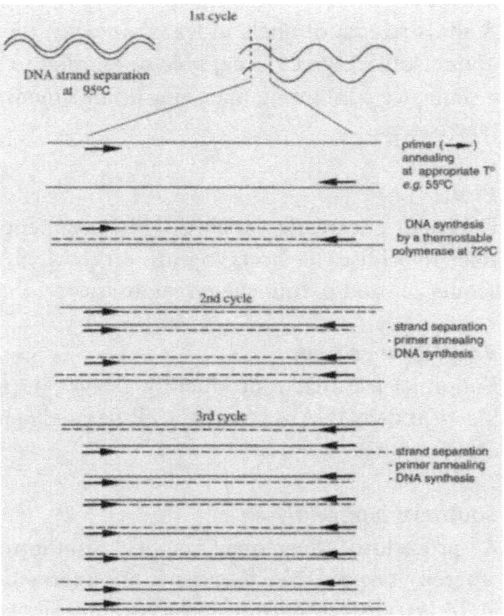

Fig. 12
The principles of PCR

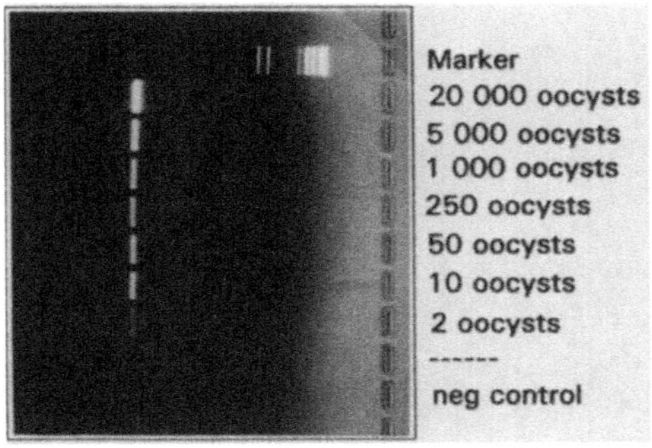

Fig. 13
Detection of *Eimeria tenella* oocysts by PCR.
DNA was extracted from decreasing numbers of E. tenella oocysts ranging from 20,000 oocysts to 2 oocysts. Sequences corresponding to the intergenic region between the 5S ribosomal genes were amplified by PCR. The amplification reactions were loaded onto an agarose gel. After electrophoresis, the amplified DNA fragments (expected size: 560 base pairs) were visualised by ethidium bromide staining. No amplification product can be observed when PCR was performed on a sample without DNA (negative control) (reproduced from Stucki et. al. *Experimental Parasitology* Vol. 76: 68-75).

one molecule, 10^9 molecules can theoretically be generated in 30 cycles. This way, using a minimal amount of parasite DNA as starting material, specific parasite DNA fragments can be amplified and little as 10 picograms of parasite DNA are now sufficient to detect the parasite (in the case of *Eimeria* this would be less than 10 oocysts). Figure 13 shows how an *E. tenella*-specific DNA fragment can be amplified from as few as two oocysts.

6.3.3 Random amplification of polymorphic DNA (RAPD)-PCR

A further method which is presently being developed in several parasite systems and which also depends on PCR is known as RAPD analysis (random amplification of polymorphic DNA). In this procedure, a single oligonucleotide primer with an arbitrary sequence can be used to amplify a set of characteristic fragments from genomic DNA by PCR. The principle of this method is that the oligonucleotide will, by chance, bind to the DNA template. If a second binding site also occurs on the complementary DNA strand within a reasonable distance (usually not more than 2-3 kilobase pairs) the stretch of DNA between them will be amplified. To increase the chances of obtaining amplification products, the PCR is performed under conditions which allow imperfect matches between the primer and the template DNA. Because there is no bias towards repetitive sequences, this method requires considerably more genomic DNA (approximately 50 ng) than when repetitive sequences are the target, but it has the advantage of being able to detect and distinguish between different strains of a particular parasite as well as different species.

Certain precautions are essential, however, when PCR technology is applied. Because of its extreme sensitivity, the risk of contamination and generating false positives are extremely high. For this reason the use of PCR for diagnostic purposes requires a special infrastructure, the implementation of strict rules and the continuous monitoring of possible contamination by including controls in all experiments.

6.4 Concluding remarks

Molecular biology has contributed considerably to the development of new diagnostic tools, often bringing sensitivity to a level where a single parasite can be detected. Molecular cloning and the production of recombinant proteins has led to an expansion of the range of parasites for which diagnostic antigens can be produced. As is the case for all diagnostic tests, however, it is important to realise that the use of specific probes or specific primers for PCR implies that they only provide a positive identification of the parasite for which the probes or the primers were designed. They provide no information on the presence of other parasites, whether related or not, which could be present in the sample. RAPD-PCR meets this requirement to some extent in that it allows the detection of different parasites or parasite strains, provided the organism is presents in the sample in sufficient numbers. Therefore, however sensitive and specific the technologies used, all results need to be interpreted with care and considered in the right context.

6.5 Glossary of terms

Cloning
Insertion of a DNA sequence into a plasmid or viral DNA vector and propagation of the recombinant DNA in a bacterial host.

Genomic DNA
The combined genetic material of an organism composed of DNA.

Hybridisation
Binding of labelled DNA (probe) to target DNA or RNA because of homology in sequence.

Polymerase chain reaction (PCR)
A process that rapidly amplifies DNA sequences; the technique relies on the separation of the DNA strands at 95°C, the annealing of specific primers to the DNA at lower temperature and the synthesis of new strands by a temperature sensitive DNA polymerase; this cycle is repeated 20 to 30 times.

Primer
A short stretch of nucleotides (also called oligonucleotide) which is capable of binding to a sequence containing matching complementary bases.

Probe
Radio- or chemically labelled DNA fragments that hybridise to homologous target DNA sequences and permit their visualisation.

Restriction enzyme
Endonuclease that reproducibly cleaves double-stranded DNA at specific, well-defined recognition sites.

Southern blot analysis
A procedure (developed by E. Southern) whereby target DNA fragments are analysed. DNA is transferred from an electrophoresis gel to a membrane by capillary action and visualised by hybridisation with a labelled DNA fragment (probe). The same technique performed with RNA is called Northern blotting.

II

Parasites of Cattle

CONTENTS

1 Stages in the gut and faeces

PROTOZOA

• Protozoa oocysts found in the faeces

Eimeria spp. Bovine coccidiosis

Location: Terminal ileum, caecum, colon

Hosts: Cattle

Species description: Of the 21 species of *Eimeria* that infect cattle, *E. bovis* and *E. zuerni* are most often associated with clinical disease. Coccidiosis is commonly a disease of young cattle and occurs especially in management systems (night holding place, limited water source, paddocks) which concentrate the hosts and the parasites within a restricted area. Bloody diarrhoea, progressive weight loss and death, especially in animals after weaning can result from heavy infections. Ruminants do normally excrete a few *Eimeria* spp. oocysts. The condition called coccidiosis includes both severe dysentery and excretion of a high number of oocysts.

Geographic distribution: World-wide

Symptoms: Diarrhoea lasting for a few hours, followed by a self cure or development of severe dysentery accompanied by a haemorrhagic and viscous diarrhoea, dehydration and paralysis. Death can occur rapidly, mainly in calves. Another form of coccidiosis is characterized by persisting, non-haemorrhagic diarrhoea with continuous weight loss until cachexia. This condition may last for several weeks. Animals that survive severe illness can have significant weight loss that is not quickly regained, or can remain permanently stunted.

Significance: *E. bovis* and *E. zuerni* are most commonly involved in clinical coccidiosis of cattle.

Diagnosis: Clinical signs and extremely high numbers of oocysts per gram of faeces (50,000–500,000).

Therapy: The drugs that are commonly used to treat clinical coccidiosis in ruminants are listed in Table 1. These include sulfonamids, nitrofurazone, amprolium (10 mg/kg po. > 10 days), monensin (1 mg/kg po. for 10–30 days) and lasalocid (0.5–1 mg/kg po. for up to 6 weeks). Sulfadimidine (33% solution for intravenous injection), sulfamethazine (50–100 mg/kg, po. daily for 4 days), sulfaquinoxaline (15 mg/kg, po. for 3 days) may be used to treat sick animals. Sulfaguanidine is less effective than the soluble sulfonamides which can be administered orally or parenterally. Sulfonamides, combined with trimethoprime can also be used to treat clinical coccidiosis. Toltrazuril (1 × 20 mg/kg) is highly effective to treat clinical coccidiosis in ruminants.

Prophylaxis: Young animals should be kept in clean and dry quarters, and watering devices should be protected from faecal contamination. Decoquinate, amprolium and ionophorous antibiotics can be used in cattle for prophylaxis (Table 3). Neonates should receive colostrum within 6 hours after birth and stress (e.g. weaning, sudden change in feed, etc.) should be minimized.

(Figures 14, 15, 16, 17, 18, 19, 20, 21, 23, Table 3)

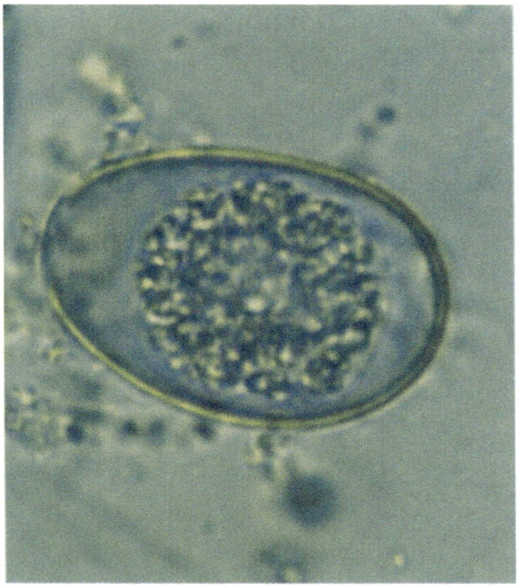

Fig. 14 Oocyst of *Eimeria bovis*
(26–32 × 18–21 µm)

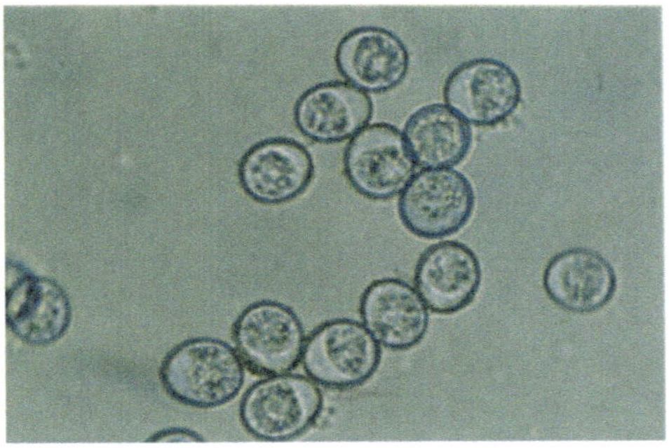

Fig. 15 Oocysts of *Eimeria zuerni*
(16–20 × 15–18 µm)

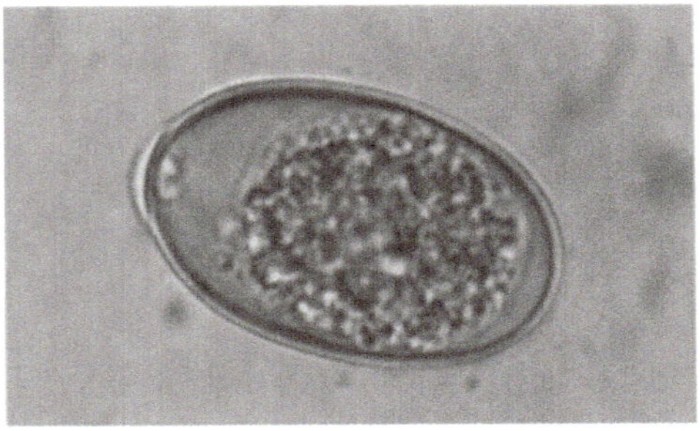

Fig. 16 Oocyst of *Eimeria brasiliensis*
(33–42 × 23–30 µm)

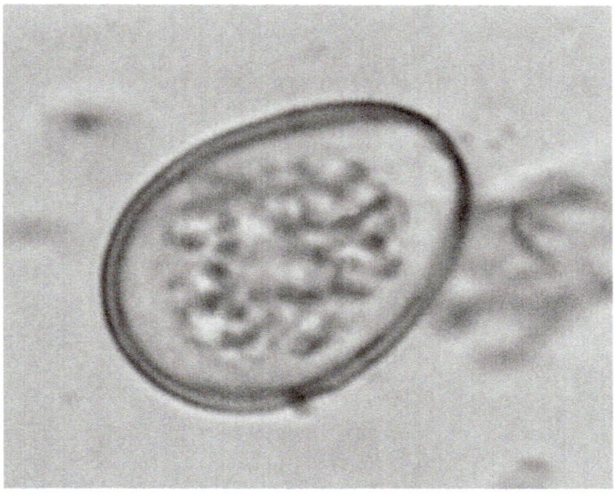

Fig. 17 Oocyst of *Eimeria alabamensis*
(16–24 × 12–16)

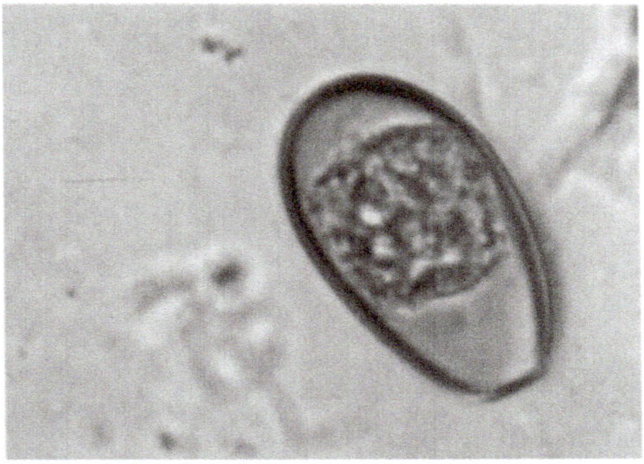

Fig. 18 Oocyst of *Eimeria auburnensis*
(36–42 × 19–26 µm)

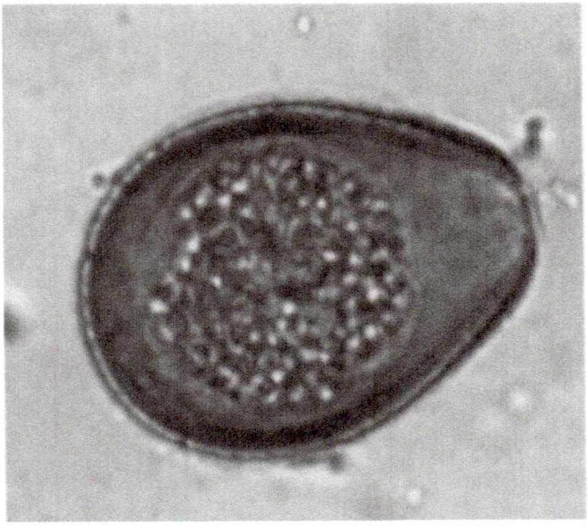

Fig. 19 Oocyst of *Eimeria bukidnonensis*
(44 × 32 µm)

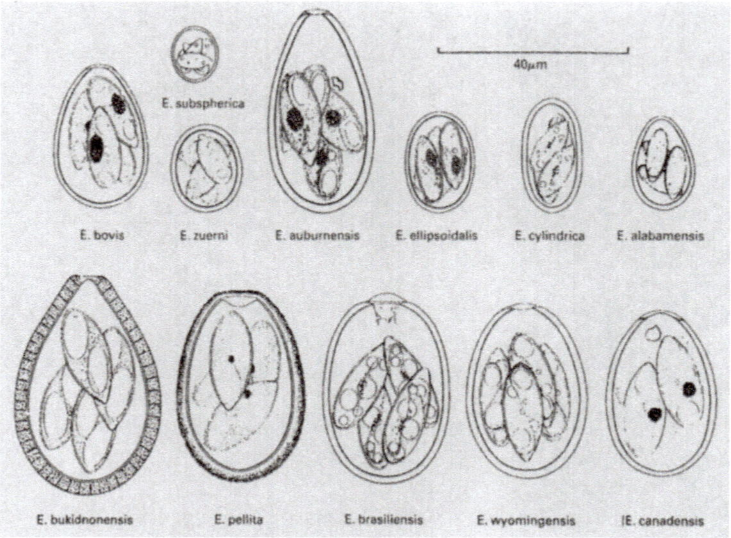

Fig. 20 Coccidia found in cattle [1]

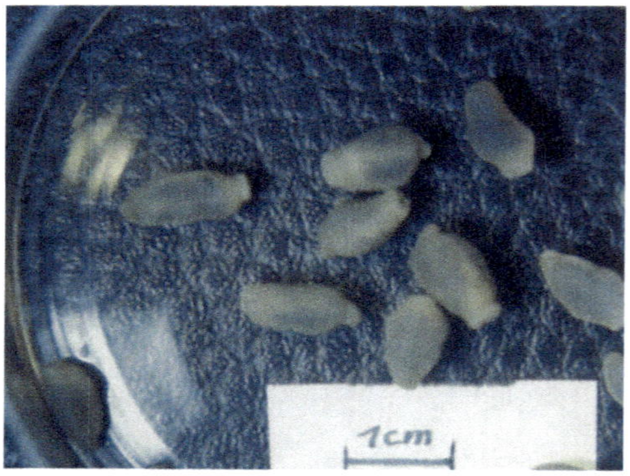

Fig. 22 Rumen flukes found in the rumen of N'Dama cattle

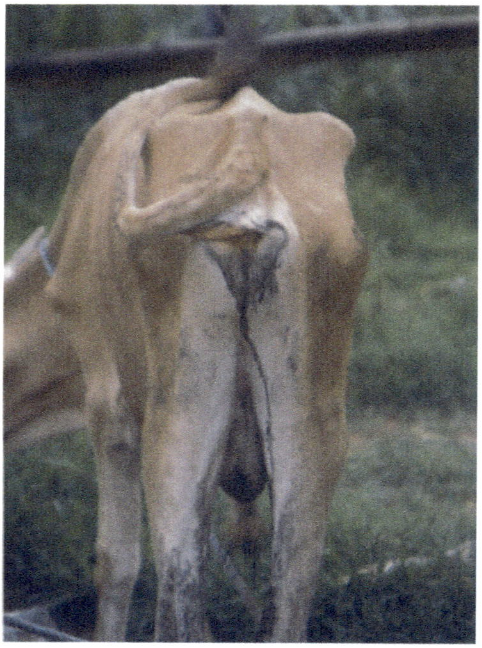

Fig. 21 Bull with an acute coccidiosis

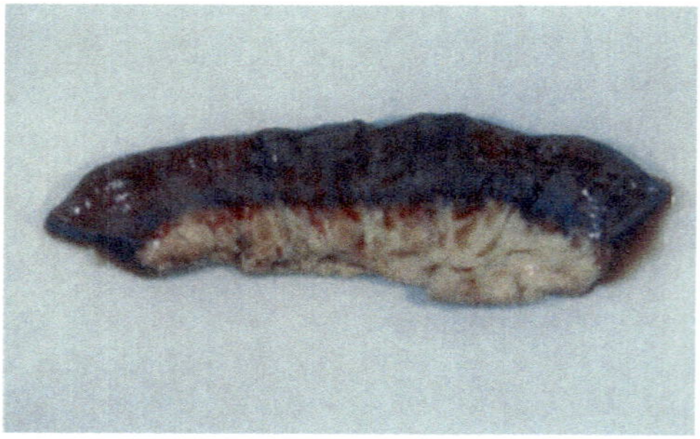

Fig. 23 Haemorrhage in the small intestine of a calf with an acute coccidiosis (*Eimeria bovis*)

Table 3 Recommended use, dosage and dosage form of anticoccidial drugs used in cattle, goats, sheep, and swine

Drug[1]	Use	Animal	Dosage	Dosage forms
Amprolium	Therapeutic	Cattle	10 mg/kg daily for 5 days	20 % soluble powder
		Sheep	50 mg/kg daily for 5 days	9.6 % solution
		Goats	100 mg/kg daily for 5 days	Feed additive crumbles
		Swine	25-65 mg/kg once or twice daily for 3-4 days	
	Prophylactic	Cattle, sheep, goats	5-10 mg/kg daily for 21 days	
		Swine	25 mg/kg in piglets for first 3-4 days of life	
Sulfonamides				
Sulfamethazine	Therapeutic	Cattle, sheep, goats	50-100 mg/kg daily for 4 days	Soluble powder or bolus
Sulfaquinoxaline	Therapeutic	Cattle, sheep, goats	15 mg/kg, po.[2] daily for 4 days	9.6 % liquid soluble powder and feed additive
Sulfaguanidine	Prophylactic	Sheep	0.5-3 g per lamb per day for 20 days	
		Swine	60 mg/kg for 7-10 days	
Ionophorous antibiotics				
Monensin	Prophylactic	Cattle, sheep & goats	1 mg/kg for 30 days	Feed additive
Lasalocid	Prophylactic	Cattle, sheep & goats	0.5-1 mg/kg per day for up to 6 weeks	Feed additive
Other compounds				
Nitrofurazone	Therapeutic	All	10-20 mg/kg daily for 5 days	88.9 % m/m
Decoquinate	Prophylactic	Cattle	0.5 mg/kg in feed for at least 28 days	6 % premix for addition to feed
Toltrazuril	Therapeutic	Sheep	20 mg/kg, single treatment	25 % liquid
Diclazuril	Therapeutic	Sheep, goats	20 mg/kg, po.	2.5 % suspension

[1] Several trade names, [2] po. = orally; [2]

Cryptosporidium parvum (syn. *C. bovis*)

Location: Small and large intestine

Hosts: All domestic animals

Species description: Spherical oocysts 4.5–5 µm in diameter are passed in the faeces. Especially calves younger than 8 weeks may be affected, showing different degrees of diarrhoea, associated with oedema and hyperplasia of the mesenteric lymph nodes. Cryptosporidial diarrhoea in both immunodeficient and non-immunodeficient human beings have been reported.

Geographic distribution: World-wide

Symptoms: Persistent diarrhoea in calves 5–35 days old that does not respond to therapy.

Significance: *Cryptosporidium parvum* is pathogenic for calves, sheep, pig, rat and man. Bovine cryptosporidiosis is a zoonosis. Diarrhoea due to *Cryptosporidium parvum* alone is often mild and self-limiting, although the severity may be related to the general strength of the calf and the density of the pathogen in the environment and the intensity of the exposure to the organism. Combination of the infection with rota- and/or coronavirus are common and result in persistent diarrhoea, emaciation and death.

Diagnosis: Oocysts may be demonstrated in Ziehl-Neelsen's carbol-fuchsin stained smears of diarrhoeic faeces (☞ METHODS, 1.10).

Therapy: No effective specific treatment known. Supportive therapy, such as rehydration and antibiotics may help in mild cases. Chemoprophylaxis of bovine cryptosporidiosis can be made experimentally with halofuginone lactate (60–120 µg/kg/day, po. for 7 days) or by paromomycin (100 mg/kg/day for 11 days).

Prophylaxis: Animals with a massive oocyst excretion should be separated from other animals and man. Contamination with faeces should be avoided. Oocysts are resistant to many disinfectants (exception 5% formalin). Emphasis should therefore be on regular removal of contaminated faecal material.

Note: Trophozoites of *Giardia bovis* (small intestine) and *Entamoeba bovis* (rumen, intestines) occur world-wide in the faeces of cattle, but are considered to be non-pathogenic.

(Figures 24, 25)

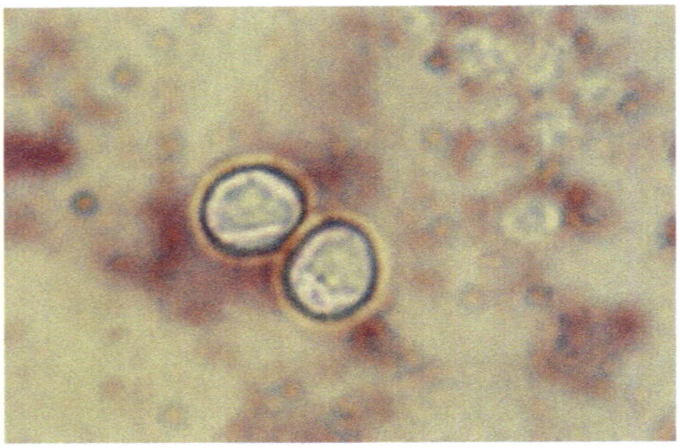

Fig. 24 Oocysts of *Cryptosporidium parvum* (4.5–5 µm) stained with carbol-fuchsine (☞ METHODS 1.10)

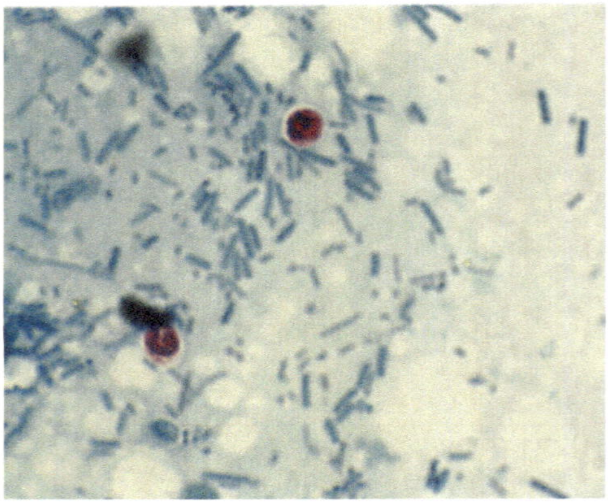

Fig. 25 Oocysts of *Cryptosporidium parvum* (4.5–5 µm) stained with the modified Ziehl-Neelsen's carbol-fuchsine (☞ METHODS, 1.10)

Buxtonella spp.

Remarks: This is a protozoan parasite found occasionally in the large intestine of cattle. Oocysts are found in the faeces. The parasite is non-pathogenic.

(Figure 26)

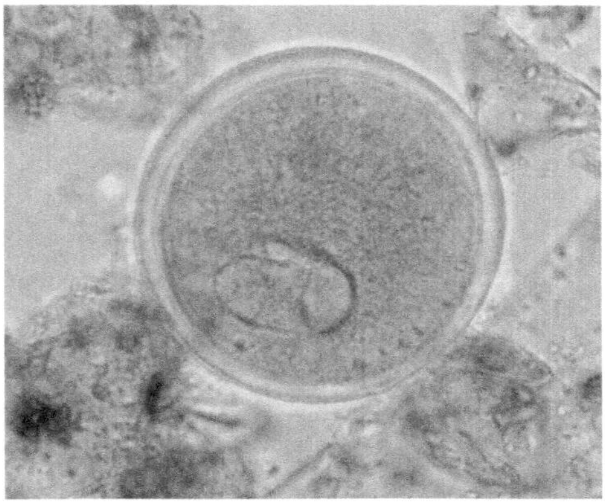

Fig. 26 Cyst of *Buxtonella* sp. (50–131 µm)

HELMINTHS

- Trematoda eggs found in the faeces and adult trematodes living in the gastrointestinal tract

PARAMPHISTOMATIDAE

Location: Adult flukes in the rumen; immature flukes in the small intestine

Hosts: Domestic and wild ruminants

Species description: A great number of species of this family has been described in Africa. Indirect life cycle with development in freshwater snails (*Bulinus* spp.; *Planorbis* spp.). The cercariae encyst on herbage which is in contact with water and develop into the infective stages (metacercariae). Infection is acquired by ingestion of herbage contaminated with metacercariae, especially around water holes. The adult flukes are generally non-pathogenic (>80% of adult cattle are infected in endemic areas). Disease occurs when masses of immature worms attach to the intestinal mucosa after excystment, causing destruction and inflammation. Peaks usually at the end of the dry season. Game animals, using the same water holes, may be a source of reinfection. Standing water, troughs and other water bodies are preferred habitats of the intermediate hosts.

Geographic distribution: World-wide

Symptoms: Enteritis with extensive diarrhoea, hypoproteinaemia, weakness during the intestinal phase, when immature worms irritate the small intestinal mucosa. Severe symptoms mainly in young stock. Irregular rumination and progressive degeneration of the animal's condition may be found. Infections with adult rumen flukes are generally inapparent, despite the high numbers of adult parasites in the rumen. Rumenitis may occur due to adult flukes, especially if *Carmyerius* spp. are involved. Adult flukes are generally non-pathogenic.

Significance: Severe diarrhoea and weakness, generally caused by the immature intestinal flukes, may lead to death.

Diagnosis: This is based on the demonstration of immature flukes in the diarrhoeic faeces and the presence of previous cases in the area.

Cave: In acute paramphistomidosis the large, clear, operculated eggs may not be found in the faeces. In many areas > 80% of the adult ruminants pass paramphistome eggs in the faeces. The presence of eggs without clinical signs does not necessarily indicate paramphistomidosis.

Therapy: Niclosamide (90 mg/kg po.), resorantel (65 mg/kg po.) and closantel are active against immature forms. Triclabendazole (12 mg/kg) and albendazole (10 mg/kg) may also be used against immature flukes. Resorantel is active only against mature flukes (☞ Table 4).

Prophylaxis: Avoiding infection by supplying the herds with clean water, e.g. bore holes or raised, snail-free troughs.

Table 4 Recommended drugs against *Paramphistomum* spp. infections in cattle

Drug	Dosage (mg/kg)	Immat. flukes	Mature flukes
Niclosamide	160.0*	+	
Oxyclozanide	18.7		
and Levamisole	19.4*	+	
Oxyclozanide	15		+
Resorantel	65		+

*at 3-day intervals

Remarks: Rumen flukes in Africa belong to the families of Paramphistomatidae (*Bothriophoron bothriophoron*; *Stephanopharynx compactus*; *Cotylophoron cotylophorum* and other *Cotylophoron* spp.; *Paramphistomum* spp. [8 species] and *Cotylophoron* spp.; [*C. daubneyi* and *C. microbothrium* are the most frequent species]) and Gastrothylacidae (*Carmyerius* spp. [*C. spatiosus; C. papillatus; C. dollfusi* [Zebu only in Madagascar]).
(Figures 27, 28, 29)

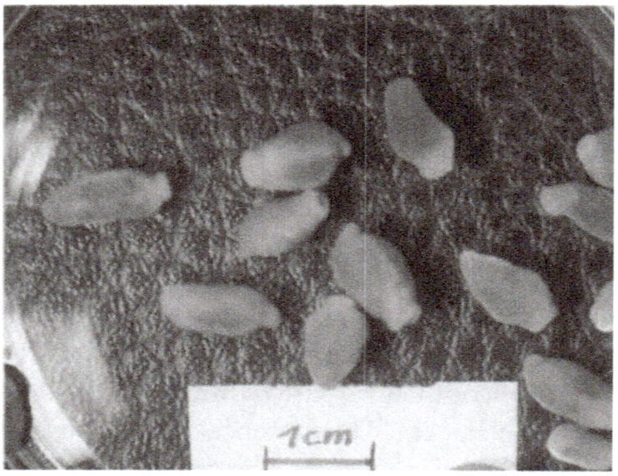

Fig. 27 Rumen flukes found in the rumen of N'Dama cattle

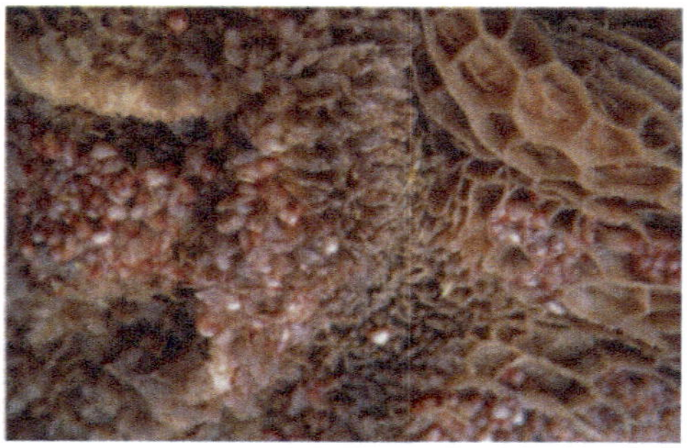

Fig. 28 *Paramphistomum* sp. attached to the rumen mucosa

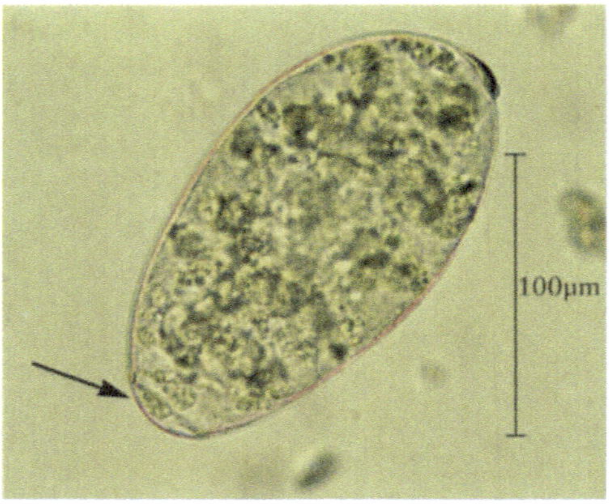

Fig. 29 Egg of a rumen fluke (Paramphistomatidae)

F. giganticca Tropical large liver fluke
(☞ CATTLE, ■ 4.2)

F. hepatica Large liver fluke of temperate areas and high altitude regions in East Africa

Location: Adult flukes in biliary ducts; eggs in the faeces (☞ CATTLE, ■ 4.2)
(Figures 30, 31)

Dicrocoelium hospes African small liver fluke
(☞ CATTLE, ■ 4.2)

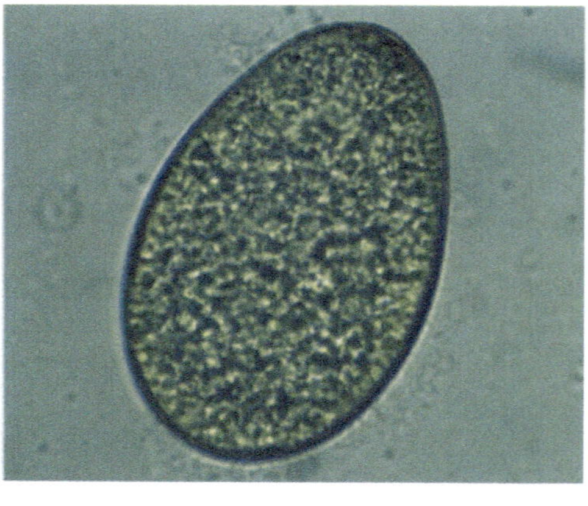

Fig. 30 Egg of *Fasciola hepatica* (130–150 × 63–90 µm)

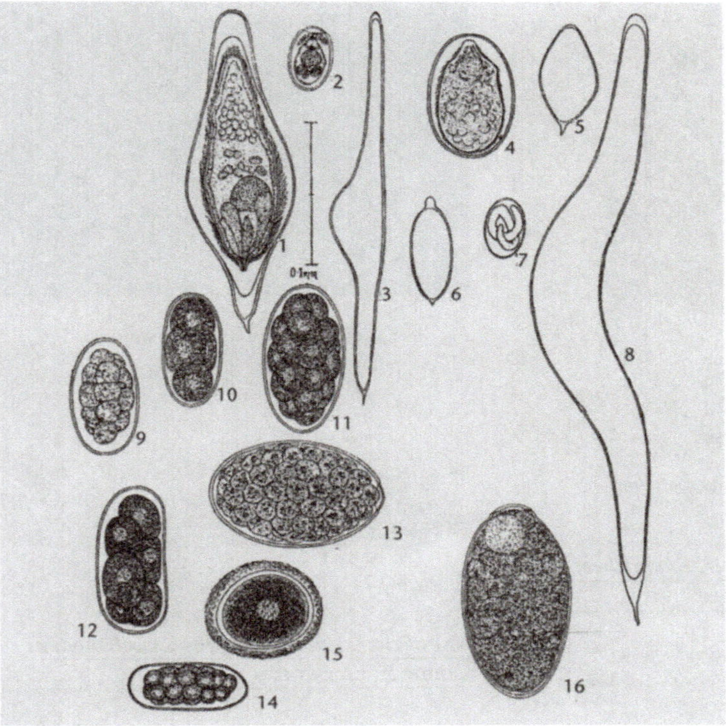

Fig. 31 Eggs of helminth parasites of cattle (not drawn completely to scale) [3]
(1) *Schistosoma bovis*, (2) *Eurytrema pancreaticum*, (3) *Schistosoma spindale*, (4) *Schistosoma japonicum*, (5) *Schistosoma indicum*, (6) *Ornithobilharzia turkestanicum*, (7) *Thelazia rhodesi*, (8) *Schistosoma nasalis*, (9) *Oesophagostomum radiatum**, (10) *Mammomonogamus laryngeus*, (11) *Mecistocirrus digitatus*, (12) *Bunostomum phlebotomum**, (13) *Carmyerius spatiosus*, (14) *Cooperia pectinata**, (15) *Toxocara vitulorum* and (16) *Fasciola hepatica*.
* Strongyle-type eggs are difficult to differentiate in routine examinations

D. dentriticum Small liver fluke

Location: Adult flukes in biliary ducts; eggs in the faeces (☞ CATTLE, ■ 4.2)

(Figures 32, 33)

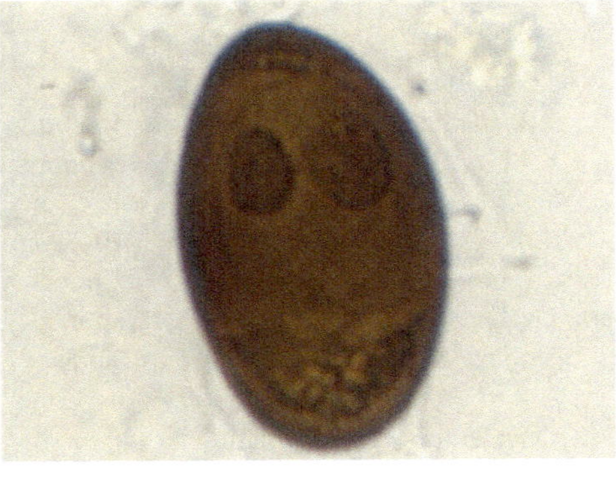

Fig. 32 Egg of *Dicrocoelium dendriticum* (36–45 × 25 µm)

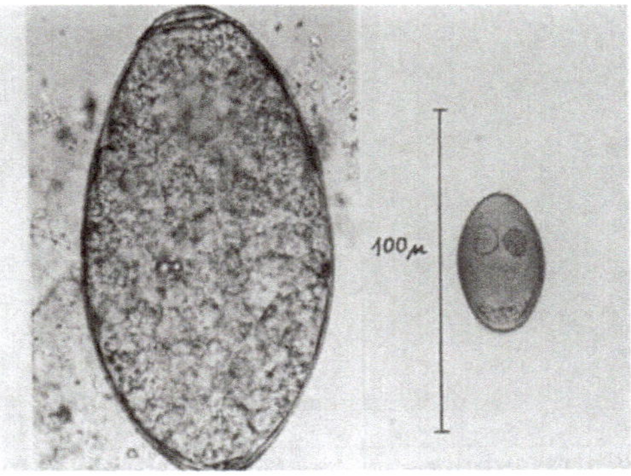

Fig. 33 Egg of *Fasciola hepatica* (a) and *Dicrocoelium dendriticum* (b) [4]

Eurytrema pancreaticum Pancreas fluke

Location: Adult flukes in pancreatic ducts; eggs in the faeces (☞ SHEEP AND GOATS, ■ 4.5)

(Figure 34)

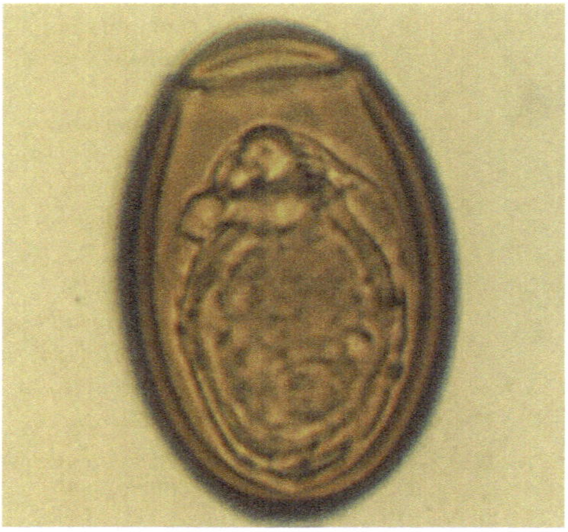

Fig. 34 Egg of *Eurytrema pancreaticum* (40–50 × 23–34 µm)

Schistosoma spp. (S. bovis, S. mattheei, S. curassoni) Blood flukes

Location: Adult flukes in mesenteric veins; eggs in the intestinal wall and faeces (☞ CATTLE, ■ 2)
(Figures 35, 36)

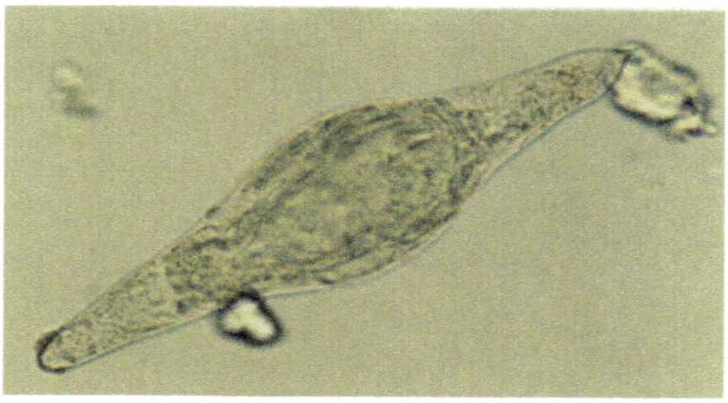

Fig. 35 Egg of *Schistosoma bovis* (180 × 60 µm)

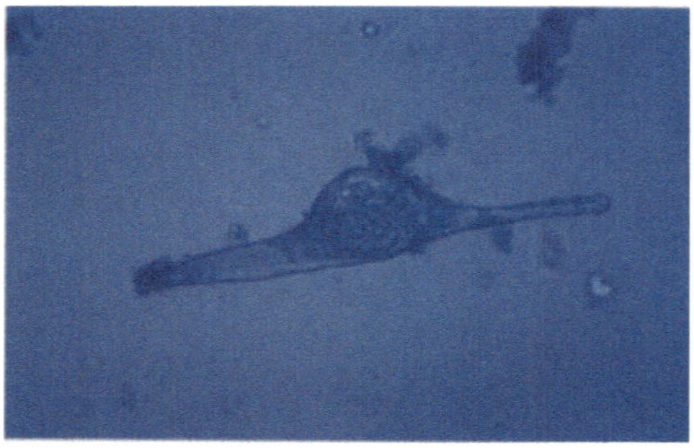

Fig. 36 Eggs of *Schistosoma spindale* (300 × 80 µm) [4]

- Cestoda eggs found in the faeces and adult cestodes living in the gastro-intestinal tract

(Figure 37)

Moniezia expansa and *Moniezia benedeni* Common tapeworms

Location: Small intestine
Hosts: Cattle, sheep, goat and many other ruminants
Species description: Worms are up to 6 m long and 1.6 cm wide (*M. expansa*). *M. benedeni* which occurs more often in cattle is broader (up to 2.6 cm). The life cycle of *Moniezia* is indirect, including many species of oribatid mites as intermediate hosts. Ruminants are infected by ingestion of the

Characteristics	*Moniezia expansa*	*Moniezia benedini*	*Avetellina spp.*	*Thysaniezia giardi*	*Stilesia hepatica*
Length	1–6 m	26 mm	3 m	2 m	20–50 cm
Width	16 mm	26 mm	3 mm	12 mm	2 mm
Egg	Semi-triangle	Diamond-shaped	Oval	Oval	Round
Genitalia	Double	Double	Single	Single	Single
Interproglottid glands	Follicular	Compact	-	-	-
Paruterine organs in gravid segment	-	-	One: lemon-shaped	Numerous: onion-shaped	Two: round

Fig. 37 Morphological identification of common cestodes in ruminants [5]

infected mites with herbage. The prepatent period is 35–40 days. Infections with *Moniezia* spp. may be found in more than 50% of a particular population. *M. expansa* eggs are triangular, contain a pyriform apparatus and measure 56 × 67 µm. *M. benedeni* eggs are cuboid, with a thick, ornamented shell and measure 75 µm in diameter.

Geographic distribution: World-wide (Figures 38, 39, 40, 41, 42)

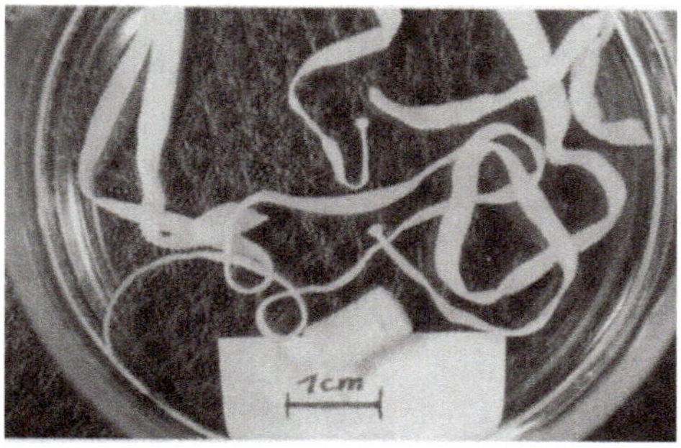

Fig. 38 *Moniezia* sp.

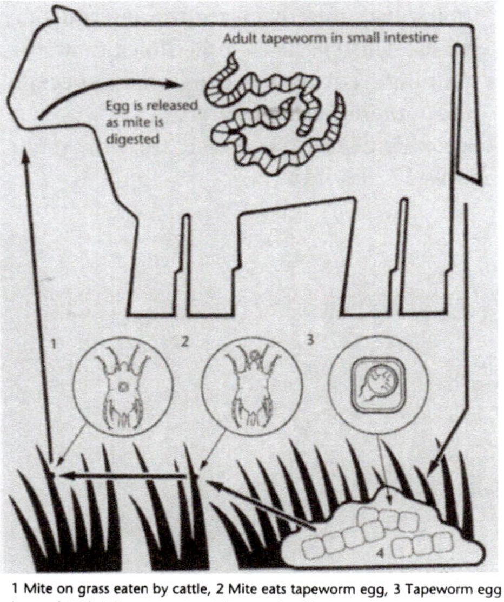

Fig. 39 Life cycle of *Moniezia* spp. [6]

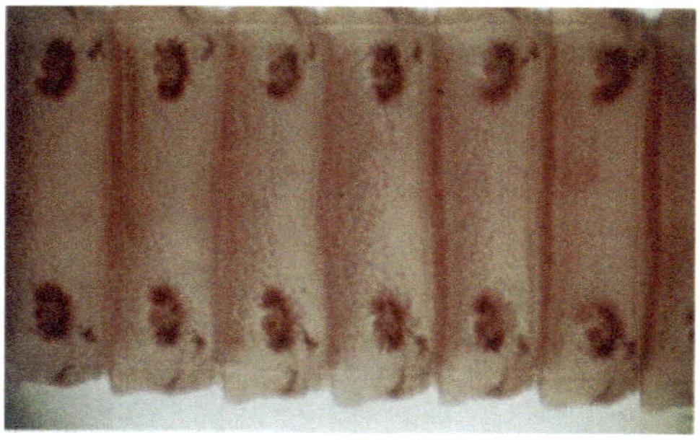

Fig. 40 *Moniezia* sp.; segments with double genitalia [4]

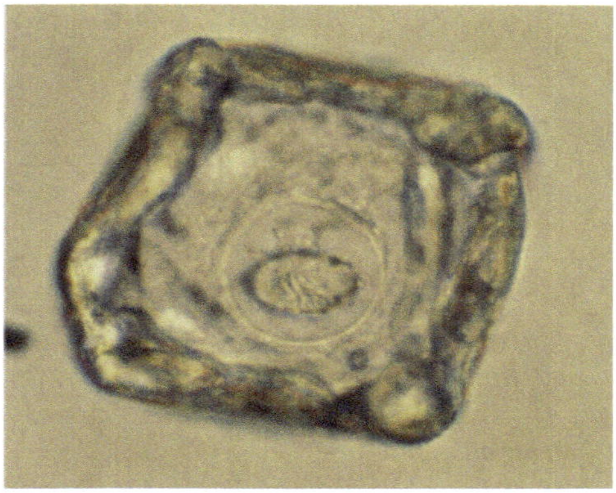

Fig. 41 Egg of *Moniezia* sp. (60–80 µm in diameter)

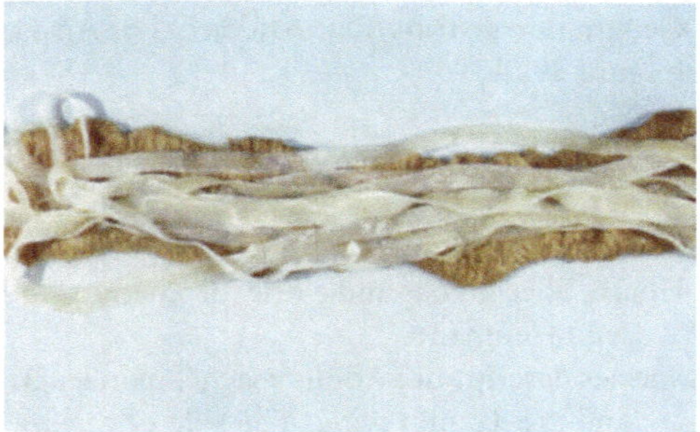

Fig. 42 *Moniezia* sp. in the small intestine of a calf

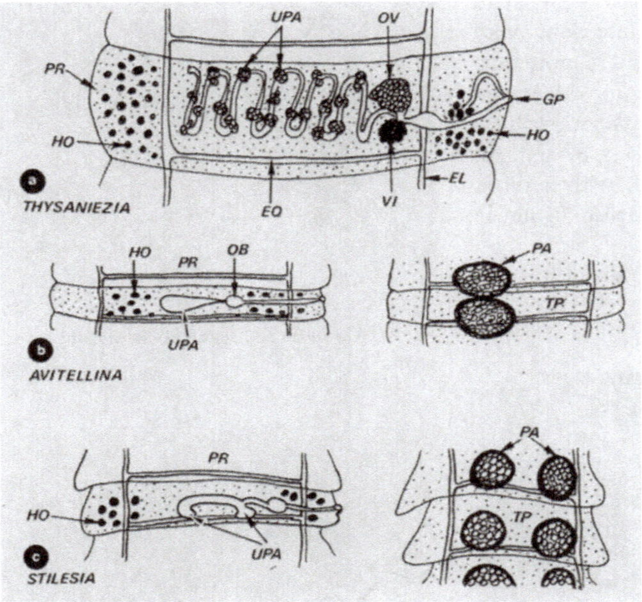

Fig. 43 Morphology (schematic) of proglottids of different tapeworms found in ruminants; EL, EQ = excretion pores, GP = genital pore, HO = testicular vesicles, OB, OV = ovary, PA = paruterine organ with eggs, PR = internal proglottis, TP = terminal proglottis, UPA = uterus with paruterine organ and VI = vitellarium [7]

Avitellina centripunctata

Location: Small intestine

Hosts: Sheep, goat, dromedary and rarely cattle

Species description: Adults reach 3 m in length and are about 3 mm wide. Proglottids appear not segmented. The uterus and the paruterine organs show an opaque line in the medial portion of the proglottids. The eggs measure 21–45 µm. This genus is non-pathogenic. Oribatid mites but also bark lice and dust lice are suspected to act as intermediate hosts.

Geographic distribution: Arid areas of Africa (Figure 37, 43)

Thysaniezia ovilla (syn. *T. giardi*)

Location: Small intestine

Hosts: Sheep, goat and cattle, dromedary and wild ruminants

Species description: Adults reach 2 m in length and are 12 mm wide. The side of the segment bulges out, giving the margin of the worm an irregular appearance. Eggs are found in groups of 10–15 in elongated paruterine organs (about 100 µm long), with a thick gray shell and a protuberance at one end. Oribatid mites and psocids (bark lice, dust lice) are the intermediate hosts. This species is not clinically important but frequently encountered, especially in southern parts of Africa.

Geographic distribution: Arid areas of Africa (Figures 37, 43, 44)

Fig. 44 *Thysaniezia ovilla*; segments with single genitalia which alternate irregularly [8]

Stilesia globipunctata

Remarks: This tapeworm occurs in the small intestine mainly of sheep, goat, dromedary and rarely of cattle and other ruminants in Europe, Africa and Asia (☞ Sheep and Goats, ■ 1).
(Figures 45, 46)

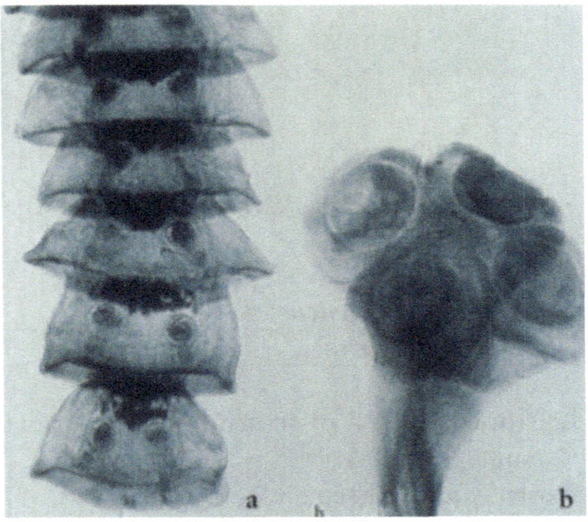

Fig. 45 *Stilesia* sp.; proglottids (a) and scolex (b); PA = paruterine organ [4]

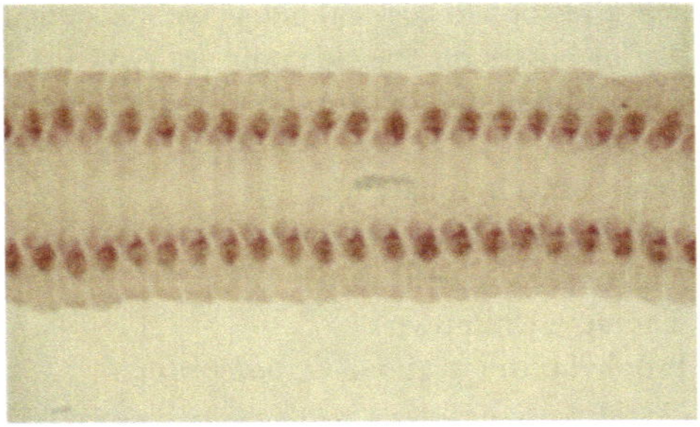

Fig. 46 *Stilesia globipunctata*; immature segments [8]

- **General features of intestinal tapeworms (*Moniezia* spp., *Thysaniezia* spp., *Avitellina* spp. and *Stilesia* spp.) of ruminants**

Symptoms: Generally inapparent infections; heavy infections are found only in young animals and can cause reduced weight gain. Masses of *Moniezia* can cause obstruction of the intestine.

Cave: Because of the large size of the tapeworms their presence is obvious and the underlying cause of parasitism, the small trichostrongylids, easily overlooked.

Significance: Tapeworms are widespread in ruminants, but their pathogenicity has not been proved conclusively and it seems that they are relatively low-pathogenic.

Diagnosis: Proglottids which look like cooked rice grains, containing typical thick-shelled or imperfectly rounded eggs, appear in the faeces. Eggs may also appear isolated in the faeces. The presence of tapeworms in the small intestine at slaughter is conclusive.

Therapy: Niclosamide (75–90 mg/kg) and praziquantel (5 mg/kg, sheep only) are specific cestodicidal drugs. In addition the following benzimidazoles are effective against tapeworms: albendazole (7.5 mg/kg), fenbendazole (5–10 mg/kg), oxfendazole (5 mg/kg), mebendazole (15–20 mg/kg, po.), netobimin (7.5–20 mg/kg, po.), febantel (5–7.5 mg/kg, po.). Special attention should be given to the control of tapeworms in lambs to avoid losses in heavily infected populations.

Prophylaxis: Reduction of the mite population is not feasible and emphasis should be given to anthelmintic treatments when losses due to tapeworms occur.

- Nematoda eggs found in the faeces, adult nematodes living in the gastrointestinal tract and first-stage larvae of *Dictyocaulus viviparus*

Gongylonema pulchrum

Gullet worm, zigzag worm

Location: Mucosa of oesophagus and forestomachs

Hosts: Sheep, goat and less frequently cattle

Species description: Eggs laid by adult worms are passed in faeces and hatch into larvae when swallowed by manure-eating beetles or cockroaches. Larvae in cattle may be liberated in the stomach and migrate towards the oesophagus. Adult worms are 6 to 14 cm in length and a number of oval cuticular thickenings appear in longitudinal rows at the anterior end. The worms are embedded in the oesophageal lining in a zigzag pattern.

Geographic distribution: World-wide

Symptoms: Rarely observed

Significance: This is a harmless parasite and mainly found at autopsy. Irritation of the oesophageal and gastric mucosae may occur in infected animals.

Diagnosis: Mainly at necropsy; eggs occur in the faeces.

Therapy: Generally not indicated

Prophylaxis: Keeping the animals on dry, well-drained grounds or concrete floors has been described to be effective in controlling infection.

(Figures 47, 48, 49)

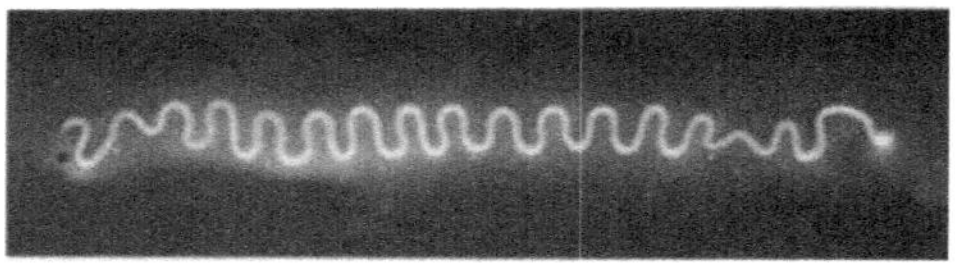

Fig. 47 *Gongylonema pulchrum*; typical zigzag pattern [4]

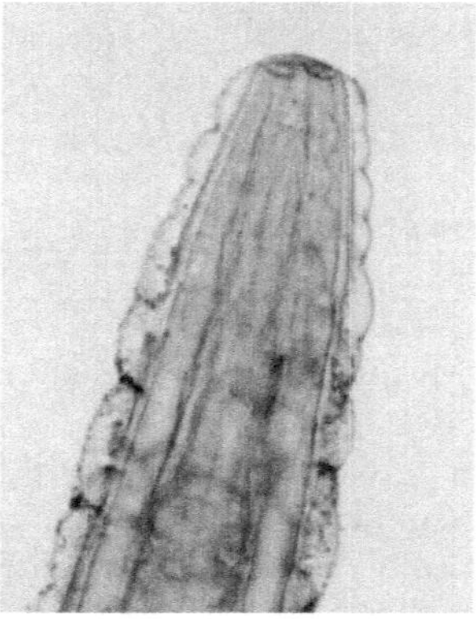

Fig. 48 *Gongylonema pulchrum*; anterior end with cuticular plaques [8]

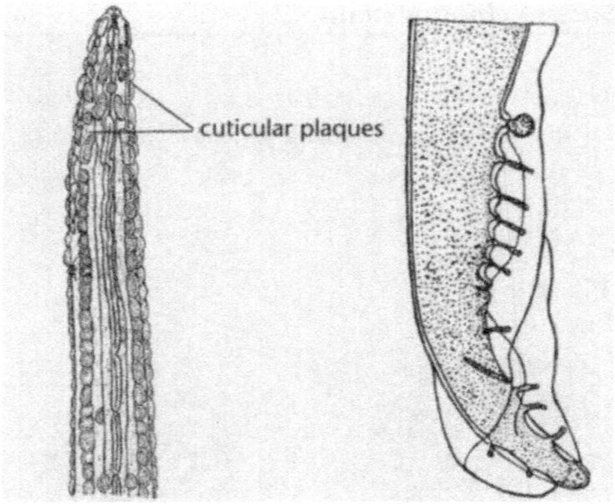

Fig. 49 *Gongylonema pulchrum*; anterior end with cuticular plaques [5]

Gongylonema verrucosum

Rumen gullet worm

Location: Mucosa of rumen, reticulum, omasum

Hosts: Cattle, sheep and goat

Species description: Not well known; dung beetles are intermediate hosts. The worms have a reddish colour when fresh. Males are 32–41 mm long and females 70–95 mm. A festooned cervical ala as well as cuticular bosses on one side only are typical.

Geographic distribution: South Africa, India, USA

Symptoms: Inapparent

Significance: Non-pathogenic

Diagnosis: Casually at necropsy

Therapy: Unknown

Prophylaxis: ☞ above *G. pulchrum*

Parabronema skrjabini

Location: Abomasum

Hosts: Cattle, sheep, goat and dromedary

Species description: This parasite belongs to the Spiruridae. *Stomoxys* spp. and *Lyperosia* spp. are intermediate hosts. Infective third-stage larvae develop in the flies and are deposited on the final host where the larvae are ingested. Males are 15–18 mm long, with one spicule measuring 600–710 µm and the other one 290–310 µm. Female

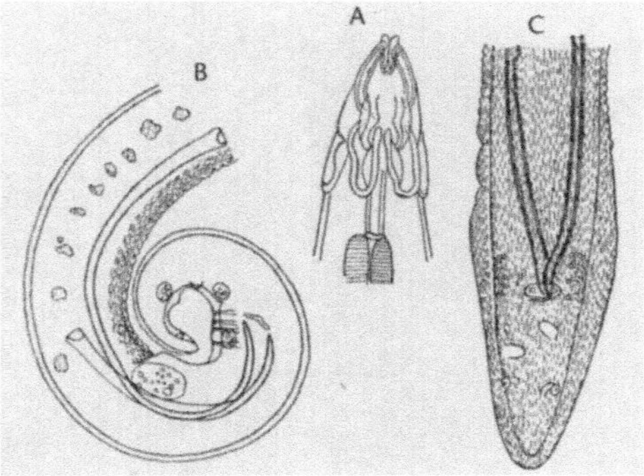

Fig. 50 *Parabronema rhodesiense*; anterior end (a), lateral view of the tail end of a male (b), ventral view of the tail of a male (c) [9]

worms are > 36 mm long and the vulva is situated at 5 mm distance to the hind end. The anterior end is characterised by pseudo-lips, which are wound around the buccal opening. Four papillae are found on these lips. The tail end of the male is reeled to a spiral and four pairs of preanal papillae are found. A group of terminal papillae is present as it is in all the spirurids.

Geographic distribution: Asia, Central and East Africa

Symptoms: Unspecific; abomasitis may be found.

Significance: Unknown; *P. skrjabini* may play a role together with other gastrointestinal nematodes

Diagnosis: At necropsy, adult worms may be found in abomasal scrapings.

Therapy and Prophylaxis: A specific therapy and prophylaxis is not described and probably also not necessary. For further information ☞ below THERAPY OF NEMATODE INFECTIONS, p. 53

(Figure 50)

Haemonchus contortus Large stomach worm, twisted wire worm, barber's pole worm

Location: Abomasum

Hosts: Cattle, sheep, goat and other ruminants

Species description: *H. contortus* is known as the "red stomach-worm" or "wire worm" of ruminants and one of their most prevalent and most pathogenic parasites. Adults are 10 to 30 mm long. Males are shorter than females and have a reddish colour and a bursa with an asymmetrical dorsal lobe and barbed spicules. Females are identified as "barber's pole worms" because their white uteri are wound around their red blood-filled intestine. The vulva flap is prominent in female worms. The life cycle is direct and typical for the strongyle nematodes. The prepatent period is 19–21 days but it can be shortened by immunosuppressive pathogens such as concomitant trypanosome infections and stress factors. In arid areas, the parasite survives the dry season as inhibited fourth-stage larvae within the abomasal mucosa of the host. The inhibited larvae resume their development a few weeks before the onset of the new rainy season. This phenomenon is accompanied by a drastic increase of the egg output of infected animals before the wet season starts ("rains rise").

Geographic distribution: World-wide

Symptoms: Anaemia, oedema ("bottle jaw"), rough coat, weight loss or retarded growth

Significance: *H. contortus* is a very common parasite and one of the most pathogenic nematodes of ruminants. Heavy infections cause death in young animals, whereas chronic infections cause anaemia, hypoproteinaemia, progressive emaciation. These effects are generally compensated during the rainy season and only appear progressively during the following dry season when previously heavily infected animals may die.

Diagnosis: Eggs of strongyle-type appear in the faeces. In acute infections anaemia and death may occur before the worms reach maturity. No eggs are found in this case in the faeces and only the examination of the abomasum at necropsy allows an exact diagnosis.

Therapy and Prophylaxis: ☞ below THERAPY OF NEMATODE INFECTIONS, p. 53

(Figures 51, 52, 53, 54, 55, 56, 57, 58, 59, 60)

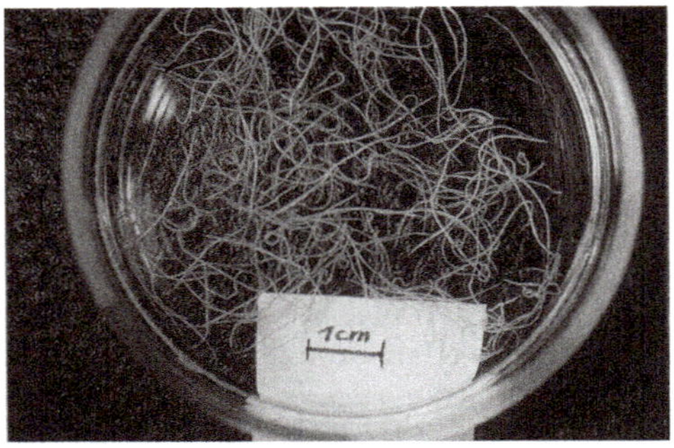

Fig. 51 *Haemonchus contortus*; adult parasites

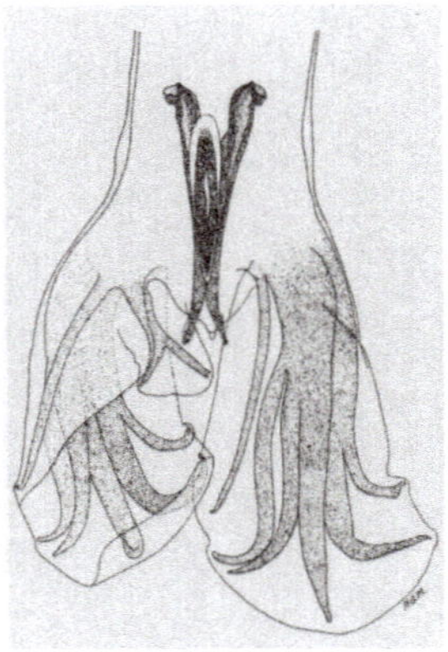

Fig. 54 *Haemonchus contortus*; bursa copulatrix (schematic) with barbed spicules (490–540 µm long) and asymmetrical dorsal lobe [3]

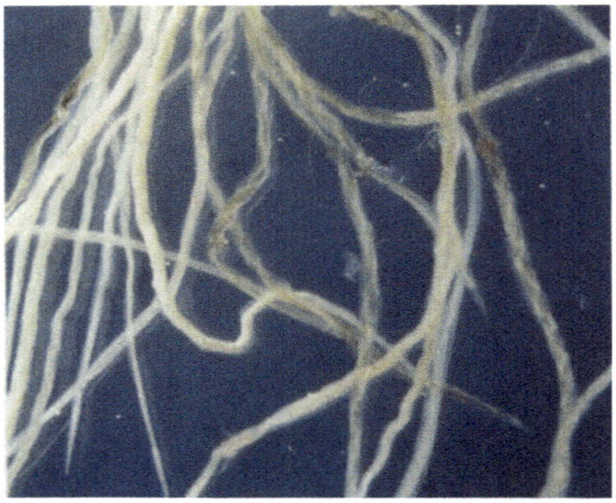

Fig. 52 *Haemonchus contortus*; twisted unteri and intesine [10]

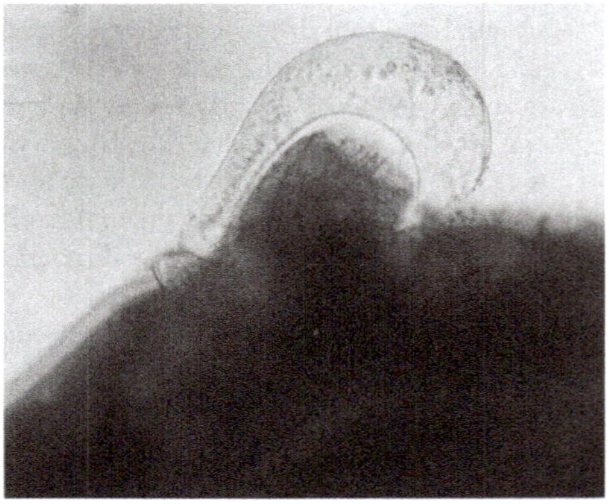

Fig. 55 *Haemonchus contortus*; vulva flap

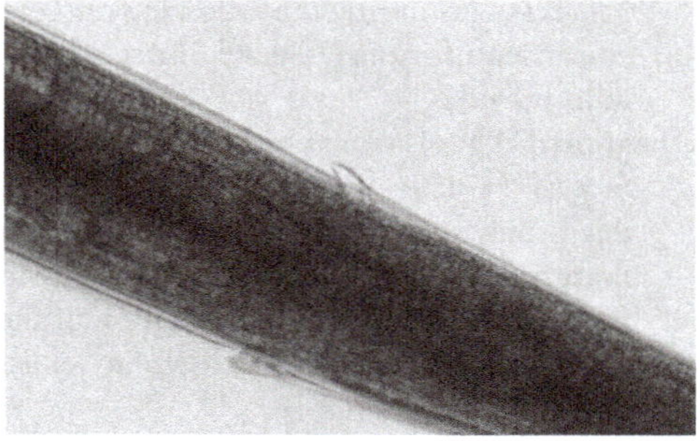

Fig. 53 *Haemonchus contortus*; prominent cervical papillae (50×)

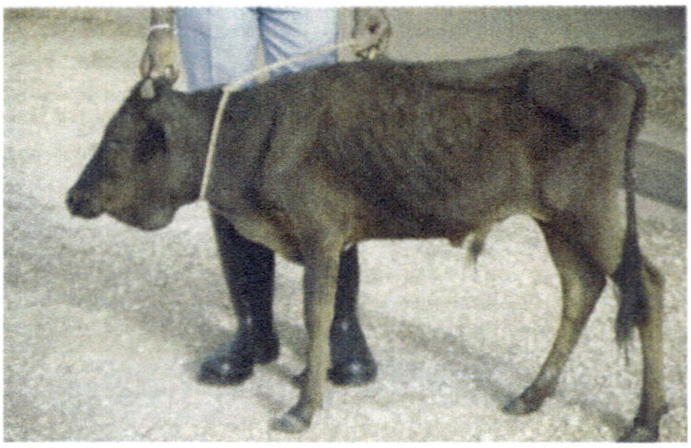

Fig. 56 N'Dama calf showing emaciation and "bottle jaw" due to a chronic haemonchosis

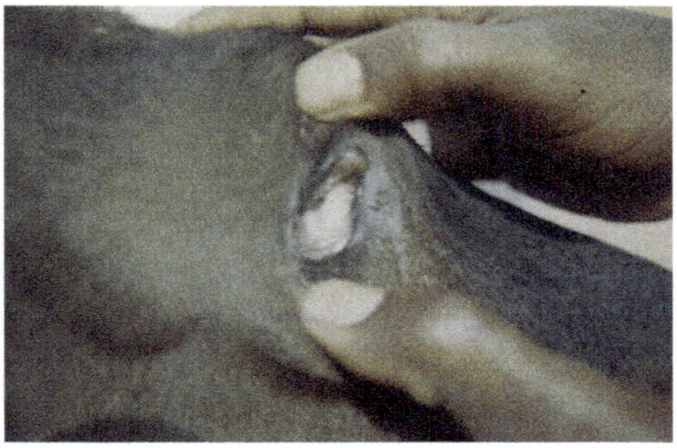

Fig. 57 Pale mucosa membranes following a heavy *Haemonchus contortus* infection

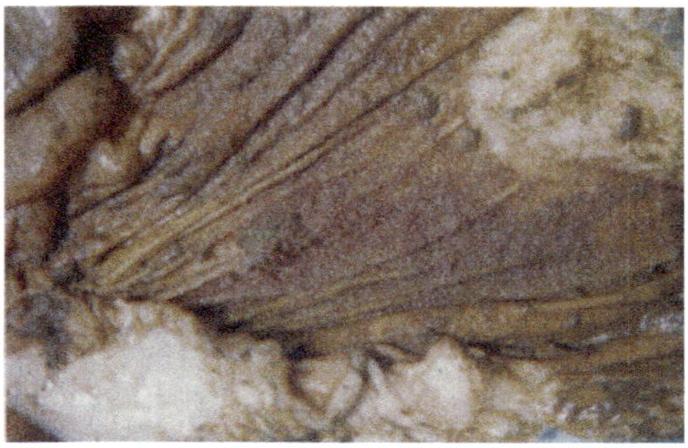

Fig. 59 *Haemonchus contort* on the abomasal mucosa of a calf

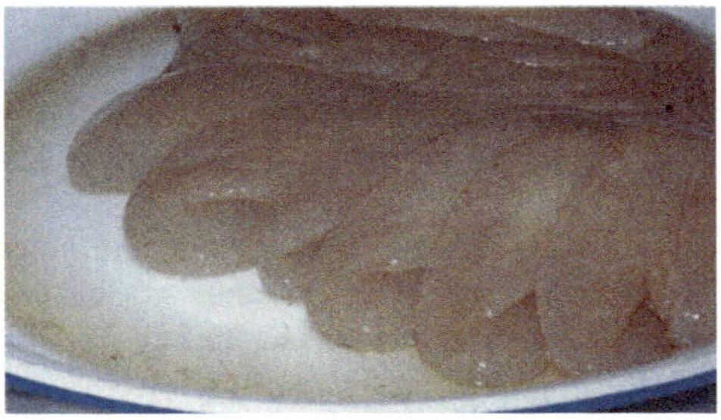

Fig. 58 Oedematous abomasal mucosa due to hypoproteinaemia [10]

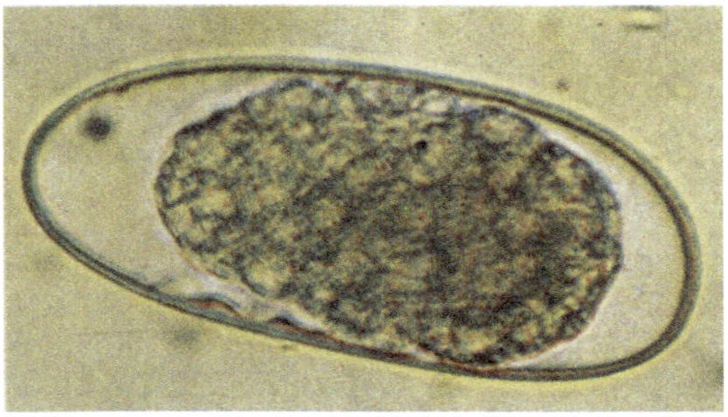

Fig. 60 Strongyle-type egg [11]

Mecistocirrus digitatus

Location: Abomasum of ruminants, stomach of pigs, rarely small intestine

Hosts: Cattle, buffalo, sheep, goat, pig and very rarely man

Species description: This nematode resembles *Haemonchus contortus*. The females also have the ovaries wound spirally around the intestine but they differ from the latter by the position of the vulva which is situated about 0.6–0.9 mm from the tip of the tail and the absence of a vulvar flap. The male bursa has a symmetrical dorsal lobe, which is very small. The spicules are long (3.8–7 mm) and united together for almost their whole length. The eggs measure 95–120 × 56–60 µm. This nematode is a blood sucker.

Geographic distribution: Widespread in Central and South America, Asia, Africa (including island of Mauritius)

Symptoms: Acute infections are associated with anaemia, weakness, poor growth and sometimes death. Chronic infections are associated with oedema, bottle jaw and progressive weight loss.

Significance: *M. digitatus* is an important parasite in endemic areas and young animals are particularly at risk. The effects are similar to those of *Haemonchus contortus*. This parasite generally occurs together with other gastrointestinal nematodes.

Diagnosis: Strongyle-type eggs appear in the faeces. Adult worms may be identified at necropsy.

Therapy and Prophylaxis: ☞ below THERAPY OF NEMATODE INFECTIONS, p. 53
(Figures 61, 62, 63)

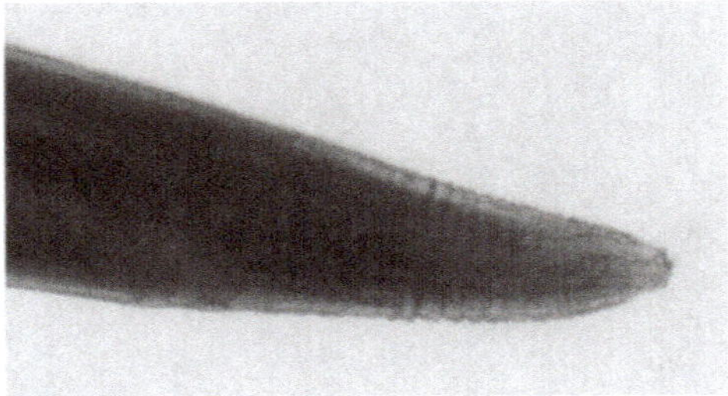

Fig. 61 *Mecistocirrus digitatus*; anterior end [8]

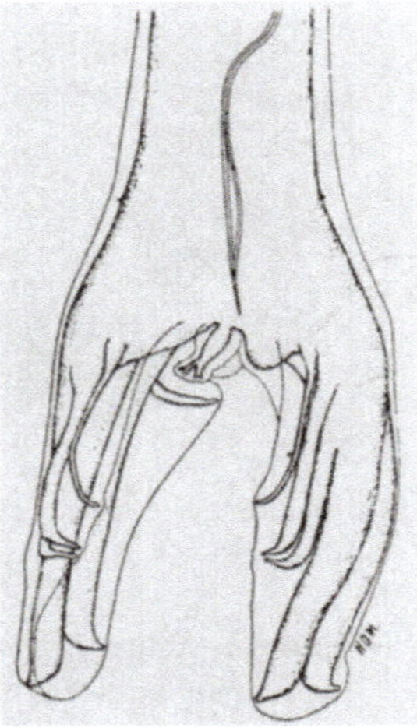

Fig. 62 *Mecistocirrus digitatus*; bursa copulatrix [3]

Trichostrongylus axei Stomach hair worm

Location: Abomasum and occasionally small intestine

Hosts: *T. axei* occurs in the abomasum of sheep, goat, cattle, wild ruminants and in the stomach of pig, horse donkey and man.

Species description: Direct nematode life cycle; males are 2.5–6 mm long and females are 3.5–8 mm long. The spicules are dissimilar: one measures 74–98 µm and the other 96–128 µm. The gubernaculum length is 50–61 µm. The eggs measure 79–92 × 31–41 µm.

Geographic distribution: World-wide

Symptoms: Weight loss and poor growth occur when animals are heavily infected especially in mixed infections with other trichostrongyles.

Significance: Serious weight loss and poor growth occur when animals are heavily infected especially in mixed infections with *Haemonchus, Ostertagia* and heavy *Cooperia* burdens.

Diagnosis: Detection of strongyle-type eggs in the sediment or flotation of faeces. An accurate diagnosis of the species can only be obtained by microscopic examimination of adult specimens at necropsy.

Therapy and Prophylaxis: ☞ below THERAPY OF NEMATODE INFECTIONS, p. 53

(Figures 64, 65, 66)

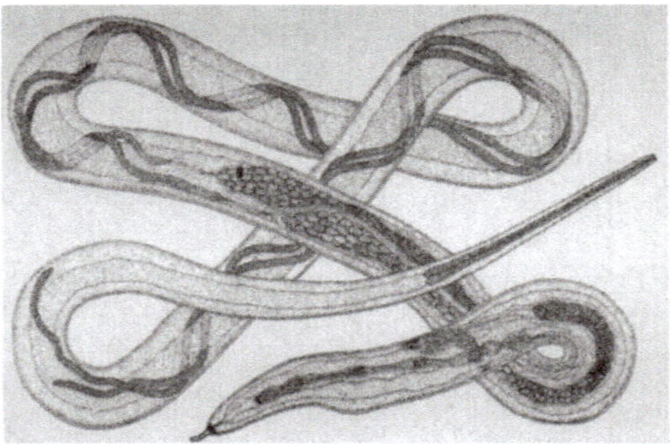

Fig. 63 *Mecistocirrus digitatus*; female worm (19–43 mm long; 470 µm in diameter) [9]

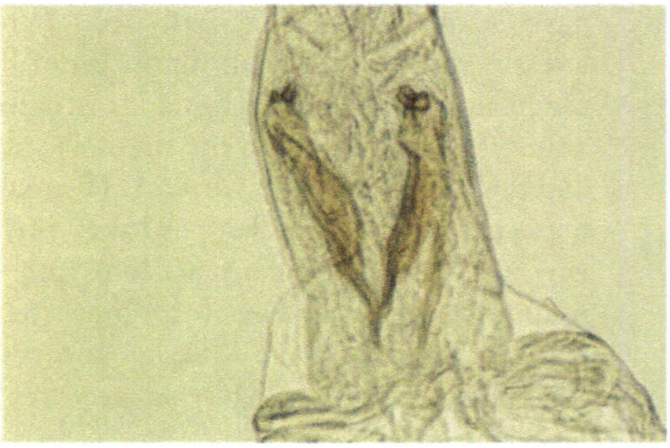

Fig. 64 *Trichostrongylus axei*; spicula (74–98µm and 96–128 µm) and gubernaculum (50–61 µm)

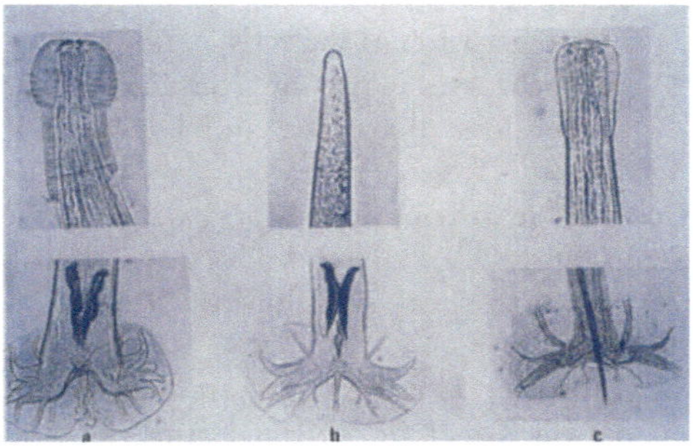

Fig. 65 (Berlin) *Cooperia* spp.; (a), *Trichostrongylus* spp. (b) and *Nematodirus* sp. (c); anterior ends (above) and bursa copulatrix (below) [4]

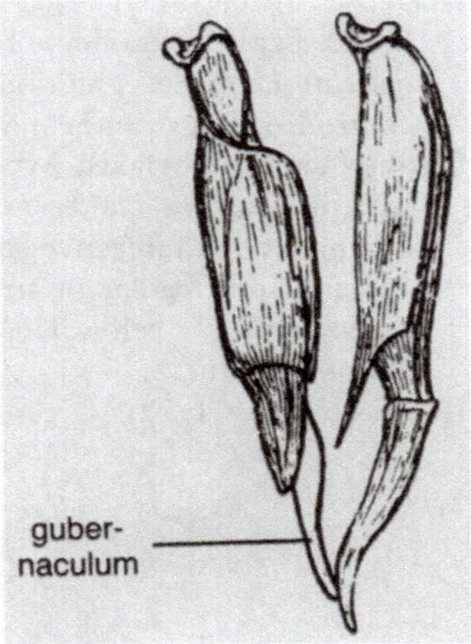

Fig. 66 *Trichostrongylus axei*; spicula (74–98 µm and 96–128 µm) and gubernaculum (50–61 µm) [5]

Trichostrongylus colubriformis and other Trichostrongylus spp. Hair worms, black scours worms

Location: Small intestine

Hosts: Cattle

Species description: ☞ above *T. axei;* the male worms are 4–4.5 mm and the females 5–7 mm long. The spicules of *T. colubriformis* are equal (135–156 µm long) and show a prominent distal end. The gubernaculum is present. Infection is acquired by ingestion of infective third stage larvae which burrow superficially into the crypts of the intestinal cells.

Geographic distribution: World-wide

Symptoms: *Trichostrongylus* spp. infections may be difficult to diagnose. The symptoms they produce are similar to those of other trichostrongylid infections. Weakness, diarrhoea or constipation and in chronic infections anaemia due to emaciation and malnutrition may be seen.

Significance: *T. colubriformis* and other small intestinal *Trichostrongylus* spp. are commonly present in mixed-species infections, so their effect is additive.

Diagnosis: Strongyle-type eggs appear in the faeces. Adult worms can be identified at necropsy.

Therapy and Prophylaxis: ☞ below THERAPY OF NEMATODE INFECTIONS, p. 53

(Figures 67, 68)

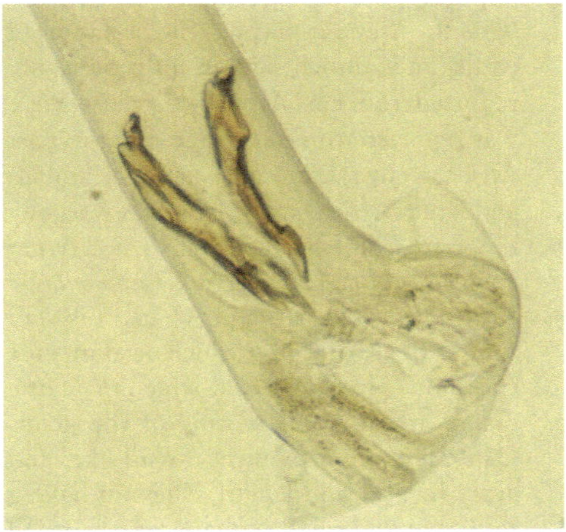

Fig. 67 *Trichostrongylus colubriformis*; bursa copulatrix with spicula (135–156 µm)

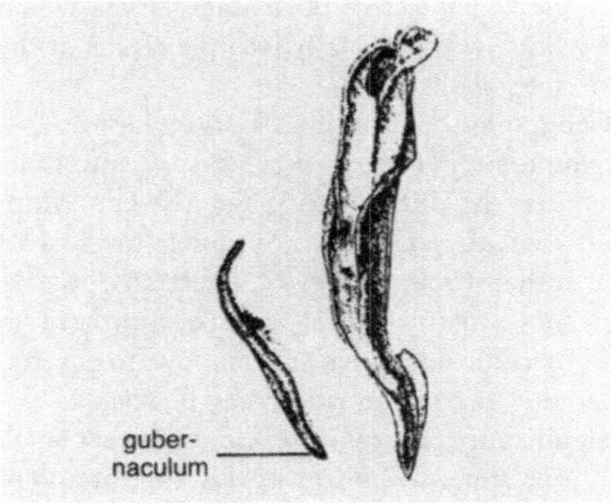

Fig. 68 *Trichostrongylus colubriformis*; spicula (135–156 μm) and gubernaculum (65–75 μm) [5]

Ostertagia spp. (O. ostertagi, O. [syn. *Skrjabinagia*] ***lyrata*** **and other species)**

Brown stomach worms

Location: Abomasum, upper small intestine

Hosts: Cattle, sheep and goat

Species description: *O. ostertagi* is the most important trichostrongylid of cattle world-wide. In Africa it plays a role in imported cattle and autochthonous infections are reported from East Africa. *O. circumcincta* was reported from sheep and goats in East Africa (Kenya, Ethiopia, Uganda, Zambia) and South Africa, and *O. pinnata* was only reported from sheep in Kenya. *O. lyrata* (syn. *Skrjabinagia lyrata* or *Grosspiculagia lyrata*) occurs in cattle in Africa. It is very similar to *O. ostertagi* which accounts for enormous losses world-wide in cattle rasing areas. Adult worms of the genus *Ostertagia* are brownish, thread-like, and grow to 9 mm in length. They all have a restricted and small cephalic vesicle, small cervical papillae projected from the body surface and pronounced longitudinal, cuticular ridges. The life cycle is direct and typical for roundworms. Environmental conditions of cold or excessive dryness may trigger a condition known as *hypobiosis*, in which larval development in the abomasal mucosa is arrested and maturation is resumed several months later. Ingested larvae enter the glands of the abomasum, causing erosion of the cells, maldigestion, protein losses with the consequence of weight loss, diarrhoea and hypoproteinaemia.

Geographic distribution: World-wide

Symptoms: Severe diarrhoea, oedema (bottle jaw or ascites), weight loss leading to emaciation.

Significance: *Ostertagia* spp. are widespread parasites of cattle. Affected cattle not only lose weight but often die of clinical ostertagiosis. *Ostertagia* spp. infections are generally accompanied by other gastrointestinal nematodes.

Diagnosis: Strongyle-type eggs appear in the faeces. Eggs per gramm > 1000 in calves indicate a harmful condition. It should be controlled with an anthelmintic treament.

Therapy and Prophylaxis: Avoid overstocking, use pasture management to avoid accumulation of infective larvae on herbage and soil; regular or strategic use of anthelmintics ☞ below THERAPY OF NEMATODE INFECTIONS, p. 53

(Figures 69, 70, 71, 72)

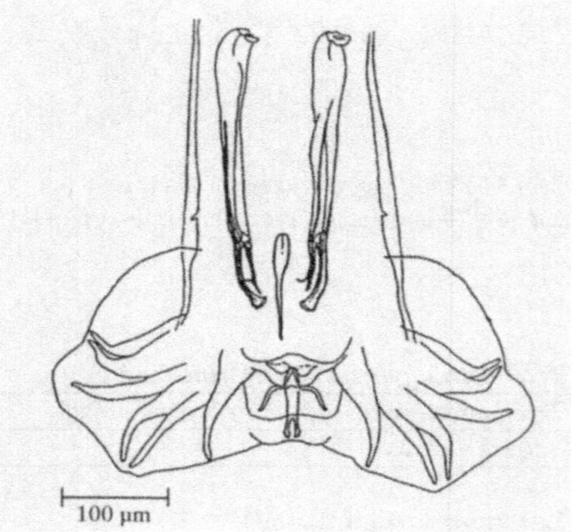

Fig. 69 *Ostertagia ostertagi*; bursa copulatrix with spiculum (200 – 280 μm) [12]

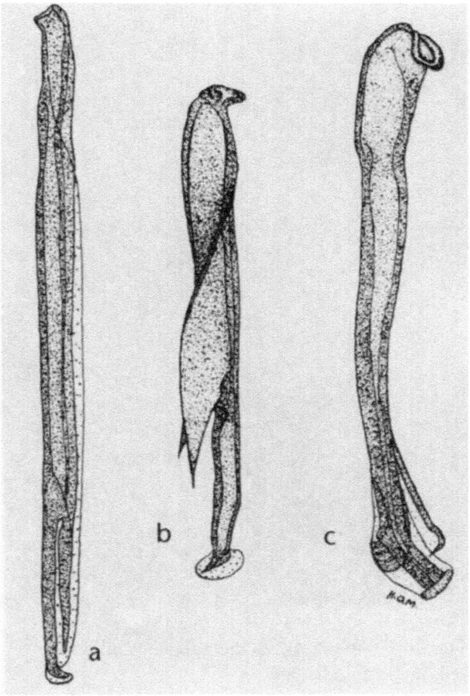

Fig. 70 Spicules of: (a) *Ostertagia circumcincta* (up to 450 µm long), (b) *Ostertagia trifurcata* (150–180 µm long) and (c) *Ostertagia ostertagi* (200–280 µm long) [3]

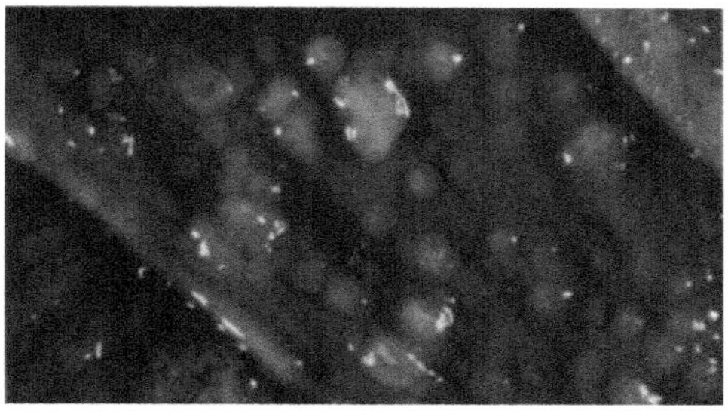

Fig. 71 *Ostertagia ostertagi*; nodules in abomasal mucosa (2–4 mm in diameter)

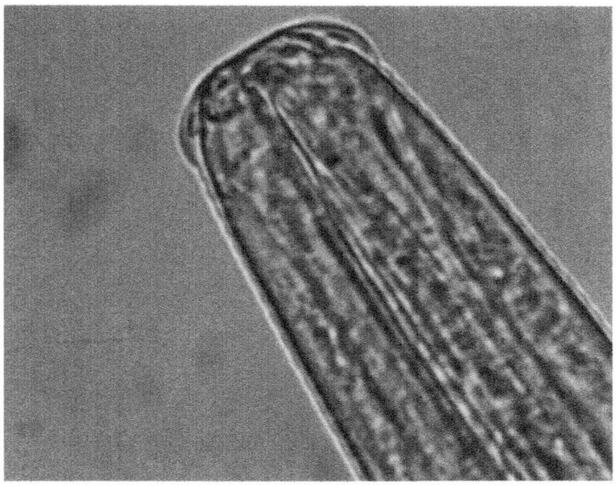

Fig. 72 *Ostertagia* sp.; anterior end with cephalic vesicle

Cooperia spp. (*C. pectinata, C. punctata, C. spatulata* and other species)

Cattle bankrupt worms

Location: Small intestine

Hosts: Cattle

Species description: Direct life cycle; infective larvae develop within 4 days after faecal deposition. Typical for all *Cooperia* spp. the "swollen" head because of a pronounced cephalic vesicle. The body cuticle bears 14–16 longitudinal ridges which appear punctuated. There are no cervical papillae. The spicules are stout, pigmented brown and usually have a ridged, winglike expansion in the middle. When present in large numbers calves may show markedly reduced weight gains. *Cooperia* spp. are generally accompanied by other trichostrongylids.

Geographic distribution: World-wide; widespread in Africa

Symptoms: Reduced weight gain, especially in calves; diarrhoea can occur, causing dehydration which can severely affect young stock.

Significance: Heavy burdens with *Cooperia* spp. result in poor utilization of feed, weight loss and transient diarrhoea. Especially in calves they can significantly contribute to the overall damage of gastrointestinal nematode infections.

Diagnosis: Strongyle-type eggs occur in the faeces. Species diagnosis only with adult specimens at necropsy.

Therapy and Prophylaxis: ☞ below THERAPY OF NEMATODE INFECTIONS, p. 53

(Figures 73, 74, 75, 76, 77, 78)

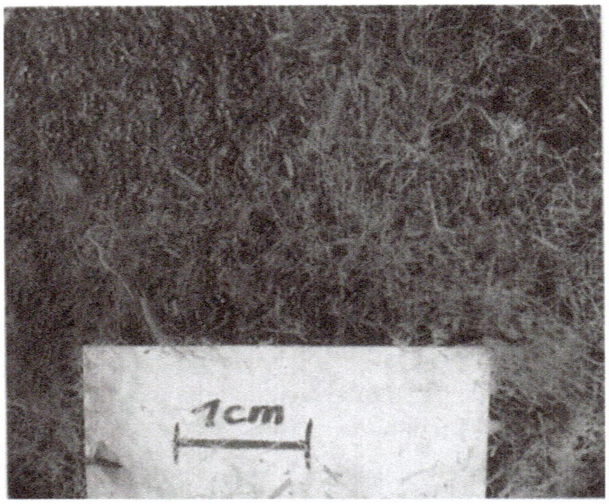

Fig. 73 *Cooperia* spp.; adult parasites [10]

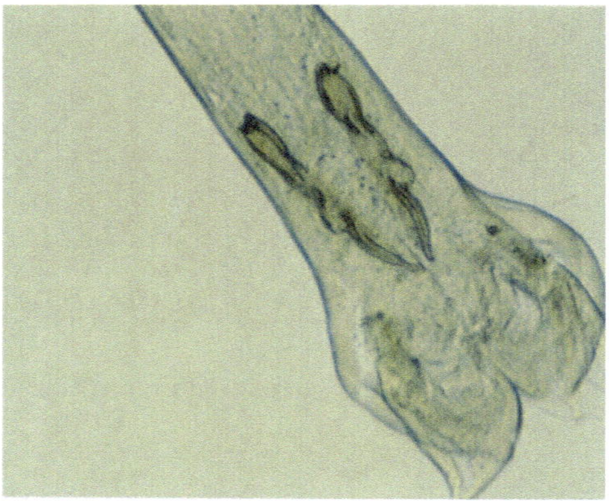

Fig. 74 *Cooperia punctata*; bursa copulatrix with spicules (123–145 μm)

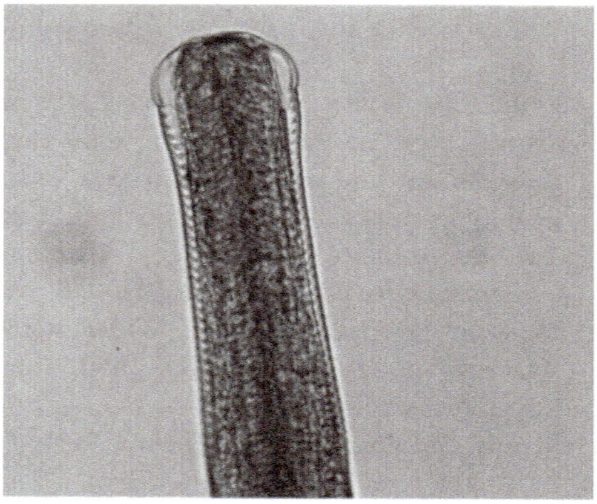

Fig. 75 *Cooperia pectinata*; anterior end with enlarged cephalic vesicle

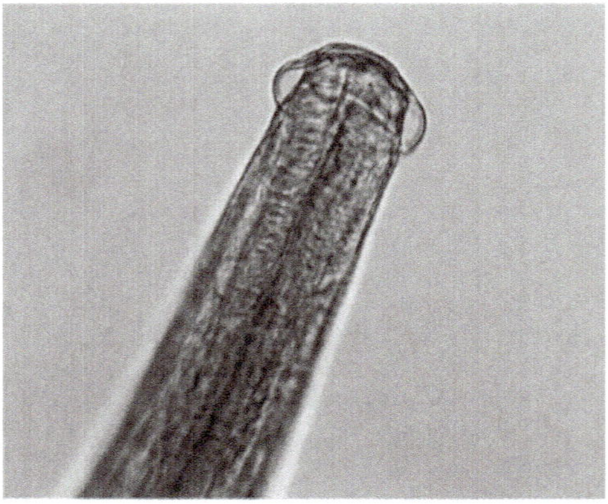

Fig. 76 *Cooperia punctata*; anterior end with enlarged cephalic vesicle

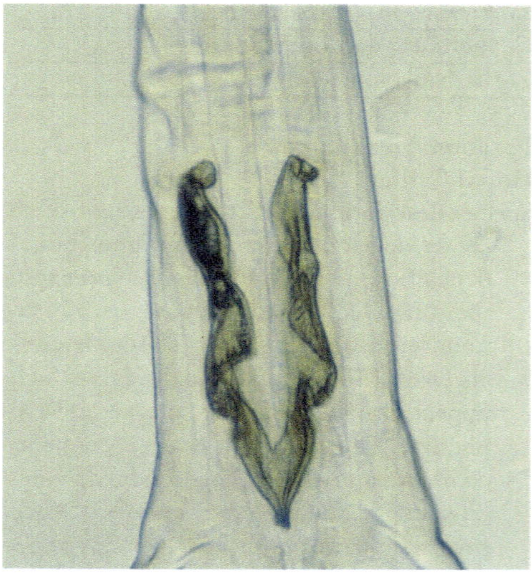

Fig. 77 *Cooperia pectinata*; spicules (240–390 μm)

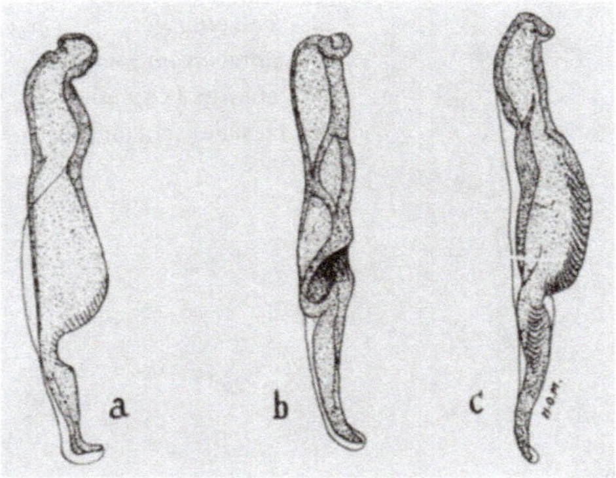

Fig. 78 Spicules of (a) *Cooperia curticei* (135–145 µm long), (b) *Cooperia punctata* (123–145 µm long) and (c) *Cooperia pectinata* (240–390 µm) [3]

Nematodirus spp. (*N. filicollis, N. spathiger, N. helvetianus, N. battus*) Thin-necked intestinal worms, thread-necked strongyles

Location: Small intestine

Hosts: Cattle (*N. helvetianus, N. filicollis,* seldom *N. spathiger*); sheep and goat (*N. spathiger, N. filicollis, N. battus*); and dromedary (*N. spathiger*)

Species description: *Nematodirus* species have an inflated cuticle (bell-glass) around their anterior end. The anterior end is clearly thinner than the posterior part. The bursa of the males has elongate lateral lobes and the spicules are long and slender and their tips are fused together. The tail of the females is short with a slender terminal appendage. The eggs are large (150–260 × 65–110 µm) and can be distinguished from those of other trichostrongylids by their large size. The life cycle is direct. Infective third-stage larvae develop within the eggs which are resistant to adverse environmental conditions. Infection occurs when infective larvae are ingested. The prepatent period is 15–28 days.

Geographic distribution: World-wide; 5–6 *Nematodirus* species are known to occur in North Africa (Maghreb) and certain regions of South Africa. Little is known about the tropical regions of Africa but it seems that *N. spathiger, N. helvetianus* and *N. filicollis* occur in tropical areas.

Symptoms: Intestinal symptoms, diarrhoea, inappetence may be associated with heavy *Nematodirus* infections.

Significance: Heavy infections together with other gastrointestinal nematodes may cause poor growth, emaciation and death. The host is harmed mainly by the larvae which may cause significant destruction of the intestinal epithelial cells.

Diagnosis: Typical eggs which are larger than most strongyle eggs appear in the faeces.

Cave: The eggs of the small ruminant hookworm *Gaigeria pachyscelis* are also large and should be differentiated from those of *Nematodirus* spp. During the prepatent period damage and symptoms of infection may be seen without the typical eggs being excreted in the faeces. Mucosal scrapings may demonstrate the immature worms in the mucosa.

Therapy and Prophylaxis: ☞ below THERAPY OF NEMATODE INFECTIONS, p. 53

(Figures 79, 80, 81, 82)

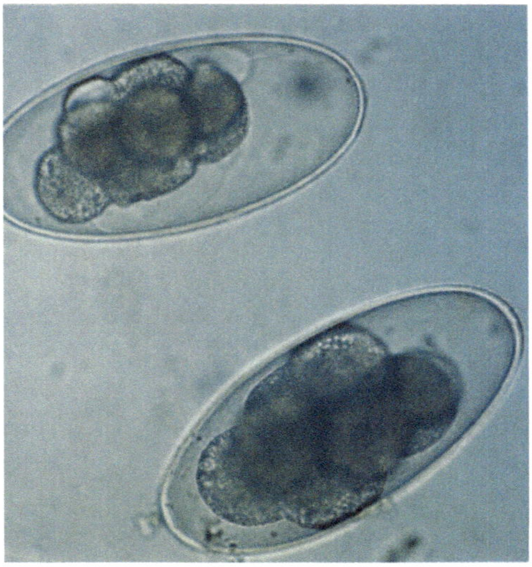

Fig. 79 Eggs of *Nematodirus* spp. (150–260 × 65–110 µm)

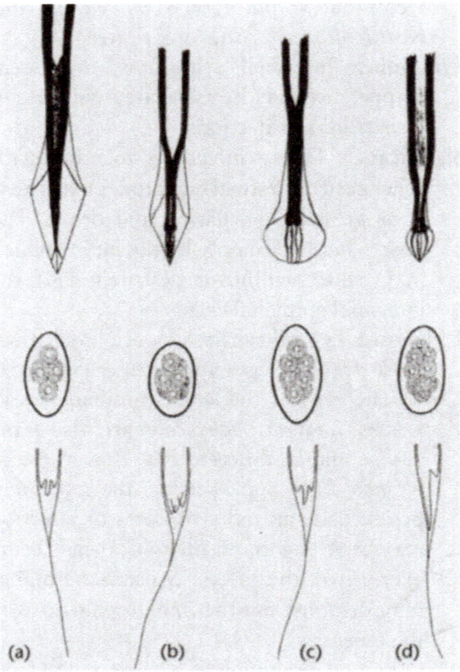

Fig. 80 Posterior end of spicules of: (a) *Nematodirus helvetianus*, (b) *N. filicollis*, (c) *N. spathiger* and (d) *N. battus* [5]

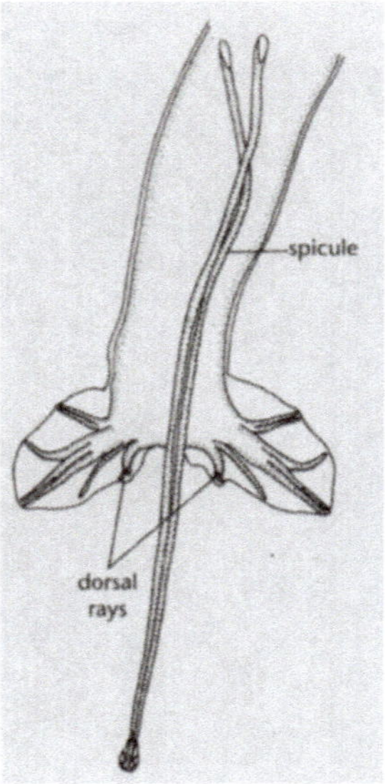

Fig. 81 *Nematodirus spathiger*; bursa copulatrix with spicules (950 µm long; tips fused together) [5]

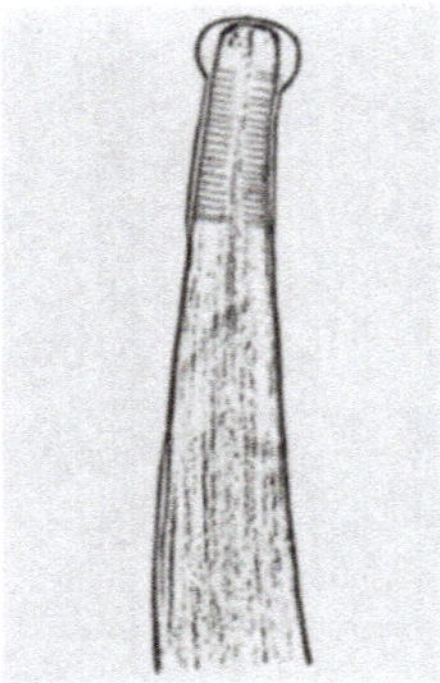

Fig. 82 *Nematodirus helvetianus*; anterior end with enlarged cephalic vesicle (schematic)

Impalaia tuberculata

Remarks: This is mainly a parasite of the dromedary, rarely of zebu, cattle and sheep in many parts of Africa. It occurs in the abomasum and upper small intestine (☞ DROMEDARIES, ■ 1).

Dictyocaulus viviparus Cattle lungworm

Remarks: The first-stage larvae of *Dictyocaulus viviparus* (☞ Cattle, ■ 4.3) is found in the faeces of infected animals. The larvae are recovered from the faeces by means of the Baermann technique (☞ METHODS, 1.7). (Figure 83)

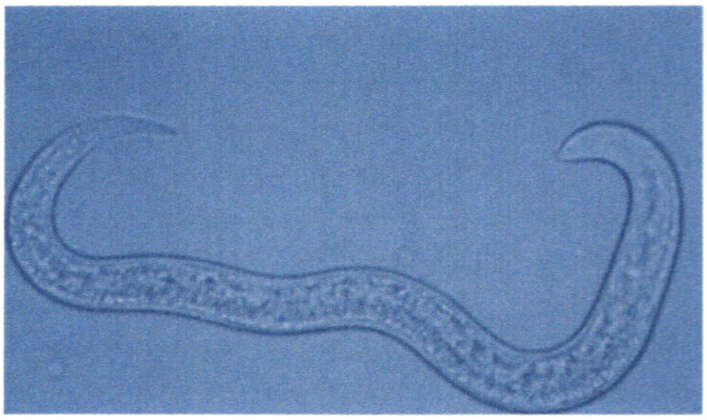

Fig. 83 First-stage larvae of *Dictyocaulus viviparus* (390–490 × 25 µm) [4]

Oesophagostomum radiatum Nodular worm

Location: Adult worms are found in the large intestine (caecum and colon ascendens). Larvae occur in nodules between small intestine and rectum.

Hosts: Cattle

Species description: Direct life cycle; ingested larvae penetrate the intestinal wall, forming nodules anywhere between the small intestine and the rectum. The head end of the adult worms is characterised by a large cephalic vesicle which is constricted behind its middle. Eggs appear in the faeces about 40 days after ingestion of the third-stage larvae.

Geographic distribution: World-wide

Significance: One of the most damaging worms to cattle when present in high numbers (> 200 adults in calves; > 1000 adults in adult cattle). Young stock may die from nodular worm infections.

Symptoms: Heavy infections are accompanied by anaemia, oedema (hypoalbuminaemia) and diarrhoea (reduced fluid absorption). *Oesophagostomum* infections occur generally with other gastrointestinal nematodes.

Diagnosis: Thin-shelled strongyle-type eggs appear in the faeces and pea-shaped nodules in the intestinal wall at necropsy indicate infection with the nodular worm. The diagnosis can be confirmed by demonstrating the typical large worms at necropsy.

Therapy and Prophylaxis: ☞ below THERAPY OF NEMATODE INFECTIONS, p. 53

(Figures 84, 85, 86, 87)

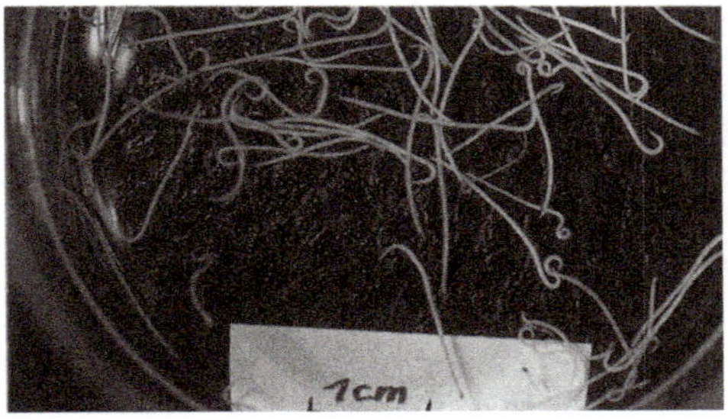

Fig. 84 *Oesophagostomum* spp.; adult parasites

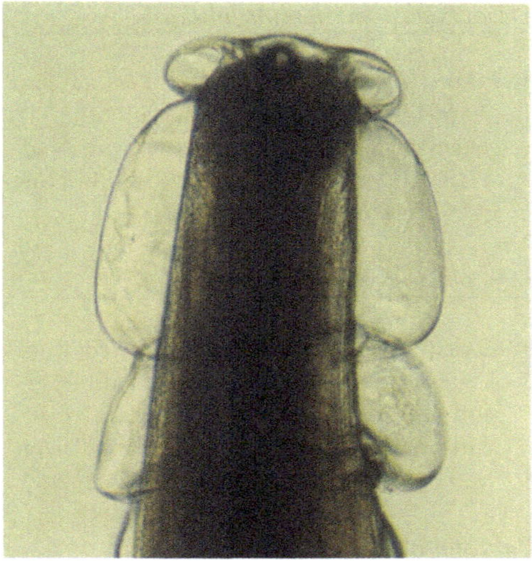

Fig. 85 *Oesophagostomum radiatum*; anterior end with large, constricted cephalic vesicle

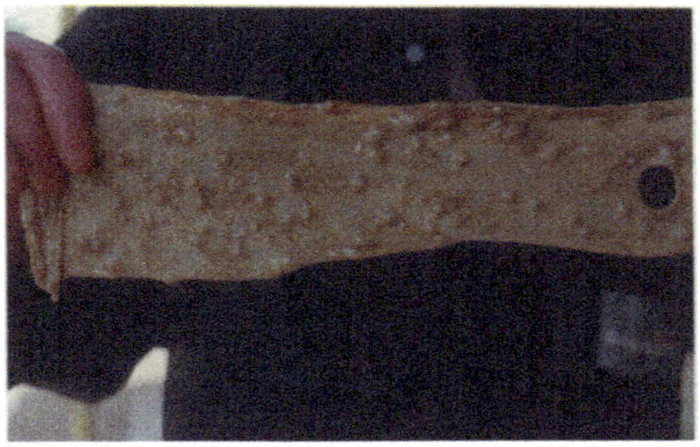

Fig. 86 Multiple nodules caused by *Oesophagostomum radiatum* in the caecal mucosa of a calf

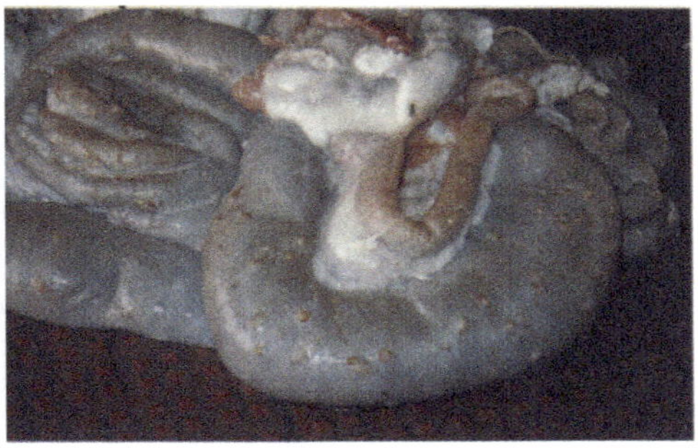

Fig. 87 Multiple nodules in the wall of the large intestine caused by *Oesophagostomum radiatum*; view from the serosa side

Oesophagostomum multifoliatum

Remarks: This is mainly a large intestinal parasite of sheep, goats but also zebu. Its occurrence has been reported from Nigeria, Kenya, Tanzania and Zimbabwe (☞ SHEEP AND GOATS, ■ 1).

Oesophagostomum columbianum

Remarks: This parasite occurs in the colon of sheep, goats, camel, a number of antelopes and occasionally of zebu. It occurs world-wide and is particularly reported from tropical Africa (☞ SHEEP AND GOATS, ■ 1).

Bunostomum phlebotomum

Cattle hookworm

Location: Small intestine

Hosts: Cattle

Species description: Adults are 10–28 mm long. There is a prominent buccal capsule with two pairs of subventral lancets. The spicules of the male measure 3.5–4 mm. The life cycle is direct. Infective larvae usually enter cattle by ingestion or by skin penetration.

Significance: *B. phlebotomum* is one of the most pathogenic helminths of cattle in warm and humid areas. Especially for suckling and freshly weaned calves, during the rainy season it can be a major pathogen causing severe anaemia. Only 50 adult specimens in the small intestine can cause severe anaemia in calves. This parasite is generally accompanied by other gastrointestinal nematodes. *Bunostomum* was found to occur focally only in certain herds of a region.

Geographic distribution: World-wide, especially in warm, humid zones

Symptoms: Penetration of the skin by larvae may cause irritation of the host: itching of the legs and feet results in cattle stamping their feet. Iron-deficiency anaemia and hypoproteinaemia, accompanied by oedma ("bottle jaw") are the predominant symptoms of cattle hookworm infections.

Significance: *B. phlebotomum* may be a serious threat to cattle, especially to calves. Because of its skin-penetrating infection mode, it can also affect suckling calves, killing them within a few days. Heavy infections cause acute anaemia and death. Chronic infections result in poor growth.

Diagnosis: Strongyle-type eggs in the faeces and severe anaemia especially in young calves during the rainy season may suggest hookworm infection.

Therapy and Prophylaxis: ☞ below THERAPY OF NEMATODE INFECTIONS, p. 53

(Figures 88, 89)

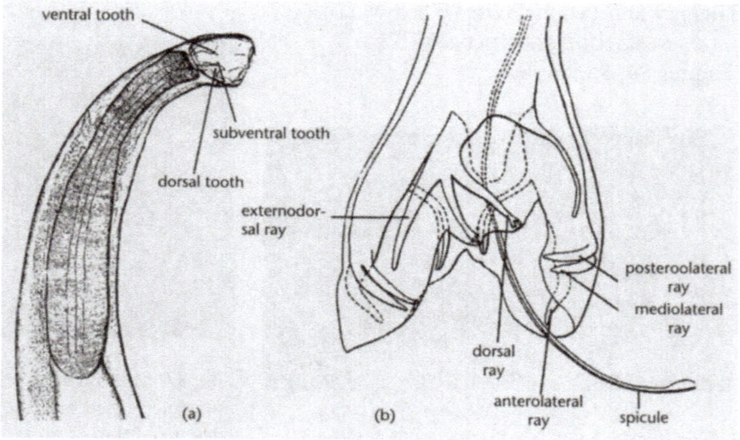

Fig. 88 *Bunostomum phlebotomum*; anterior end (a) and bursa copulatrix (b) [5]

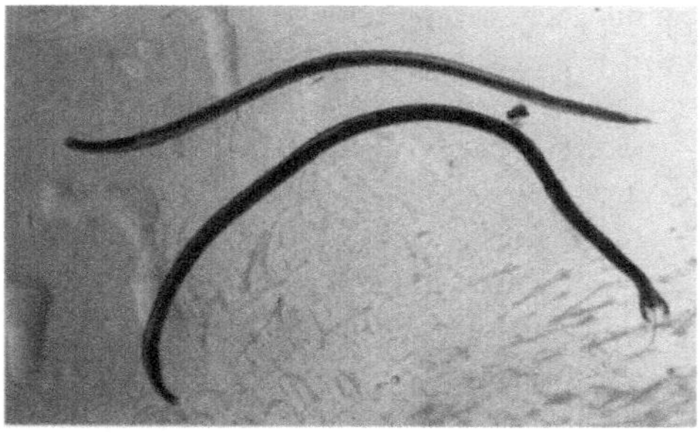

Fig. 89 *Bunostomum phlebotomum*; adult male (10–18 mm) and female (25–28 mm)

Toxocara (syn. *Neoascaris*) ***vitulorum***
Large cattle roundworm

Location: Small intestine
Hosts: Cattle
Species description: Large white worms with blunt ends, up to 30 cm long and 5 mm in diameter. The head end is characterised by three lips without papillae. The cuticle is thin and these worms therefore have a soft, translucent appearance. Adults are almost exclusively found in young calves. Adult females produce enormous numbers of eggs (8×10^6 eggs per day).
The patency is low and 4–6 months after birth no adults remain in calves. Eggs become infective within 15 days and may survive for extended periods. Infection is acquired by ingestion of embryonated eggs (containing second-stage larvae). The larvae hatch in the intestine of the host and penetrate the intestinal wall and either migrate via liver, lungs, trachea, oesophagus to the intestines where they develop to adults or they migrate to several tissues, including mammary glands. These larvae may remain dormant until they are mobilized during the late pregnancy to pass via the milk to the calves. These larvae may reach maturity about three weeks after the calf is born. *Toxocara* larvae can also cross the placenta. *T. vitulorum* is found almost exclusively in calves and prenatal and trans-mammary infections constitute the major sources of infection of young calves.
Geographic distribution: World-wide
Symptoms: Unspecific; intermittent diarrhoea, steatorrhoea, colic due to intestinal obstruction, weight loss and death.
Significance: In tropical and subtropical regions of Africa *T. vitulorum* is considered as a serious parasite with high mortality rates among neonatal calves. In temperate areas this parasite occurs without producing great losses.
Diagnosis: Eggs with thick, pitted shells (75–95 × 60–75 µm) appear in the faeces of calves which are around 4–6 weeks old. Sometimes adult, almost transparent worms appear on the faeces. An increased antibody titer of the pregnant cow close to birth may indicate a risk of prenatal infection of the foetus.
Therapy: Several of the anthelmintics commonly used for trichostrongyle infections in cattle are also effective against *T. vitulorum* in calves. These include albendazole, fenbendazole, oxfendazole, febantel, mebendazole and levamisole. Piperazine (70–150 mg, po.) also eliminates *T. vitulorum* (☞ below THERAPY OF NEMATODE INFECTIONS).
Prophylaxis: In endemic areas pregnant cows and neonatal calves should be treated with compounds which are effective especially against immature stages such as levamisole (7.5 mg/kg po. or pour on), pyrantel (10–20 mg/kg po.) or fenbendazole (7.5 mg/kg po.).
(Figures 90, 91)

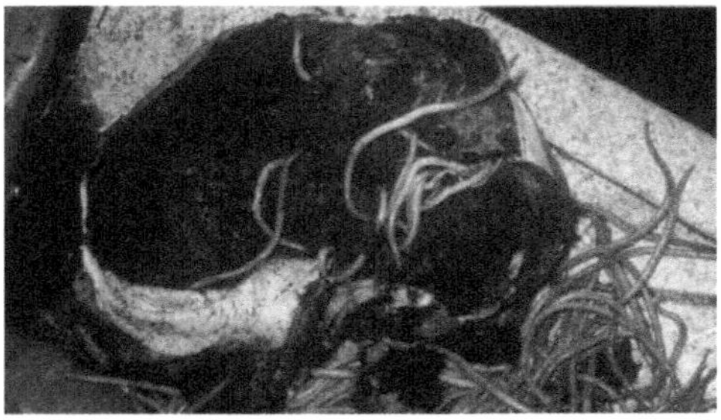

Fig. 90 *Toxocara vitulorum*; adult worms (up to 30 cm long) found in the small intestine at slaughter [8]

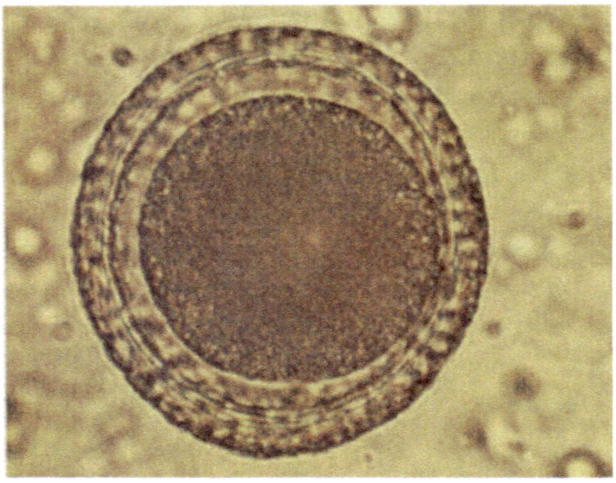

Fig. 91 Egg of *Toxocara vitulorum* (69–95 × 60–77 µm) [11]

Trichuris ovis, Trichuris globulosa and *Trichuris discolor* Whipworms

Location: Caecum and colon

Hosts: Cattle, sheep, goat and many other ruminant species

Species description: Whip worms are 3–8 cm long and easily identified by their long filamentous anterior portion and a thick shorter posterior portion. The male posterior end is usually tightly coiled and there is a single spicule. Direct roundworm life cycle. Infective larvae (second-stage larvae) develop within the eggs after at least 3 weeks on pasture. Eggs may remain infective for several years. Animals become infected by ingesting embryonated eggs, and the larvae penetrate the anterior small intestine for 2–10 days before they move to the caecum where they develop to adults. Prepatent period is 50–84 days and varies markedly among the species. High numbers of preadult and adult worms cause irritation and inflammation of the caecum and colon.

Geographic distribution: World-wide

Symptoms: Mild infections (up to 50 adult *Trichuris* spp. in cattle or small ruminants) do not cause symptoms. Heavy infections (> 500 adult *Trichuris* spp.) may cause colitis, diarrhoea, progressive weight loss. Oedema may occur in the neck and thoracic region.

Significance: Whipworms are widespread but the naturally acquired infections in cattle, sheep and goats usually do not cause clinical disease. Sheep older than 8 months show an age resistance, resulting in a resistance to reinfection 2–3 weeks after a primary infection. However, animals kept in poor condition and carrying multiple infections (e.g. trypanosomes and trichostrongylids) are often heavily parasitised by *Trichuris* spp.

Diagnosis: Demonstration of the characteristic, brown, barrel-shaped eggs with a transparent plug at either pole.

Therapy: Some of the modern benzimidazoles (at increased dose rates) may be used to treat *Trichuris* spp. and *Capillaria* spp. infections in ruminants. These include albendazole, fenbendazole, netobimin and oxfendazole. Ivermectin (200 µg/kg, sc.) is effective.

Prophylaxis: Difficult because of the tenacity of the infective eggs. Regular removal of faeces in the surroundings of the animals may drastically reduce the infection risk.

(Figures 92, 93, 94)

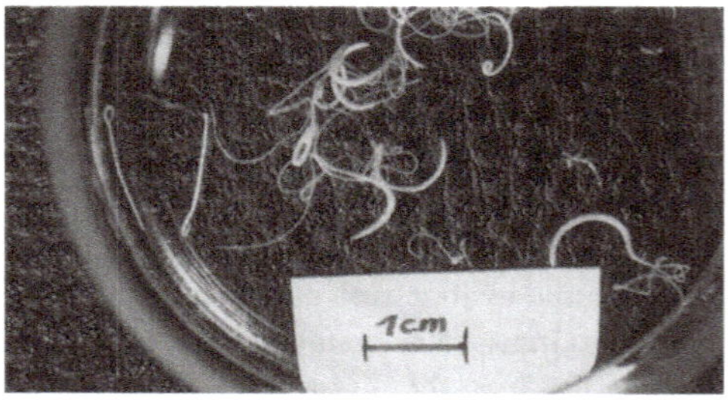

Fig. 92 *Trichuris* spp.; adult parasites

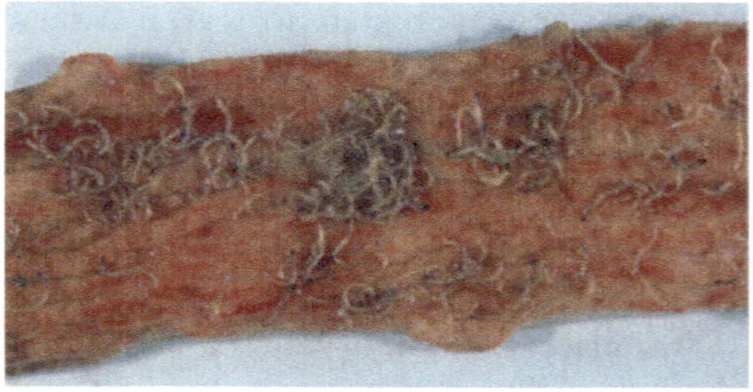

Fig. 93 *Trichuris* spp.; masses of worms in the large intestine of a calf

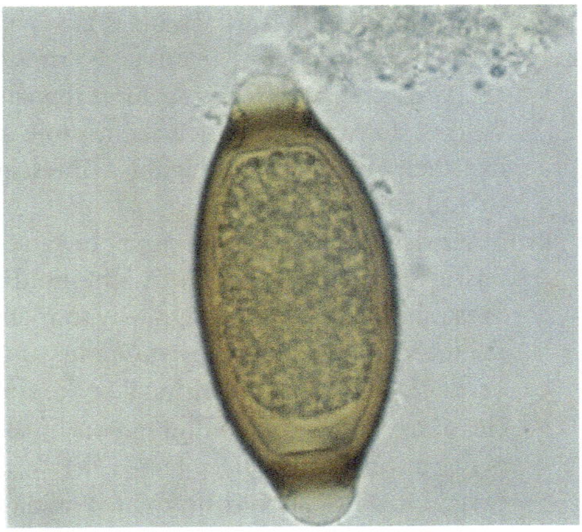

Fig. 94 Egg of *Trichuris* spp. (70–80 × 25–40 µm) [4]

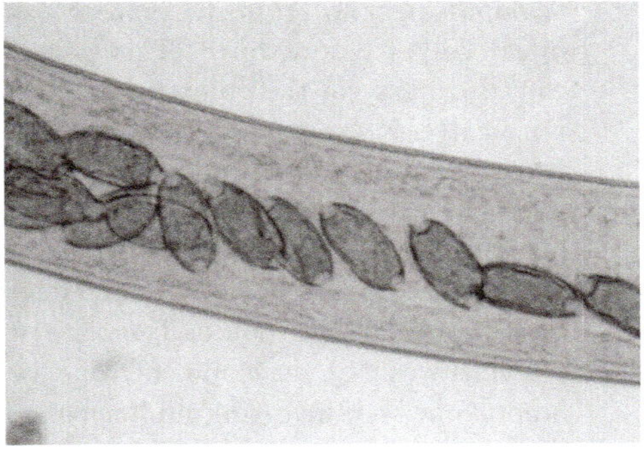

Fig. 95 *Capillaria bovis*; adult parasite containing eggs

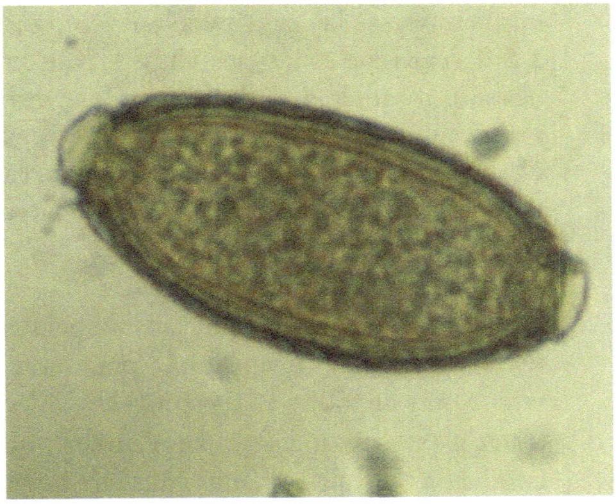

Fig. 96 Egg of *Capillaria bovis* (40–50 × 22–25 µm)

Trichuris skrjabini

Remarks: This parasite occurs in dromedaries and may occasionally be found in cattle (☞ DROMEDARIES, ■ 1).

Capillaria bovis

Location: Small intestine

Hosts: Cattle, sheep, goat and other ruminants

Species description: *C. bovis* occurs in the gastrointestinal tract of cattle, sheep and goats. The males are 8–13 mm and the females are 12–20 mm in length. The eggs measure 45–50 µm × 22–25 µm. The life cycle is direct.

Geographic distribution: Temperate climates but via imports also in Africa

Symptoms: Low or no pathogenic effect in ruminants

Significance: Little is known about *Capillaria* spp. except that they occur frequently.

Diagnosis: Detection of *Capillaria* eggs by the flotation or sedimentation method.

Therapy and Prophylaxis: ☞ *Trichuris* spp.

(Figures 95, 96)

Strongyloides papillosus

Intestinal threadworm

Location: Small intestine

Hosts: Cattle, sheep, goat, dromedary and other ruminants

Species description: *S. papillosus* is a hair-like nematode which is 3.5–6 mm long and only 0.05–0.06 mm wide. Only the parthenogenetic females are parasitic. They are embedded in the mucosa of the upper small intestine. Free-living males and females reproduce sexually outside the host. Infection is acquired by ingestion of infective third-stage larvae and skin penetration.

S. papillosus can cross the placenta and infect calves before birth. This parasite can also pass via the colostrum to newborn calves.

After ingestion or skin penetration of infective larvae they migrate via blood to the lungs. After penetration of the alveoli they are coughed up and swallowed, and develop within 9 days into adults. There are two possible ways of development; one is a homogonic cycle involving adult females in the host producing eggs that do not require fertilisation to develop. These eggs are passed in the faeces and then develop to infective third-stage larvae.

In the heterogonic cycle adult threadworms in the intestine lay eggs which develop into a different type of larvae. These larvae can develop to adult males and females which can live outside the host. The fertilised eggs of this population produce infective larvae that are ingested by the host. The prepatent period is about 10 days!

Geographic distribution: World-wide

Symptoms: The migratory phase is associated with coughing, fever and pneumonia which may be followed by secondary infections, especially in calves kept under poor conditions. Adult parasites cause irritation and severe inflammation of the small intestine. Catarrhal enteritis, digestive disturbances and intermittent diarrhoea may be seen. Death may occur in suckling calves.

Significance: Intestinal threadworms are widespread in warm and humid areas. They may cause great losses, particularly in young calves.

Diagnosis: Small, embryonated, thin-shelled eggs appear in the faeces. The adult, parasitic females are difficult to recognise at necropsy. Microscopical examination of mucosa scrapings is necessary to discover them.

Therapy: Not all the anthelmintics are effective against the intestinal threadworms. Albendazole, febantel and fenbendazole, oxfendazole are effective and proven against *S. papillosus*. Most of the modern benzimidazoles are effective against *S. papillosus* (Table 5). Thiabendazole (75 mg/kg, po.) is very effective. Ivermectin (200 μg/kg, sc.) is effective against the adult worms. Levamisole and mebendazole are insufficiently effective against intestinal threadworm infections.

Prophylaxis: Special attention must be paid to pasture management. The night holding areas should be rotated regularly to reduce the infection risk in the surroundings of the herds. Suckling calves should be kept on clean, dry areas to avoid infection by skin penetration. In heavily infected herds, the pregnant cows should be treated with an anthelmintic to avoid transplacental infection of the unborn calf. Treatments must be repeated more frequently than with other nematodes because of the extremely short prepatent period.

(Figures 97, 98)

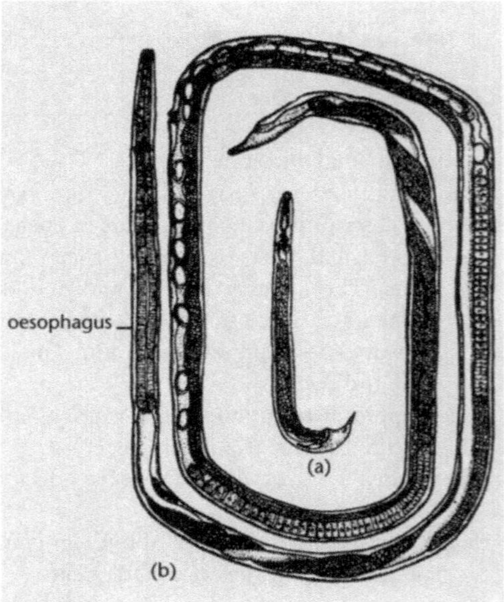

Fig. 97 *Strongyloides papillosus*; free living male (a) and parthenogenetic parasitic female (3.5–6 mm long) with elongated oesophagus (b) [5]

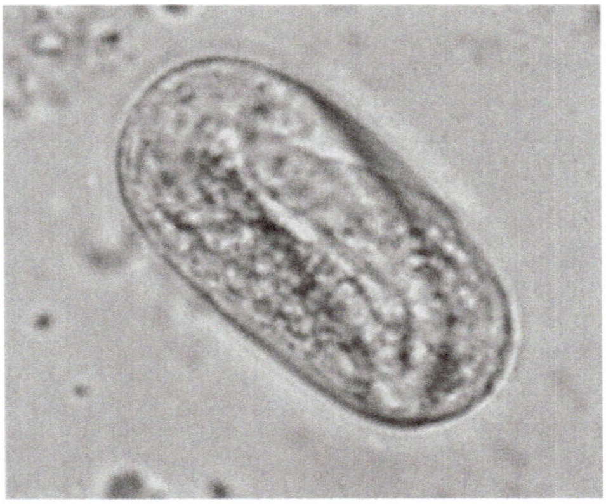

Fig. 98 Embryonated egg of *Strongyloides papillosus* (45–65 × 25 μm)

- **Therapy of nematode infections**

Species of *Haemonchus, Mecistocirrus, Parabronema, Trichostrongylus, Ostertagia, Cooperia, Impalaia, Nematodirus, Bunostomum,* and *Oesophagostomum*

Gastrointestinal nematodes occur wherever ruminants are raised. Attempts to control nematode infections should concentrate on a reduction of the worm load rather than on an eradication of these parasites. The risk to acquire a harmful infection is high where the stocking rate is high (fenced paddocks, correos, night holding places, etc.) or when the daily grazing time is short at the time when animals should put on body weight (e.g. rainy season in mixed farming-systems of sub-Saharan regions). Priority should be given to strategic control rather than to a regular dosing of anthelmintics. Animals at risk (weaned calves) should be treated repeatedly during the first grazing season. Strategic control programs of first season grazing animals in temperate areas are described extensively (☞ FURTHER READING). In semiarid areas first season calves should be treated at least twice during the rainy season, 4 weeks after the onset of the rains and at the end of the rains with an anthelmintic listed below, in order to make animals use the great food resources of the wet season. An additional treatment at the culmination of the wet season may markedly increase the growth rate. Regular rotation of the heavily contaminated pastures or night holding places and long daily grazing periods during the rainy season are effectively reducing the risk of nematode infections. Rainy season treatment is more effective than dry season treatment.
(Figures 99, 100, 101, Table 5)

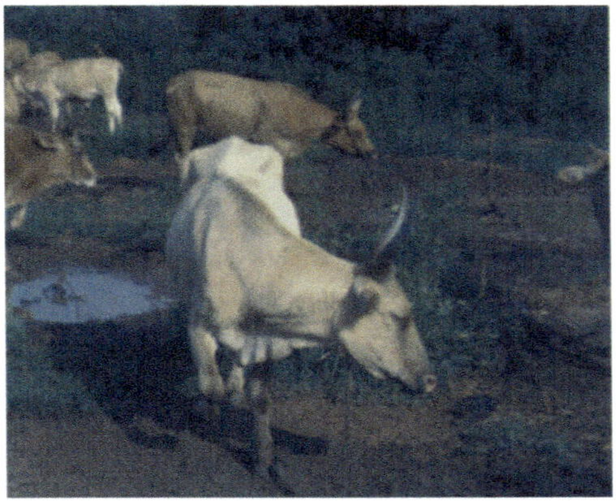

Fig. 99 N'Dama cattle tethered on a "correo". The night holding areas may represent an important source of infections with gastrointestinal nematodes

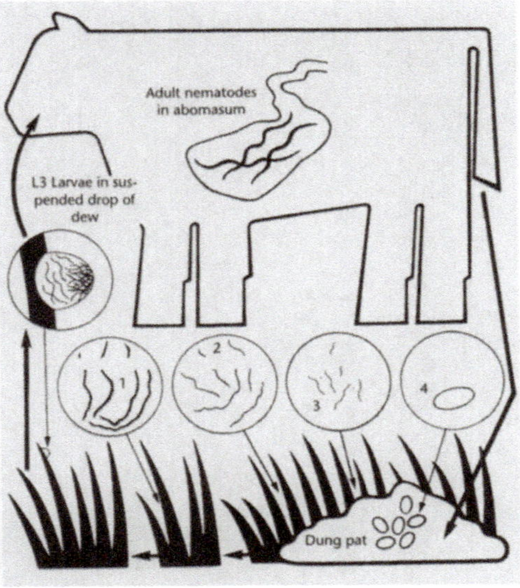

1 L3 Larvae in grass, 2 L2 Larvae in dung, 3 L1 Larvae in dung pat, 4 Nematode egg in dung pat

Fig. 100 Direct life cycle of a typical round worm

Table 5 Anthelmintics recommended for cattle and sheep

Anthelmintics	Spectrum	Dosage (mg/kg)		
		Cattle	Sheep	AM
Albendazole	Nematodes, cestodes, trematodes	7.5	5.0	po.
Coumaphos	*Trichostrongylid* spp.	2 (6x)		po.
Febantel	Nematodes	7.5	5	po.
Fenbendazole	Nematodes, cestodes	7.5	5.0	po.
Ivermectin	Nematodes, arthropods	0.2	0.2	po. or sc.
Ivermectin and Clorsulon	Nematodes, trematodes, arthropods	0.2/7		po.
Ivermectin	Nematodes, trematodes, arthropods	0.5		pour on
Levamisole	Nematodes	5 0	5.0	sc. or im.
Levamisole	Nematodes	7.5	7.5	po.
Levamisole	Nematodes	10	10	pour on
Mebendazole	Nematodes	20		po.
Netobimin	Nematodes, cestodes	7.5	7.5	po.
Morantel tartrate	Nematodes	10	10	po.
Morantel tartrate	Nematodes	SRB*		ir.
Oxfendazole	Nematodes, cestodes	4.5	5	po.
Phenothiazine	Nematodes	220[1]		po.
Pyrantel tartrate	Nematodes	12.5	25	po.
Thiabendazole	Nematodes	44–75		po.
Moxidectin	Nematodes, arthropods	0.2	0.2	po.

*Slow Release Bolus (rumen retention device releases about 200 mg/day for 60 days)

[1] safety index very low (= 1); AM = application method, po. = orally, sc. = subcutaneously, im. = intramuscularly and ir. = intraruminal

PROTOZOA

TRYPANOSOMATIDAE

Trypanosoma congolense, Trypanosoma vivax, Trypanosoma brucei Tsetse-transmitted trypanosomosis, Nagana, sleeping sickness

Hosts: Cattle, sheep, goat and many other domestic and wild animal species

Vector: Several species of tsetse flies: *Glossina morsitans* (savanna areas), *Glossina palpalis* (areas around rivers and lakes) and *Glossina fusca* (high forest areas). All three species transmit trypanosomosis and feed on a wide spectrum of mammals.

Species description: The most important trypanosomes affecting cattle, sheep and goats are as follows (in order of importance): *T. congolense, T. vivax* and *T. brucei*. These three species belong to the Salivaria (Table 6). The differentiation and the morphological characteristics of these pathogenic trypanosomes are listed in Table 7. All three species are transmitted by tsetse flies. Most tsetse-transmission is cyclic and begins when blood from a trypanosome infected animal is ingested by the fly. The trypanosomes lose their surface coat, multiply in the fly, re-acquire a new surface coat and become infective. The life cycle within the tsetse fly varies among the different trypanosome species. The infective form for animals in the tsetse fly is referred to as the metacyclic form. The development in the tsetse flies may be as short as 1 week with *T. vivax* or extend to a few weeks for *T. brucei*. Mechanical transmission requires blood containing trypanosomes being transferred from one animal to another. Tsetse flies inoculate metacyclic trypanosomes into the skin of animals, where the trypanosomes multiply and cause swellings (chancres). They enter the blood stream either directly or through the lymph nodes, then the bloodstream where they divide rapidly by binary fission. *T. congolense* attach to endothelial cells and localize in capillaries. *T. brucei* and *T. vivax* invade tissues and cause tissue damage in several organs. The necropsy findings vary and are not specific. Extensive petechiae of the serosal membranes, especially in the peritoneal cavity may occur in acute, fatal cases. The lymph nodes and the spleen are usually swollen. Chronic cases are associated with atrophy of body and organ fat, severe anaemia and swollen lymph nodes.

The immune response of infected animals is vigorous, and immune complexes cause inflammation, which contributes to the clinical signs and lesions of trypanosomosis. Trypanosomes have multiple genes that code for different surface-coat glycoproteins. The number of different antigenic types of glycoprotein that can be made is unknown but exceeds several hundred. The antigenic variation results in persistence of the organisms in the host and is a way of the parasite to evade the host's immune system. Antigenic variation has prevented the development of a vaccine and permits reinfections when animals are exposed to a new antigenic type of the same trypanosome species. Animals infected with trypanosomes show some degree of immunodepression and are more susceptible to a.o. gastrointestinal helminth infections. *Haemonchus contortus* shows a reduced prepatent period and causes a markedly increased mortality in animals that are chronically infected with trypanosomes.

Some *bos indicus* (Zebu) are very sensitive to trypanosomosis and they are generally

Table 6 Pathogenicity[1] of salivarian trypanosomes in livestock

Trypanosome subgenus	Trypanosome species	Cattle	Sheep and Goats	Pigs	Camels	Equines
Trypanozoon	*T. brucei*[2]	+	+ +	+	+ + +	+ + +
	T. evansi[3]	+ +	+	+ +	+ + +	+ + +
	T. equiperdum[4]	-	-	-	-	+ + +
Nannomonas	*T. congolense*	+ + +	+ +	+	+ +	+ +
	T. simiae	-	+	+++	+++	-
Duttonella	*T. vivax*	+ + +	+ +	-	+ +	+ +
Pycnomonas	*T. suis*[5]	-	-	+ +	-	-

- = not pathogenic; + = mildly pathogenic; + + = moderately pathogenic; + + + = severely pathogenic;
[1]under usual field conditions, but which is modified by many factors; [2]*T. brucei gambiense* and *T. brucei rhodesiense* cause human sleeping sickness in West and East Africa, respectively, and have animal reservoirs, in which pathogenicity is low; *T. brucei brucei* is not infective to humans; [3]mechanical transmission by biting flies other than tsetse; [4]venereal transmission; [5]rarely encountered

Table 7 Morphological characteristics of trypanosomes

Species	Free flagellum	Kinetoplast	Undulating membrane	size in µm	Size and motility in dark ground
T. vivax	present	large, terminal	not prominent	20-26	large,extremely active, transverses the whole field quickly
T. brucei	present in all but stumpy forms central	small, subterminal	prominent	12-35*	large, rapid movements in confined areas
T. congolense	absent	medium, subterminal, marginal	not prominent	9-18	small, adheres to red blood cells by anterior end

* polymorphic: slender, intermediate and stumpy forms; *T. theileri* is frequently found in cattle and may be distinguished by its large size; *T. theileri* is more than twice the size of the pathogenic African trypanosomes

not raised within the tsetse-belt. The most pathogenic species for cattle is *T. congolense*, which causes an acute, lethal disease in zebu cattle. Some pure taurine cattle breeds are less susceptible and succumb less to the disease. *T. vivax* causes a less acute disease than *T. congolense*. In East Africa, however, *T. vivax* can cause an acute hemorrhagic syndrome. Development of clinical symptoms is slower but remissions are frequent. *T. brucei* causes a chronic infection without distinct symptoms.

A number of indigenous African taurine cattle breeds (e.g. N'Dama, Baoulé, West African Shorthorn and many others) are less susceptible to trypanosomosis (often referred to as "trypanotolerance"). These breeds are adapted to a certain environment and tsetse-challenge and may be an alternative way to control losses due to trypanosomosis. However, "trypanotolerance" is not an absolute trait and refers to a lower susceptibility of an indigenous breed to its innate environment. If such animals are kept under heavy trypanosomosis challenge they may equally succumb like other non-tolerant breeds. Many indigenous breeds of sheep and goats from western and Central Africa are also resistant to trypanosome infections.

Geographic distribution: *T. congolense* and *T. brucei* occur mainly within the tsetse-belt (area from latitude 15°N to 29°S) of Africa. *T. vivax* occurs in Africa within the tsetse-belt where it is transmitted by tsetse flies but also in non-tsetse areas (Central and South America, West India, Mauritius) where it may be transmitted by Tabanids and biting flies.

Symptoms: The primary clinical signs are intermittent fever, anaemia and weight loss. Cattle usually have a chronic course with a high mortality, especially if there are other stress factors such as poor nutrition or other diseases. Mortality rates are increased if çoncomitant infections with gastrointestinal helminths are present. Blood sucking nematodes (e.g. *Haemonchus contortus, Bunostomum* spp. and *Gaigeria* spp.) may severely aggravate the anaemia. Ruminants generally recover gradually if the number of infected tsetse flies is low. However, stress results in relapse.

Significance: Tsetse-transmitted trypanosomosis is one of the major constraints for cattle rearing within the tsetse-belt of Africa. Trypanosomes render their host more susceptible to other diseases (e.g. worm infections) which then may contribute to the high mortality.

Diagnosis: A presumptive diagnosis is based on finding an animal in poor condition in an endemic area. Confirmation depends on demonstrating trypanosomes in a wet mount of the buffy coat area of a PCV tube after centrifugation (☞ METHODS, 3.4). Other infections that cause anaemia and weight loss, such as gastrointestinal nematodes, babesiosis, anaplasmosis and theileriosis should be eliminated by further examinations. Various serological tests are suitable for herd and area screening rather than for individual diagnosis. Tests for the detection of circulating trypanosome species-specific antigens in peripheral blood may be useful for both individual and herd diagnosis.

Therapy: Most of the drugs commonly used to treat trypanosomosis (Table 8) have a narrow therapeutic index. Therefore the administration of the correct dosing is essential. Resistance to trypanocidal drugs is widespread and should be considered in refractory cases. The following compounds may be used in ruminants: Diminazene aceturate (3.5–7 mg/kg, im.), homidium bromide (1 mg/kg, im.), isometamidium (0.5–1 mg/kg, im.) and quinapyramine sulfate (5 mg/kg, sc.) (☞ Table 8). Concomitant gastrointestinal nematode infections should be treated at the same time and supportive treatment (e.g. iron dextrane) may help recovery (☞ CATTLE, ■ 1).

Prophylaxis: Control can be carried out at several levels. Attempts to eradicate tsetse flies have failed and are no longer justifiable. Tsetses can be partially controlled in the surrounding of a herd by spraying or dipping of animals. The strategic use of insecticide-impregnated screens may drastically reduce the tsetse population in the surrounding of herds and thus the infection risk. Pour-on application of insecticides on a herd level is an effective way of controlling both tsetse flies and fly nuisance (☞ CATTLE, ■ 5). Losses due to trypanosomosis are often drastically increased by other opportunistic infections (mainly gastrointestinal nematodes) and other stress fac-

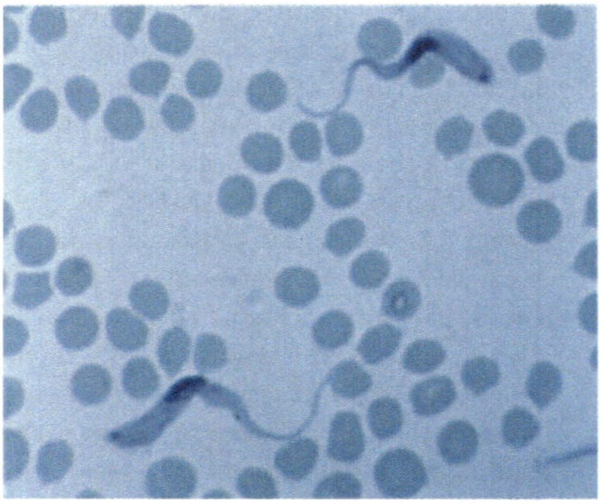

Fig. 101 *Trypanosoma vivax* (20–26 μm); Giemsa-stained bloodsmear [4]

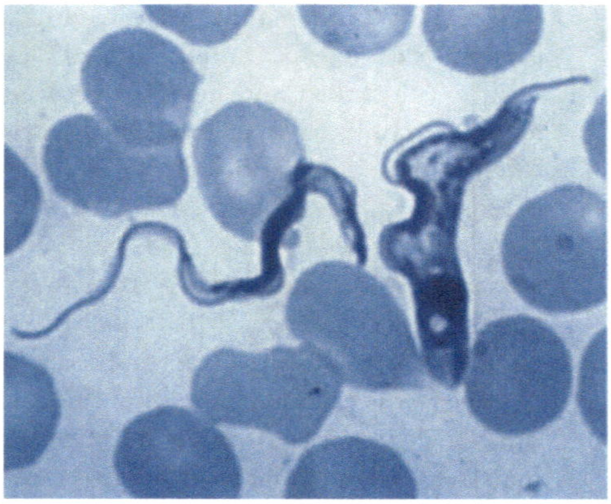

Fig. 102 *Trypanosoma brucei* (12–35 μm); Giemsa-stained bloodsmear; this species is polymorphic: slender form (left), stumpy form (right) [13]

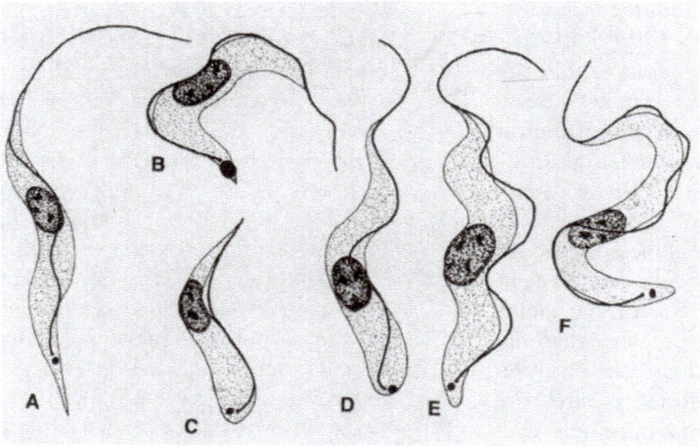

Fig. 103 Important *Trypanosoma* species of livestock: (a) *Trypanosoma theileri* (60–70 μm), (b) *T. cruzi*, (c) *T. congolense* (9–18 μm), (d) *T. vivax* (20–26 μm), (e) *T. equiperdum* (25 μm) and (f) *T. brucei* (12–35 μm, polymorphic) [14]

tors. Control measures should also include these factors. The prophylactic use of trypanocidal drugs requires a regular application of the drug and includes the risk of creating resistance. It should therefore be limited to emergencies, such as cattle trekking through infested areas and herds seasonally exposed to high trypanosomosis risk. Isometamidium (1–2 mg/kg, im.) protects cattle for 2 to 6 months. Prophylactic use of trypanocidal drugs should be avoided in cattle prior to slaughtering, since drug residues may be detrimental to human health. Proper nutrition is essential in all cases and the strategic application of crop residues at the late dry season may significantly improve the nutritional status and thus the resistance of animals in endemic areas. The exploitation and propagation of indigenous breeds can be a promising way of animal production in endemic areas.
(Figures 101, 102, 103, 104, 105, Table 6, Table 7, Table 8)

Table 8 Generic and trade names of trypanocides for the the treatment and prevention of animal trypanosomosis

Compound generic name	Trade name	Manufacturer	Action	Range of dosage Rates (mg/kg)	Route of administration	Remarks
Diminazene aceturate	Berenil	Hoechst AG, Germany	T	3.5-7.0	IM SC	Also babesiacidal; toxic to horses, donkeys, dogs, and camels
	Ganasag	Squibb, USA	T	3.5-7.0	IM or SC	
Homidium bromide	Ethidium	CAMCO Animal Health, UK	T(P)	1.0	IM	
Homidium chloride	Novidium	Rhône-Merieux, France	T(P)	1.0	IM	
Isometamidium	Samorin	Rhône-Merieux, France	P/T	0.25-1.0	IM, IV[3]	Toxic above 2 mg/kg; highly irritant; avoid SC administration
	Trypamidium	Rhône-Poulenc Sante France	P/T	0.25-1.0	M, IV[3]	
Ouinapyramine sulfate[1]*	Antrycide	Coopers Animal Health Ltd, UK	T	3.0-5.0	SC	Rest animals before and after treatment
Ouinapyramine prosalt[1]	Antrycide[2] R.F.	Coopers Animal Health Ltd, UK	PT	3.0-5.0	SC	Dosage calculated as sulfate
Suramin*	Naganol Antrypol	Bayer AG, Germany	T	10.0	IV	Severe local reactions by other routes
Melaminophenylarsine dihydrochloride	Cymelarsan	Rhône-Merieux, France	T	0.25-0.5	IM, SC	The IM route is preferred in equines. *T. evansi* and *T. brucei*

Many of these preparations are sold under a variety of trade names. Consult publications such as *Veterinary Pharmaceuticals and Biologicals*, 6th ed. Lenexa, KS, Veterinary Medicine Publishing Co, 1989/1990;
[1]Reintroduced in 1985 to treat mainly *T. evansi* infections;
[2]Prosalt. This is a mixture of sulfate and chloride salts of quinapyramine;
[3]Given by very slow injection of 1% W/V solution at 0.5 mg/kg;
T = therapeutic action; P = prophylactic action; (P) = short prophylactic activity; IM = intramuscular; IV = intravenous; SC = subcutaneous;
* no longer commercially available

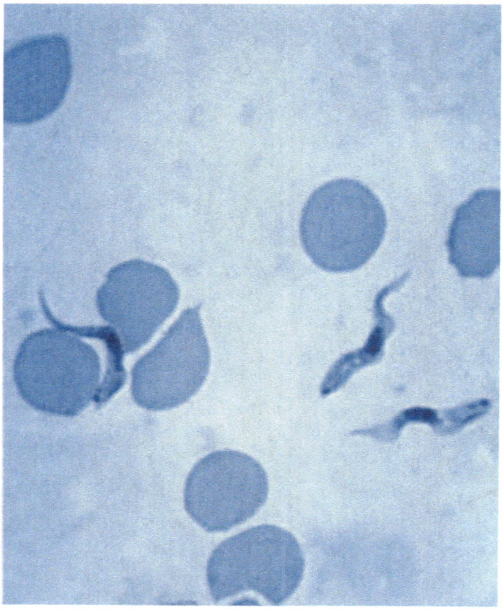

Fig. 104 *Trypanosoma congolense* (9–18 µm); Giemsa-stained bloodsmear [15]

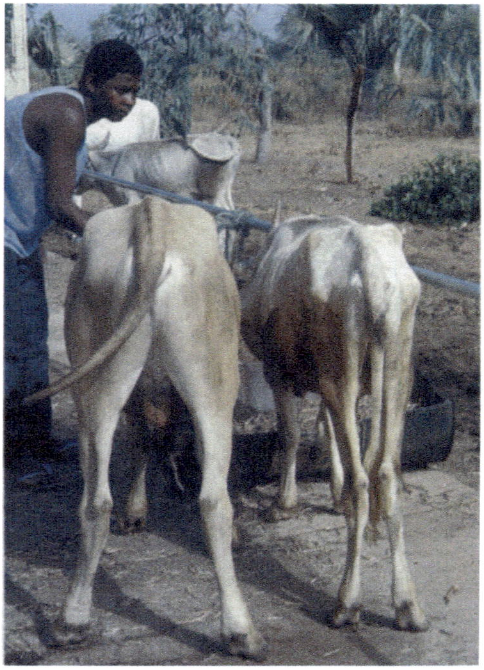

Fig. 105 Comparison of a trypano-tolerant N'Dama cattle (left) and susceptible zebu (right) after 15 weeks' exposure to a middle-grade tsetse challenge. Both animals were chronically infected with *Trypanosoma congolense* [36]

Trypanosoma evansi (syn. *T. brucei evansi*)
Surra

Remarks: *T. evansi* occurs in dromedaries, equines, buffaloes, carnivores and many other mammalian species. It occurs in North Africa, Asia, Middle and South America. The pathogenicity of *T. evansi* strains varies considerably but the highest pathogenicity is commonly observed in camels and equines (☞ DROMEDARIES, ■ 2). Several species of blood-sucking flies act as vectors. *T. evansi* is not transmitted by tsetse flies. No developmental stages have been demonstrated in the vectors which differentiate the parasite from *T. brucei*. *T. evansi* is 15–35 µm long and 1.5–2.5 µm wide. *T. evansi* is morphologically identical with *T. brucei* and other members of the subgenus Trypanozoon (☞ DROMEDARIES, ■ 2).

Trypanosoma theileri

Hosts: Cattle

Vector: Tabanid flies (*Tabanus* spp. and *Haematopota* spp.)

Species description: This is a large species (60–70 µm, sometimes up to 120 µm in length=twice the size of the pathogenic trypanosomes) and belongs to the Stercoraria. The undulating membrane is well developed and the free flagellum is well defined. Although the parasite is considered as non-pathogenic it may assume increased significance when stress conditions arise or when concurrent infections with other pathogens are present.

Geographic distribution: World-wide
Symptoms: Infections are often asymptomatic.
Significance: This species may be very prevalent but it seems to be nonpathogenic.
Diagnosis: ☞ above *T. congolense*, *T. vivax*, *T. brucei*
Therapy and Prophylaxis: Generally not indicated
(Figure 106)

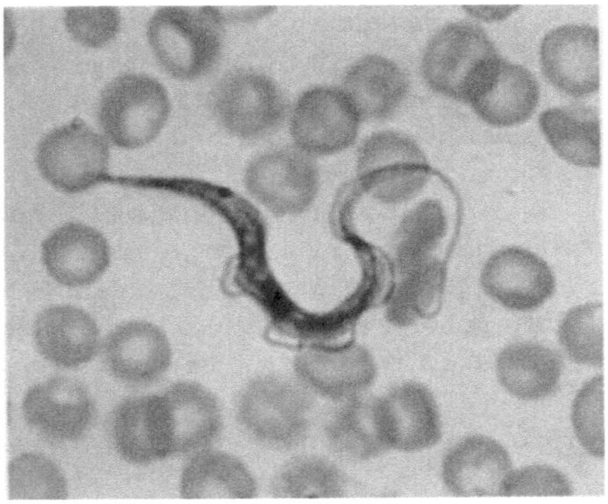

Fig. 106 *T. theileri* (60–70 µm, sometimes up to 120 µm); Giemsa-stained bloodsmear [4]

BABESIIDAE

Babesia bovis

Redwater, tropical bovine babesiosis

Hosts: Cattle
Vector: *Boophilus* spp. (*B. microplus, B. annulatus*) and possibly *Rhipicephalus bursa*.
Species description: This is a small form, 2.4 × 1.5 µm and slightly larger than *B. divergens*. The organisms (merozoites) are usually found in the centre of the erythrocytes. Vacuolated "signet-ring" forms are especially common. Transovarian transmission occurs in the ticks.
Geographic distribution: Tropical Africa, Madagascar, Mediterranean basin and southern Europe
Significance: The disease caused by *B. bovis* is similar to that caused by *B. bigemina*. Affected animals may die. The strains vary in virulence. In some regions *B. bovis* is more virulent than *B. bigemina*.
(Figures 107, 108)

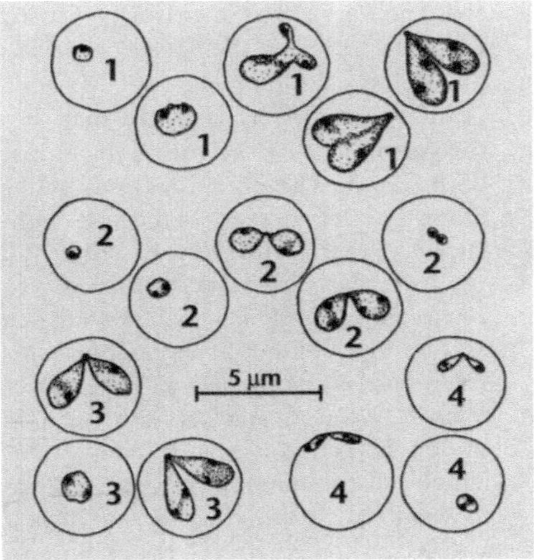

Fig. 107 Morphology of bovine *Babesia* spp. 1 *Babesia bigemina* , 2 *Babesia bovis* , 3 *Babesia major* and 4 *Babesia divergens* [16]

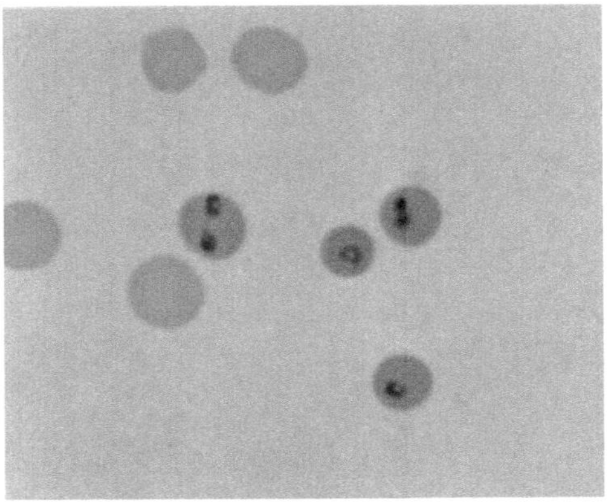

Fig. 108 *Babesia bovis* (2.4 × 1.5 µm, "small form"); Giemsa-stained bloodsmear [4]

Babesia divergens
European bovine babesiosis

Hosts: Cattle
Vector: *Ixodes ricinus* and possibly other ticks
Species description: This species is smaller than *B. bovis*. The merozoites usually occur as paired, club-shaped organisms about 1.5 × 0.4 µm. The angle between the pair is relatively large, so that they diverge more from each other than those of *B. bovis*. The organisms tend to lie along the circumference of the host erythrocyte. Other forms may be stout and pyriform, measuring 2 × 1 µm; some may be circular and others may be vacuolated and up to 2 µm in diameter. Transovarian transmission occurs in the vector. Highest parasitaemia levels are found during the period of high fever.
Geographic distribution: Northwestern Africa in woodlands at altitudes above 1000 m. It also occurs in northern and central Europe.
Significance: The disease entity produced by *B. divergens* is less severe than that caused by *B. bigemina*. In severe infections death may occur.
(Figure 109)

Babesia bigemina (syn. *Piroplasma bigeminum*), Redwater, tropical bovine piroplasmosis, tick fever, "Texas fever"

Hosts: Cattle
Vector: *Boophilus* spp. (*B. microplus, B. decoloratus, B. calcaratus*), *Rhipicephalus* spp. (*R. evertsi, R. bursa* and *R. appendiculatus*), and *Haemaphysalis* spp. (*H. punctata*)
Species description: This is a large form, 4–5 µm by 2 µm wide. Round forms are 2–3 µm in diameter. The organisms are characteristically pear-shaped and lie in pairs forming an acute angle in the erythrocyte. Round, oval or irregularly shaped forms may occur, depending on the stage of development. Transovarian transmission occurs in the ticks. *B. bigemina* is one of the most pathogenic *Babesia* species known.
Geographic distribution: Tropical Africa, Madagascar, Mediterranean basin and many other parts of the world
Significance: *B. bigemina* is one of the most important diseases of cattle in some tropical and subtropical areas.
(Figure 110)

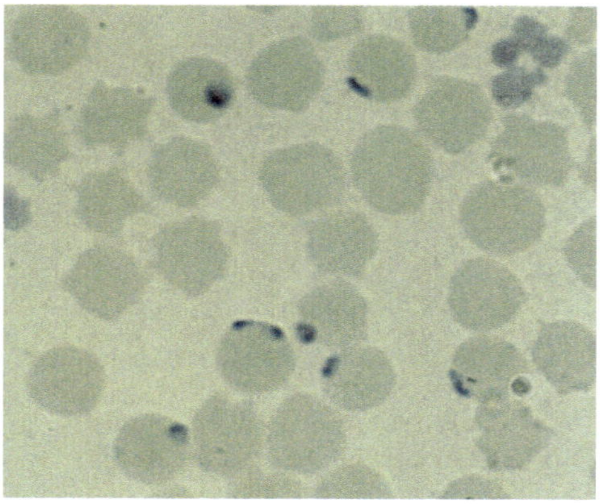

Fig. 109 *Babesia divergens* (1.5 × 0.4 µm); Giemsa-stained bloodsmear [4]

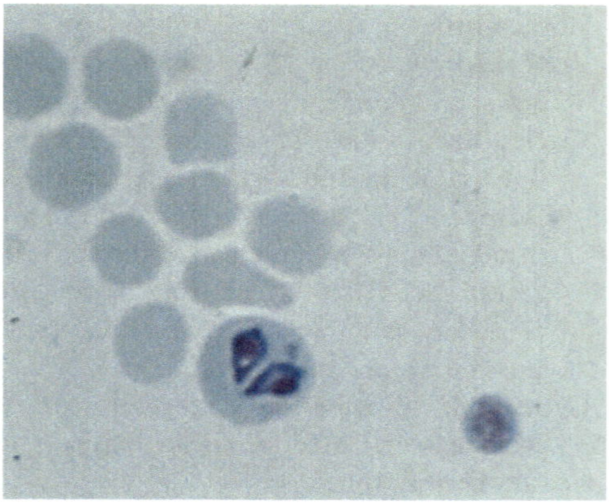

Fig. 110 *Babesia bigemina* (4–5 × 2 µm, "large form"); Giemsa-stained bloodsmear [4]

Babesia major (syn. *Piroplasma major*)

European bovine piroplasmosis

Hosts: Cattle

Vector: *Haemaphysalis punctata*

Species description: This species resembles *B. bigemina* except that it lies in the centre of the erythrocyte. The pyriform bodies are 2.6 × 1.5 µm and the angle formed by the organisms is less than 90°. Round forms are about 1.8 µm in diameter. Transovarian transmission may occur in the tick vector.

Geographic distribution: North Africa, Europe, UIS, South America

Significance: *B. major* is less pathogenic than *B. bovis*. Clinical signs are moderate and sometimes infections are inapparent.

(Figure 111)

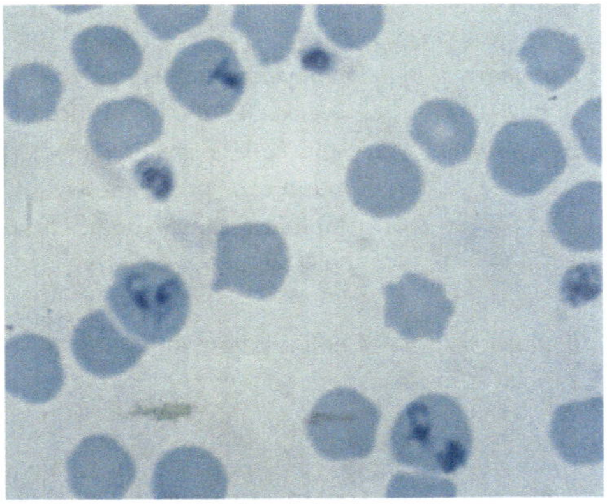

Fig. 111 *Babesia major* (2.6 × 1.5 µm); Giemsa-stained bloodsmear [15]

- **General features of bovine babesiosis**

Symptoms: Infections with *B. bigemina*, *B. major* and *B. divergens* are characterised by a haemolytic syndrome (haemolytic babesiosis), including continuous fever (40–41°C), high parasitaemia (2.5–10%), anaemia, icterus (intense yellow-brownish ocular, gingival and vaginal mucosae) and haemoglobinuria (dark brown, frothy urine) and general depression. Abortion and agalactia in dairy cows are early signs. The symptoms are less pronounced in the subacute form. *B. bovis* infections are dominated by a shock syndrome, leading to death following a steep rise in temperature in the peracute form. Acute disease is accompanied by fever, ataxia, pedalling movements and overt agressivity (attacks). Haemolysis, icterus and haemoglobinuria are less apparent than in other babesioses.

Significance: Widespread throughout the tropics, causing heavy losses in non-resistant (often imported) livestock. Without treatment mortality rates are very high (30% for *B. bigemina*, 70–80% for *B. bovis*). *B. bigemina* is one of the most important diseases of cattle in some tropical and subtropical areas.

Diagnosis: Clinical diagnosis is difficult and can be confused with leptospirosis (peracute disease), anaplasmosis (chronic in nature) or cowdriosis (no movements). Splenomegaly, icterus and haemoglobinuria and thickened bile in the gall bladder are characteristics of haemolytic babesiosis. Petechiae and microinfarcts suggest infections with *B. bovis*. The presence of Babesia parasites in the blood smears of animals without clinical symptoms does not necessarily support the diagnosis of babesiosis. It can be a resurgence of a chronic infection following an immunosuppression due to another disease. In *B. bigemina* infections the severity of the disease can be deducted from the percentage of parasitized red blood cells (< 0.1% mild, 0.5–1% subacute, 5–10% severe infection), whereas in *B. bovis* infections the presence of parasites indicates babesiosis, because parasite concentration in the peripheral blood is considerably lower than in the organs. In acute *B. bovis* infections impression smears of congested organs show punctiform babesial bodies in agglutinated erythrocytes. Serological techniques (IFAT, ☞ METHODS, 5.1) are available and should be used especially in epidemiological studies. For the individual

Table 9 Drugs used in the treatment of babesiosis in cattle

Drug	Dosage	AM	Parasite	Remark
Trypan blue*	2-3 mg/kg	IV	*B. bigemina*	Not effective against small babesias; discouloration of animal's flesh; can cause severe tissue sloughing if not given IV
Acridine derivatives				
Euflavine[1]*	4-8 ml/100 kg as 5% solution	IV	*B. bigemina* *B. bovis* *B. divergens*	Highly irritant if not given IV
Diamidine derivatives				
Amicarbalide Diampron[1]	5-10 mg/kg	IM	*B. bigemina* *B. divergens* *B. bovis*	
Diminazene Berenil[2]	3-5 mg/kg	IM	*B. bigemina* *B. bovis* *B. divergens*	
Imidocarb	1-3 mg/kg Imizol[3]	SC or IM	*B. bigemina* *B. bovis* *B. divergens*	Prophylactic activity up to 8 weeks depending on dose and *Babesia spp.* involved; nephrotoxic; cholinesterase inhibitor; slowly metabolized and eliminated–tissue
Phenamidine Lomadine[1]	8-13.5 mg/kg	SC or IM	*B. bigemina* *B. bovis*	Cholinesterase inhibition
Quinoline derivatives				
Quinuronium Babesan[4]	1 mg/kg	SC	*B. bigemina* *B. bovis* *B. divergens*	Low therapeutic index Slow effect against *B. bovis* Side effects associated with the stimulation of the parasympathetic nervous system

Many of these preparations are sold under a variety of trade names; * no longer commercially available; IM = intramuscular; IV = intravenous; SC = subcutaneous; AM = application method;

[1] May & Baker Ltd., Dagenham, England. [2] Hoechst AG, Frankfurt, Germany. [3] Burroughs Wellcome & Co., London, England. [4] ICI-, Macclesfield, Cheshire, England

diagnosis the demonstration of the parasite in the bloodsmear or with the QBC method (☞ METHODS, 3.1 and 3.3) is more adequate.

Therapy: Diminazene aceturate (3.5 mg/kg, im.), Imidocarb dipropionate (1.2–2.4 mg/kg, sc.), quinuronium sulfate (1–2 mg/kg, sc. or im.) and amicarbalide diisethionate (5–10 mg/kg, im.) can be used against the pathogenic *Babesia* species of cattle (☞ Table 9).

Two points should be considered: 1) For serious clinical attacks the dose should be split to avoid shock due to massive destruction of *Babesia*. 2) Most babesicidal drugs are toxic to the host, so caution is required in their use. The commonly used babesicidal compounds are listed in Table 9. In endemic areas it is preferable to support immunity within the population, as such animals can withstand repeated infections. The aim of therapy is therefore to reduce but not to eradicate the parasite concentration within the host. In severely affected animals emphasis should also be given to supportive treatment (electrolytes, rehydration, iron-dextran, etc.) and rich nutrition during the convalescence.

Prophylaxis: Several methods are used in endemic areas to control or prevent babesiosis.

- Controlled immunisation, using babe sicidal-drugs:
  Application of a babesicidal drug (e.g. diminazene aceturate, 3.5 mg/kg, im.) following inoculation of a non-attenuated *Babesia* strain.
- Imidocarb (2 mg/kg) is administered to an animal prior to the introduction onto an infected pasture. The delayed action of imidocarb controls clinical infection (up to 60 days for *B. bigemina* and up to 21 days for *B. divergens* and *B. bovis*) without blocking the immune response.
- Immunization with attenuated *B. bovis* and *B. bigemina* strains:
  Inoculation of a attenuated *Babesia* strains. Several research teams are presently working on the development of *Babesia* vaccines in cattle. In some countries vaccines are available.
- Prophylaxis through tick control:
  In tropical Africa and the Mediterranean region tick control is essential (☞ CATTLE, ■ 5) and should be made weekly during periods of adult tick activity.

(Figure 112, Table 9)

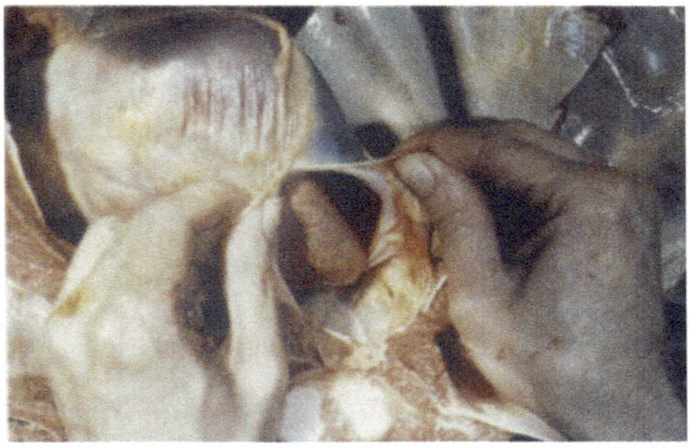

Fig. 112 Icterus and hydropericardium caused by *Babesia bigemina* infection [8]

THEILERIIDAE

Theileriosis is caused by protozoan parasites of the genus *Theileria*. In cattle, there are two highly pathogenic species. *Theileria parva* is the cause of East Coast Fever in East and Central Africa. A variant regarded as either a subspecies, *T. parva lawrencei*, or a type, *T. parva* (*lawrencei* type), is a common benign parasite of the African buffalo (*Syncerus caffer*), which, when transmitted to cattle, causes a condition called corridor disease. *T. parva* (*bovis* type) causes the "January disease" in Zimbabwe. *Theileria annulata* causes tropical theileriosis, which is widespread through the Mediterranean basin, the Middle East and Asia. Other species that infect cattle in Africa are *T. mutans*, *T. taurotragi* and *T. velifera*. They are usually benign, although *T. mutans* may be pathogenic under some circumstances. *T. orientalis* is a generally benign species found in the Mediterranean basin, the Middle

East, Asia and Australia which may cause disease in imported cattle.
(Figures 113, 114, 115)

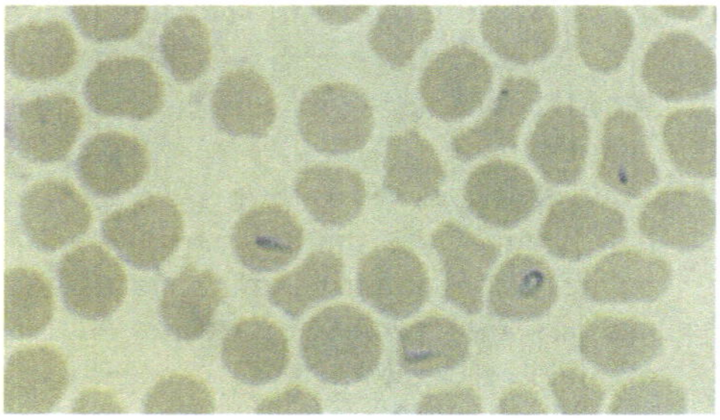

Fig. 113 *Theileria orientalis*; Giemsa-stained blood smear; this species occurs outside of Africa and is lowly pathogenic [4]

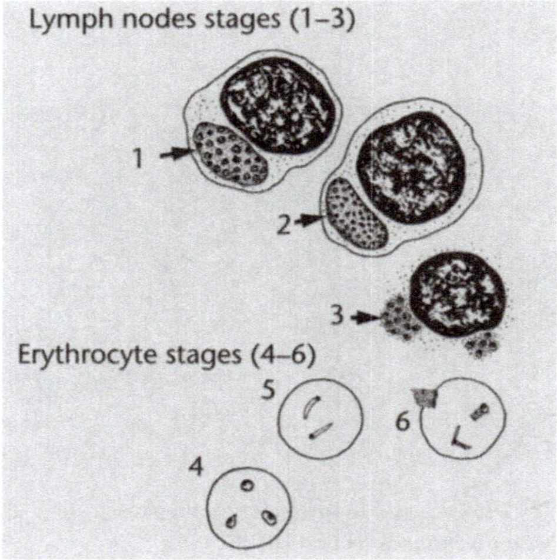

Fig. 114 Morphology of *Theileria* spp. stages in mammals; stages found in the lymph nodes: (1) Macroschizont with medium-sized nuclei (0.4–2 µm; Koch's blue bodies), (2) Microschizont with small nuclei (0.3–0.8 µm) and (3) Merozoites (0.7–1 µm); stages found in the erythrocytes: intra-erythrocytic stages may be (4) circular, oval or piriform (0.8 x1.5 µm; 80%) or (5) comma-shaped (0.5 × 2 µm; 20%); (6) some parasites appear to have a velum [16]

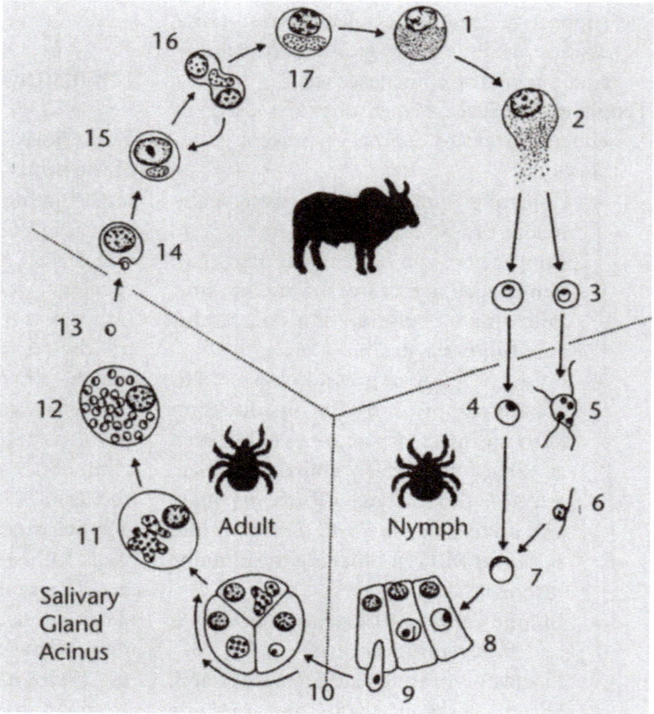

Fig. 115 Life cycle of *Theileria parva* [17]
(1) Merogony, (2) Merozoites (3) Piroplasm in erythrocyte, (4) Macromete, (5) Syngamy, (6) Microgamete, (7) Zygote in gut lumen, (8) Gut epithelial cells, (9) Kinete, (10) Moult, (11) Sporogony, (12) Sporozoites, (13) Sporozoite in saliva, (14) Sporozoite enters lymphocyte, (15) Schizont in lymphoblast, (16) Clonal expansion, (17) Schizont

Theileria parva (syn. *T. bovis, T. lawrencei*)
East Coast Fever, bovine theileriosis, Corridor Disease, Rhodesian tick fever

Hosts: Cattle, water buffalo, African buffalo

Vector: *Rhipicephalus appendiculatus* (equatorial East Africa and southern Africa above 1200 m) and *Rhipicephalus duttoni* (Angola plateau). Other vectors are *Rhipicephalus zambeziensis, Hyalomma excavatum, H. dromedarii, H. truncatum* and some other *Rhipicephalus* spp.

Species description: *T. parva* causes a disease called East Coast Fever (ECF), which is responsible for high mortality among susceptible and imported stock. The zebu in endemic areas has a high natural resistance, but animals imported into endemic areas are highly susceptible. Transmission of the parasite in all is on a stage to stage basis (trans-stadial transmission). There is no transovarial transmission in the tick vector as in *Babesia* spp. The organisms occur both in erythrocytes and in lymphocytes. The forms in the red blood cells are mainly rod-shaped, 1.5–2 × 0.5–1 µm, but round, oval, comma- and ring-shaped forms may also occur (Fig. 114, 4–6). Several parasites may occur in individual erythrocytes but there is no multiplication in the red cells. The multiplying forms of the parasite occur in the cytoplasm of lymphocytes and occasionally in the endothelial cells of the lymphatic glands and the spleen. These are schizonts, being circular or irregularly shaped structures about 8 µm in diameter. Two forms of schizonts are recognized. Those which contain large chromatin granules, 0.4–2 µm in diameter, are termed macroschizonts and produce macromerozoites, 2–2.5 µm in diameter (Fig. 114, 1). The other forms contain smaller chromatin granules, 0.3–0.8 µm in diameter, and are referred to as microschizonts and produce micromerozoites (Fig. 114, 2). The latter invade the red blood cells and may represent sexual stages of the parasite. After the intraerythrocytic stages are ingested by ticks, merozoites are liberated and differentiate into sexual stages. There is a sexual development of *T. parva* in the tick vector which results in infective sporozoites. Cattle are infected when vector ticks engorge on an animal and these infective particles (sporozoites) are transmitted. Most recovered animals remain carriers of infection.

Geographic distribution: East, Central and South Africa according to the distribution of the main vector *Rhipicephalus appendiculatus*.

Symptoms: High fever, swelling of the lymph nodes, dyspnoea and death. Fever occurs 7–10 days after the tick bite and continues throughout the course of the disease and may reach > 42°C. Lymph node swelling becomes pronounced and generalized. Anorexia, loss of condition, lacrimation and nasal discharge may occur. Terminally, dyspnoea is common. Just before death, a sharp fall in temperature occurs and pulmonary exsudate pours from the nostrils. Anaemia is not a major diagnostic sign as it is in babesiosis.

Significance: ECF is a serious disease with high mortality in susceptible stock.

Diagnosis: Lymphoblasts in Giemsa-stained lymph node biopsy smears (☞ METHODS, 3.1) during the acute febrile phase contain multinuclear schizonts. Lymph node enlargement and massive pulmonary oedema and hyperaemia are the most striking post-mortem lesions. Haemorrhages are common on the serosal and mucosal surfaces of many organs.

Therapy: Cattle with clinical ECF may be treated with parvaquone (2 × 10–20 mg/kg, im. at 48 h intervals),buparvaquone (2 × 2.5 mg/kg, im. at 48 h intervals) or with the coccidiostat halofuginone (2 × 1.2 mg/kg, po. at 48 h intervals). Chlortetracycline and oxytetracyline are relatively ineffective. None of these drugs will sterilize infections, and recovered animals may be carriers.

Prophylaxis: Immunization of cattle using an infection-and-treatment procedure is practical and relatively effective. The components for this procedure are cryopreserved sporozoite stabilates of the appropriate strains of *Theileria* derived from infected ticks and a single dose of either long-acting oxytetracycline or buparvaquone given simultaneously or of parvaquone given 1 week after infection. Cattle should be immunized 3–4 weeks before being turned out onto infected pasture. The incidence of ECF can be reduced by regular tick control, but in many areas this means biweekly acaricidal treatments. The use of pour-on acaricides is a promising way of tick control in endemic areas (☞ CATTLE, ■ 5.1) (Figures 116, 117, 118, 119, 120, 121, 122, 123)

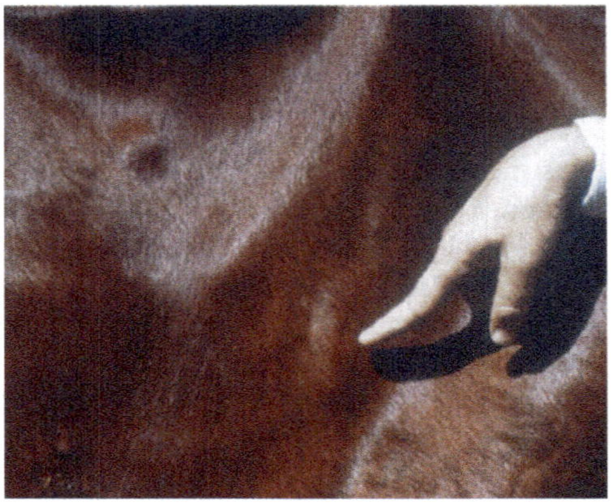

Fig. 118 Lymph node swelling in a *Theileria parva* infected cattle [4]

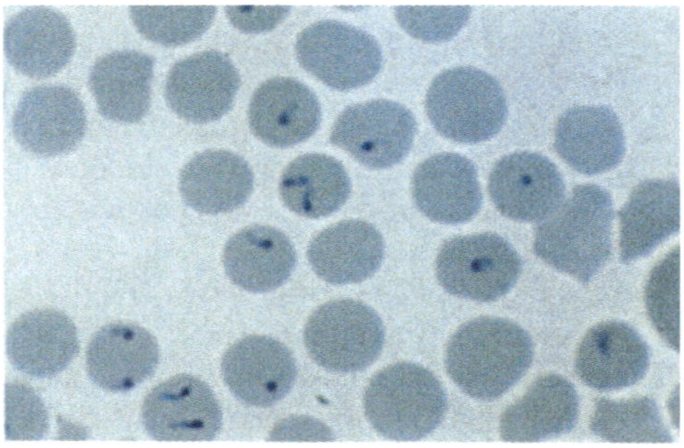

Fig. 116 *Theileria parva*; erythrocyte forms [4]

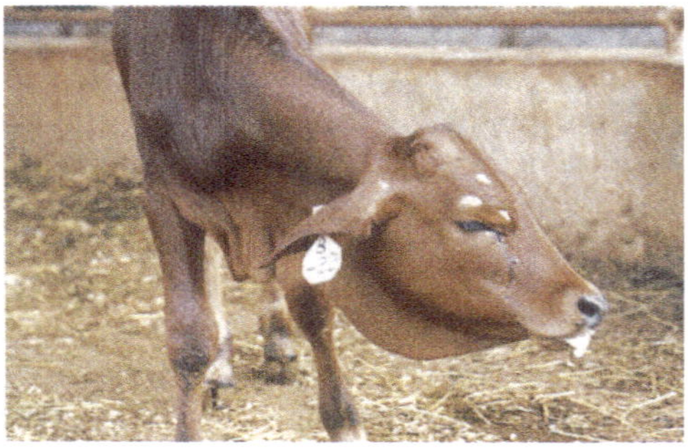

Fig. 119 Lacrimation and nasal discharges in a *Theileria parva* infected cattle [8]

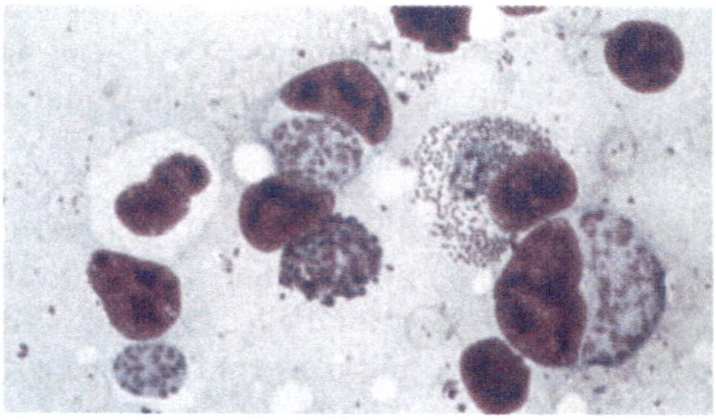

Fig. 117 *Theileria* sp.; macroschizonts ("Koch's blue bodies"and microschizonts in lymph node smears [4]

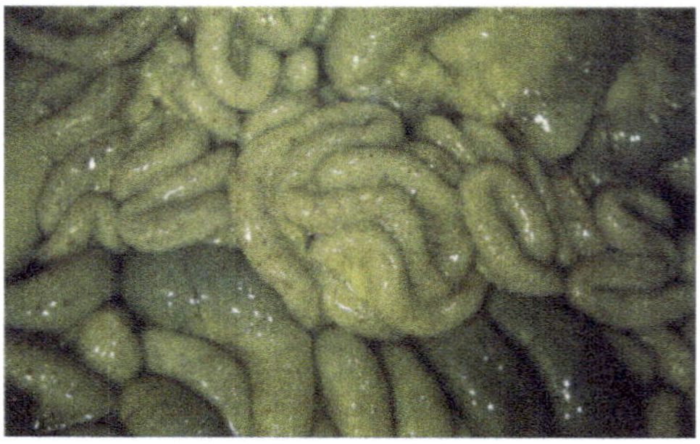

Fig. 120 *Theileria parva*; petechial haemorrhage on the intestinal serosa [8]

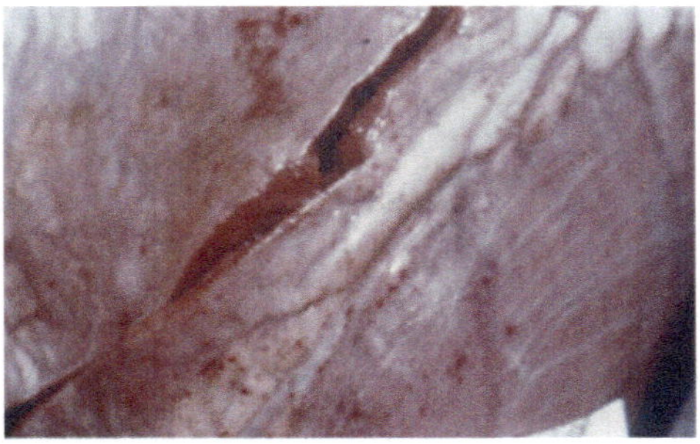

Fig. 121 *Theileria parva*; petechial haemorrhage on the surface (epicard) of the heart [8]

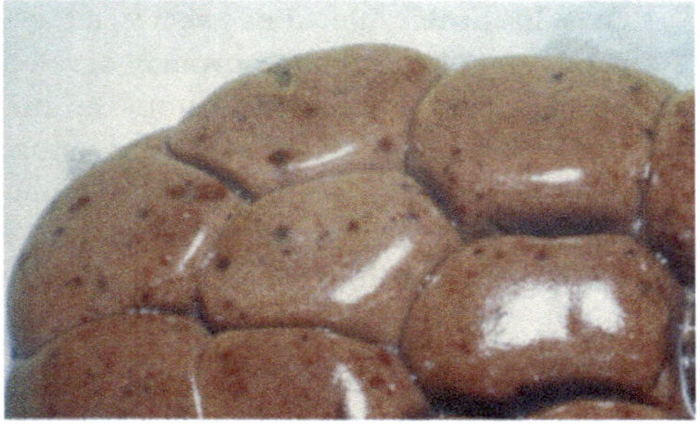

Fig. 123 *Theileria parva*; petechial haemorrhage on the kidneys [15]

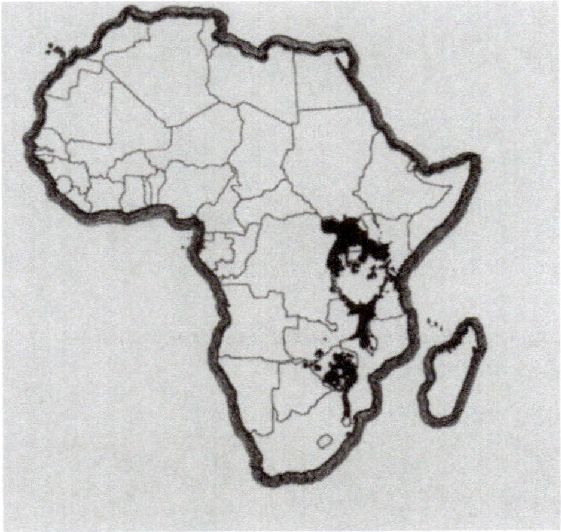

Fig. 122 The reported distribution of *Theileria parva* [17]

Theileria annulata Mediterranean Coast Fever, Tropical theileriosis, Egyptian ever

Hosts: Cattle, water buffalo

Vector: *Hyalomma* spp. (*H. detritum, H. truncatum, H. anatolicum* and other *Hyalomma* spp.)

Species description: *T. annulata* produces a highly fatal disease of cattle in North Africa. Mortality rates may be up to 90% in some regions. This species occurs commonly in the lymphocytes and erythrocytes of bovine species. The organisms in the red blood cells are more or less indistinguishable from those of *T. parva*. They occur more commonly as round, oval- or ring-shaped (0.5–1.5 µm) forms. Rod shapes, commas (1.6 µm) and anaplasma-like organisms may also occur. Macroschizonts and microschizonts are found in the lymphocytes of the spleen and lymph nodes. *T. annulata* is transmissible by blood passage, and schizonts are numerous in the circulating blood. The development cycle in the vertebrate host is comparable to that of *T. parva*. The disease may be acute (duration: 3–4 days) or more chronic (duration: 2–3 weeks) in nature. The incubation period is 9–25 days. Animals that recover from *T. annulata* infections are resistant to reinfection. There is no cross-immunity between *T. annulata, T. parva* and *T. mutans*. The multiplication of *Demodex* sp. and *Besnoitia besnoiti* cysts in the subcutis is favoured by the immunosuppression produced by *Theileria* infections.

Geographic distribution: North Africa, Sudan, Mauretania, Ethiopia, southern Europe, southern UIS and Asia.

Symptoms: Fever (40–41.5°C), depression, lacrimation, nasal discharge and swelling of the superficial lymph nodes; emaciation rapidly occurs. A few days after the initial symptoms marked anaemia, jaundice (bilirubinaemia) develop. Haemoglobinuria may occur, but is not always present. In acute cases animals may die within 1–2 days. In chronic infections a very heterogeneous complex of symptoms may develop over the period of 2 months until the animal recovers. Decreased milk production, digestive disturbances (cessation of rumination, diarrhoea or constipation) and infertility (abortion) may be seen. The severity of the disease does not necessarily correspond to the level of parasitaemia. Similarities with babesiosis may occur and must be differentiated.

Significance: *T. annulata* may cause mortalities of up to 90% in certain areas. It causes one of the most important diseases of cattle in endemic regions.

Diagnosis: This is based on the demonstration of parasites in the red blood cells or in stained smears (☞ METHODS, 3.1) taken from lymph node or spleen biopsies. The differentiation between *T. parva* and *T. annulata* organisms is difficult but the geographic spread of these two diseases is quite different. *T. annulata* often occurs together with *Babesia* spp. and/or *Anaplasma* spp. At necropsy the mucosa membranes of the abomasum and the small intestine show characteristic ulcers (2–12 mm in diameter), surrounded by an inflammation. Multiple petechiae may be found on the epi- and endocardium. The spleen, liver and lymph nodes are markedly enlarged.

Therapy: Tetracyclines have both prophylactic and therapeutic activity against *T. annulata*. Rolitetracycline (4 mg/kg, im.) administered daily during 4 days moderated the clinical signs markedly. Similar results were achieved by a single injection of a long-acting oxytetracycline formulation (20 mg/kg).

Prophylaxis: Immunization of cattle using an infection- and -treatment procedure is very effective and widely used. The application of 2 × 10^6 parasitised lymphoblasts obtained from subcultured *T. annulata* strains were inoculated into animals prior to exposure. No clinical signs developed and the animals were able to withstand heavy natural challenge. Another possibility is to apply a single injection of a long-acting oxytetracycline formulation (20 mg/kg) prior to exposure. Regular tick control of herds in endemic areas may markedly reduce the disease incidence (☞ CATTLE, ■ 5.1 THERAPY AND PROPHYLAXIS OF ECTOPARASITES, p. 141).
(Figures 124, 125)

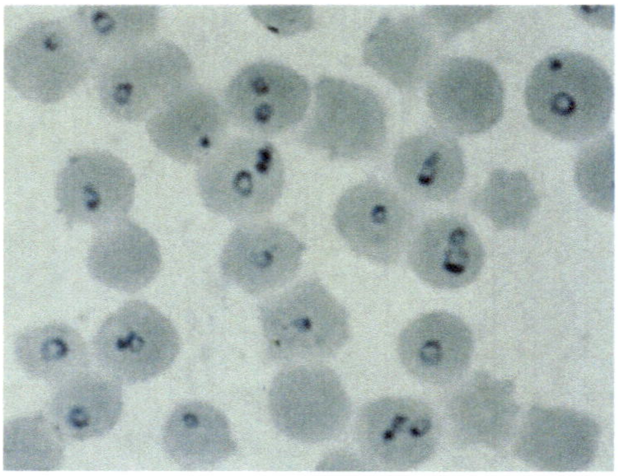

Fig. 124 *Theileria annulata*; erythrocyte forms (experimental infection) [4]

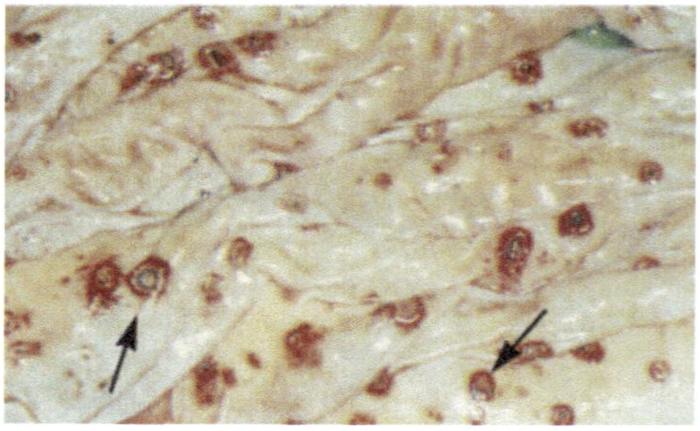

Fig. 125 Abomasal ulcerations caused by *Theileria parva* and *Theileria annulata* [15]

Theileria mutans Benign bovine theileriosis

Hosts: Cattle

Vector: *Amblyomma variegatum* and *Amblyomma hebraeum*

Species description: *T. mutans* causes a mild bovine theileriosis which is usually nonfatal. Morphologically it is not distinguishable from the pathogenic *T. parva* and *T. annulata*. The forms in the erythrocytes are round, oval, piriform, comma-shaped or *Anaplasma*-like. The round forms are 1–2 µm in diameter and the oval forms measure 1.5 × 0.6 µm. Binary fission occurs in the erythrocytes. The incubation period is 10–20 days.

Geographic distribution: Throughout Africa, Madagascar, Réunion, Mauritius, southern Europe, Asia, Australia, UIS, Caribbean

Symptoms: Similar to a mild form of *T. annulata* infection. Anaemia is the major clinical sign. Icterus and lymph node swellings may occur.

Significance: *T. mutans* is usually only slightly- or non-pathogenic for indigenous cattle in endemic areas. An acute form may develop in cattle imported into an endemic area. The mortality is generally less than 1%.

Diagnosis: Same as for other *Theileria* species

Therapy: Unknown; the same drugs as for the pathogenic *Theileria* species may be used.

Prophylaxis: Tick control and immunisation as for the pathogenic *Theileria* species.

(Figures 126, 127, 128)

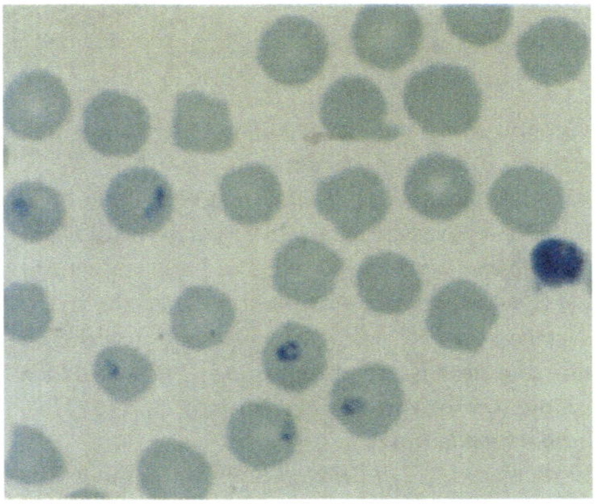

Fig. 126 *Theileria mutans*; erythrocyte forms [4]

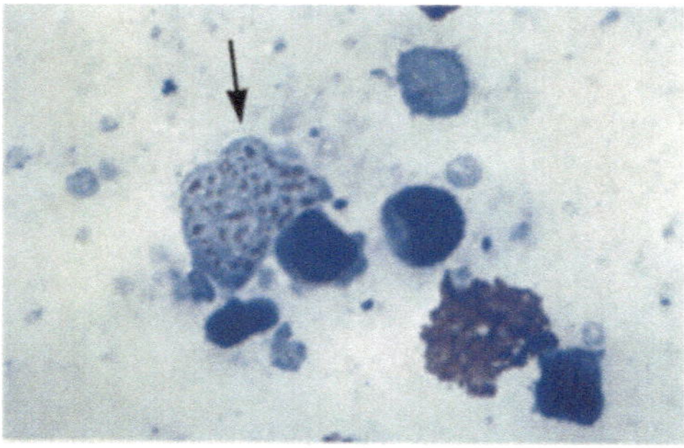

Fig. 127 *Theileria mutans*; macroschizont (rarely encountered) [15]

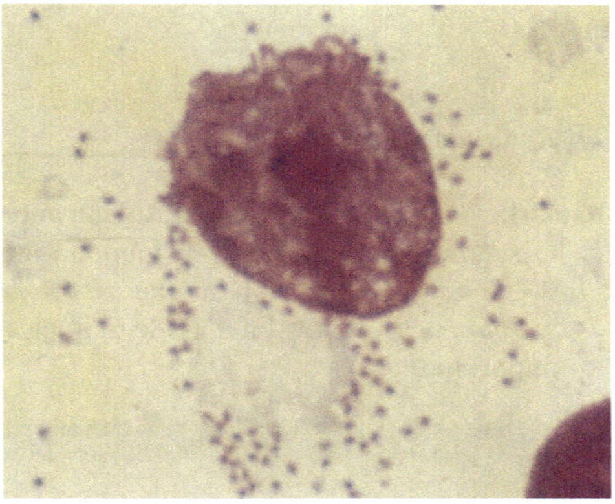

Fig. 128 *Theileria mutans*; microschizonts (rarely encountered) [15]

Theileria velifera

Remarks: This is another mild *Theileria* species of cattle in Africa and in the Caribbean. Its distribution coincides with that of the vector *Amblyomma variegatum* (Africa and Madagascar) and *Amblyomma lepidum* and *Amblyomma hebraeum* elsewhere. The parasites occur as pleomorphic or rod-shaped bodies in the erythrocytes and presumably lymphocytes. Most are 1–2 µm long. The great majority have a rectangular "veil" 1.0–3.5 µm long, extending out from the side. This species is nonpathogenic.

(Figure 129)

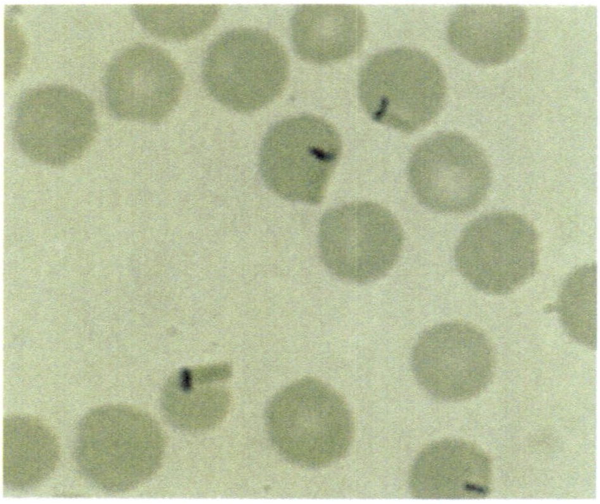

Fig. 129 *Theileria velifera*; erythrocyte forms [4]

Theileria taurotragi

Remarks: This species is found in African antelopes and can occasionally be found in cattle. It can also develop in the vector of *T. parva*. It is of low epidemiological importance.

RICKETTSIALES

ANAPLASMATACEAE

Anaplasma spp.

Anaplasmoses are infectious diseases, virulent, inoculable and not directly transmitted, that affect domestic and wild ungulates. The causative agent is a Rickettsia of the genus *Anaplasma*, usually transmitted by ticks, but which may also be transmitted mechanically by biting Diptera (*Tabanidae, Stomoxys*). The pathological signs are progressive anaemia (acute or slow) ending in cachexia and death. *Anaplasma* are exclusively found within erythrocytes. They are located intracellularly and surrounded by a vacuolar invagination of the host cell. The infection starts with an initial body that grows to become an elementary body. This multiplies by doubling or binary fission to produce new initial bodies. After several binary fissions, initial bodies accumulate in the vacuole to leave the host cell in order to parasitize other erythrocytes. The different *Anaplasma* species are morphologically indistinguishable. The criterion used is the location of the organism in the erythrocyte (marginal or central). (Figure 130)

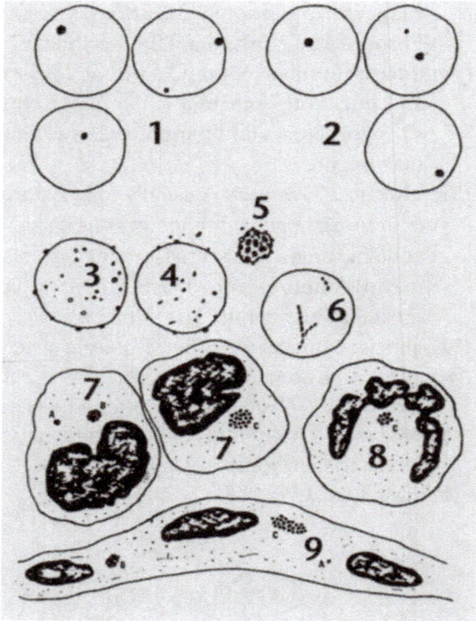

Fig. 130 Morphology (schematic) of various Rickettsiales found in ruminants;
Anaplasmataceae: (1) *Anaplasma marginale* (80–90% parasites marginal or peripheral); (2) *Anaplasma centrale* (80–90% of parasites central); (3) *Eperythrozoon wenyoni*, (on the erythrocyte surface); (4) *Eperythrozoon teganodes* (on the surface and near the erythrocyte); (5) *Eperythrozoon tuomii* (on the thrombocyte surface) and (6) *Haemobartonella bovis*;
Ehrlichiaceae: (7) *Ehrlichia bovis* (in monocytes); (8) *Ehrlichia phagocytophila* (in granulocyte) and (9) *Cowdria ruminantium* (in the vascular endothelium);
development stages: A = elementary body, B = initial body amd C = mass of elementary bodies [16]

Anaplasma marginale The malignant anaplasmosis of cattle, Gallsickness

Remarks: 80–90% of the organisms are peripheral. *A. marginale* is distributed throughout the tropics corresponding to the distribution area of *Boophilus decoloratus* and *Boophilus microplus* usually considered as the main vectors. Transplacental infection occurs.
(Figures 130, 131)

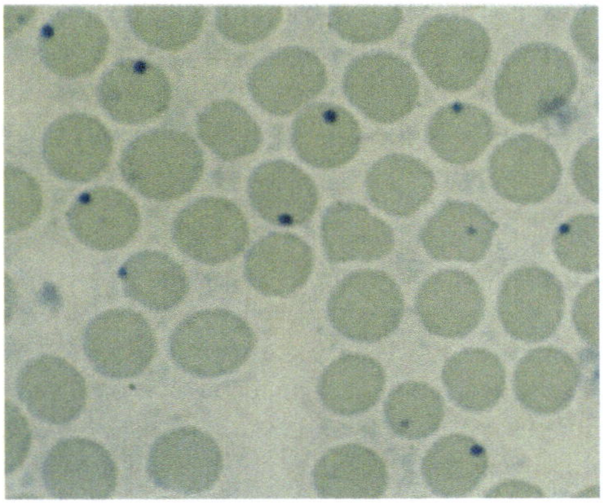

Fig. 131 *Anaplasma marginale*; Giemsa-stained bloodsmear [4]

Anaplasma centrale Mild anaplasmosis of cattle, Gallsickness

Remarks: *A. centrale* is predominantly located in the centre of the erythrocytes. The distribution and vectors are the same as in *A. marginale*. Anaplasmosis due to *A. marginale* is generally mild and often clinically inapparent.
(Figures 130, 132, 133)

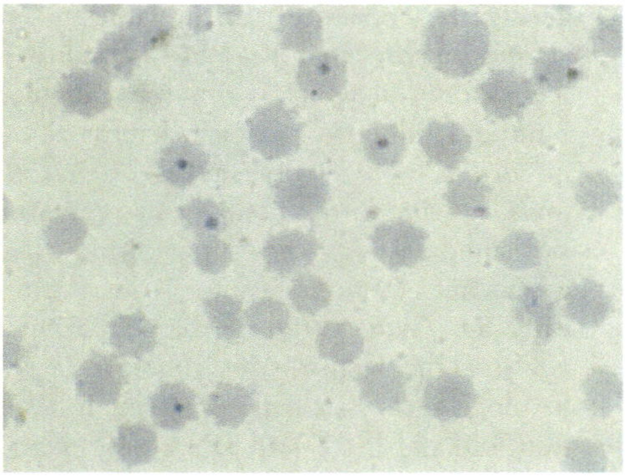

Fig. 132 *Anaplasma centrale*; Giemsa-stained bloodsmear [4]

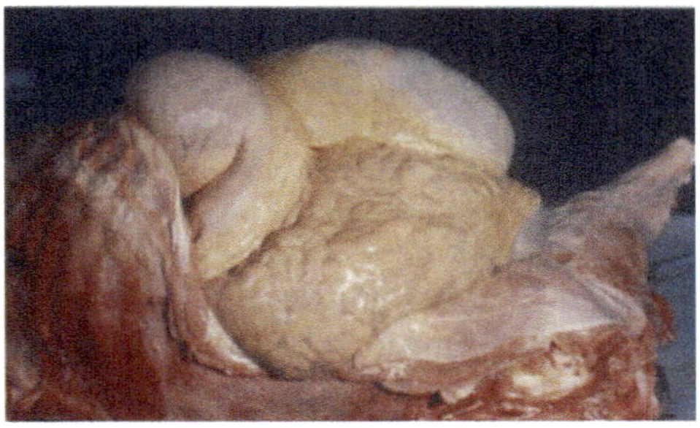

Fig. 133 Icterus associated with anaplasmosis (yellow abdominal fat) [15]

- **General features of bovine anaplasmosis**

Symptoms: Calves undergo mild infections, with little or no mortality. In yearlings the disease is more severe but most animals recover. In adult cattle, the disease is more severe, anaemia is marked and mortality may reach 50%. The disease starts with general depression, indolence, fever (40–41°C). Milk production falls rapidly. Weight loss and progressive anaemia, dehydration and icterus occurs. Affected animals often succumb to hypoxia when moved or handled for treatment. Recovered animals often remain carriers for life.
Significance: *Anaplasma marginale* causes severe losses in endemic areas.

Diagnosis: In endemic areas, anaplasmosis should be suspected in adult cattle showing chronic anaemia without haemoglobinuria, leading to cachexia. Icterus is an important sign. Anaplasmosis often follows an acute form of babesiosis or theileriosis and appears to be a prolonged convalescence. Demonstration of the organisms in Giemsa-stained blood smears confirms the diagnosis (☞ METHODS, 3.1). Serological tests such as complement fixation and the IFAT and DNA probes are useful tools for diagnostic purposes. Anaemia due to helminth infections should be excluded by coprological examination.

Therapy: Acute anaplasmosis is most effectively treated with tetracyclines (oxytetracycline, 5–10 mg/kg, im. or iv.) or chlortetracycline (1.5 mg/kg, po.), especially if administered early in the course of infection. Long-acting oxytetracycline formulations may give sustained blood levels. Imidocarb dipropionate (1.2–2.4 mg/kg., sc.) may also be used for *Anaplasma* infections. Symptomatic and supportive treatment is important. Transfusion of 4–6 l of normal blood is often indicated and should be repeated in 48 h intervals, until the animal appears stronger. Oral and parenteral rehydration with isotonic saline and glucose solution is vital for dehydrated animals. Handling and disturbances should be avoided, since even mild exertion can produce hypoxia and death. Animals should be kept in shade with free access to fresh water.

Prophylaxis: Regular dipping, spraying of animals during the vector season drastically reduces the incidence of the disease. Several methods exist to immunize animals in endemic areas. Inoculation of blood containing *A. centrale* which gives rise to a mild infection that protects against a subsequent infection with the virulent and very pathogenic *A. marginale*. The use of virulent and attenuated *A. marginale* isolates to induce immunity or a chronic carrier status in calves is a widely accepted technique throughout the tropics where anaplasmosis is endemic. The use of virulent organisms in adult cattle is hazardous, and treatment at the onset of the patent infection with tetracyclines is recommended to temper the course of infection.

Eperythrozoon spp.

Organisms found on the surface of erythrocytes or near thrombocytes, occasionally they are located near erythrocytes. They multiply by binary fission. In general the size of *Eperythrozoon* is 0.4–1 µm. The most important vectors of *Eperythrozoon* spp. are sucking lice, infected through trans-stadial transmission. *Hyalomma anatolicum* possibly transmits *E. wenyoni*. *Eperythrozoon* spp. are generally not very pathogenic in spite of sometimes high infection levels. They may assume increased significance together with other protistan infections (*Babesia* spp., *Theileria* spp., *Anaplasma* spp. or *Trypanosoma* spp.). The only pathogenic *Eperythrozoon* species which produces a disease entity is *E. suis*. The disease is characterised by a slow development of anaemia, comparable to anaplasmosis. Oxytetracyclines (5–10 mg/kg, im. or iv.) are effective against all *Eperythrozoon* spp. Prophylaxis requires lice and tick control.

In cattle the following species are present in tropical Africa: *Eperythrozoon wenyoni* occurs on the erythrocyte surface; *Eperythrozoon teganodes* occurs on the erythrocyte surface or near to it and *Eperythrozoon tuomii* occurs on the thrombocyte surface.

(Figures 130, 134)

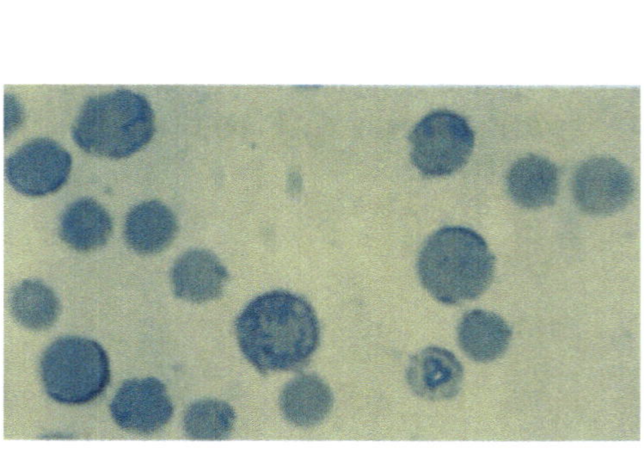

Fig. 134 *Eperythrozoon wenyoni*; Giemsa-stained bloodsmear [13]

Haemobartonella spp.

These are organisms found on the surface of erythrocytes which form branched chains and multiply by binary fission. The organisms are coccoid (0.1–1 µm) or bacilliform (1–5 × 0.7–1.5 µm). They cause a defined disease entity in dogs and cats and rats. *Haemobartonella* spp. are often detected as resurgent parasites during concomitant infections or following splenectomy. Tetracyclines are the drugs of choice for treating *Haemobartonella* infections, but therapy is rarely indicated (☞ also above ANPLASMATACAE, Fig. 130).

Haemobartonella bovis

Remarks: It occurs on the erythrocyte surface. These coccoid or bacilliform organisms occur on the erythrocyte surface of cattle in Mediterranean regions. Vectors are sucking lice and ticks (species unknown). *Haemobartonella bovis* is relatively non-pathogenic. In rare cases the parasite may be associated with slow anaemia and symptoms similar to anaplasmosis. *Haemobartonella* spp. and *Eperythrozoon* spp. are difficult to distinguish reliably by light microscopy (☞above ANPLASMATACAE, Fig. 130).

EHRLICHIACEAE

Ehrlichia bovis Tropical bovine ehrlichiosis, "Nofel" or "Nopel"

Hosts: Cattle

Vector: Ticks of the genera *Amblyomma, Hyalomma* and *Rhipicephalus*

Species description: *Ehrlichia bovis* occurs in mononuclear cells of cattle. The syndrome corresponds to the disease called "Nofel" (Fulani/Peule in West Africa; ear = nopi in peul) or "Nopel" (Bororos in Central Africa), because of the ears being kept low at the beginning of an acute infection. The clinical signs vary greatly ranging from inapparent forms to serious fatal forms, dominated by nervous signs, ataxic gait, stiff legs, walking in circles, phases of excitement followed by somnolence, epileptic crisis with falls, rolling eyes and salivation. Death may occur in an epileptic attack. The disease is always serious in imported cattle. The nervous signs are similar to those of cowdriosis.

Geographic distribution: North and Central Africa, Middle East, Ceylon

Symptoms: Anorexia, fever, incoordination and enlargement of lymph nodes

Significance: *Ehrlichia bovis* is of low significance for indigenous cattle. However, it is a serious problem for imported or newly introduced cattle in many tropical areas.

Diagnosis: Microscopic examination of peripheral blood smears demonstrates *E. bovis* in monocytes or macrophages. For differential diagnosis infections with *Cowdria ruminantium* have to be excluded. *C. ruminantium* is located exclusively in the endothelial cells (brain and other tissues) and not in the peripheral blood leucocytes, whereas *E. bovis* is found in monocytes and macrophages.

Therapy: Oxytetracyclines (5 mg/kg, im., for 4 days) or streptomycin-penicillin (3 g and 3 mio. units per day, im.); other tetracyclines may be used in emergencies.

Prophylaxis: This consists of regular tick control. There are no immunization procedures described.

(Figures 130, 135)

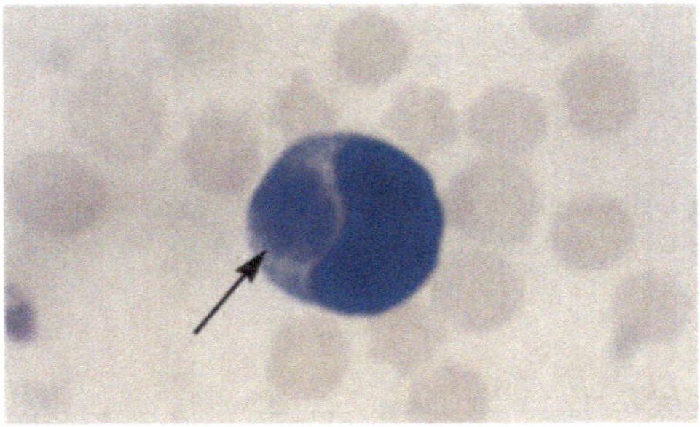

Fig. 135 *Ehrlichia bovis*; mass of elementary bodies in a monocyte [15]

Ehrlichia phagocytophila
European ehrlichiosis

Remarks: *E. phagocytophila* occurs in the neutrophilic and eosinophilic granulocytes of cattle, sheep and other domestic and wild ruminants in Europe. Goats are not very susceptible. *Ixodes ricinus* transmits the disease by trans-stadial infection. The disease is characterized by fever which occurs after an incubation period of 4–11 days. The infection causes a state of immunosuppression and is therefore a predisposing factor to a variety of secondary infections. The animals usually recover after this febrile phase. However, the most characteristic problems are abortion in pregnant ewes and cattle, and progressive weight loss following infection may occur. At necropsy hypertrophy of the spleen and lymph nodes may be seen. The diagnosis is made by demonstrating the organisms in stained blood smears (☞ METHODS, 3.1). Serological tests such as IFAT (☞ METHODS, 5.1) may be used for epidemiological studies.
Therapy: Long acting oxytetracyclines (5 mg/kg, im.) have a certain curative effect.
Prophylaxis: ☞ above *Ehrlichia bovis*
(Figures 130, 136)

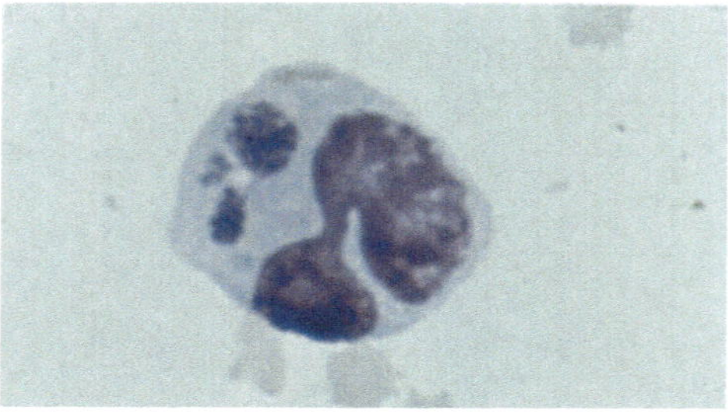

Fig. 136 *Ehrlichia phagocytophila*; mass of elementary bodies in a granulocyte [4]

Ehrlichia ondiri

Remarks: This parasite occurs in granulocytes of cattle in high-altitude grassland regions of East Africa. Members of the genus *Haemaphysalis* and other genera are suspected to be vectors of the disease. The incubation period is 1–2 weeks. The disease starts with a fever attack which is accompanied by a petechial exanthema of the mucosae of the mouth, nose, vulva, eyes (poached egg eye), digestive tract, urinary bladder, pericardium and endocardium. Extended haemorrhage in the gastrointestinal tract and the pulmonary oedema cause death.
Diagnosis is made by microscopic examination of blood smears. Organisms of *E. ondiri* are found in granulocytes.
Therapy and Prophylaxis: ☞ above *Ehrlichia bovis*

Cowdria ruminantium Heartwater, Tyewde

Hosts: Cattle, sheep, goat and other ruminants
Vector: Several species of the tick genus *Amblyomma* transmit the disease: *Amblyomma variegatum* in open savannas from equatorial Africa to Madagascar; *Amblyomma gemma* in East Africa (Massai and Somalian steppes); *Amblyomma pomposum* has limited geographic distribution and occurs in the Angolan plateau, Zambia, southwestern Tanzania; *Amblyomma lepidum* in East Africa (Massai steppes, Sahelian steppes of the Nile in Sudan) and *Amblyomma tholloni* in the Zambezi region. *C. ruminantium* is also present on the Caribbean islands.
Species description: Cowdriosis is specific to ruminants of the family Bovidae and is most severe in sheep and goats but also causes great losses in cattle. Imported ruminants are much more susceptible to cowdriosis than indigenous breeds. They may suffer heavy losses. But also indigenous ruminants are affected especially when they are in poor general condition (endoparasitism, malnutrition, chronic infections, etc.) or with weakened defence (lactation, gestation). This applies especially to the early rainy season in the Sahel-Sudanese region when animals are weakened by the long food shortage of the dry season and when there is a drastic

proliferation of the *Amblyomma* ticks. Cowdriosis can then become a great problem. The incubation period is 8–15 days. Endothelial cells are the preferred sites of the proliferation of this pathogen, especially of the nervous system, kidney, spleen, lymph nodes, salivary glands and heart muscle. Young calves (< 6 weeks), lambs and kids (< 1 week) are fairly resistant and may recover spontaneously.

Geographic distribution: The distribution of heartwater corresponds to that of all its vectors.

Symptoms: The symptoms are almost identical in both cattle and small ruminants, except that the nervous symptoms are rarer in cattle and not as distinct (e.g. posture of pushing against a wall, ataxia, haggard eye, aggressiveness). Digestive signs are more constant in cattle than in sheep and goats. Diarrhoea may occasionally be seen. Several forms of cowdriosis can occur, ranging from a peracute form (death within 2–3 hours; tyewde of the Fulani) to inapparent infections. There are no pathognomonic signs. In the peracute form an animal may abruptly drop to the ground, struggle, start to pedal, indicating serious nervous disorders. Death follows rapidly. The acute form can last for up to 5 days and is accompanied by initial hyperthermia, breathlessness and dyspnoea. Nervous signs may occur, often at the end of the disease, suggesting tetanus or poisoning. Fluttering of the eyelids and acute gastroenteritis may also occur. The subacute form is rare (12–15 days), developing sometimes pulmonary complications. Attenuated forms are frequent. Animals recover after a short febrile phase. Sometimes, hyperthermia is the only clinical sign.

Significance: Cowdriosis is a serious problem in areas infested by the ticks *Amblyomma* spp.

Diagnosis: In acute forms diagnosis can be based on clinical signs. Demonstration of colonies of the organisms in the cytoplasm of capillary endothelial cells is necessary for definitive diagnosis. This is done with Giemsa-stained "squash" smears of cerebral gray matter. An indirect IFAT (☞ METHODS, 5.1) test may be used to detect antibodies of animals that have recovered from infection. In sheep and goats these antibodies persist for several years, and their presence correlates well with their resistance to reinfections. Seropositive cattle are resistant to challenge, although antibodies disappear within 12 months after infection.

At necropsy hydropericardium is the predominant sign. The exudate is clear, usually amber or yellow. It is a consistent sign of heartwater. It may be as much as 700 ml in small ruminants. Hydrothorax, ascites and splenomegaly are often found. The gall bladder is usually distended. Extensive congestion of the viscera and petechiae on the serous membranes and mucosae of the digestive tract may be seen. Microscopically the deformation of endothelial cells by rickettsial masses is the most striking finding. Smears are made either with material scraped from the internal wall of a major artery, or with a fragment of cerebral cortex crushed between two slides. May-Grünwald/Giemsa staining usually reveals masses of elementary bodies, appearing as blue granules in the cytoplasm of endothelial cells. The initial bodies are dark blue.

Therapy: Oxytetracycline (5–10 mg/kg, im. or iv.) usually effects a cure if administered early. Later in the febrile phase, when clinical signs appear, a higher dose level (10–20 mg/kg) is required.

Prophylaxis: There is no vaccine yet. Several immunization schedules have been applied successfully ("controlled immunization": infection with a laboratory-maintained strain followed by antibiotic treatment) but they require a very careful monitoring of the infected animals and laboratory maintenance of parasite strains.

These methods are expensive and should therefore be reserved for valuable animals (e.g. breeding stock, drought animals, etc.). Tick control is a substantial part of heartwater prophylaxis.

Remarks: Merozoites of *Toxoplasma gondii*

and *Sarcocystis* spp. may occur in the blood stream during the acute phase.
(Figures 130, 137, 138, 139, 140)

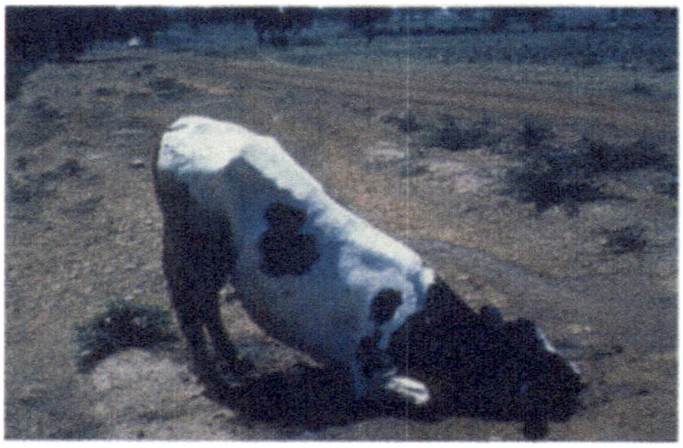

Fig. 137 Nervous symptoms associated with *Cowdria ruminantium* [15]

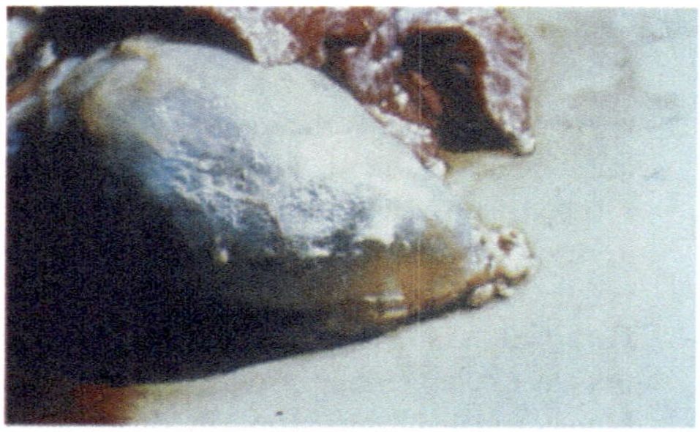

Fig. 138 Hydropericardium (heart water) caused by *Cowdria ruminantium* [15]

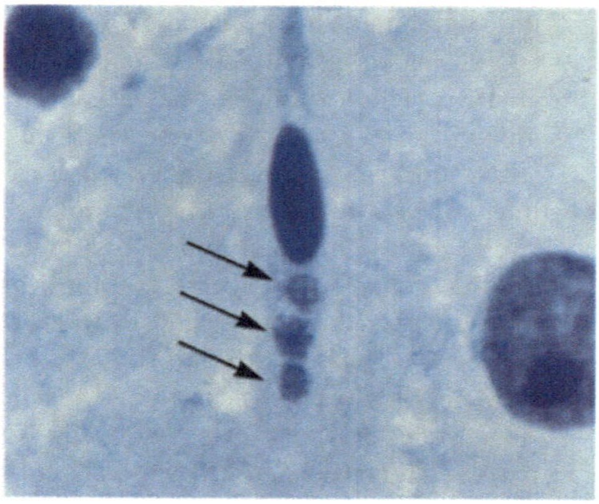

Fig. 139 *Cowdria ruminantium* organisms in the capillary endothelial cells [4]

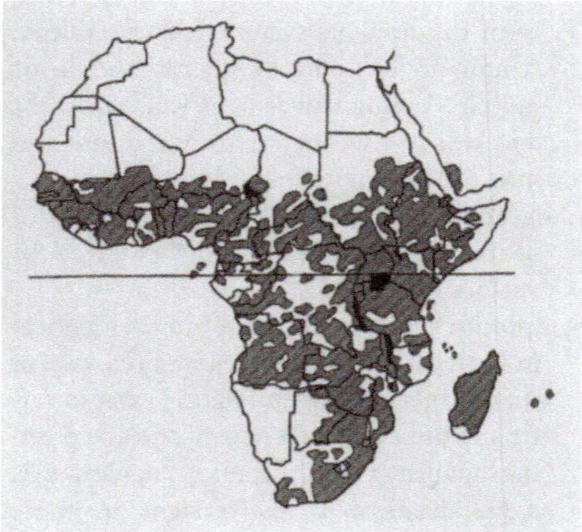

Fig. 140 The known distribution of the known vectors of heartwater in the African region [13]

HELMINTHS

- Trematoda found in the blood and circulatory system

Schistosoma bovis Blood fluke, Bilharziosis

Location: Mesenteric veins

Hosts: Cattle, sheep, goat, equine and dromedary

Species description: *S. bovis* occurs in the portal and mesenteric veins of cattle, sheep, goats, equines, camels and rarely in man. The males of *S. bovis* are 9–22 mm long and 1–2 mm wide. The females are 12–28 mm long. The eggs are spindle-shaped and passed in the faeces. The size of the eggs is 132–247 µm × 38–60 µm.

Geographic distribution: Central, East and West Africa

(Figures 141, 142)

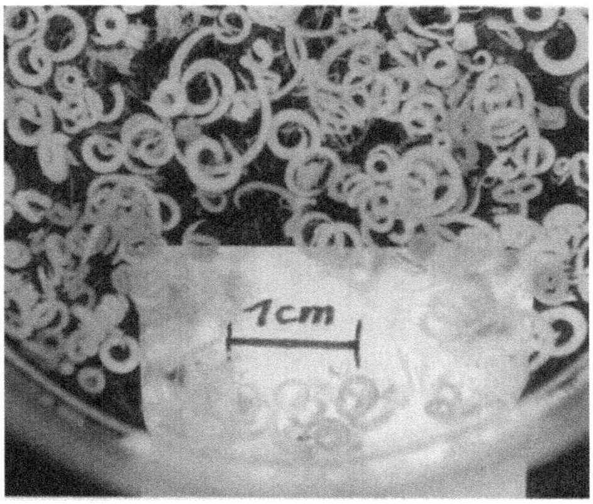

Fig. 141 *Schistosoma bovis*

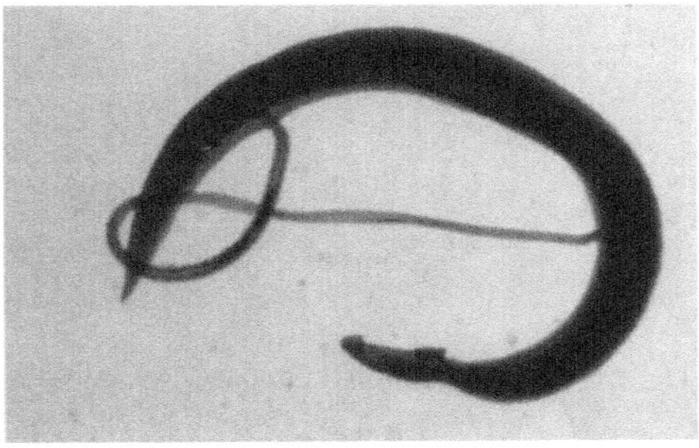

Fig. 142 *Schistosoma bovis*; male (thick) and female (slender)

Schistosoma mattheei

Location: Portal and mesenteric veins and less frequently cystic and lung veins
Hosts: Cattle, sheep, goat, wild ruminants, equine and man
Species description: Females measure 18–25 mm and males 9–14 mm. The eggs measure 170–280 × 70–85 µm and have a terminal spine. The prepatent period is 7 weeks. The life cycle is similar to *Schistosoma bovis*. Intermediate hosts are *Bulinus africanus*, *Bulinus globosus* and other *Bulinus* spp.
Geographic distribution: Southern Africa, Mozambique, Zambia, Malawi, Zimbabwe, Tanzania; Central Africa (Tchad)

Schistosoma intercalatum

Remarks: This species occurs mainly in man and primates in Central Africa. Sheep and goats and other domestic and wild ruminants may accidentally acquire infection. *S. intercalatum* is found in the portal and mesenteric veins. The eggs measure 140–240 µm × 50–85 µm.

Schistosoma curassoni

Location: Portal and mesenteric veins
Hosts: Cattle, sheep and goat
Species description: Intermediate hosts are snails of the genus *Bulinus*. Eggs are similar to those of *S. mattheei.*
Geographic distribution: West Africa (Senegal, Mauretania, Mali)

- **General features of *Schistosoma* spp. infections**

Life cycle: Aquatic snails (*Bulinus* spp.) act as intermediate hosts in the life cycle of *Schistosoma* spp. In the case of *S. bovis*, *S. mattheei* and *S. intercalatum* snails of the genus *Bulinus* spp. act as intermediate hosts. The eggs hatch after contact with water. The miracidia infect aquatic snails and cercariae emerge 38–126 days after infection from the snail and actively penetrate the skin or the rumen of the definite host. Schistosomosis (bilharziosis) occurs near permanent fresh water bodies (pools, backwaters, ponds, lakes and marshy pastures). To become infected, the final host needs the contact with water. This might occure during drinking in these areas, passing through water or grazing in swamps.
Symptoms: These are rarely seen even in heavy infections. Symptoms are mainly caused by the eggs which are deposited by the adult flukes in the wall of the intestines. Intermittent diarrhoea which may contain specks of blood, anaemia and progressive weakness may occur. Both diarrhoea and constipation can be seen and blood and mucus are sometimes found in the faeces together

with the eggs. A chronic hepatic syndrome has been described with neurological signs like ataxia, hypermetria, disorientation, leaning against walls, coprophagy, etc. Sheep are more susceptible than cattle and can die in large numbers while cattle survive, unless they have very heavy burdens.

Significance: Although specific clinical signs are often overlooked, blood flukes may constitute a serious problem in endemic areas.

Diagnosis: This is made by faecal examination. Spindle-shaped eggs are found in the sediment. In chronic cases, it may not be possible to find eggs in the faeces and the diagnosis must be confirmed by a post-mortem examination. At necropsy adult flukes can be found in the mesenteric veins or in the portal system.

Therapy: The therapy of schistosomosis is not easy. Highly efficient anthelmintics may have fatal consequences because dead worms may cause massive thrombus formation in the liver. Therapy should aim to kill the worms over a long period of time rather than risk the massive damage caused by the simultaneous death of all worms. In general treatment of schistosomosis is uneconomical since a large number of repeated doses at intervals of 2–3 days is required. Praziquantel at 25 mg/kg body weight is effective, although two treatments, 3–5 weeks apart are required. Other drugs which have some schistosomicidal properties are stibophen (7.5mg/kg, im. 6 ×), lucathone hydrochloride (50 mg/kg for sheep and 30 mg/kg for cattle; both every other day until three treatments have been given), hycanthone (6 mg/kg, im.) and trichlorfon (10–12 mg/kg, im. 11 × at intervals of 3–5 days).

Prophylaxis: In areas where schistosomosis is of great importance, grazing in swamps, rice fields, ponds (habitat of the intermediate host) should be avoided. Water from bore holes should be used for drinking purposes. Infection can be reduced by fencing off contaminated bodies of water and providing clean drinking water. These measures not only reduce the incidence of schistosomosis, but they also control other trematodes such as *Fasciola* spp. and paramphistomes which frequently occur in the same localities as schistosomes. If the drinking water is contaminated with intermediate snail hosts the use of molluscicides may be indicated. An ecologically justifiable way will probably be the use of molluscicidal plants which can be cultured in water bodies containing the snail-intermediate host.

(Figures 31, 35, 36, 143, 144)

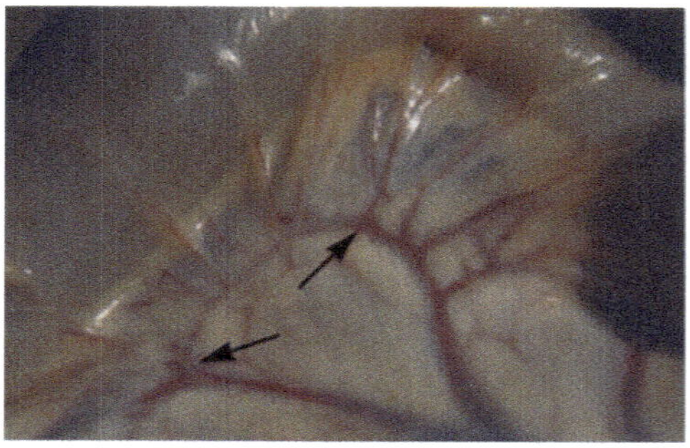

Fig. 143 *Schistosoma bovis* in the mesenteric veins

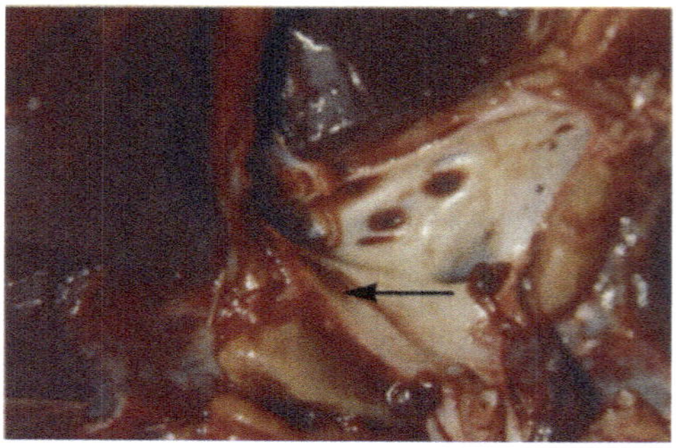

Fig. 144 *Schistosoma bovis* in the portal vein of the liver

- Nematoda larvae (microfilariae) found in the blood and adult nematodes living in the circulatory system

Onchocerca armillata Aortic filariosis

Location: Adult worms are found within tunica media of the aorta. Microfilariae are found in the blood stream (transiently) and in the skin of the dorsal parts of the body (definitively).

Hosts: Cattle, rarely small ruminants and camel

Species description: Adults are found in the aorta. Males are about 7 cm long and females up to 70 cm. The microfilariae are unsheathed, measure 346–382 μm × 5.5–6.8 μm and are mainly found in and under the skin on the dorsal parts of the animal (hump, wither, neck, rarely dewlap and lower parts). In chronic infections the aortic wall is thickened and the intima shows tortuous tunnels and there are numerous nodules containing yellow caseous fluid and coiled worms. Infection is transmitted by bites of insects of the families Simuliidae and Ceratopogonidae. The infection is very common (up to 90%) in some areas.

Geographic distribution: Throughout Africa

Symptoms: Clinically mostly inapparent; calcification of the aortic wall and aneurysm may cause cardiovascular symptoms.

Significance: Weakly pathogenic but prevalent in some regions (80–90% of all animals examined)

Diagnosis: Microfilariae appear in the blood stream and in the skin. Typical nodular lesions in the aortic wall may be found at necropsy.

Therapy: This is rarely indicated. Diethylcarbamazine is microfilaricid (5–8 mg/kg daily for 21 days). Ivermectin (200 μg/kg) was found to be highly effective against the microfilariae of many *Onchocerca* spp.

(Figures 145, 146, 159)

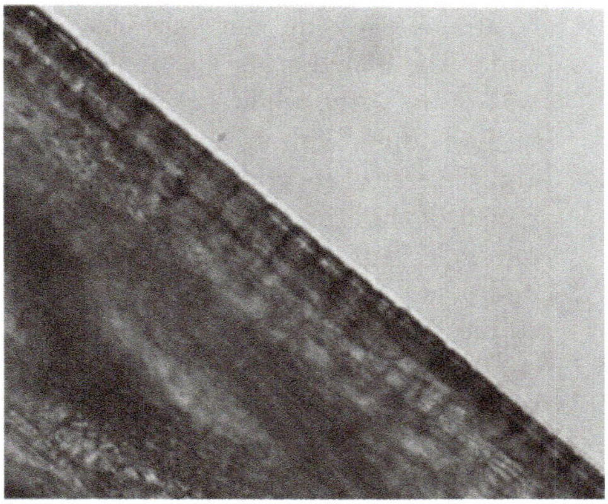

Fig. 145 *Onchocerca armillata*; typical striated cuticula

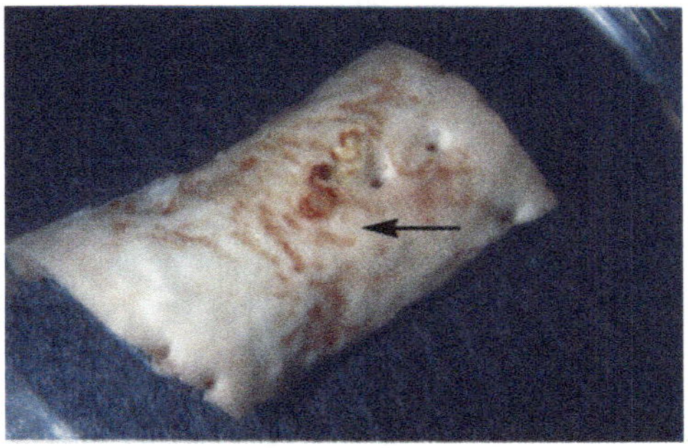

Fig. 146 *Onchocerca armillata*; aortic nodules containing the coiled adult worms (arrow)

Onchocerca spp., *O. gutturosa, O. dukei* and *O. ochengi*

Remarks: These species are found in the nuchal ligament or in/under the skin on several parts of the body (☞ CATTLE, ■ 4.1.2 and ■ 5.1). Microfilariae may occasionally be found in the circulating blood during their migration to their predilection site.

Elaeophora poeli Large aortic filaria

Location: Thoracic portion of the aorta

Hosts: Cattle, water buffalo

Species description: Males are 45–70 mm long and females 40–300 mm. The microfilariae are 340–360 µm long and 7.0–7.5 µm wide. The male occurs in nodules in the wall of the aorta, while the female is fixed in the nodules with its anterior extremity and the rest of its body hangs free in the lumen of the vessel. The females are 350 µm wide in the intranodular part of the body and 1.5–1.8 mm wide in the free parts of the body. The life cycle is unknown. Affected vessels are swollen and less elastic. The intima is uneven and rised by nodules which are 8–13 mm in diameter.

Geographic distribution: Central and East Africa, South East Asia, Philippines

Symptoms: There is no evidence that the parasite causes clinical signs.

Significance: Unknown

Diagnosis: Nodules in the aorta, unsheathed microfilariae may occur in the blood stream.

Therapy and Prophylaxis: Not indicated (Figure 147)

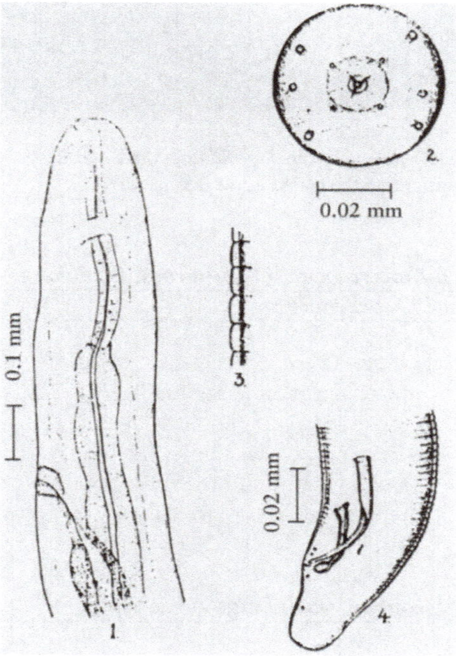

Fig. 147 *Elaeophora poeli*; anterior end of a female (1); anterior end (2), cuticular structure (3) and tail end (4) of a male [18]

Setaria labiatopapillosa

Location: Adult worms occur in the abdominal cavity (☞ CATTLE, ■ 4.4).
Microfilariae are sheathed, 140–230 µm long and appear in the peripheral blood. (Figure 148)

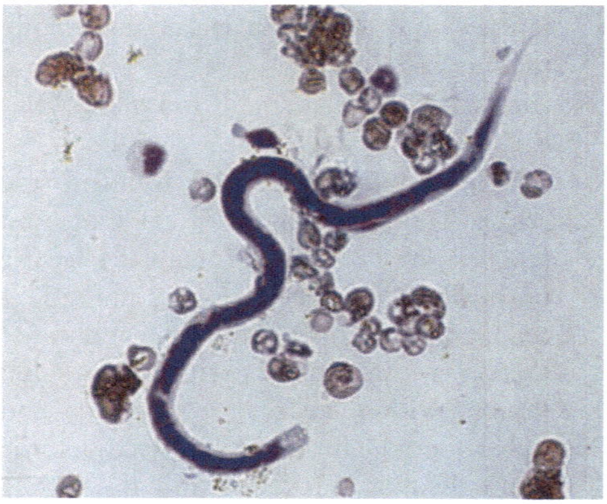

Fig. 148 *Setaria labiatopapillosa*; sheathed microfilariae are 140–230 µm long; Giemsa-stained bloodsmear

3 Stages in the urogenital system

PROTOZOA

Tritrichomonas foetus (syn. *Trichomonas foetus*) Bovine trichomonad abortion

Location: In the bull the parsites are found in the preputial cavity. In cows trichomonads are found in the vagina and uterus.

Hosts: Cattle

Species description: This is a venereal protozoal disease of cattle characterized by early foetal death and infertility, associated with greatly extended calving intervals. It is reported from many tropical countries. The organism is ordinarily 10–15 × 5–10 μm, but there is considerable pleomorphism. At the anterior end there are three flagella about the same size as the parasite. An undulating membrane runs the full length of the body and is bordered by a filament which continues beyond the membrane as a posterior flagellum. Multiplication is by longitudinal binary fission. Under natural conditions the infection is transmitted during coitus from the bull to the cow or vice versa. It may also be transmitted mechanically, e.g. by gynaecological examination of cows with contaminated tools. The organisms are found only in the genital tract of the cow and bull. Most bulls remain permanently infected after a primary infection. The bull is usually the source of initial and continuous infection within a herd. Infected cows usually recover spontaneously after mean durations of 20 weeks (primary exposure) and 10 weeks (secondary exposure). Cows can remain infected throughout pregnancy and discharge trichomonads from the genital tract following calving.

Geographic distribution: World-wide

Symptoms: Purulent vaginitis, metritis, placentitis and abortion are commonly found in infected cows and can cause enormous losses. Prolonged sterility and extended calving intervals are predominant features (*cave:* differential diagnosis: *Brucella abortus*!). There is a persistent uterine discharge containing large numbers of the parasites. Bulls are usually carrier of the parasite without clinical symptoms.

Significance: Venereal disease of cattle characterised by abortion and infertility in cows. *T. foetus* can cause considerable losses in infected herds. In many countries the incidence has greatly been reduced by the artificial insemination using a bull known to be free of the disease.

Diagnosis: History of abortions in a herd and demonstration of the organism in the vaginal or uterine discharges or in the foetus (mainly stomach). In bulls the organisms are in the prepuce, frequently in small numbers. Microscopical examination of the preputial smegma for trichomonads is the most common method to confirm a herd diagnosis. Preputial fluid may be collected with a pipette (e.g. AI pipette) which is introduced into the prepuce, and smegma is collected with a combination of scraping and aspiring via an attached rubber bulb or syringe. The same procedure may be used to collect vaginal fluid. It is important to avoid contamination with faecal material, as such material contains masses of protozoa similar in appearance to *T. foetus*. The organisms may not be numerous and careful, systematic examination is necessary. Diagnosis is based on the size and shape of the organisms as well as the characteristic aimless, jerky motion on a warmed slide. Only living organisms are useful for diagnostic purposes. Confirmation depends on finding the organisms in at least one animal in a suspected herd. The organisms may be cultured in special media (e.g. Diamond's Trichomonad Medium). The diagnosis can be confirmed by the Polymerase Chain Reaction (PCR) which is the most sensitive and specific diagnostic method nowadays. Serological examinations on a herd level may be used for epidemiological purposes but are of little value for individual animals.

Therapy: This is extremely difficult and does not eliminate the parasites. Compounds which have been reported to be effective against trichomonads are dimetridazole, ipronidazole and metronidazole. Thorough rinsing out of affected genital organs with acridine and iodine preparations may reduce the number of parasites but it does not clear the infection. The only effective and sustainable way to control bovine trichomonosis is strict prevention.

Prophylaxis: Control measures are based on the assumption that transmission occurs only during coitus and that infected cows that undergo 3 months of sexual rest after calving with normal uterine involution are free of infection. Animals with pyometra or genital abnormalities should be culled. Artificial insemination (AI) with semen free of trichomoads is the most effective way of controlling the disease. However, if AI is not possible, the exposed animals should be treated repeatedly for recognizable uterine disease and allowed 3 months of sexual rest. For breeding, a young, not infected bull should be used. Bulls and cows should be examined for reinfection. Control may be supported by eliminating all bulls > 3 years old and using younger bulls for mating. This is based on the relative lack of susceptibility of young bulls to trichomonad infection. Slaughter, rather than treatment, of bulls is generally recommended.

(Figures 149, 150)

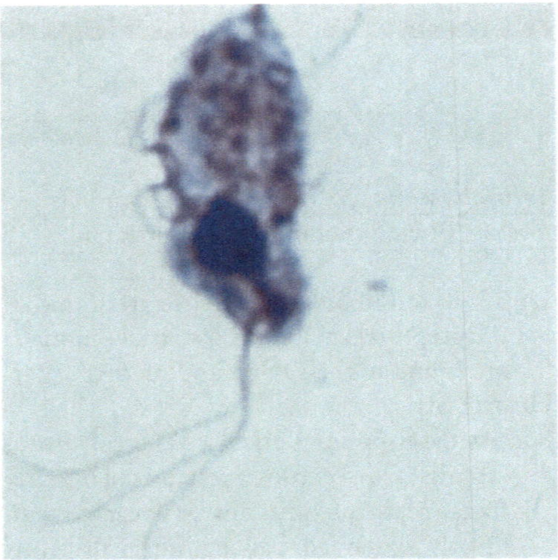

Fig. 149 *Tritrichomonas foetus* (12–18 × 6–10 μm); Giemsa-stained bloodsmear [4]

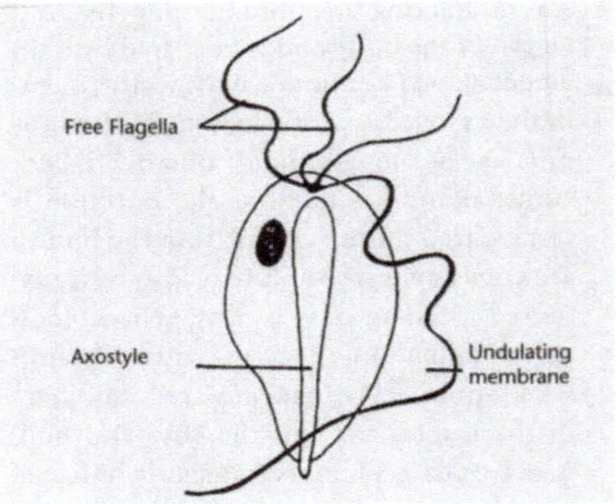

Fig. 150 Morphology of *Tritrichomonas foetus* (schematic) [19]

4.1 Locomotory system

4.1.1 Muscles

PROTOZOA

Sarcocystis bovicanis (syn. *S. cruzi*), ***Sarcocystis bovifelis*** (syn. *S. hirsuta*) **and**
Sarcocystis bovihominis (syn. *S. hominis*)
Bovine Sarcosporidiosis

Location: Cysts, containing the infective stage, called bradyzoites, occur in the striated musculature of cattle.

Hosts: Cattle are intermediate hosts of three *Sarcocystis* species of which the dog (*S. bovicanis*), the cat (*S. bovifelis*) or man (*S. bovihominis*) are final hosts.

Species description: Cysts of several *Sarcocystis* species are found in the muscles of cattle. Cattle always act as intermediate hosts. *S. bovicanis* is the most pathogenic species for cattle. Infection is acquired orally by ingestion of sporocysts from the faeces of infected hosts. Tissue cysts in cattle are infectious for at least 1 year. The life cycle of *Sarcocystis* spp. is as follows: infective sporocysts, excreted by the final host (cat, dog, man) are ingested, sporozoites are released in the intestine and invade many tissues via blood stream. Schizogony occurs in the endothelial cells of blood vessels in most organs, preceding the development of typical cysts in the striated musculature. Cysts may occasionally also be found in the brain. Cysts vary in size, depending on the species, from a few mil-

Table 10 *Sarcocystis* species found in muscles of cattle

Species	Synonym	Definite host	Pathogenicity IH*	DH**
S. bovicanis	*S. cruzi*	Dog, coyote, wolf	+++	0
S. bovifelis	*S. hirsuta*	Cat	0	0
S. bovihominis	*S. hominis*	Man, rhesus monkey, baboon, chimpanzee	0	+

*IH = Intermediate Host; **DH = Definitive Host; 0 = non-pathogenic; + = mildly pathogenic; +++ = severely pathogenic

limetres to several centimetres in length. The peripheral region of a cyst contains globular forms (metrocytes), which produce two daughter cells by endodyogeny and these after further replication give rise to banana-shaped bradyzoites. Infection of the final host is by ingestion of muscle cysts, containing bradyzoites. *S. bovifelis* is nonpathogenic for cattle and produces microscopic cysts of 12 × 1 µm. *S. bovihominis* has man and some primates as definitive hosts and the sarcocysts are compartmented, with a wall of about 6 µm tick that appears radially striated by light microscopy. The pathogenicity of *S. bovihominis* for cattle is still in debate. The following description refers to this species. Following ingestion of sporulated oocysts or sporocysts by cattle (excreted by dogs, wolves, coyotes, raccoons, foxes, hyenas) several generations of schizonts occur in the endothelial cells of blood vessels and metrocytes are found in the striated musculature about 1 month after infection. Fully developed muscle cysts, containing the infective bradyzoites occur 2–3 months after infection.

Geographic distribution: World-wide

Symptoms: Anorexia, intermittent fever attacks, anaemia, weight loss were observed after experimental infection of calves. Deaths occurred about 30 days after a heavy infection with 10^5–10^6 sporocysts. Reduced milk yield, loss of condition, dyspnoea and abortion were observed in adult cattle.

Significance: *Sarcocystis* infection occurs throughout the world. Economic losses during a fresh infection may be higher than expected. Once muscle cysts are formed the infection is inapparent.

Diagnosis: This is very difficult in the acute phase (1 month post infection). During this period schizonts may be demonstrated in vascular endothelial cells by means of stained-scrapings taken from the blood vessels or by histopathological examination. Detection of meronts in Giemsa-stained blood smears (☞ METHODS, 3.1) or biopsy for detection of schizonts. At necropsy artificial digestion of affected muscles might reveal the muscle cysts. Serological tests (IFAT, ELISA; ☞ METHODS, 5.1 and 5.2) are indicated after the acute phase. The PCR (☞ METHODS, 6.3.2) may be used as a highly sensitive method to detect *Sarcocystis* infections.

Therapy: This is extremely difficult in cattle and rarely indicated. Amprolium (100 mg/kg, po., daily during 30 days) was effective to avoid clinical signs in cattle (endothelial schizogony) during experimental infections. Amprolium and halofuginone (0.66 mg/kg, po., 2 × on consecutive days) may be used in sheep and goats to avoid clinical disease after infection.

Prophylaxis: The contamination of cattle food with faeces of dogs, cats and man as well as the feeding of raw cattle meat to dogs should be avoided.

(Figures 151, 152, 153, Table 10)

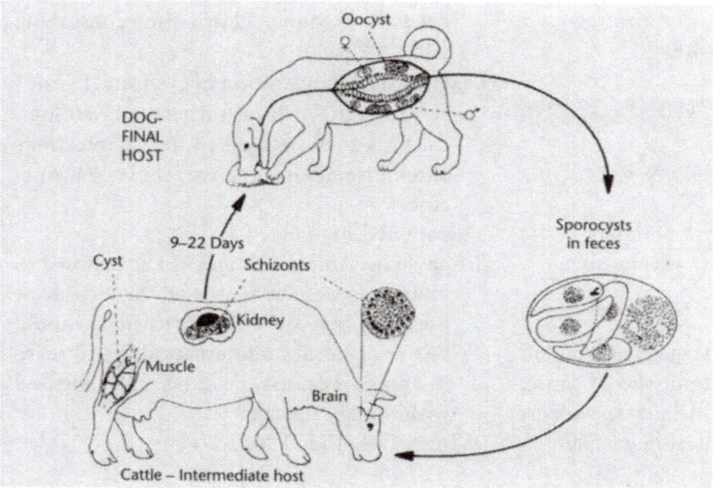

Fig. 151 Life cycle of *Sarcocystis bovicanis* [3]

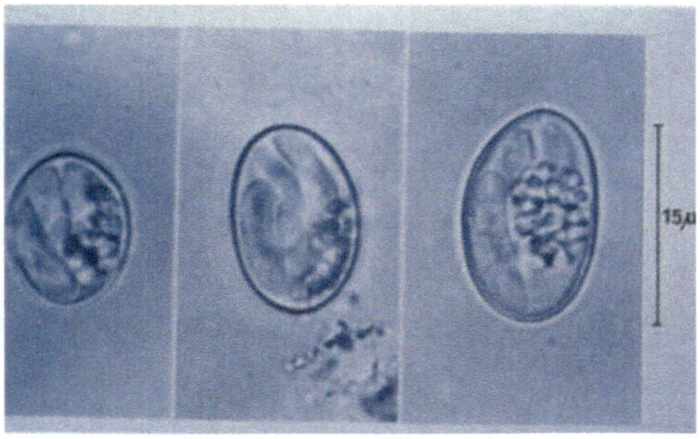

Fig. 152 Sporozoites of *Sarcocystis suicanis* (left), *Sarcocystis ovicanis* (middle) and *Sarcocystis bovicanis* (right) [4]

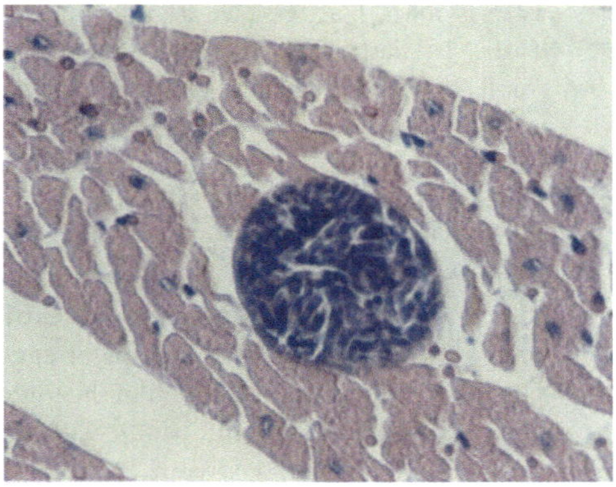

Fig. 153 *Sarcocystis bovicanis* (syn. *S. cruzi*); tissue cyst (70 µm in diameter) [10]

Toxoplasma gondii

Remarks: Tissue cysts of *T. gondii* may also occur in ruminants as they do in pigs (☞ Swine, ■ 4.1). A diagnosis based on clinical signs is not possible. Cysts may be seen in histopathological examinations. High antibody titers by the Sabin-Feldman-test, IFAT or ELISA (☞ Methods, 5.1 and 5.2) may indicate an infection. The PCR technique (☞ Methods, 6.3.2) may be used for the sensitive detection of *T. gondii* infections in all domestic animals species and will thus provide an important epidemiological tool. Tissue cysts of *T. gondii* in cattle may constitute an infection risk of minor importance for man.

Neospora sp.

Remarks: Cysts of *Neospora* sp. are found in the muscles of cattle. The entire life cycle is still unknown. Until 1988 the parasite was diagnosed as *T. gondii*. *N. caninum* causes neuromuscular disorders in dogs and is the main cause of abortion in cattle in the

USA. Tachyzoites and tissue cysts are the only stages so far known. For diagnosis and treatment ☞ CATTLE, ■ 4.6.

HELMINTHS

• Cestoda larvae found in the muscles

Cysticercus bovis Larvae of the human tapeworm ***Taenia saginata*** cysticercosis, "beef measles"

Location: Cysticerci (larval stage) are found in striated and non-striated muscles of cattle, anywhere in the body. Adult tapeworms are found in the small intestine of man.

Intermediate hosts: Cattle

Species description: The final host of this parasite is man. Cattle serve as intermediate hosts. In cattle the parasite appears as small, fluid-filled cysts (10 mm × 4.5 mm) which give a spotty or measle-like appearance to the beef muscle. These cysts contain 1 protoscolex and occur predominantly in the heart muscle, diaphragm, tongue and masseters. In infected man proglottids are passed in the faeces. Infection of cattle occurs by ingestion of proglottids or eggs. The larvae (oncospheres) hatch in the intestine and penetrate the intestinal wall and are carried via blood stream to muscles where they become bladder worms 8–20 weeks after ingestion. Some of the cysticerci may become calcified and are no longer infective. Man is infected by eating uncooked measly meat of cattle containing viable cysticerci. Adult tapeworm develop in man in 3–5 weeks.

Geographic distribution: World-wide

Symptoms: Cysticercosis in cattle is usually inapparent, except if vital structures in organs are affected (e.g. heart, diaphragm). Infections with *Taenia saginata* in man may be associated with loss of appetite and diarrhoea but they are usually inapparent.

Significance: Carcasses containing beef measles are condemned at meat inspection. Consumption of infected, inadequately cooked meat may infect man. Therefore consequent inspection of cattle carcasses needs to be done. This is time-consuming and expensive.

Diagnosis: Demonstration of cysticerci in muscles of cattle at meat inspection. Serological tests may be used to detect infections antemortem but some are relatively unspecific.

Therapy: Not indicated

Prophylaxis: Animals should not be exposed to human faeces. Water used for livestock purposes (e.g. drinking, irrigation) should be free of faecal contamination. The disease is spread because pastures are irrigated with human sewage.

(Figures 154, 155, 156, 157)

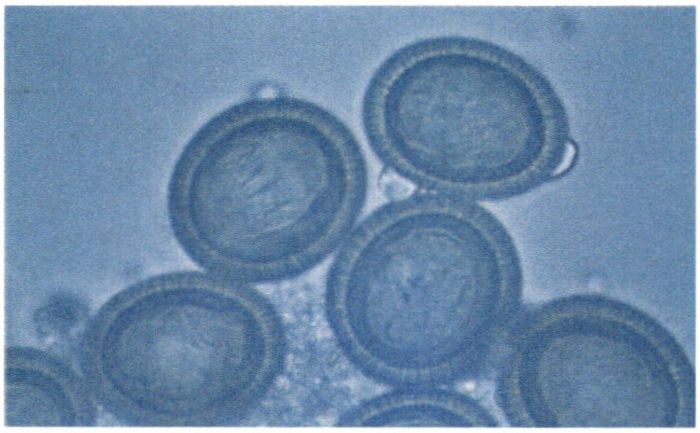

Fig. 154 *Taenia* sp. eggs (34–39 × 31–38 μm) containing oncospheres [4]

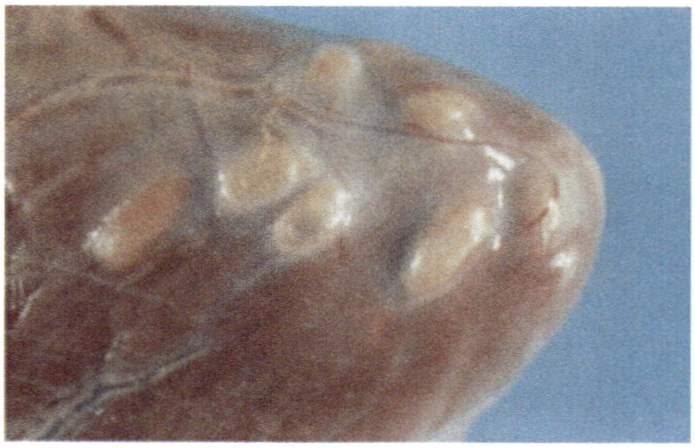

Fig. 155 Cysts of *Cysticercus bovis* (10 × 4–5 mm) in the heart of a cattle [4]

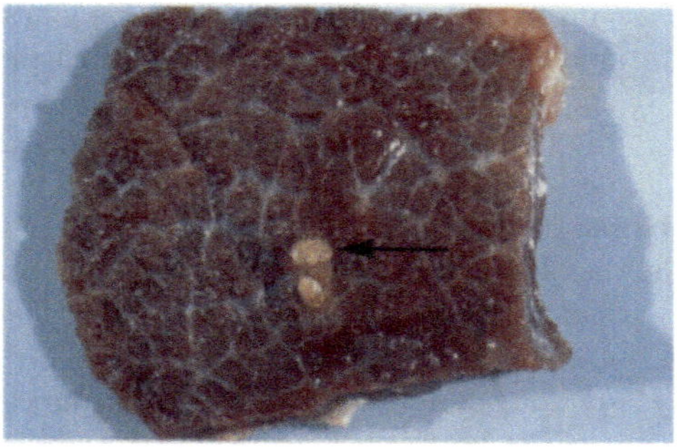

Fig. 156 Calcified tissue cyst of *Cysticercus bovis* in the masseter muscle of a cattle

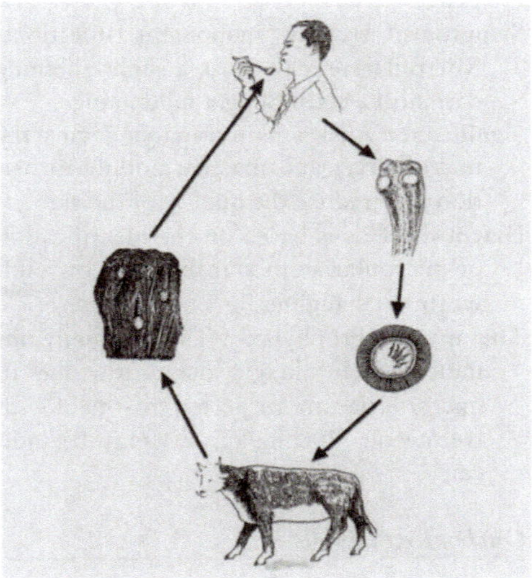

Fig. 157 Life cycle of *Taenia saginata/Cysticercus bovis*

Cysticercus dromedarii (syn. *C. cameli*)

Remarks: The larva (*Cysticercus dromedarii*) of a hyena tapeworm (*Taenia hyaenae*) is frequently found in the muscles of the dromedary, cattle and goats (☞ DROMEDARIES, ■ 4.1.1). It is rarely found in sheep. *C. dromedarii* cysts are twice as large as *C. bovis*, measuring 12–18 mm in length. They are pearly white and the lateral invaginated protoscolex has a double row of hooks. Although they are not dangerous to man, their presence is repugnant, and parasitized meat should be condemned and not fed to dogs or other caniidae.

• Nematoda larvae and adult nematodes found in the muscles

Onchocerca dukei Muscular and subcutaneous onchocercosis of cattle

Remarks: Adult worms of this species are found in the subcutaneous, perimuscular and muscular tissue of cattle in tropical Africa (☞ CATTLE, ■ 5.1). It is very frequent in West Africa where sometimes up to 100% of the cattle are infected. *O. dukei* forms intramuscular and subcutaneous nodules. These nodules are fibrous reactions of the host, yellow or grayish-white in colour. They are oval (3–6 mm in diameter) with a raised contour. These nodules are hard to touch, and when sliced one or several worms appear, surrounded by pus. This is the major difference to *Cysticercus bovis*. The intramuscular nodules can be completely embedded in the muscles or only partly covered. The entire musculature may be involved, especially the flank, intercostal and limb muscles. Subcutaneous nodules may be found almost everywhere (☞ CATTLE, ■ 5.1).
(Figures 158, 159)

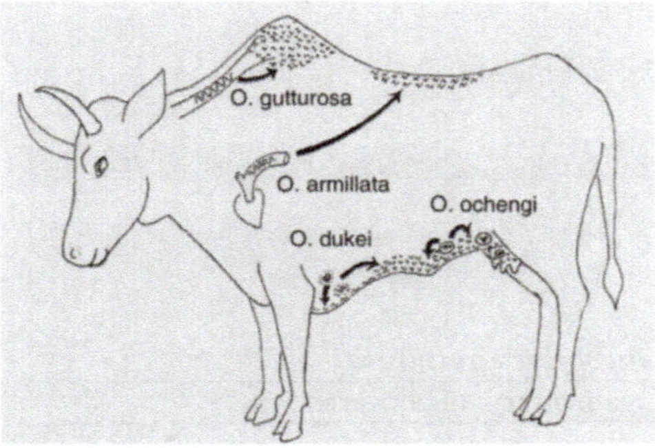

Fig. 158 Sites of occurrence of some *Onchocerca* species found in cattle in Africa [20]

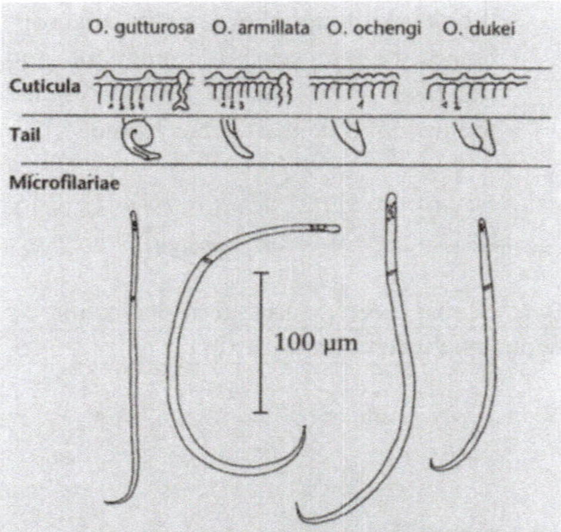

	O. gutturosa	O. armillata	O. ochengi	O. dukei
Lenght	263/249	382/346	298/277	240/217
Diameter	4.4/3.4	6.8/5.5	7.9/5.9	6.7/4.8
n	26/13	15/13	22/13	22/8

Fig. 159 Key for the identification of *Onchocerca* species of cattle in Africa [20]

ARTHROPODS

- Insecta larvae found in the muscles

Hypoderma bovis* and *Hypoderma lineatum
Larvae of the warble flies

Remarks: Larvae of the warble flies may sometimes occur in the muscles during their migratory period. *Hypoderma lineatum* migrates through the wall of the oesophagus (☞ CATTLE, ■ 5.1).

4.1.2 Tendons

HELMINTHS

- Nematoda larvae and adult nematodes found in the tendons

Onchocerca gutturosa
Ligamentary onchocercosis

Location: Adult worms of this species occur in the ligamentum nuchae and also in the ligaments of the hip, elbow, stifle, knee joints and the external side of the scapular cartilage. Microfilariae are found in the skin of the hump and back, sometimes ears and neck of cattle.
Hosts: Cattle
Species description: Males are 2–3 cm long and females are up to 60 cm long or more. The microfialriae are unsheathed and 249–263 µm long and 3.4–4.4 µm wide. The intermediate hosts are members of the family *Simuliidae*.
Geographic distribution: Probably worldwide, extremely common throughout Africa.
Symptoms: Usually inapparent infections. Microfilariae may cause a slightly itching dermatitis, resembling a mild mange.
Significance: Allergic skin reactions against the microfialriae and massive nodule formation may reduce the quality of the skin.
Diagnosis: This is based on the identification of microfilariae in skin biopsies or adult worms at slaughter.
Therapy and Prophylaxis: This is usually not indicated. If allergic dermatitis due to microfilariae are suspected treatment with ivermectin (200 µg/kg, sc.) may be indicated.

Onchocerca lienalis

Remarks: Adults are found in the ligamentum abomaso-lienale. Microfilarieae occur in the skin. The infection is asymptomatic.

4.2 Liver

HELMINTHS

- Trematoda found in the liver

***Fasciola gigantica* Giant liver fluke**

Location: Bile ducts
Hosts: Cattle, sheep, goat, dromedary, horse, pig and many other animal species
Species description: *F. gigantica* is the common liver fluke of livestock in Africa and South

Asian countries. *F. gigantica* resembles *F. hepatica*. Its size is larger, being 25–75 mm in length and up to 12 mm in breadth. The size of the eggs is 156–197 μm × 90–104 μm. The most frequently involved intermediate hosts are *Lymnaea auricularia* and *L. natalensis*. These are aquatic snails living in fairly large permanent bodies of water. The snail vectors can survive an amphibious existence but can only aestivate for very short periods. Metacercariae (the cyst stage of cercariae formed after the tail is cast off) encyst on plants under water such as rice plants, etc. Metacercariae may survive for up to 4 months on stored plants and thus infection may be transmitted by feeding rice straw. *F. gigantica* adults reach the bile ducts 12 weeks after infection. The immature stages migrate through the liver parenchyma. Infections with *F. gigantica* can occur extremely focal, revealing high prevalences in some regions and low prevalences in others. Infection is acquired by eating herbage which is contaminated with metacercariae. The prepatent period is 9–12 weeks.

Geographic distribution: Throughout Africa and Asia

Symptoms: In sheep an acute and a chronic form can occur whereas in cattle only the chronic form seems to play a role. The pathogenesis is essentially the same as in *F. hepatica*.

Significance: *F. gigantica* causes mainly a chronic fasciolosis in cattle and an acute, often fatal, syndrome in sheep.

Diagnosis: Detection of typical operculated eggs with the sedimentation method. *Cave: F. gigantica* eggs are similar to the eggs of some rumen fluke species! *F. gigantica* eggs only appear 15 weeks after infection! Adult flukes are found in the bile ducts at necropsy.

Therapy: ☞ *F. hepatica*

Prophylaxis: ☞ *F. hepatica* in many parts of Africa it is not possible to avoid grazing around lakes, swamps especially if these places are used for watering. The use of bore holes for watering cattle is an effective means to reduce infections with *F. gigantica*.

(Figure 160)

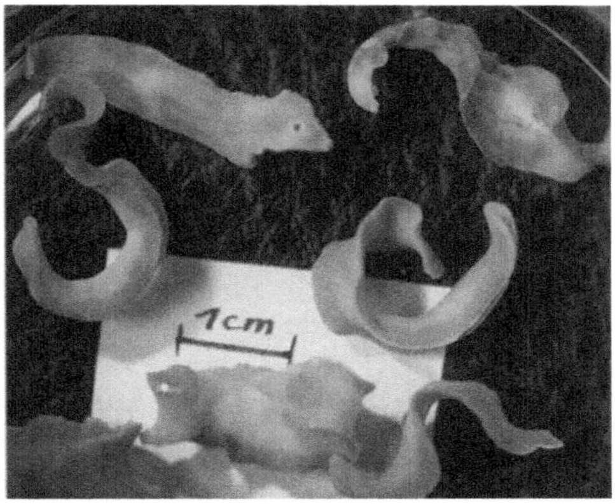

Fig. 160 *Fasciola gigantica*; the giant liver fluke

Fasciola hepatica Common liver fluke

Location: Bile ducts of the liver, sometimes gall bladder

Hosts: Cattle, sheep, goat, horse, donkey, pig and many other animal species

Species description: *F. hepatica* is occurs world-wide – except in Africa and South Asia where it is replaced by *F. gigantica* – and affects especially cattle and sheep. Its size is 30 by 15 mm. The eggs measure 130–150 × 65–90 μm. *F. hepatica* eggs hatch within 10–12 days after deposition and the miracidium, the first larval stage, penetrates actively into the intermediate host which is generally an amphibious snail of the genus *Lymnaea*. Cercariae leave the snail 4–7 weeks after infection and settle on plants just below water level. After casting off the tail they form a cyst about 0.2 mm in diameter (metacercariae). The metacercariae are infective. Ingested metacercariae penetrate the small intestinal wall and reach the liver via abdominal cavity. The duration of the migration within the liver parenchyma is 6–8 weeks after which the young flukes reach maturity in the bile ducts. Infection occurs orally by ingestion of metacercariae on herbage. The incubation period is 2–4 weeks. First symptoms may be seen 5–7 days after infection in acute fasciolosis.

Geographic distribution: Temperate areas world-wide and high altitude regions in East and South Africa.

Symptoms: *F. hepatica* causes a wide range of clinical symptoms, depending on the number of metacercariae ingested but none of the symptoms is pathognomonic. Chronic fasciolosis is the most common form in cattle, sheep and other hosts. The symptoms of chronic fasciolosis are generally associated with hepatic fibrosis and hyperplastic cholangitis. Anaemia, oedema (bottle jaw), digestive disturbances (constipation, diarrhoea) and cachexia develop gradually.

Acute fasciolosis is less common than the chronic disease and occurs mainly in sheep. It is basically a hepatitis caused by the simultaneous migration of large numbers of immature flukes. Sudden death may occur in acute fasciolosis.

Significance: *F. hepatica* is the most important trematode of domestic ruminants and the most common cause of liver fluke disease in temperate areas.

Diagnosis: The oval, operculated, golden-brown eggs (130–150 × 65–90 µm) appear in the faeces 10 weeks after infection. The sedimentation is the most reliable method for the detection of *Fasciola* spp. eggs (☞ METHODS, 1.5). Eggs are expelled intermittently, depending on the evacuation of the gall bladder. *Fasciola* spp. eggs are very similar to eggs of the rumen flukes (family Paramphistomidae). Rumen flukes are very prevalent in ruminants in most parts of Africa whereas fasciolosis is rather focal. The differentiation between *Fasciola* spp. eggs and eggs of Paramphistomidae is not easy. The detection of the adult flukes in the liver at necropsy or slaughter is the most reliable method to confirm fasciolosis. Prevalence studies should be based on abattoir surveys rather than on coproscopic investigations.

Therapy: A number of compounds is available to treat fasciolosis in cattle. These are oxyclozanide (10 mg/kg, po.), rafoxanide (7.5 mg/kg, po.), nitroxynil (10 mg/kg, sc.), albendazole (10 mg/kg, po.), closantel (5 mg/kg, po.), triclabendazole (12 mg/kg, po.), netobimin (20 mg/kg, po.) and clorsulon (7 mg/kg, po.). Some of these diamphenethide (100 mg/kg, po.), nitroxynil (15 mg/kg, sc.), closantel (10 mg/kg, po.), triclabendazole (12 mg/kg, po.) and clorsulon (7 mg/kg, po.) are active against immature flukes. The treatment interval for strategic control should be chosen according to the local epidemiological situation.

Prophylaxis: The snail intermediate host may be controlled by drainage of land, fencing off water pools to exclude animals from the snail habitats. The use of plant molluscicides offers new prospects for future snail control.

(Figures 30, 31, 32, 161, 162, 163, 164, 165)

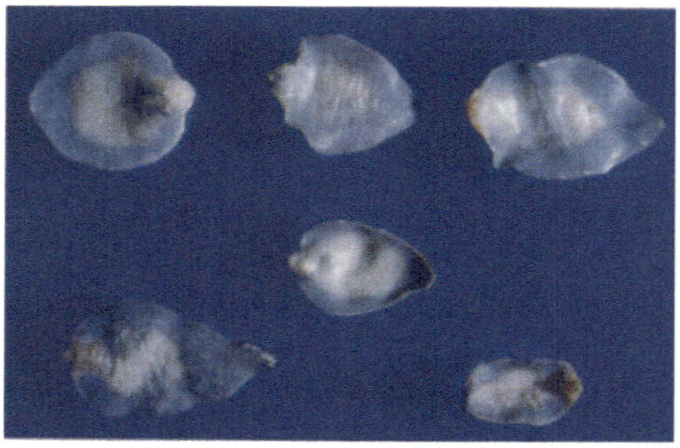

Fig. 161 *Fasciola hepatica*; the common liver fluke (30 × 15 mm)

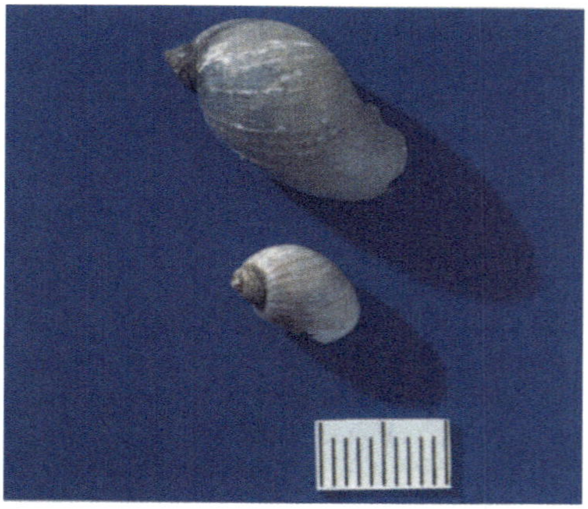

Fig. 162 *Lymnaea truncatula*; the intermediate host of *Fasciola hepatica* [10]

Fig. 163 Life cycle of *Fasciola hepatica* [6]

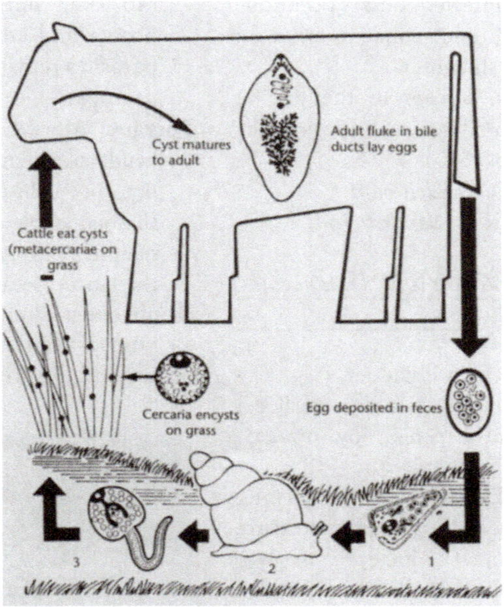

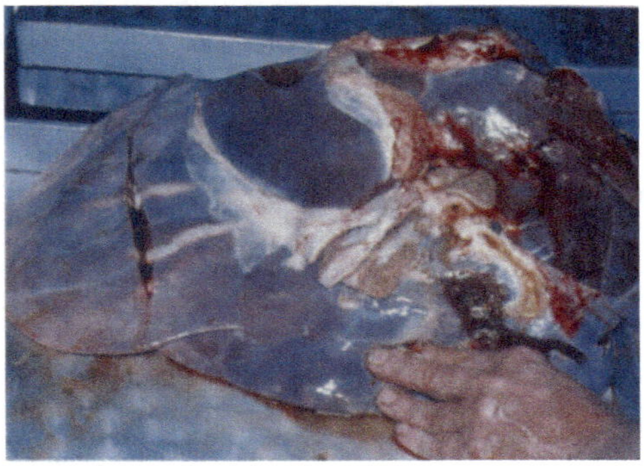

Fig. 164 *Fasciola hepatica* infection; cholangitis and calcification of the bile ducts [4]

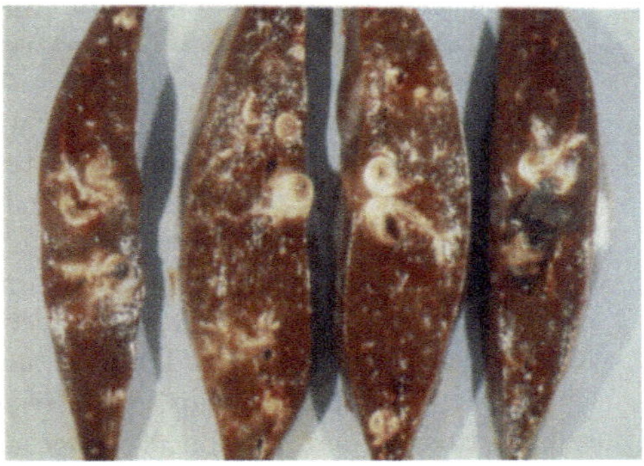

Fig. 165 *Fasciola hepatica* infection causing cholangitis and calcification of the bile ducts

Dicrocoelium hospes **African lancet fluke**

Location: Bile ducts and gall bladder

Hosts: Sheep, goat, cattle and other ruminants

Species description: *D. hospes* is 6–10 mm long and 0.8–1 mm wide. The eggs measure 36–45 µm × 25 µm. The life cycle involves two intermediate hosts. The first is a land snail (*Limicolaria* spp., *Achatina* spp. and probably others) and the second an ant (*Dorylus* spp., *Cematogaster* spp. and other genera). *D. hospes* is closely related to *D. dendriticum*. Infection is acquired by ingestion of infected ants (containing metacercariae) via herbage. Migration of immature flukes from the intestine via ductus choledochus into the biliary system. The prepatent period is up to 97 days.

Geographic distribution: North, Central and West Africa

Symptoms: Generally clinically inapparent; heavy infections cause diarrhoea, cholangitis and weight loss.

Significance: In some regions a high percentage of animals is infected. Losses occur due to poor growth and condemnation of infected livers at slaughter.

Diagnosis: Adult *D. hospes* in the bile at necropsy; detection of parasite eggs in the sediment of faeces.

Therapy: ☞ below *D. dendriticum*

Prophylaxis: ☞ below *D. dendriticum*

Dicrocoelium dendriticum (syn. *D. lanceolatum)* Common lancet fluke

Location: Bile ducts or gall bladder

Hosts: *D. dendriticum* occurs mainly in sheep, goat, cattle but also in pig, dog, donkey, rabbit and rarely in man.

Species description: The fluke is 6–10 mm long and 1.5–2.5 mm wide. The eggs measure 36–45 × 20–30 µm. The life cycle involves two intermediate hosts, a land snail as the first (*Zebrina* spp., *Cionella* spp. and 29 other species are described) and ants of the genus *Formica* and *Lasius* as the second intermediate hosts. Ants infected with metacercariae attach to herbage overnight and are available to grazing animals in the early morning. Infection occurs by ingestion of infected ants (containing metacercariae) via herbage. Migration of immature flukes from the intestine via ductus choledochus into the biliary system. The prepatent period is 47–54 days. Cirrhosis of the liver and thickening of the bile ducts may occur in heavy infections.

Geographic distribution: Europe, Asia, the Americas, North Africa, occasionally in imported ruminants in other parts of Africa; autochthonous infections seem not to occur in Africa.

Symptoms: Often without clinical symptoms. Heavy infections may produce weight loss, anaemia and hypoproteinaemia.

Significance: Lancet flukes may cause extensive liver damage, causing the host to "do poorly". Condemnation of livers at slaughter may cause severe economic losses among cattle herds.

Diagnosis: Demonstration of typical eggs in the sediment of faeces. The eggs are small (40 × 25 µm), thick walled, yellowish-brown and contain a miracidium. Adult parasites may be found in the bile ducts at necropsy.

Therapy: Albendazole (20 mg/kg, po.), fenbendazole (50 mg/kg, po.), netobimin (20 mg /kg, po.) thiophanate (50 mg/kg, po.), thiabendazole (200 mg/kg, po.) and praziquantel (50 mg/kg, po.) are effective against the lancet fluke.

Prophylaxis: Elimination of the intermediate hosts is not feasible.

(Figures 32, 33, 166, 353)

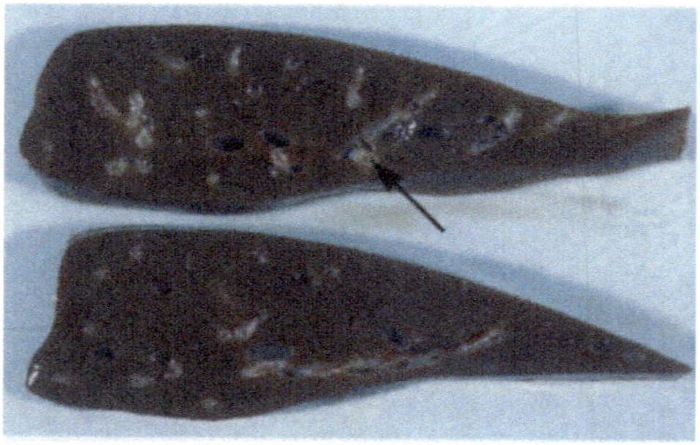

Fig. 166 *Dicrocoelium dendriticum* found in the bile ducts

***Schistosoma* spp.**

Remarks: Schistosomes may often be found at necropsy in the portal veins of the liver (☞ CATTLE, ■ 2).

- **Cestoda found in the liver**

Echinococcus granulosus (syn. *E. unilocularis)* Hydatid tapeworm, hydatidosis

Location: Larvae (hydatid cysts) of *E. granulosus* are found in the liver and the lungs of cattle, sheep, goats, swine, horse, dromedary and other domestic animals and man (= intermediate hosts). Adult tapeworms are found in the small intestine of the dog and other related carnivores (= final hosts).

Hosts: Canids are the final hosts of *E. granulosus*. Intermediate hosts are ungulates and man.

Species description: *E. granulosus* is a small tapeworm with 3–4 proglottids and a total length of 2–6 mm. It occurs in the small intestine of the dog and other canids (hyaena, coyote, fox, etc.). Adult tapeworms in the dogs pass proglottids or eggs in the faces. When ingested by cattle or other intermediate hosts, these eggs hatch in the intestine. The oncospheres (hexacanths) penetrate the gut wall, enter the portal vein and reach the liver, which is the first capillary filter for the larvae and subsequently the lungs, which are the second capillary filter. The remaining oncospheres may reach via the arteries other organs. In all these organs hydatid cysts (bladder worms) develop. These are large cysts filled with fluid and tapeworm heads (protoscolices). The hydatid cysts develop slowly over several months. They are commonly 5–10 cm in diameter and contain a liquid. The hydatid cyst is composed of a thick outer, concentrically laminated membrane. About 5 months after infection brood capsules, each containing several protoscolices develop from the inner part of the capsule (germinal membrane). The brood capsules may become detached and float free in the cyst fluid, being termed "hydatid sand". At this time the cyst is infective for the definitive host. The life cycle is completed when a dog ingests protoscolices. Hydatid cysts are usually found in the lungs of sheep and cattle, but primarily in the livers of horses. In pigs, hydatid cysts are found in both the liver and the lungs. The hydatid cysts may be multilocular (sheep, cattle, pigs) or unilocular (horse). In man hydatid cysts may be found in many organs. The significance of the hydatid cyst depends on the severity of the infection and the organ in which it is situated. In domestic animals clinical signs are not commonly seen despite heavy infections. Human hydatidosis is often associated with clinical signs and the function of the affected organ is often impaired. This is especially true if the heart or the brain are involved. Adult tapeworms are harmless to the dogs and seldom cause clinical symptoms.

Geographic distribution: World-wide

Symptoms: Hydatid cysts do not usually cause clinical symptoms unless the cysts are numerous or become very large.

Significance: Hydatidosis in cattle is not usually a problem, but infected organs are condemned at slaughter. In man hydatidosis is a serious problem. Infected dogs are a reservoir for both infection of domestic animals and man.

Diagnosis: Usually the diagnosis of hydatidosis is made at slaughter or necropsy. Infected dogs pass eggs in the faeces which cannot be differentiated from those of *Taenia* spp. Immundiagnostic tests (ELISA, Immunoblotting; ☞ METHODS, 5.2 and 5.3) are widely used in medical parasitology and may assume significance in epidemiological studies. *E. granulosus* eggs, excreted by dogs are very similar to those of *Taenia* spp. The differentiation may be carried out by means of monoclonal antibodies.

Therapy: Treatment of hydatidosis in cattle and other intermediate hosts is rarely indicated. Control of hydatidosis is based on prophylaxis.

Prophylaxis: Dogs should not be fed with uncooked meat in general and infected organs in particular. In endemic areas where human hydatidosis is of great importance special attention should be paid to the safe destruction of affected organs, the reduction of stray dogs and the anthelmintic treatment of domestic dogs. Praziquantel (5 mg/kg, po. or 5.7 mg/kg, sc. or im.), bunamidine hydrochloride (25–50 mg/kg, po.) and the combination of febantel/praziquantel/pyrantel are sufficiently effective against adult *E. granulosus* tapeworms in dogs.

(Figures 167, 168, 169, 170)

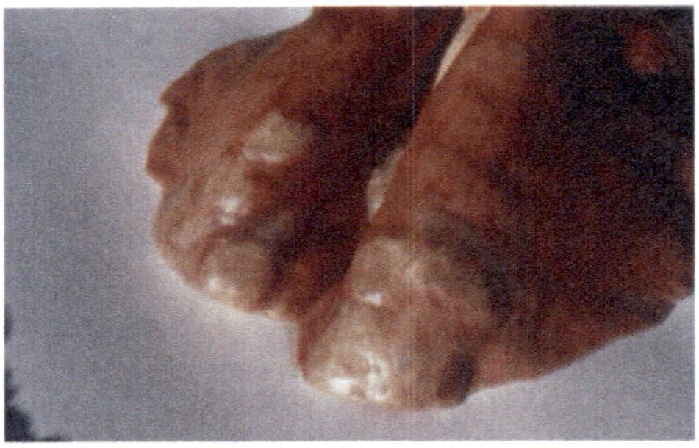

Fig. 167 *Echinococcus granulosus*; hydatid cyst in the lungs of a cattle [4]

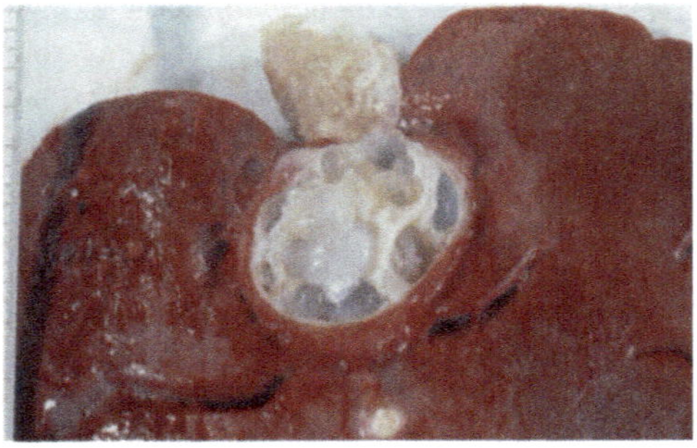

Fig. 169 *Echinococcus granulosus*; hydatid cyst [42] opened [4]

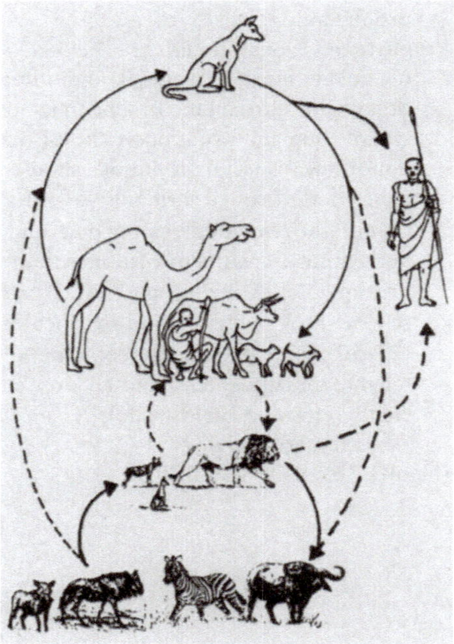

Fig. 168 Life cycle of *Echinococcus granulosus* in sub-Saharan Africa [21]

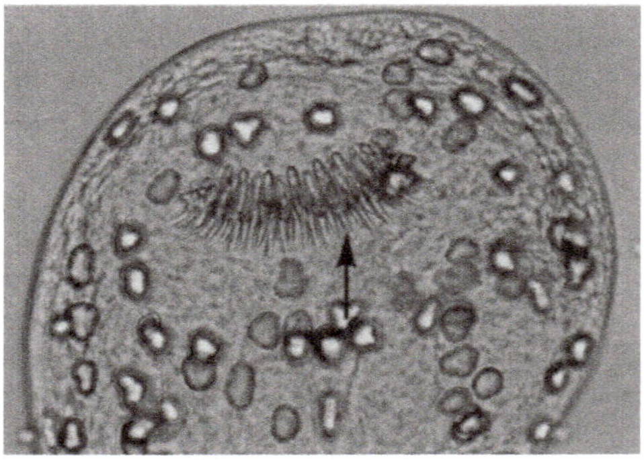

Fig. 170 *Echinococcus granulosus*; protoscolex (100 × 160 in diameter) with typical hook collar

Stilesia hepatica

Remarks: This parasite occurs in the bile ducts and small intestine of sheep and goats (☞ SHEEP AND GOATS, ■ 4.2). In endemic areas wild ruminants and rarely cattle may also be affected. This parasite is very prevalent in tropical and southern Africa. *S. hepatica* is non-pathogenic but extremely prevalent (in 90–100% of sheep) in many parts of Africa. It is non-pathogenic and does not require treatment.

Cysticercus tenuicollis

Remarks: Migrating post-oncospheral stages may occasionally be found in the liver parenchyma and thin-necked cysts may be found on the serosa of the liver (☞ CATTLE, ■ 4.4 and SHEEP AND GOATS, ■ 4.4).

POROCEPHALIDA

Linguatula serrata "tongue worm"

Remarks: This is a cosmopolitan parasite and it occurs in the nasal and respiratory passages of the dog and other canids, snakes, very rarely in man, horse, goat and sheep. The parasite is tongue-shaped and the cuticle is transversely striated. Males are 1.8–2 cm, females are 3–13 cm long. The eggs measure about 90–70 µm. The eggs are ingested by a herbivorous intermediate host (horse, sheep, goat, cattle, rodents, rabbit, etc.) and hatch in the alimentary canal and the larvae migrate to the mesenteric lymph nodes, in which they develop to the infective nymphal stage. The larva is up to 500 µm long and undergoes about six to 9 moults. It usually lies in a cyst surrounded by a viscid fluid. These cysts may be found at necropsy in the intestinal lymph glands, the liver or in other organs. Dogs become infective by eating the infective viscera, especially of sheep and cattle. Infected dogs show sneezing and discharge from the nostrils. The infection in cattle is clinically inapparent.
(Figures 171, 172)

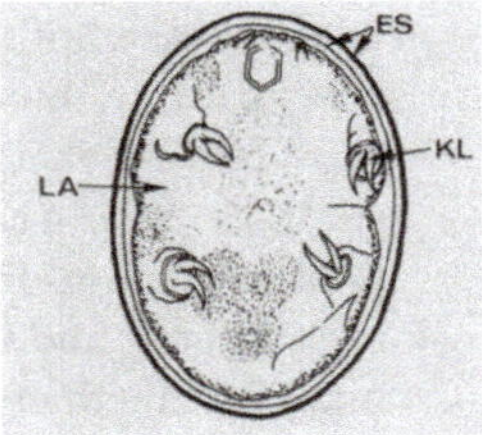

Fig. 171 *Linguatula serrata*; embryonated egg (90 × 70 µm); [47]; ES = egg shell; KL = claw; LA = larva [7]

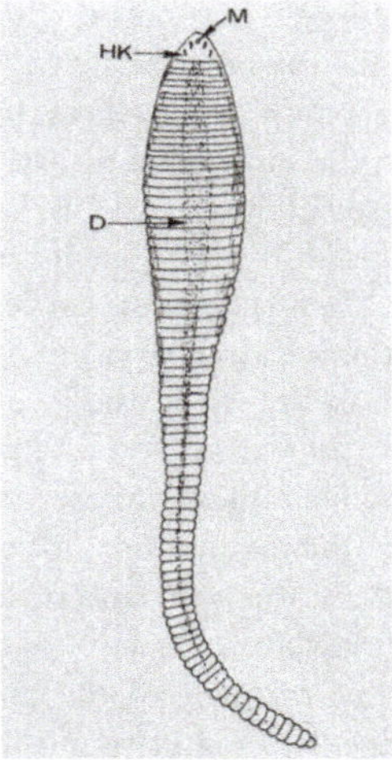

Fig. 172 *Linguatula serrata*; adult female (up to 13 cm long); M = mouth opening; HK = hooks; D = intestine [7]

4.3 Respiratory system

HELMINTHS

• Cestoda found in the lungs and trachea

Echinococcus granulosus (syn. *E. unilocularis)* Hydatid tapeworm, hydatidosis

Remarks: Larvae (hydatid cysts) of *E. granulosus* are often found in the lungs and liver of cattle and other domestic animals (☞ CATTLE, ■ 4.2).

• Nematoda found in the lungs and trachea

Dictyocaulus viviparus Cattle lungworm, parasitic bronchitis

Location: Trachea, bronchi and bronchioles
Hosts: Cattle, camel and some deer species
Species description: Males are 4–5 cm long and the females 6–8 cm. The eggs measure 82–88 × 33–38 µm. The adult worms live

in the airways and produce eggs which contain larvae. These eggs are moved with respiratory secretions towards the larynx. They are then coughed up and swallowed. Hatching occurs in the intestine and first-stage larvae are passed in the faeces. On the pasture the larvae moult twice to reach the third stage which is infective for cattle. When swallowed the infective larvae penetrate the gut wall and move to the local lymph nodes, where they moult to become fourth-stage larvae. Then they migrate via the thoracic duct to the jugular vein, after that to the right side of the heart and then to the lungs where they are arrested in the capillaries and break through to the air passages. Development to maturity in the bronchi of the host takes about 4 weeks. Larval stages remain inhibited for several months. Irritation of the respiratory mucosa by larvae and adult worms cause increased respiratory secretions and lung congestion with blockage of air passages. Aspiration of eggs and larvae into the alveoli leads to consolidation of lobules. Severe epithelialization and peribronchial fibrosis usually occur a few weeks after the infection has started. These chronic lung alterations may be the cause of the unthriftiness, commonly observed in animals after a heavy infection. Immunity is built up as quickly as 10 days after an initial infection but it wanes in the absence of reinfection.

Geographic distribution: World-wide

Symptoms: Parasitic bronchitis is characterized by severe coughing, rapid breathing, dyspnoea and rapid loss of condition. Severe cases lead to emphysema and pneumonia. Death may occur in heavy infections.

Significance: Parasitic bronchitis due to *D. viviparus* may cause great losses in endemic areas. Even animals after a moderate initial infection show retarded growth for prolonged periods of time. In Africa *D. viviparus* has been frequently found in imported animals. Autochthonous infections occur sporadically.

Diagnosis: This is based on the clinical signs, rapid and heavy breathing, coughing, nasal discharges and the demonstration of larvae in the faeces by the Baermann method (☞ METHODS, 1.7 and CATTLE, ■ 1). However, coughing may occur in the prepatent period before larvae are found in the faeces. Usually parasitic bronchitis is a herd problem, seen especially in young calves which have recently been exposed to an infected pasture.

Therapy: Levamisole (5 mg/kg, sc. or 7.5 mg/kg, po.), the benzimidazoles (fenbendazole, 7.5 mg/kg, po.; oxfendazole, 4.5–5 mg/kg, po.; albendazole, 7.5 mg/kg, po.; febantel, 7.5 mg/kg, po.) netobimin (12.5 mg/kg, po.) and ivermectin (200 µg/kg, sc.) are highly effective against all stages of *D. viviparus*. These drugs are also effective against lungworms in sheep, horses and pigs. In calves, aggravated coughing a few minutes after treatment (especially with levamisole, sc.) is characteristic for the infection and often regarded as a confirmation of the diagnosis. Heavily affected calves should be moved inside and supportive treatment should be administered.

Prophylaxis: Pastures with a recent history of lungworm infection are highly dangerous for young calves. Lungworm infections may be controlled in several ways. Calves may be vaccinated with X-radiated *Dictyocaulus* larvae (Dictol®), in countries where the vaccine is available, twice (4 weeks apart) prior to exposure. The animals should be housed during the vaccination period and for another 2 weeks after the second dose to allow time to build up an adequate level of immunity before release on pasture. Another approach is the strategic control of infections. In first-season cattle, a first treatment is applied 2–3 weeks after turn-out and, depending on the infection risk and the duration of the drug, repeated treatments are required during the period of high challenge (benzimidazoles monthly, ivermectin 3 and 10 weeks after turn-out). A sustained release device (anthelmintic with a prolonged activity)

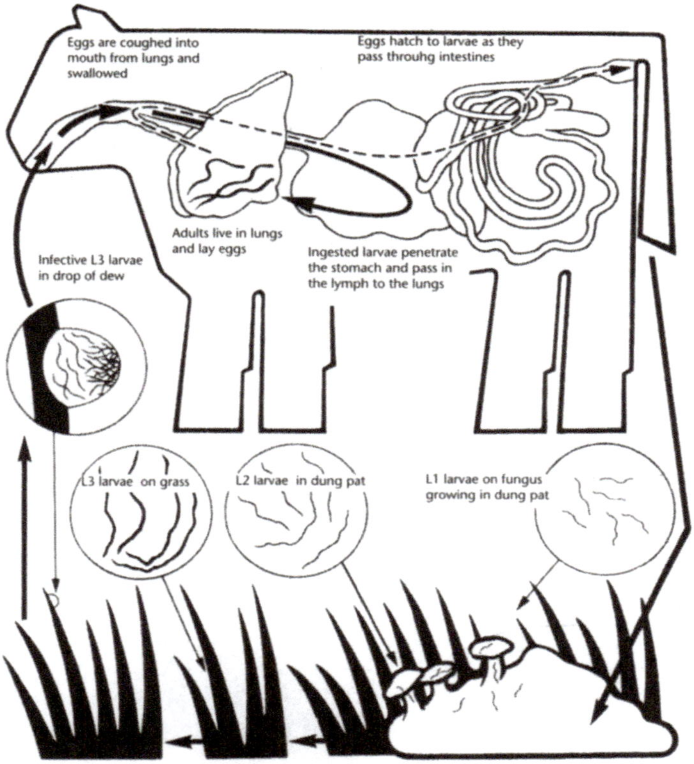

Fig. 173 Life cycle of *Dictyocaulus viviparus*; the third-stage larvae penetrate the intestinal mucosa and not the mucosa of the stomach [6]

may also be applied about 2–3 weeks after turn-out or prior to the period with the highest infection risk.

(Figures 83, 173, 174)

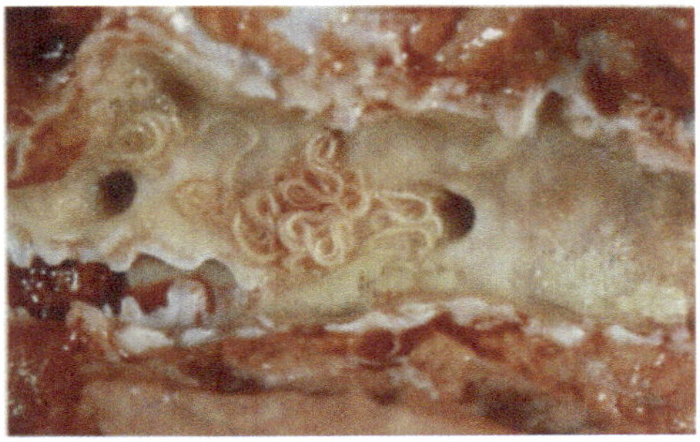

Fig. 174 *Dictyocaulus viviparus*; adult worms in trachea

Mammomonogamus laryngeus

Location: Larynx

Hosts: Cattle, water buffalo, occasionally sheep, goat and rarely man

Species description: *M. laryngeus* is not very pathogenic for cattle. The worms are attached to the mucosa of the larynx. The males and females are found in permanent copulation. The life cycle is unknown.

Geographic distribution: Caribbean Islands, South America, Asia, Central Africa (Cameroon)

Symptoms: Affected animals may cough and sometimes lose condition. Calves may develop bronchitis. Pneumonia due to respiratory secretions which are aspirated, causing pulmonary reactions have been observed.

Significance: Heavy infections in endemic areas may cause losses due to massive irritation of the larynx by the parasites. Bronchitis and pneumonia may occur.

Diagnosis: This is made by finding the eggs in the faeces or adult worms at necropsy.

Therapy: Unknown. Nitroxynil (10mg/kg, sc.), which is used against *Syngamus* spp. of poultry may also be used against *Mammomonogamus laryngeus*. Modern benzimidazoles and ivermectin (200 µg/kg. sc.) may be used in heavily infected cattle.

Prophylaxis: Unknown
(Figures 175, 176, 177)

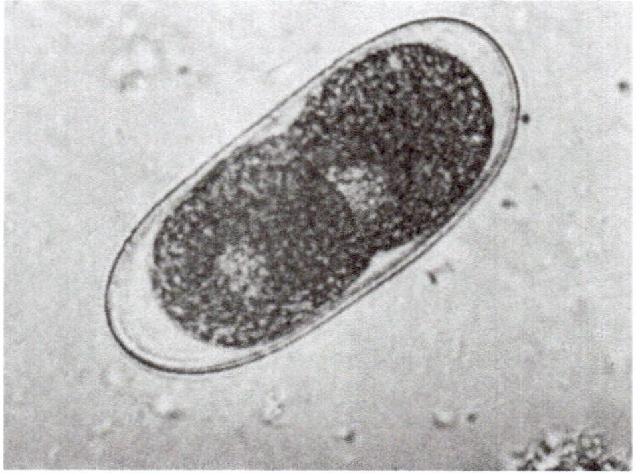

Fig. 176 Egg of *Mammomonogamus laryngeus* (323 × 50 µm) [8]

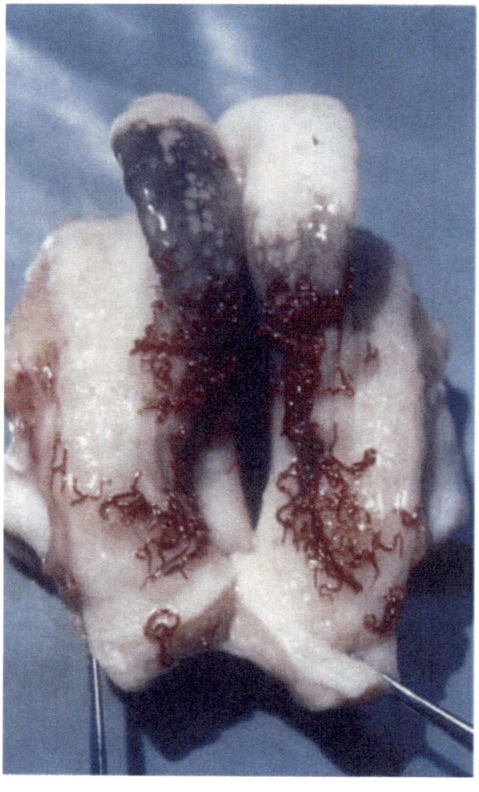

Fig. 175 *Mammomonogamus laryngeus* (males are 3–3.5 mm long, females are 8.5–10 mm long) [8]

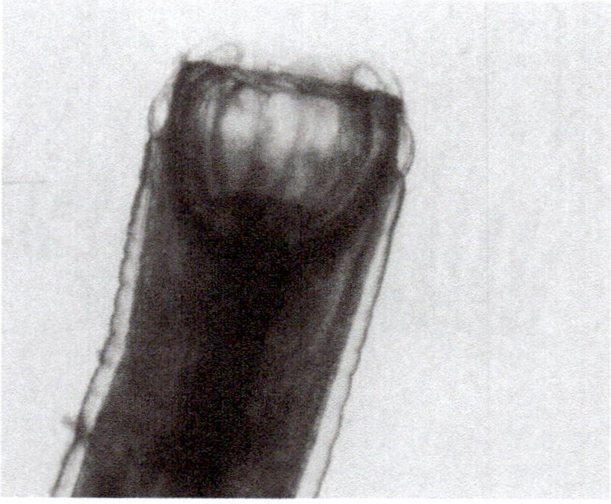

Fig. 177 *Mammonogamus laryngeus*; head end [8]

Mammomonogamus nasicola

Location: Nasal cavities

Hosts: Cattle, sheep and goat

Species description: The males and females of this parasite are permanently joined in copulation. Males are 4–6 mm long and females 11–23 mm. Eggs are 54 × 98 µm and have only a few blastomeres. Life cycle and pathogenesis are unknown. An optional reservoir host (e.g. earthworm or snail) is being suspected. After oral ingestion of infective larvae the parasite reaches the respiratory tract through the blood stream. The parasites suck blood and are bright red in fresh samples.

Geographic distribution: Central and South America, West Indies, Central Africa.

Symptoms: Heavy infections cause irritation of the nasal mucosa, sneezing and nasal discharges. *M. nasicola* may be differentiated from *Schistosoma* infection of nasal passages.

Significance: ☞ above *M. laryngeus*

Diagnosis: ☞ above *M. laryngeus*

Therapy: Unknown

Prophylaxis: Unknown

(Figure 178)

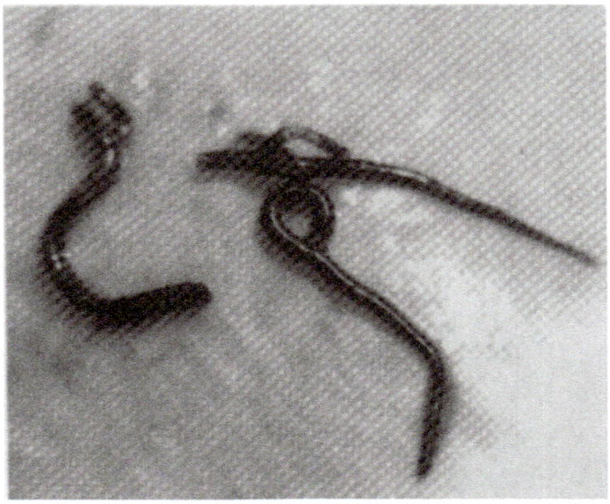

Fig. 178 *Mammomonogamus nasicola* [18]

4.4 Abdominal cavity

HELMINTHS

• Cestoda found in the abdominal cavity

Cysticercus tenuicollis Larval stage of the canine tapeworm *Taenia hydatigena*

Remarks: The thin-necked larvae (*Cysticercus tenuicollis*) of *Taenia hydatigena* are often found attached to the omentum, the intestinal mesentery and to the serosal surface of abdominal organs, especially the liver of cattle, sheep and other herbivores. Cysticerci are often found at meat inspection without any previous clinical signs. The feeding of condemned material to dogs should be avoided (☞ SHEEP AND GOATS, ■ 4.4).

(Figures 179, 180)

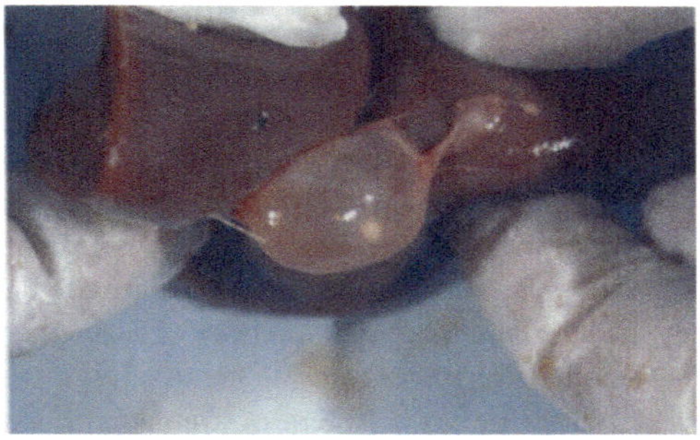

Fig. 179 *Cysticercus tenuicollis*; thin-necked cyst attached to the liver of a sheep. The protoscolex can be seen through the cyst wall

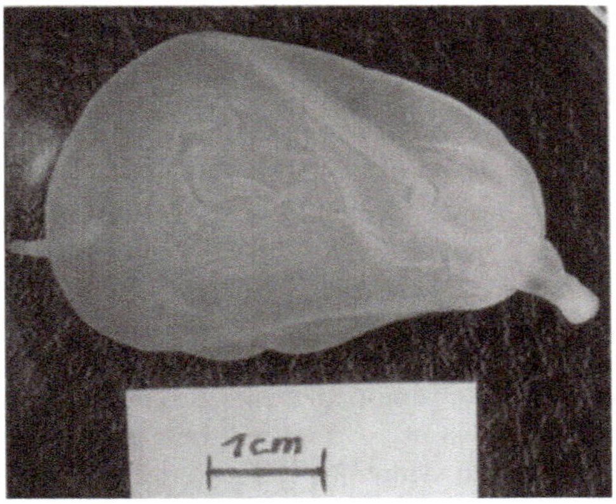

Fig. 180 *Cysticercus tenuicollis*; thin-necked stage found in cysts

• Nematoda found in the abdominal cavity

Setaria labiatopapillosa Bovine abdominal filariosis

Location: Peritoneal cavity

Hosts: Cattle, deer, giraffe and other ruminants

Species description: Males are up to 4–6 cm long and females 6–12 cm. There is a distinct peribuccal ring with dorsal and ventral prominences. The tail of the female terminates in a marked button which is divided into a number of papillae. The microfilariae are sheathed, measure 240–260 µm and appear in the peripheral blood (☞ CATTLE, ■ 2). Several species of mosquitoes act as vectors (*Aedes* spp., *Culex* spp. and *Anopheles gambiae* and other *Anopheles* spp.). Infective larvae are produced in the vector in 12–16 days. Adult worms in the peritoneal cavity are non-pathogenic. The major pathogenic effect occurs when immature stages migrate erratically in the central nervous system of abnormal hosts (e.g. *Setaria digitata* or *S. labiatopapillosa* microfilariae introduced by vectors in horses, sheep and goats). The affected animals suffer from an acute, focal encephalomyelomalacia. The lesions are usually single tracks left by migrating larvae and may be found in any part of the CNS.

Geographic distribution: World-wide

Symptoms: Adult worms in the peritoneal cavity do not cause clinical signs. Erratic larvae in the CNS may cause nervous signs, depending on the location of the lesions. Muscular weakness, ataxia, paralysis and death may occur.

Significance: Adult worms in the peritoneal cavity are non-pathogenic. Erratic larvae in the CNS of an abnormal host may cause nervous symptoms and even death.

Diagnosis: This is made by demonstrating the microfilariae in stained blood smears or with the dark ground/buffy coat method (☞ METHODS, 3.1 and 3.4) or by finding the adult worms in the abdominal cavity. The antemortem diagnosis of immature worm-associated CNS disturbances under field conditions is impossible. Histopathological examination of stained brain sections may result in an aetiological diagnosis.

Therapy: Chemotherapy is difficult because adult worms are very resistant to most drugs. Ivermectin (200–500 µg/kg, sc.) and diethylcarbamazine (25–100 mg/kg/day during several days, sc.) are effective against the microfilariae.

Prophylaxis: Unknown (Figures 148, 181, 182)

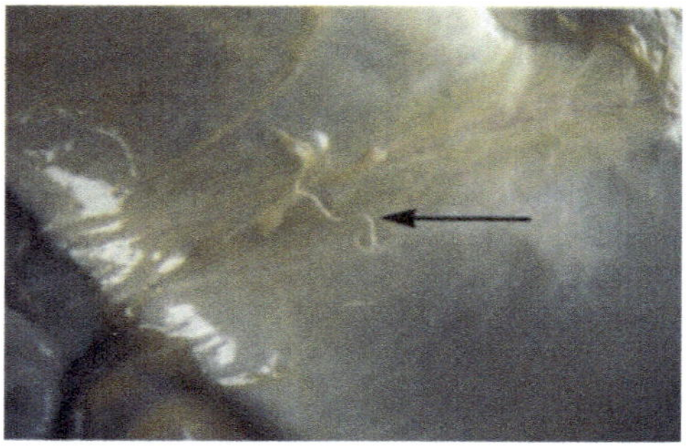

Fig. 181 *Setaria labiatopapillosa*; adult worm on the intestinal serosa; males are 4–6 cm long and and females are 6–12 cm long

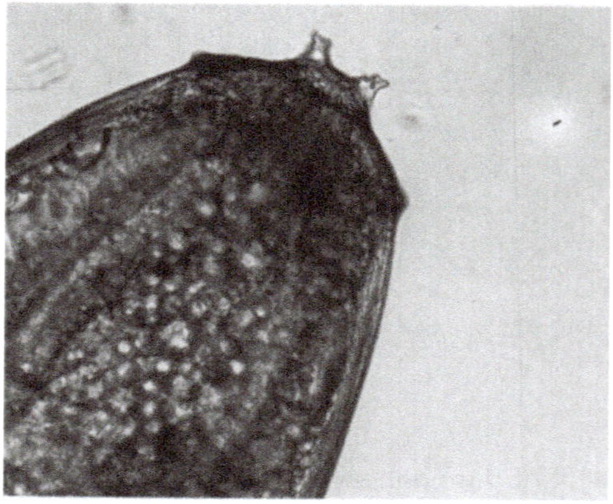

Fig. 182 *Setaria labiatopapillosa*; anterior end

4.5 Pancreas

HELMINTHS

- Trematoda found in the pancreas

Eurytrema pancreaticum **Pancreatic fluke**

Remarks: This parasite occurs in the pancreatic ducts, bile ducts, occasionally duodenum of sheep, goats (☞ SHEEP AND GOATS, ■ 4.5) and occasionally cattle in Asia, Brazil,

Madagascar and Réunion. There are no obvious clinical signs unless heavy infections are present. However, recent reports suggest that in areas with a high prevalence and intensity of infection, *Eurytrema pancreaticum* may be responsible for chronic wasting and mortality, especially in sheep.
(Figures 34, 183)

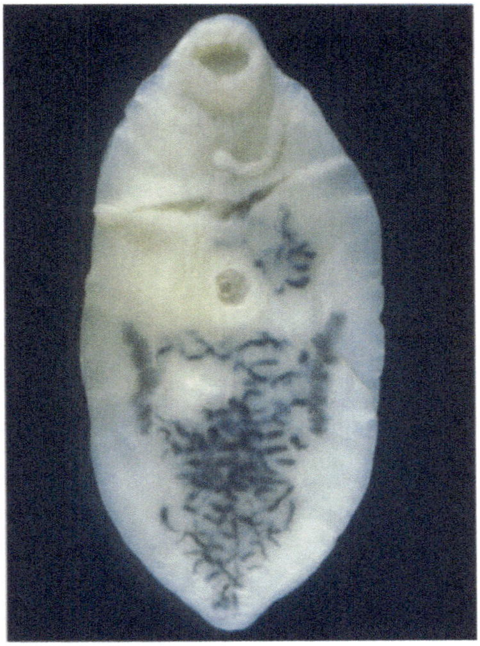

Fig. 183 *Eurytrema pancreaticum*; (8–16 mm long and 5–8. 5 mm wide) [8]

4.6 Central nervous system

PROTOZOA

Toxoplasma gondii

Remarks: Tissue cysts of this parasite may occasionally be found in the brain of sheep and cattle. These cysts contain merozoites (6–8 μm long) and are infective for the final host (cat) (☞ also SWINE, ■ 4.1 and 4.6).

Neospora sp.

Remarks: *Neospora caninum* is a recently recognized new parasite species. It resembles *T. gondii* and causes neuromuscular disorders (polyradiculoneuritis, myositis, paralysis) in dogs and abortion in cattle. *Neospora* sp. is suspected to be responsible for up to 20% of cattle abortion in some parts of the USA. The entire life cycle is unknown. No final host has been found so far in which the sexual development occurs. The only stages of this parasite are tachyzoites and tissue cysts. These are thick-walled (1–4 μm) as compared to *T. gondii* which produces thin-walled (< 0.5 μm) cysts. *Neospora*-like organisms were found in the central nervous system of dogs, cats, lambs, calves and foals. Transplacental transmission has been demonstrated in all these cases. The diagnosis is based on the demonstration of parasites in stained tissue sections or isolation from freshly aborted foetuses. Positive IFAT titres (☞ METHODS, 5.1) in neonatal calves prior to colostrum application is a strong indication of a prenatal infection. The main location of tissue cysts in cattle is the central nervous system. Sulfonamids combined with trimethoprime, pyrimethamine (1mg/kg, daily po. for 4 weeks) and clindamyzine (13.5 mg/kg, 3 × daily po. during 10 days) are used in dogs for treatment. No specific treatment is yet available for ruminants.
(Figures 184, 185)

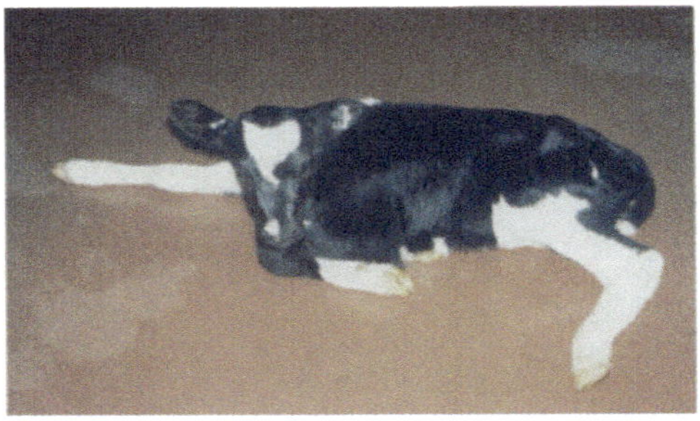

Fig. 184 A weak-born calf with neuromuscular disorders due to a congenital *Neospora caninum* infection [22]

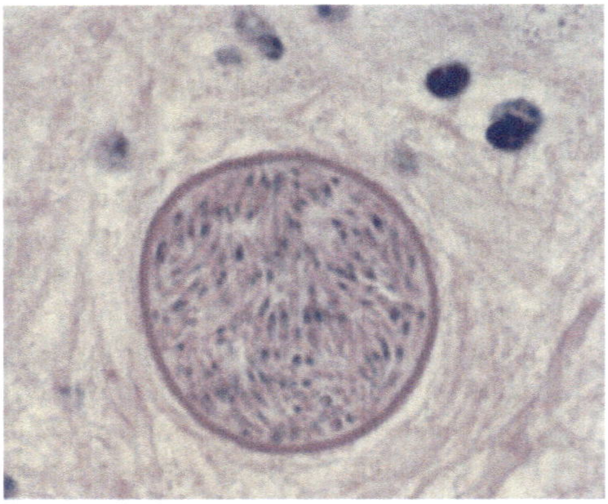

Fig. 185 *Neospora caninum*; thick walled cyst (1–4 µm thick; 70–120 µm in diameter) in the brain of a calf [22]

HELMINTHS

- Cestoda cysts found in the central nervous system

Coenurus cerebralis Larval stage of the canine tapeworm *Taenia multiceps* (syn. *Multiceps multiceps*) "gid", "stuggers", "sturdy"

Remarks: The intermediate stage of the canine tapeworm *Taenia multiceps*, a coenurus, develops in the brain and spinal cord mainly of sheep and goats and less commonly in cattle (☞ SHEEP AND GOATS, ■ 4.6).

5.1. Skin and coat

5.2 Eyes

5.1. Skin and coat

PROTOZOA

Besnoitia besnoiti (syn. *Sarcocystis besnoiti*)
Elephant skin disease

Location: *Besnoitia* cysts are found in the dermis, subcutaneous tissue, fasciae, laryngeal, nasal and other mucosae.

Hosts: Domestic and wild cats act as definitive hosts. Intermediate hosts are cattle, goat, wildebeest, impala and kudu. Sheep, rabbit and some rodents may be experimental intermediate hosts.

Species description: This is a protozoan disease of the skin, subcutis, blood vessels and mucous membranes. These *Toxoplasma*-like organisms multiply in endothelia, histiocytic and other cells and produce characteristic large, thick-walled cysts filled with bradyzoites. The *Besnoitia* cysts may reach up to 600 µm in diameter. They are usually spherical and packed with crescentic trophozoites (bradyzoites) each 2–7 µm in length. Parenteral application of blood, taken from an infected animal may transmit the disease to other animals. Unsporulated oocysts (15 × 13 µm) are shed in the faeces of the final host (Felidae). The mode of transmission is not completely known. In particular the transmission from infected cattle to cats remains to be substantiated. Biting flies (e.g. *Glosssina palpalis* and other biting flies) and ticks may transmit *B. besnoiti* mechanically to cats. Needle inoculation of tissues that contain cysts can transmit some *Besnoitia* spp. to other hosts. It has also been suggested that contaminated water troughs may be an important source of infection. The mortality is usually below 10% although animals may lose condition. Pregnant animals may abort. Bulls may become sterile and hides are of little value for leather-making purposes. Animals of all ages, from 6 months upwards may be infected.

Geographic distribution: Southern Europe, Africa, Asia, South America

Symptoms: The initial stage of the disease starts with fever after an incubation period of 6–10 days. Cyst formation in the skin starts 1–4 weeks after the start of the temperature rise. Inappetence, photophobia, enlargement of the lymph nodes and oedematous swellings on the limbs and the lower parts of the body, orchitis and rhinitis may accompany the febrile stage. Animals are reluctant to move, respiration is rapid and diarrhoea and abortion may occur during this phase. In mild infections recovery may occur in this stage. In the second stage of the disease, the skin becomes hard, thick and wrinkled and develops cracks that allow secondary bacterial infections and myiasis to develop. Movement is painful. A serosanguineous fluid oozes from the cracks. The skin is scurfy and folded and the whole appearance is one of extensive mange. There is hair loss over the swollen skin. Severe infections cause emaciation and death may occur. Cysts may appear in the scleral conjunctiva and nasal mucosa. Although mortality is low, convalescence is slow in severe cases. Severely affected bulls may remain permanently sterile. Previously infected animals may be carriers for life. The hairless condition may remain for several months.

Significance: Besnoitiosis may be a severe problem in endemic areas. Although the mortality is low, affected animals may be emaciated and sick for months.

Diagnosis: This is based on the clinical signs with the typical skin lesions following a febrile phase. Microscopical examination of affected skin by means of stained biopsies may reveal the typical cysts, containing the bradyzoites. Spherical, encapsulated pseudocysts are pathognomonic. The best method of diagnosis is the examination of the scleral conjunctiva. The cysts can be seen in the scleral conjunctiva with the naked eye, revealing many chronic cases without signs.

Therapy: There is no satisfactory treatment. Affected animals should be separated and treated symptomatically (antibiotics, insect-repellants, etc.). Sulfonilamide application prevented cyst development in experimental studies. Antimony (1%, 0.6 ml/kg, po.) cured besnoitiosis in a goat.

Prophylaxis: This is difficult until the exact mode of transmission is known. In some countries, a tissue-cultured vaccine is available and quite effective. Separation of cattle from cats, and of domestic cattle from wild ruminants, and the elimination or isolation of infected animals should help to prevent transmission of this parasite.

(Figures 186, 187, 188)

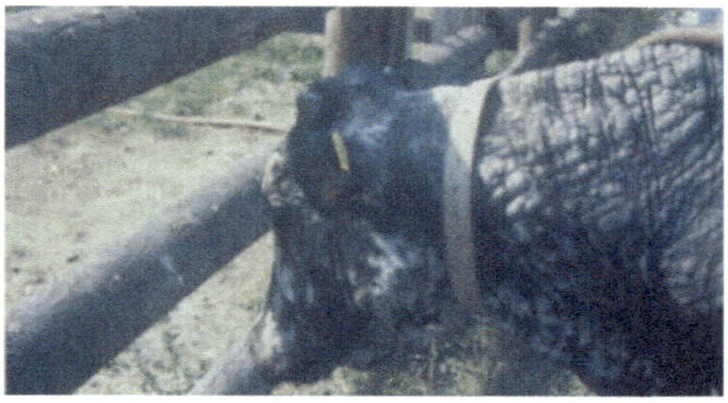

Fig. 186 Thickened skin ("elephant hide disease") following a *Besnoitia besnoiti* infection [4]

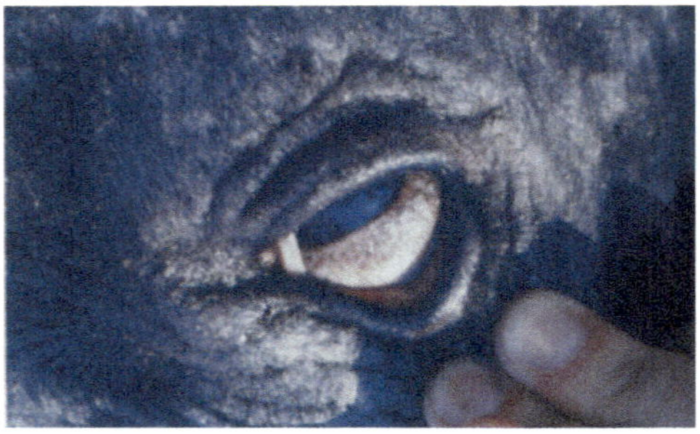

Fig. 187 *Besnoitia besnoiti*; cysts can be seen in the scleral conjunctiva with the naked eye [4]

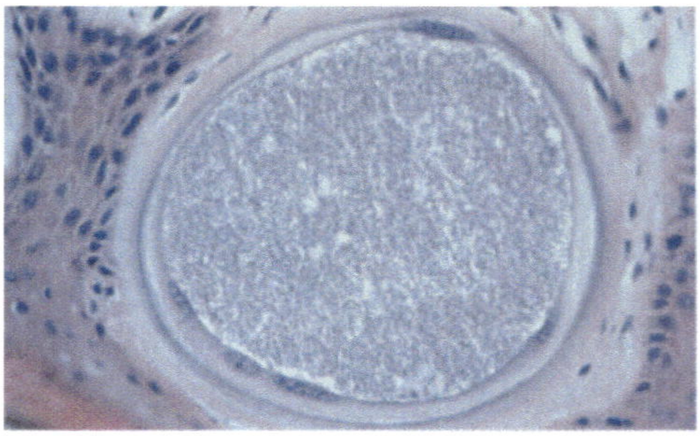

Fig. 188 *Besnoitia besnoiti*; thick-walled cyst found in the subcutaneous tissue, the cysts may be up to 600 µm in diameter [4]

HELMINTHS

• Nematoda found in the skin

Parafilaria bovicola "Verminous nodules", "verminous haemorrhagic dermatitis"

Location: Adults are found in subcutaneous nodules on the upper side of the body. Microfilariae are found in the bloody excretions of the skin nodules.

Hosts: Cattle

Species description: Males are 2–3 cm and females are 4–5 cm in length. The eggs measure 45 × 30 µm and contain microfilariae. Development occurs in *Musca* spp. which become infected when they feed on the skin lesions. When feeding on lacrimal secretions or wounds they transmit the microfilariae to the next definitive host. The verminous nodules are likely to break and ooze blood, causing a haemorrhagic dermatitis.

Geographic distribution: World-wide, especially many parts of Africa

Symptoms: Subcutaneous nodules on the upper side of the body; these nodules are painful and contain the worms. Nodules are likely to break when the gravid female starts with the excretion of eggs. These haemorrhages and nodules are typical signs of the infection with *P. bovicola*.

Significance: Nodules are painful and irritating, and the carcasses at slaughter are downgraded.

Diagnosis: Verminous nodules, haemorrhage, microfilariae in the exudate

Therapy: Ivermectin (0.2 mg/kg, sc.) is fully effective against adults. Nitroxynil (20 mg/kg, sc.) is also effective but must be repeated 3 days later. High doses of levamisole and fenbendazole (50 mg/kg, po.) daily for 5 days were effective.

Prophylaxis: Fly (and tick) control may reduce the entrance points of infective larvae.

(Figure 189)

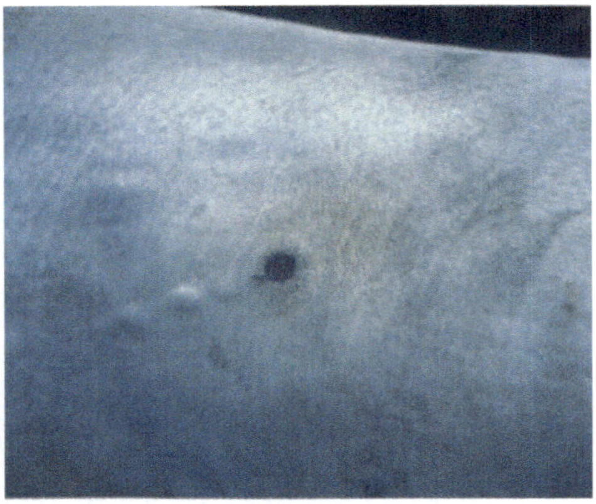

Fig. 189 *Parafilaria bovicola* causing "bleeding spots" and nodules on the skin of cattle; "bleeding spots" are markedly seasonally

Onchocerca dukei Muscular onchocercosis

Location: Adult worms of this species are found in the subcutaneous, perimuscular and muscular tissue of cattle in Africa.

Hosts: Cattle

Species description: The nodules are found in the ventral thorax region, abdomen, diaphragm and thighs. These nodules may be confused with the cysts of *Cysticercus bovis* (*Taenia saginata*). Microfilariae are 240–217 µm long and 4.8–6.7 µm wide and their predilection site is the subcutis of the lower thorax and the umbilical region. The parasite is transmitted by species of the genus *Simulium*.

Geographic distribution: Tropical Africa and also in sub-Saharan West Africa

Symptoms: Infections are usually clinically inapparent.

Significance: Losses occur mainly by condemnation of carcasses when a lot of subcutaneous and intramuscular nodules are seen during meat inspection. Such meat is repugnant.

Diagnosis: This is often made at meat inspection. Nodules are found particularly in the thorax, abdomen and diaphragm and may be confused with the cysts of *Cysticercus bovis* (☞ CATTLE, ■ 4.1). Skin biopsies soaked for 12 hours in physiological saline may be investigated after staining with Giemsa (☞ METHODS, 3.1). Typical microfilariae may be seen.

Therapy: This is not usually indicated.

Prophylaxis: This is generally not feasible in endemic areas (☞ Cattle, ■ 4.1.1).

Onchocerca gibsoni

Location: The adult worms are found in subcutaneous nodules on the brisket, shoulders and external surfaces of the hind-limbs. Microfilariae are found intradermally around the nodules with a predilection to the brisket region.

Hosts: Cattle

Species description: Adult worms cause nodular swellings in the skin but infected animals are not clinically ill. Infected carcasses must be trimmed to remove the nodules. The adults lie in groups or "worm nests" in the subcutaneous tissue and a nodule is formed around them. The worm nests may be up to 5 cm in diameter. There is a fibrous capsule around the nodules which becomes thicker as the nodule ages. This capsule may eventually become calcified. The males are 30–53 mm and the females 140–190 mm long (sometimes up to 500 mm). The tail of the male is curved and it bears lateral alae and 6–9 papillae on either side. The spicules are unequal in size and measure 0.14–0.22 and 0.047–0.094 mm, respectively. The microfilariae are not sheathed and 240–280 µm long. The intermediate hosts are members of the genus *Culicoides* (e.g. *Culicoides pungens* and probably others).

Geographic distribution: Asia, Australia, southern Africa

Symptoms: The infections do not usually cause clinical signs. Nodules may be found at the predilection sites.

Significance: Infected carcasses may be trimmed or even condemned at slaughter.

Diagnosis: This is based on finding the adult worms in subcutaneous nodules or microfilariae in the skin of the brisket. Microfilariae are not evenly distributed in the skin, but occur in irregularly distributed "nests". A number of small skin biopsies (2 mm in diameter) may be placed in a drop of physiological saline solution for 1–2 hours. Microfilariae then migrate into the solution and can be examined.

Therapy: ☞ below *Onchocerca ochengi*

Prophylaxis: Unknown; insect repellents may reduce the attacks by the vectors.

Onchocerca ochengi (syn. *Onchocerca dermata)* "Intradermal onchocercosis of cattle"

Location: This species is found in subcutaneous and intradermal nodules on the ventral regions and flanks, primarily the udder and scrotum.

Hosts: Cattle

Species description: In endemic areas up to 50% of the cattle are infected. The intermediate host has not been identified yet but a biting insect is suspected. Small nodules occur deep in the hide. Microfilariae occur intradermally around the nodules. The microfilariae of *O. dukei* and *O. ochengi* are concentrated in the skin of the posterior and anterior belly.

Geographic distribution: East and West Africa

Symptoms: Intradermal nodules may be formed mainly in the abdominal region, on the udder and scrotum and sometimes in other parts of the body. Microfilariae can cause allergic reactions and local hyperkeratosis.

Significance: The value of leather, which is often perforated by these nodules, is markedly decreased by this parasite.

Diagnosis: Intradermal nodules can be detected by palpation. At slaughter they are visible on the internal surface of the hide.

Therapy: This is generally not indicated. However, the microfilariae may be killed by diethylcarbamazine (5–8 mg/kg, po. during 3 weeks), ivermectin (200 µg/kg, sc.), but also levamisole at increased dosage rates.

Prophylaxis: Unknown; insect repellents may reduce the attacks by the vectors.

(Figures 159, 190)

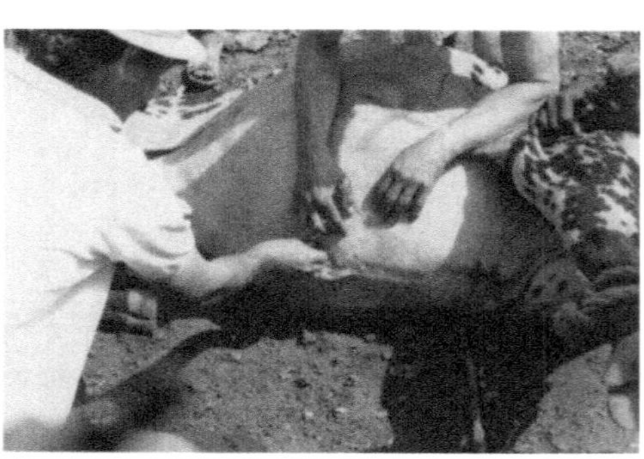

Fig. 190 *Onchocerca ochengi*; skin nodules [23]

Dipetalonema dermicola* and *Dipetalonema ruandae

Remarks: These filariid worms are rarely found in cattle. The former occurs in the skin and the latter in the connective tissue of the oesophagus. They are non-pathogenic and the life cycle is unknown.

Setaria labiatopapillosa Bovine abdominal filariosis

Remarks: Microfilariae of this filariid worm which occurs in the abdominal cavity of cattle (☞ CATTLE, ■ 4.4) may occasionally be found in the skin. The microfilariae are sheathed, measure 240–260 µm and appear usually in the peripheral blood. Several species of mosquitoes act as vectors (*Aedes* spp., *Culex* spp. and *Anopheles gambiae* and other *Anopheles* spp.).

***Stephanofilaria* spp. (*S. stilesi, S. assamensis* and other *Stephanofilaria* spp.)**

Remarks: *Stephanofilaria* spp. are small filarial parasites responsible for circumscribed dermatitis. *S. stilesi* causes a dermatitis along the ventral midline (between the brisket and the navel) of cattle. Adult worms are 3–6 mm long and usually found in the dermis, just beneath the epidermal layer. Microfilariae are 50 µm long and are enclosed in a spherical, semi-rigid vitelline membrane. The intermediate host for *S. stilesi* is the female horn fly *Haematobia irritans* and a *Musca* sp. for *S. assamensis*. The infective larvae are introduced into the skin as the horn fly feeds. For diagnosis, deep skin scrapings are macerated in isotonic saline and examined microscopically for adults and microfilariae must be differentiated from the microfilariae of *Onchocerca* spp. and *Setaria* spp. which are much larger (200–250 µm). No effective treatment is known yet for *S. stilesi*, but topical application of organophosphates (trichlorfon, 6–10%, daily for 7 days) have proved effective against other species of *Stephanofilaria*. Ivermectin (200 µg/kg, sc.) is effective against adult worms of *S. assamensis*.

(Figure 191)

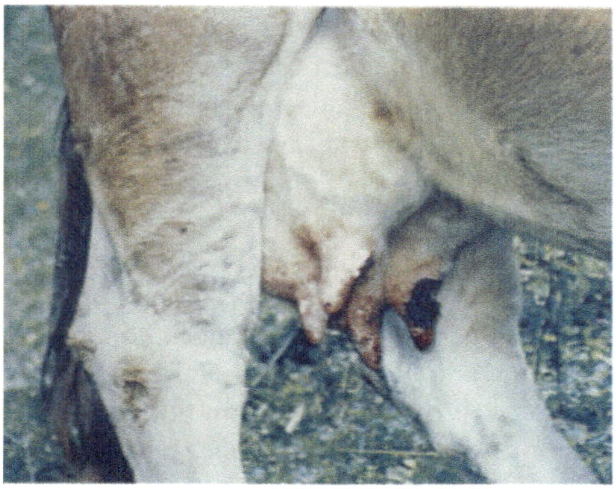

Fig. 191 *Stephanofilaria* sp., circumscribed dermatitis on the udder [15]

ARTHROPODS

Arthropods are divided into two main groups:

Arachnida
- *Ticks*
- *Mites*

Insecta
- *Lice*
- *Fleas*
- *Dipterida*

• Arachnida found in/on the skin

– Ticks

(Figure 192)

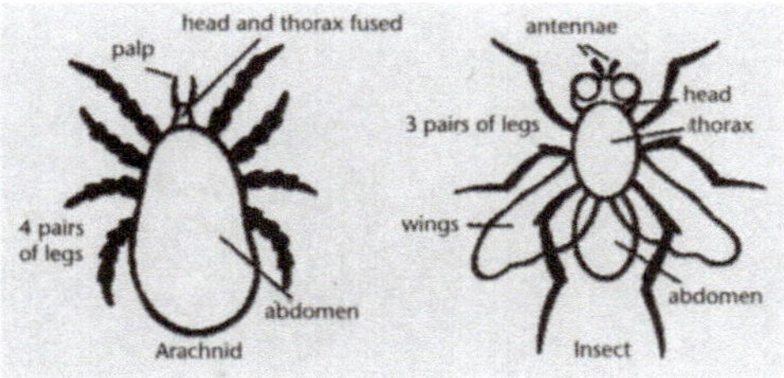

Fig. 192 Principle differences in the morphology of arachnids and insects [6]

Ticks may impair cattle health in 3 different ways:

- **Direct noxious effects**

Attachment to the host causes irritation of the skin with subsequent ulceration and secondary infections. The wounds are attracted by screw-worms and other flies and myiasis may develop. Heavy infestations are associated with anaemia, since adult female ticks imbibe up to 10 ml of blood. Furthermore the presence of large numbers causes annoyance and animals become anxious and restless which may be a cause of loss of weight and condition. The life cycle of ticks may involve one, two or three hosts (Figures 193, 194, 195, 196).

In cattle the following ticks have a direct noxious effect:

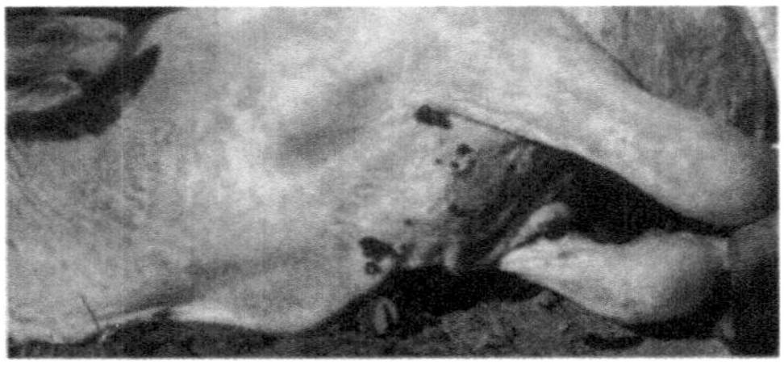

Fig. 193 Skin wounds: noxious effects of tick infestation

IXODIDAE ("hard ticks")

Amblyomma spp. *(A. variegatum, A. hebraeum)*
Boophilus spp. *(B. decoloratus, B. microplus)*
Dermacentor spp.
Haemaphysalis spp.
Hyalomma spp.
Ixodes spp.
Rhipicephalus spp. *(R. appendiculatus, R. sanguineus, R. evertsi, R. parvus, R. pulchellus, R. sinus)*

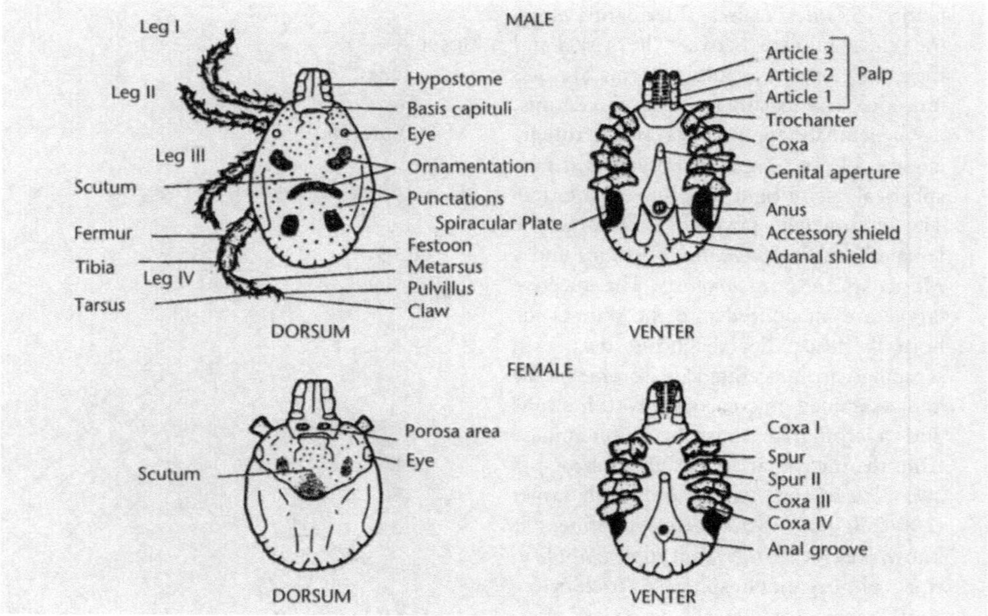

Fig. 194 Characteristics of hard ticks (Ixodidae) [24]

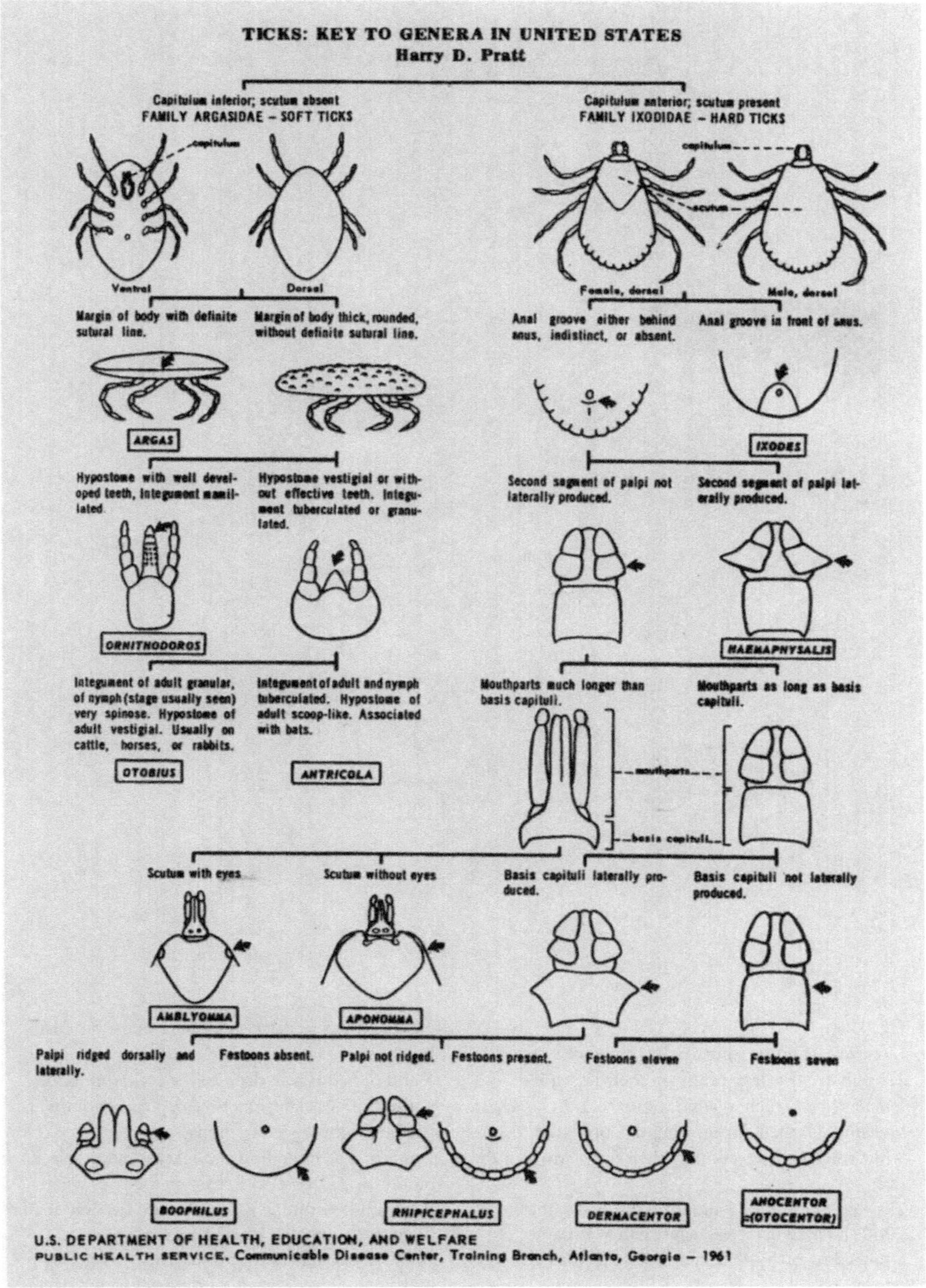

Fig. 195 Key for the identification of tick genera [25]

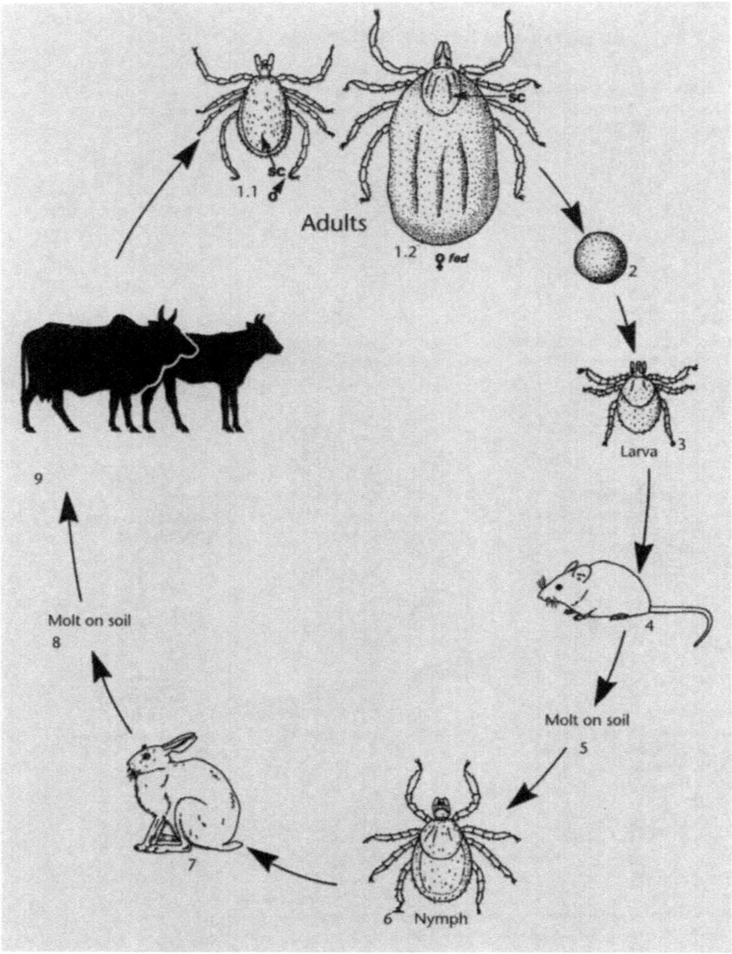

Fig. 196
Life cycle of a three-host tick (*Ixodes ricinus*)
1.1 and 1.2: Eyeless adults on their hosts; fed females (1.2) reach a length of up to 1.5 cm. Their scutum (SC) then appears small. Copulation occurs while the females feed; they then drop down to the soil;
2: Over a period of 1 month females lay about 2000 spherical to ovoid eggs, which become attached to each other and thus appear as clusters on the soil;
3 and 4: Larvae hatch from the eggs after 3–36 weeks (depending on the temperature) and creep onto the tops of grass, from where they attach to passing hosts (mostly small mammals, but also humans);
5 and 6: Fed larvae drop to the soil, and moult within 5–7 weeks (sometimes up to 5 months) to become eight-legged nymphs;
7 and 8: The nymphs attack larger mammals, suck blood for 2–7 days and drop to the soil, where they moult within 2–8 months and become sexually mature adults (1.1 and 1.2);
9: Mostly in spring the adults attack larger mammals including a variety of domestic animals and man, where especially females suck for 5–14 days. The whole development is temperature-dependent and in Europe needs about 3 years [26]

ARGASIDAE ("soft ticks")
– ***Otobius megnini*** Spinose ear tick
(Figures 197, 198)

- **Transmission of diseases**

One of the most damaging effects of ticks is their ability to transmit diseases to their hosts. Some of these are serious with fatal consequences. Transovarian transmission from one tick generation to another via the eggs is possible and contributes to spreading the disease.

The following pathogens are transmitted by ticks:

Babesia bovis	Redwater, tropical bovine babesiosis

Remarks: This is transmitted by *Boophilus microplus*, the pantropical blue tick (☞ CATTLE, ■ 2).

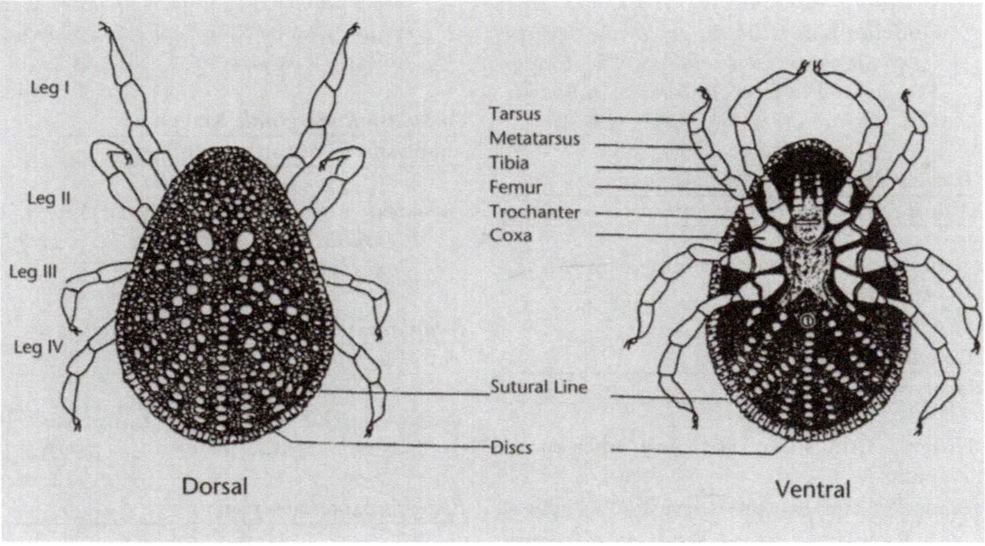

Fig. 197 Characteristics of soft ticks (Argasidae, *Argas* sp.) [26]

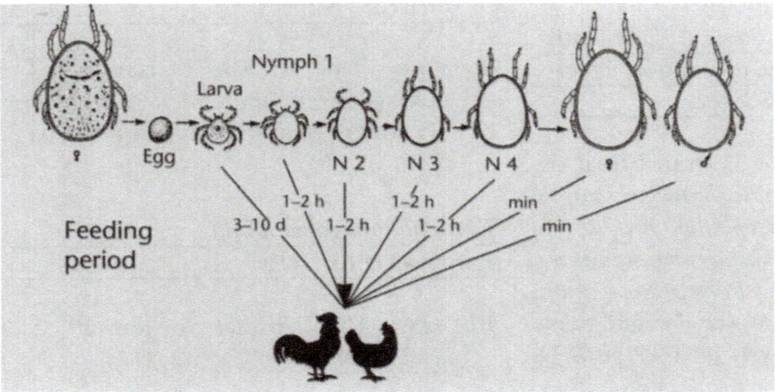

Fig. 198 Example of a typical argasid life cycle; development stages of *Argas* sp., which need about 3–36 months to mature (depending on the temperature); except for larvae, which suck blood for 3–10 days, all stages feed several times but only for a few minutes each time [24]

Babesia divergens
European bovine babesiosis

Remarks: *B. divergensis* transmitted by *Ixodes ricinus* (☞ CATTLE, ■ 2).

Babesia bigemina (syn. *Piroplasma bigeminum*) Redwater, tropical bovine piroplasmo sis, tick fever, "Texas fever"

Remarks: This parasite is transmitted by *Boophilus microplus; B. decoloratus* (the common blue tick), *B. calcaratus, Rhipicephalus* spp. (*Rh. evertsi, Rh. bursa, Rh. appendiculatus*) and *Haemaphysalis* spp. (*H. punctata*) (☞ CATTLE, ■ 2).

Babesia major (syn. *Piroplasma major*)
European bovine piroplasmosis

Remarks: *B. majoris* transmitted by *Haemaphysalis punctata* (☞ CATTLE, ■ 2).

Cowdria ruminantium
Heartwater, Tyewde

Hosts: Cattle, sheep, goat and other ruminants

Remarks: This parasite is transmitted by several species of the tick genus *Amblyomma*, particularly by *Amblyomma variegatum* (the tropical bont tick) and *A. hebraeum* (the South African bont tick). Other species which may be involved are *A. gemma, A. pomposum, A. lepidum* and *A. tholloni* (☞ CATTLE, ■ 2).

Theileria parva (syn. *T. bovis, T. lawrencei*)
East Coast Fever, bovine theileriosis, Corridor disease, Rhodesian tick fever

Remarks: This parasite is transmitted by *Rhipicephalus appendiculatus* (the brown ear tick) and *Rhipicephalus evertsi* (the red-legged tick) and *Rhipicephalus duttoni*. Other vectors are *Hyalomma excavatum, H. dromedarii, H. truncatum* and some other *Rhipicephalus* spp. (☞ CATTLE, ■ 2).

Theileria annulata Mediterranean Coast Fever, Tropical theileriosis, Egyptian Fever

Remarks: This parasite is transmitted by *Hyalomma detritum, H. truncatum* and *H. anatolicum* (☞ CATTLE, ■ 2).

Theileria mutans Benign bovine theileriosis, mild gallsickness

Remarks: This parasite is transmitted by *Amblyomma variegatum, A. hebraeum* and possibly also by *Rhipicephalus appendiculatus* and *R. evertsi* (☞ CATTLE, ■ 2).

Anaplasma marginale Malignant anaplasmosis of cattle, gallsickness

Remarks: This parasite is transmitted by *Boophilus decoloratus* and *B. microplus* (☞ CATTLE, ■ 2).

Anaplasma centrale Mild anaplasmosis of cattle, gallsickness

Remarks: This parasite is transmitted by *Boophilus decoloratus* (☞ CATTLE, ■ 2).

Eperythrozoon wenyoni

Remarks: This parasite is transmitted by *Hyalomma anatolicum.* The pathogen occurs on the erythrocyte surface (☞ CATTLE, ■ 2).

Ehrlichia bovis Tropical bovine ehrlichiosis, "Nofel" or "Nopel"

Remarks: This parasite is transmitted by tick species of the genera *Amblyomma, Hyalomma* and *Rhipicephalus* (☞ CATTLE, ■ 2).

Ehrlichia phagocytophila
European ehrlichiosis

Remarks: This parasite is transmitted by *Ixodes ricinus* (☞ CATTLE, ■ 2).

Ehrlichia ondiri

Remarks: This parasite occurs in granulocytes of cattle in high altitude grassland areas of East Africa. The exact vector is unknown but ticks of the genus *Haemaphysalis* are suspected (☞ CATTLE, ■ 2).

Borrelia theileri Tick Spirochaetosis

Remarks: This is transmitted by *Boophilus decoloratus* and *Rhipicephalus evertsi*. Tick spirochaetosis occurs in cattle, sheep, goats and horses.

- **Tick toxicosis**

Tick paralysis

43 tick species belonging to 10 genera are known to induce tick paralysis in man and a variety of mammals. These ticks are capable of releasing a toxin into the host which causes a condition associated with progressive, ascending, afebrile, symmetrical paralysis, with hind legs being affected first followed by the forelegs.

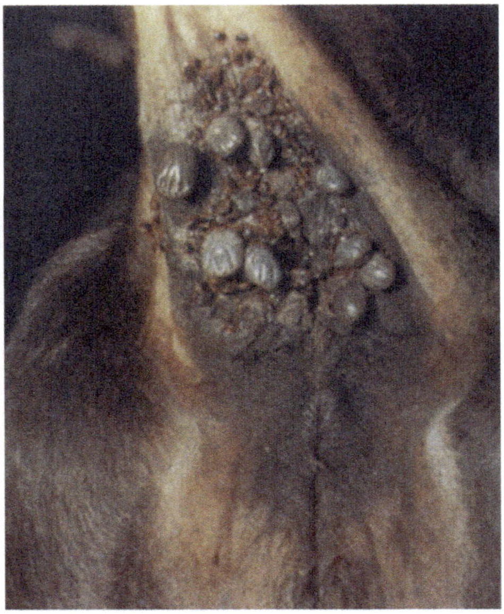

Fig. 199 *Rhipicephalus evertsi*; the red-legged tick, an important cause of tick paralysis [10]

Animals may die. Paralysis is relieved if ticks are removed in time. Most domestic animal species appear to be susceptible to tick paralysis.
Lambs and calves and to a lesser extent adult cattle are susceptible to tick paralysis. *Ixodes rubicundus* (the karoo paralysis tick) mainly affects sheep and goats in South Africa and *Rhipicephalus evertsi* causes the "spring lamb paralysis" in lambs but also in calves.
(Figure 199)

Sweating sickness

An acute, febrile tick-borne toxicosis characterised by a profuse, moist eczema and hyperaemia of the skin and visible mucous membranes. Watering of the eyes and nose, salivation and a extremely sensitive skin with a sour odour are other typical signs. Eventually the skin becomes cracked and predisposed to secondary infections (incl. screw-worm infections and myiasis). Often the course is acute and death may occur within a few days. In less acute cases recovery may occur.
It is mainly a disease of young calves but also sheep in eastern, central and southern Africa. The causative agents are certain strains of *Hyalomma truncatum* which produce an epitheliotropic toxin. Calf mortality may reach 70%.

Symptoms: Generalized hyperaemia with subsequent desquamation of the superficial layers of the mucous membranes of the upper respiratory, gastrointestinal and external genital tracts and profuse moist dermatitis. For diagnosis it is essential to determine the presence of the vector. Clinical signs appear 4–11 days after the tick bite.

Therapy: Ticks must be removed quickly. Antibiotics and anti-inflammatory agents are useful to combat secondary infections. Immune serum may be used.

Prophylaxis: Control of tick infestations is the only effective measure. Removal of ticks, symptomatic treatment and good nursing are indicated.

(Figures 200, 201)

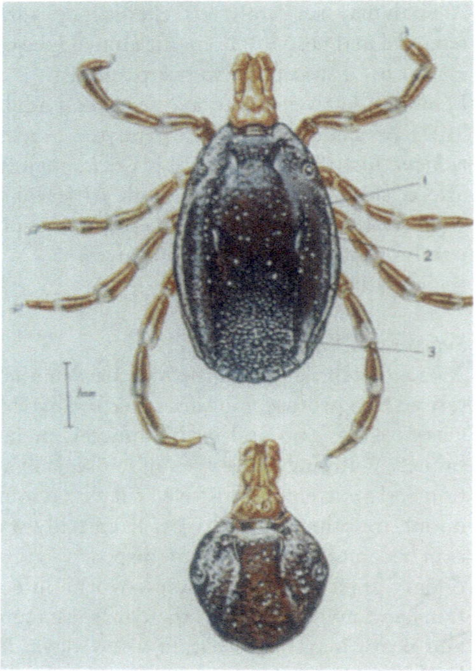

Fig. 200 *Hyalomma truncatum*; an important cause of sweating sickness; (1) marginal groove, (2) scutum and (3) pronounced punctuation [4]

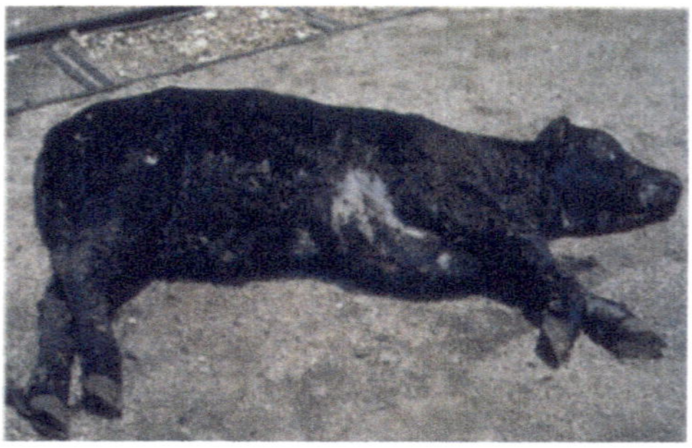

Fig. 201 Sweating sickness, an acute, febrile tick-borne toxicosis characterised by a profuse, moist eczema and hyperaemia of the skin. This condition is often caused by *Hyalomma truncatum* [4]

General toxicosis

Tick toxicosis is a general aggravation of the toxic effect of the parasite's saliva. Certain toxins have a suppressive effect on the animals and occasionally this may reactivate chronic infections. Infections with *Babesia* spp. and *Anaplasma* spp. may occur during massive *Rhipicephalus appendiculatus* infestations. Toxicosis, associated with general disorders, occurs with *Ornithodoros savignyi* (sand tampan) in young calves and lambs, especially when there are many bites. Animals show cutaneous oedema, haemorrhage, rapidly progressing weakness and prostration. Death can occur within 6 hours. Toxicosis may occur in recumbent animals, during rest.
(Figure 202)

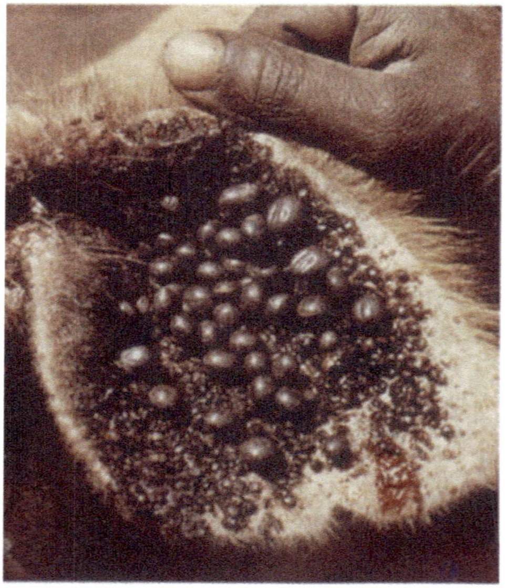

Fig. 202 *Rhipicephalus appendiculatus* (the brown ear tick); an important cause of tick toxicosis [10]

- **Description of ticks affecting cattle**

IXODIDAE (**"hard ticks"**)

***Amblyomma* spp.**

Hosts: All domestic livestock species
Species description: 3-host ticks. *Amblyomma*

spp. are large ticks and have ornate (patterned) upper body surfaces. Festoons (= rectangular division of the rear body edge) are present. *Amblyomma* ticks have long, prominent mouth parts, easily distinguished from the short mouth parts of *Dermacentor*. *Amblyomma variegatum* (the tropical bont tick) is the vector of heartwater and produces skin wounds with its large mouth parts. These wounds may become secondarily infected and may develop into abscesses. Tick paralysis may also occur due to the bont tick. The bont tick occurs mainly on the perineum, udder and in the axillae and inguinal areas. Some *Amblyomma* species, notably *Amblyomma hebraeum* (the South African bont tick) are often resistant to chemicals now in use.

Geographic distribution: *Amblyomma* spp. occur in central and southern Africa and many other parts of the world.

(Figures 203, 204, 205, 206, 207)

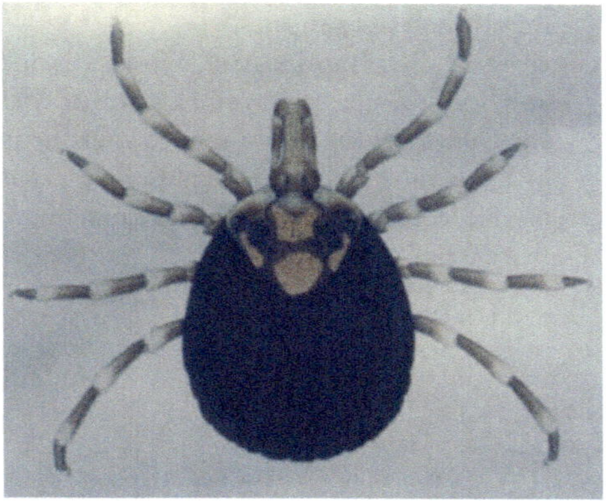

Fig. 203 *Amblyomma variegatum*; female [13]

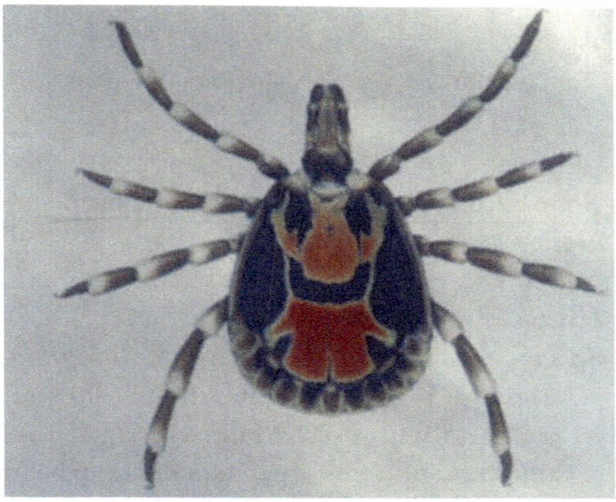

Fig. 205 *Amblyomma variegatum*; male [13]

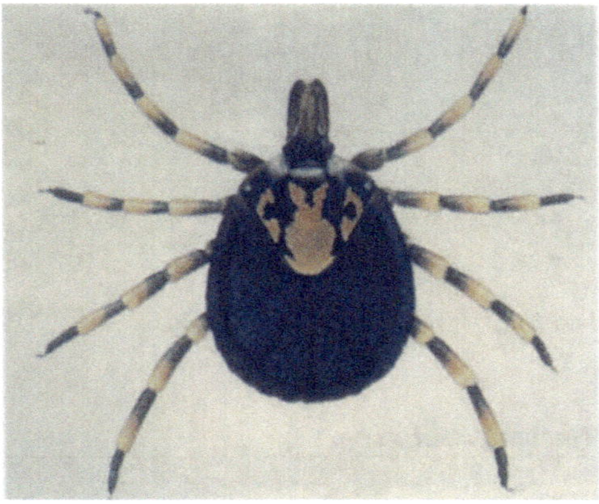

Fig. 204 *Amblyomma hebraeum*; female [13]

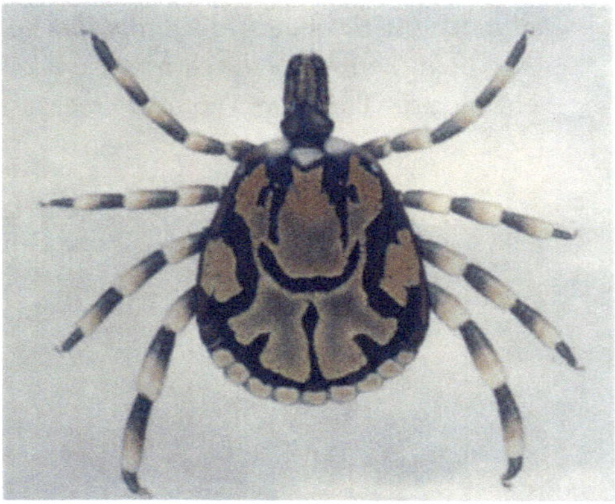

Fig. 206 *Amblyomma hebraeum*; male with bright festoons [13]

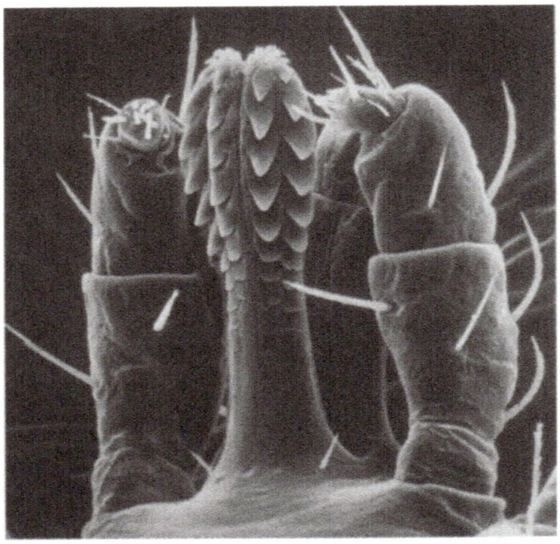

Fig. 207
Amblyomma variegatum; chelicera and palpes

Boophilus spp. Cattle fever tick, tropical cattle tick

Hosts: Horse and cattle

Species description: 1-host ticks. *Boophilus* spp. are plain brown in colour. They are inornate with eyes. Males are small (3–4 mm) and fully engorged females may be up to 12 mm in length. Members of *Boophilus* transmit several diseases and cause skin irritation which leads to licking and scratching and to secondary bacterial infections. Large numbers may cause anaemia. 1-host ticks such as *Boophilus* spp. are often the first to develop resistance to chemicals. Therefore control measures have to be changed frequently. *Boophilus decoloratus* (the blue tick) is one of the most important species of this genus and is found mainly on the neck, thorax, back and udder.

Geographic distribution: Throughout the world in warm climates

(Figure 208)

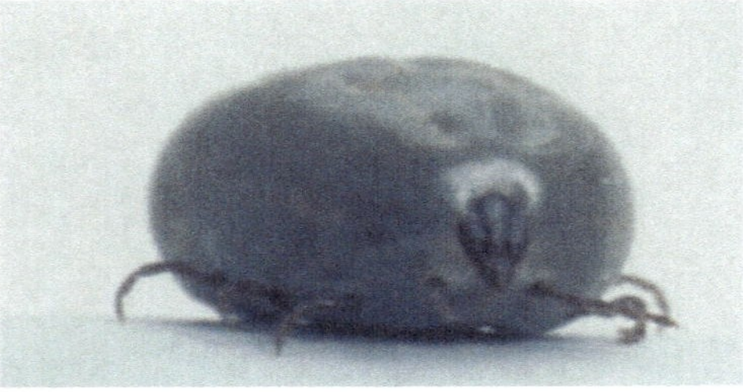

Fig. 208 *Boophilus* sp.; engorged female (up to 2 cm in diameter) [10]

Dermacentor spp.

Hosts: Many wild and domestic mammals

Species description: Some species are 1-host ticks while others are 3-host ticks. *Dermacentor* ticks have ornate (patterned) upper body surfaces. Festoons are present. The mouth parts are short.

Geographic distribution: Asia, Europe, North and South America and some parts of Africa; *Dermacentor* may damage their hosts by transmitting diseases (e.g. Q fever, tularemia), causing tick worry and anaemia.

(Figure 209)

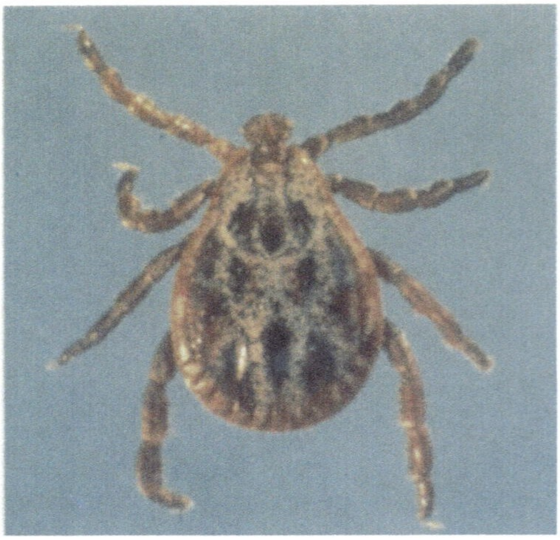

Fig. 209 *Dermacentor marginatus*; male [4]

Haemaphysalis spp.

Hosts: Dogs, birds and in Africa to a lesser extent cattle

Species description: 3-host ticks which are

small, inornate without eyes. Festoons are present. They may be found on the skin on all parts of the body. In addition to annoying cattle they may transmit cattle tick fever, anaplasmosis, and Q fever. They may also produce paralysis and anaemia in heavy infestations.

Geographic distribution: World-wide

(Figure 210)

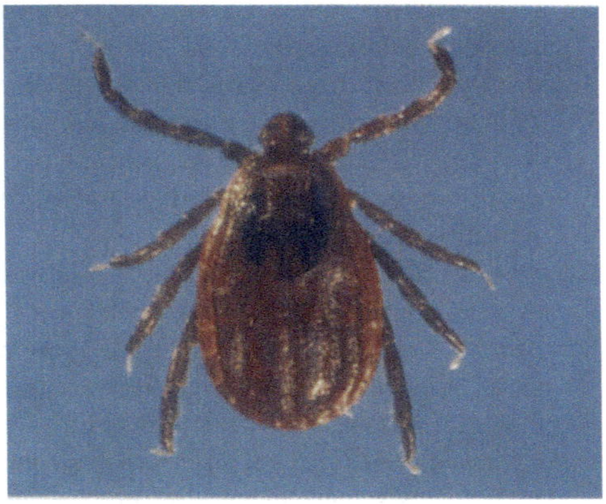

Fig. 210 *Haemaphysalis punctata*; female [4]

Hyalomma spp. The bont-legged tick

Hosts: Horse, domestic ruminants and camel

Species description: Usually 2-host ticks, although three hosts may be used by some species. Inornate (sometimes ornate) eyes are present and festoons may be absent or present. Hypostome and palps are long. *Hyalomma truncatum* causes sweating sickness. Predilection sites are the distal parts of the legs, udder, tip of the tail and perianal region.

Geographic distribution: *Hyalomma* spp. occur in many parts of Africa, depending on the particular species.

(Figure 200)

Ixodes spp. *Paralysis ticks*

Hosts: Cattle, horse and many other animal species

Species description: 3-host tick. *Ixodes* ticks are plain brown in colour and the only eyeless species. The paralysis tick (*Ixodes rubicundus*) has a 2-year life cycle with specific requirements of temperature and humidity. *Ixodes* spp. are found anywhere on the skin of their host. *I. rubicundus* prefers lower parts of legs and abdomen. *Ixodes* spp. are a primary cause of tick paralysis in sheep and goats but they may also transmit diseases.

Geographic distribution: Europe, North America, South Africa

(Figures 211, 212)

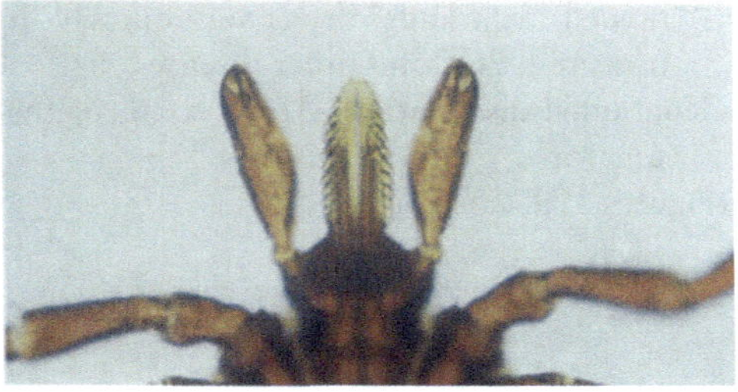

Fig. 211 *Ixodes ricinus*; mouth parts [4]

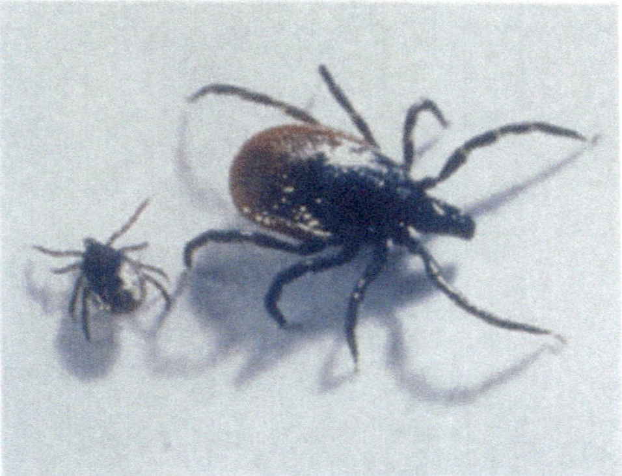

Fig. 212 *Ixodes ricinus*; female (large) and male (small) [4]

Rhipicephalus spp.

Hosts: Cattle, sheep and goat and many other animal species

Species description: 2- or 3-host ticks; festoons are present. *Rhipicephalus appendicula-*

tus (the brown ear tick) is a 3-host tick, plain brown in colour and occurs in the ears of the host. It is the chief vector of ECF and other diseases. Brown ear ticks are impossible to control by pasture rotation because they can survive up to 2 years on the pasture without feeding and they can feed on a large number of different species of wild and domestic animals.

Rhipicephalus evertsi (the red-legged tick) is a 2-host tick and has red legs. The adults typically occur around the anus and the nymphae are found deep in the ears. The red-legged tick is known to develop resistance to acaricidal drugs very quickly. It transmits ECF and other diseases.

Geographic distribution: Africa south of the equator

(Figures 199, 202, 213)

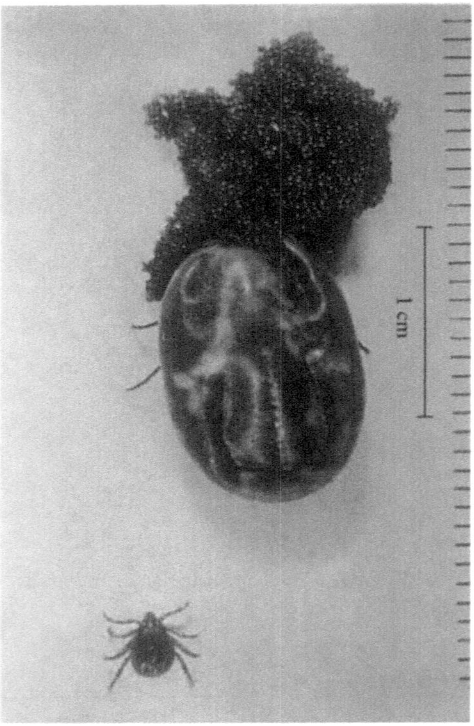

Fig. 213 *Rhipicephalus appendiculatus*; male (small) and egg excreting female (1 cm in diameter) [8]

ARGASIDAE ("soft ticks")

Otobius megnini *Spinose ear tick*

Location: Larvae and nymphae feed deep in the external ear canal. Adults are non-parasitic and live on the ground.

Hosts: Horse, donkey, mule, cattle, sheep, goat

Species description: 1-host tick. Free-living adult females lay eggs on the ground which hatch within 3 weeks. Larvae and nymphs live and feed on one host for up to 7 months. Infestations of this species usually build up in kraals and stables, where the host densities are high. *O. megnini* can persist in empty kraals and stables for more than 2 years.

Geographic distribution: Arid and semi-arid areas of South and South West Africa

Symptoms: Infested animals shake their heads. Loss of appetite, debilitation and anaemia may be present. Irritation in the ear associated with secondary infections (incl. myiasis) may dominate the clinical picture. Ulceration (ear canker) may occur and ticks may clog the ears, causing deafness. Waxy and oily material is discharged from the ear. Larvae and nymphs may sometimes be seen in masses. Infested animals hold their head to one side and feeding is impaired. Weight loss may occur.

Significance: Heavy infestations cause otitis externa, great annoyance and blood loss. *O. megnini* may cause severe problems in livestock in many parts of Africa.

Diagnosis: Ticks may be found by swabbing the ear or by direct inspection of heavily infected ears. Larvae and nymphs are found inside the ear. The adult ticks are difficult to find as they breed in hidden cracks of barns, fences and trees.

(Figures 214, 215)

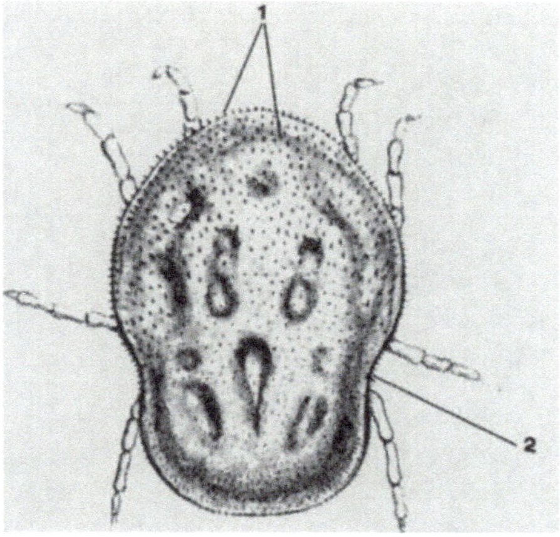

Fig. 214 *Otobius megnini* (the spinose ear tick); nymph (3–8 mm long): (1) integument covered with short, sharp spines and (2) posterior part of the body constricted [27]

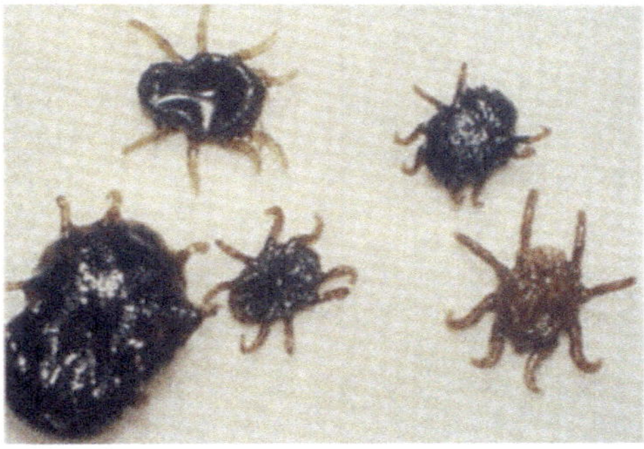

Fig. 215 *Otobius megnini*; nymphs (up to 8 mm long) [6]

Ornithodoros savignyi The sand tampan

Remarks: This tick may be a serious pest of cattle. It may cause death in calves and tick toxicosis in adult cattle (☞ SHEEP AND GOATS, ■ 5.1).

- **Tick control in cattle**
  ☞ THERAPY AND PROPHYLAXIS OF ECTOPARASITES, p. 141

– Mites

(Figures 216, 217)

Chorioptes bovis Chorioptic mite, foot mange, leg mite

Location: On the legs, base of tail and upper rear surface of the udder

Hosts: Cattle

Species description: The tarsal suckers have unjointed and short pedicels. Typical mite life cycle. Chorioptic mange feed on skin debris and lymph.

Geographic distribution: World-wide

Symptoms: Scabs or scales develop on the skin of the lower parts of the body. There is some exudation and crust formation on the lower body and legs, but this does not spread over a wide area. Cattle may stamp and scratch infected areas.

Significance: The disease is not as serious as sarcoptic or psoroptic mange but it is very prevalent.

Diagnosis: Demonstration of mites in skin scrapings taken from the edge of the lesions (☞ METHODS, 4.1).

Therapy: These mites are superficial and are therefore not very sensitive to Ivermectin (200 µg/kg, sc.) but it may be an aid in controlling the foot mange. Dips and sprays may be used (☞ below *Psoroptes ovis*). Ivermectin applied topically (500 µg/kg)

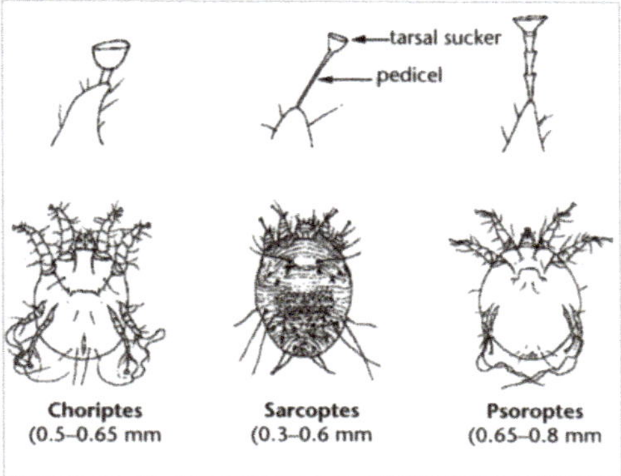

Fig. 216 *Chorioptes*, *Sarcoptes* and *Psoroptes* mites with genus-specific morphology of pedicels and tarsal suckers (schematic)

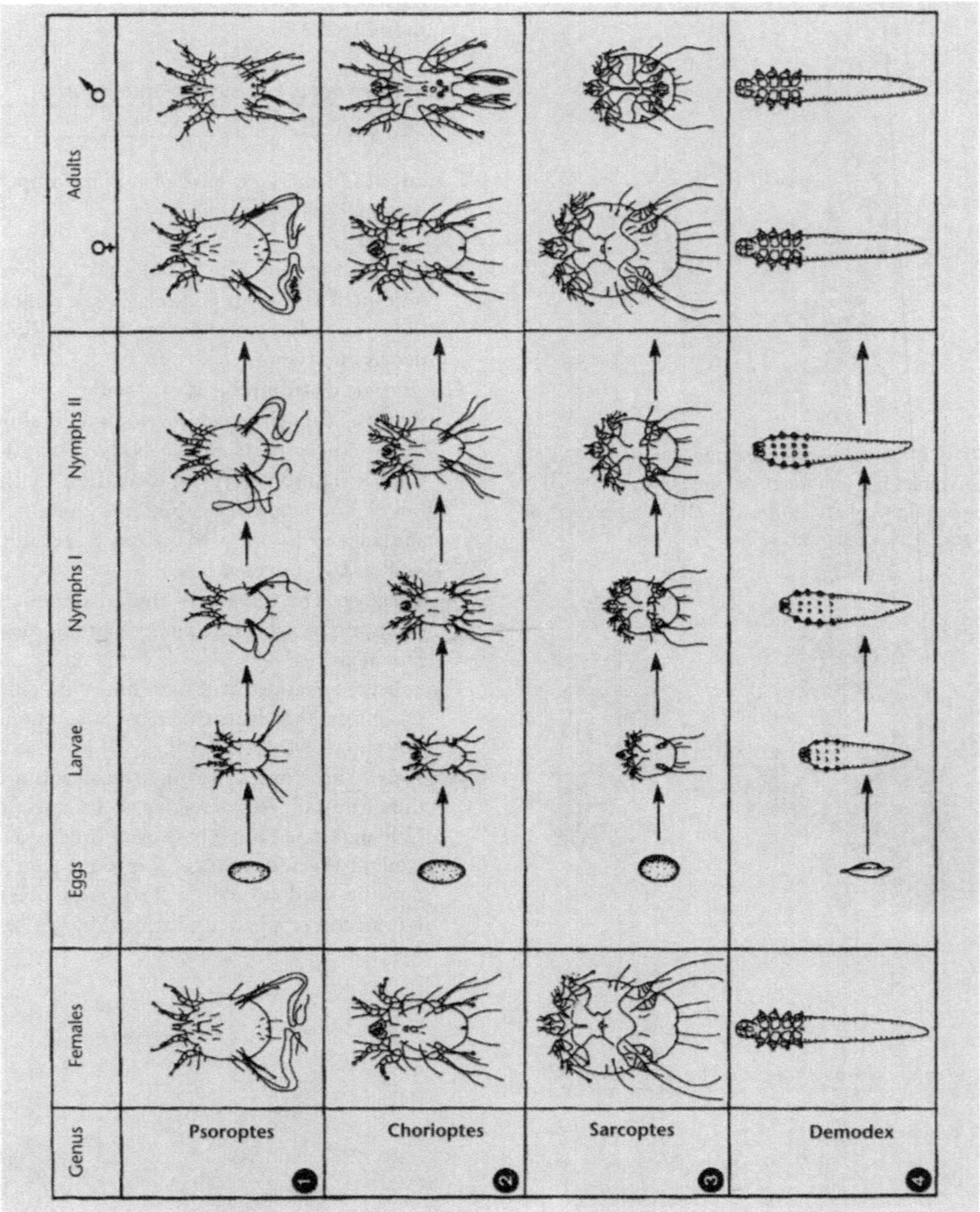

Fig. 217 Developmental stages in the life cycle of important groups of mites. All stages live on/in the skin of their hosts. Larvae have only three pairs of legs. Feeding larvae and nymphs increase in size and moult. In some species there is clear sexual dimorphism; (1) *Psoroptes* spp. feed (as piercing mites) on the lymph fluid and occasionally on the blood of their hosts, (2) *Chorioptes* spp. feed (as chewing mites) on the epidermal products, (3) *Sarcoptes* spp. penetrate the epidermis, forming canals and (4) *Demodex* spp. feed on hair follicles or on sebaceous glands [26]

is effective against chorioptic mange. Crotoxyphos (0.25%) applied as a spray can also be used against the leg mite.

Prophylaxis: ☞ below *Psoroptes ovis*
(Figures 218, 219)

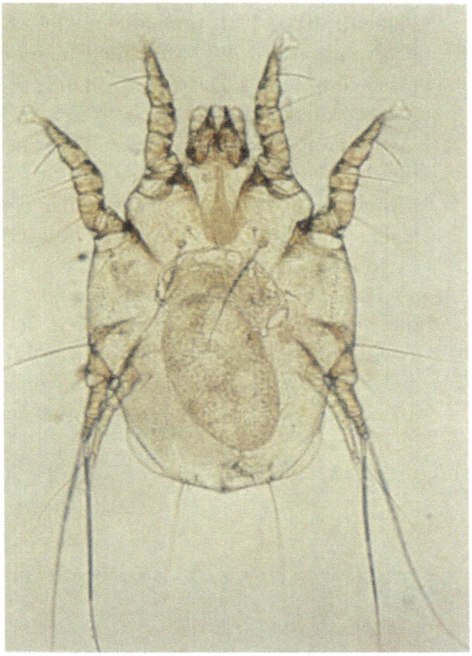

Fig. 218 *Chorioptes bovis*, adult female (max. 650 µm long) with short, unjointed pedicels [4]

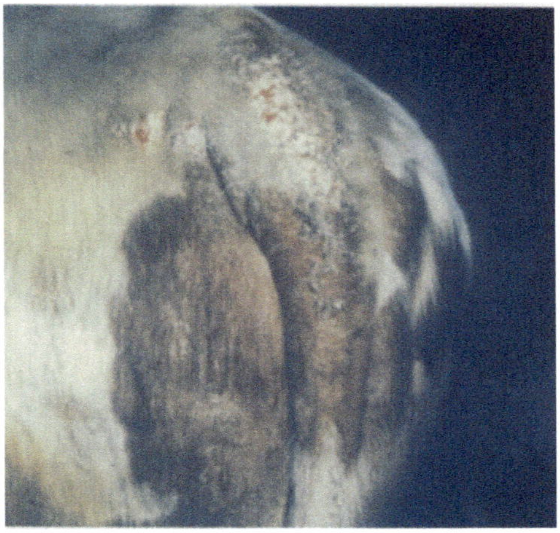

Fig. 219 *Chorioptes bovis* infestation [4]

Sarcoptes bovis Itch mite, mange mite

Location: Neck, the back in front of the tail, inner surface of the thighs and the udder and sometimes the whole body surface

Hosts: Cattle

Species description: This is a minute parasite in outline. The tarsal suckers have unjointed and long pedicels. Females have a number of spines on the upper surface. The life cycle is typical for mites, the entire period of development is spent on the host. (☞ SWINE, ■ 5.1) The mange may occur very seasonally in temperate zones (late winter). *Sarcoptes* mites prefer areas of thin hair but the lesions may spread to other parts. *Sarcoptes* mites puncture the skin to feed on lymph and skin debris.

Geographic distribution: World-wide

Symptoms: Intense itching is caused by irritation. Animals scratch which may result in dermatitis, accompanied by an exudate that coagulates and dries to form crusts. The skin is thickened, wrinkled and hair is lost.

Significance: Irritation to the host causes weight loss and emaciation. Skins of carcasses are of poor quality. Animals in poor condition due to mite attacks are subject to other diseases.

Diagnosis: Demonstration of mites of deep skin scrapings taken from the edge of the lesions (☞ METHODS, 4.1). *Sarcoptes* mites are usually found deep in the skin whereas *Psoroptes* mites are more superficial.

Therapy: This mite is very sensitive to Ivermectin (200 µg/kg, sc.). After one treatment no living mites were recovered. Dips and sprays may also be used to reduce the clinical effects (☞ below *Psoroptes ovis*).

Prophylaxis: ☞ below *Psoroptes ovis*
(Figures 220, 221)

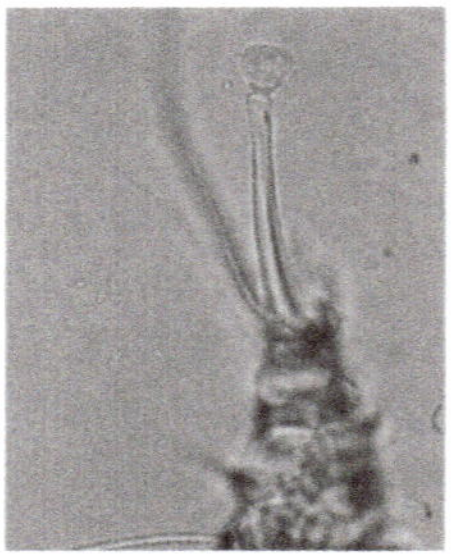

Fig. 220 *Sarcoptes* sp.; mite with unjointed, long pedicels (30–35 µm long) [4]

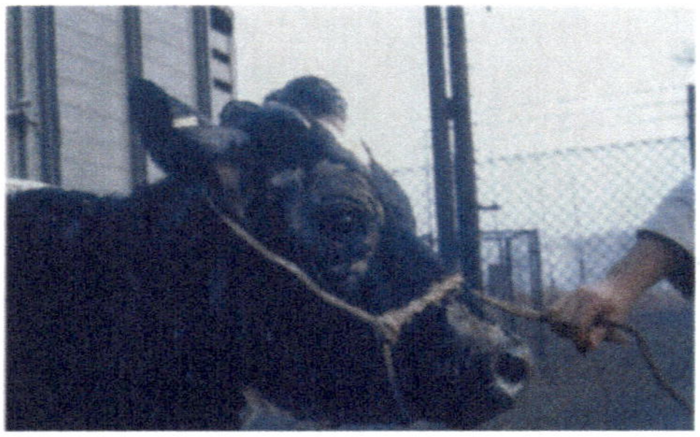

Fig. 221 *Sarcoptes* sp. infestation of a cattle [4]

Psorpotes ovis (syn. *Psoroptes communis var. bovis)* Psoroptic mite

Location: Any part of the body, especially areas of dense hair such as withers, back and root of tail

Hosts: Cattle, sheep

Species description: The mites are oval in shape and the tarsal suckers have long, jointed pedicels. Typical mite life cycle, taking 9 days. This is a notifiable and quarantinable disease in many parts of the world.

Geographic distribution: World-wide

Symptoms: Affected skin is covered with exudate. This dries to form a scab. Massive loss of hair usually occurs. Lesions may cover the entire body. Deaths in untreated calves are not uncommon. The course may be acute in young calves and chronic nature may also be found. The prognosis is usually favourable following early treatment.

Significance: Psoroptic mange is a widespread and serious disease of cattle. Infested animals lose weight and the skins are of lower quality.

Diagnosis: Demonstration of mites in skin scrapings taken from the edge of the lesions (☞ METHODS, 4.1).

Therapy: Infested cattle should be dipped, not sprayed. The following compounds may be used for dips: toxaphene (0.5–0.6%), coumaphos (0.3%), phosmet (0.2–0.25%), diazinon (0.025%), flumethrine (1 l of a 6% solution in 1500 l of water) and many other compounds. Depending on the product, repeated treatments are required (label instructions should be checked). Ivermectin (200 µg/kg, sc.) is effective against *Psoroptes ovis*. One treatment resulted in clinical healing, but a second treatment is indicated in eradication programs.

Prophylaxis: Newly introduced animals are the main source of infection for a herd. These animals must be checked carefully and possibly treated before being introduced into the new herd. A quarantine may be indicated.

(Figures 222, 223, 224)

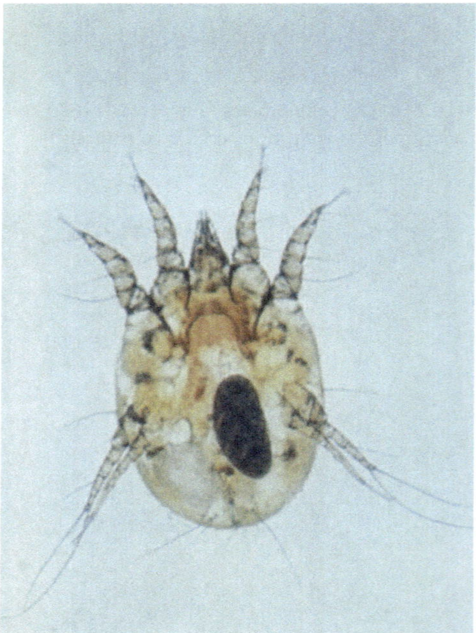

Fig. 222 *Psoroptes* sp. female mite (max. 800 µm long) with egg [4]

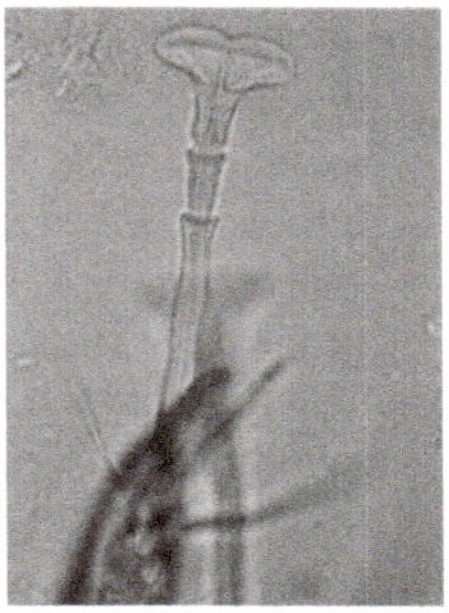

Fig. 223 *Psoroptes* sp.; mite, jointed, long pedicels (68 µm long) [4]

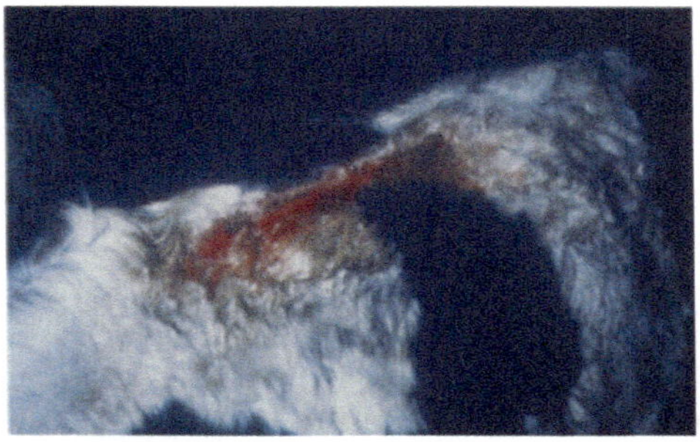

Fig. 224 *Psoroptes* sp. infestation of a cattle [4]

Demodex bovis

Demodectic or follicular mite

Location: Neck, brisket, shoulder, face
Hosts: Cattle
Species description: *Demodex* mites are cigar-shaped, elongated mites, about 0.25 mm long. The thorax bears 4 pairs of stout, short legs and the abdomen is transversely striated. The life cycle is not clearly understood. *Demodex* is transmitted from the cow to the calf while nursing and may cause considerable damage to hides. Lesions are pronounced in young dairy cattle but are rarely visible or palpable on beef cattle. Rarely the lesions may appear over the entire body.
Geographic distribution: World-wide
Symptoms: Small papules and nodules may be seen. They are red and thick and a waxy, white material can be expressed from them. This material contains numerous mites. Nodules may also be filled with pus and abscesses covered with small scales may be seen. The course of bovine demodectic mite infection is usually mild but may extend over many months.
Significance: Damage to skin may affect the production of leather. Demodectic mange is not considered to be a major parasite of cattle but it may open the skin for secondary problems (bacterial and fungal infections, myiasis, etc.).
Diagnosis: Microscopical examination of the cheesy, waxy fluid from the nodules which may contain many mites. Long-standing nodules of the skin are characteristic.
Therapy: There is no satisfactory treatment. Systemic and topical applications of chemical compounds have given some relief.
Prophylaxis: Unknown
(Figures 225, 226)

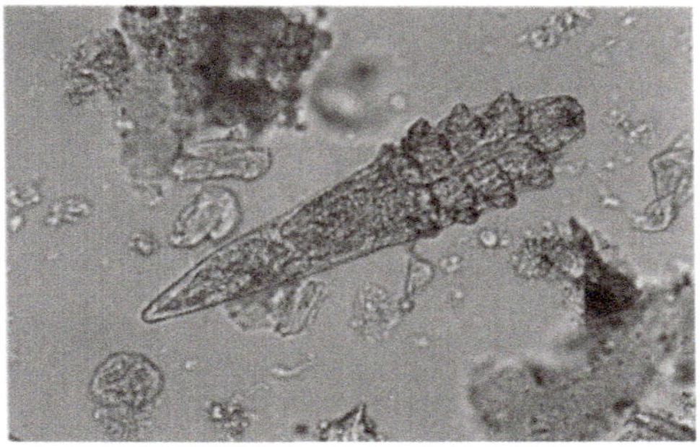

Fig. 225 Cigar-shaped *Demodex bovis* mite, (250–400 × 70 µm)

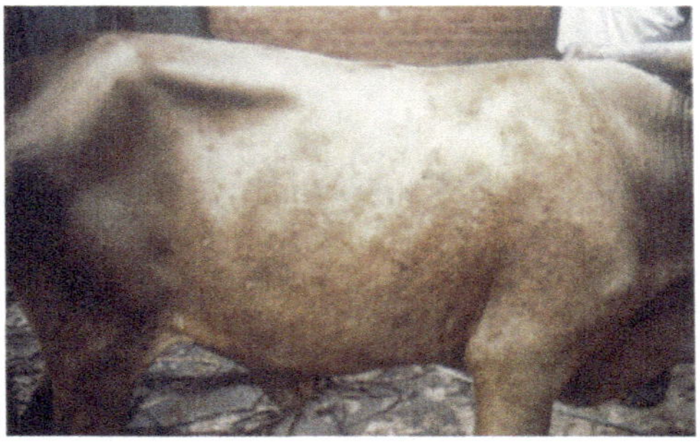

Fig. 226 *Demodex bovis* causing multiple skin nodules [8]

Psoregates bos Itch mites of cattle, "Australian itch"

Remarks: Itch mites occur in Canada, Australia and South Africa. These mites are minuscule (189 × 189 µm) and difficult to collect. They are spherical and have paired claws and legs which are arranged radially. Alopecia and desquamation occur, but the lesions lack the scab formation associated with mange mite infestations. Lime-sulfur spray or dip applied twice, with a 2-week interval, is indicated to be the acaricide of choice.
(Figure 227)

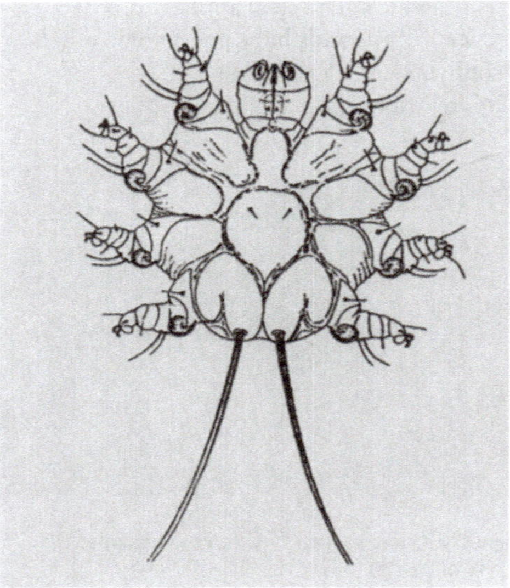

Fig. 227 *Psoregates* sp.; female mite [28]

Raillietia spp. (*R. auris* and *R. caprae*)

Location: Middle and inner ear
Hosts: Cattle, sheep (*R. auris*) and goat (*R. caprae*)
Species description: The mites feed on epidermal cells and wax but not on blood.
Geographic distribution: North America, Australia, East Africa, Europe.
Symptoms: Infestations are usually inapparent but otitis media and interna with nervous signs, including head shaking, head rotation to the affected side, circling, and general incoordination, can be found in a progressive stage of the infestation.
Significance: *Raillietia* spp. infections can cause signs similar to those of other CNS infections and should therefore be excluded.
Diagnosis: It is almost impossible to diagnose *Raillietia* spp. antemortem. Demonstration of the mites in the middle or inner ear at necropsy.
Therapy: Ivermectin may eliminate the mites. Acaricides, applied topically may also be effective.
Prophylaxis: Unknown
(Figures 228, 229)

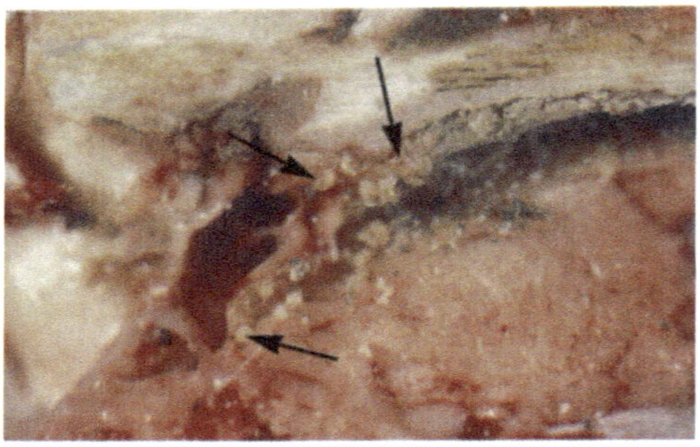

Fig. 228 *Raillietia auris* causing otitis media and interna

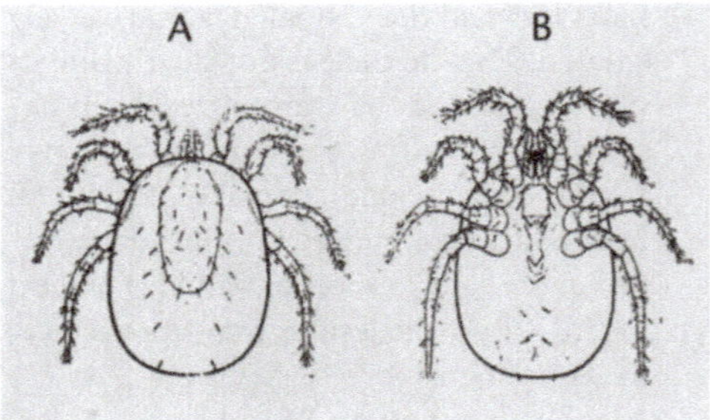

Fig. 229 *Raillietia auris*; dorsal view (A) and ventral view (B) [29]

• Insecta found on the skin

– Lice

(Figure 230)

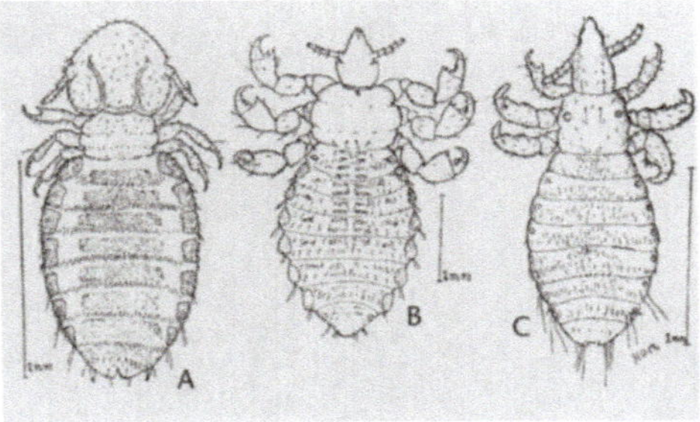

Fig. 230 Cattle lice: *Bovicola bovis* (A), *Haematopinus eurysternus* (B) and *Linognathus vituli* (C) [3]

MALLOPHAGA Chewing lice

Bovicola bovis *(syn. Damalinia bovis)*

Red louse, "chewing louse"

Location: Skin surface, especially the neck, withers and root of tail

Hosts: Cattle

Species description: These lice belong to the Mallophaga and are 1–2 mm long and wingless. They have a broad head with mouth parts adapted for chewing. The entire life is spent on the host. The infestations are heaviest in winter when the coats are dense.

Geographic distribution: World-wide, primarily in cooler areas

Symptoms: Intense itching associated with these lice may be observed. Animals show typical parasite worry (not feeding, not sleeping). Scratching may produce skin wounds or bruises and the coat becomes rough.

Significance: Biting lice are widespread and important parasites. Losses such as reduced growth and secondary skin infections due to intense itching may occur.

Diagnosis: Lice may be seen on skin. The eggs occur as white specks attached to the hairs.

Therapy: ☞ below THERAPY AND PROPHYLAXIS OF ECTOPARASITES

Prophylaxis: ☞ below THERAPY AND PROPHYLAXIS OF ECTOPARASITES, p. 141

(Figure 231)

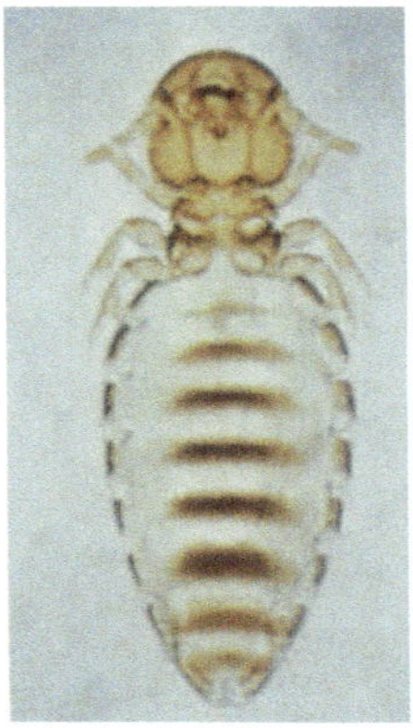

Fig. 231 *Bovicola bovis* (1.5–2 mm long); the cattle chewing louse [4]

ANOPLURA Blood sucking lice of cattle

Haematopinus eurysternus

Short-nosed cattle louse

Remarks: This species occurs world-wide. It is 3.4–4.8 mm long. The louse is fairly broad and the head is short.

(Figures 232, 233, 234)

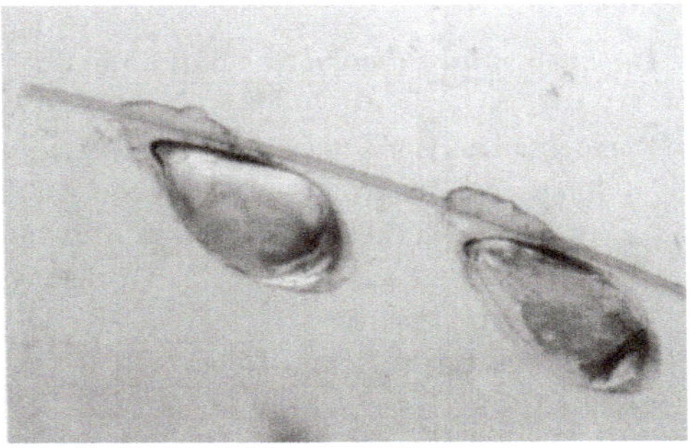

Fig. 232 *Haematopinus eurysternus;* eggs attached to the hair of a cattle

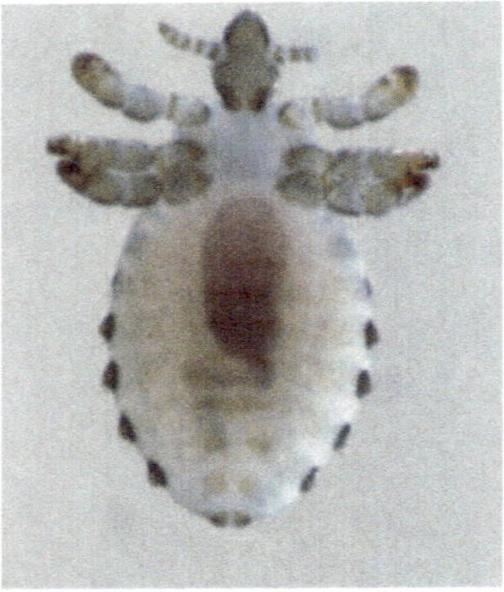

Fig. 233 *Haematopinus eurysternus* (3.4–4.8 mm long); the short-nosed cattle louse

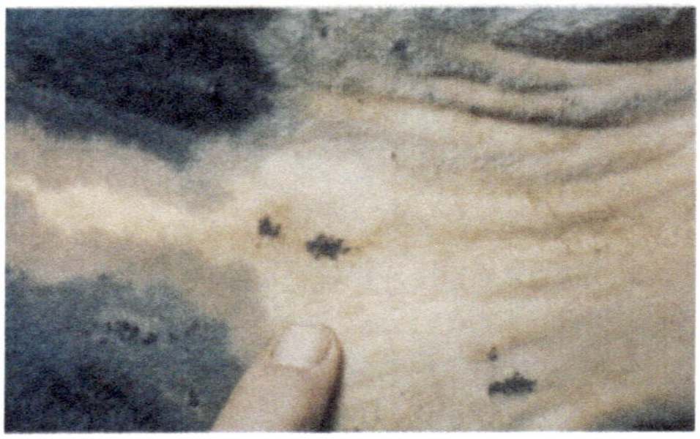

Fig. 234 *Haematopinus* sp.; on the skin of a cattle [15]

Haematopinus quadripertusus
Tail louse of cattle

Remarks: This species occurs on cattle in North America, Queensland, Papua-New Guinea and tropical Africa.

Haematopinus tuberculatus Buffalo louse

Remarks: This is a large species (up to 5.5 mm long) and occurs in Asia and the Pacific area. It also occurs on camels in Australia.

Linognathus vituli
Long-nosed cattle sucking louse

Remarks: This species has a long narrow head and a slender body. It is 2.5 mm in length.
(Figure 235)

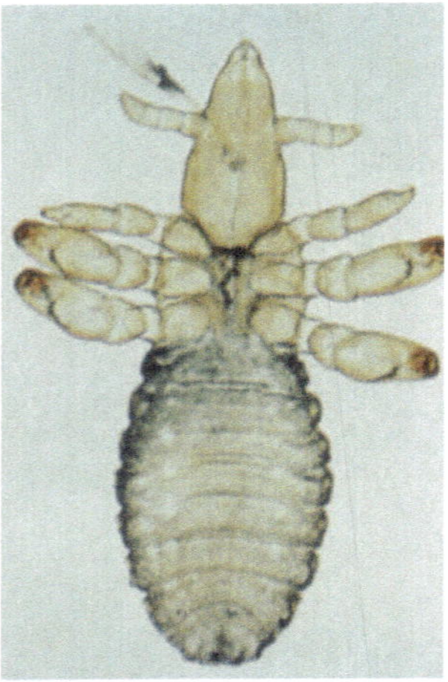

Fig. 235 *Linognathus vituli* (up to 2.5 mm long); the long-nosed cattle sucking louse [4]

Solenopotes capillatus

Remarks: This is the smallest of the sucking lice of cattle and occurs in conspicuous clusters on the neck, head, shoulders, dewlap, back and tail.
(Figure 236)

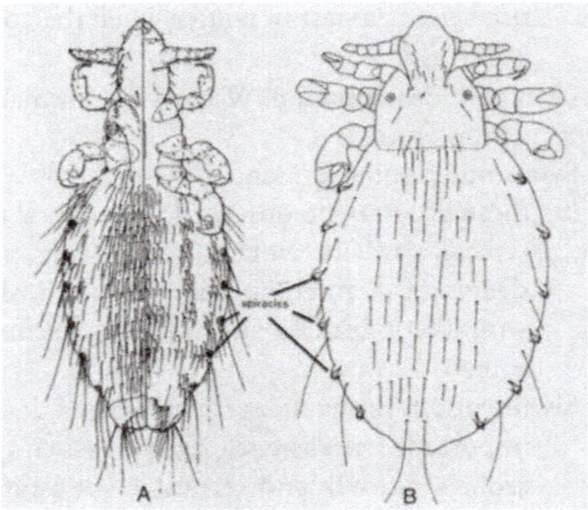

Fig. 236 (A) *Linognathus ovillus* (2.0– 2.5 mm) and (B) *Solenopotes capillatus* (1.3–1.7 mm) [29]

- **General features of blood sucking lice of cattle**

Location: These lice are often found on protected areas of the skin such as side of the neck, brisket, back, head and between the legs.
Hosts: Cattle
Species description: Wingless insects with long mouthparts adapted for sucking. The life cycle takes 1 month. Heavy infestations may occur in immunosuppressed animals (e.g. calves following trypanosome infections).
Geographic distribution: World-wide. Some species are restricted to certain regions.
Symptoms: Louse worry is characterized by licking, scratching and rubbing. The coat becomes rough and secondary infections may occur. Heavy infestations may cause anaemia. Such animals may be more susceptible to other infectious diseases and environmental stress.
Significance: These are common parasites of cattle which can cause severe problems if present in large numbers.
Diagnosis: Lice and their eggs may be found on the skin.
Therapy: A wide variety of insecticides and application modi may be employed. Dipping is being replaced by delivery systems such as "pour-on" and "low-volume spray" for pyrethroid insecticides. Low tolerance for insecticides in milk limits the insecticides that may be used on dairy cattle and goats. Effective compounds include crotoxyphos, crotoxyphos combined with dichlorvos, coumaphos, fenvalerate, stirofos, coumaphos, dioxathion, malathion, methoxychlor, phosmet and permethrin. Label instructions should be considered. Dipping and spraying provides excellent coverage, and usually two treatments 2 weeks apart will effectively control lice. Ivermectin (200 µg/kg, sc.) is effective against sucking lice.
Prophylaxis: This is difficult wherever direct contact between the animals of the herd is possible.

- Fleas

No fleas have been found on the body surface of cattle.

- Dipterida

CULICIDAE Mosquitoes

***Aedes* spp., *Anopheles* spp. and *Culex* spp.**

Remarks: They belong like flies to the order Dipterida, with a single pair of wings. The main genera are *Anopheles, Culex* and *Aedes.*
They are slender with small spherical heads and large eyes. Both sexes live on fluids which are derived from organic sources, such as jus of fruits and vegetables. Females are capable to suck blood which appears to be necessary for the laying of eggs. Eggs are laid either on water or on vegetation floating on the surface of water. Therefore mosquitoes are found near stagnant pools. Because of their dependence on water their numbers generally become less during the dry season.
Significance: Mosquitoes can cause considerable distress to livestock but their main importance is their ability to act as intermediate hosts or vectors of viral (Rift Valley Fever, Equine encephalomyelitis, African Horse Sickness, Fowl pox, Blue tongue, Lumpy skin disease), bacterial (avian spirochaetosis), protozoan (Avian and human malaria) and filarial (*Setaria equina, Setaria labiatopapillosa*) and probably other diseases.
(Figures 237, 238, 239)

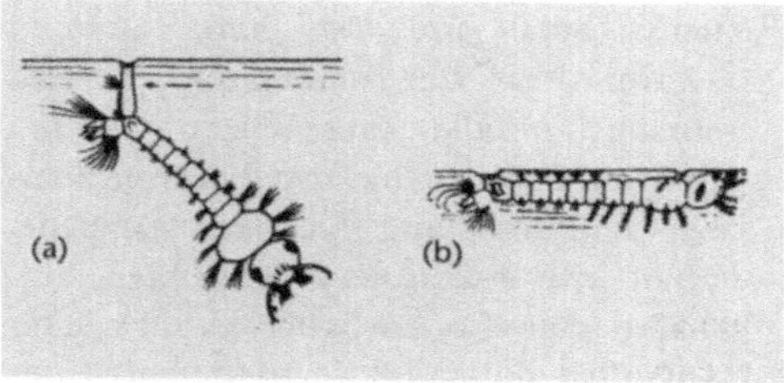

Fig. 237 *Culex* sp. larva (a) and *Anopheles* sp. larva (b) showing their feeding position in water

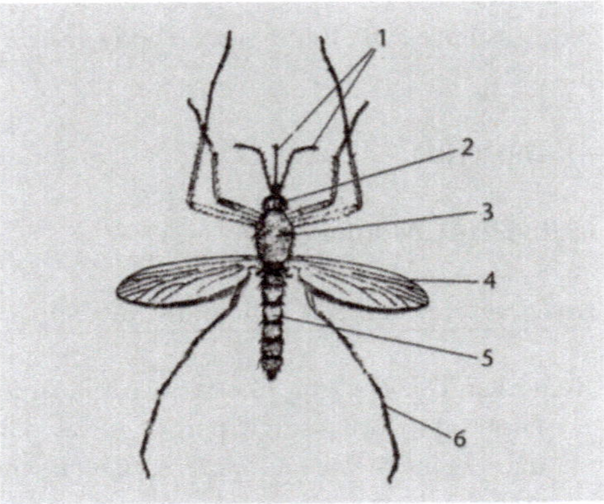

Fig. 238 Culicidae (schematic): adult mosquito with antennae and proboscis long (1), small head with large eyes (2), thorax (3), wings long and narrow (4), abdomen elongate (5) and legs long and slender (6) [27]

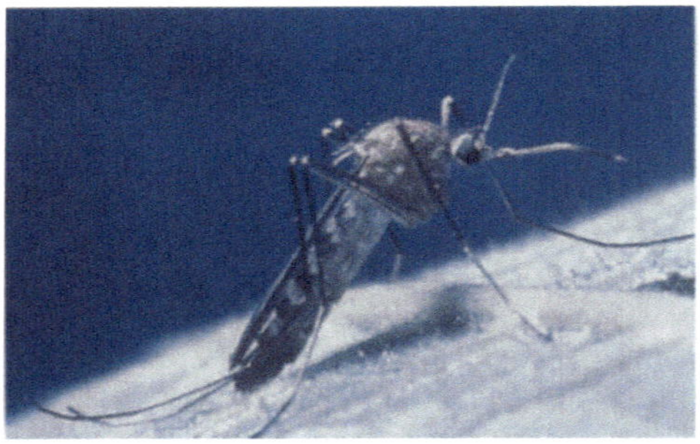

Fig. 239 *Culex* sp.; female in feeding position

SIMULIIDAE

Simulium spp. Black flies, midges

Remarks: Small size (1–5 mm), found in swarms near free-running well aerated streams. *Simulids* cause severe irritation to livestock when they occur in large numbers and herds and flock will stampede, often with disastrous results. Man, animals and poultry are liable to attack. Bites are inflicted on all parts of the body, giving rise to vesicles which burst exposing the underlying flesh. Skin wounds caused by simulids heal very slowly. Certain areas of the tropics are rendered uninhabitable by simulids.

Significance: Irritation of livestock; skin wounds with secondary infections and myiasis; transmission of *Onchocerca volvulus* in man

(Figures 240, 241, 242, 243, 244, 245)

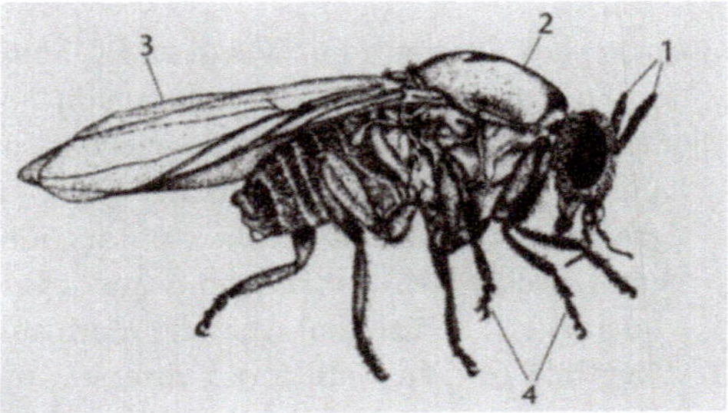

Fig. 240 *Simulium* sp. (blackfly) adult; (1) antennae short and horn-like, (2) humped thorax, (3) wings broad and clear and (4) legs short [27]

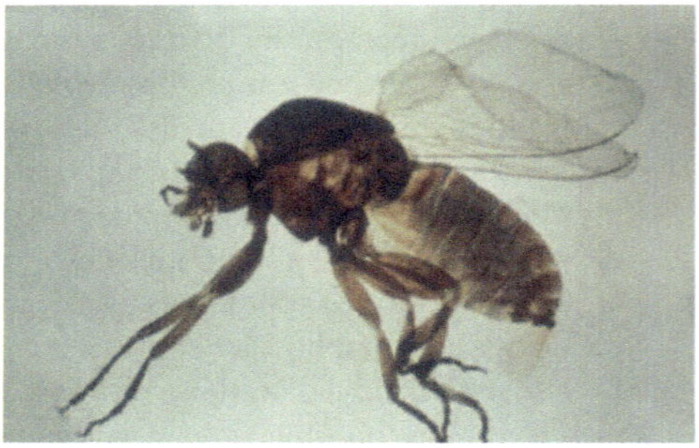

Fig. 241 *Simulium* sp., female (5 mm) [4]

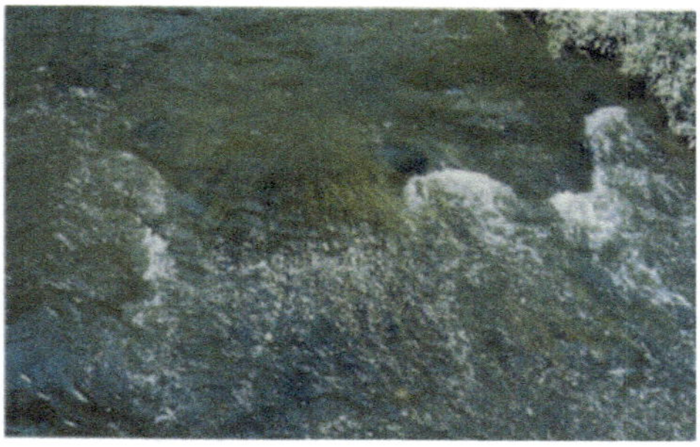

Fig. 242 *Simulium* larvae develop in free-running, well-aerated streams [30]

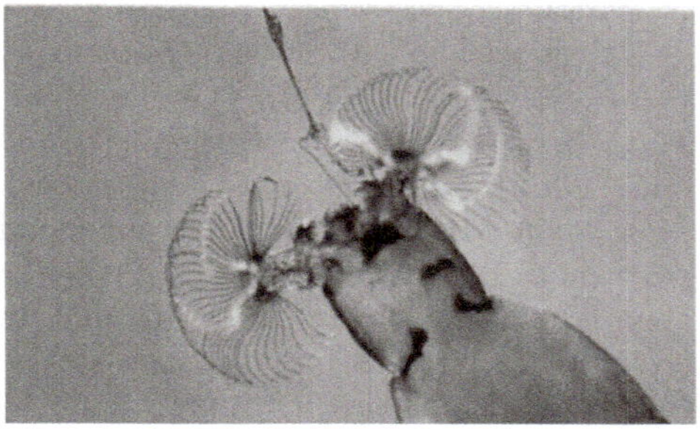

Fig. 243 *Simulium* sp. larva with typical mouth brushes [30]

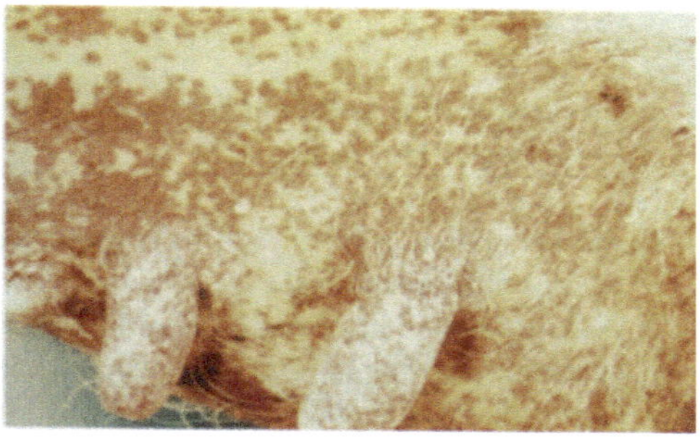

Fig. 244 Erythema and massive skin irritation on the udder due to *Simulium* bites [30]

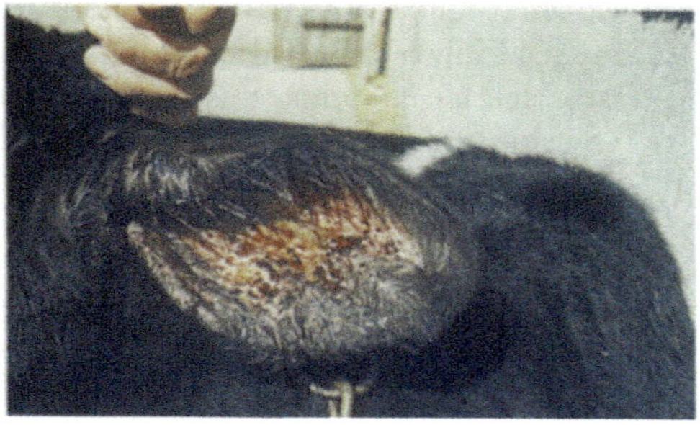

Fig. 245 Moist eczema-like skin alterations on the ear of a cattle following *Simulium* bites [30]

CERATOPOGONIDAE

Culicoides spp. Biting midges, seasonal dermatitis, sweet itch

Remarks: They are very small (1–3 mm long). Adult female midges attack cattle, sheep, poultry, horse, man and other species, causing marked irritation by penetration of the skin with their proboscis. The bites cause intense itching. Only the females suck blood mainly during the twilight periods and at night. *Culicoides* occur often in large swarms a few hundred metres around the breeding sites. These are moist areas such as fresh or brackish water or seepages from decaying vegetable or dung heaps.

Significance: 1) Massive irritation of livestock, itching, allergic skin reactions (sweet-itch, seasonal dermatitis) in horses (☞ HORSES AND DONKEYS, 5.1), and 2) transmission of *Onchocerca gibsoni* and other *Onchocerca* spp. in cattle and horses, African Horse Sickness, Blue tongue of sheep. (Figure 246)

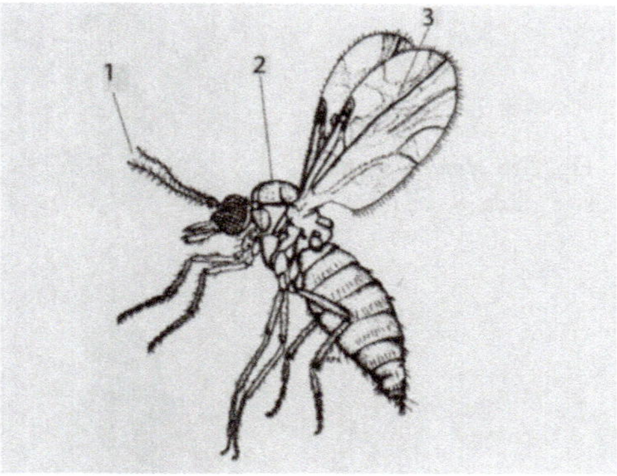

Fig. 246 *Culicoides* sp. (biting midge); adult (1–3mm long); (1) antennae long, (2) humped thorax and (3) mottled wings [20]

TABANIDAE

Tabanus spp. *Haematopota* spp. and *Chrysops* spp. Horse flies

Remarks: These robust flies have powerful wings and breed on leaves of plants in the vicinity of water. Female tabanids attack mammals to suck blood. They cause deep, painful, irritating bites. They generally bite several times for one blood meal because they are disturbed by the host's defense. A number of diseases (besnoitiosis, anaplasmosis, trypanosomosis and anthrax, hog cholera, equine infectious anaemia) are mechanically transmitted by tabanids. This is of special importance especially when horseflies are numerous among a crowded livestock population.
(Figures 247, 248, 249)

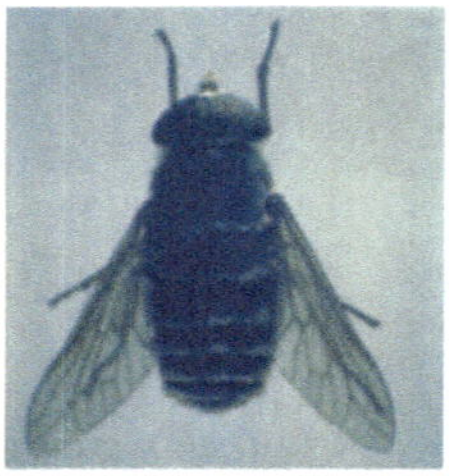

Fig. 247 *Tabanus* sp.; adult (17–25 mm) [13]

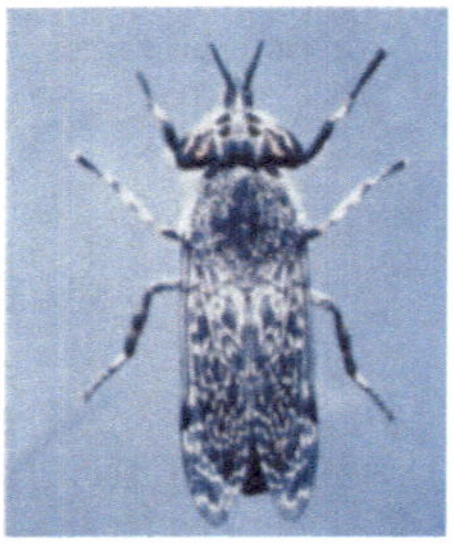

Fig. 248 *Haematopota* sp.; adult (8–13 mm)

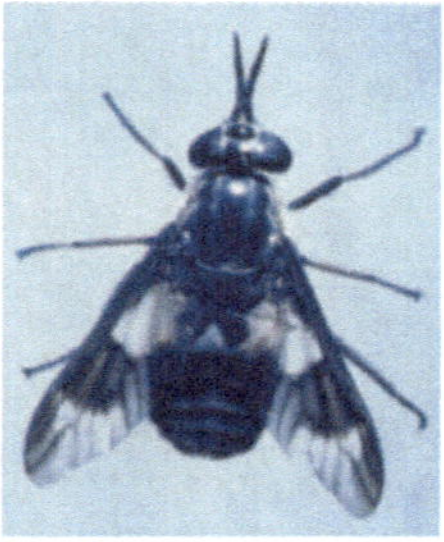

Fig. 249 *Chrysops* sp.; adult (9–12 mm)

MUSCIDAE

Musca spp., *Lyperosia* spp. and *Haematobia* spp. Muscid flies

Remarks: Muscid flies are annoying livestock especially during the summer or rainy season. They are swarming around farm livestock. The resulting irritation is incessant and much of the energy of the animals is lost to defend against fly attacks. In addition to the nuisance the flies often carry pathogens on their feet and bodies. Some also act as intermediate hosts for other parasites. Two genera need to receive special attention: *Musca* and *Haematobia.*

Musca domestica (the common house fly) and other *Musca* spp. are non-biting muscid. *Musca autumnalis* is attracted to wounds and other moist parts of the body, especially the eyes. It may provoke conjunctivitis and an ulcerative dermatitis. The infectious keratoconjunctivitis ("pinkeye") mainly caused by *Moraxella bovis* may be transmitted by muscid flies, especially *M. autumnalis*. *M. domestica* is known to transfer pathogenic bacteria mechanically from one wound to another. It is also capable of transmitting numerous pathogenic agents of medical and veterinary importance (*Salmonella, Shigella, Entamoeba histolytica*, cestodes of poultry, *Habronema* spp., *Thelazia* spp., *Parafilaria bovicola* and others). The preferred breeding place is in the faeces of animals or in decaying organic matter.
(Figures 250, 251, 252)

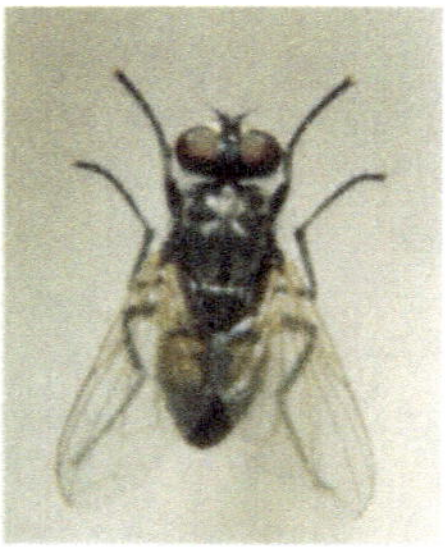

Fig. 250 *Musca domestica*; adult (6–7 mm) [12]

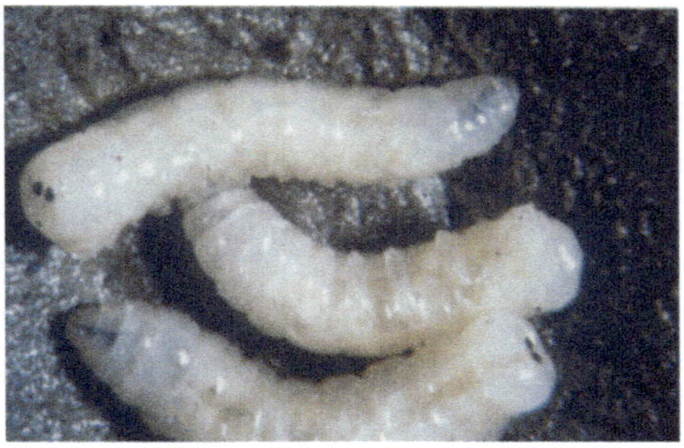

Fig. 251 *Musca domestica*; larvae [4]

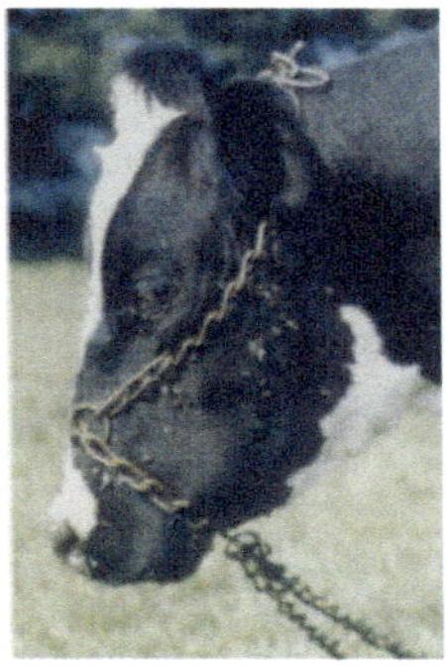

Fig. 252 *Musca autumnalis*; adult flies in situ

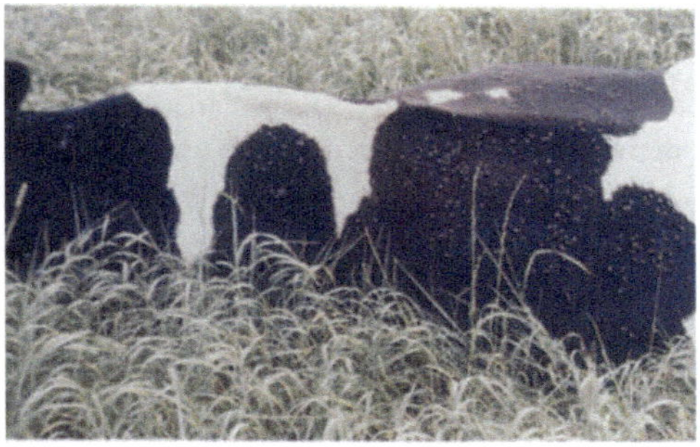

Fig. 253 *Haematobia* sp.; adult flies on the back of a cattle

Haematobia minuta and other *Haematobia* spp. (the horn flies, buffalo flies) are biting muscids and act as vectors of *Stephanofilaria stilesi* in cattle and *Parafilaria multipapillosa* in horses. The adults of this fly live almost permanently on cattle, buffalo, sheep and other animals. They congregate along the backs where their bites cause severe irritation so that the cattle rub themselves raw. The female only leaves her host briefly to lay her eggs in fresh cattle or buffalo dung. The larval development requires a high relative humidity of nearly 100%. The fly is therefore widely distributed in Central, East and southern Africa. The horn flies are obligatory parasites of cattle and a serious pest wherever they occur. *Haematobia* spp. cause intense worry and irritation to animals, the bite being very painful. Serious blood loss may occur when large numbers attack and loss of condition, reduced performance is a common result. The flies cause sores at the base of the horns, on the poll, ears, neck, withers and tail root.
(Figures 253, 254, 255)

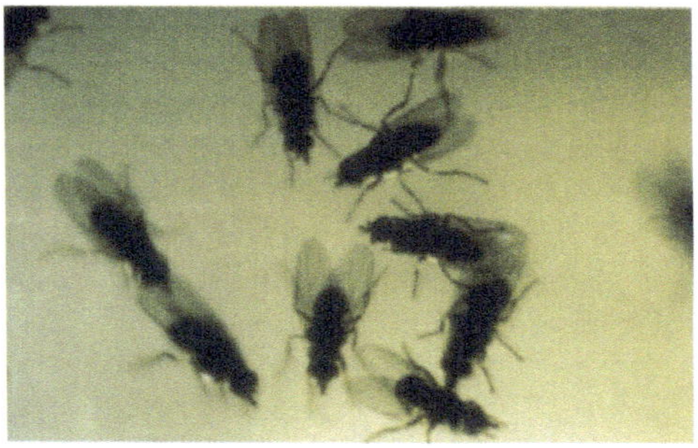

Fig. 254 *Haematobia irritans*; adult flies (5–6 mm) [10]

Stomoxys calcitrans* and *Stomoxys nigra

Stable fly

Remarks: *S. calcitrans* also belongs to the muscids. It attacks almost all livestock species. *Stomoxys* breeds in manure (preferably horse manure) or in decaying organic matter. They require a very damp situation (heaped-up decaying vegetable matter). It is a biting muscid and occurs world-wide. Both sexes of this fly are bloodsuckers and can become extremely irritating pests of man and domestic animals. On cattle the flies prefer to feed on the legs while on dogs the ears may be so bitten that they become sore and scabby. Their salivary secretions cause toxic reactions with an immunosuppressive effect, rendering the host more susceptible to diseases.

Significance: *S. calcitrans* acts as intermediate host of *Habronema microstoma* (☞ HORSES AND DONKEYS, ■ 1), *Trypanosoma evansi, Anthrax, Dermatophilus congolensis*, agents of the lumpy wool in sheep and probably many other pathogens. Its painful bite causes intense worry and irritation to animals. It may produce toxic reactions and immunosuppression. Blood loss may be marked following continuous, heavy attacks.

Control: Sanitation is the most important control measure in stable fly control. Manure, straw and decaying matter should be kept away from the environment of cattle, since this provides the development medium for the flies. If good sanitation procedures are practiced, then chemical control is less likely to be needed. Without sanitation chemical control measures are likely to fail.

(Figures 255, 256, 257)

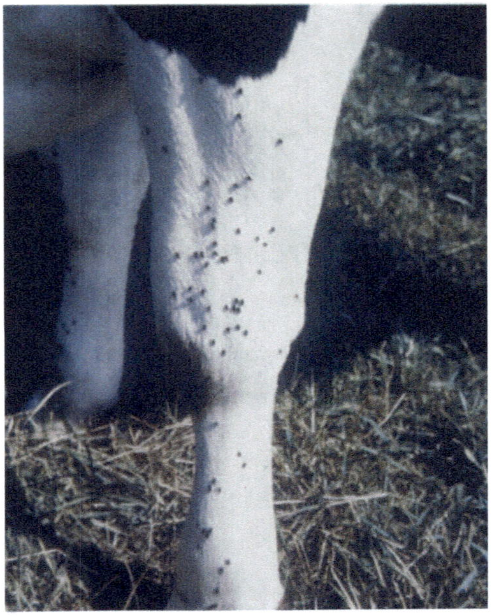

Fig. 257 *Stomoxys calcitrans*; adult flies in situ

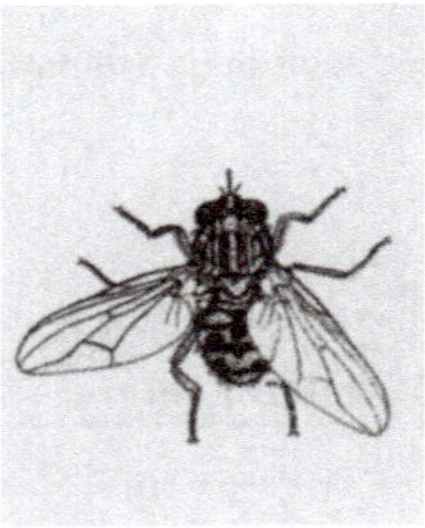

Fig. 255 *Stomoxys calcitrans* (the stable fly); adult fly (4–6 mm) with a prominent and rigid proboscis; the maxillary palps are shorter than the proboscis and the thorax has longitudinal stripes [27]

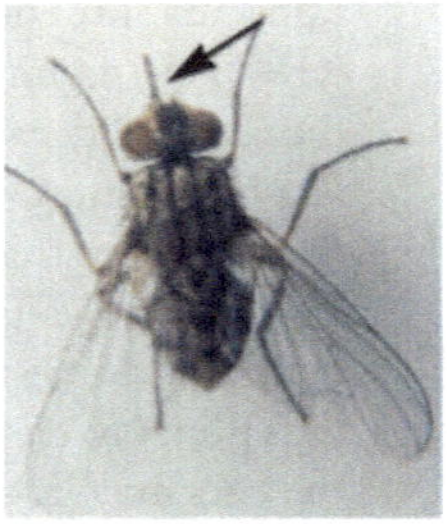

Fig. 256 *Stomoxys calcitrans*; adult fly (4–6 mm) with prominent biting mouthparts (arrow) [10]

GLOSSINIDAE

Glossina spp. Tsetse flies, "flies that are destructive of cattle" from Sechuana

Remarks: Most tsetse flies are active during the daytime and hunt by sight and smell and feed every 2 to 3 days. Both sexes suck blood and are equally capable of transmitting trypanosomes. The female is larviparous, producing one larva at a time and an estimated total of 8–12 larvae during her life. Apart from two species in south-western Arabia, tsetse flies are confined to the African continent, where they infest around 7.5 million square kilometres, mainly tropical regions on either side of the equator. Wherever these bloodsucking flies are, they render the area unsuitable for man and his livestock.

(Figures 258, 259)

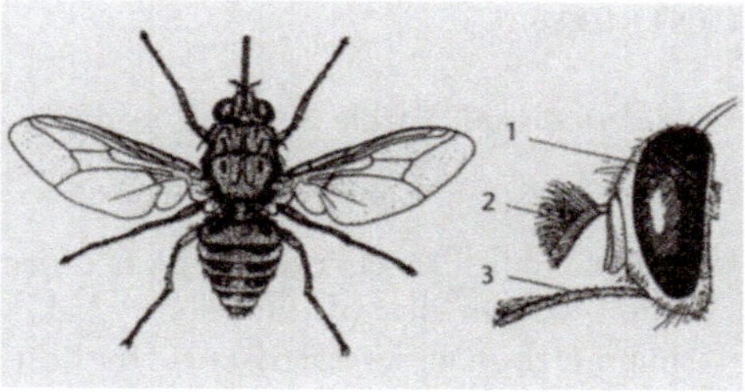

Fig. 258 *Glossina* sp. (tsetse fly); adult flies are robust insects, ranging in size from 6–16 mm and can be distinguished from other flies by their wing venation; the head shows prominent eyes (1), charactersitic antennae (2) and a prominent piercing proboscis [27]

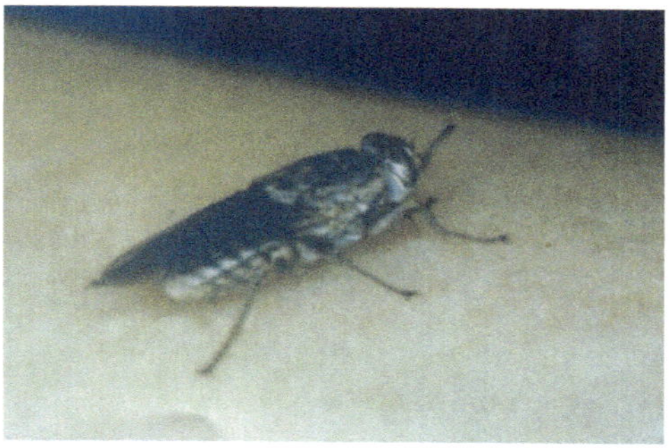

Fig. 261 *Glossina palpalis*; adult in feeding position [4]

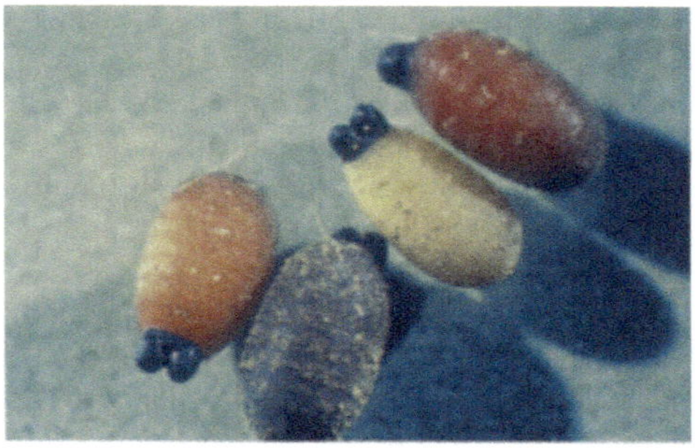

Fig. 259 Pupae (6–7 mm long) of tsetse flies (*Glossina* spp.) [13]

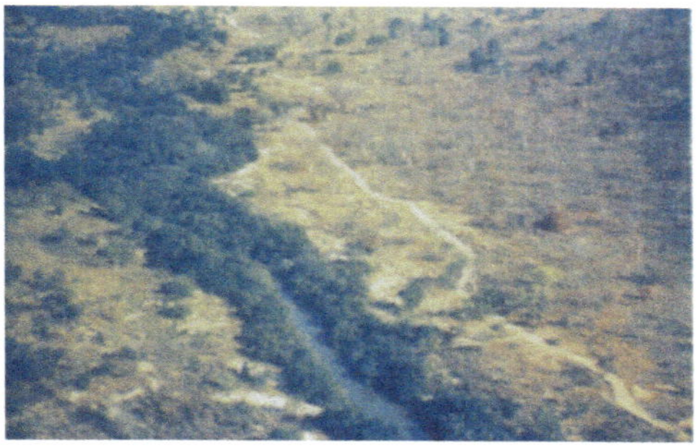

Fig. 262 Riverine habitat of *Glossina palpalis* [13]

Some 31 species of tsetse flies are known which can be divided into three groups, each with different habits and requirements: 1. Flies of the *Glossina palpalis* group are riverine species and feed on reptiles and ungulates. 2. Flies of the *Glossina morsitans* group are savannah and dry thorn-bush species which feed mainly on large animals. 3. Members of the *Glossina fusca* group occur in the rainforest and have require-ments between the first 2 groups, preferring dense shade and riverine thickets.

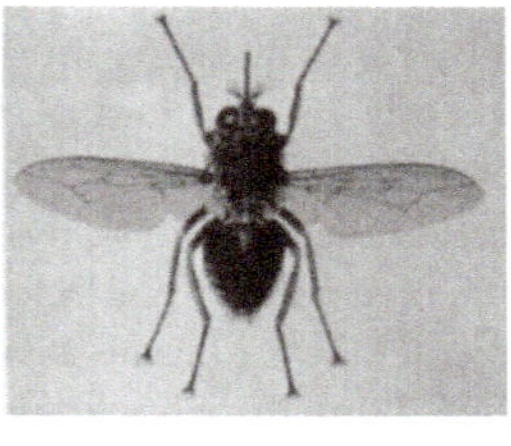

Fig. 260 *Glossina palpalis*; adult [13]

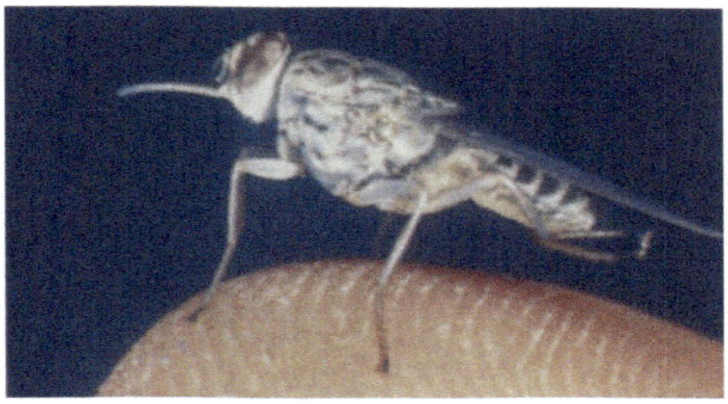

Fig. 263 *Glossina morsitans* with a prominent piercing proboscis [13]

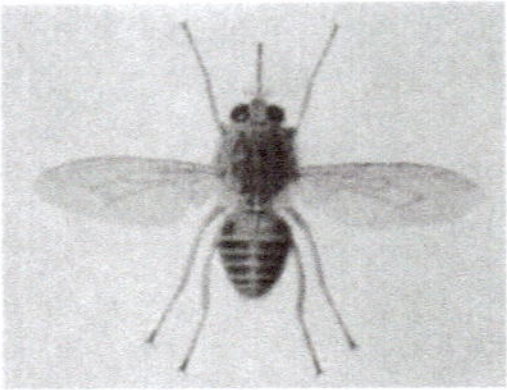

Fig. 264 *Glossina morsitans*; adult (8–11 mm) [13]

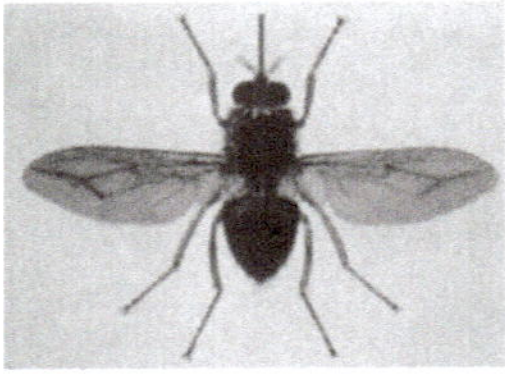

Fig. 265 *Glossina fusca*; adult [13]

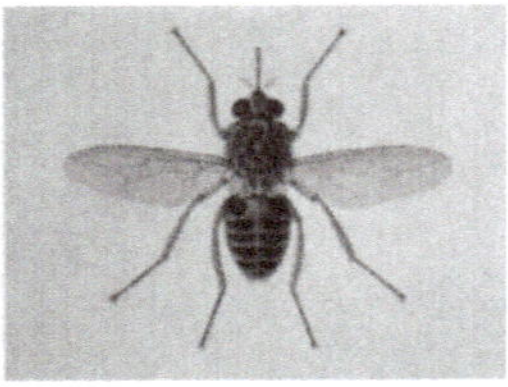

Fig. 266 *Glossina tachinoides*; adult [13]

Significance: Tsetse flies are vectors of human and animal trypanosomosis. Trypanosomosis of domestic animals is caused mainly by *T. congolense*, *T. vivax*, *T. brucei* and *T. simiae*. (☞ CATTLE, ■ 2). The most important vectors are *Glossina morsitans*, *G. palpalis*, *G. tachinoides*, *G. fusca*, *G. brevipalpis* and *G. pallidipes*.

(Figures 260, 261, 262, 263, 264, 265, 266, 267)

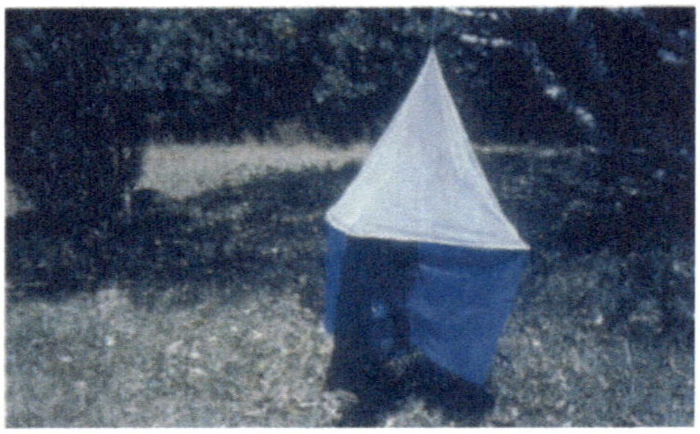

Fig. 267 Biconical tsetse trap [4]

OESTRIDAE

Hypoderma spp. Warble fly, cattle grubs, heel flies

Location: Adult flies lay eggs on hairs of legs and occasionally of the body. Larvae migrate through several tissues of the host's body and appear in the subcutaneous tissue of the back.

Hosts: Cattle

Species description: Adult warble flies are hairy insects like bumble-bees. They do not feed and only live for a few days. The females lay their eggs on the hind legs of cattle and occasionally horses. The eggs of *Hypoderma bovis* are attached singly to an individual hair and the hatched larvae penetrate the skin and migrate along nerves to the spinal cord and then through the dorsal muscles till they come to lie below the skin on the back. *H. lineatum* eggs are attached in rows of 7–20 eggs per hair. Larvae penetrate the skin, migrate first to the oesophageal region and thence to the back. In spring the larvae leave through the holes, drop to the ground and burrow into soil to pupate.

Geographic distribution: Many countries of the northern hemisphere. Warble flies are reported from northern and southern Africa and are not widespread in tropical areas.

Symptoms: Clinical symptoms are rarely seen during the migratory phase, except if larvae are killed during their passage through the spinal cord. Paralysis may then occur. Nodules with an opening are usually seen in the skin of the back. These cysts contain a larva. When the adult flies attack cattle, stampeding may occur.

Significance: The adult flies severely disturb cattle which become apprehensive and attempt to escape by running away, often aimlessly. Consequently feeding and performance is reduced. In addition, warble flies cause extensive damage to the skin of cattle and the commercial value of the hides is markedly reduced. *H. bovis* larvae may cause paralysis when dying or being killed during their migration through the spinal canal. Severe oedema may occur when larvae of *H. lineatum* are killed during their migration through the oesophageal region.

Diagnosis: Larvae in cysts or lumps under the skin of the back indicate warble infestation. Eggs may be found on hair of the animal's legs.

Therapy: Cattle, especially calves, in areas where grub numbers are high, should be treated as soon as possible after the end of the warble fly season. They should not be treated later than 8–12 weeks before the anticipated first appearance of grubs in the backs, since adverse reactions may occur when migratory larvae are killed in the spinal cord. Pour-on treatments of coumaphos, famphur, fenthion, phosmet, trichlorfon or ivermectin may be used and poured evenly along the midline of the back. Sprays containing coumaphos or phosmet also control cattle grubs. The entire surface of the skin should be wet for sufficient absorption. Coumaphos and phosmet may also be used as dips. Ivermectin (200 µg/kg, sc.) is highly effective against cattle grub. Oral application is also effective.

Prophylaxis: Attacks by adult warble flies are difficult to avoid and entail excessive use of insecticides. Early treatment in endemic areas is indicated.

(Figures 268, 269, 270, 271)

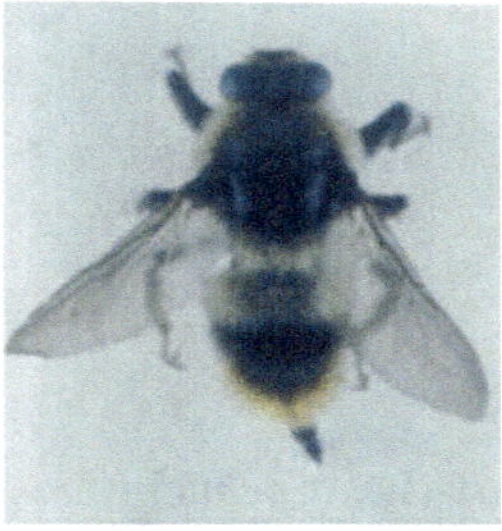

Fig. 268 *Hyporderma bovis* (warble fly); adult (15 mm long) [4]

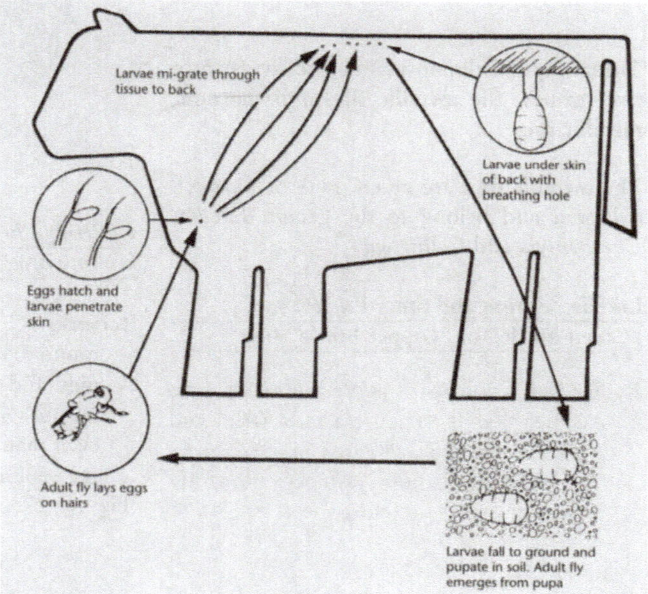

Fig. 269 Life cycle of *Hyporderma* spp. [6]

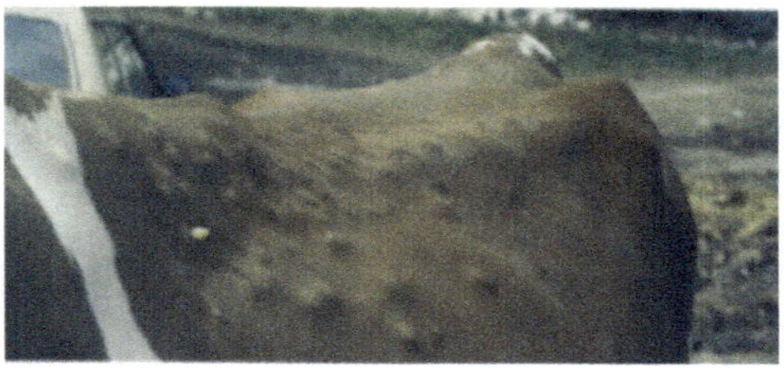

Fig. 270 *Hyporderma bovis* larvae causing nodules on the back

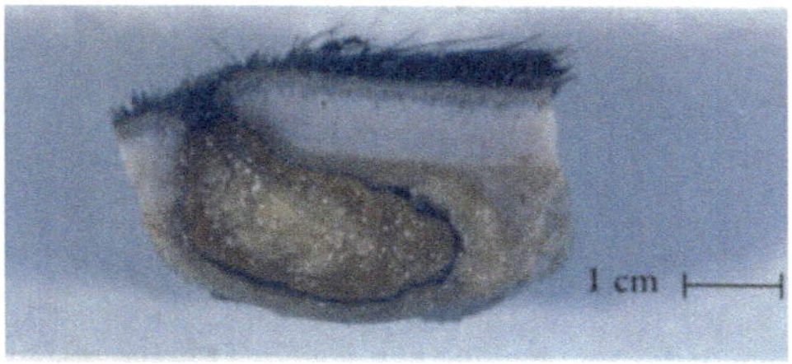

Fig. 271 *Hypoderma bovis*; section through a skin nodule containing a larva

CALLIPHORIDAE The blowflies and their allies

Remarks: They are highly important in many domestic animal species and man. The adults are free-living and the larvae are parasitic maggots which develop in the tissue of their host, causing a condition called myiasis. The larvae may be laid into pre-existing wounds. Myiasis is often a secondary skin problem.
(Figure 272)

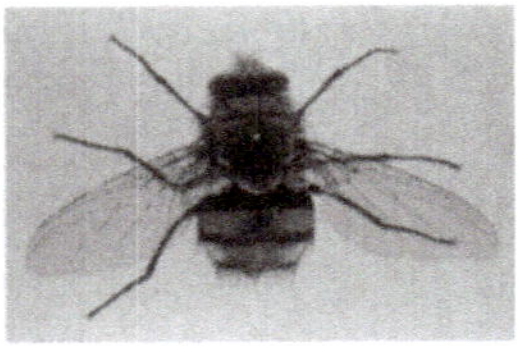

Fig. 272 *Calliphora* sp.; adult (12 mm long) [4]

The family of Calliphoridae can be divided into two groups, the **metallic flies** and the **non-metallic flies.**

The **metallic flies** are green, blue or purplish coloured and belong to the genera *Lucilia, Chrysomyia* and *Callitroga*

***Lucilia cuprina* and other *Lucilia* spp.** "Green-bottle" or "copper-bottle" flies

Remarks: *L. cuprina* is the predominant cause of sheepblow fly strike in South Africa and Australia. It causes myiasis in sheep. It is the most important primary blow fly initiating strikes on living sheep (☞ SHEEP AND GOATS, ■ 5.1).
(Figure 273)

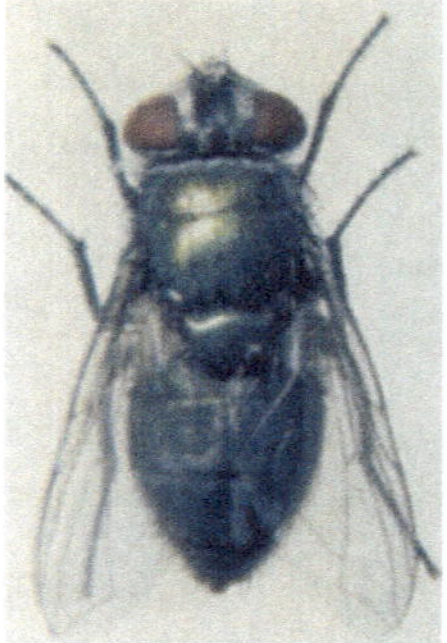

Fig. 273 *Lucilia sericata* (the green-bottle flies); adult (8–9 mm)

Chrysomya bezziana Cattle screwworm, the Old World screwworm, blow fly strike of cattle

Remarks: *C. bezziana* infests cattle but also horses, sheep, dogs and sometimes man. It occurs in tropical and southern Africa and oriental regions. *C. bezziana* causes severe myiasis and toxins produced by the larvae result in retarded healing of wounds. Death may occur in severe cases.
(Figure 274)

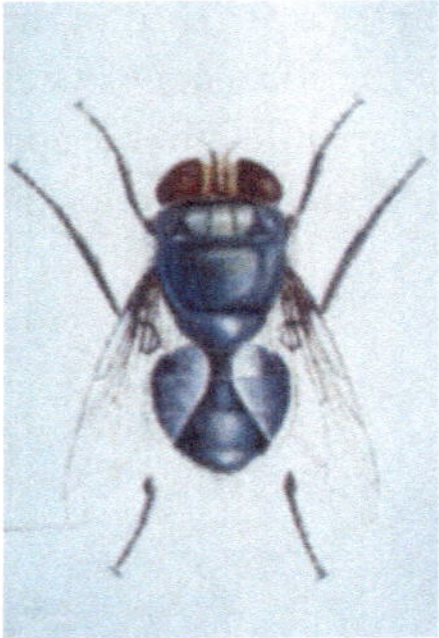

Fig. 274 *Chrysomya bezziana* (the cattle screwworm); adult (8–10 mm) [20]

Callitroga hominivorax (syn. *Cochliomyia hominivorax)* "American screwworm"

Remarks: *C. hominivorax* has recently been found to occur also in North Africa. Cattle, pigs and equines suffer most frequently, but other animals, including fowls and even man may also be affected. Pathology is essentially the same as in *C. bezziana.*
(Figures 275, 276)

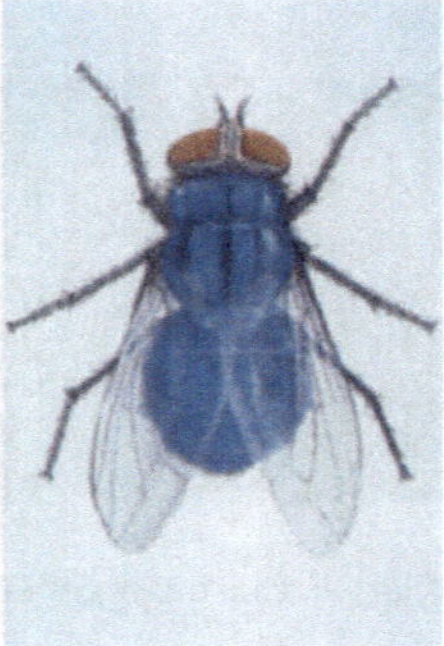

Fig. 275 *Callitroga hominivorax* (syn. *Cochliomyia hominivorax*) the "screwworm"; adult (8–10 mm long) [19]

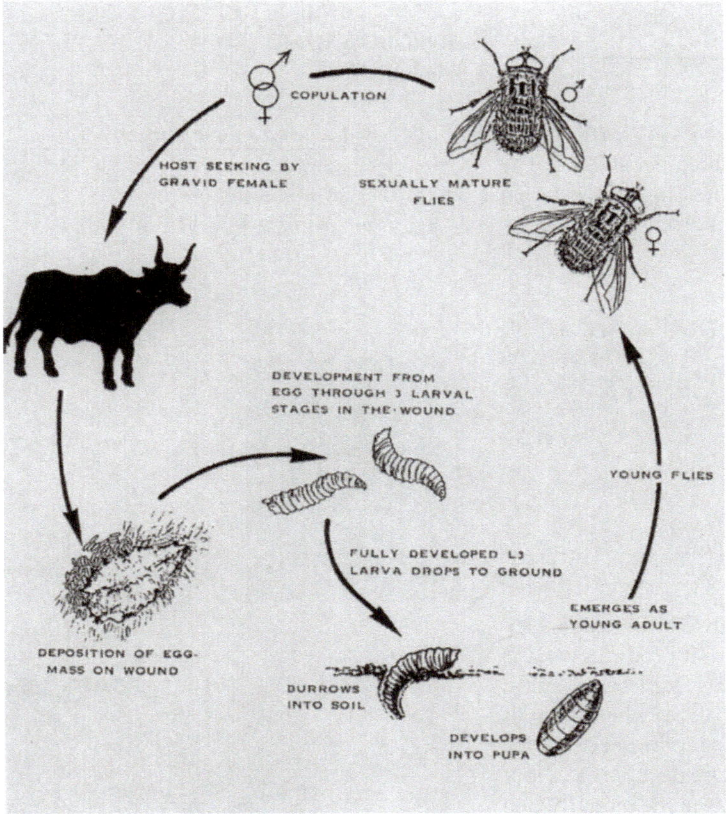

Fig. 276 Life cycle of *Callitroga hominivorax* [31]

The **non-metallic flies** are dull grey, yellow-brown or black and belong to the genera *Wohlfartia*, *Sarcophaga* and *Cordylobia*

Sarcophaga haemorrhoidalis

Red-tailed fleshfly

Remarks: The fly is very common in Africa south of the Sahara and is frequently found around human habitations. Flies of this species are larviparous and may lay their larvae in wounds or sores although larvae may also be deposited on faeces, carrion or fresh meat. Several animal species and man may be affected. The fly may cause myiasis, especially in sheep in some parts of the world.
(Figures 277, 278)

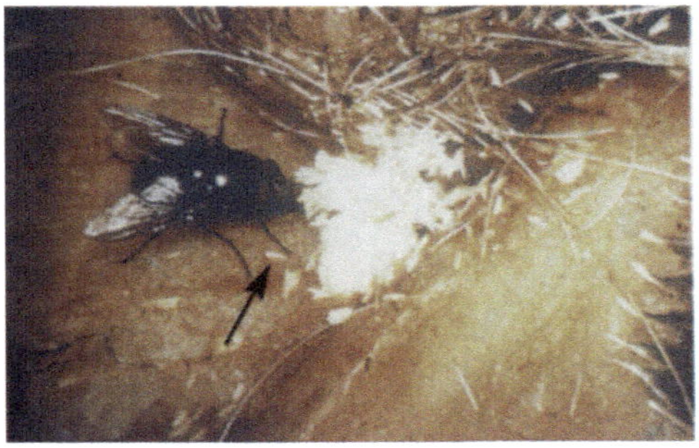

Fig. 277 *Sarcophaga* sp.; adult fly depositing its larvae on the skin of a cattle [8]

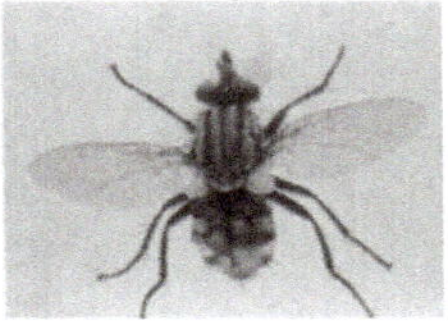

Fig. 278 *Sarcophaga* sp.; adult fly (13–15mm long) [4]

Wohlfartia magnifica
Old World fleshfly

Remarks: This species occurs in North Africa. The fly attacks man and other animals. The larvae may be deposited into the external ear of man or in sores around the eyes.
(Figure 279)

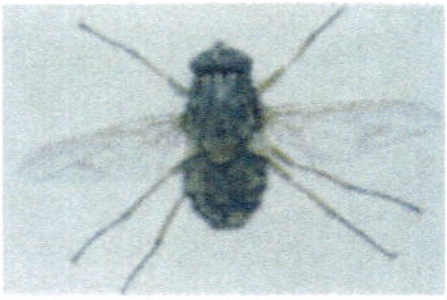
Fig. 279 *Wohlfartia* sp.; adult fly (8–14 mm long) [4]

Cordylobia anthropophaga
Tumbu fly or "skin maggot fly"

Remarks: The fly is widely distributed in Africa south of the Sahara. It produces myiasis in man, dogs and other domestic animals. Eggs are laid around places where animals lie. After hatching the larvae penetrate the skin of the host, producing a boil of about 1 cm across with a hole in the centre. When mature the larvae wriggle out of the hole and pupate on the ground. Tumbu boils are found commonly on the ventral parts of the body but also on any other area of the body.
(Figures 280, 281)

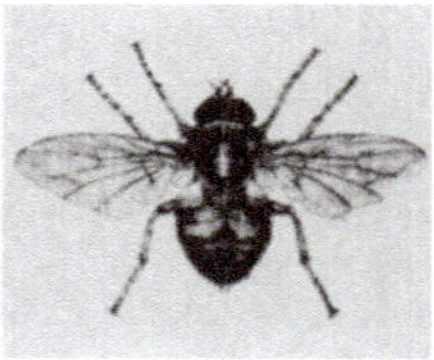
Fig. 280 *Cordylobia anthropophaga* (Tumbu fly); stout fly with two black marks on the thorax; the face and legs are yellow (8–12 mm long) [27]

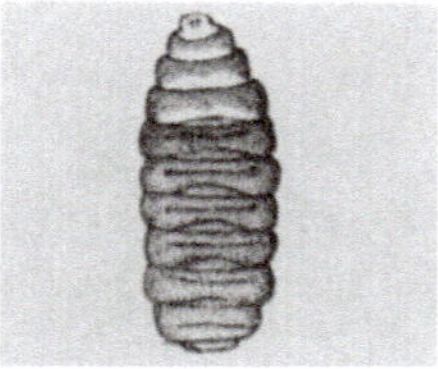
Fig. 281 *Cordylobia anthropophaga*; third-stage larva (12–28 mm long) [27]

HIPPOBOSCIDAE
The louse flies

Hippobosca equina Horse louse fly

Hosts: Horse and cattle
Geographic distribution: World-wide
(☞ Horses and Donkeys, 5.1)
(Figures 282, 283)

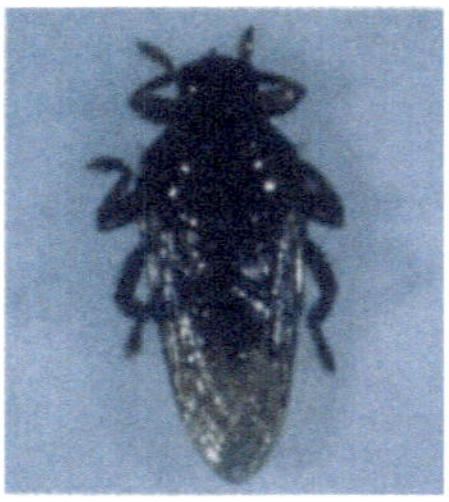
Fig. 282 *Hippobosca equina* (horse louse fly; 7–9 mm long)

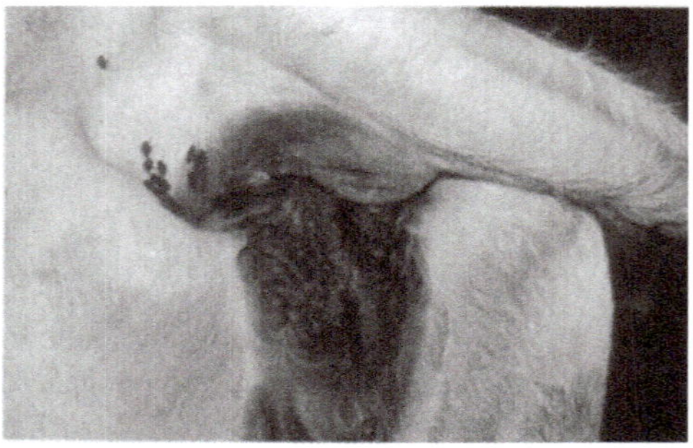
Fig. 283 *Hippobosca* sp.; adult louse flies on a cattle [4]

Hippobosca variegata

Hosts: Horse and cattle
Geographic distribution: Tropical Africa and oriental regions

Hippobosca rufipes Cattle louse fly

Hosts: Mainly wild and domestic Bovidae, less frequently horses
Geographic distribution: Tropical Africa (arid and semi-arid areas of Africa)
(Figure 284)

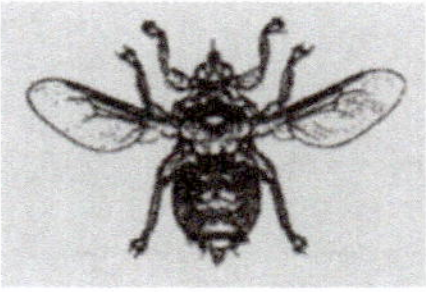

Fig. 284 *Hippobosca rufipes* (cattle louse fly); this fly is very hard-bodied and difficult to squash. It has well-developed wings and strong legs ending in well-developed claws (8–11 mm long) [27]

Hippobosca maculata

Hosts: Horse and cattle
Geographic distribution: Tropical and subtropical areas of Africa
(Figure 285)

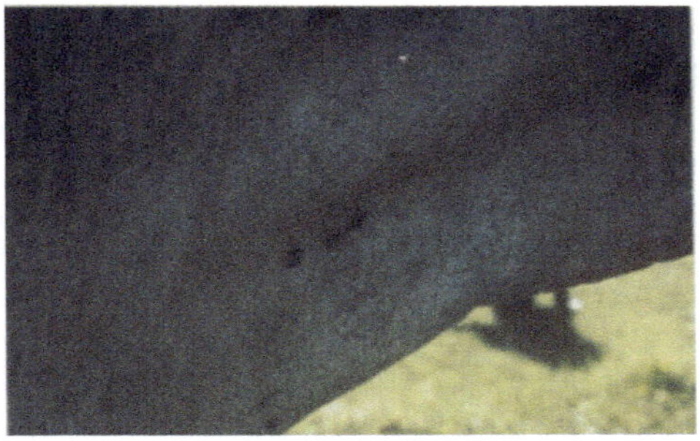

Fig. 285 *Hippobosca maculata*; adults (8 mm long) attached to the jugular vein region of a cattle [8]

Hippobosca camelina Camel louse fly

Hosts: Camel, horse and occasionally cattle
Geographic distribution: Northern Africa and Middle East

- **General features of *Hippobosca* spp.**

Location: The adult louse flies remain for long periods on their host and cluster in the perineal region, between the hindlegs to the pubic region, but may also bite on other parts of the body.
Species description: The flies live permanently on their host and feed on blood. Mainly cattle and horses are affected. They rarely fly and then usually not more than a few metres. They spend their whole time on the host and are strongly attached to their host and therefore difficult to dislodge. When disturbed they can quickly move sideways.
Symptoms: Infested animals scratch and rub, and skin-trauma are often seen as a consequence of heavy infestations.
Significance: These flies are a source of great irritation. They transmit the non-pathogenic *Trypanosoma theileri*, anthrax and other bacterial infections to cattle.
Diagnosis: Identification of flies located under the tail and between the hindlegs.
Therapy: ☞ below, THERAPY AND PROPHYLAXIS OF ECTOPARASITES, p. 141
Prophylaxis: Regular grooming may be helpful to reduce louse fly infestations.

- **Therapy and prophylaxis of ectoparasites** (for arachnids and insects)

A great number of insecticides is used to control both arachnids and insects (Table 11). Methods of application include whole-body sprays, dips, dusts and topical application to the dermis and ears. Dips are more effective for ticks. Thorough treatment of the infested area is required, especially when ticks infest the ears or underside of the tail or mites infest localized patches on the skin. Impregnated ear tags, containing pyrethroids or organophosphates, are of increasing importance in fly control. Elimination of parasites or stages in the environment is difficult because many ectoprasites are capable of surviving in the environment for prolonged periods (e.g. some ticks can live on the ground up to 300 days without feeding). In areas where many ticks exist reinfection of the host occurs continuously and treatment therefore must be repeated regularly. Some ticks are not strictly species-specific and ticks normally adapted to horses can occasionally also affect cattle or other animals and they must be treated, too, if attempts are made to reduce tick infestations.
In subhumid areas the period of highest tick activity is the wet season and only few ticks are found on animals during the dry season. Con-

sequently tick control is focussed to the wet season. In tropical areas most ticks are active throughout the year and must be controlled continuously.

Table 11 Some common compounds to control external parasites of cattle

Compound	Pest
Organophosphates	
Chlorpyrifos	Lice, horn flies
Coumaphos	Horn flies, lice, ticks, grubs, screw worms, mites
Crotoxyphos and dichlorvos	Horn flies, face flies, stable flies, house flies,lice, ticks
Dichlorvos	Horn flies, face flies, stable flies, house flies
Dichlorvos and tetrachlorvinphos	Horn flies, face flies, lice, ticks
Diazinon	Horn flies (including pyrethroid-resistant flies), spinose ear ticks, lice, mites, *Hypobosca* spp.
Dioxathion	Horn flies, lice, mites
Fenthion	Horn flies, lice, *Hypoderma* spp.
Malathion	Lice, keds, mites
Phoxim	Mites, lice, flies, myiasis, ticks
Phosmet	Grubs, lice, horn flies, ticks, mites
Stirofos	Horn flies, face flies, house flies, stable flies
Tetrachlorvinphos	Horn flies, lice, ticks
Trichlorfon (metrifonat)	Grubs, lice, mites
Carbamates	
Carbaryl	Mites, lice, ticks, flies
Promacyl	Mites, lice, ticks, flies
Chlorinated Hydrocarbons*	
Lindane	Screwworm larvae, mites, lice, ticks, flies
Methoxychlor	Mites, lice, ticks, flies
Toxaphen	Mites, lice, ticks, flies
Pyrethrins and Pyrethroids	
Cyfluthrin	Horn flies, horse flies
Cypermethrin	Horn and face flies, ticks
Deltamethrin	Flies, including tsetse flies
Fenvalerate	Horn and face flies, spinose ear ticks
Flumethrin	Flies, including tsetse flies, ticks
Permethrin	Horn flies, face flies, mites, ticks, lice
Pyrethrin	Horn flies, face flies, mites, lice
Avermectins	
Doramectin	Mites, lice, ticks, *Hypoderma* spp.
Ivermectin	Mites, lice, *Hypoderma* spp.

* some are no longer approved by some governments

5.2 Eyes

Thelazia rhodesi Cattle eyeworm

Location: Conjunctival sac

Hosts: Cattle, rarely sheep and goat

Species description: Milky-white worms, males 8–12 mm long and females 12–18 mm. The cuticle is transversely striated. The spicules are 0.75–0.85 and 0.115–0.13 mm long. Intermediate hosts are *Musca larvipara* and *Musca amica*. Infected flies transmit the infective larvae via saliva to calves. Adult *Thelazia* appeared 20–25 days after infection. In some regions a high percentage of calves is infected but lesions are often absent.

Geographic distribution: World-wide

Symptoms: Conjunctivitis, clouded cornea, marked lacrimation. The affected eyes may be swollen and covered with exsudate and pus. Without treatment progressive keratitis and ulceration of the cornea may occur.

Significance: Infections with eyeworms may be very prevalent in some regions. Heavy infections may cause marked irritation, keratitis and weight loss of affected animals.

Diagnosis: This is made by the detection of worms in the conjunctival sacs. Examination of the lacrimal secretions may reveal eggs or first-stage larvae.

Therapy: Levamisole (5 mg/kg, sc.) and ivermectin (200 µg/kg, sc.) are active against *Thelazia* spp. Concurrent use of antibiotic ointment for secondary invaders is recommended.

Prophylaxis: Fly control measures against the face fly aid in the control of thelaziosis in both cattle and horses.

(Figures 286, 287, 288)

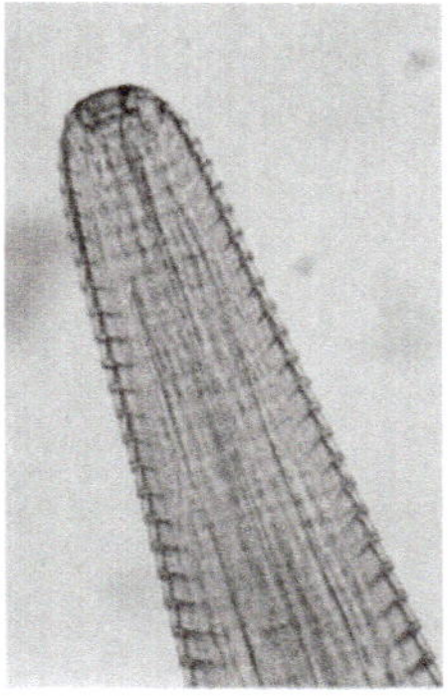

Fig. 286 *Thelazia rhodesi* (eyeworm); anterior end with typical cuticular striation

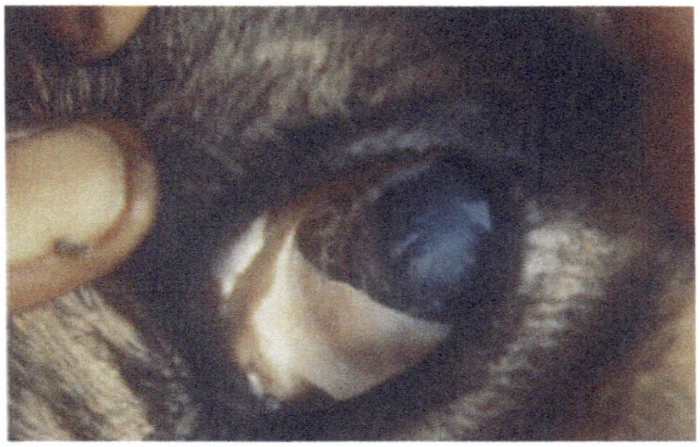

Fig. 287 *Thelazia rhodesi* in the eyes of a cattle

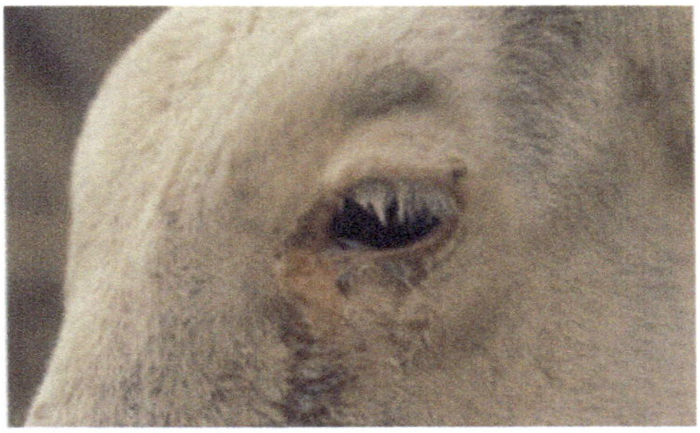

Fig. 288 N'Dama cattle with lacrimation due to *Thealzia rhodesi* infection

III

Parasites of Sheep and Goats

CONTENTS

1 Stages in the gut and faeces

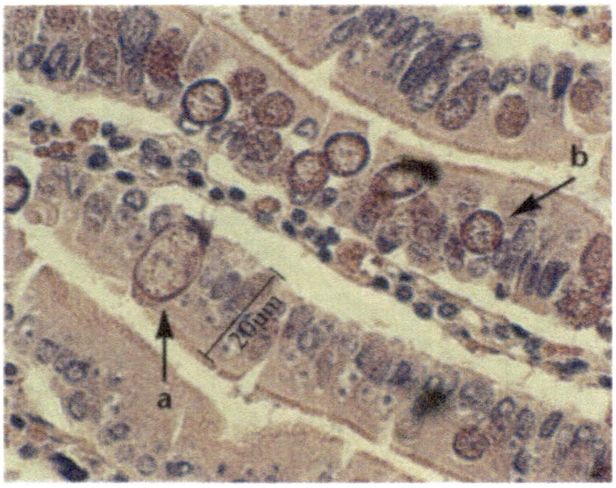

Fig. 289 *Eimeria* spp.; intestinal tissue section (sheep); heavy infection showing (a) oocysts (approx. 20 µm) and (b) gametocytes

PROTOZOA

- **Coccidiosis in sheep and goats**

Sheep and goats have their own species of Coccidia. Cross-transmission is not possible. Out of a spectrum of more than 10 species which occur world-wide in sheep and goats, generally only a few are highly pathogenic and only if predisposing factors increase the susceptibility of the host animal (stress at weaning, malnutrition, other diseases, etc.) or if the management conditions are such that animals are exposed to a very high infection risk (using highly contaminated feedlot confinements).

All the *Eimeria* spp. produce unsporulated oocysts which are passed in the faeces. Within 1–4 days sporulation occurs (oocysts with four sporocysts each containing two sporozoites). The sporulated oocyst represents the infective stage of *Eimeria* spp. The further development occurs in the epithelial cells and the cells of the lamina propria at species specific sites within the intestines. Oocysts occur 6–35 days after infection. Disease due to *Eimeria* spp. mainly occurs in young animals.
(Figures 289, 290)

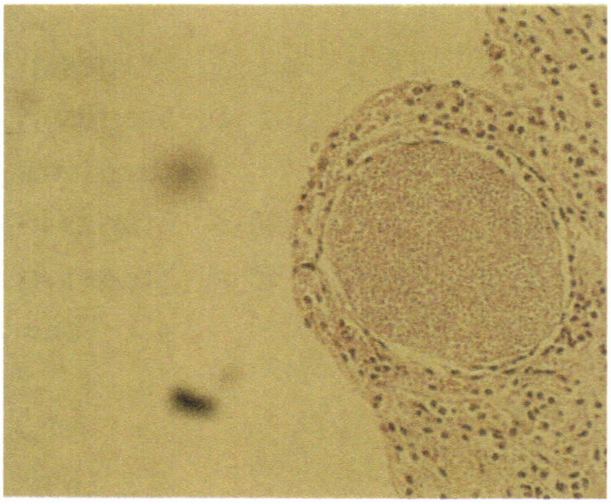

Fig. 290 *Eimeria* spp.; intestinal tissue section (sheep); macroschizont (100 µm in diameter)

Eimeria ovinoidalis (syn. *E. ninakohlyakimovae*), ***Eimeria ahsata, Eimeria bakuensis*** (syn. *E. ovina*) **and other *Eimeria* spp.**
Coccidiosis of sheep

Remarks: 15 species of *Eimeria* spp. have been described for sheep. Oocysts of similar appearance affect goats, but cross-transmission studies have confirmed their separate identity. *E. ovinoidalis* is the most pathogenic species. It affects the caecum and colon, causing severe enteritis, which may become haemorrhagic. Suckling lambs 4–7 weeks old are most commonly

affected. *E. ahsata* is also highly pathogenic for sheep. The intestines of infected lambs are thickened and oedematous and the Peyer's patches and lower parts of the small intestine are inflated. Deaths may occur. Other *Eimeria* oocysts (e.g. *E. crandalis*) are often produced in large numbers by lambs without causing disease. *E. bakuensis* causes white patches on the mucosa and sometimes polyps but its pathogenic role is in debate.
(Figures 291, 292, 293)

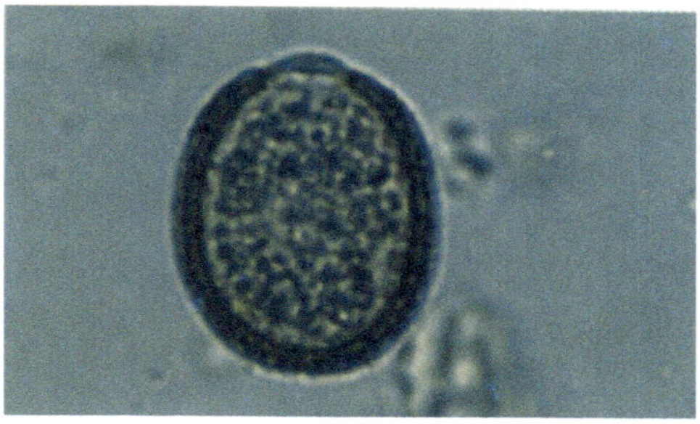

Fig. 291 Oocyst of *Eimeria intricata*

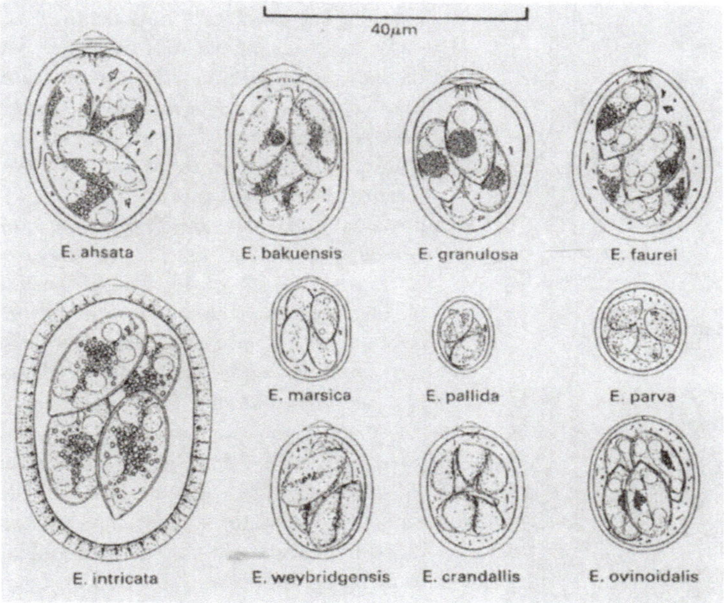

292 *Eimeria* species found in sheep (schematic) [1]

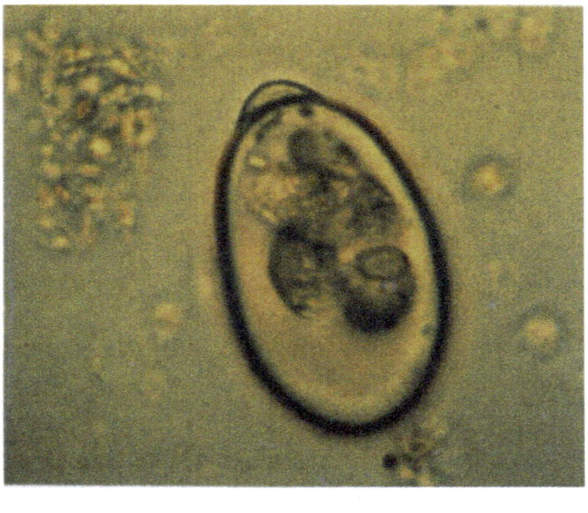

Fig. 293 Oocyst of Eimeria ahsata (39 × 25 μm) [15]

Eimeria arloingi, Eimeria christenseni, Eimeria ninakohlyakimovae and other *Eimeria* spp. Coccidiosis of goats

Remarks: Young goats commonly harbour a number of species of Coccidia and frequently produce oocysts at the rate of 10^5–10^6 per g of faeces without showing any clinical symptoms. Disease may occur following stress such as weaning, changes in diet, weather stress or regrouping, etc. *Eimeria arloingi, Eimeria christenseni* and *Eimeria ninakohlyakimovae* are the most pathogenic species in goats world-wide.
(Figures 294, 295)

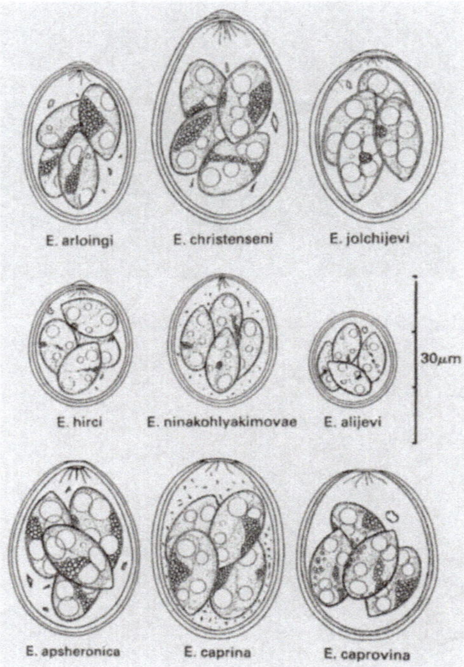

Fig. 294 *Eimeria* spp. found in goats [1]

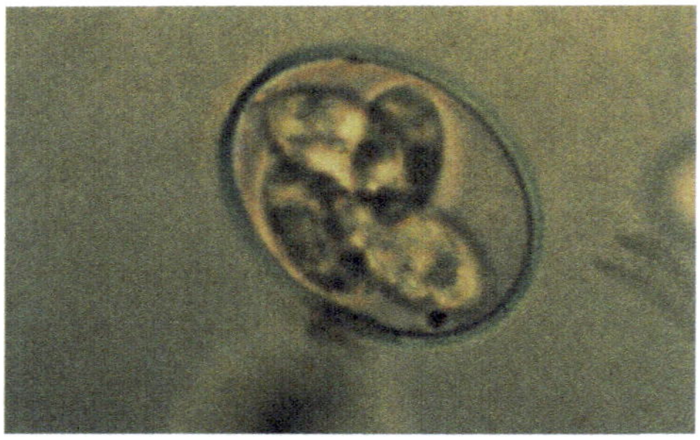

Fig. 295 Sporulated oocyst of *Eimeria ninakohlyakimovae* (24 × 19 µm) [15]

- **General features of coccidiosis in sheep and goats**

Symptoms: Diarrhoea (not always), dysentery, tenesm, exsiccosis; heavy infections cause fever, general depression, muscular spasms, CNS symptoms and finally death may occur. Secondary bacterial infections often aggravate the disease.

Significance: Coccidiosis may cause severe losses in small ruminants.

Diagnosis: This is difficult. Oocyst output can be very misleading because healthy lambs may produce more than 10^6 oocysts per g of faeces, whereas lambs dying of coccidiosis sometimes show very few oocysts. A satisfactory diagnosis can be made based on clinical history of the flock and autopsy lesions. Scrapings from the intestinal lesions usually reveal large numbers of gametocytes and oocysts. High oocyst counts of *E. ovinoidalis* from a number of scouring lambs support the diagnosis.

Therapy: Acute coccidiosis may be treated with trimethoprime/sulfonamide combinations. Lasalocid (15–70 mg/head/day, po.) may be used in sheep; amprolium can be used for clinical coccidiosis in sheep and goats; toltrazuril (15–20 mg/kg, po.).

Prophylaxis: Lasalocid (22–33 ppm, po.) and Monensin (1 mg/kg, po., daily during several days or 10–20 mg/kg feed) are highly effective against ovine coccidiosis. Amprolium (55 mg/kg, po. twice daily during 10 days) protects lambs against severe clinical disease. Sulfaguanidine (3 g/lamb daily or 0.1 mg/kg, po.), sulfaquinoxaline (2.5–4 g/kid daily or 8–70 mg/kg), sulfamerazine (65–130 mg/kg, po.) and nitrofurazon (70.4 mg/kg, po. daily for 7 days) control coccidiosis in lambs and goat kids. Decoquinate (0.5 kg/kg, po.) can be used in goats (☞ Cattle, 1, Table 3, p.27).

Cryptosporidium parvum

Remarks: Diarrhoea in neonatal lambs and goat kids may occur due to *C. parvum* infections. Appropriate colostrum supply is of great importance to avoid cryptosporidial diarrhoea. (☞ Cattle, 1).

Giardia duodenalis (syn. *G. caprae, G. ovis* and *G. quadrii*)

Remarks: This parasite occurs in sheep and goats and has been associated with diarrhoeic episodes in lambs and goat kids.

Cysts measure 14 × 8 μm and may be demonstrated in faeces by the flotation or SAF method (☞ METHODS, 1.4 and 1.12). Vegetative forms (trophozoites) may be found in fresh faeces of diarrhoeic animals. (Figure 296)

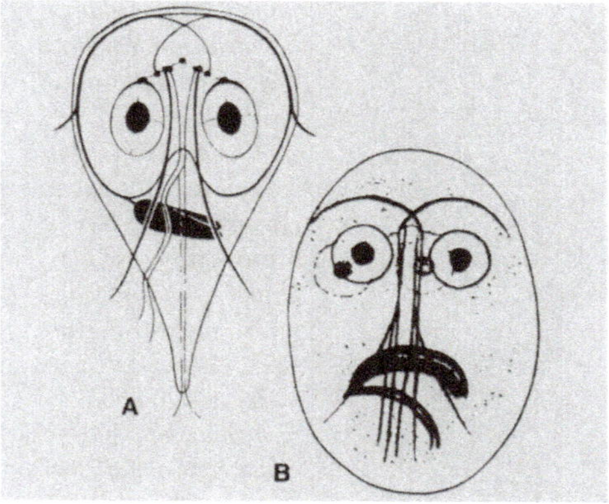

Fig. 296 (A) *Giardia* sp. trophozoite and (B) *Giardia bovis* cyst (16 × 10 μm) [14]

***Entamoeba* spp. (*E. ovis, E. dilimani* and *E. wenyoni*)**

Remarks: Several *Entamoeba* species are common in the intestine of sheep, goats and other ruminants. Little is known about their significance. They seem to be of low pathogenicity.

HELMINTHS

- Trematoda eggs found in the faeces and adult trematodes living in the gastrointestinal tract

Rumen flukes belong to the families of Paramphistomatidae and Gastrothylacidae each of which containing several species (☞ CATTLE, ■ 1). *Bothriophoron bothriophoron, Calicophoron microbothrium, Calicophoron daubneyi, Cotylophoron cotylophorum, Carmyerius spatiosus* and *Carmyerius papillatus* are the most frequent rumen flukes in small ruminants in Africa. Adult flukes do not cause clinical disease although they are commonly found in the rumen and sometimes in large numbers. The immature worms attach to the duodenal mucosa by means of their large posterior sucker and may cause severe enteritis, necrosis and haemorrhage. Affected animals exhibit anorexia, polydipsia, unthriftiness and severe diarrhoea. Extensive mortality may occur, especially in lambs. For diagnosis and control ☞ CATTLE, ■ 1.

Table 12 Recommended drugs against *Paramphistomum* spp. infections in sheep

Drug	Dosage (mg/kg) sheep	Immature flukes	Mature flukes
Niclosamide	90	+	
Rafoxanide	15	+	
Resorantel	65	+	+
Oxyclozanide	17	+	+

F. gigantica **Tropical large liver fluke**
(☞ CATTLE, ■ 1 and ■ 4.2)

F. hepatica **Large liver fluke of temperate areas and high altitude regions in East Africa**

Location: Adult flukes in biliary ducts; eggs in the faeces (☞ CATTLE, ■ 1 and ■ 4.2)

Dicrocoelium hospes **African small liver fluke and *Dicrocoelium dendriticum* Small liver fluke**

Location: Adult flukes in biliary ducts; eggs in the faeces (☞ CATTLE, ■ 1 and ■ 4.2)

Eurytrema pancreaticum **Pancreas fluke**

Location: Adult flukes in pancreatic ducts; eggs in the faeces (☞ CATTLE, ■ 1 and SHEEP AND GOATS, ■ 4.5)

***Schistosoma* spp. (*S. bovis, S. mattheei* and *S. curassoni*) Blood flukes**

Location: Adult flukes in mesenteric veins; eggs in the intestinal wall and faeces (☞ CATTLE, ■ 1 and SHEEP AND GOATS, ■ 2).

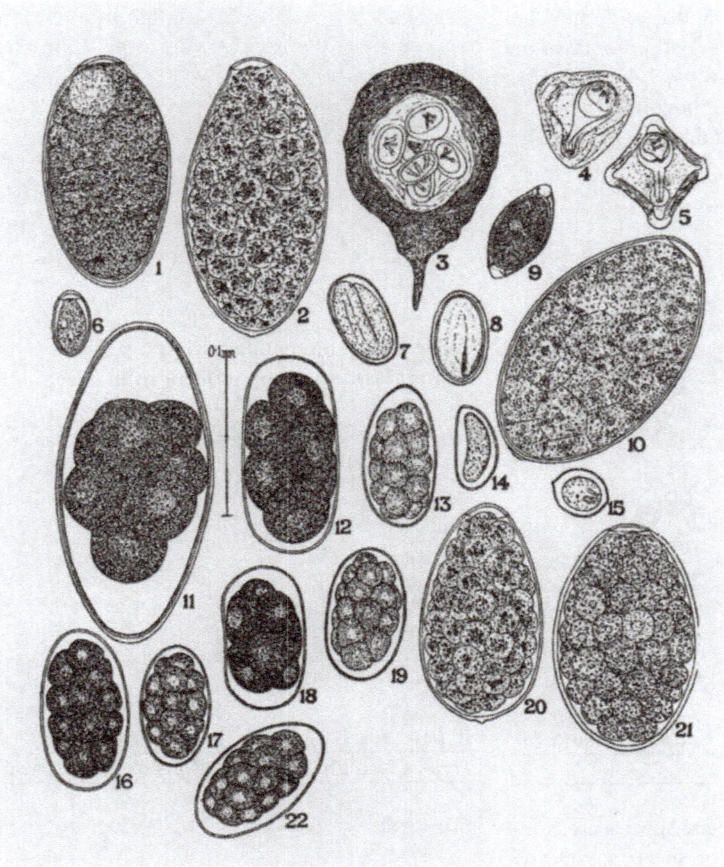

Fig. 297 Helminth eggs of sheep (schematic, not drawn to scale), (1) *Fasciola hepatica*, (2) *Paramphistomum cervi*, (3) *Thysaniezia ovilla*, (4) *Moniezia expansa*, (5) *M. benedeni*, (6) *Dicrocoelium dendriticum*, (7) *Strongyloides papillosus*, (8) *Gongylonema pulchrum*, (9) *Trichuris globulosa*, (10) *Fasciola gigantica*, (11) *Nematodirus spathiger*, (12) *Gaigeria pachyscelis*, (13) *Trichostrongylus* sp.*, (14) *Skrjabinema ovis*, (15) *Avitellina centripunctata*, (16) *Chabertia ovina**, (17) *Haemonchus contortus**, (18) *Bunostomum trigonocephalum**, (19) *Oesophagostomum columbianum**, (20) *Cotylophoron cotylophorum*, (21) *Fascioloides magna* and (22) *Ostertagia circumcincta**; * Strongyle-type eggs are difficult to differentiate in routine examinations [3]

- Cestoda eggs found in the faeces and adult cestodes living in the gastro-intestinal tract

Moniezia expansa and *Moniezia benedeni*

Common tapeworms

Remarks: *Moniezia* spp. infections in sheep are prevalent but are of relatively low pathogenicity. Heavy infections may result in unthriftiness and gastrointestinal disturbances. *Moniezia* spp. are easily seen at necropsy because of their size, but often the much smaller and much more pathogenic trichostrongylids (e.g. *Trichostrongylus colubriformis*) can not be seen with the naked eye. Therefore, many earlier observations which associated tapeworm infections with diarrhoea, emaciation and weight loss

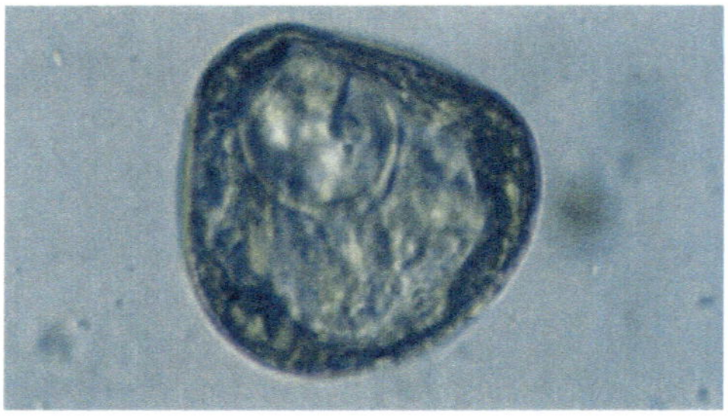

Fig. 298 Egg of *Moniezia* sp. (60–80 µm in diameter)

did not accurately consider the underlying infections with nematodes (☞ CATTLE, ■ 1). For diagnosis, therapy and prophylaxis ☞ CATTLE, ■ 1.
(Figures 298, 299, 300)

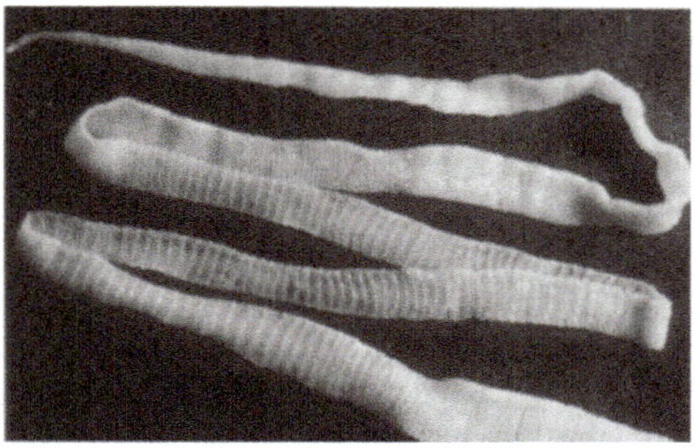

Fig. 299 *Moniezia* sp.; tapeworm with pronounced segments [32]

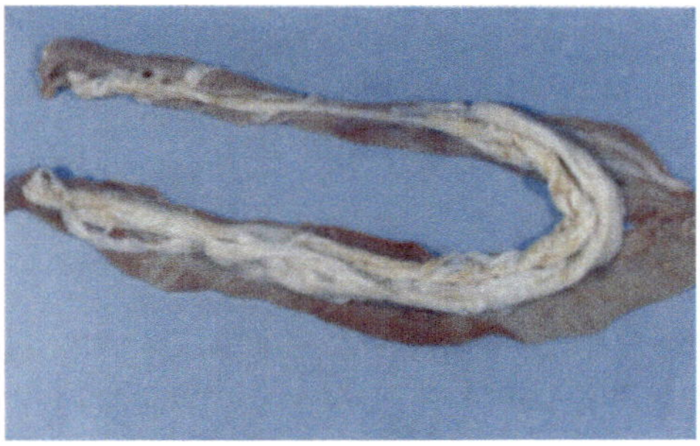

Fig. 300 *Moniezia* sp. found in the small intestine of a sheep [11]

Avitellina centripunctata

Remarks: This is a very common tapeworm of small ruminants and cattle in semi-arid and arid areas of Africa and Asia. Lambs acquire infections but many months elapse before the worms are adult. Adults are common in yearlings and older sheep. Lambs and kids may carry heavy burdens but often no obvious clinical signs may be found. However, clinical observations of pot-bellied suckling animals which improve after treatment are frequently reported. For diagnosis and control ☞ CATTLE, ■ 1.
(Figure 301)

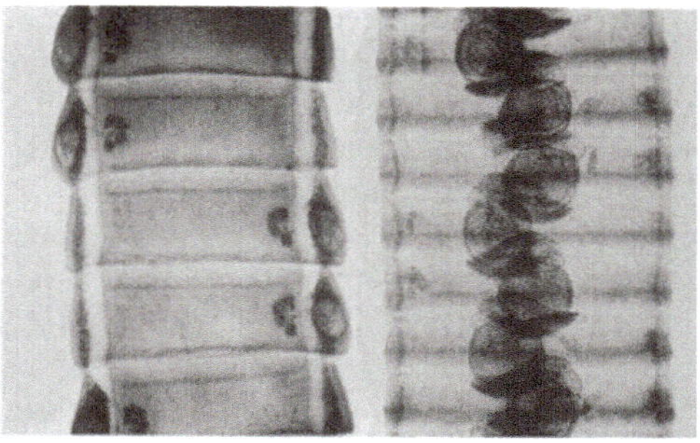

Fig. 301 Stained segments of *Thysaniezia ovilla* (left) and *Avitellina centripunctata* (right) [4]

Thysaniezia ovilla (syn. *T. giardi*)

Remarks: This species is frequently encountered in sheep and goats in many parts of Africa, especially in those with low rainfall. It occurs in the small intestine and is not very pathogenic but heavy infections occasionally produce clinical signs. For diagnosis and control ☞ CATTLE, ■ 1.

Stilesia globipunctata

Location: Small intestine, duodenum and upper jejunum (☞ CATTLE, ■ 1)
Hosts: Sheep, goat, dromedary, rarely cattle and other ruminants
Species description: Adults are 45–60 cm long and up to 2.5 mm wide. The scolex of the adult worm penetrates the mucosa of the duodenum and jejunum and causes a proliferative inflammation. The scolex is embedded in the mucosa while the posterior proglottids are free in the lumen. Heavy infections can cause death.
Geographic distribution: Arid areas of Africa

Stilesia hepatica

Remarks: This parasite occurs in the bile ducts (☞ CATTLE, ■ 1 and SHEEP AND GOATS, ■ 4.2) and occasionally small intestine of sheep and goats in tropical and southern Africa. It is non-pathogenic but extremely prevalent (in 90–100% of sheep) in many parts of Africa. The condemnation of a large proportion of sheep livers at meat inspection is the major loss due to this parasite. The ovoid eggs measure 16–19 × 26 µm. These eggs or the proglottids may appear in the faeces of infected animals.

- **Preventive measures to control intestinal tapeworms**

(*Moniezia* spp., *Avitellina* spp., *Thysaniezia* spp. and *Stilesia* spp.) of ruminants

Therapy: Niclosamid (45–75 mg/kg, po.) and praziquantel (3.75 mg/kg, po., sheep only) are specific cestocidal drugs. In addition the following benzimidazoles are effective against tapeworms: albendazole (3.8–5mg/kg, po.), fenbendazole (10 mg/kg, po.), oxfendazole (5 mg/kg, po.), mebendazole (10–20 mg/kg, po.), netobimin (20 mg/kg, po.), febantel (5–15 mg/kg, po.). Special attention should be given to the control of tapeworms in lambs to avoid losses in heavily infected populations (☞ CATTLE, ■ 1).

- Nematoda eggs found in the faeces, adult nematodes living in the gastrointestinal tract and first-stage larvae of lungworms

Gongylonema pulchrum Gullet worm or zigzag worm

Remarks: This parasite occurs in the mucosae of the oesophagus and forestomachs of sheep, goats, less frequently cattle (☞ CATTLE, ■ 1).

G. verrucosum Rumen gullet worm

Remarks: This is an apathogenic nematode, found in the mucosa of the forestomachs. This parasite may occasionally be found at necropsy (☞ CATTLE, ■ 1).

Parabronema skrjabini

Remarks: This spirurid worm occurs occasionally in the abomasum of small ruminants. The life cycle includes *Stomoxys* spp. and *Lyperosia* spp. as intermediate hosts (☞ CATTLE, ■ 1). For therapy and prophylaxis ☞ CATTLE, ■ 1; THERAPY OF NEMATODE INFECTIONS

Haemonchus contortus Large stomach worm, "twisted wire worm", "barber's pole worm"

Location: Abomasum

Hosts: Cattle, sheep, goat and other ruminants

Species description: *H. contortus* is one of the most prevalent and most pathogenic parasites of ruminants, particularly sheep (life cycle and morphology ☞ CATTLE, ■ 1). It can rapidly kill young sheep. When high numbers of infective larvae are ingested at once, deaths can occur suddenly while the sheep still appear to be in good health. This is termed "acute prepatent disease" when eggs are not yet found in the faeces but high numbers of preadult *Haemonchus* specimens have started to suck blood. In this case the host was killed before the parasites were mature. Haemonchosis is always associated with anaemia as both fourth-stage larvae and adult worms suck blood. Chronic infections which result from continuous ingestion of third-stage larvae may produce oedema ("bottle jaw"), iron-deficiency anaemia, progressive wool breaks and death. *H. contortus* usually occurs together with other gastrointestinal nematodes. Sometimes, sheep infected with *H. contortus* may exhibit self-cure which is a sudden loss of the worm load. This phenomenon is rarely seen in animals kept under poor nutritional and hygienic conditions. Ingested larvae may arrest their development at the end of the rainy season (or summer) and survive the dry season (or winter) as inhibited larvae within their host. This phenomenon is also termed hypobiosis. This is an adaptation of the parasite to adverse environmental conditions, when the preparasitic development from the egg to the third-stage larva is impossible.

Geographic distribution: World-wide, especially in warm areas

Symptoms: Anaemia, oedema ("bottle jaw"), rough coat, weakness, weight loss or retarded growth

Significance: *H. contortus* is a common parasite of sheep that may kill lambs rapidly. Chronic infections cause weakness, anaemia, making sheep raising uneconomical.

Diagnosis: Eggs of strongyle-type appear in faeces. However, in prepatent diseases, clinical signs (anaemia) and death occur before the worms are mature. Species identification only by identification of adult worms at necropsy.

Therapy and Prophylaxis: ☞ CATTLE, ■ 1; THERAPY OF NEMATODE INFECTIONS

(Figures 302, 303, 304, 305)

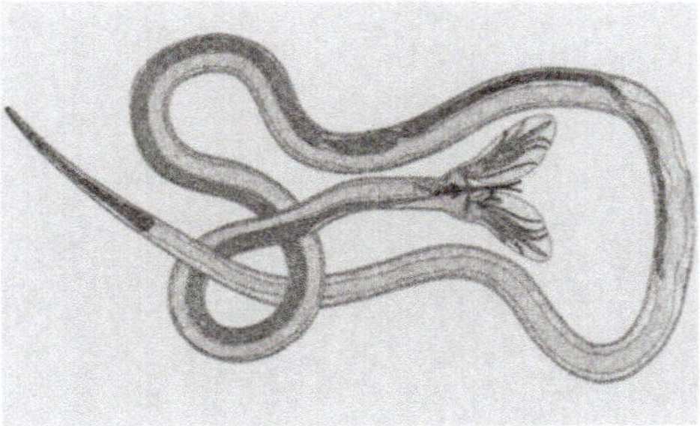

Fig. 302 *Haemonchus contortus*; male (10–20 mm × 400 μm) [9]

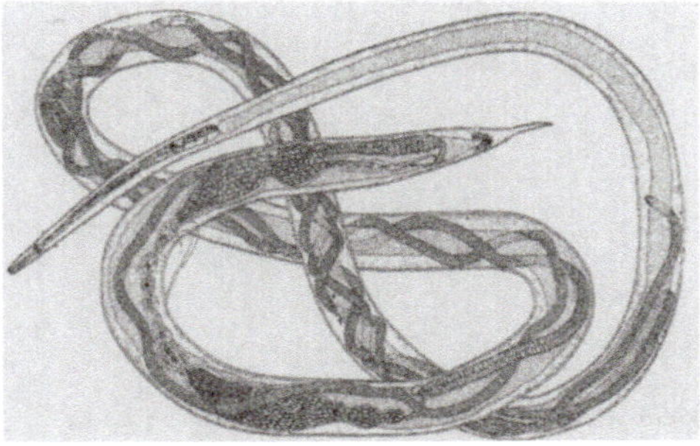

Fig. 303 *Haemonchus contortus*; female (18–30 mm × 500 μm) [9]

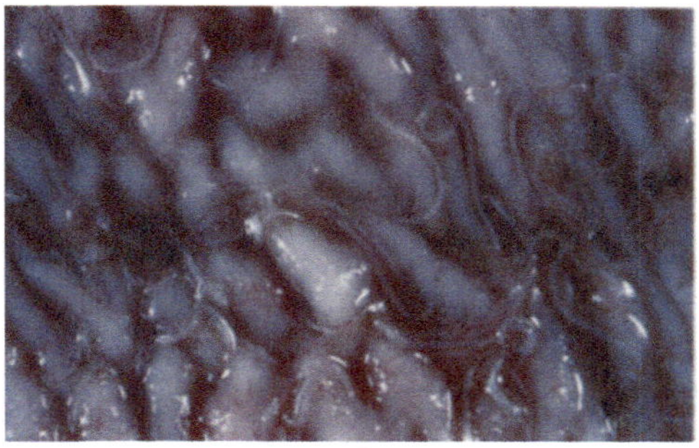

Fig. 304 *Haemonchus contortus*; adult worms on the abomasal mucosa

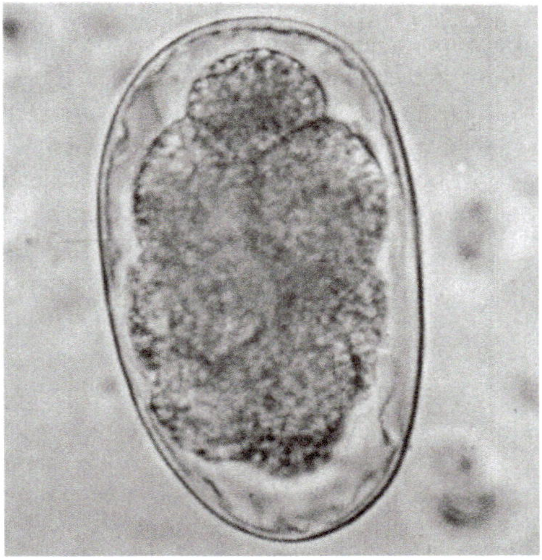

Fig. 305 Strongyle-type egg (74 × 44 μm) [11]

Mecistocirrus digitatus

Remarks: This is mainly a parasite of cattle and occurs occasionally in the abomasum of goats and very rarely of sheep (☞ CATTLE, ■ 1). For therapy and prophylaxis ☞ CATTLE, ■ 1; THERAPY OF NEMATODE INFECTIONS

Trichostrongylus axei Stomach hair worm

Remarks: This trichostrongylid species occurs world-wide in the abomasum of sheep and goats. It is often found in mixed infections with other gastrointestinal nematodes (e.g.

Ostertagia spp., or *Haemonchus contortus*). Adult worms penetrate the lining of the abomasum, causing irritation and inflammation. Wart-like swellings may occur and cause diarrhoea, weight loss and reduce appetite (☞ CATTLE, ■ 1). For therapy and prophylaxis ☞ CATTLE, ■ 1, p. 41; THERAPY OF NEMATODE INFECTIONS

***Trichostrongylus* spp. (*T. colubriformis, T. probolurus, T. vitrinus, T. capricola* and other *Trichostrongylus* species)** Small intestinal hair worm, bankrupt worm, black scours worm

Location: Small intestine
Hosts: Sheep and goat
Species description: These nematodes are small (up to 5.5 mm long), reddish-brown and without a specially developed head-end. There is no buccal capsule. A typical structure for all *Trichostrongylus* spp. is the excretory pore, situated near the anterior extremity. Males have bursae with large lateral lobes and the morphology of the spicules and the gubernacula is species-specific. Typical direct nematode life cycle. Infection occurs by ingestion of third-stage larvae. The prepatent period is 20–25 days.
Geographic distribution: World-wide
Symptoms: Weakness, progressive weight loss, depressed appetite, digestive troubles such as diarrhoea or constipation
Significance: *Trichostrongylus* species commonly occur with other gastrointestinal nematodes. Therefore losses due to *Trichostrongylus* spp. are not easy to measure. and their effects are additive. If coccidiosis accompanies trichostrongylosis, enteritis may occur.
Diagnosis: Strongyle-type eggs appear in the faeces. Adult worms may be found at necropsy.
Therapy and Prophylaxis: ☞ CATTLE, ■ 1; THERAPY OF NEMATODE INFECTIONS
(Figure 306, 307)

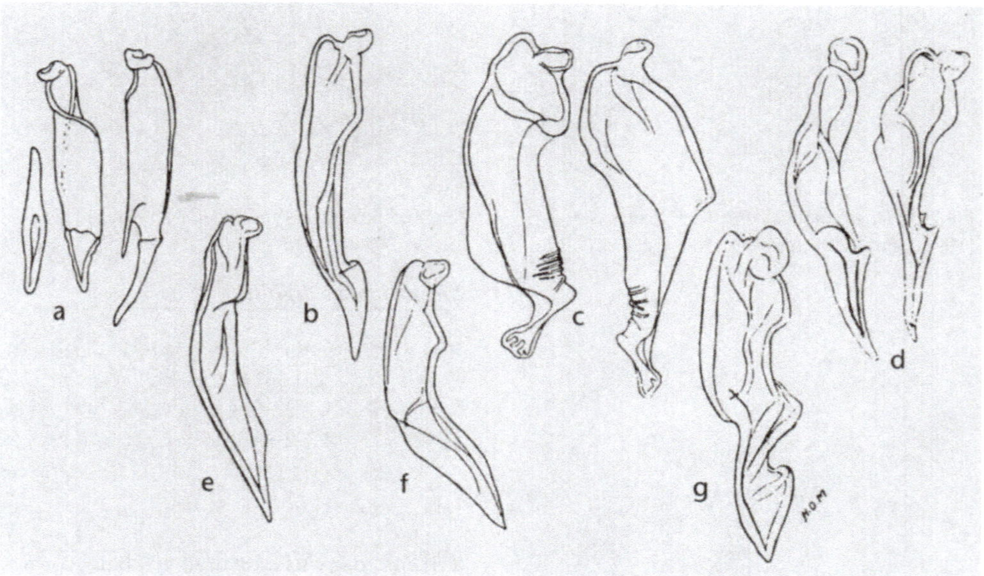

Fig. 306 Morphology and length of spicules of some *Trichostrongylus* species: (a) *T. axei* (85–95 and 110–150 µm), (b) *T. colubriformis* (135–156 µm), (c) *T. rugatus* (137–145 and 141–152 µm), (d) *T. falculatus* (100 µm), (e) *T. vitrinus* (160–170 µm), (f) *T. capricola* (130–145 µm) and (g) *T. probolurus* (126–134 µm) [3]

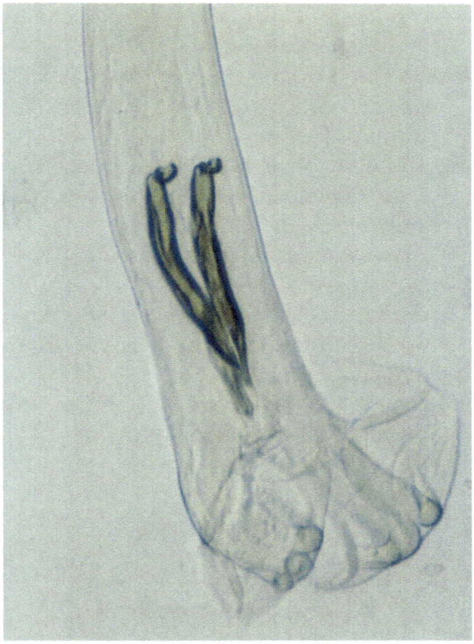

Fig. 307 *Trichostrongylus vitrinus*; bursa copulatrix and spicules (160–170 µm)

Ostertagia (syn. *Teladorsagia*) *circumcincta*, *Ostertagia* (syn. *Teladorsagia*) *trifurcata*, *Ostertagia pinnata* and other *Ostertagia* spp. Brown stomach worms

Location: Abomasum and rarely in the small intestine

Hosts: Sheep and goat

Species description: These species are brownish, thread-like nematodes up to 12 mm in length. Males are smaller with straight, slender spicules. All members of the genus *Ostertagia* have a small cephalic vesicle, cervical papillae and longitudinal cuticular ridges. The morphology of the bursa copulatrix and the spicules varies among the particular species. Typical direct nematode life cycle; infection is acquired by ingestion of infective third-stage larvae which may develop to adults within 17 days; arrested development (hypobiosis) occurs.

Geographic distribution: Widespread in moist, temperate regions; autochthonous infections are focal in Africa but *Ostertagia* spp. infections have repeatedly been reported from imported sheep and goats.

Symptoms: Profuse watery diarrhoea, progressive weight loss associated with hypoproteinaemia; death may occur.

Significance: These nematodes cause serious losses world-wide by producing weight loss and decreased wool production.

Diagnosis: Strongyle-type eggs appear in the faeces.

Therapy and Prophylaxis: ☞ CATTLE, ■ 1, p. 42; THERAPY OF NEMATODE INFECTIONS

Pseudomarshallagia elongata

Remarks: This species was found in the abomasa of sheep and goats in Ethiopia. It is similar to *Ostertagia* spp. For therapy and prophylaxis ☞ CATTLE, ■ 1 THERAPY OF NEMATODE INFECTIONS

Cooperia curticei, *Cooperia pectinata*, *Cooperia punctata* and other *Cooperia* spp.

Location: Small intestine

Hosts: Sheep and goat

Species description: GENERAL FEATURES OF COOPERIA spp. ☞ CATTLE, ■ 1; *Cooperia* spp. have a direct life cycle; prepatent period is 15–20 days.

Geographic distribution: World-wide

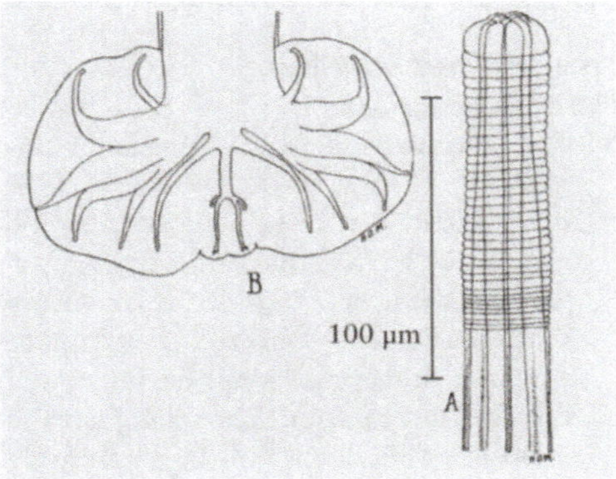

Fig. 308 *Cooperia* sp.; anterior end with enlarged cephalic vesicle (A) and bursa copulatrix (B) [3]

Symptoms: Diarrhoea, weight loss and decreased wool growth

Significance: The effects of *Cooperia* spp. are additive to those of other gastrointestinal nematodes. Diarrhoea in lambs caused by heavy *Cooperia* infections may be fatal due to dehydration.

Diagnosis: Strongyle-type eggs appear in the faeces. Adult worms may be found at necropsy.

Therapy and Prophylaxis: ☞ CATTLE, ■ 1; THERAPY OF NEMATODE INFECTIONS

(Figure 308)

Paracooperia daubneyi

Location: Small intestine

Hosts: Sheep only

Species description: This genus resembles *Cooperia* spp. but differs in that the spicules are divided distally into three processes: one is serrate, one is winged and large and the third is slender and difficult to see. The gubernaculum is absent.

Geographic distribution: East Africa, Central Africa

Symptoms, Significance and Diagnosis: ☞ above *Cooperia* spp.

Therapy and Prophylaxis: ☞ CATTLE, ■ 1; THERAPY OF NEMATODE INFECTIONS

Nematodirus spathiger, Nematodirus filicollis, Nematodirus battus and other *Nematodirus* spp. Thread-necked strongyles

Location: Small intestines

Hosts: Sheep and goat

Species description: General features of this genus ☞ CATTLE, ■ 1. The life cycle is direct and typical for nematodes. Infection is acquired by ingestion of third-stage larvae, free-living or in eggs. Larval stages are the primary cause of disease. They damage the lining of the small intestine. Erosion of the intestinal mucosa occurs and pieces of it may become loose and be shed in the faeces.

Geographic distribution: *N. spathiger* and *N. filicollis* occur world-wide including East and Central Africa; *N. helvetianus* occurs in Europa, USA and in (Africa).

Symptoms: Loss of appetite, diarrhoea and weight loss. Wool growth is reduced in chronic infections.

Significance: *Nematodirus* infections may cause significant mortality in lambs, when present in high numbers.

Diagnosis: Characteristic large strongyle-type eggs appear in the faeces.

Cave: the eggs of the small ruminant hookworm *Gaigeria pachyscelis* are similar to those of *Nematodirus* spp.!

Therapy and Prophylaxis: ☞ CATTLE, ■ 1; THERAPY OF NEMATODE INFECTIONS

(Figures 309, 310, 311)

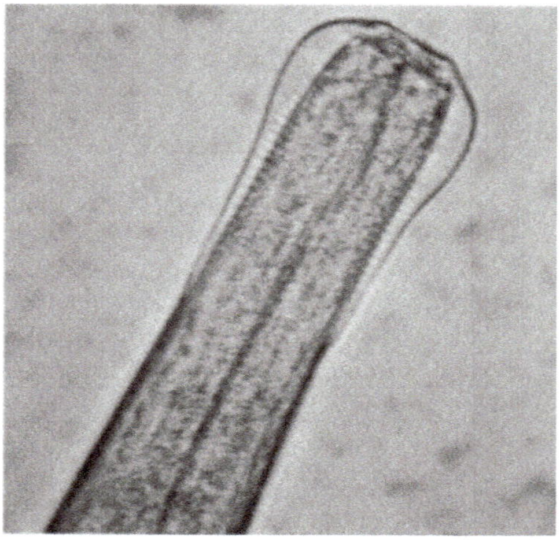

Fig. 309 *Nematodirus* sp.; anterior end with cephalic vesicle [32]

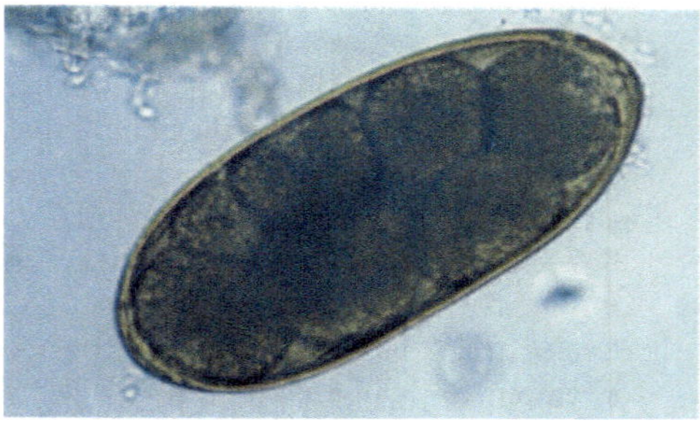

Fig. 310 Egg of *Nematodirus battus* (152–182 × 67–77 µm)

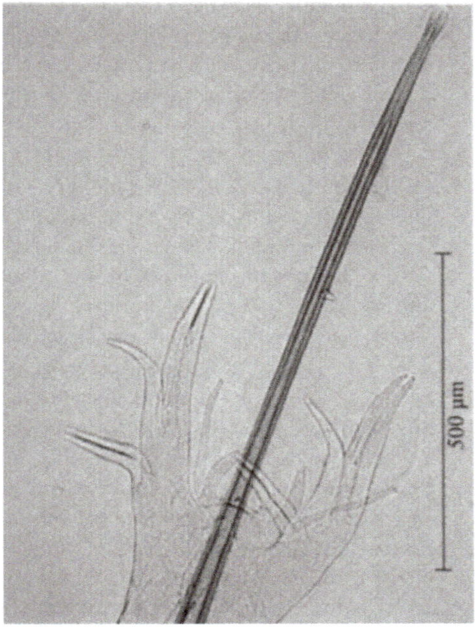

Fig. 311 *Nematodirus* sp.; bursa copulatrix with long spicula [32]

Impalaia tuberculata

Location: Abomasum and small intestine
Hosts: Dromedary, rarely sheep and cattle
Species description: These parasites belong to the Nematodirinae.
Geographic distribution: Central, eastern and southern Africa
Symptoms, Significance and Diagnosis: ☞ *Nematodirus* spp.
Therapy and Prophylaxis: ☞ CATTLE, ■ 1; THERAPY OF NEMATODE INFECTIONS; ☞ DROMEDARIES, ■ 1.

Impalaia nudicollis

Location: Small intestine
Hosts: Sheep
Species description: The male is 5–9 mm long. The female is 11–13 mm long.
Geographic distribution: East Africa
Symptoms, Significance and Diagnosis: ☞ above, *Nematodirus* spp.
Therapy and Prophylaxis: ☞ CATTLE, ■ 1; THERAPY OF NEMATODE INFECTIONS (Figure 312)

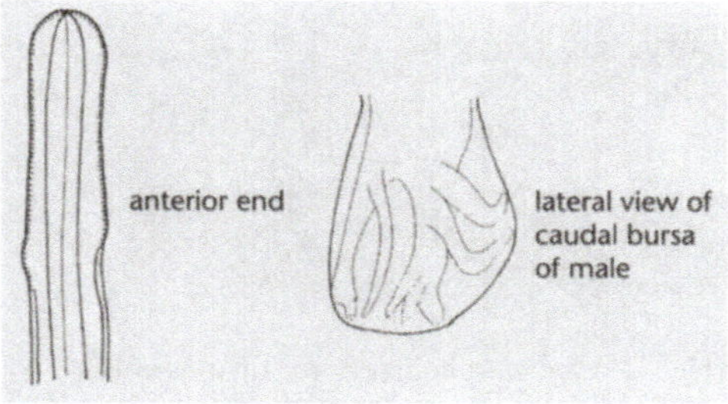

Fig. 312 *Impalaia nudicollis* (schematic) [16]

First-stage larvae of the following lungworms may be found in the faeces of sheep and goats:

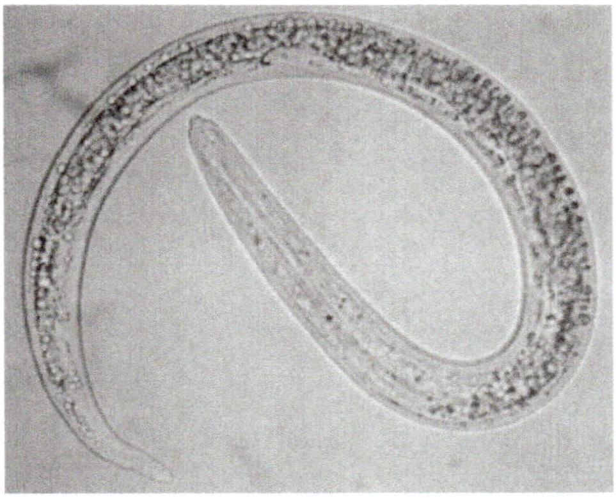

Fig. 313 *Dictyocaulus filaria*; first-stage larva (550–580 µm) [11]

DICTYOCAULIDAE Large lungworm

Dictyocaulus filaria Common lungworm

(☞ SHEEP AND GOATS, ■ 4.3; Fig. 313)

PROTOSTRONGYLIDAE Small lungworms

Protostrongylus rufescens Red lungworm

(☞ SHEEP AND GOATS, ■ 4.3)

Muellerius capillaris Hair lungworm

(☞ SHEEP AND GOATS, ■ 4.3)

Neostrongylus linearis

(☞ SHEEP AND GOATS, ■ 4.3)

Cystocaulus ocreatus

(☞ SHEEP AND GOATS, ■ 4.3)
(Figures 314, 315, 316)

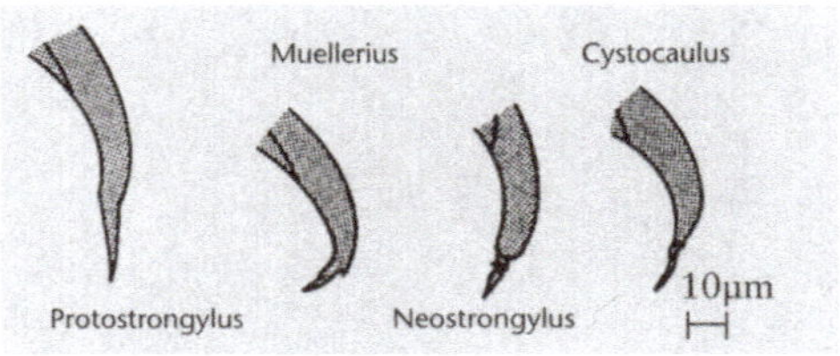

Fig. 314 The morphology of the tip (posterior end) of the lungworm larvae is relevant for the diagnosis [33]

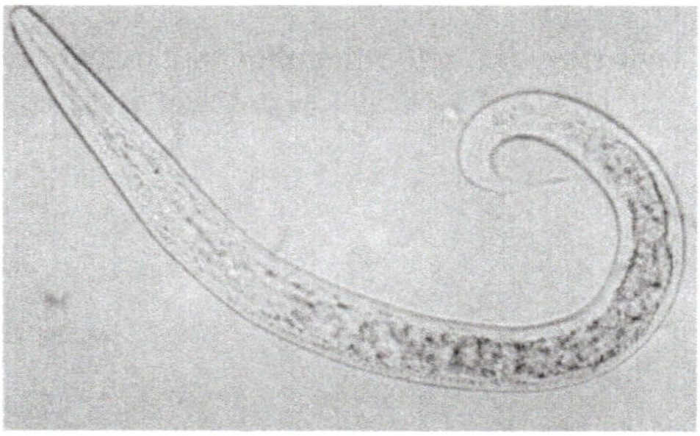

Fig. 315 *Protostrongylus rufescens*; first-stage larva (320–400 µm) [11]

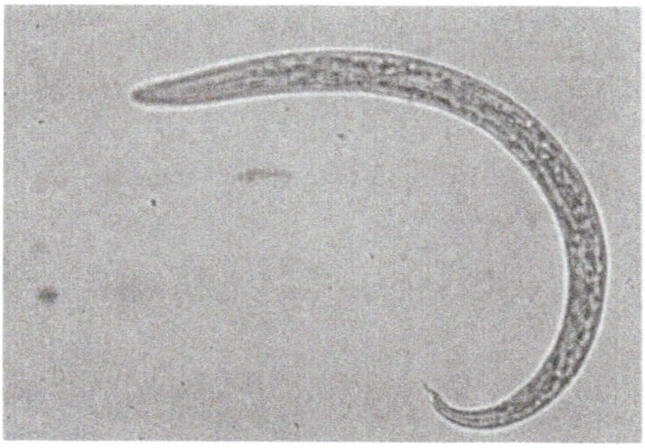

Fig. 316 *Muellerius capillaris*; first-stage larva (300–320 µm) [15]

Oesophagostomum columbianum

Nodular worm

Location: Colon

Hosts: Sheep, goat, camel and antelope

Species description: The male is 12–16.5 mm long and the female 15–21.5 mm and about 0.45 mm wide. The large cervical alae produce a marked dorsal curvature of the anterior part of the body. The cuticle forms a mouth collar which is separated from the rest of the body by a constriction. The anterior extremities of the cervical alae are pierced by marked cervical papillae. The male bursa contains two equal spicules, 0.77–0.86 mm long. The tail of the female is 500–600 µm long and ends in a fine point and the vulva is situated about 0.8 mm anterior to the anus. The eggs measure 73–89 × 34–45 µm. The life cycle is direct. After ingestion of the third-stage larvae they burrow into the wall of the gut anywhere between the small intestine and the rectum. Here they molt to the fourth-stage before leaving the gut wall and migrating to the large intestine, where they undergo their final molt and develop to the adult stage. Sometimes a number of larvae may remain in the mucosa for extended times. The prepatent period is about 41 days. *O. columbianum* larvae cause extensive nodule formation in the gut wall which impairs the ability of the intestine to absorb fluid and nutrients. Diarrhoea and weight loss may occur. Diarrhoea usually starts on the 6th day after a severe infection and coincides with the larvae leaving the nodules.

Geographic distribution: World-wide, particularly common in tropical and subtropical areas

Symptoms: In lambs the first sign is a persistent diarrhoea, which results in exhaustion and death unless the animals are treated. The faeces contain much mucus and sometimes blood. In chronic infections the animals show progressive emaciation, general weakness, and the skin becomes dry and the wool is unthrifty. The chronic oesophagostomosis in sheep is characterized by extreme emaciation, cachexia ending in complete prostration and death.

Significance: *O. columbianum* is a serious pathogen of sheep. 200–300 adult worms constitute a severe infection for lambs. Extensive nodule formation in the small and large intestine seriously affects the

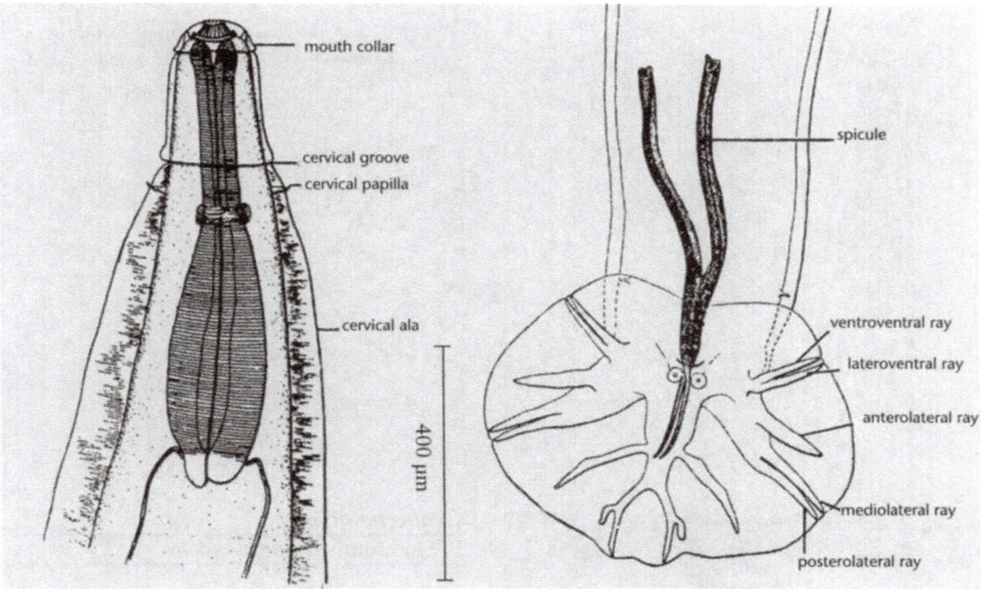

Fig. 317 *Oesophagostomum columbianum*; anterior end (left) and bursa copulatrix (right) [5]

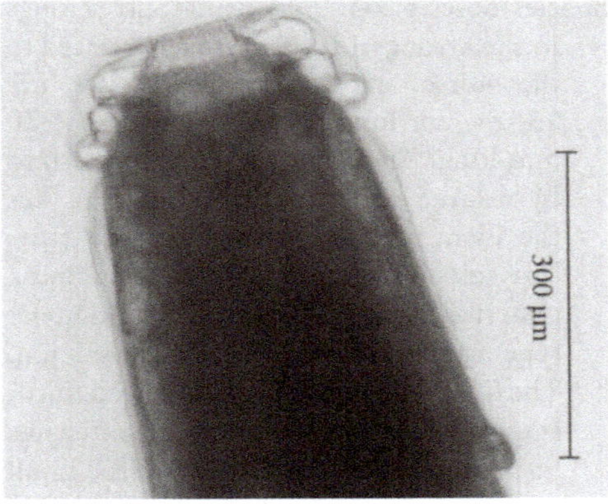

Fig. 318 *Oesophagostomum columbianum*; anterior end [8]

absorption, bowel movement and digestion. The nodules may rupture to the peritoneal surface causing peritonitis and peritoneal adhesions.

Diagnosis: Examination of diarrhoeic faeces may show fourth-stage larvae in acute cases or strongyle-type eggs in more chronic infections. Chronic infections without adult parasites are difficult to recognize and autopsy of a selected animal may be indicated.

Therapy and Prophylaxis: ☞ CATTLE, ■ 1; THERAPY OF NEMATODE INFECTIONS (Figures 317, 318)

Oesophagostomum venulosum

Nodular worm

Remarks: This occurs in the colon of sheep, goat, deer and camel. The male is 11–16 mm and the female 13–24 mm long. There are no lateral cervical alae and the cervical papillae are behind the oesophagus. The spicules of the male are 1.1–1.5 mm long. The life cycle is similar to that of *O. columbianum* but the pathogenic effect is different. *O. venulosum* is relatively nonpathogenic and seldom causes nodules. Even in heavy infections the parasite does not cause significant clinical signs. Fog diagnosis, therapy and prophylaxis: ☞ CATTLE, ■ 1; THERAPY OF NEMATODE INFECTIONS (Figures 319, 320)

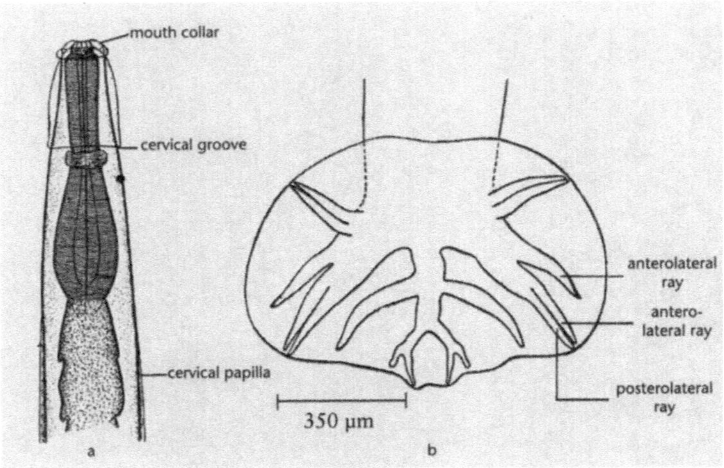

Fig. 319 *Oesophagostomum venulosum*; anterior end (a) and bursa copulatrix (b) [5]

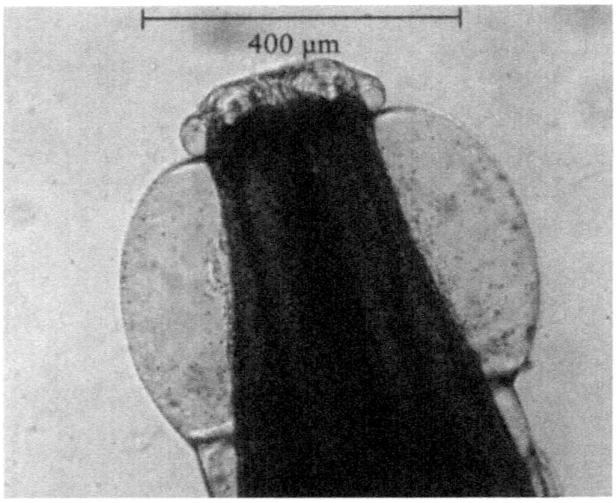

Fig. 320 *Oesophagostomum venulosum*; anterior end

Oesophagostomum multifoliatum

Remarks: This is a large-intestinal parasite of sheep and goats in eastern Africa. It has been reported from Nigeria, Kenya, Tanzania and Zimbabwe. The males are 12–14 mm and the females 14–17 mm long. This species differs from *O. columbianum* in that the cervical papillae are located just anterior to the end of the oesophagus and that the tail of the female is only 250–300 µm long. The eggs are large (150–170 × 68–80 µm) and similar to those of *Nematodirus* spp. No information is available on the life cycle and pathogenic effect of this species.

Chabertia ovina

Large-mouthed bowel worm

Location: Colon

Hosts: Sheep and goat

Species description: This nematode belongs to the Strongylidae and closely related to the horse strongyles. The males are 13–14 mm long and females are 17–20 mm long. The head end is characterized by a large buccal capsule which makes the identification of this parasite easy. The spicules are 1.3–1.7 mm long and a gubernaculum is present. The strongyle-type eggs measure 90–105 × 50–55 µm. The life cycle is direct. The ingested third-stage larvae undergo an extensive histiotropic phase in the wall of the small intestine prior to the third moult. 26 days after infection the larvae 4 may reach the colon. Fourth-stage larvae develop mainly in the lumen of the caecum and after the 4th moult immature adults then pass to the colon where patency occurs about 50 days after infection. The adult worms attach to the mucosa of the colon by means of their buccal capsule and then draw in a plug of mucosa. The worms suck blood only accidentally when a blood vessel is ruptured. The mucosa is inflamed, congested and swollen and covered with mucus in severe cases.

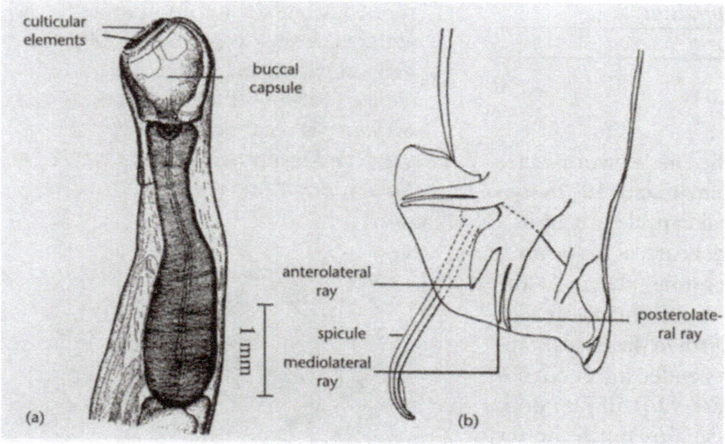

Fig. 321 *Chabertia ovina*; anterior end (a) and bursa copulatrix (b) [5]

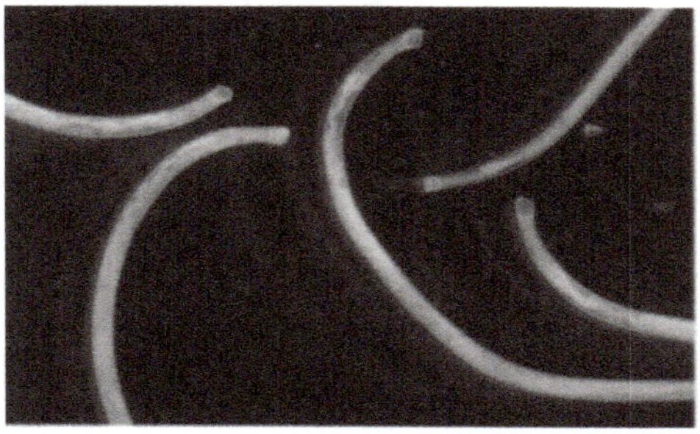

Fig. 322 *Chabertia ovina*; adults (13–20 mm long)

Geographic distribution: World-wide

Symptoms: Marked diarrhoea with blood and mucus may be seen in severely affected animals. Sheep lose condition, become anaemic and die following heavy infections.

Significance: *Chabertia* is significant only in heavily infected animals. Weight loss and reduced wool growth are the major results.

Diagnosis: Strongyle-type eggs appear in the faeces. Diagnosis can be confirmed either by identification of third-stage larvae following faecal culture or by demonstrating the adult worms in the colon at necropsy.

Therapy: Most of the benzimidazoles commonly used to treat gastrointestinal nematodes of ruminants are effective against *Chabertia ovina* (☞ CATTLE, ■ 1 THERAPY OF NEMATODE INFECTIONS)

Prophylaxis: ☞ CATTLE, ■ 1; THERAPY OF NEMATODE INFECTIONS

(Figures 321, 322, 323, 324)

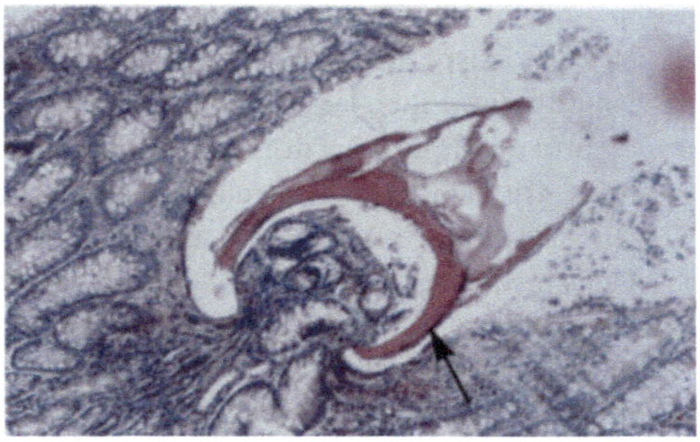

Fig. 323 *Chabertia ovina*; buccal capsule attached to the intestinal mucosa

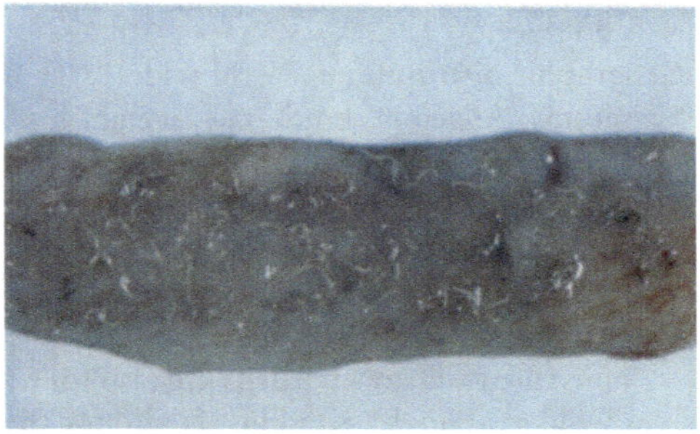

Fig. 324 *Chabertia ovina* attached to the colon of a lamb

Bunostomum trigonocephalum
Small ruminant hookworm

Location: Small intestine

Hosts: Sheep and goat

Species description: The male worms are 12–17 mm and the females are 19–26 mm long. The large buccal capsule is bent in a dorsal direction and bears at its ventral margin a pair of chitinous plates. At the base there is a pair of subventral lancets. There are no dorsal teeth in the buccal capsule. The spicules are slender and about 0.6 mm long. The eggs are 92 × 50 µm. Both the spicules and the eggs are much shorter than those of *Gaigeria pachyscelis*; direct life cycle; infection percutaneously or per os. Larvae migrate through the lungs and via the trachea to the oesophagus where they are swallowed to develop further in the small intestine. Prepatent period is 30–60 days. This parasite occurs in warm moist areas with a rainfall of more than 500 mm per year. Percutaneous infection is common. 4000 infective larvae can kill sheep without any previous clinical signs. At necropsy multiple haemorrhage may be found in the lungs. Adult worms cause anaemia and hypoalbuminaemia with oedema ("bottle-jaw"). 200–300 adult worms are fatal. In the small intestinal mucosa ulcers and erosions may be found which bleed after the worms have moved to another site of attachment. Usually the infection occurs together with other gastrointestinal nematodes, so the effect is additive.

Geographic distribution: World-wide

Symptoms: Anaemia, bottle jaw, weight loss. Chronic infections with only a few worms cause unthriftiness and thus great indirect losses within infected herds.

Significance: This is a prevalent and very pathogenic parasite of sheep in humid and moist areas. Heavy burdens are also found in older animals. Kraaling facilitates the spread of this parasite.

Diagnosis: This may be suspected from the clinical signs and the presence of strongyle-type eggs but the infection must be differentiated from other nematode infections that cause anaemia. However, only the demonstration of the adult parasites at necropsy is conclusive.

Therapy and Prophylaxis: ☞ CATTLE, 1; THERAPY OF NEMATODE INFECTIONS

(Figure 325)

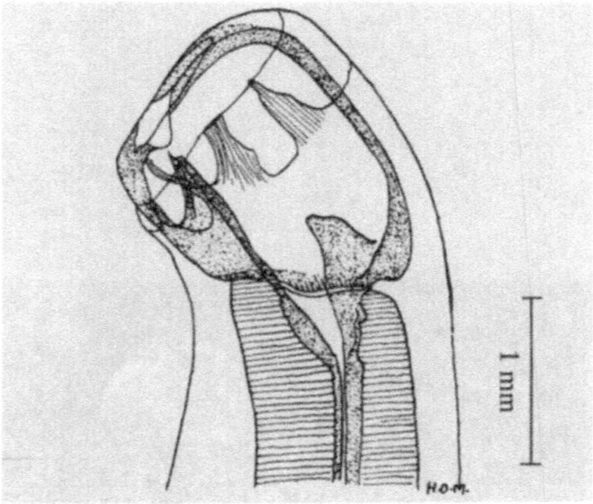

Fig. 325 *Bunostomum trigonocephalum*; anterior end with buccal capsule containing a pair of subventral lancets [3]

Gaigeria pachyscelis Hookworm

Location: Small intestine

Hosts: Sheep and goat

Species description: This parasite resembles in general *Bunostomum trigonocephalum*. Males are up to 20 mm long and females up to 30 mm. The buccal capsule contains a large dorsal cone, but no dorsal tooth and a pair of subventral lancets which have several cusps each. The male bursa has small lateral lobes joined together ventrally and a voluminous dorsal lobe. The spicules are slender with recurved unbarbed ends. They are 1.25–1.33 mm long. The eggs measure 105–129 × 50–55 µm (much larger than the eggs of *B. trigonocephalum*). The life cycle is direct and similar to those of other hookworms. Infection occurs through the skin but also by ingestion of infective larvae. Migration of the larvae via blood through the lungs, trachea, oesophagus and finally intestines where they mature about 10 weeks after infection. This is a very potent anaemia-causing pathogen. About 100 adult worms were found to be sufficient to cause death. The worms are usually found to be attached to the mucosa of the first part of the small intestine, frequently in groups of two to three. The worms are often surrounded by fresh blood. After primary infections there is a good immunity which prevents from reinfections.

Geographic distribution: India, Indonesia, Africa

Symptoms: Anaemia and sudden death may occur in heavy infections. In more chronic infections the usual signs of hookworm infection are seen.

Significance: The worms are potent bloodsuckers and may be of great significance in endemic areas. The skin-penetrating larvae were suspected to introduce the organisms of footrot into the feet of sheep.

Diagnosis: This is made by demonstrating the characteristic large eggs in the faeces. These eggs are at first sight similar to *Nematodirus* spp. eggs. Demonstration of adult worms in the small intestine.

Therapy and Prophylaxis: ☞ CATTLE, ■ 1; THERAPY OF NEMATODE INFECTIONS

(Figure 326, 327)

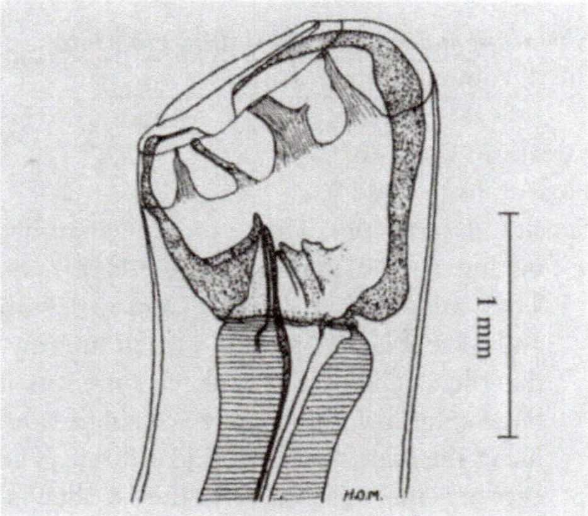

Fig. 326 *Gaigeria pachyscelis*; anterior end with buccal capsule [3]

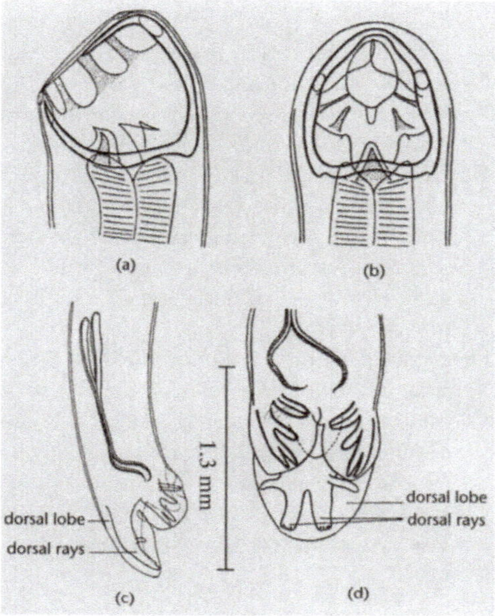

Fig. 327 *Gaigeria pachyscelis*; anterior end lateral (a), dorsal (b), tail end of a male lateral (c) and ventral view (d). The tail end shows prominent dorsal lobes compared with *B. trigonocephalum* [5]

Trichuris ovis and *Trichuris globulosa*

Whipworm

Location: Caecum

Hosts: Sheep, goat, camel, cattle and other ruminants

Species description: Nematodes with a long, slender neck and a much thicker hind end, giving them the appearance of a whip. Males are 50–80 mm long and have a curled tail. Females are 35–70 mm long. Direct nematode life cycle. Infective larvae develop within the eggs and infection is acquired by ingestion of eggs containing infective larvae (second-stage larvae). These infective eggs are very resistant to adverse conditions and may remain viable for years. Prepatent period is 1–3 months and varies markedly among the various species. Larval penetration into the intestinal wall may cause irritation, haemorrhage and may be instrumental for secondary bacterial infections. Heavy infections produce thickening of the caecal wall and normal fluid absorption is impaired.

Geographic distribution: World-wide

Symptoms: Colitis, secondary infections and diarrhoea may occur in heavy infections.

Significance: Importance in sheep is unknown. High numbers of larvae cause haemorrhages and localised oedema when they penetrate the gut. The pathogenic effect of adult worms is low and generally additive to other worms.

Diagnosis: Demonstration of the characteristic, brown, barrel-shaped eggs with a transparent plug at either pole. Disease produced by immature stages may only be recognised at necropsy.

Therapy and Prophylaxis: ☞ CATTLE, ■ 1; THERAPY OF NEMATODE INFECTIONS

(Figures 328, 329, 330)

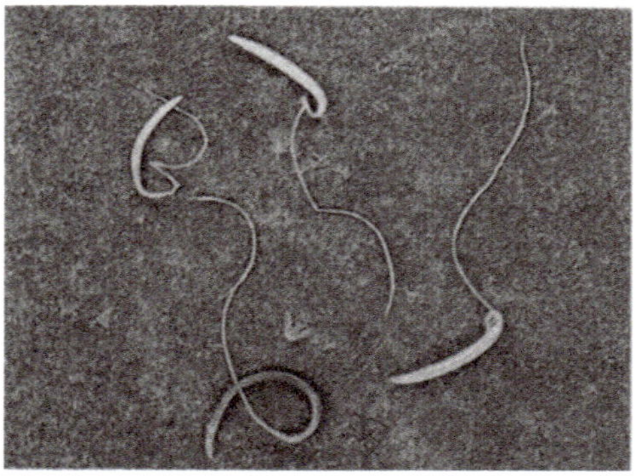

Fig. 328 *Trichuris* sp. (female: 35–70 mm and male: 50–80 mm) [32]

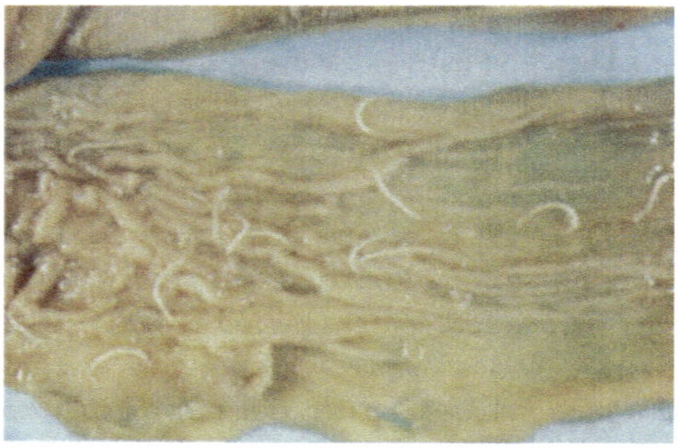

Fig. 329 *Trichuris* sp. attached to the large intestinal mucosa of a sheep [4]

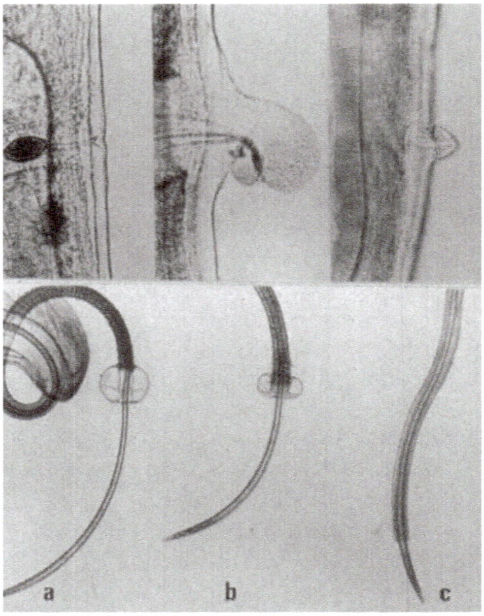

Fig. 330 *Trichuris* sp. of small ruminants; vulva (above) and spiculum (below) of *T. globulosa* (a), *T. ovis* (b) and *T. skrjabini* (c) [4]

Capillaria bovis

Remarks: This parasite occurs world-wide in the gastrointestinal tract of cattle, sheep and goats. The pathogenic role has not yet been defined conclusively, but it seems to be non-pathogenic (☞ CATTLE, ■ 1).

Skrjabinema ovis and *Skrjabinema alata*

Small ruminant pinworms

Location: Caecum

Hosts: Sheep and goat

Species description: These small nematodes belong to the family of the *Oxyuridae*. They are small, about 3–8 mm in length and have 3 large lips and 3 small intermediate lips. The oesophagus terminates in a large spherical bulb. There is a single spicule in the male. The life cycle is direct. The eggs are embryonated when they are deposited by the female in the perianal region. Eggs drop off and are ingested. Larvae hatch in the small intestine and migrate to the large intestine where they mature in about 25 days after infection.

Geographic distribution: World-wide; in Africa: Kenya, Nigeria, Tchad, Réunion

Symptoms: Unknown

Significance: *Skrjabinema* spp. are non-pathogenic. They may be mistaken for other dangerous nematodes such as *Oesophagostomum columbianum*.

Diagnosis: Eggs containing larvae may be found on the skin surrounding the anus. Adult worms may be seen in the colon at necropsy. The typical oesophagus of *S. ovis* distinguishes it from fourth-stage larvae of *O. columbianum*.

Therapy and Prophylaxis: ☞ CATTLE, ■ 1; THERAPY OF NEMATODE INFECTIONS
(Figures 331, 332)

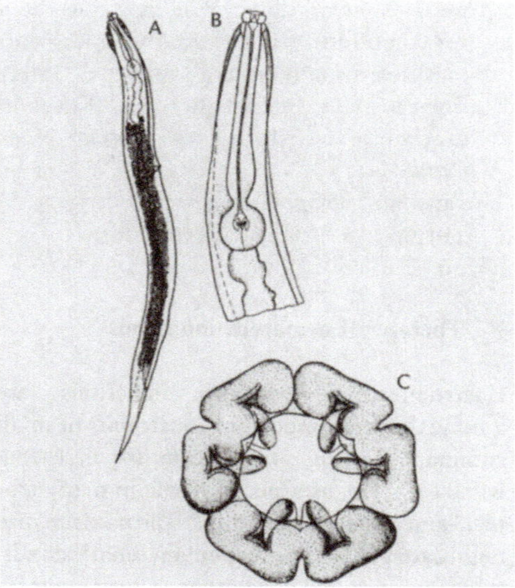

Fig. 332 *Skrjabinema ovis*; adult female (A), anterior end (B) and anterior view (C) [34]

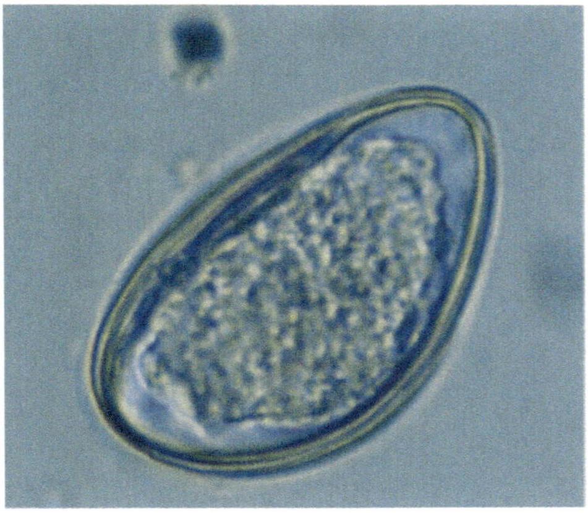

Fig. 331 Egg of *Skrjabinema ovis* (54–57 × 32–34 µm)

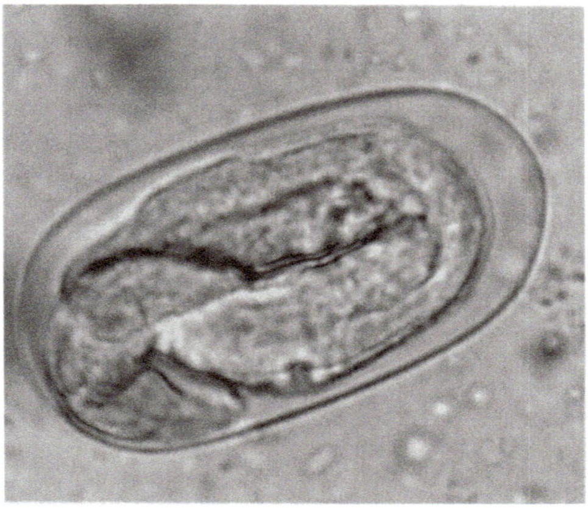

Fig. 333 Egg of *Strongyloides papillosus* (47–65 × 25–26 µm)

Strongyloides papillosus

Intestinal threadworm

Remarks: General description ☞ CATTLE, ■ 1. Transmammary infection occurs. Larvae are present in the ewe's milk from the 8th to the 19th day after lambing. Eggs of *S. papillosus* may occur in the lamb's faeces as early as 21 days after birth. An infection dose of 11,000 larvae were found to be lethal to lambs and kids. Enteritis with diarrhoea or constipation followed by secondary bacterial infections were found in heavily infected sheep and goats. Anaemia due to the reduced absorption of proteins which are essential for haematopoiesis and low calcium, magnesium and phosphate levels were also observed in heavy infections. General depression and paralysis was found just prior to death. Young animals are usually severely affected. Infections in older animals are rare. Kraaling facilitates the spread of *Strongyloides papillosus*.

Therapy and Prophylaxis: ☞ CATTLE, 1; THERAPY OF NEMATODE INFECTIONS

(Figure 333)

- **Therapy of nematode infections**

Gastrointestinal helminth infections are among the most important constraints of small ruminant rearing world-wide (☞ FURTHER READING). This is especially true in many tropical and subtropical regions. The parasites are highly adapted to the particular climatic conditions (e.g. arrested development during winter or dry season) and this should be considered for the control. As a rule sheep and goats have their own parasites, a feeding pattern which is different from cattle and therefore a different epidemiology as far as gastrointestinal helminths are concerned. The following basic health prevention should be carried out in both traditional and intensified sheep rearing: Vaccinations against the endemic viral and bacterial diseases (mainly: Peste des Petits Ruminants (PPR), Pasteurellosis, Anthrax, Blackleg (*Clostridium chauvoei*)). All the animals of a flock should further be treated with an anthelmintic during the rainy season either regularly every month when stocking rates are high or 3 weeks after the onset of the rains and once around 3–4 weeks before the end of the rains. At the end of the rainy season a high proportion of ingested nematode larvae tend to remain arrested in their development. These arrested larvae may be responsible for "dry season outbreaks" and early outbreaks in the following rainy season. For the last treatment of the rainy season an anthelmintic should be used which is also effective against the inhibited larvae. Most modern bendzimidazoles (fenbendazole, albendazole, oxfendazole, etc.) and probenzimidazoles (netobimin) and ivermectin are highly effective against inhibited larvae. Thiabendazole, levamisole, pyrantel tartrate are not effective against inhibited larvae. As a rule, animals should be kept worm-free during the rainy season so that they can make best use of the food resources in order to survive the dry season. (☞ CATTLE, 1; THERAPY OF NEMATODE INFECTIONS and Table 5 p. 54)

PROTOZOA

TRYPANOSOMATIDAE

Trypanosoma congolense, Trypanosoma vivax and *Trypanosoma brucei* Tsetse-transmitted trypanosomosis

Remarks: *T. congolense, T. vivax* and *T. brucei* may cause a chronic disease in sheep and goats, and may last from several weeks to several months. These three species belong to the *Salivaria*. The symptoms are mild and not very specific. Infected animals show fever attacks, rough and dull coat. Reproduction may be seriously impaired. The chronic trypanosome infection may render animals more susceptible to other diseases, especially when the animals live under poor nutritional conditions. The Sahelian breeds are very susceptible to trypanosomes but they avoid tsetse-infested areas. The indigenous dwarf breeds in the Guinean zone seem to be resistant to trypanosome infections and the disease is rarely detected in these breeds. A high percentage of animals kept in high tsetse-challenge areas are generally found to carry trypanosomes but these parasites are often of minor importance for the anaemia, weakness and unthriftiness. Very often these animals carry heavy burdens of gastrointestinal parasites and viral and bacterial diseases (Peste des Petits Ruminants (PPR), Pasteurellosis and other endemic diseases). Regular anthelmintic treatments during the rainy season and prophylactic vaccination against PPR are essential for a successful small ruminant production. The prophylactic use of trypanocidal drugs is generally not indicated in indigenous small ruminant breeds (☞ CATTLE, ■ 2). For therapy and prophylaxis ☞ Table 6 p. 56, Table 8 p. 59.

Trypanosoma melophagium

Remarks: This non-pathogenic trypanosome infects sheep. It is 50–60 µm in length and resembles *T. theileri* (☞ CATTLE, ■ 2). It belongs to the Stercoraria and is transmitted by the sheep ked, *Melophagus ovinus*, a pupiparous bloodsucking insect that permanently infests sheep. Infection occurs by contamination of the skin and if a ked is eaten by the sheep, the metacyclic stages penetrate the buccal mucosa. *T. melophagium* is widespread and usually demonstrable only by culture techniques but it may be also demonstrated microscopically in the peripheral blood.
(Figure 334)

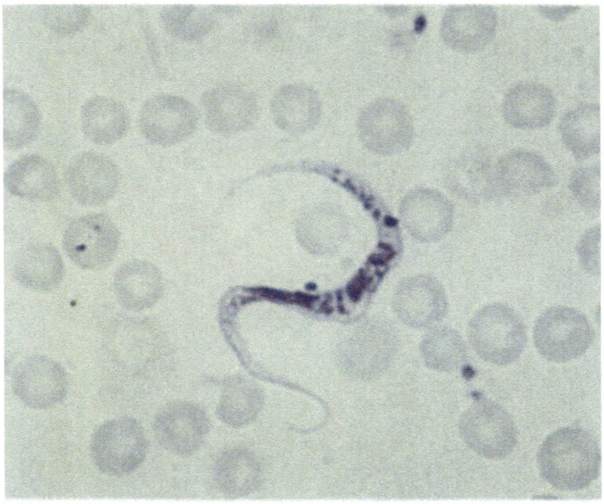

Fig. 334 *Trypanosoma melophagium* (50–60 µm long) [8]

BABESIIDAE

Babesia motasi (syn. *Piroplasma motasi*) European piroplasmosis of small ruminants

Hosts: Sheep and goat

Vector: *Haemaphysalis* spp. (*H. punctata; H. sulcata* and *H. parva*) in Europe, Mediterranean basin and northwestern Africa, *Dermacentor* spp. and *Rhipicephalus bursa* may also be involved.

Species description: This is a large form, measuring 2.5–4 × 2 µm, the pyriform stages resembling those of *Babesia bigemina*. The angle between the parasites is acute. The organisms occur singly or in pairs. The development cycle is similar to that of *B. bigemina*. Both transovarian and stage to stage transmission occur in *Rhipicephalus bursa*. Recovered animals are immune against *B. motasi* but not against *B. ovis* infections.

Geographic distribution: Southern Europe, Middle East, UIS, Southeast Asia, northwestern Africa

Symptoms: In the acute form high fever, haemoglobinuria, severe anaemia and prostration occur. Death is common. In the chronic form there are no characteristic signs and death is unusual.

Significance: *B. motasi* is a serious infection and frequently fatal in the acute form.

Diagnosis: This is based on clinical signs and the demonstration of the parasites in the peripheral blood. Highest parasitaemia levels are found during the time of acute fever.

Therapy: Diminazene aceturate (3.5 mg/kg, im.), imidocarb dipropionate (1.2–2.4 mg/kg, sc.) and quinuronium sulfate (1–2 mg/kg, sc. or im.) can be used against *B. motasi* infections.

Prophylaxis: The control of *Babesia* spp. in sheep and goats is similar to that in cattle and depends on regular tick control, the therapeutic and prophylactic use of drugs and attempts to immunize young animals with blood from older infected animals followed by a treatment with a babesiacidal drug (☞ CATTLE, ■ 2).

(Figures 335, 336)

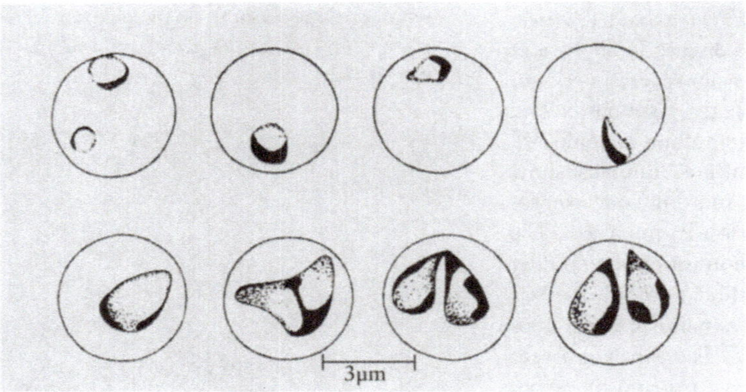

Fig. 335 *Babesia* species of sheep; *Babesia ovis* (upper row) and *Babesia motasi* (lower row) [3]

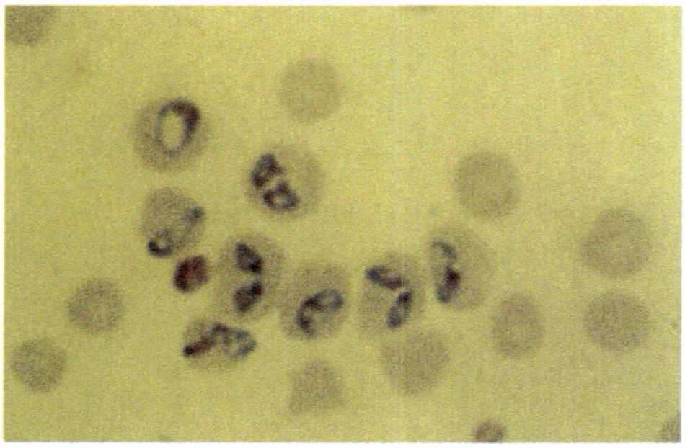

Fig. 336 *Babesia motasi*; stained bloodsmear [13]

Babesia ovis Tropical babesiosis of small ruminants

Hosts: Sheep and goat

Vector: *Rhipicephalus bursa* (Mediterranean basin and central-western Asia) and *Rhipicephalus evertsi* (tropical Africa) and probably other *Rhipicephalus* spp.

Species description: *B. ovis* is much smaller than *B. motasi*, being 1–2.5 µm in length. The majority of the organisms are round, occuring at the margin of the red cell. Pyriform

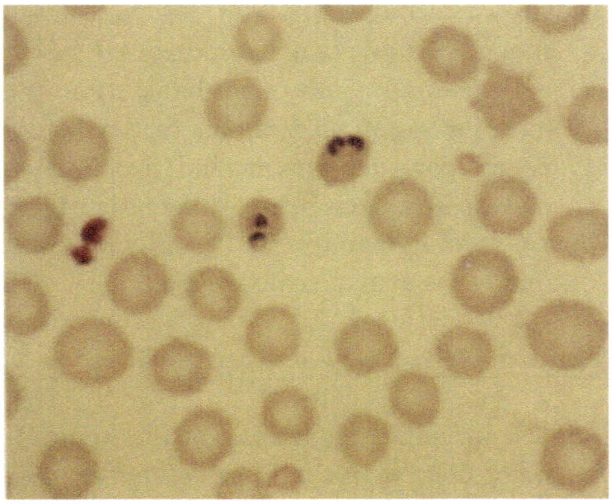

Fig. 337 *Babesia ovis*; stained bloodsmear [15]

organisms are comparatively rare. *B. ovis* is morphologically similar to that of *Babesia bovis*. *Rhipicephalus bursa* is a 2-host tick and transovarian and stage to stage transmission occurs in *R. bursa*. Recovered animals are immune to reinfection and there is no cross-immunity with *B. motasi*

Geographic distribution: Southern and central Europe, northern and tropical Africa, central-western Asia

Symptoms: Fever, jaundice, haemoglobinuria and anaemia may be seen in acute cases. The effects are usually less severe than those seen in *B. motasi* infections.

Significance: *B. ovis* may be an important cause of anaemia and icterus of small ruminants in endemic areas. It is considerably less pathogenic than *B. motasi*. In traditional management systems in endemic zones the disease passes often unnoticed.

Diagnosis: Demonstration of the organisms in stained blood smears and the clinical signs. In chronic infections about 1% of the erythrocytes are infected.

Therapy: Imidocarb dipropionate (1.2–2.4 mg/kg, sc.) is effective against *B. ovis* infections. Diminazene aceturate (3.5 mg/kg, im.) is only partially effective against *B. ovis*.

Prophylaxis: The control of *Babesia* spp. in sheep and goats is similar to that in cattle (☞ CATTLE, ■ 2 and *B. motasi*).

(Figure 337)

THEILERIIDAE

Theileria hirci (syn. *T. lestoquardi*)
Malignant theileriosis of small ruminants

Hosts: Sheep and goat

Vector: *Rhipicephalus bursa* and *Hyalomma anatolicum* and other species to be determined

Species description: This species is found in lymphocytes and erythrocytes of sheep and goats. The majority of the erythrocytic forms is round to oval (0.6–2 µm in diameter), about 20% are rod-shaped and a small percentage are *Anaplasma*-like. Binary or quadruple fission occurs in the erythrocytes. Schizonts occur in the lymphocytes of the spleen and lymph nodes. They range in size from 4–10 µm and contain up to 80 chromatin granules, 1–2 µm in diameter. Both macroschizonts and microschizonts occur. The disease may be highly fatal, mortality ranging from 50–100%. The infection is mild in young lambs and kids, due to maternal immunity. An acute form is more common, but subacute and chronic forms have been observed. The acute form resembles ECF.

Geographic distribution: North and East Africa, southern Europe, southern UIS, Asia.

Symptoms: In the acute form, high fever, listlessness, nasal discharge, jaundice, petechial haemorrhage in submucous, subserous and subcutaneous tissues may occur. The lymph nodes, spleen and kidneys are markedly enlarged. Haemoglobinuria may occur.

Significance: *T. hirci* is a very pathogenic species causing severe losses among small ruminant populations, mainly in the Mediterranean and North African regions.

Diagnosis: Is based on the detection of the organisms in blood smears or lymph nodes or spleen smears.

Therapy and Prophylaxis: ☞ CATTLE, ■ 2 (*T. parva*), parvaquone (1 × 20 mg/kg, im.), buparvaquone (2 × 2.5 mg/kg, im.) or the coccidiostat halofuginone (1 × 1.2 mg/kg, po.) may also be used to treat theileriosis

in small ruminants. Chlortetracycline and oxytetracyline are relatively ineffective. Tick control is an essential part of the prophylaxis.
(Figures 114, 115, 338)

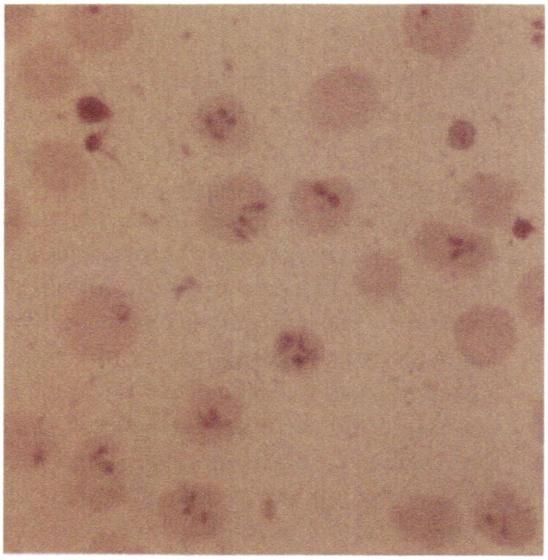

Fig. 338 *Theileria hirci*; erythrocyte forms (round forms 0.6–2 μm) [15]

Theileria ovis Benign theileriosis of small ruminants

Hosts: Sheep and goat

Vector: *Rhipicephalus bursa* in the Mediterranean basin and *Rhipicephalus evertsi* in tropical Africa

Species description: This species is found in lymphocytes and erythrocytes of sheep and goats and is much more widely distributed than *T. hirci*. The erythrocytic stages resemble those of *T. hirci* in shape and size but are much more sparse in infected animals, with less than 2% of the erythrocytes infected.

Geographic distribution: Africa, Asia, India, UIS, parts of Europe

Symptoms: The infection is usually mild and clinically inapparent.

Significance: The pathogenicity of this *Theileria* species is low and there is seldom mortality but the prevalence may be very high in endemic areas.

Diagnosis: Demonstration of the parasites in stained blood or lymph node smears. *T. ovis* is structurally indistinguishable from the more pathogenic *T. hirci*, but the small number of parasites present and their lack of pathogenicity may help to differentiate them.

Therapy and Prophylaxis: ☞ *T. hirci*; but therapy is generally not indicated.

Theileria separata Mild ovine theileriosis

Remarks: A mild theileriosis has be found in sheep. The vector is *Amblyomma variegatum*. It is distinguished from *T. ovis* by the presence of vela on some trophozoites. This species causes a mild and often clinically inapparent theileriosis in sheep.
(Figure 339)

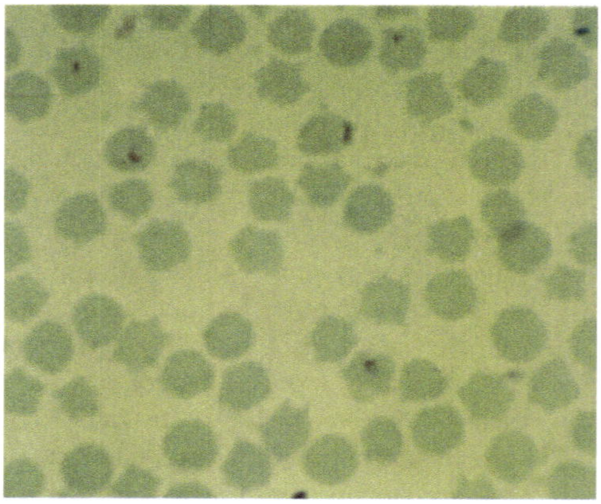

Fig. 339 *Theileria separata*; erythrocyte forms [13]

RICKETTSIALES

ANAPLASMATACEAE

Anaplasma **spp.**

Remarks: ☞ CATTLE, ■ 2 ANAPLASMATACEAE

Anaplasma ovis Tropical anaplasmosis of small ruminants

Remarks: It is comparable to *A. marginale* with 70% located marginally or peripherally. Its distribution corresponds to the most important vectors, *Rhipicephalus bursa* in the Mediterranean basin and *Rhipicephalus evertsi* in tropical Africa. Transplacental infection occurs.

Symptoms: Similar to those of *A. marginale* (☞ CATTLE, ■ 2)

Therapy and Prophylaxis: ☞ CATTLE, ■ 2 *A. marginale*

(Figure 340)

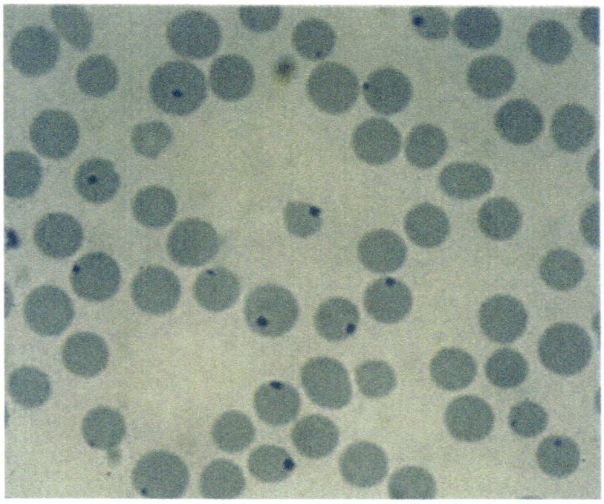

Fig. 340 *Anaplasma ovis*; stained bloodsmear [15]

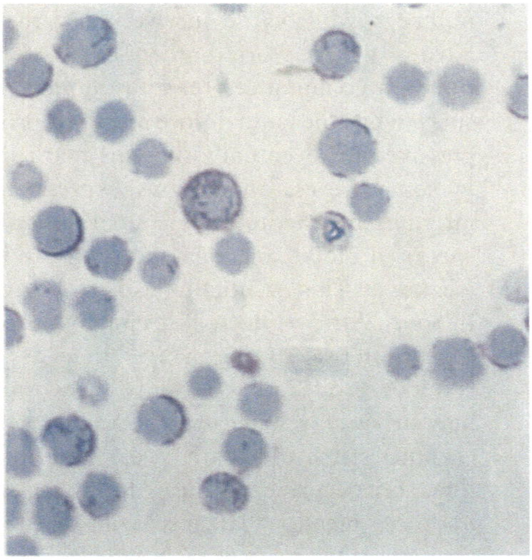

Fig. 341 *Eperythrozoon* sp.; stained bloodsmear [15]

Eperythrozoon ovis

Remarks: This species occurs on the erythrocyte surface. It is a nonpathogenic form but it sometimes occurs frequently in sheep (☞ CATTLE, ■ 2). *Linognathus ovillus* and possibly also ticks (*Hyalomma marginatum* and *Rhipicephalus bursa*) are vectors of *E. ovis*.

(Figure 341)

EHRLICHIACEAE

Ehrlichia ovina Tropical ehrlichiosis of small ruminants

Remarks: The parasite occurs in mononuclear cells of sheep in North and Central Africa. Vectors are *Rhipicephalus bursa* in Mediterranean basin and *Rhipicephalus evertsi* in tropical Africa. Despite sometimes heavy parasitaemia *E. ovina* usually causes a mild disease similar to that of *E. bovis*.

Therapy and Prophylaxis: ☞ CATTLE, ■ 2 *E. bovis*.

(Figure 342)

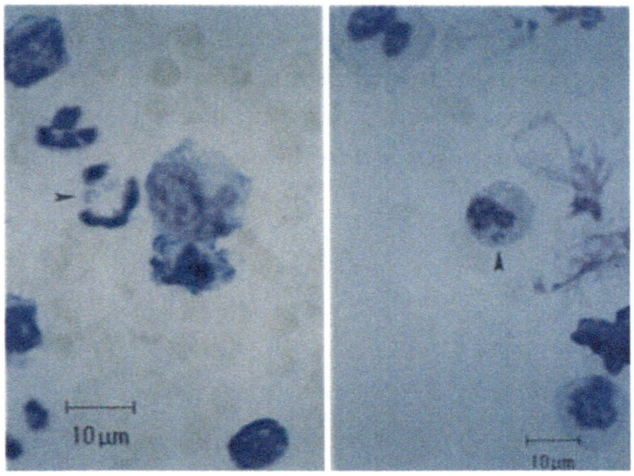

Fig. 342 *Ehrlichia* sp.; mass of elementary bodies (left) and initial body (right)

Ehrlichia phagocytophila
European ehrlichiosis

Remarks: *E. phagocytophila* occurs in the neutrophilic and eosiniphilic granulocytes of cattle, sheep and other domestic and wild ruminants in Europe. Goats are not very susceptible. *Ixodes ricinus* transmits the disease by transstadial infection. The disease is characterized by fever which occurs after an incubation period of 4–11 days. The animals usually recover after this febrile phase. However, the most characteristic problems are abortion in pregnant ewes and cattle and progressive weight loss following infection may occur. *Ehrlichia phagocytophila* increases the susceptibility to secondary infections. At necropsy hypertrophy of the spleen and lymph nodes may be seen. The diagnosis is made by demonstrating the organisms in stained blood smears. Serological tests (IFAT) may be of value for epidemiological studies.

Cowdria ruminantium Heartwater, Tyewde

Remarks: The infection caused by *Cowdria ruminantium* is virulent, inoculable, and noncontagious. It is specific to ruminants and causes great losses in sheep, goats and cattle. The disease can only be transmitted by ticks. Its symptoms are characterised by gastroenteritis associated with exudative pericarditis, often followed by nervous disorders. The symptoms are almost identical in both cattle and small ruminants, except that the nervous symptoms are rarer in cattle and not as distinct. Digestive signs are more constant in cattle than in sheep and goats. Young calves (< 6 weeks), lambs and kids (< 1 week) are fairly resistant and may recover spontaneously. For symptoms, diagnosis, therapy and prophylaxis ☞ CATTLE, ■ 2.
(Figure 343)

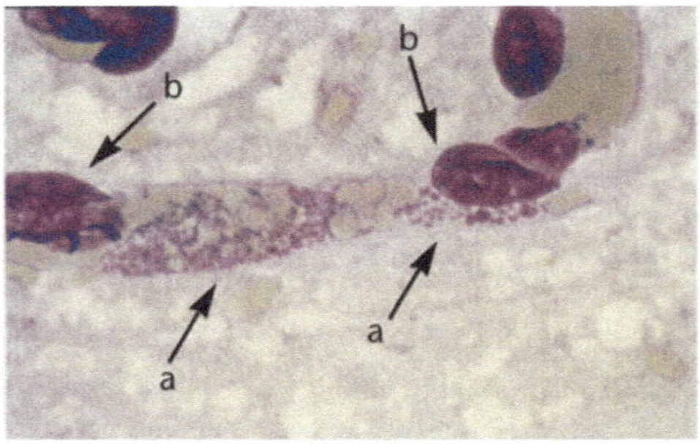

Fig. 343 *Cowdria ruminantium*; stained smear of a brain capillary; masses of organisms in endothelial cells (a) and nuclei of endothelial cells (b) [15]

Toxoplasma gondii **and** *Sarcocystis* **spp.**

Remarks: Merozoites may occur in the blood stream during the acute phase (☞ CATTLE, ■ 2).

HELMINTHS

• Trematoda found in the blood and circulatory system

***Schistosoma* spp.** Blood fluke, Bilharziosis

Remarks: The following *Schistosoma* species are found in small ruminants in Africa: *S. bovis, S. mattheei,* and *S. curassoni.*
Sheep are considerably more susceptible to schistosomosis than cattle and die in large numbers, while cattle survive unless they have very large worm burdens. The infection may go unnoticed for some months in sheep while the animals lose mass at a progressive rate, eventually showing markedly sunken eyes, an anxious expression, intermittent diarrhoea which may contain specks of blood, anaemia and progressive weakness. This eventually leads to death. In South Africa, infected sheep may die of schistosomosis during winter time as a result of respiratory infections. The worms may survive for many years in the sheep. A chronic course and death 4 years after the infection occurred in sheep following *S. mattheei* infection. The disease in sheep is characterized by anorexia, muscle wasting, haemorrhage and plasma-leaking into the gastrointestinal tract and impaired diges-

tion and food absorption. Low serum albumin and haemoglobin may be found following heavy infection. For therapy and prophylaxis ☞ CATTLE, ■ 2.

- Nematoda found in the blood and circulatory system

Onchocerca armillata

Remarks: This filarial worm may occasionally be found in the aorta of small ruminants. It is non-pathogenic (☞ CATTLE, ■ 2).

3 Stages in the urogential system

No pathogenic parasites have been found so far in the urogential system of sheep and goats.

4 Stages in internal organs

4.1 Locomotory system

4.1.1 Muscles

PROTOZOA

***Sarcocystis* spp.** Sarcosporidiosis of small ruminants

Location: Cysts, containing the infective stage, called bradyzoites, occur in the striated musculature of sheep and goat.

Hosts: Sheep are intermediate hosts of four *Sarcocystis* species of which either the dog (*S. ovicanis* and *S. arieticanis*) or the cat (*S. ovifelis*) are final hosts. Goats are intermediate hosts of three *Sarcocystis* species in two of which the dog (*S. capracanis* and *S. hircicanis*) acts as final host.The final host of *S. moulei* is probably the cat. Details of the life cycle of *Sarcocytis* species are still unknown.

Species description: Cysts of several *Sarcocystis* species are found in the muscles of sheep and goats. (For general description and life cycle ☞ Cattle, ■ 4.1.1). *S. ovifelis* produces big cysts, about 1 cm in length which are macroscopically visible. This species is non-pathogenic. Only those species in which the dog acts as final host are pathogenic. *S. ovicanis* is highly pathogenic for lambs and pregnant ewes. *S. capracanis* is equally pathogenic for kids and adult goats.

Geographic distribution: World-wide

Symptoms: Anorexia, weakness and death may occur in lambs infected with *S. ovicanis*. A high proportion of pregnant ewes aborted, became anaemic and lost weight during heavy infections.

Significance: *Sarcocystis* spp. are common among small ruminant populations throughout the world. Economic losses during a fresh infection may be higher than expected. Once muscle cysts are formed the infection is usually inapparent.

Diagnosis: At necropsy of acutely ill animals the heart was the most severely affected organ, schizonts were found in epithelial cells. *S. ovicanis* stages have not been found in the placenta, fetus or uterine tissues following abortion (☞ CATTLE, ■ 4.1.1).

Therapy and Prophylaxis: ☞ bovine *Sarcocystis* spp. (☞ CATTLE, ■ 4.1.1)

(Figures 344, 345, 346, 347, Table 13)

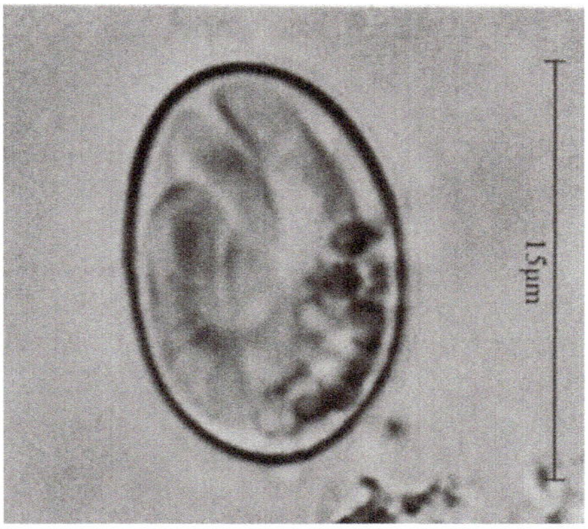

Fig. 345 Sporocyst of *Sarcocystis ovicanis* [4]

Table 13 Sarcocystis species found in the muscles of sheep and goat

Species	Synonym	Pathogenicity			
		IH	DH	IH	DH
S. ovifelis	*S. gigantea**	sheep	cat	0	
S. ovicanis	*S. tenella*	sheep	dog	+++	0
S. arieticanis		sheep	dog	+++	0
S. medusiformis		sheep	cat	+	0
S. capracanis		goat	dog	+++	0
S. hircicanis		goat	dog	+	0
S. moulei		goat	cat	0	0

IH = intermediate host; DH = definitive host; *= macroscopic; 0 = non-pathogenic; + = low; ++ = moderate and +++ = high pathogenicity

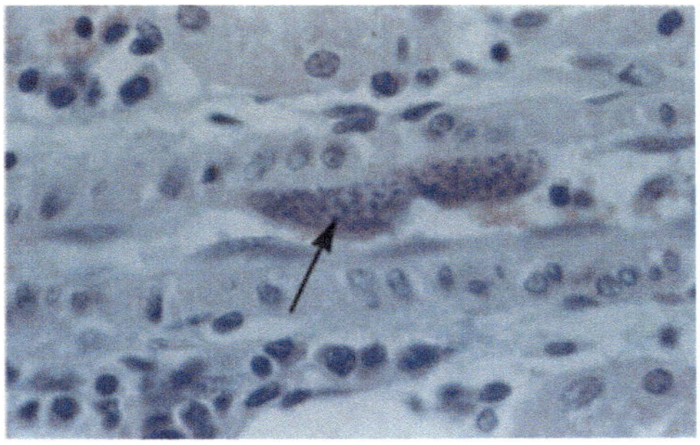

Fig. 346 *Sarcocystis capracanis*; schizonts with merozoites in endothelial cells (400×) [4]

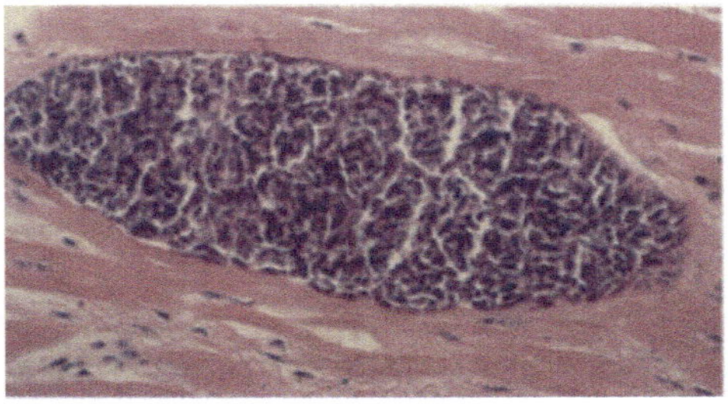

Fig. 344 *Sarcocystis* sp. HE-stained muscular cyst (150 µm long)

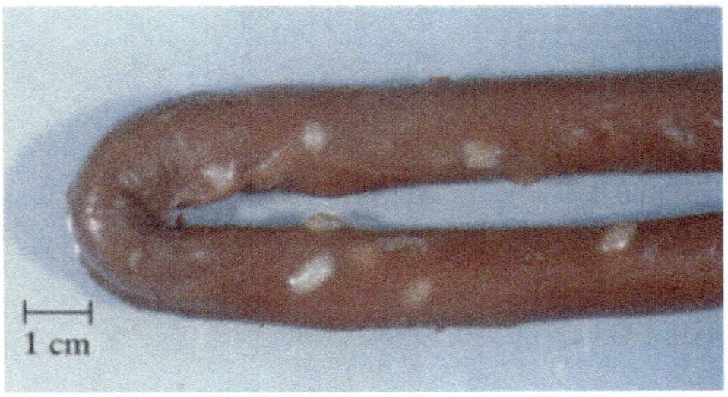

Fig. 347 *Sarcocystis ovifelis* (syn. *S. gigantea*); cysts on the outside of the oesophagus of a sheep

Toxoplasma gondii

Remarks: *T. gondii* is an important cause of abortion in sheep and goats and responsible for high mortalities in lambs and young goats (> 10% of mortalities in lambs). Transmission occurs via infective oocysts from cats, congenitally and galactogenically. Abortion occurs mainly when pregnant goats and sheep acquire first infection during pregnancy. Animals normally do not show any clinical signs during the abortion. Infections are more serious in goats than in sheep. The placenta shows numerous yellowish-white necrotic foci in the villi. Tissue cysts of *T. gondii* may also occur in ruminants as they do in pigs (☞ SWINE, ■ 4.1). Muscle cysts are about 100 µm in diameter, containing merozoites which are 6–8 µm in diameter. Encephalomyelitis due to *T. gondii* infections may occur in sheep. Affected sheep have myelomalacia and schizonts appear in astrocytes. Infection is most often acquired orally by ingestion of sporulated oocysts from the faeces of cats.

Cave: Uncooked meat (mainly meat of pigs but also of sheep) is a potential source of Toxoplasma infection in man.

(Figure 348, 349)

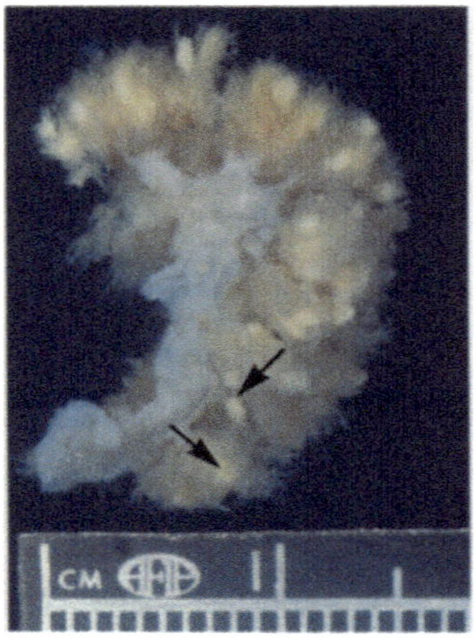

Fig. 348 *Toxoplasma gondii*; placenta of sheep showing cotyledon with numerous yellowish-white necrotic foci in villi [22]

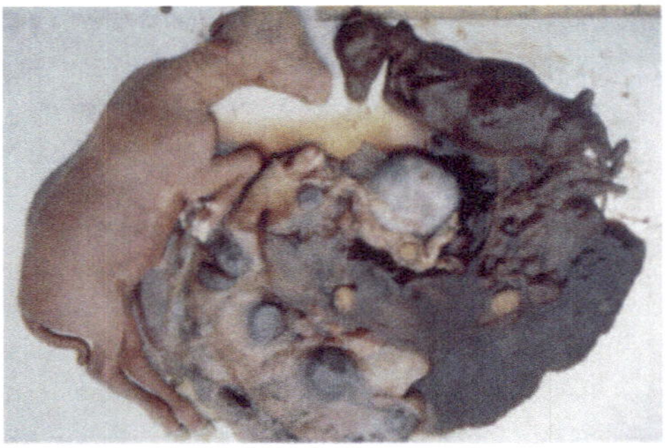

Fig. 349 *Toxoplasma* abortion of sheep; lesions characteristic of *Toxoplasma* are found in cotyledons of both lambs [22]

HELMINTHS

• Cestoda larvae found in the muscles

Cysticercus ovis *Larvae of the canine tape worm Taenia ovis*

Location: Cysticerci are found in the heart, diaphragm, masseters and other musculature.

Intermediate Hosts: Sheep and goat

Species description: The life cycle of *Taenia ovis* is similar to that of *Taenia saginata* (☞ CATTLE, ■ 4.1.1). Larvae (oncospheres) are disseminated with the blood and develop in skeletal and cardiac musculature. Mature cysticerci measure 10 × 5 mm and contain 1 protoscolex.

Geographic distribution: World-wide

Symptoms: Clinical signs are not usually seen.

Significance: This parasite is of importance as a cause of financial loss to the meat industry. Infected carcasses are unaesthetic and usually condemned at meat inspection.

Diagnosis: Detection of cysticerci in the striated musculature at meat inspection. *Cysticercus ovis* (possesses hooks) is macroscopically not distinguishable from *Cysticercus bovis* (no hooks).

Therapy: This is generally not indicated in the intermediate host. A consequent treatment of all dogs within a population would inevitably reduce the incidence of cysticerosis in small ruminants, but this is generally not feasible.

Prophylaxis: Infected meat should not be fed to dogs. A highly protective recombinant vaccine may soon be available. The vaccination of small ruminants against *T. ovis* will then be the prophylactic measure of choice.
(Figure 350, 351)

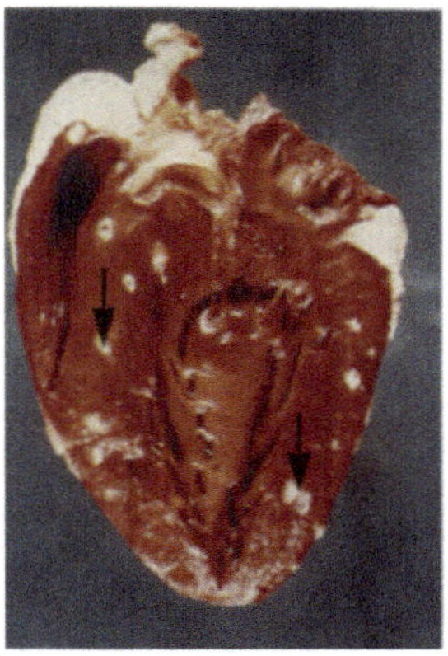

Fig. 350 *Cysticercus ovis*; heart muscle with cysts [10]

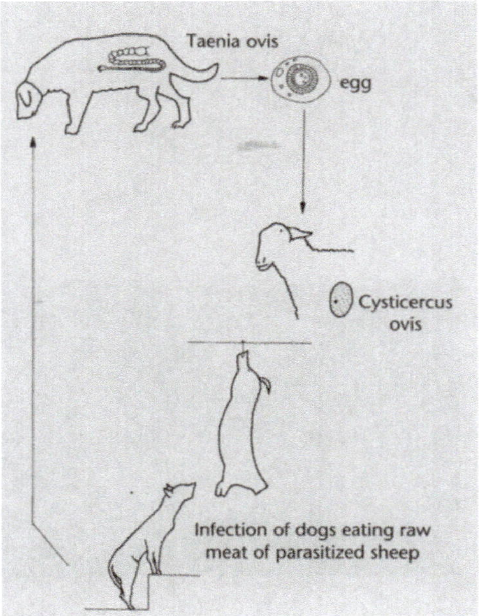

Fig. 351 Life cycle of *Cysticercus ovis* [16]

4.1.2 Tendons

HELMINTHS

- Nematoda larvae and adult nematodes found in the tendons

Onchocerca gutturosa (syn. *O. lienalis*)

Remarks: This parasite may sometimes be found in sheep (☞ CATTLE, ■ 4.1.2).

4.2 Liver

HELMINTHS

- Trematoda found in the liver

Fasciola gigantica Giant liver fluke

Remarks: This is the common liver fluke of domestic stock in Africa. It also occurs in Asia, the Pacific islands, southern USA, southern Europe and the Middle East. In Africa the parasite occurs in the bile ducts of cattle, sheep, goats, dromedary, horse, pigs and many other animal species (☞ CATTLE, ■ 4.2).

Fasciola hepatica Common liver fluke, liver fluke disease, liver rot

Remarks: This parasite occurs in the bile ducts of sheep, goat, cattle, horse, donkey, pig and many other animal species. The fluke is cosmopolitan in its distribution and the cause of fasciolosis, especially in sheep and cattle (☞ CATTLE, ■ 4.2). *F. hepatica* is a world-wide problem in sheep rearing systems. Fasciolosis in sheep is characterized by decreased wool growth, weight loss and liver condemnation at slaughter. *F. hepatica* may cause an acute form in sheep, associated with sudden deaths.

Dicrocoelium spp. Lancet flukes

Remarks: *D. hospes* occurs in the bile ducts and gall bladder of sheep, goat, cattle and other ruminants from Egypt to Angola, particularly in the western half of the African continent. This parasite is closely related to *D. dendriticum*. In heavy infections, extensive hepatic cirrhosis and distension of the bile ducts may occur. Such sheep may be unthrifty (☞ CATTLE, ■ 4.2).
(Figures 352, 353, 354, 355)

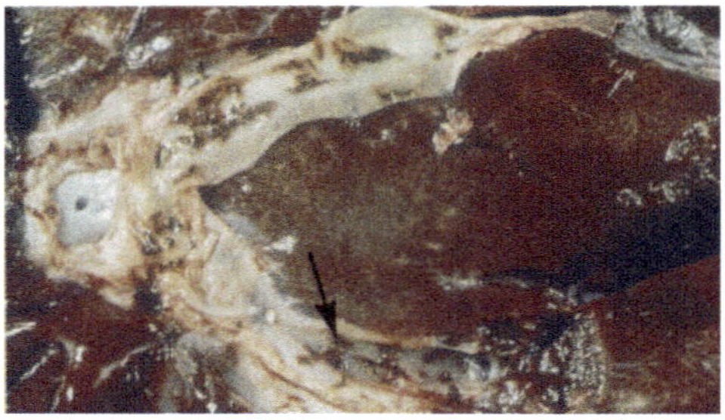

Fig. 352 *Dicrocoelium dendriticum*; adult flukes in bile ducts of a sheep

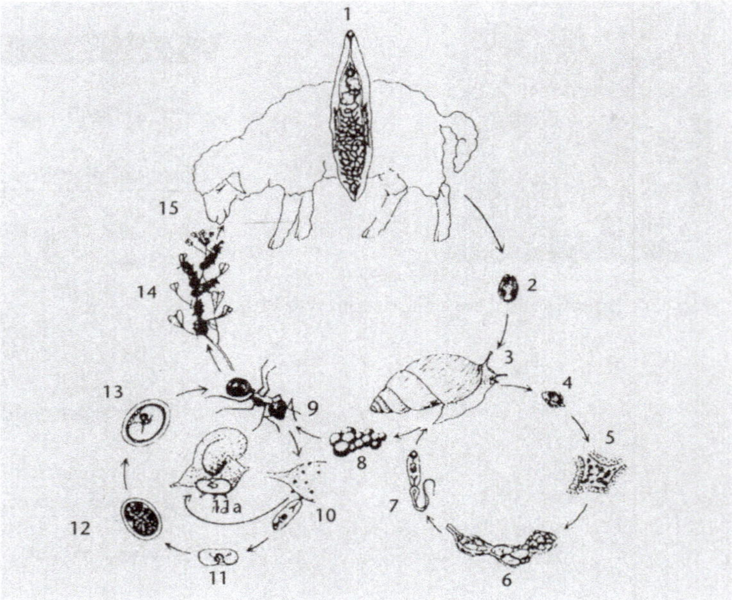

Fig. 353 Life cycle of *Dicrocoelium dendriticum*; (1) adult flukes in the liver of sheep, (2) eggs excreted with the faeces, (3)–(8) development in snails (first intermediate hosts), (9)–(13) development in ants (second intermediate hosts) and (14) ants containing the infective metacercariae in the brain attach to herbage

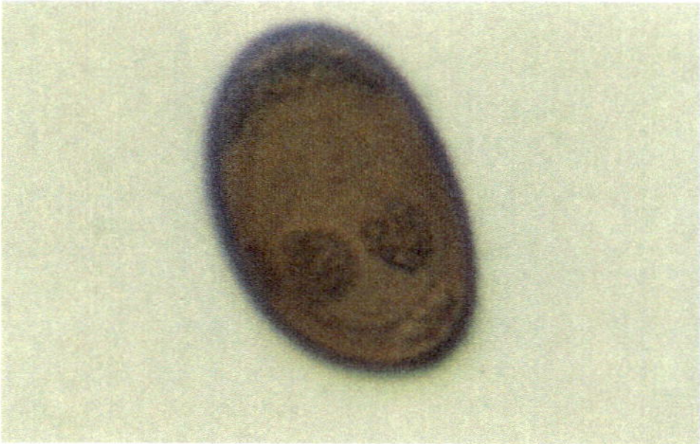

Fig. 354 Egg of *Dicrocoelium dendriticum* (36–45 × 25 μm)

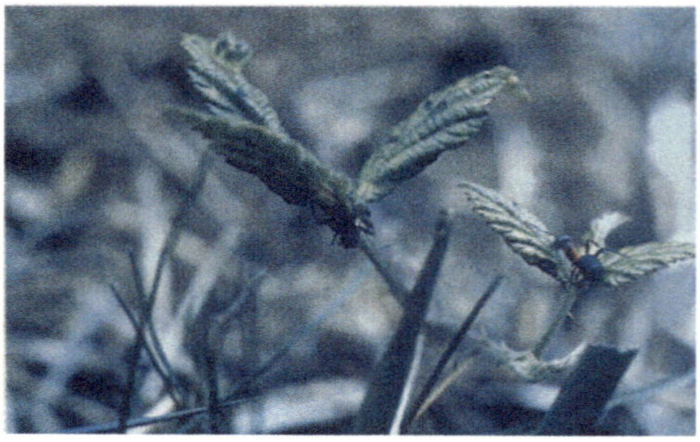

Fig. 355 *Dicrocoelium dendriticum* infected ants remain attached to herbage

• Cestoda found in the liver

Echinococcus granulosus (syn. *E. unilocularis*) Hydatid tapeworm, hydatidosis

Remarks: Hydatid cysts are often found in the liver and lungs of sheep where they are often multivesicular. Infected sheep usually do not show any clinical signs but constitute a major reservoir for new infections. Infected organs should never be fed to dogs, which are the principal hosts of *E. granulosus*. Sheep and goats and many other ungulates and man may act as intermediate hosts. Infection of the intermediate hosts are usually inapparent, except in man where hydatidosis is a severe condition and the function of the affected organ is frequently impaired (☞ CATTLE, ■ 4.2).
(Figure 356)

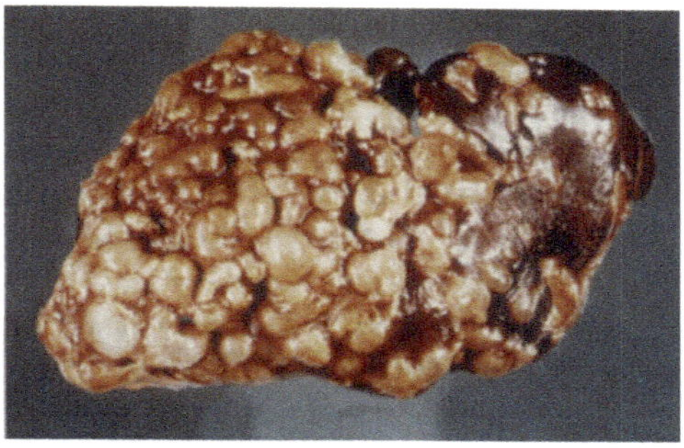

Fig. 356 *Echinococcus granulosus*; hydatid cyst in the liver of a sheep [10]

Stilesia hepatica

Location: Bile ducts and small intestine
Hosts: Sheep, goat, wild ruminants and rarely cattle
Species description: The life cycle is not known but probably involves oribatide mites. It is non-pathogenic. Heavy infections are often seen in apparently perfectly healthy sheep. Affected livers may sometimes show cirrhosis and thickened walls of the bile ducts. Although the bile ducts may be almost occluded, or even form sac-like occlusions, no icterus or clinical signs are seen. Adults have a large scolex with prominent suckers and measure 20–50 cm in length and up to 2 mm in width.
Geographic distribution: Tropical and southern Africa, Asia
Symptoms: Infections are often clinically inapparent.
Significance: The condemnation of a large proportion of sheep livers at meat inspection is the major loss due to this parasite. The parasite itself does not impair the raising of sheep.
Diagnosis: Proglottids or ovoid eggs may appear in the faeces. The proglottids are short and the eggs measure 16–19 × 26 µm.
Therapy: Praziqunatel (15 mg/kg, po.) can be used for treatment.
Prophylaxis: Unknown
(Figures 37, 43, 357, 358)

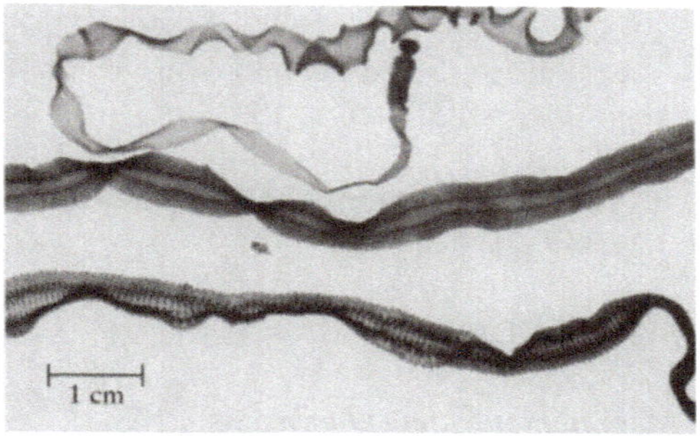

Fig. 357 *Stilesia hepatica*; scolex and proglottids (20–50 cm × 2 mm) [8]

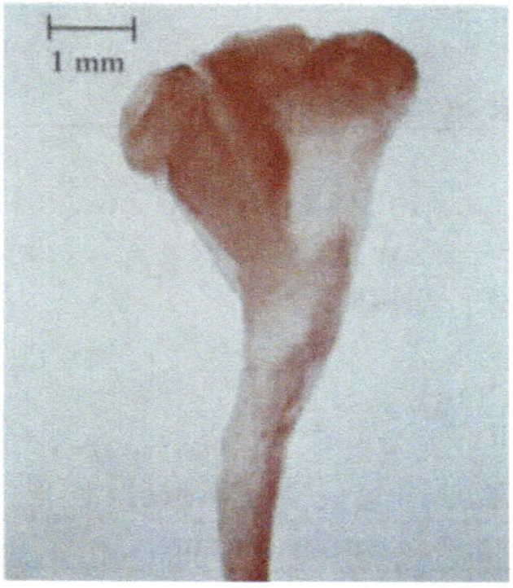

Fig. 358 *Stilesia hepatica*; scolex [4]

Cysticercus tenuicollis

Remarks: Migrating oncospheres may occasionally be found in the liver parenchyma and thin necked cysts may be found on the serosa of the liver (☞ SHEEP AND GOATS, ■ 4.4).

Linguatula serrata "tongue worm"
(☞ CATTLE, ■ 4.2)

4.3 Respiratory system

HELMINTHS

- Cestoda found in the respiratory system

Echinococcus granulosus (syn. *E. unilocularis*)
Hydatid tapeworm, hydatidosis

Remarks: Larvae (Hydatid cysts) of *E. granulosus* are often found in the lungs and liver of cattle and other domestic animals (☞ CATTLE, ■ 4.2).

- Nematoda found in the lungs and trachea

SYNGAMIDAE

Mammomonogamus laryngeus

Remarks: This parasite may occasionally be found in the larynx of small ruminants (☞ CATTLE, ■ 4.3).

Mammomonogamus nasicola

Remarks: This parasite may occasionally be found in the nasal cavities of small ruminants (☞ CATTLE, ■ 4.3).

DICTYOCAULIDAE

Dictyocaulus filaria Large lungworm of small ruminants, parasitic bronchitis

Location: Bronchi and bronchioles

Hosts: Sheep, goat, dromedary and some wild ruminants

Species description: The male is 3–8 cm long and the female is 5–10 cm long. The worms have a milk-white colour and the intestine shows as a dark line. There are very small lips and a very small, shallow buccal capsule. The spicules of the male bursa are stout, dark-brown, boot-shaped and 0.4–0.64 mm long. The eggs measure 112–138 × 60–90 μm. The life cycle is direct and similar to that of *D. viviparus* (☞ CATTLE, ■ 4.3). The prepatent period is 24–28 days. In infected animals the bronchial mucosa and the peribronchial tissue are inflamed and infiltrated with mononuclear cells. Localized pneumonia, atelectasis and compensatory emphysema may be seen.

Geographic distribution: World-wide, especially in warm moist areas; *D. filaria* was reported from Tchad, Sudan, Ethiopia, Kenya, Mozambique, Zimbabwe, Malawi and South Africa

Symptoms: Infected animals may cough and show nasal discharge. Dyspnoea, rapid respiration and abnormal lung sounds can be heard on auscultation. Young animals are mainly affected, but the disease may occur at all ages and is usually chronic. The body temperature is not elevated unless pneumonia and secondary infection develops.

Significance: Lungworm infections may cause serious losses in sheep in endemic areas. Lung damage often persists for long periods and animals are unthrifty and susceptible to secondary infections.

Diagnosis: This is made by demonstrating first-stage larvae in fresh faeces. Eggs or larvae may be found in the sputum or nasal discharge, but during the prepatent period their absence is not significant. At necropsy atelectatic areas of variable size may be seen in the lungs. The bronchi in the affected parts contain the worms and large amounts of mucus, which are mixed with blood and desquamated epithelial cells, leucocytes and eggs of the worms.

Therapy: ☞ CATTLE, ■ 4.3 THERAPY OF *DICTYOCAULUS VIVIPARUS*

Prophylaxis: In endemic areas, young sheep must be kept off areas where infected sheep have been grazing. Infected animals should be treated with anthelmintics. For further prophylactic measures ☞ also CATTLE, ■ 4.3. The prophylactic use of irradiated *D. filaria* larvae has been successfully used in some countries but the vaccine is not commercially available.

(Figures 313, 359)

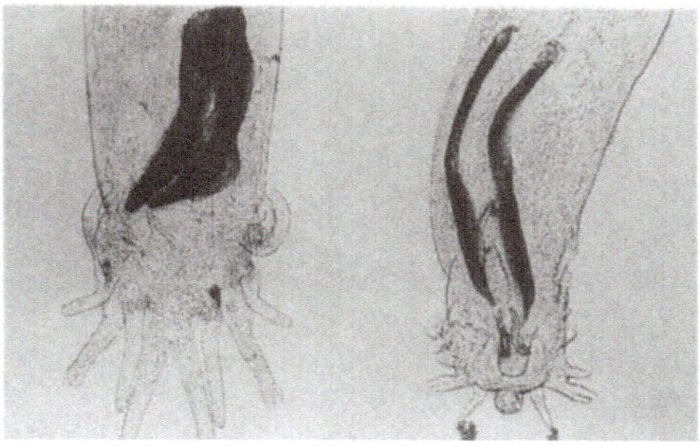

Fig. 359 *Dictyocaulus filaria* (left) and *Protostrongylus rufescens* (right); posterior end of males [4]

PROTOSTRONGYLIDAE

Protostrongylus rufescens Red lungworm;
Muellerius capillaris Hair lungworm;
Neostrongylus linearis* and *Cystocaulus ocreatus

These four species are generally referred to as small lungworms of small ruminants.

Location: Adult worms occur in small air passages (small bronchioles, bronchioli) and in some species even in the alveoli and the pulmonary parenchyma and the subpleural tissue (e.g. *Muellerius capillaris*). The eggs are found in the bronchioli and alveoli.

Hosts: Sheep, goat and some wild ruminant species

Species description: The life cycle of all small lungworms includes an intermediate host which may be one species of land snails of the genera *Helicella, Theba, Abida, Zebrina, Arianta, Succinea, Helix, Cepaea, Monacha,* etc. or nude slugs such as *Limax, Agriolimax, Arion*, etc. The first-stage larvae which are passed in the faeces penetrate the foot of the snail to develop to the infective third-stage in about 12–14 days. The final host becomes infected by swallowing the snail with its food. The larvae are liberated in the gut of the ruminant host and penetrate the intestinal wall and pass via the mesenteric lymphatic glands to the lungs. Further development is similar to that of *Dictyocaulus* species. *Muellerius capillaris* and *Protostrongylus rufescens* are frequently encountered in Europe but they are also found in many parts of Africa. Differentiation can easily be made by the examination of the first-stage larvae which are passed in the faeces of animals with patent infections. As a general rule, small lungworms cause extensive alterations of the lungs but generally little or no clinical signs. In some areas almost 100% of the adult sheep and goats are infected and show massive lung reactions. These are not easily distinguishable between the different lungworm species. The worms live in the small air passages and cause inflammation. The resulting exudate fills the alveoli and the inflammatory and allergic process spreads to the peribronchial tissue. The alveolar epithelium is desquamated and infiltration with round cells and proliferation of the surrounding connective tissue occurs. The result is a small focus of lobular pneumonia and the number of such foci depends on the number of parasites present. In *Muellerius capillaris* infections, greyish nodules up to 2 cm in diameter may be seen on the pleural surface. These "brood nodules" consist of necrotic masses, resulting from leucocytes and pulmonary tissue and masses of eggs, and they are surrounded by a wall of connective tissue and giant cells. These nodules may calcify. An adenoma-like proliferation of the bronchial epithelium and a hypertrophy of the smooth muscles around the alveoli and bronchioli is often seen. *Muellerius capillaris* is usually not found in lambs or kids under six months of age. Thereafter the prevalence increases with age and may reach 100% in goats older than 3 years. *Muellerius capillaris* may cause interstitial pneumonia and clinical signs. It seems that this species is relatively pathogenic for goats.

Geographic distribution: Europe, Africa, Australia, North America

Symptoms: Animals show no definite clinical signs, but heavy infections affect the general health, and the weakened lungs are susceptible to secondary infections which may produce pneumonia.

Significance: Small lungworms are extremely prevalent and often not associated with clinical disease. However, if the lesions are large and animals kept under poor conditions severe problems may result due to secondary infections.

Diagnosis: This is based on the identification of first-stage larvae in the faeces by means of the Baermann apparatus. The larva of *P. rufescens* is 0.25–0.32 mm long. The tip of its tail has a wavy outline but no dorsal spine. The larva of *M. capillaris* is 0.23–0.3 mm long. The tail of the larva has an undulating tip and a dorsal spine. At necropsy the nodules in the lungs are typical and may support the diagnosis (☞ Fig. 314, p. 158).

Therapy: The therapy of the small lungworms in sheep and goats is difficult. Most of the modern benzimidazoles (albendazole 5 mg/kg, po., fenbendazole 5 mg/kg, po., febantel 5 mg/kg, po., mebendazole 10–20 mg/kg, po., oxfendazole 5 mg/kg, po., netobimin 7.5 mg/kg, po. and levamisole 5.0 mg/kg, sc., are partially effective against the adult worms. Ivermectin (200 µg/kg, sc.) is highly effective against adults of *Protostrongylus rufescens*.

Prophylaxis: This is difficult because of the ubiquitous presence of the intermediate hosts. Often, regular anthelmintic treatment with a broad spectrum compound controls both gastrointestinal and heavy lungworm infestations. Snail control on pastures with molluscicides is ineffective and ecologically not justifiable.

(Figures 360, 361, 362, Table 14)

Table 14 Comparison of prepatent periods and patency periods of different lung worm species

Genus	Prepatent period	Patency
Protostrongylus spp.	4–5 weeks	2 years
Neostrongylus spp.	2 months	2 years
Cystocaulus spp.	1 month	5–6 years
Muellerius spp.	1 month	5–6 years
Dictyocaulus spp.	24–28 days	2–3 months

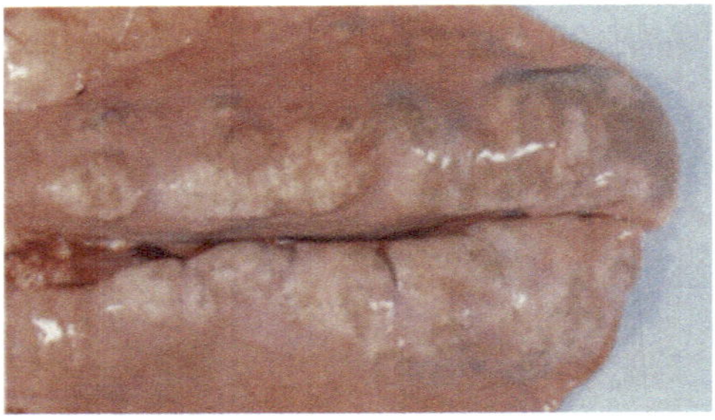

Fig. 360 *Muellerius capillaris*; brood nodules in the lungs (dorsal view)

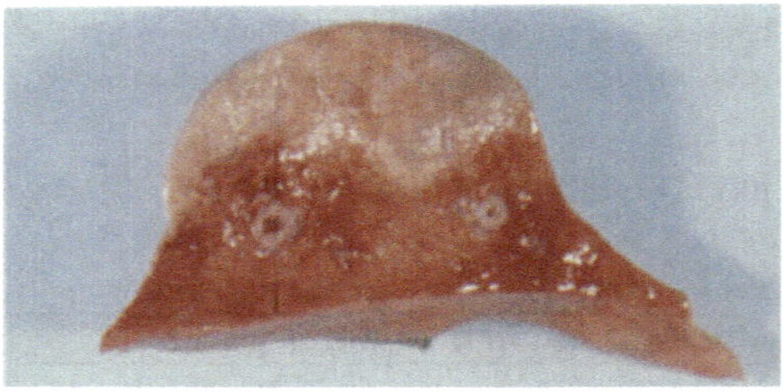

Fig. 361 *Muellerius capillaris*; brood nodules in the lungs (section)

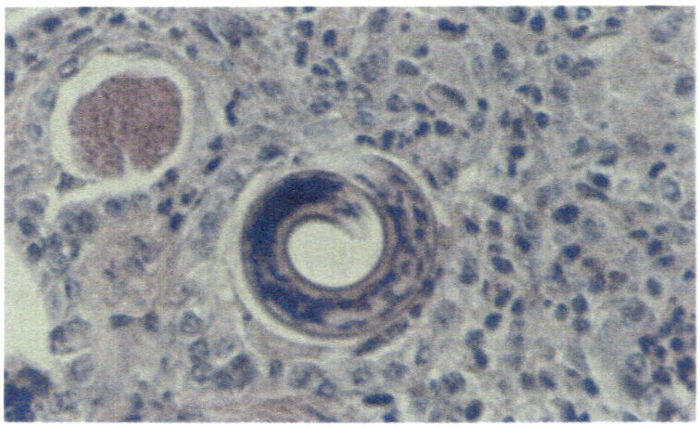

Fig. 362 *Muellerius capillaris*; tissue section showing the parasites and the massive cellular infiltration of the lungs (250 ×)

- Insecta larvae found in the respiratory system

Oestrus ovis Sheep nasal flies, sheep nasal bot, nasal myiasis

Location: Larvae live in nasal passages and frontal and nasal sinuses

Hosts: Sheep and goat

Species description: Adult flies are about 12 mm long. The body is greyish-brown, with many small black spots on the thorax, which is covered with fine, light brown hair. The female flies produce live larvae which are deposited around the nostrils of sheep and occasionally goats. These larvae crawl into the nasal passages where they remain for a variable period, ranging from 2 weeks in summer to 9 months during the colder part of the year. They attach themselves with the oral hooks to the mucous membranes, causing irritation, and then enter the frontal sinuses where they develop into second- and third-stage larvae. The mature larvae are sneezed out by the host and pupate on the ground for 3–9 weeks before becoming adults. The mature flies live for about 2 weeks. Usually 4–15 larvae are present in infested sheep.

Geographic distribution: World-wide

Symptoms: Sneezing and nasal discharges and fly worry are the consequences of *O. ovis* infestations. Decreased appetite, restlessness and poor gains are the results of nasal bot fly strikes. Respiration may be impaired by the larvae and the thickening of the nasal mucosa. Occasionally the larvae may penetrate the bones of the skull and enter the cerebral cavity. These sheep show a characteristic behavior (stagger).

Significance: The larvae cause irritation and excessive secretion. Infected sheep sneeze frequently and secondary bacterial infections are common. Sheep try to avoid attacks by the adult fly by pressing their noses between other sheep or they may run from place to place, stamping their feet and shaking their heads continuously. Consequently their time spent with feeding is considerably reduced.

Diagnosis: Clinical signs may help, but must be differentiated from other conditions with sneezing and nasal discharges. Sometimes larvae may be found on the ground after a severe sneezing attack. Very often the diagnosis can only be made at necropsy when the skull is opened longitudinally. Nasal myiasis often produces clinical signs which are similar to those seen in CNS disorders (restlessness, shaking of the head, etc.).

Therapy: Ivermectin (200 µg/kg, sc.) is highly effective. Ruelene (110 mg/kg, po.) administered as a drench should afford good control. Rafoxanide (7.5–10 mg/kg, po.) as a drench or bolus, trichlorfon (75 mg/kg, po. or as a drench) and nitroxynil (15–20 mg/kg, sc.) have been reported to be effective.

Prophylaxis: Fly repellents may be used but are not very effective.

(Figures 363, 364, 365)

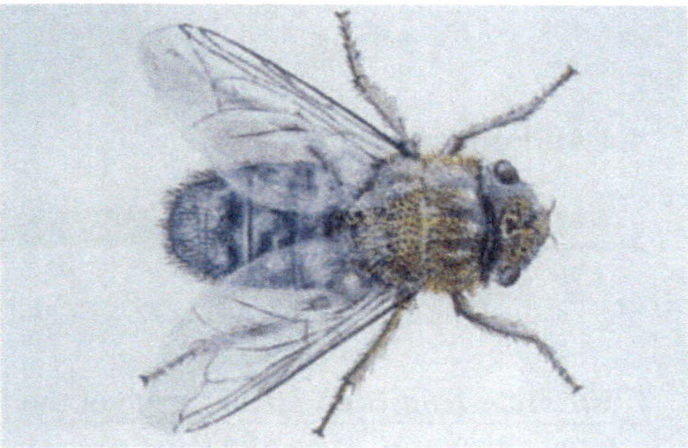

Fig. 363 *Oestrus ovis;* the sheep nasal fly (10–12 mm) [19]

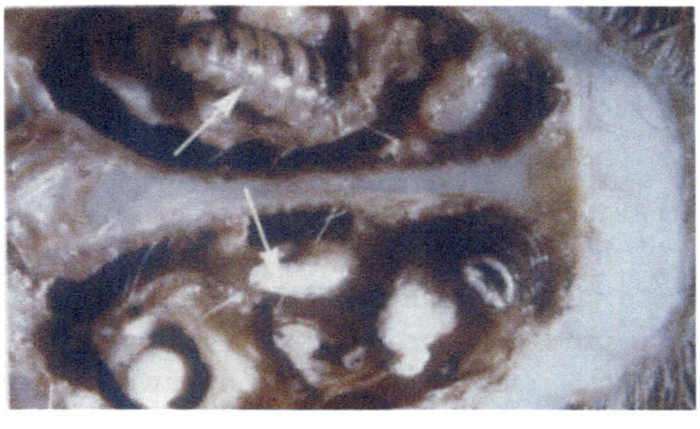

Fig. 364 Conchae of a sheep with *Oestrus ovis* larvae (20–30 mm × 7–10 mm) [8]

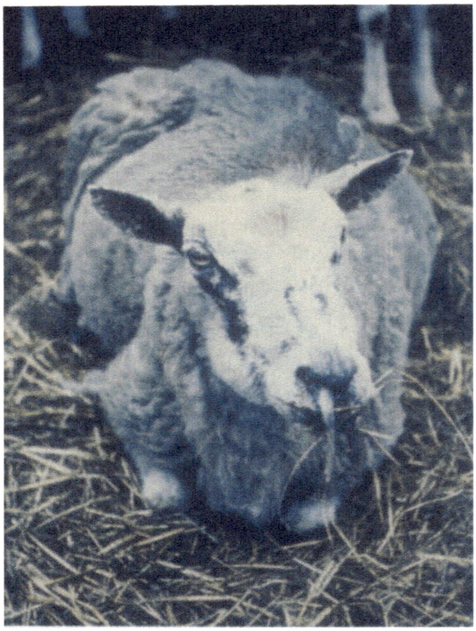

Fig. 365 *Oestrus ovis* infestation causing nasal discharge [15]

4.4 Abdominal cavity

HELMINTHS

- Cestoda found in the abdominal cavity

Cysticercus tenuicollis Larval stage of the canine tapeworm *Taenia hydatigena*

Location: Cysticerci are found attached to the omentum, the intestinal mesentery and to the serosal surface of abdominal organs, especially the liver. Adult tapeworms occur in the small intestine of dogs and other Canidae.

Hosts: Sheep and other domestic and wild herbivores including pig and horse, act as intermediate hosts. Dog, wolf, hyaena and other wild carnivores are the final hosts.

Species description: Adult tapeworms are 75–500 cm long and have two rows of 26 and 46 rostellar hooks. Gravid proglottids measure 12 × 6 mm. The eggs are oval and 36–39 × 31–35 µm. Infections of the dogs are usually inapparent. Infections of the intermediate hosts are acquired by ingestion of proglottids or eggs passed in the faeces of the dog. Ingested eggs hatch in the small intestine and oncospheres reach the liver via the portal vein. Here the embryos break out of the portal system and migrate through the liver parenchyma and towards the serosal surface for up to 30 days. They cause haemorrhagic tracts. The cysticerci develop subserosal from about 18 –28 days after infection. They reach maturity between 34 and 53 days and are found attached to the greater omentum, mesentery, liver and other serosal surfaces of abdominal organs. Mature cysticerci are up to 6 cm long and have a thin, long neck. They contain a single scolex. The life cycle is closed, if carnivores ingest cysticerci. The prepatent period in the dog is 51 days and dogs may remain infected for more than one year. The prevalence of infection in sheep is high. In some regions more than 80% of the slaughtered sheep and goats show cysticerci. Migration of young cysticerci through the liver parenchyma causes haemorrhagic and later fibrotic tracts.

Geographic distribution: World-wide

Symptoms: Infections in intermediate hosts are usually inapparent. Heavy infections may cause traumatic hepatitis when large numbers of larvae migrate through the liver. Death may result often due to haemorrhage. This may occasionally occur in young lambs and pigs. Animals during that time often show unthriftiness. Mature cysticerci in the peritoneal cavity usually cause no harm.

Significance: Losses occur through condemned livers and organs.

Diagnosis: This is based on finding the cysticerci at slaughter. Cysticerci are covered by a layer of serosa. If this layer is broken the typical thin-necked organism appears. The diagnosis antemortem is difficult. Serological tests may be unspecific. Haemorrhagic tracts may be seen in the liver when masses of larvae have passed through the parenchyma.

Therapy: This is not indicated in intermediate hosts. Dogs may be treated as described in *Echinococcus granulosus* (☞ CATTLE, ■ 4.2).

Prophylaxis: Removed cysticerci at slaughter should not be fed to dogs. Dogs should in general not be allowed to feed on condemned meat and organs.

(Figures 179, 180, 366)

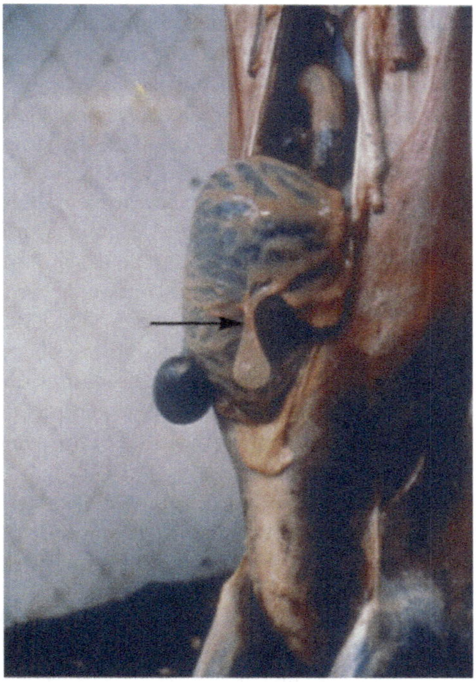

Fig. 366 *Cysticercus tenuicollis*; thin-necked cysts attached to the serosa [10]

- Nematoda found in the abdominal cavity

Setaria labiatopapillosa

Remarks: This parasite occurs in the peritoneal cavity of cattle, deer, giraffe and other ruminants. Sheep and goats may occasionally be abnormal hosts in which erratic microfilariae may invade the CNS and produce nervous symptoms. The diagnosis of microfilariae-associated (mainly *S. digitata*) neurological disturbances can only be made at necropsy by microscopical examination of CNS sections (☞ CATTLE, ■ 4.4).

4.5 Pancreas

HELMINTHS

- Trematoda found in the pancreas

Eurytrema pancreaticum

Pancreatic fluke

Location: Pancreatic ducts, bile ducts, occasionally duodenum

Hosts: Sheep, goat and cattle

Species description: These flukes are 8–16 mm long and 5–8.5 mm wide. The bodies are thick with large suckers. The eggs measure 40–50 × 23–34 µm. The life cycle is indirect with two intermediate hosts. Land snails of the genera *Bradybaena* and *Cathaica* serve as first intermediate hosts. Grasshoppers of different genera act as second intermediate hosts. Infective metacercariae develop in 3 weeks after infection of the grasshopper. Sheep and goats are infected by eating infected grasshoppers. After ingestion the immature flukes migrate via the pancreatic duct into the pancreas. The prepatent period in sheep and cattle is 80–100 days. Infection produces a catarrhal inflammation with destruction of the duct epithelium. Eggs may penetrate into the walls of the ducts causing granuloma. Occasionally fibrosis may produce atrophy of the parenchyma.

Geographic distribution: Eastern Asia, Brazil, Madagascar, Réunion

Symptoms: Severely infected animals may be poor in condition. Heavily infected sheep show chronic wasting condition and increased mortality.

Significance: This parasite is not a serious threat unless a herd is heavily infected.

Diagnosis: There are no obvious clinical signs. *Dicrocoelium*-like eggs appear in the faeces (☞ Cattle, ■ 1).

Therapy: The therapy is is difficult. Praziquantel (20 mg/kg, po. for 2 days) has been reported to be effective.

Prophylaxis: As for *Dicrocoelium*, the control of intermediate hosts is not feasible.

(Figure 367)

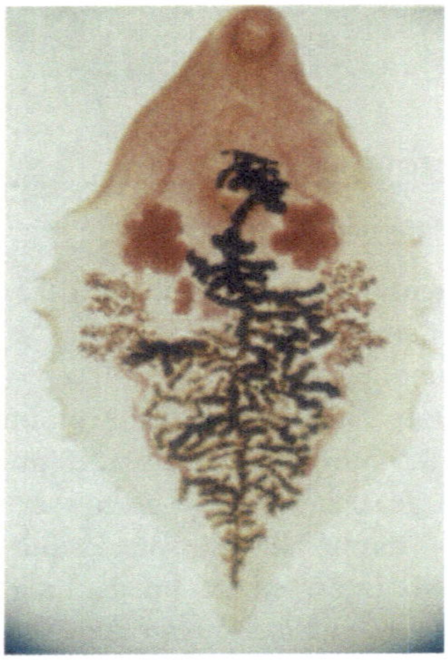

Fig. 367 *Eurytrema pancreaticum*; adult fluke (8–16 × 5–8.5 mm; stained) [4]

4.6 Central nervous system

HELMINTHS

Toxoplasma gondii

Remarks: Tissue cysts of this parasite may occasionally be found in the brain of sheep and cattle (☞ CATTLE, ■ 4.6). These cysts contain merozoites (6–8 µm long) and are infective for the final host (cat). Encephalomyelitis due to *T. gondii* infections may occur in sheep. Affected sheep have myelomalacia and schizonts appear in astrocytes (☞ SWINE, ■ 4.1).

Neospora caninum

Remarks: Thick-walled tissue cysts of this parasite may occasionally be found in the brain of sheep and cattle (☞ CATTLE, ■ 4.6).

PROTOZOA

• Cestoda cysts found in the central nervous system

Coenurus cerebralis

Larval stage of the canine tapeworm *Taenia multiceps* (syn. *Multiceps multiceps*) "gid", "stuggers", "sturdy"

Location: The larval stage, a coenurus, develops in the brain and spinal cord of sheep and goats. In the goat the cysts may also reach maturity in other organs, intramuscularly and subcutaneously.

Hosts: Sheep and goat; adult *Taenia multiceps* occurs in the small intestine of the dog, fox, coyote, hyaena and other Canidae.

Species description: Adult tapeworms in dogs are 40–100 cm in length. Eggs measure 29–37 µm in diameter. Larvae develop in the brain into a large fluid-containing cyst, measuring 5–6 cm in diameter. The cyst contains several hundred protoscolices invaginated in clusters on the cyst wall. *Coenurus* cysts cause increased intracranial pressure which is the cause of the neurological symptoms.

Geographic distribution: World-wide; in Africa *C. cerebralis* was reported from Kenya, Ethiopia, Sudan, Angola, Tchad, Zaire, Congo, Senegal, northern and southern Africa.

Symptoms: Ataxia, hypermetria, blindness, head deviation, stumbling and paralysis. In sheep, palpation of the skull caudal to the horn buds may reveal rarefaction of the skull.

Significance: *C. cerebralis* may account for remarkable losses among small ruminants in endemic areas. The disease must be differentiated from other conditions associated with nervous signs.

Diagnosis: Clinical symptoms are not specific. Diagnosis is often made at necropsy.

Therapy: The therapy is difficult. However, surgery to remove the cysts which are located on the surface of the brain, has a reasonable chance of success and may be justified in valuable animals.

Prophylaxis: Dogs associated with livestock should not be fed the heads of infected animals and should be dewormed regularly. Praziquantel (5 mg/kg, po. or 5.7 mg/kg, sc. or im.), bunamidine hydrochloride (25–50 mg/kg, po.), nitroscanate (50 mg/kg, po.) and the combination of febantel/praziquantel/pyrantel are sufficiently effective against adult *Taenia multiceps* in dogs. Some benzimidazoles administered for a few days may eliminate both nematodes and cestodes: fenbendazole (50 mg/kg, po. during 3 days) or mebendazole (2 × 100 mg/animal/day during 5 subsequent days for dogs > 2 kg body weight).
(Figure 368)

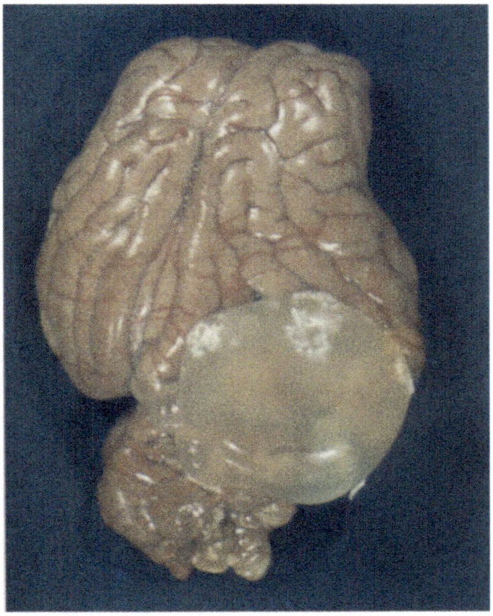

Fig. 368 *Coenurus cerebralis*; cyst in the brain of a sheep

5 Stages on the body surface

5.1 Skin and coat

5.2 Eyes

5.1 Skin and coat

PROTOZOA

Besnoitia besnoiti (syn. *Sarcocystis besnoiti)*

Remarks: *Besnoitia* cysts are found in the dermis, subcutaneous tissue and fascia and in the laryngeal and nasal mucosae of cattle, goat, wildebeest, impala and kudu. Sheep may be experimental intermediate hosts. Definitive hosts are domestic and wild cats. *Besnoitia besnoiti* is a protozoan disease of the skin, subcutis, blood vessels and mucous membranes. These *Toxoplasma*-like organisms multiply in endothelial cells and produce characteristic large, thick-walled cysts filled with bradyzoites. The *Besnoitia* cysts may reach up to 600 μm in diameter (☞ CATTLE, ■ 5.1).

HELMINTHS

• Nematoda found in the skin

Onchocerca **spp.**

Remarks: Very little is known about filarial worms of the subcutaneous tissue of sheep and goats but there is some evidence that several species may occur. They seem to be of little significance and do not require control.

ARTHROPODS

Arthropods are divided into two main groups:

Arachnida
- *Ticks*
- *Mites*

Insecta
- *Lice*
- *Fleas*
- *Dipterida*

• Arachnida found in/on the skin

– Ticks

Sheep ticks are of great economic importance, but not to the extent that they are in cattle. These parasites cause tick worry, blood loss and damage at feeding sites. Wounds left from tick bites are susceptible to additional attack by blowflies. Infested sheep itch, bite and scratch causing self-inflicted wool damage and skin trauma which may become secondarily infected. Heavy tick burdens may result in anaemia, loss of appetite and weight loss (☞ Directly Noxious Effects). Some tick species cause tick paralysis (☞ Tick Toxicoses). Apart from the direct noxious effects ticks may act as vectors of a number of diseases in sheep such as louping ill, rickettsial tick-borne fever, Nairobi sheep disease, spirochaetosis, heartwater and Q fever. Ticks may therefore provoke disease in 3 different ways:

• **Direct noxious effects**
In sheep and goats ticks of the following genera and species have a direct noxious effect (☞ CATTLE, ■ 5.1):

IXODIDAE ("hard ticks")
Amblyomma spp.
Boophilus spp.
Dermacentor spp.
Haemaphysalis spp.
Hyalomma spp.
Ixodes spp.
Rhipicephalus spp.

ARGASIDAE ("soft ticks")
Otobius megnini The spinose ear tick

• **Transmission of diseases**
Some of the tick-borne parasitic infections are as follows (☞ SHEEP AND GOATS, ■ 2; general aspects ☞ CATTLE, ■ 5.1).

Babesia ovis
Tropical babesiosis of small ruminants

Remarks: It is transmitted by *Rhipicephalus bursa* and *Rhipicephalus evertsi.*

Babesia motasi *(syn. Piroplasma motasi)*
European piroplasmosis of small ruminants

Remarks: It is transmitted by *Haemaphysalis* spp. (*H. punctata, H. sulcata* and *H. parva*), *Dermacentor* spp. and *Rhipicephalus bursa.*

Theileria hirci *(syn. T. lestoquardi)*
Malignant theileriosis of small ruminants

Remarks: It is transmitted by *Rhipicephalus bursa* and *Hyalomma anatolicum* and other species to be determined.

Theileria ovis Benign theileriosis of small ruminants

Remarks: It is transmitted by *Rhipicephalus bursa* and *Rhipicephalus evertsi.*

Anaplasma ovis Tropical anaplasmosis of small ruminants

Remarks: It is transmitted by *Rhipicephalus bursa* and *Rhipicephalus evertsi* in tropical Africa; transplacental infection occurs.

Eperythrozoon ovis

Remarks: This species occurs on the erythrocyte surface. It is transmitted by *Linognathus ovillus* and possibly also by ticks (*Hyalomma marginatum* and *Rhipicephalus bursa*).

Cowdria ruminantium Heartwater, Tyewde

Remarks: The infection is transmitted by *Amblyomma hebraeum* and *Amblyomma variegatum* (☞ CATTLE, ■ 2).

Ehrlichia ovina Tropical ehrlichiosis of small ruminants

Remarks: The parasite is transmitted by *Rhipicephalus bursa* in Mediterranean basin and *Rhipicephalus evertsi* in tropical Africa.

Ehrlichia phagocytophila European ehrlichiosis

Remarks: *Ixodes ricinus* transmits the disease by trans-stadial infection.

• **Tick Toxicosis**

Tick paralysis
Lambs and calves are particularly susceptible to tick paralysis. *Ixodes rubicundus* (the Karoo paralysis tick) mainly affects sheep and goats and *Rhipecephalus evertsi* causes the "spring lamb paralysis" in lambs but also in calves. Worldwide several species of the genera *Amblyomma, Dermacentor* and *Ixodes* are associated with tick paralysis in sheep (Table 15). This condition can be fatal within several days if the parasites are not removed. The paralysis is caused by toxins injected by female ticks while they suck blood. Cases of tick paralysis are reported from most regions

of the world. The most common tick species which cause tick paralysis are listed in Table 15 (☞ CATTLE, ■ 5.1)
(Figures 369, 370)

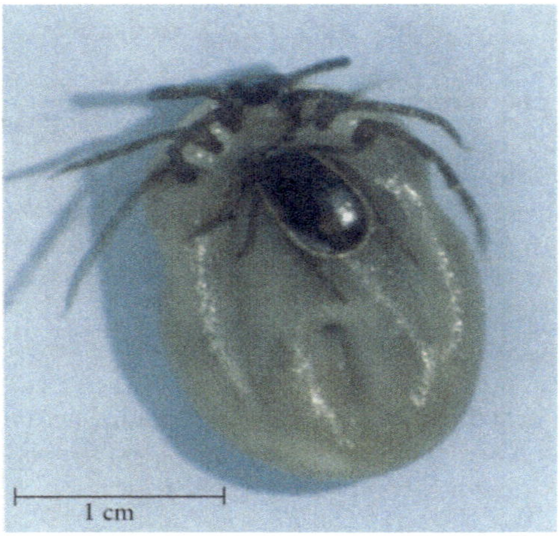

Fig. 369 *Ixodes ricinus*; engorged female and male [4]

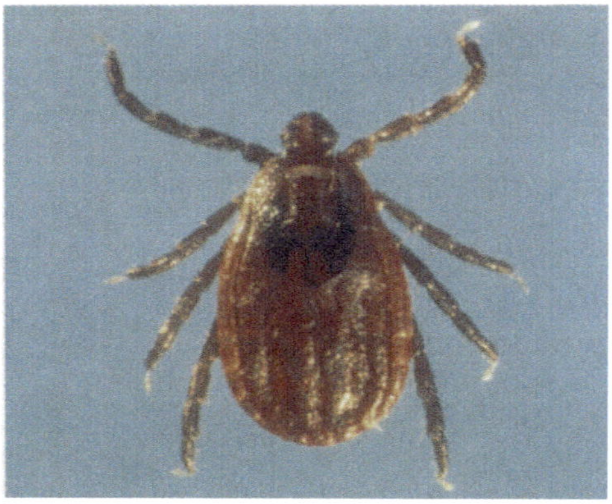

Fig. 370 *Haemaphysalis punctata*; female (3 × 2 mm) [4]

Table 15 The most common tick species causing tick paralysis in sheep

Tick species	Occurrence
Ixodes rubicundus	dry regions,southern Africa
Ixodes ricinus	Western Europe
Ixodes gibbosus	Mediterranean basin
Haemaphysalis punctata	Mediterranean basin
Haemaphysalis sulcata	Mediterranean basin
Rhipicehalus evertsi	East and southern Africa

Sweating sickness
It is mainly a disease of young calves but also sheep in eastern, central and southern Africa. The causative agents are certain strains of *Hyalomma truncatum* which produce an epitheliotropic toxin. Calf mortality may reach 70% (☞ Cattle, ■ 5.1).

General toxicosis
Toxicosis, associated with general disorders occurs with *Ornithodoros savignyi* (sand tampan) in young calves and lambs, especially when there are many bites. Animals show cutaneous oedema, haemorrhage, rapidly progressing weakness and prostration. Death can occur within 6 hours. Toxicosis may occur in recumbent animals, during rest (☞ Cattle, ■ 5.1).

- **Description of ticks affecting sheep and goats**

IXODIDAE (**"hard ticks"**)

A general description of each genus is made in CATTLE, ■ 5.1.

Table 16 Hard tick genera which are important for small ruminants:

Tick species	Geographic distribution
Amblyomma spp.	Central and southern Africa
Boophilus spp.	Warm climates throughout the world
Dermacentor spp.	North and southern Africa
Haemaphysalis spp	Throughout Europe, Asia, Africa
Hyalomma spp.	Southern UIS, Iran, Palaearctic region
Ixodes spp.	North and southern Africa
Rhipicephalus spp.	Africa south of the equator

ARGASIDAE (**"soft ticks"**)

Ornithodoros moubata The eyeless tampan

Remarks: This tick causes much trouble by feeding on sheep at their resting place in the pastures. It lives in the native huts and in the sand under trees where animals and human beings frequently seek shelter. In huts they live in cracks in the floor or under loose soil, from which they emerge at night to feed. In burrows they bury themselves in the earth lining, coming out to feed when a suitable host is available. Adult females lay batches of about 100 eggs and brood over the eggs in the sand. Development includes a larval stage which remains quiescent until it has moulted to the nymphal stage. Several nymphal stages are passed through and the nymphs, like the adults, attack their host for short periods to feed. This tampan sucks blood on its hosts. It is extremely resistant to both starvation and desiccation (survival time off the host up to 5 years).

Significance: In sheep *O. moubata* mainly causes irritation. It is also known to transmit the following diseases: *Borrelia duttoni* (relapsing fever of man), African swine fever, Q fever, *Borrelia anserina* and *Aegyptianella pullorum* in fowls.

(Figure 371)

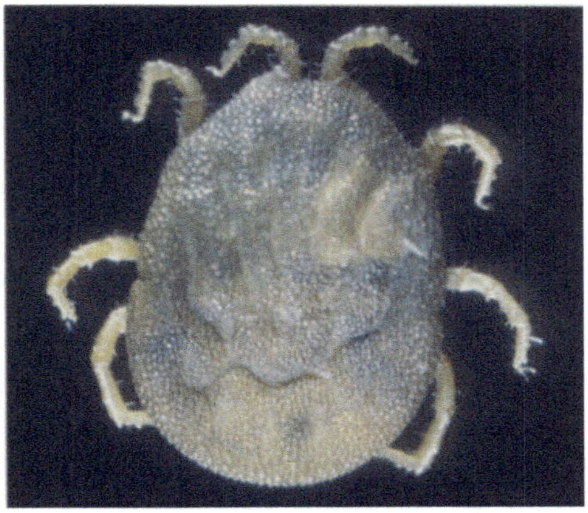

Fig. 371 *O. moubata*; dorsal view (8 mm long) [8]

Ornithodoros savignyi The sand tampan

Remarks: Its habits are similar to those of *O. moubata*. To the naked eye it is indistinguishable from the eyeless tampan. It occurs on man, camel, cattle, sheep and goats and many other animals (including birds). On standing cattle it feeds on the legs, especially, just above the hoofs.

Significance: *O. savignyi* is a major pest of domestic stock in areas in which it occurs. Its bites are extremely painful and it secretes toxins in its saliva that frequently cause death especially of calves, kids and lambs (tick toxicosis). Adult animals may also die from these toxic effects, especially when they have been attacked by large numbers of ticks. The sand tampan may cause severe allergic reactions in man.

Otobius megnini Spinose ear tick

Remarks: Larvae and nymphae feed deep in the external ear canal. Adults are non-parasitic and live on the ground. The spinose ear tick is a serious threat to sheep. Damage caused by the blood-sucking larvae and nymphs on the inside of the ears may result in marked debilitation, depressed appetite, restlessness and massive loss of weight in sheep. Weakness and anaemia may occur in heavy infestations. A waxy exudate is found in the ears (☞ CATTLE, ■ 5.1).

- **Tick control in sheep and goat**

(☞ CATTLE, ■ 5.1 THERAPY AND PROPHYLAXIS OF ECTOPARASITES [arachnids and insects])

– **Mites**

Psoroptes ovis The sheep scab mite

Location: Most areas of the body, especially those heavily wooled and haired such as shoulders, sides and back are affected.

Hosts: Sheep

Species description: The *Psoroptes* spp. occurring on domestic animals are all morphologically very much alike (☞ CATTLE, ■ 5.1). Mites pierce the skin to obtain lymph and cause an inflammatory reaction, resulting in the exudation of serum which coagulates on the skin surface. The irritation caused by the mites also makes the sheep bite and pull at the skin, thus aggravating the condition. In many countries sheep scab is a notifiable disease and controlled by the national veterinary authorities.

Geographic distribution: World-wide

Symptoms: Continuous scratching and rubbing occurs in affected flocks. Wool breaks may occur, leaving the skin exposed. Depression, loss of appetite, weight loss and death can occur in heavy infestations.

Significance: Psoroptic mange is highly contagious and spreads rapidly in flocks. Wool loss, weight loss and death may cause enormous losses throughout the world in sheep rearing enterprises.

Diagnosis: The diagnosis is based on identification of mites in skin scrapings.

Therapy: Ivermectin (200 µg/kg, sc.) is effective against psoroptic mange in sheep, although 2 injections with 7-day interval are required to eliminate mites. One injection is effective against *Sarcoptes* spp. and *Psorergates* spp. A single dipping in toxaphene (0.5–0.6%) eliminates all mites that affect sheep except *Psoroptes ovis*. Other approved dips effective against *Psoroptes ovis* and *Chorioptes ovis* are coumaphos (0.3%) and phosmet (0.2–0.25%), diazinon, fenvalerate and flumethrin. It is of fundamental importance that the entire flock is treated.

Prophylaxis: ☞ CATTLE, ■ 5.1 *Psoroptes bovis*

(Figures 372, 373)

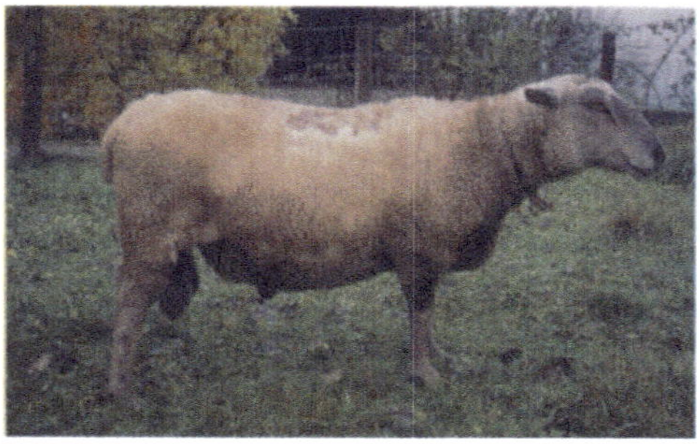

Fig. 372 infested with *Psoroptes ovis*; initial lesions on the back

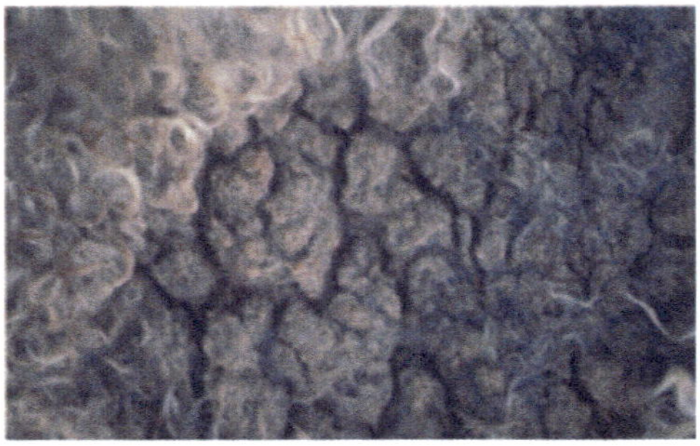

Fig. 373 Skin fissures caused by *Psoroptes ovis*; these wounds are often complicated by myiasis

Psoroptes caprae

Remarks: Some authors consider *P. caprae* to be a valid species of goats. Psoroptic mange of goats (ear mange of goats) especially of some breeds (Angora goats) in some parts of the world is considered to be *Psoroptes cuniculi*, which is known to infest the ears of domestic rabbits. Any of the acaricides approved for use as sheep dips will eliminate ear mange of goats.

Chorioptes ovis Chorioptic mange, "leg mange", "foot scab"

Location: Chorioptic mange is most often found on the hindlegs and between the toes, or on the scrotum of rams.

Hosts: Sheep

Species description: This is the most frequent type in sheep. General genus description is given in CATTLE, ■ 5.

Geographic distribution: World-wide

Symptoms: Infested sheep scratch and rub their feet. Localized scabs may be seen. The lesions are less severe and localized than in *Psoroptes ovis* infections.

Significance: Foot scab is not a major problem in sheep raising, but chronic infections of flocks may cause considerable indirect losses, due to restlessness, scratching, weight losses and secondary skin infections.

Diagnosis: The diagnosis is based on identification of mites in skin scrapings.

Therapy: ☞ above *Psoroptes ovis*

Prophylaxis: ☞ above *Psoroptes ovis*
(Figure 374)

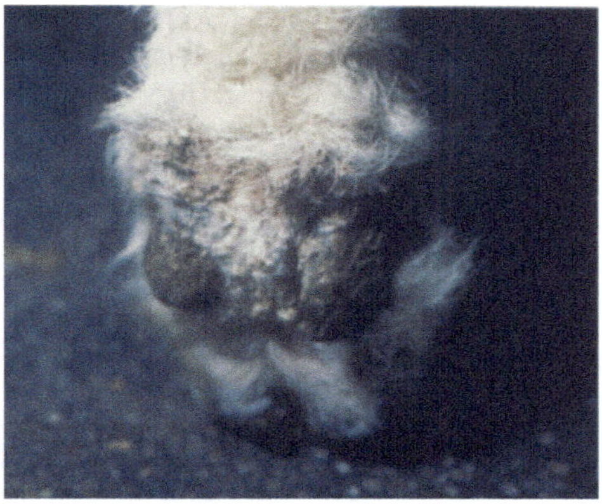

Fig. 374 Foot of a sheep infested with *Chorioptes ovis*; posterior view [15]

Sarcoptes ovis Sarcoptic mange

Location: This mite occurs mainly on non-wooly skin, starting usually at the head and face.

Hosts: Sheep

Species description: This species is rarely found. Genus description ☞ Cattle, ■ 5; *Sarcoptes bovis*. Female adults burrow tunnels in skin and lay eggs. All stages of sarcoptic mites are very susceptible to drying and can survive for only a few days off sheep.

Geographic distribution: World-wide

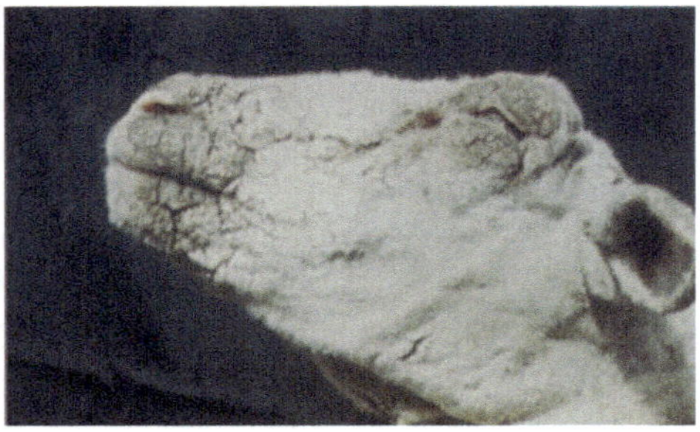

Fig. 375 Head of a sheep infested with *Sarcoptes ovis* [4]

Symptoms: Affected skin is thickened and crusts may be seen. Scratching and rubbing followed by wool loss may occur.

Significance: Sarcoptic mange is rarely a serious problem in wooled sheep.

Diagnosis: This is based on identification of mites in skin scrapings.

Therapy: ☞ above *Psoroptes ovis*

Prophylaxis: ☞ above *Psoroptes ovis*
(Figure 375)

Psorergates ovis Itch mite, "Australian-itch"

Location: Skin all over the body

Hosts: Sheep

Species description: This is a very minute mite, one-third the size (189 × 189 µm) of psoroptic mites. The mite is spherical and has paired claws and legs which are arranged radially. Especially fine-wooled sheep are affected. The adult mites spread by contact and are most often transferred between shorn sheep.

Geographic distribution: Australia, USA, New Zealand, South Africa

Symptoms: These mites cause severe irritation, leading to rubbing and biting at the fleece of sheep. Newly infected animals show more signs than chronically infested animals.

Significance: Itch mite is a serious problem in Merino sheep in Australia, causing great losses in wool production due to fleece derangement and low wool quality and quantity. Itch mites are also of great significance in South Africa.

Diagnosis: This is difficult because of the small size of the mites. Microscopical examination of skin scrapings may reveal these small mites. Sodium hydroxide liquefies debris in scrapings and may be helpful to detect the mites.

Therapy: Ivermectin (200 µg/kg, sc.) is highly effective against *Psorergates ovis*. A single injection usually kills all the mites. Dipping and spraying (☞ above *Psoroptes ovis*), especially after shearing is an important control measure.

Prophylaxis: Yearly dipping after shearing for

the control of the parasites will normally suppress the itch mite population. This will keep the infestation rate low but eradication is difficult to be achieved.
(Figure 376)

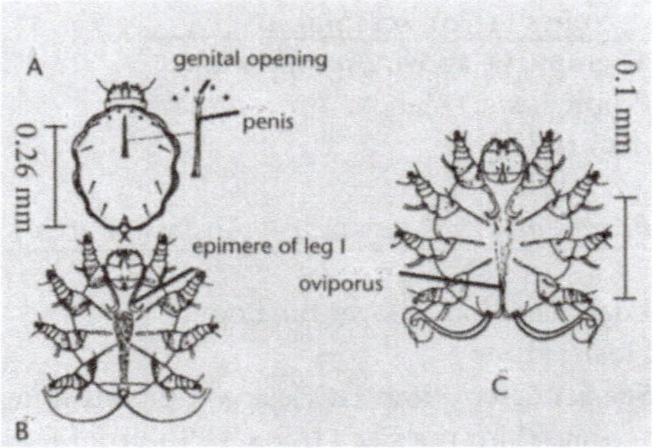

Fig. 376 *P. ovis* (schematic); (A) dorsal view of male with enlargement of penis and genital opening; (B) ventral view of a male; (C) ventral view of female [29]

***Demodex* spp. (*D. ovis* and *D. caprae*)**
Demodectic mite

Location: Hair follicles and sebaceous glands of skin. Favoured areas are eyelid, prepuce of male and vulva of female. Often-affected areas are also skin of the neck, shoulder, thorax, and flank.

Hosts: Sheep and goat

Species description: The nodules produced by this cigar-shaped mite (genus description ☞ CATTLE, ■ 5.1) range in size from pinhead to hazelnut, contain a thick, waxy, greyish material that can easily be expressed. Numerous demodectic mites are found in this material. There is some evidence that *Demodex* are normally found in and on the healthy skin and that they may resume increased significance when the host animal is immunosuppressed.

Geographic distribution: World-wide

Symptoms: Nodules occur in the skin. The nodules of goats appear as cysts with mild inflammation in the surrounding tissue.

Significance: Demodectic mange in goats may cause considerable losses due to damage of the hides.

Diagnosis: Numerous demodectic mites are found in the contents of skin nodules. However, there is some evidence that *Demodex* may be present in normal healthy skin without apparent signs.

Therapy: There is no satisfactory treatment. Incision of the nodules and disinfection with tincture of iodine was described to give the best therapeutic results in valuable goats. Organophosphates may also be used.

Prophylaxis: Unknown
(Figure 377)

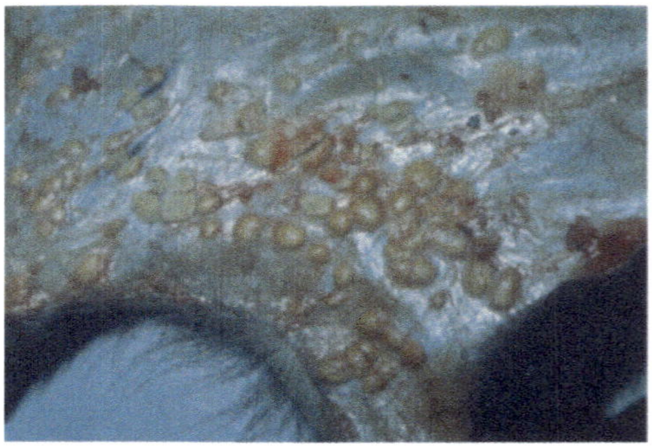

Fig. 377 *Demodex caprae* in subcutaneous nodules of a goat (0.5–1.5 cm in diameter) [4]

***Raillietia* spp. (*R. auris* and *R. caprae*)**

Location: Middle and inner ear

Hosts: Sheep (*R. auris*), goat (*R. caprae*) and cattle

Species description: The mites feed on epidermal cells and wax but not on blood.

Geographic distribution: North America, Australia, East Africa, Europe.

Symptoms: Infestations are usually inapparent but otitis media and interna with nervous signs, including head shaking, head rotation to the affected side, circling, general incoordination, can be found in a progressive stage of the infestation.

Significance: *Raillietia* spp. infections can cause signs similar to those found in other CNS infections and should therefore be excluded.

Diagnosis: It is almost impossible to diagnose *Raillietia* spp. antemortem; demonstration of the mites in the middle or inner ear at necropsy.

Therapy: Ivermectin may eliminate the mites but the diagnosis is difficult. Acaricides, applied topically, may also be effective.

Prophylaxis: Unknown (☞ CATTLE, ■ 5.1)

• Insecta found on the skin

– Lice

MALLOPHAGA Chewing lice

Lepikentron ovis Ovine chewing louse **and *Bovicola*** (syn. *Damalinia*) ***caprae*** Caprine chewing louse

Hosts: Sheep and goat

Location: Skin of the neck, withers and root of the tail

Species description: *Lepikentron ovis* is a small, wingless insect, 1–2 mm long. The head is broad and flat with mouth parts adapted to chewing. *Bovicola caprae* parasitises the common goat and *Bovicola crassipes* and *Bovicola limbatus* are found mainly on Angora goats.

Geographic distribution: World-wide

Symptoms: Infested sheep bite, scratch and show a poor body condition. Louse worry may produce low fleece quality.

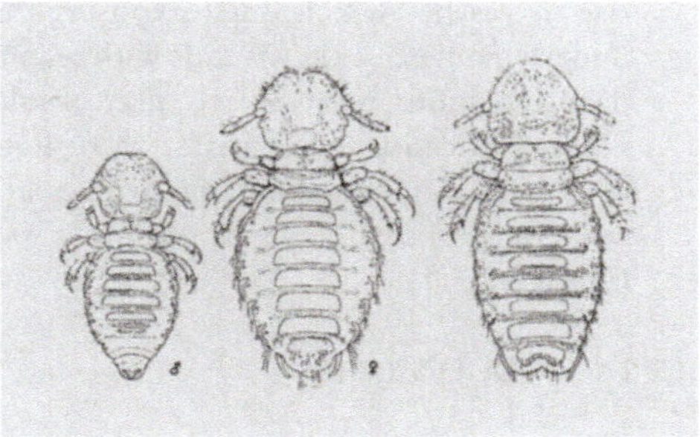

Fig. 378 Chewing lice (Mallophaga) of sheep and goats; (left) *Bovicola caprae* male (1 mm) and female (1.5–2 mm) and (right) *Bovicola bovis* (1.5–2 mm) [35]

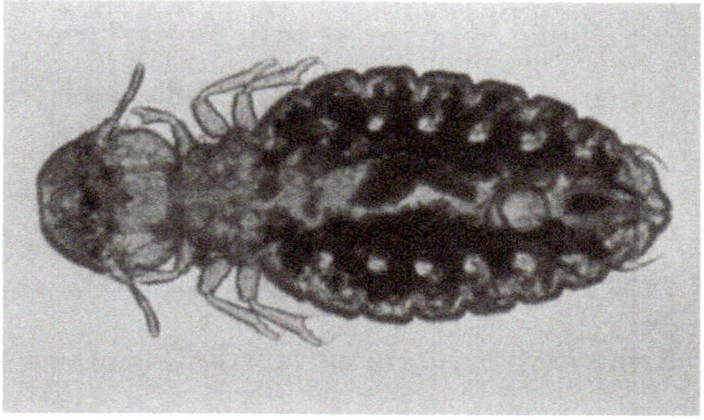

Fig. 379 *Bovicola caprae* (1–2mm) [4]

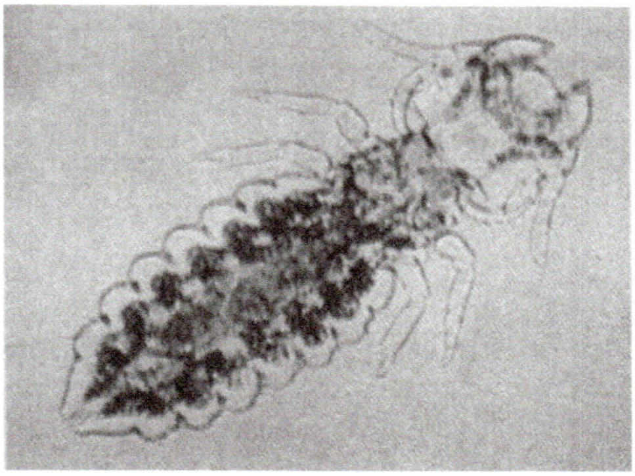

Fig. 380 *Lepikentron ovis* (1–2 mm) [32]

Significance: Louse worry may cause decreased food intake, reduced wool growth and the overall profitability may significantly be reduced.

Diagnosis: Nits and adults may be seen in fleece and on skin.

Therapy: ☞ CATTLE, ■ 5.1 THERAPY OF CHEWING LICE OF CATTLE

Prophylaxis: ☞ CATTLE, ■ 5.1

(Figures 378, 379, 380)

ANOPLURA Blood sucking lice of sheep and goats

Linognathus ovillus The sheep body louse, face louse

Remarks: It occurs chiefly on the face of sheep in Australia, New Zealand and probably many other parts of the world (☞ CATTLE, ■ 5.1).

Linognathus pedalis The sheep foot louse

Remarks: It occurs on legs, belly and feet where no wool exists.

Linognathus africanus The African sheep louse, the blue louse

Remarks: It occurs mainly on the face of sheep.

Linognathus stenopsis The goat sucking louse

Remarks: It occurs mainly on goats. (Figure 381)

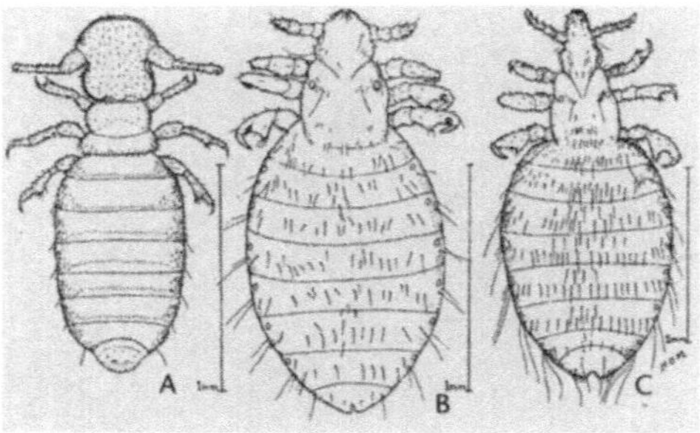

Fig. 381 Sheep lice; (A) *Lepikentron ovis*, (B) *Linognathus pedalis* and (C) *Linognathus africanus* [3]

- **General features of blood sucking lice of sheep and goats**

Species description: These are wingless insects with mouth parts adapted for piercing skin and sucking blood. The head is long and narrow. The entire life cycle is spent on the host. Lice may survive in warm environments for up to 25 days in the absence of their host.

Geographic distribution: *Linognathus* spp. occur in many parts of the world.

Symptoms: Scratching, rubbing and biting are seen in heavy infestations. Wool breaks and general unthriftiness, matted, dull fleece with tufts of loose wool may indicate lice infestation.

Significance: Heavily infested animals have markedly reduced weight gain and wool growth.

Diagnosis: Presence of nits on wool and adult lice on skin.

Therapy: ☞ ■ CATTLE, 5.1 THERAPY OF SUCKING LICE OF CATTLE p. 129

Prophylaxis: This is difficult wherever direct contact between the animals of the herd is possible. If sheep and goats are kept in sheds these may also be fumigated.

– Fleas

No fleas have been found on the body surface of sheeps and goats.

– Dipterida

CULICIDAE Mosquitoes

Remarks: With a single pair of wings, they belong, like flies, to the order Diptera. The main genera are *Anopheles, Culex* and *Aedes.* They are important vectors of diseases of sheep (e.g. Rift Valley fever, Lumpy skin disease, Blue tongue) (☞ CATTLE, ■ 5.1).

SIMULIIDAE

Simulium spp. Black flies, midges

Remarks: Simulids cause severe irritation to livestock when they occur in large numbers and herds and flocks will stampede, often with disastrous results. Bites are inflicted on all parts of the body, giving rise to vesicles which burst exposing the underlying flesh. Skin wounds with secondary infections and myiasis may result. Black flies cause severe irritation of livestock and certain areas of the tropics are rendered uninhabitable by simulids. (☞ Cattle, ■ 5.1)

CERATOPOGONIDAE

Culicoides spp. Biting midges

Remarks: Very small size (1–3 mm long). Adult female midges attack cattle, sheep, poultry, horse, man and other species, causing marked irritation by penetration of the skin with their proboscis. The bites cause intense itching. Biting midges cause massive irritation of livestock and transmit the Blue tongue virus to sheep (☞ CATTLE, ■ 5.1).

TABANIDAE

Tabanus **spp.,** ***Haematopota*** **spp. and** ***Chrysops*** **spp.** Horse flies

Remarks: Several species of horse flies attack sheep and goats. They may cause irritation (stampeding of flocks may result) and transmit a number of diseases to livestock (besnoitiosis, anaplasmosis, trypanosomosis and anthrax; ☞ ■ CATTLE, 5.1).

MUSCIDAE

Musca **spp.,** ***Lyperosia*** **spp. and** ***Haematobia*** **spp.** Muscid flies

Remarks: Muscid flies annoy livestock especially during the summer or rainy season. They swarm around farm livestock. The resulting irritation is incessant and much of the energy of the animals is lost to defend against fly attacks. In addition to the nuisance the flies often carry pathogens on their feet and bodies. Some also act as intermediate hosts for other parasites. Two genera need to receive special attention: *Musca* and *Haematobia*.

Musca domestica Common house fly

Remarks: This is a non-biting muscid. It is attracted to wounds and other moist parts of the body, especially the eyes where it may provoke an ulcerative dermatitis. *M. domestica* is known to transfer pathogenic bacteria mechanically from one wound to another (☞ CATTLE, ■ 5.1).

Haematobia minuta **and other** ***Haematobia*** **spp.** Horn flies, buffalo flies

Remarks: These are biting muscids. The adults of this fly live almost permanently on cattle, buffalo sheep and other animals. They congregate on the back where their bites cause severe irritation so that the cattle rub themselves raw. *Haematobia* spp. cause intense worry and irritation to animals, the bite being very painful. Serious blood loss may occur when large numbers attack and loss of condition, reduced performance is a common result. The flies cause sores at the basis of the horns, on the poll, ears, neck, withers and tail root (☞ CATTLE, ■ 5.1).

Stomoxys calcitrans Stable fly

Remarks: *S. calcitrans* also belongs to the muscids. It attacks almost all livestock species. It is a biting muscid and occurs worldwide. Both sexes of this fly are bloodsuckers and can become extremely irritating pests of man and domestic animals. Their salivary secretions cause toxic reactions with an immunosuppressive effect, rendering the host more susceptible to diseases. *S. calcitrans* acts as vector of *Trypanosoma evansi*, *Anthrax*, *Dermatophilus congolensis*, the "lumpy wool" in sheep and other pathogens (☞ ■ CATTLE, 5.1). Its painful bite causes intense worry and irritation to animals. It may produce toxic reactions and immunosuppression. Blood loss may be marked following continuous, heavy attacks.

GLOSSINIDAE

Glossina **spp.** Tsetse flies

Remarks: Tsetse flies are active during the day time and hunt by sight and smell. Both sexes suck blood and are equally capable of transmitting trypanosomes. Trypanosomosis in domestic animals is caused by *T. congolense*, *T. vivax*, *T. brucei* and *T. simiae* (☞ CATTLE, ■ 5.1).

Oestrus ovis Sheep nasal bot, nasal myiasis (☞ SHEEP AND GOATS, ■ 4.3).

CALLIPHORIDAE The blowflies and their allies

They are highly important in many domestic animal species and man. The adults are free-living and the larvae are parasitic maggots which develop in the tissue of their host, causing a condition called myiasis. The larvae may be laid into preexisting wounds. Myiasis is often a secondary skin problem. Calliphoridae can be divided into groups: **metallic** and **non-metallic flies**.

Metallic flies are green, blue or purplish coloured and belong to the genera *Chrysomya*, *Lucilia* and *Calliphora* (blowflies, bottle flies).

Lucilia cuprina and other *Lucilia* spp. Green-bottle or copper-bottle flies

Remarks: *L. cuprina* is the predominant cause of sheep blowfly strike in South Africa and Australia. It causes myiasis in sheep. It is the most important primary blowfly initiating strikes on living sheep. Sheep are only attacked by primary blowflies if moisture is present in the fleece with resulting bacterial decomposition of the wool and superficial skin layers known as "fleece-rot". The odour arising from such processes attracts the primary blowflies, which liquefy the tissue and extend the process. The larvae of the primary blowflies, which initiate the attack, create conditions attractive to secondary blowflies.
(Figures 382, 383)

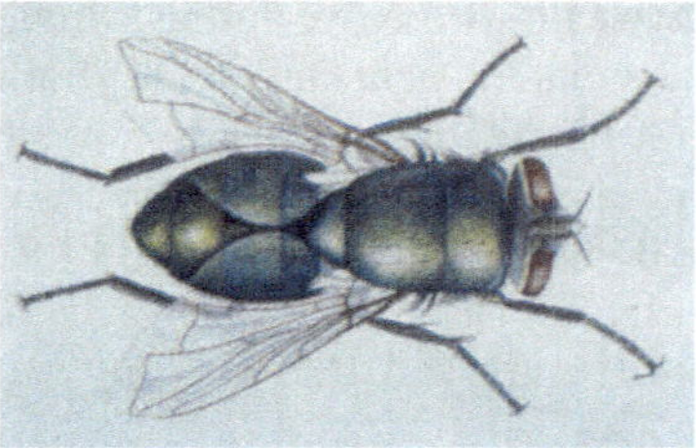

Fig. 382 *Lucilia cuprina*; adult (8–10 mm) [27]

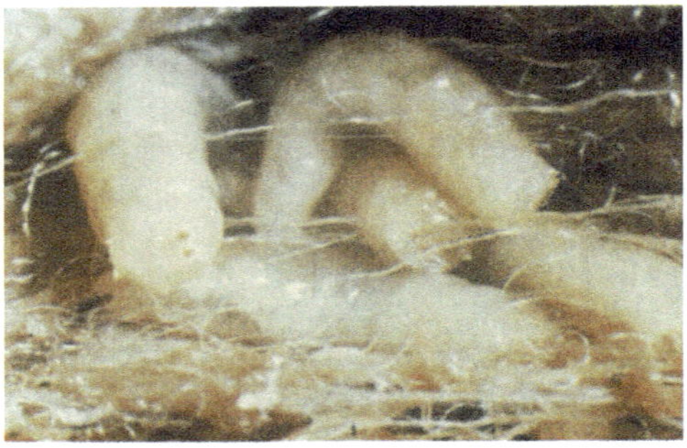

Fig. 383 *Lucilia cuprina*; praepupae in a skin wound of a sheep (10–20 mm)

Lucilia sericata Green bottle fly

Remarks: *L. sericata* is the predominant cause of sheep blowfly strike world-wide. *Lucilia* spp. lay eggs in areas of skin with constant moisture (the breech and tail). *Lucilia* spp. are the first flies to strike living sheep. Prolonged wet weather may cause

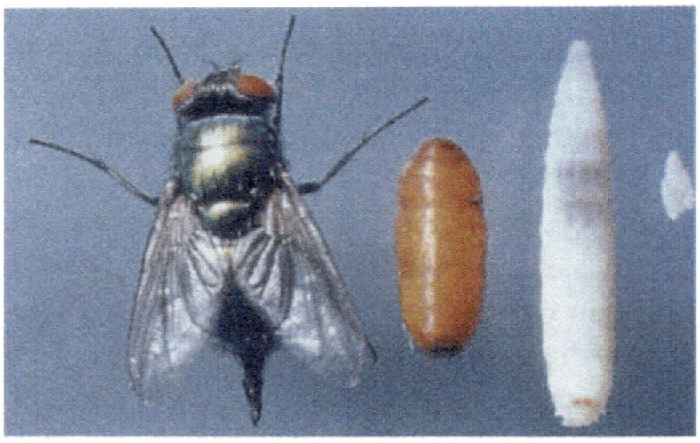

Fig. 384 *Lucilia sericata*; adult (8–9 mm; left) and pupa, larva, eggs (right) [4]

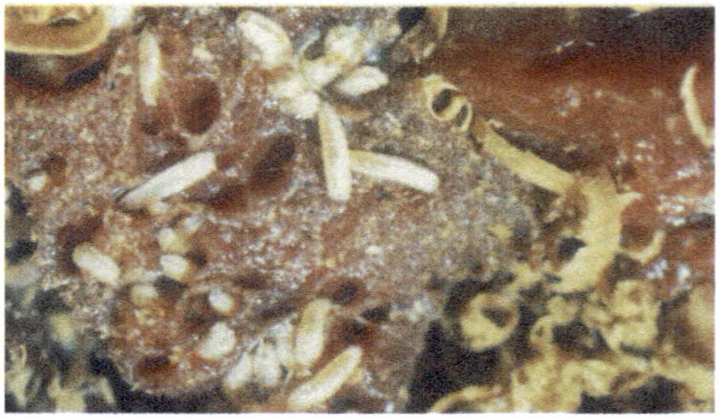

Fig. 385 *Lucilia sericata*; larvae (1.5–2 cm) in a skin wound

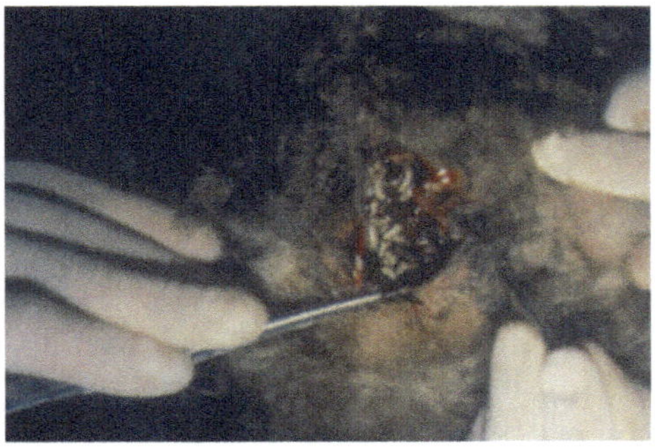

Fig. 386 *Lucilia sericata*; myiasis of a skin wound [11]

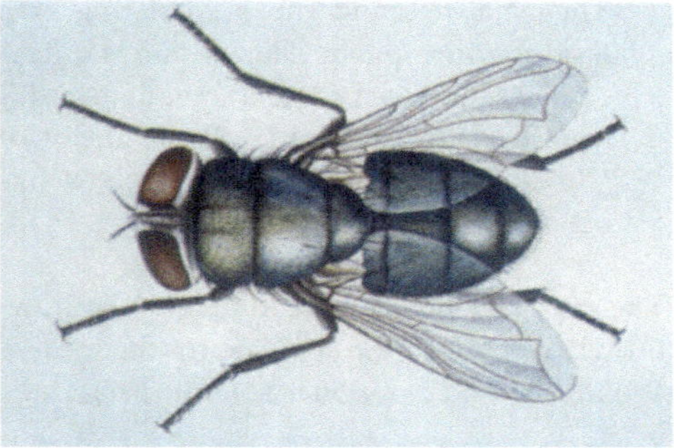

Fig. 388 *Chrysomya albiceps* [27]

Lucilia to strike sheep in the wool of the back. These flies are responsible for more losses than any other single parasite of sheep.
(Figures 384, 385, 386)

Chrysomya chloropyga Green-tailed blowfly

Remarks: This is probably the second important primary blowfly of sheep in South Africa. *Chrysomya marginalis* may also act as a primary blowfly.
(Figure 387)

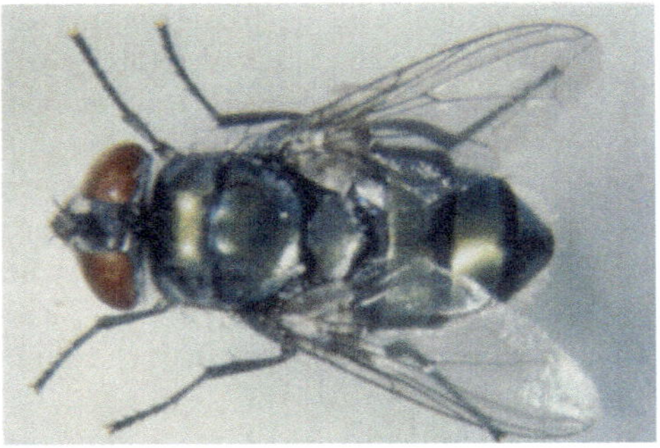

Fig. 387 *Chrysomya chloropyga*; adult (10–12 mm) [10]

Chrysomya albiceps **and other** ***Chrysomya*** **spp.**
(Figure 388)

Calliphora **spp.** Bluebottle flies

Remarks: Large flies (12 mm) metallic blue in colour with stout bodies. Adult flies attack existing skin wounds, e.g. from castration, tail docking or wounds affected by primary blowflies. They may extend these wounds in which bacterial infections have already started. They cause severe myiasis. *Calliphora* blowflies may kill sheep and cause great losses world-wide.

Callitroga hominivorax (syn. *Cochliomyia hominivorax*) "American screwworm"

Remarks: *C. hominivorax* has recently been found to occur also in North Africa. Cattle, pigs and equines suffer most frequently, but other animals, including fowls and even man may also be affected. Pathology is essentially the same as in *C. bezziana* (☞ CATTLE, ■ 5.1).

Chrysomyia rufifacies Screwworm fly, carrion fly

Remarks: Flies are 8–10 mm long and bluish-green. Larvae are up to 14 mm long with thorn-like spines. This blowfly strikes sheep after primary infestations which are established by *Lucilia* spp. and *Calliphora* spp. They may weaken and kill sheep. If sheep are struck by *Chrysomyia* spp., death will usually follow.

They may expand the pre-existing skin lesions enormously. The wound is infected by secondary bacterial invaders and is usually foul-smelling. Resistance of *Chrysomyia* to several insecticides has been reported.

The non-metallic flies are dull grey, yellow-brown or black and belong to the genera *Wohlfartia* and *Sarcophaga* (flesh-flies).

Sarcophaga haemorrhoidalis Red-tailed flesh-fly

Remarks: The fly is very common in Africa south of the Sahara and is frequently found around human habitations. Flies of this species are larviparous and may lay their larvae in wounds or sores although larvae may also be deposited on faeces, carrion or fresh meat. Several animal species and man may be affected. The fly may cause myiasis, especially in sheep.

Wohlfartia magnifica Old World flesh-fly

Remarks: It occurs in North Africa. The fly attacks man and other animals. The larvae may be deposited into the external ear of man or in sores around the eyes.

Cordylobia anthropophaga Tumbu fly or "skin maggot fly"

Remarks: The fly is widely distributed in Africa south of the Sahara. It produces myiasis in man, dogs and domestic animals. Eggs are laid around places where animals lie. After hatching the larvae penetrate the skin of the host, producing a boil of about 1 cm across with a hole in the centre. When mature the larvae wriggle out of the hole and pupate on the ground. Tumbu boils are found commonly on the ventral parts of the body but also on any other area of the body.

HIPPOBOSCIDAE The louse flies

Melophagus ovinus Sheep ked

Location: Skin on the neck, shoulders and belly
Hosts: Sheep
Species description: The sheep ked is a wingless fly living permanently on sheep. The legs are strong with claws at the end. Adult females deposit larvae on wool using an adhesive material. Larvae remain in place and molt to the pupal stage. Pupae last 19–23 days in summer and 36 days in winter. These pupae are resistant to treatment. The ked is a blood sucker and can cause anaemia if it is present in high numbers. They cause severe irritation so that infested sheep rub, bite and scratch themselves continuously. The piercing mouth parts of keds open wounds susceptible to further bacterial and parasitic (myiasis) infections. *Trypanosoma melophagium* is a non-pathogenic trypanosome which infects sheep. It belongs to the Stercoraria and is transmitted by the sheep ked, *Melophagus ovinus*. Infection occurs by contamination of the skin and if a ked is eaten by the sheep, the metacyclic stages penetrate the buccal mucosa.
Geographic distribution: World-wide
Symptoms: Intense itching from irritation causes sheep to rub, bite and scratch themselves and tearing the fleece. Heavy infestation may cause anaemia.
Significance: The sheep ked causes marked irritation with reduced grazing and fleece quality. It may further cause anaemia when present in high numbers.
Diagnosis: Adults and pupae may be seen on sheep.
Therapy: Insecticides which are also used to treat lice infestations may be applied. Dips, sprays, pour-on formulations may be used. Organophosphates and pyrethroids applied as dips, sprays or pour on are highly effective. (☞ CATTLE, ■ 5.1 THERAPY AND PROPHYLAXIS OF ECTOPARASITES, p. 141.

Prophylaxis: Shearing removes pupae and adults and should be carried out before lambing. A subsequent insecticidal treatment may eliminate the remaining ked (☞ CATTLE, ■ 5.1 THERAPY AND PROHYLAXIS OF ECTOPARASITES p. 141).
(Figure 389)

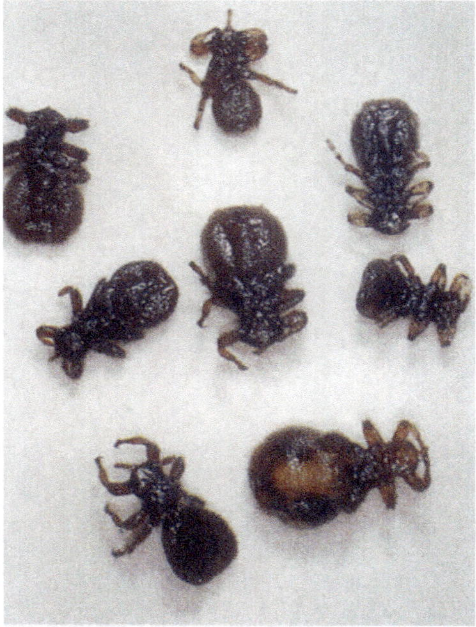

Fig. 389 *Melophagus ovinus* (3–5 mm) [32]

5.2 Eyes

Thelazia rhodesi Eyeworm

(☞ CATTLE, ■ 5.2)

IV

Parasites of Horses and Donkeys

CONTENTS

1 Stages in the gut and faeces

PROTOZOA

Eimeria leuckarti (syn. *Globidium leuckarti*)
Globidiosis

Location: Small intestine
Hosts: Horse and donkey
Species description: *E. leuckarti* oocyst is one of the largest of the genus *Eimeria* (80–88 × 55–59 µm) oval, thick wall, dark brown, distinct micropyle. Sporulation time is 20–22 days at 20°C.
Geographic distribution: World-wide
Symptoms: Acute and chronic diarrhoea
Significance: Little is known but serious diarrhoeic episodes have been attributed to massive infection with this parasite mainly in foals.
Diagnosis: *E. leuckarti* is too dense to rise in the flotation fluid usually used in the diagnostic laboratory and must be looked for by the sedimentation technique.
Therapy: Sulfonamids such as sulfadimidine (sulfamethazine, 220 mg/kg, po. or iv.), sulfadimethoxine (55 mg/kg, po.), sulfathiazole (66 mg/kg, po.) and the poorly soluble sulfaguanidine can be used against globidiosis.
Prophylaxis: Regular change of the feeding and holding area or disinfection of the stable reduces the infection risk.
(Figure 390, Table 1)

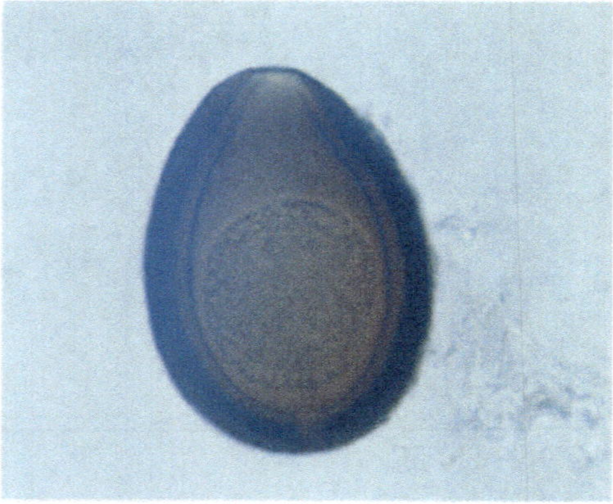

Fig. 390 Oocyst of *Eimeria leuckarti* (80–88 × 55–59 µm) [4]

Cryptosporidium parvum

Remarks: This species has only been found in immunodeficient foals (☞ CATTLE, 1).

HELMINTHS

(Figure 391)

- Trematoda eggs found in the faeces and adult trematodes living in the gastro-intestinal tract

Gastrodiscus aegyptiacus
Equine intestinal fluke

Location: Colon and small intestine
Hosts: Equine, pig and warthog
Species description: *G. aegyptiacus* belongs to the family Paramphistomatidae. Intermediate hosts are snails of the genus *Bulinus* and *Cleopatra*. Infection is acquired by eating metacercariae with vegetation.
Geographic distribution: Throughout Africa and India

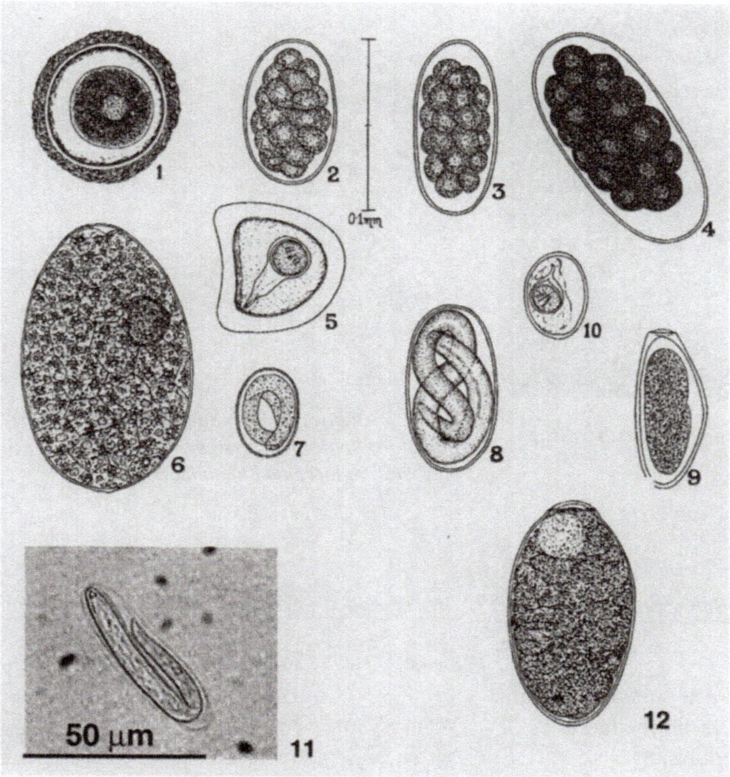

Fig. 391 Eggs of helminths found in equines [3]:

1 *Parascaris equorum*
2 *Strongylus* spp.
3 *Trichonema* spp.
4 *Triodontophorus tenuicollis*
5 *Anoplocephala* spp.
6 *Gastrodiscus aegyptiacus*
7 *Strongyloides westeri*
8 *Dictyocaulus arnfieldi*
9 *Oxyuris equi*
10 *Paranoplocephala mamillana*
11 *Habronema* spp.
12 *Fasciola hepatica*

Symptoms: Heavy infections are accompanied by diarrhoea, anaemia, oedema, emaciation and marked weakness. With the usual chronic mild infection there is no apparent effect on the host.

Significance: Adults have a relatively low level of pathogenicity. High numbers of immature flukes can cause severe problems. High numbers of *G. aegyptiacus* were found in horses in Central Africa.

Diagnosis: The diagnosis is based on the presence of eggs or immature flukes in the fluid faeces, and history of being kept on marshy pastures.

Therapy: The following compounds are effective against trematodes and can be considered for treatment: oxyclozanide, diamphenethide, rafoxanide, nitroxynil, albendazole, closantel, triclabendazole, netobimin and clorsulon. Some of these are active against immature flukes: diamphenethide (100 mg/kg), nitroxynil (15 mg/kg), closantel (10 mg/kg), triclabendazole (10 mg/kg) and clorsulon (7 mg/kg).

Prophylaxis: In addition to treatment of infected horses, wet pastures and swamps should be avoided. Horses should be watered with fresh water at bore holes.

(Figure 392)

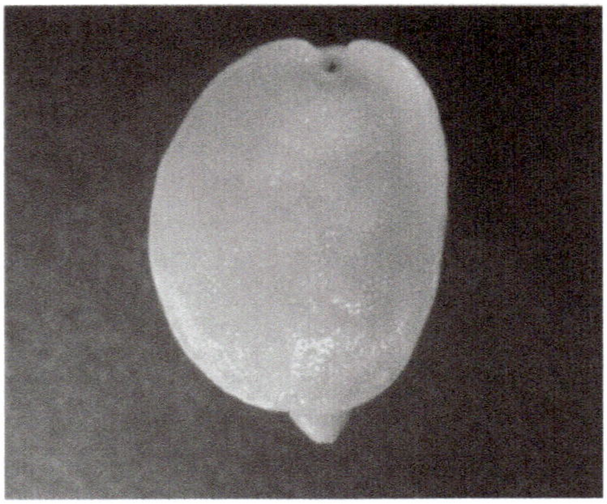

Fig. 392 *Gastrodiscus aegyptiacus*; ventral view (9–17 mm long)

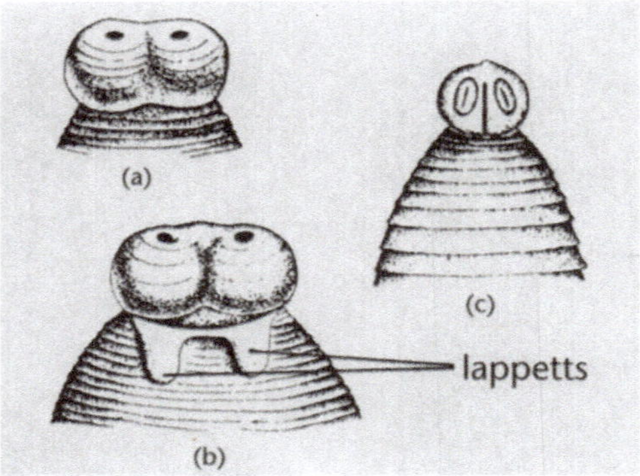

Fig. 393 Anterior end of equine tapeworms (schematic): *Anoplocephala magna* (a), *A. perfoliata* (b) and *Paranoplocephala mamillana* (c) [5]

Schistosoma bovis and *Schistosoma mattheei*
Blood flukes

Location: Adult flukes in the mesenteric and portal veins, eggs occur in the faeces. (☞ Horses and Donkeys, 2)

Characteristics	*A. magna*	*A.perfoliata*	*P.mamillana*
Length	80 cm (long)	8 cm (short)	0.6–5.0 cm (minute)
Width	2 cm	0.8–1.4 cm	0.5 cm
Sucker	Round	Round	Slit-like
Ear-shaped lappets posterior to suckers	Absent	Present	Absent

Fig. 394 Description of equine tapeworms [5]

- Cestoda eggs found in the faeces and adult cestodes living in the gastrointestinal tract

Anoplocephala magna Equine tapeworm

Location: Small intestine
Hosts: Horse and donkey
Species description: *A. magna* is the largest tapeworm of equines. It is up to 80 cm long and 2 cm wide and has a typical tapeworm shape.
Significance: *A. magna* in high numbers can cause a catarrhal or haemorrhagic enteritis.
(Figures 393, 394, 395, 396, 397)

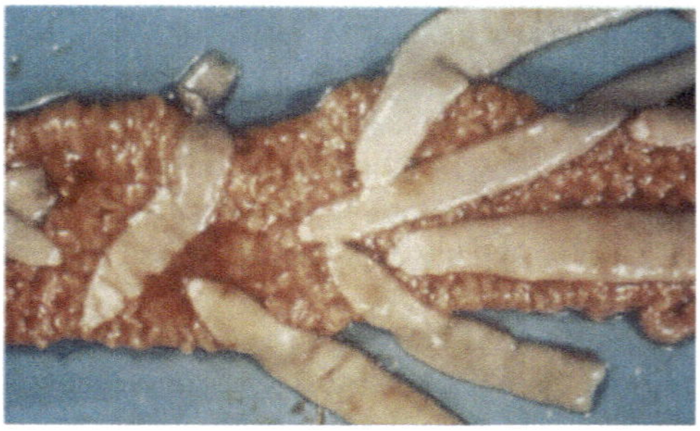

Fig. 395 *Anoplocephala magna*; adult tapeworms in the small intestine of a horse [15]

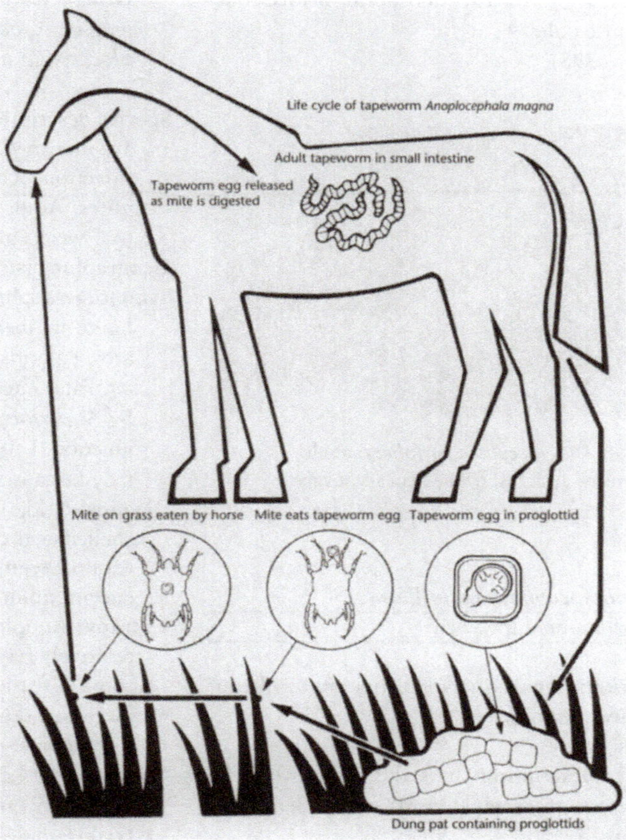

Fig. 396 Life cycle of equine tapeworms [36]

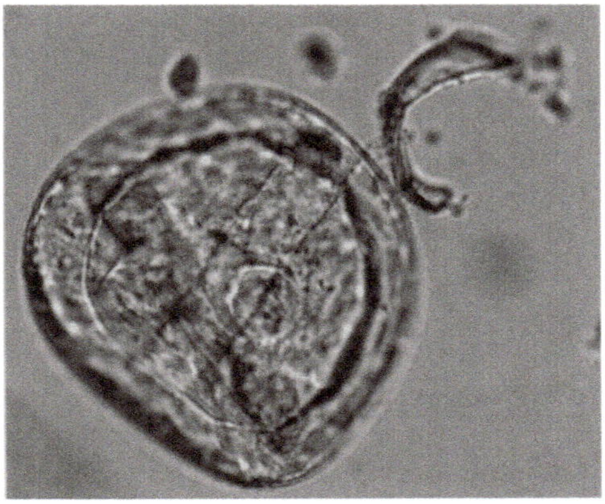

Fig. 397 Egg of *Anoplocephala* spp. (70–80 μm)

Anoplocephala perfoliata

Tapeworm of the ileocaecal-valve

Location: Large intestine, ileocaecal valve (found on either side)

Hosts: Horse and donkey

Species description: *A. perfoliata* varies from a few mm to 8 cm in length (some authors indicate length up to 30 cm) and looks at first sight more like a trematode. Closer inspection shows that the body is segmented, but the proglottids (segments) are crowded together. The scolex of *A. perfoliata* differs from the others in that there are prominent swellings (lappets) behind the suckers (Figure 393).

Significance: *A. perfoliata* normally causes little clinical effect but the site of attachment is often inflamed and ulcerated. Partial

occlusion of the ileocaecal orifice may cause colic.
(Figure 398)

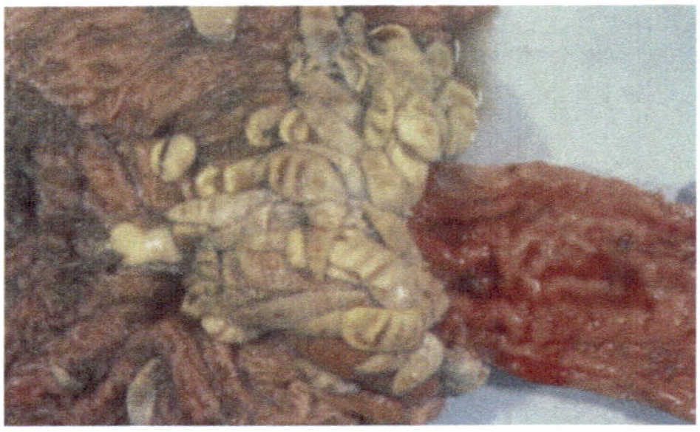

Fig. 398 *Anoplocephala perfoliata*; adult tapeworms attached to the ileocaecal valve

Paranoplocephala mamillana
Dwarf equine tapeworm

Location: Small intestine (jejunum, ileum) rarely stomach
Hosts: Horse
Species description: It is the smallest of the three equine tapeworms with a length of only 4 cm.
Significance: *P. mamillana* is seldom responsible for ill health.
(Figures 391, 393, 399)

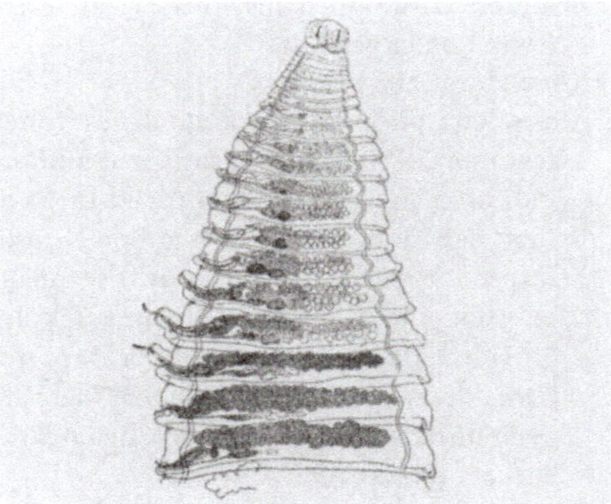

Fig. 399 *Paranoplocephala mamillana*; head and immature proglottids [9]

- **General features of *Anophocephala magna, A. perfoliata* and *Paranoplocephala mamillana***

Species description: Life cycle: Oribatid mites are intermediate hosts of all three species. Infection occurs via ingestion of infected mites. Adult tapeworms develop within 4 to 6 weeks after infection (Figure 396).
Geographic distribution: World-wide
Symptoms: Light infections are not apparent. Large numbers cause haemorrhagic or ulcerative enteritis, seen especially with *A. magna*. Fatal intestinal blockage may be caused by *A. perfoliata*, clustering at the ileocaecal junction. Unthriftiness, colic and diarrhoea may be caused by heavy infections.
Diagnosis: Identification of square, thick-shelled eggs containing the pyriform apparatus or segments in the faeces, or the presence of adult worms at necropsy.
Therapy: Anoplocephalidae are known to be relatively resistant to treatment. However, some of the modern anthelmintics, at increased dosage rates, are partially effective against equine tapeworms. Pyrantel pamoat (13.2 mg/kg, po.) at twice the label dosage is effective against *A. perfoliata*. Niclosamide (88 mg/kg, po.), fenbendazole (3 × 10 mg/kg, po.), resorantel (65 mg/kg, po.) and dichlorphen (20 mg/kg, po.), bithionol (7 mg/kg, po.) or mebendazole (20 mg/kg, po.) are safe and can also be used to treat equine tapeworms.
Prophylaxis: Prophylaxis is difficult as oribatid mites occur everywhere with densities of up to 20,000 per m^2.

- **Nematoda eggs found in the faeces, adult nematodes living in the gastrointestinal tract and first-stage larvae of *Dictyocaulus arnfieldi* and *Probsmayria vivipara***

Gongylonema pulchrum Gullet worm

Location: Mucosa of the oesophagus
Hosts: Horse, donkey and ruminants
Species description: *G. pulchrum* lies embed-

ded in the oesophageal mucosa in a zigzag fashion and reaches 14.5 cm in length. Eggs are passed in the faeces and hatch after being eaten by dung beetles in which the larvae develop to the infective stage. Infection of the horse occurs by eating the infected beetles (☞ CATTLE, ■ 1).

Geographic distribution: World-wide

Symptoms: Generally inapparent infections although chronic irritation of the mucosa occurs.

Significance: *G. pulchrum* is of little clinical importance.

Diagnosis: Eggs in the faeces or adults are seen at necropsy in longitudinal rows of circular raised thickenings on the worm's forward end.

Therapy: Not indicated

Prophylaxis: Manure removal and normal sanitary measures are sufficient to reduce the infection risk.

Parascaris equorum Horse roundworm

Location: Small intestine

Hosts: Horse and donkey

Species description: Typical direct nematode life cycle. Within the egg the second-stage larvae develop to infectivity on pasture in 6 weeks. When swallowed, larvae hatch and penetrate the intestinal wall and are carried by the blood to the lungs, where they migrate up to the trachea. They are then coughed up and swallowed again and mature in the small intestine. *P. equorum* are whitish worms up to 30 cm long with 3 prominent lips. The principal source of infection for young foals is contamination of pasture, paddock or stall with eggs from foals of the previous year.

Geographic distribution: World-wide

Symptoms: Adult worms in heavy infections can cause bile duct and intestinal obstructions and occasionally gut perforation. Damage is more pronounced in foals. Acute parascariasis is also accompanied by severe enteritis, resulting in alternating constipation and foul-smelling diarrhoea. Large numbers of larvae breaking into the lungs cause a "summer cold" with coughing, fever and anorexia. Mature horses rarely show clinical signs, as previous infections confer good resistance.

Significance: Highly important, mostly in foals younger than 6 months in which parascariosis causes severe debilitation, retarded growth and even death.

Diagnosis: Identification of round, pitted, thick-walled eggs in the faeces.

Therapy: Piperazine (88 mg/kg, po.) and thiabendazole (100 mg/kg, po.) are effective against adult worms. Cambendazole (20 mg/kg), febantel (6 mg/kg), fenbendazole (7.5 mg/kg), mebendazole (10 mg/kg), pyrantel pamoat (19 mg/kg) and ivermectin (0.2 mg/kg) for oral administration are effective against adult and larval stages of *P. equorum.*

Prophylaxis: As foals become infected with *P. equorum* soon after birth, treatment and/or prophylaxis should start when foals are about 8 weeks old and repeated at 6–8- week intervals, until they are yearlings.

(Figures 400, 401)

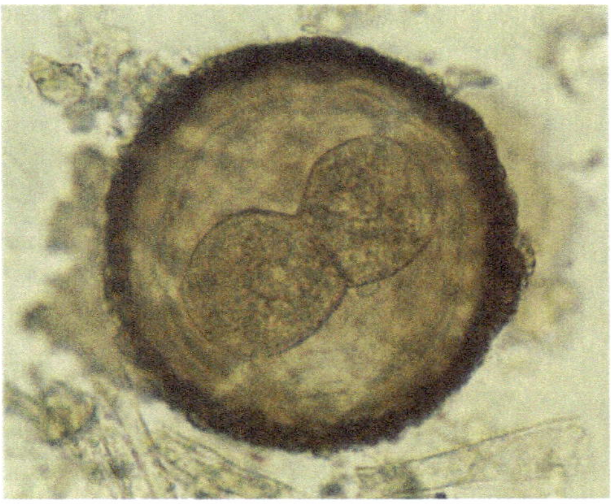

Fig. 400 Egg of *Parascaris equorum* (90–100 µm in diameter), partially developed

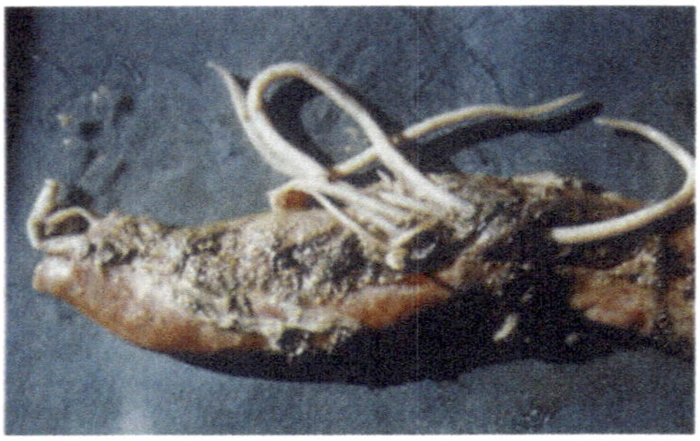

Fig. 401 *Parascaris equorum*; adult worms (males are 15–28 cm long, females are 16–50 cm long) found in the small intestine of a foal at necropsy

Strongyloides westeri

Equine intestinal threadworm

Location: Small intestine

Hosts: Horse and donkey

Species description: *S. westeri* is a hair-like, 8–9 mm long nematode. Only the parthenogenic females are parasitic. Free-living males and females reproduce sexually outside the host. Infection is acquired by ingestion of larvae, skin penetration or via the milk of the mare. Ingestion of larvae and skin penetration involves migration to the lungs. There are two possible ways of development, a homogonic cycle involving adult females in the host producing eggs that do not require fertilisation to develop. These eggs are passed in the faeces and then develop to infective third-stage larvae.
In the heterogonic cycle adult threadworms in the intestine lay eggs which develop into a different type of larvae. These larvae can develop to adult males and females which can live outside the host. The fertilized eggs of this type yield in infective larvae wich are ingested by the host. Migrating larvae can cross the mammary glands to infect nursing foals.

Geographic distribution: World-wide

Symptoms: Foals with heavy burdens show acute diarrhoea, weakness and emaciation. Older animals may harbour large burdens without clinical manifestations. Migration of *S. westeri* larvae through the lungs can cause severe haemorrhage and respiratory distress. Skin penetration may result in irritation and dermatitis.

Significance: Highly important in neonatal foals. Severe diarrhoea which can be so severe as to cause death in foals. The most important route of transmission is galactogenic.

Diagnosis: Identification of thin-shelled eggs (45 × 38 µm) containing a larva.

Therapy: Cambendazole (20 mg/kg, po.), thiabendazole (75 mg/kg, po.), ivermectin (0.2 mg/kg), fenbendazole at increased dosage rate (50 mg/kg, po.), oxibendazole (15 mg/kg, po.) and other benzimidazoles generally at increased dosage rates.

Prophylaxis: Reduction of densities of the free-living larvae by removal of the faeces and provision of dry quarters. Pre-foaling treatments to the mare reduce transmammary infection.

(Figures 402, 403, 404)

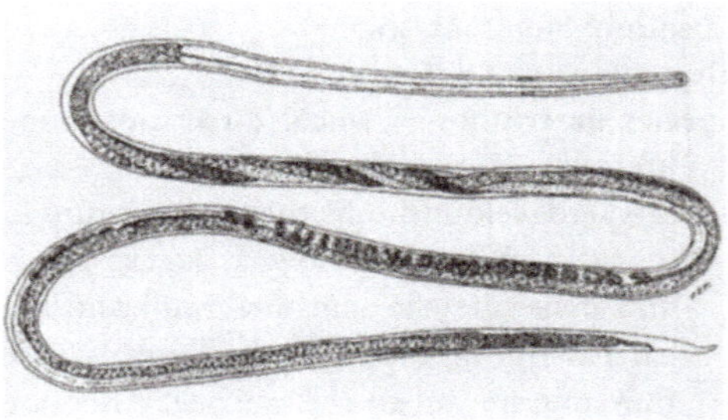

Fig. 402 *Strongyloides westeri*; adult parasitic female (0.1–9 mm long) [3]

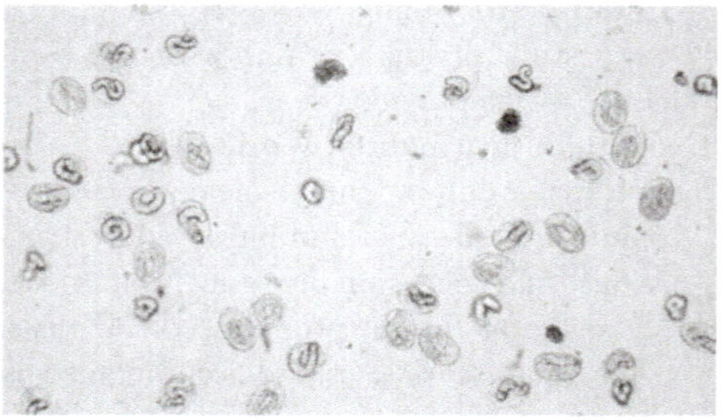

Fig. 403 Eggs of *Strongyloides westeri* (40–50 × 30–40 µm) [15]

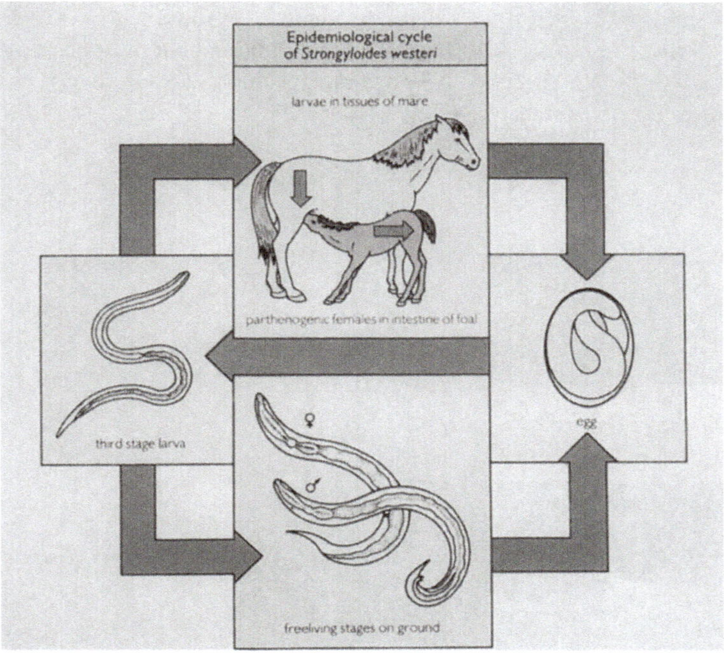

Fig. 404 Life cycle *Strongyloides westeri*; infection may also be acquired galactogenically and percutaneously (not shown on this figure) [37]

Oxyuris equi Equine pinworm

Location: Large intestine (caecum, colon)

Hosts: Horse and donkey

Species description: Adult female worms migrate out of the anus and lay eggs on the perianal skin. The eggs are covered with sticky fluid. Infective larvae develop within 3–5 days inside the eggs. The horse may be infected accidentally by licking the eggs with the itchy fluid or by ingesting embryonated eggs with feed or water. Adult pinworms are of little significance in the intestine, but cause perineal irritation and intense pruritus following egg laying.

Geographic distribution: World-wide

Symptoms: Loss of condition, poor appearance, biting and scratching at the perineal region are often seen in horses infected with *O. equi*. Irritation in the perineal region causes wounds open to secondary infections and myiasis. Dull hair coat and loss of hair is known as "rat-tail".

Significance: Most of the clinical significance results from the intense itching caused by the sticky fluid with which the eggs are attached to the rump.

Diagnosis: Presence of masses of whitish-yellow eggs around the anal region.

Therapy: Most of the broad-spectrum drugs recommended for the strongyles (☞ below) and trichlorfon (35 mg/kg, po.) are effective against pinworms.

Prophylaxis: Regular treatment will eliminate the intestinal worms and frequent change of bedding will restrict reinfection.

(Figures 405, 406, 407)

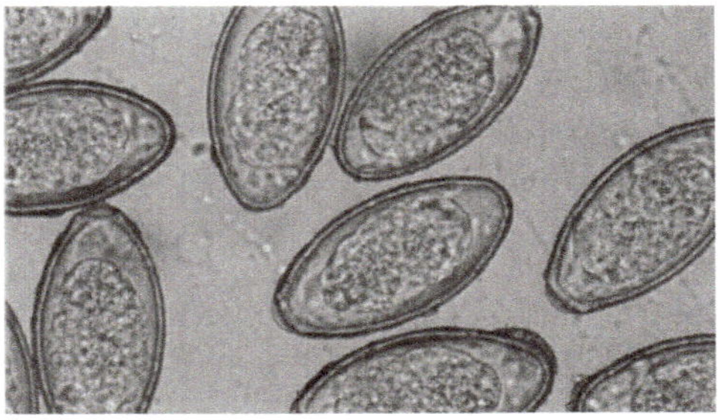

Fig. 405 Eggs of *Oxyuris equi* (85–95 × 40–45 μm)

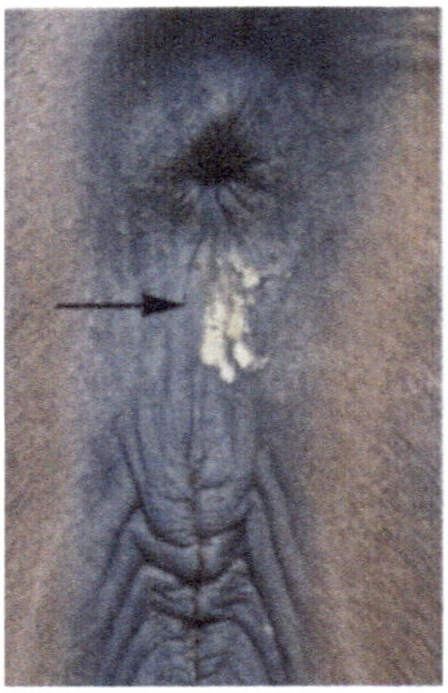

Fig. 406 Masses of yellowish eggs of *Oxyuris equi* around the perineum of a horse

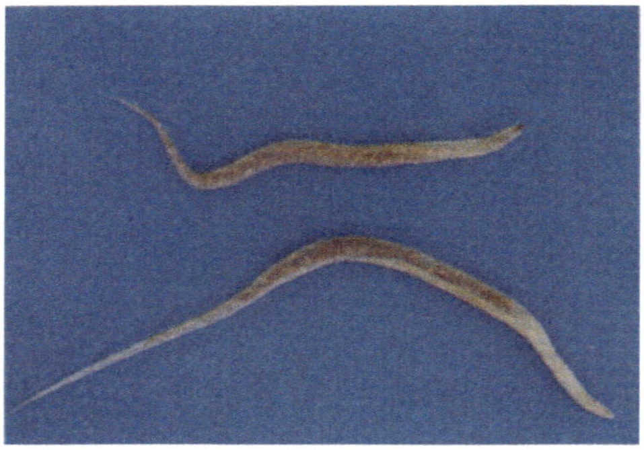

Fig. 407 *Oxyuris equi*; adults (males are 0.9–1.2 cm long, females are 4–12 cm long) [37]

Probstmayria vivipara Small pinworm

Location: Colon
Hosts: Horse and donkey
Species description: It is a tiny pinworm only 2–3 mm long. Complete life cycle takes place in the host.
Geographic distribution: World-wide, except some Western European regions
Symptoms: Inapparent infections are common.
Significance: It is not clinically important. Millions of this pinworm may be present in infected horses with no clinical signs.
Diagnosis: First-stage larvae may be found in the faeces. Larvae may be collected with the Baermann apparatus. *P. vivipara* may also be found at necropsy.
Therapy: Is not indicated but most benzimidazoles and dichlorvos are effective.
(Figure 408)

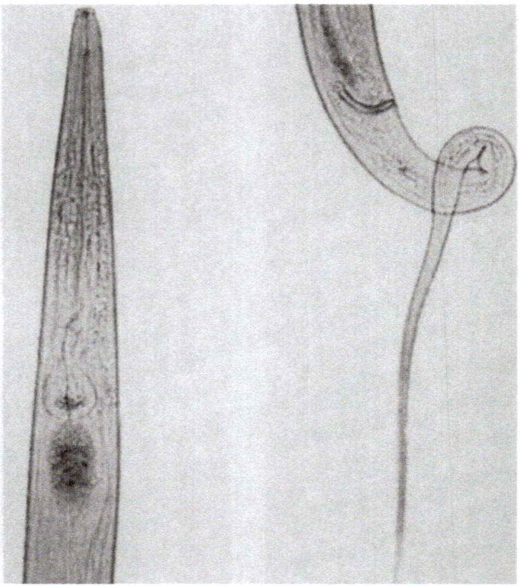

Fig. 408 *Probstmayria vivipara*; anterior end (left), posterior (right) of an adult female (2.2–3.8 mm) [38]

- **Stomach worms**

Habronema muscae,
H. majus (syn. *H. microstoma*) **and**
Draschia megastoma (syn. *H. megastoma*)
Equine stomach worms, summer sores

Location: Adult worms of *H. muscae* and *H. majus* occur on the horse stomach mucosa under a layer of mucus. *D. megastoma* is in tumour-like swellings of the stomach wall. Larvae may be found in non-healing skin wounds (☞ HORSES AND DONKEYS, ■ 5.1).
Hosts: Horse and donkey
Species description: Adult worms are found in the stomach. Larvae or embryonated eggs produced by the adult worms are passed in

the faeces and ingested by the housefly (*Musca* spp.) or stablefly (*Stomoxys* spp.) maggots which develop in manure. Larval development occurs within the maggot and the infective third-stage larvae is reached at the time the adult fly emerges from the pupa. Infective third-stage larvae are deposited by the intermediate hosts on preexisting wounds (cutaneous habronemosis) or on moisture of the genitalia or eyes (ocular habronemosis) and migrate into the host's tissue. These irritations cause a granulomatous reaction. Larvae are deposited by the flies around the nostril, lips and wounds of horses as the flies feed. The cycle is closed when larvae or infected flies are ingested by the horse.

In temperate areas cutaneous wounds tend to heal during the winter but often recur in subsequent warm seasons (summer sores) when flies are active again. In hot, humid zones *D. megastoma* is mainly responsible for both, gastric tumour-like lesions and cutaneous habronemosis.

Geographic distribution: World-wide

Symptoms: Mild digestive disorders may result from gastric habronemosis. Granulomatous lesions on the skin and eyes resistant to conservative wound treatment are characteristic for cutaneous habronemosis (☞ Horses and Donkeys, ■ 5.1)

Significance: Adult *Habronema* are of little concern but ocular or cutaneous larvae cause annoyance and wounds with a protracted healing, open for subsequent problems (e.g. myiasis). *D. megastoma* produces tumour-like swellings in the stomach (up to 10 cm in diameter) which may rupture and cause fatal peritonitis or block the passage.

Diagnosis: Antemortem diagnosis is difficult since the thin-shelled eggs or larvae are easily missed in faecal examinations. Worms and eggs may be found in gastric lavage. The almost transparent adult worms can be found during postmortem examination. Non-healing, reddish brown, greasy skin granuloms that contain rice-grain-sized, calcified material is indicative for cutaneous habronemosis. Larvae in lesion scrapings can sometimes be found.

Therapy: High dosages of the following benzimidazoles cured gastric habronemosis: thiabendazole (3 × 75 mg/kg), oxfendazole (3 × 15 mg/kg), fenbendazole (1 × 30–60 mg/kg) and oxibendazole (10 mg/kg, po.). Ivermectin (200 µg/kg, po.) is highly effective. Two intramuscular dosages of ivermectin (200 µg/kg) cured summer sores within 5 weeks.

Prophylaxis: Fly prevention by stacking manure and using insecticides where horses are kept during the day. Skin breaks should be avoided during the fly season and existing wounds should be treated with fly repellents or a combination of an antiseptic and insecticide.

(Figures 409, 410, 411)

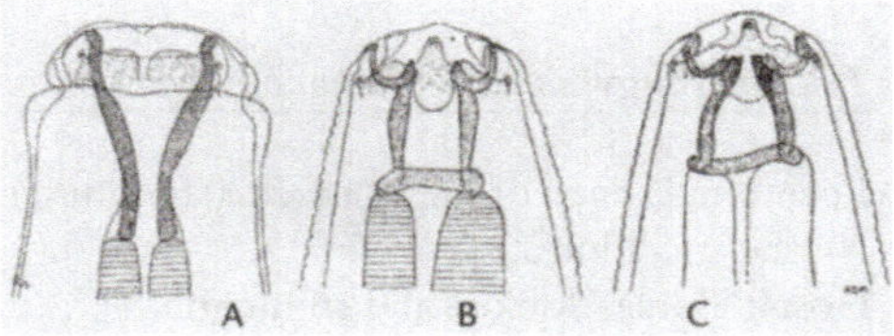

Fig. 409 Lateral views of anterior ends of equine species of *Habronema* spp. and *Draschia* spp. (schematic): (A) *D. megastoma* (males are 7–10 mm, females are: 10–13 mm), (B) *H. muscae* (males are 8–14 mm, females are 12–22 mm) and (C) *H. majus* (males are 9–16 mm, females are 15–25 mm) [3]

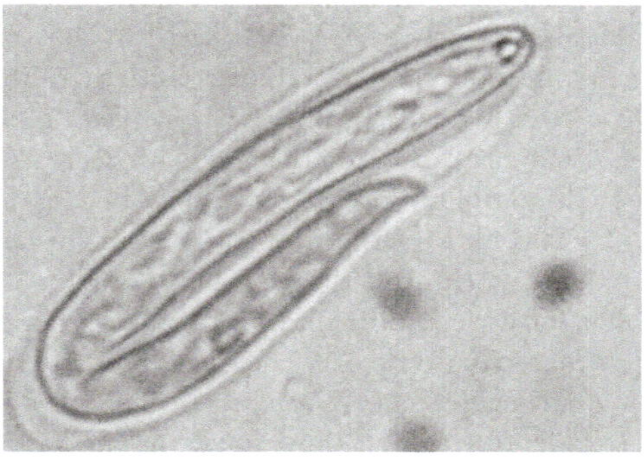

Fig. 410 Egg of *Habronema* spp. (40–50 × 10–16 µm) [11]

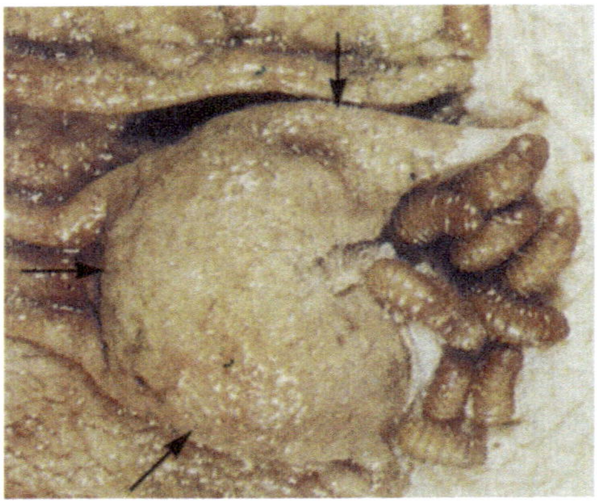

Fig. 411 Large fibrous granuloma in the stomach mucosa caused by *Draschia meagastoma*. The botfly larvae which are present in the illustration do not contribute to the pathological process [37]

Trichostrongylus axei Stomach hair worm

Location: Lumen of the stomach glands and in the small intestine

Hosts: Horse, donkey and ruminants (☞ CATTLE, 1)

Species description: Direct life cycle, typical for nematodes. *T. axei* has an exceptionally wide host-range and is common in many ruminant and equine species. The adults are slender and up to 8 mm long.

Geographic distribution: World-wide

Symptoms: Oedema, dark, foul-smelling diarrhoea and rapid loss of condition

Significance: *T. axei* is usually part of a mixed infection and therefore additive to the overall "worm-damage". Leakage of plasma proteins into the gut and decreased digestibility occurs in heavy infections. Chronic catarrhal gastritis is caused by larvae penetrating the gastric mucosa.

Diagnosis: It is difficult to rely only on faecal examination because the eggs are similar to strongyle eggs. The species can only be identified via third-stage larvae after copro-culture or adult worms at necropsy.

Therapy: ☞ below, LARGE AND SMALL STRONGYLES

Prophylaxis: As *T. axei* is primarily a parasite of cattle and sheep, grazing management is important. Overcrowding must be avoided and brood mares should be treated as foals are very susceptible. Removal of faeces and regular stool check is a helpful aid in strongyle control.

- **Large strongyles**

Strongylus vulgaris, Strongylus equinus* and *Strongylus edentatus Large strongyles

Location: Adult worms are found in the large intestine.

Hosts: Horse and donkey

Species description: Life cycle: adults of all 3 species live in the large intestine. Eggs develop into infective third-stage larvae within 3 days under moist and warm conditions. Infection is acquired by ingestion of larvae which drop their protective sheath in the small intestine. After this stage the *Strongylus* species have different somatic migration patterns which are mentioned under the individual species descriptions.

Geographic distribution: World-wide

Significance: Large strongyles are the most important parasites of equines. Of the three species, *S. vulgaris* is the most pathogenic.

(Figures 412, 413)

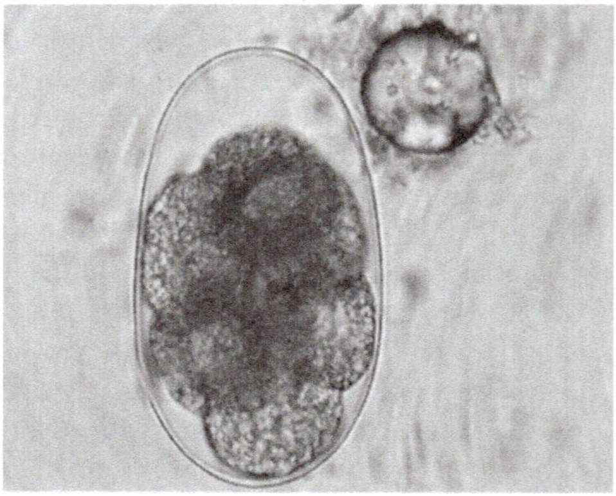

Fig. 412 Strongyle-type egg (72–93 × 40–54 µm) found in equines

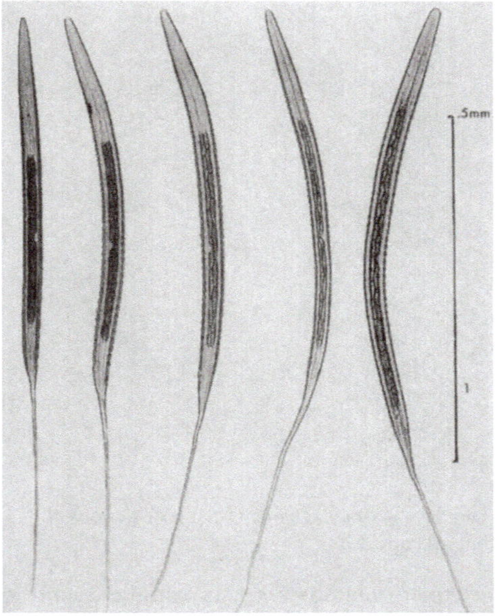

Fig. 413 Third-stage larvae of equine strongyles (850–1000) μm [38]

Strongylus vulgaris Bloodworm, Verminous endarteritis

Species description: *S. vulgaris* is the smallest of the large strongyles, reaching 2 cm in length and has typically ear-shaped teeth set in the deep of the buccal cavity. Third-stage larvae penetrate the intestinal mucosa, moult into fourth-stage larvae and penetrate further nearby blood vessels and wander through the arteries for 2 weeks before reaching the cranial mesenteric artery, where they remain for 4 months. After moulting to immature adults *S. vulgaris* returns via the arteries to the large intestine and burrows into the lumen. 6–8 months after the infection eggs are passed in the faeces. The colic associated with this parasite is not provoked by the adult worms in the gut but by the larvae during their migration through the arteries. As the larvae migrate they damage the endothelial lining of the vessels, thereby stimulating thrombus production. These clots are swept away to lodge in smaller vessels leading to thromboembolic colic.

Symptoms: *S. vulgaris* is especially important because of the damage the larvae do to the cranial mesenteric artery and its branches. Colic of various degrees, temporary lameness, gangrenous enteritis, intestinal stasis, possibly rupture and other effects depending on the location of the infarct may follow.

Diagnosis: Very difficult during the migratory, prepatent phase of the infection. Postmortem examination is indicated and larvae can be used for species identification. Adults may be found in the large intestine and eggs are present in the faeces.

(Figures 414, 415, 416, 417, 418)

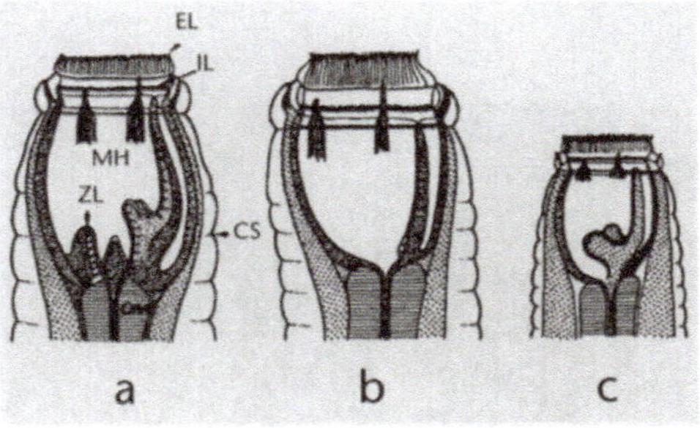

Fig. 414 Dorsolateral view of the anterior end of various *Strongylus* spp.: (a) *Strongylus equinus*, (b) *S. edentatus* and (c) *S. vulgaris*; EL = external leaf crown, IL = internal leaf crown, CS = cuticular striation and ZL = tooth [33]

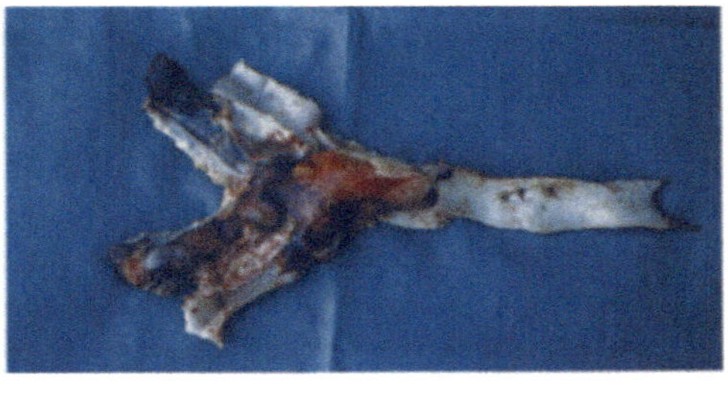

Fig. 415 Mesenteric artery with thrombosis due to migrating larvae of *Strongylus vulgaris*

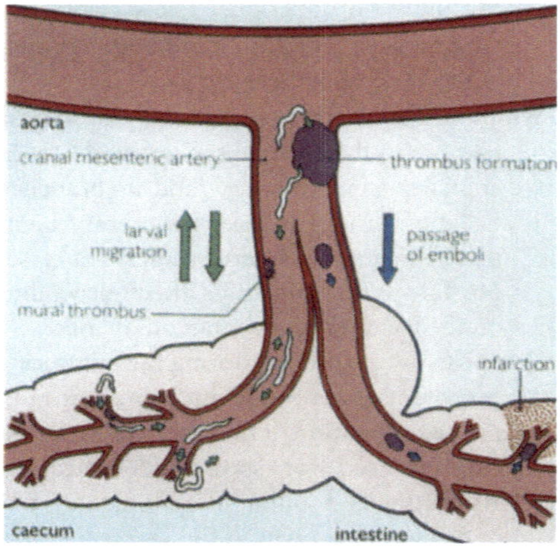

Fig. 416 Migratory route of *Strongylus vulgaris*. Note that the third-stage larvae migrate within the intima and not in the lumen of blood vessels [37]

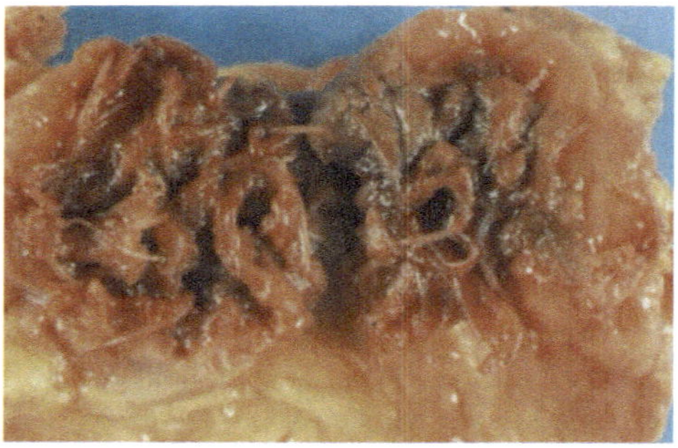

Fig. 417 *Strongylus vulgaris* larvae in a thrombus [4]

Strongylus edentatus

Species description: *S. edentatus* reaches 4 cm in length. Larvae penetrate the intestine and migrate via the portal vein to the liver, where moulting occurs and nodule formation takes place. After 9 weeks the fourth-stage larvae wander to the peritoneum, causing the formation of nodules. Migrating to the large intestine, larvae form caseous nodules in the gut wall, which they rupture to enter the colon lumen almost a full year after infection. Aberrant larvae or

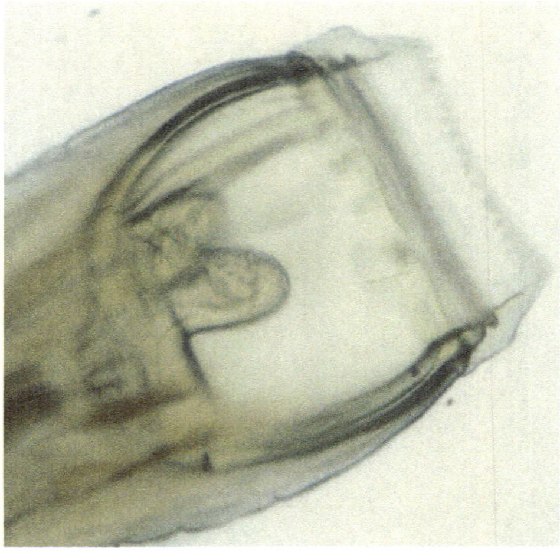

Fig. 418 *Strongylus vulgaris*; anterior end with buccal capsule

their migratory tracts can be found in unexpected sites such as the pleural cavity and testis.

Symptoms: Adult large strongyles (*S. vulgaris, S. equinus* and *S. edentatus*) are "plug-feeders", ingesting plugs of mucosa as they move about in the intestine. Heavy feeding of this type produces intestinal damage, blood and protein loss into the intestine. Intestinal damage causes diarrhoea, fever, oedema, anorexia, depression, weight loss and dehydration.
The attendant blood loss may lead to anaemia, especially in *S. equinus* infections. *S. equinus* and *S. edentatus* larvae rarely cause damage of clinical consequence during their migratory phase which is in contrast to *S. vulgaris* larvae which cause great problems during migration within the arteries and hardly any damage as adult worms in the gut.

Diagnosis: Diagnosis of mixed strongyle infections is based on demonstration of eggs in the faeces (*Strongylus* spp.). Differential diagnosis can be made by identifying the infective larvae after copro-culture. Colic due to verminous arteritis can be associated with a palpable, painful enlargement at the root of the mesentery.

(Figures 419, 420, 421)

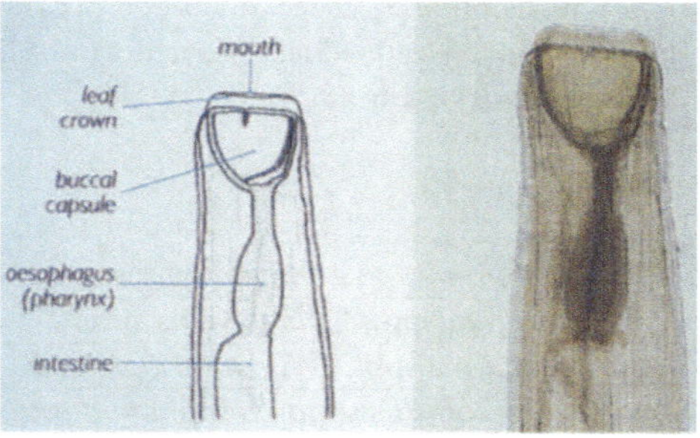

Fig. 419 *Strongylus edentatus*; anterior end [37]

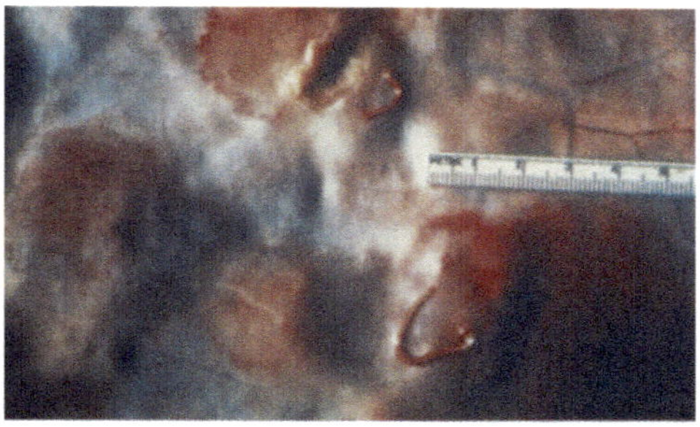

Fig. 420 Migratory pathway of *Strongylus edentatus* [37]

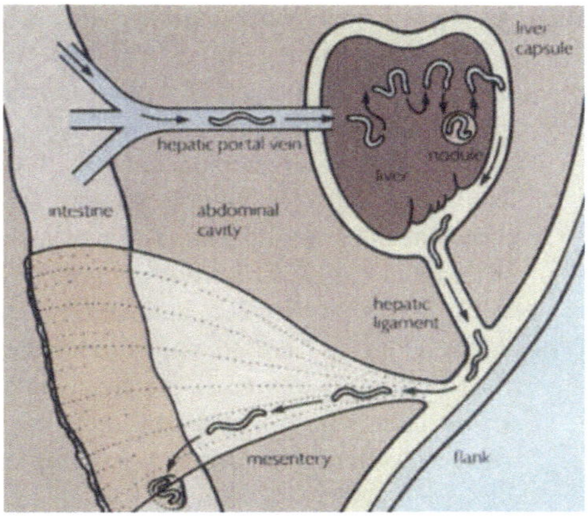

Fig. 421 *Strongylus edentatus* larvae from the parietal peritoneum of the flank [15]

Strongylus equinus

Species description: *S. equinus* reaches 5 cm in length. After burrowing into the submucosa of the small intestine and moulting to the fourth-stage larvae *S. equinus* forms a nodule on the intestine. After that larvae wander to the liver where they meander through the liver parenchyma for 6–7 weeks without nodule formation. Emerging from the liver they moult to immature adults and migrate in various abdominal organs (incl. pancreas) then return to the large intestine. Passage to and from the liver occurs directly across the peritoneal cavity. Prepatent period is about 9 months. *S. equinus* rarely causes damage of clinical consequence during its migratory phase. *S. equinus* suck up to 10 ml of blood per day. Heavy infections are associated with anaemia.

Symptoms and Diagnosis: ☞ above Symptoms and diagnosis of *S. edentatus*

(Figures 422, 423)

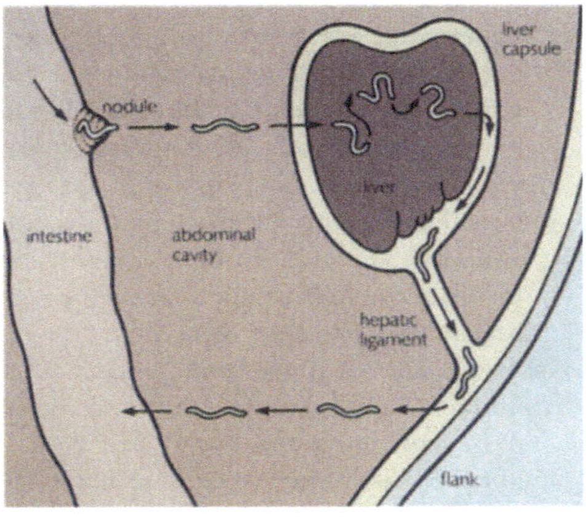

Fig. 422 Migratory pathway of *Strongylus equinus* [37]

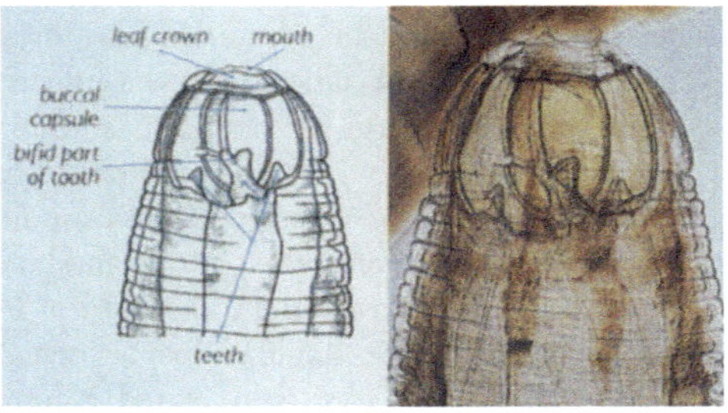

Fig. 423 *Strongylus equinus*; anterior end [37]

• **Control of large strongyles**

Therapy: Ivermectin (0.2 mg/kg) is effective against both adult and larval stages of *S. vulgaris* and *S. edentatus* and only against adult *S. equinus* worms. Fenbendazole (10 mg/kg, po. during 5 days) and oxfendazole (15 mg/kg, po.) at dosages higher than for the adult worms are also effective against larval infections. Most of the modern broad-spectrum anthelmintics such as cambendazole, mebendazole, oxfendazole, oxibendazole are effective against adult large and small strongyles. Pyrantel (19 mg/kg, po.) is efficacious against adult small and large strongyles and larvae of most of the small strongyles. Febantel (6 mg/kg, po.) is effective against adult large and small strongyles. Dichlorvos (31–41 mg/kg, po.) is highly effective against *S. vulgaris* and *S. equinus* and against small strongyles. Haloxon (60–75 mg/kg,po.) is only effective against *S. vulgaris*. Trichlorfon (40 mg/kg, po.) combined with mebendazole, fenbendazole, oxfendazole or pyrantel (each at its regular therapeutic dosage) is highly effective against ascarids, pinworms, small and all the three large strongyles.

Prophylaxis: Grazing horses are likely to be infected, therefore a control program attempts to minimize the level of pasture contamination and reduce the risks associated with the migrating larvae. All horses kept in the same feeding-community should be treated and preferably at the same time. Newly acquired horses should be de-wormed before admittance to the herd. Whatever program is used, faecal samples should be examined periodically to maintain surveillance of the effectiveness. Horses kept in arid areas should be treated at least twice during the rains (midway and end of rains) with a compound which is effective against adults and larvae in order to increase the utilization of feed during that time. Regular dosing (generally every 4–8 weeks) is indicated in humid areas. Colic may be associated with the use of anthelmintics, especially when organophosphorous products (trichlorfon or dichlorvos) are used.

• **Small strongyles**

***Triodontophorus* spp., *Trichonema* spp., *Cyathostomum* spp., *Cylicocyclus* spp., *Cylicostephanus* spp., *Cylicodontophorus* spp., *Gyalocephalus* spp., *Oesophagodontus* spp. and *Craterostomum* spp.**

Location: Large intestine

Hosts: Horse and donkey

Species description: More than 25 species of small strongyles are found in the caecum and colon. Apart from *Triodontophorus* spp. which are almost as large as *S. vulgaris*, most of them are smaller than the large strongyles. *Triodontophorus* spp. are also known as the "non-migratory" large strongyles. One species, *Triodontophorus tenuicollis*, causes severe ulcers in the wall of the colon. There is no extra-intestinal migration of the larvae within the host. Small strongyles undergo a typical direct nematode life cycle and larvae develop within the wall of the large intestine. Larvae may undergo hypobiosis and remain dormant in the intestinal wall during periods of adverse environmental conditions (dry season, winter). Small strongyles usually appear as mixed infections. Damage is mainly caused by the adult worms which are plug feeders, ingesting plugs of intestinal mucosa and blood vessels. Larvae within the gut wall may also suck blood. Animals under three years of age are more susceptible particularly if kept on overcrowded pastures. Several species of small strongyles are resistant to many of the benzimidazoles which is a heritable trait and not reversible.

Geographic distribution: World-wide

Symptoms: Loss of condition, anaemia, weakness, acute or chronic diarrhoea

Significance: Small strongyles are extremely prevalent and cause considerable economic loss and severe disease wherever horses are raised.

Diagnosis: Species identification is impossible solely based on the egg morphology. Larval identification following faecal culture is indicated. Strongyle eggs passed by foals of 6 months or less are those of the small strongyles as the prepatent period of *Strongylus* spp. is longer.

Therapy: ☞ above LARGE STRONGYLES. Benzimidazole-resistant strains are susceptible to piperazine (88 mg/kg, po.), pyrantel-pamoat (19 mg/kg, po.), dichlorvos (31–41 mg/kg, po.), ivermectin (0.2 mg/kg, sc.) haloxon (60–75 mg/kg, po.) and oxibendazole (10 mg/kg, po.).

Prophylaxis: ☞ above LARGE STRONGYLES

Remarks: The "horse strongyles" consist of more than 40 species many of which are distributed world-wide. They are responsible for a variety of clinical syndromes, including the well-known loss of condition, often associated with anaemia, that characterizes the "wormy-horse" and acute or chronic diarrhoea.

(Figures 424, 425, 426, 427, 428, 429, 430)

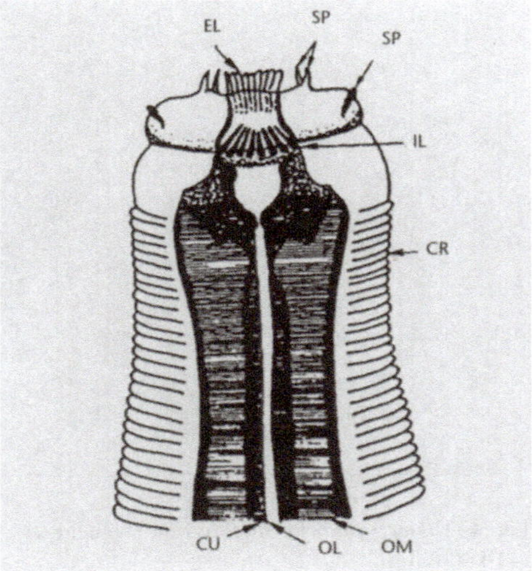

Fig. 424
Dorsolateral view of the anterior end of a small strongylid (*Cylicostephanus* sp.); EL = external leaf crown, IL = internal leaf crown, CR = cuticular striation, SP = papillae, CU = cuticula, OL = oesophagus and OM = oesophageal muscle [33]

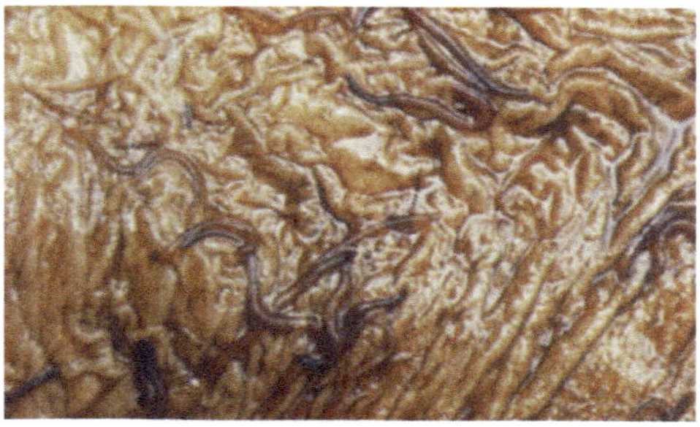

Fig. 425 Small strongyles (females up to 25 mm; males up to 15 mm) in the colon of a horse [10]

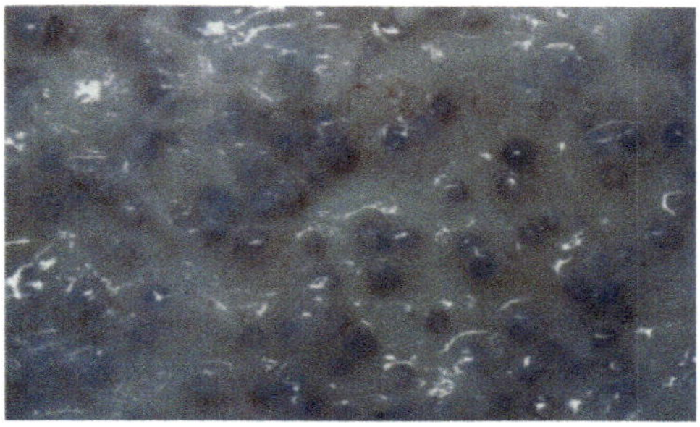

Fig. 426 Developing small strongyle larvae in the mucosa of the caecum

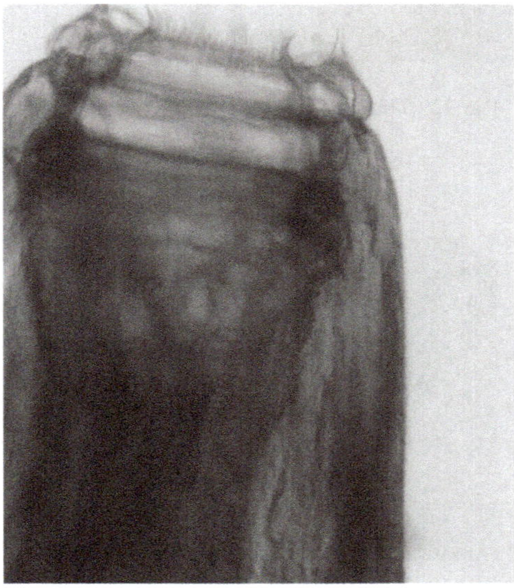

Fig. 427 Small strongyle with a well-developed leaf crown and a pronounced buccal capsule

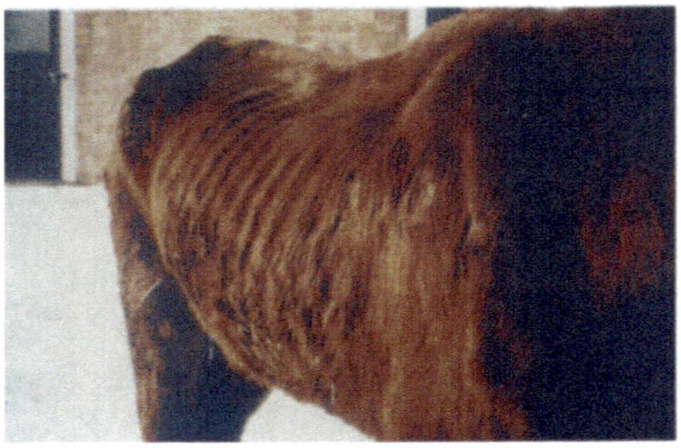

Fig. 428 A wormy horse due to winter cyathostominosis [15]

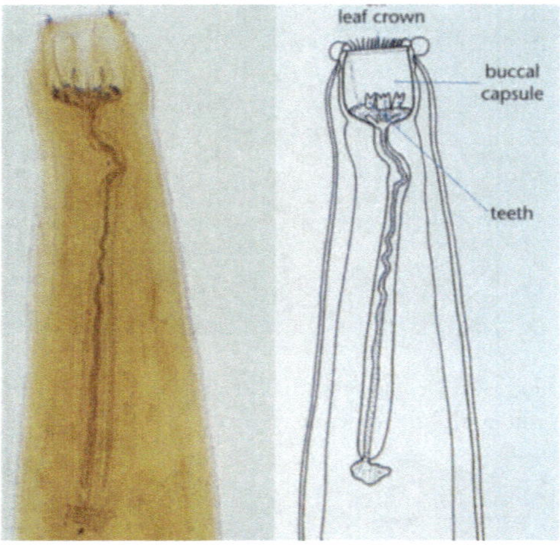

Fig. 429 *Triodontophorus* sp.; anterior end [37]

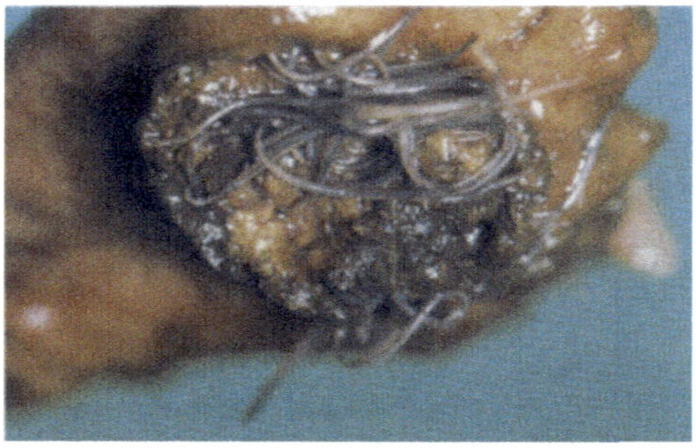

Fig. 430 *Triodontophorus* sp. group of adults forming a large ulcer in the large intestine (17–26 mm long) [37]

Dictyocaulus arnfieldi Equine lungworm

Location: Adult worms in the bronchi and bronchioles of donkeys and horses, embryonated eggs and larvae in fresh faeces (☞ HORSES AND DONKEYS, ■ 4.3). (Figures 431, 432)

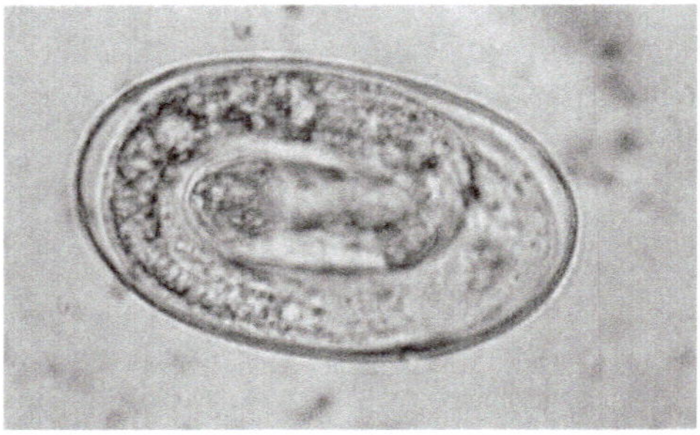

Fig. 431 *Dictyocaulus arnfieldi*; egg containing a larva (74–96 × 46–58 µm) [11]

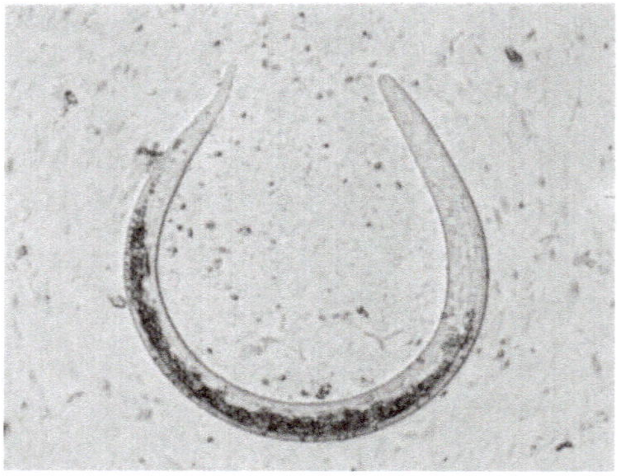

Fig. 432 *Dictyocaulus arnfieldi*; first-stage larva (420–480 µm)

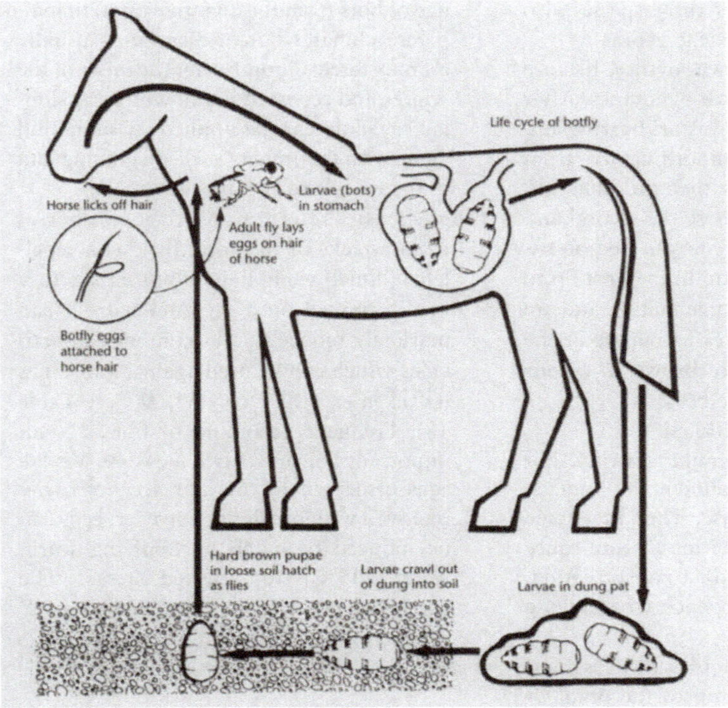

Fig. 433 Life cycle of horse botflies [36]

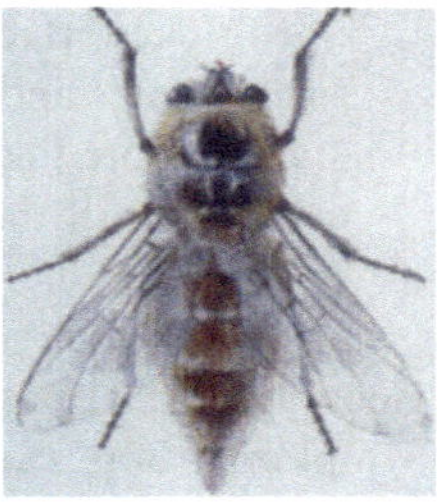

Fig. 434 *Gasterophilus* sp.; the horse bot fly (8–18 mm) [19]

- Insecta found in the gut

***Gasterophilus* spp.** Horse bot flies

Gasterophilus intestinalis (syn. *G. equi*) Common horse bot fly

Location: Eggs are deposited mainly on forelegs, between the knee and the hoof but also in the scapular region where they are licked by the host which stimulates hatching. Larvae are found in the cardiac portion of the stomach.

Gasterophilus nasalis The throat bot fly

Location: Eggs are laid in the intermandibulary space in numbers of up to 500 and usually 1 per hair. Larvae are found in the pylorus region of the stomach and duodenum.

Gasterophilus haemorrhoidalis The nose or lip bot fly or rectal bot fly

Location: Eggs are laid on hairs of the lips and around the mouth.
Third-stage larvae attach to the stomach but also to the hosts rectum, sometimes in great numbers.

Gasterophilus pecorum The plant bot fly

Location: Eggs are deposited on the leaves of plants and its larvae are ingested by grazing animals.
Second-stage larvae and sometimes third-stage larvae are found in the pharynx and the upper part of the oesophagus but third-stage larvae is normally attached to the fundus of the stomach.
Geographic distribution: Africa, Old World

- **General features of the horse bot flies**

Hosts: *G. intestinalis* occurs in horses and donkeys whereas the other three species also parasitize other equids (e.g. zebras).

Species description: The larvae of these flies are gastrointestinal parasites of equines. After hatching the first larval instars burrow into dermal layers of the mouth cavity, from which they move to either the pharynx, stomach or rectum, where the second and third-stages attach. The larvae feed on tissue exudates and remain in the host up to 1 year before they become mature and are excreted with the faeces to pupate in the soil. The adult flies are brown in colour and hairy and resemble bees.

Geographic distribution: Global

Symptoms: Bots cause a mild gastritis, but large numbers can be found in the stomach without clinical signs. The first-stage instars migrating to the mouth can cause stomatitis and may produce pain on eating. Adult flies cause annoyance when laying eggs.

Significance: 1) The adult flies distress their equine host markedly up to the point of causing stampeding. 2) Irritation by the larvae during migration, e.g. dermatitis, inflammation of the pharynx, oesophagus, stomach or rectum (rectum prolapse). 3) Large numbers in the pyloric region may interfere with the sphincter function.

Diagnosis: Specific diagnosis of *Gasterophilus* infection is difficult and can be made only by demonstrating larvae in the faeces. Observation of the cream-white bot eggs (1–2 mm) on the animal's hair may help.

Therapy: In temperate areas it is assumed that most animals are infected by the end of the summer. A single treatment at a time when the adult flies have disappeared is usually adequate. Oral application (gel or pellet via feed, solutions via stomach tube) of trichlorfon (10 mg/kg, po. for bots only; 40 mg/kg, po. for bots and nematodes), dichlorvos (adults: 31–41 mg/kg, foals: 20 mg/kg for treatment of bots and ascarids; 10/mg/kg at 3–4 weeks intervals during fly season for bot control) and ivermectin (200 µg/kg, po.) is effective against all stages of bots and removes a high percentage of bots from the digestive tract. In temperate climates bot medication is usually administered 1 month after the onset of the winter and repeated in midwinter. A similar schedule can be applied to subhumid areas with treatments at the beginning and in the middle of the dry season.

Prophylaxis: Protection of exposed horses from attacks of the adult flies with repellents (dimethyl phtalate) is not satisfactory but if applied on a regional basis it can markedly reduce the fly numbers. Insecticides which can be used against adult flies (☞ HORSES AND DONKEYS, ■ 5.1, Table 18). Frequent grooming of horses is an important bot preventive measure. Visible eggs cemented to the hair are not easily removed with brushing; however, eggs can be induced to hatch by applying warm water (45°C) to affected areas. The hatched larvae can then be washed away easily.

(Figures 433, 434, 435, 436, 437, 438, 439)

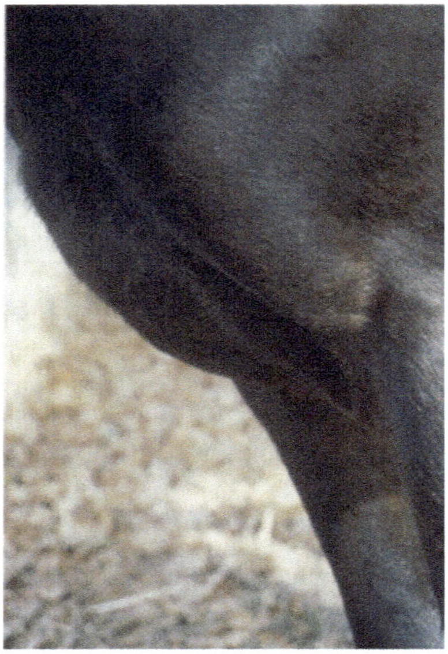

Fig. 435 *Gasterophilus* eggs deposited on the skin of the chest

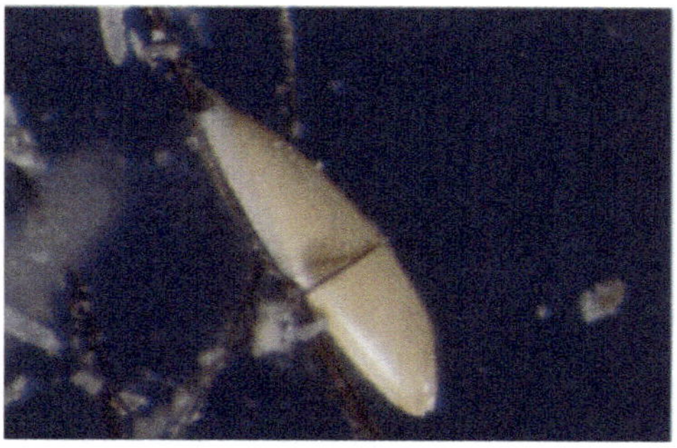

Fig. 436 *Gasterophilus* egg attached to a hair (up to 2 mm long)

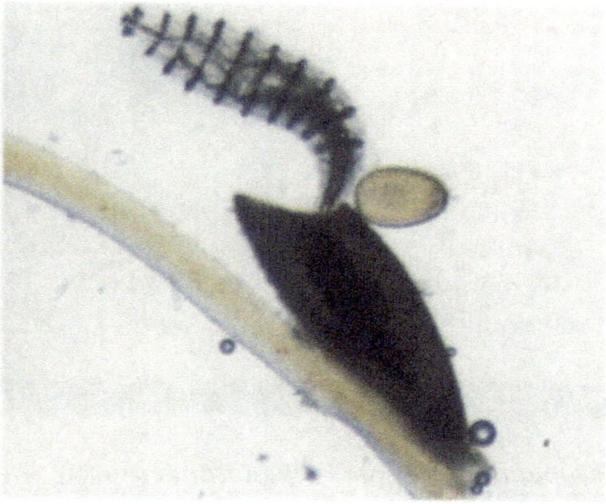

Fig. 438 *Gasterophilus* egg with a hatching larva

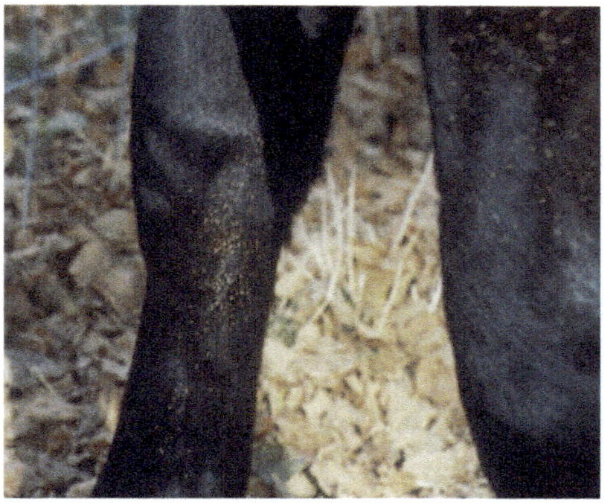

Fig. 437 *Gasterophilus* eggs deposited on the skin of the forelegs

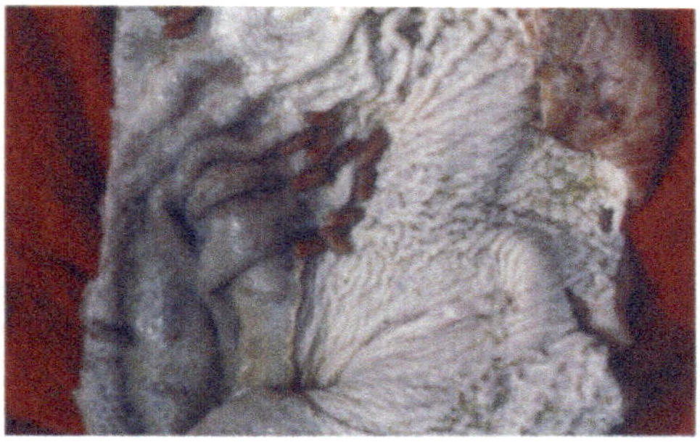

Fig. 439 *Gasterophilus* larvae (up to 2 cm long) attached to the gastric mucosa

2 Stages in the blood and circulatory system

PROTOZOA

Trypanosoma spp. *(Trypanosoma brucei, Trypanosoma congolense* and *Trypanosoma vivax)* "Nagana", "Sannare", sleeping sickness

Hosts: Horse, donkey and many other domestic and wild animals (☞ CATTLE, ■ 2)

Vector: Various tsetse flies of the genus *Glossina* (☞ CATTLE, ■ 5.1)

Species description: Tsetse-transmitted trypanosomosis is one of the major constraints for horse breeding in Africa south of the Sahara and within the tsetse belt. Donkeys are less susceptible and suffer significantly less from trypanosomosis than horses. *T. brucei* is very virulent in horses and can cause an acute infection with death within 15 days after disease onset. A subacute form may last for up to 3 months after the infection. *T. congolense* and *T. vivax* are usually chronic infections with progressive anaemia and weakness.

Geographic distribution: Africa, south of the Sahara

Symptoms: Acute *T. brucei* infections cause hyperthermia, rapid emaciation, oedema of the lower parts of the thorax and abdomen, joints and genitalia, keratitis and nasal discharge. Locomotory ataxia may develop to general paralysis or paresis. *T. congolense* and *T. vivax* infections are usually more protracted with progressive anaemia and emaciation, irregular fever attacks, corneal opacity and nasal discharge. Oedema is rare at the beginning of infection and "self-cure" may occur, especially if the animal is kept under good conditions. However, when animals are overworked or suffer from other conditions, the disease can become more acute or can render the animal more susceptible to other diseases.

Significance: Tsetse-transmitted trypanosomosis (mainly *T. brucei* but also *T. congolense* and *T. vivax*) is a major constraint for equines, especially horses in tsetse-infested regions of Africa. Both the direct noxious effect of trypanosomes on the host and their immunosuppressive effect are of great significance.

Diagnosis: A presumptive diagnosis is based on finding an anaemic animal in poor condition in an endemic area. Confirmation by demonstrating trypanosomes in stained bloodsmears or wet mounts. The most sensitive rapid method is a wet mount of the buffy coat area of a PCV tube after centrifugation. Other infections that cause anaemia and weight loss are babesiosis, anaplasmosis and should be excluded by examining a stained bloodsmear. African Horse Sickness and Equine Infectious Anaemia should be excluded as underlying viral infections.

Therapy: The most effective but often poorly tolerated compound against *T. brucei* and *T. evansi* (☞ below) is quinapyramine (5 mg/kg, sc.). The dosage should be split in three portions and administered at 6-hour intervals. Suramin sodium (7–10 mg/kg, im. or iv.) was highly effective but it is no longer commercially available. Isometamidium is effective against *T. vivax* (0.5 mg/kg, im.) and *T. congolense* and against *T. brucei* (0.5–1 mg/kg, im.), provided that the dosage is divided over several injection sites. Diminazene aceturate (3.5 mg/kg, im.) is highly effective against *T. brucei*, *T. vivax* and *T. congolense,* half of the dosage is administered immediately and the other half 6 hours later.

Prophylaxis: Isometamidium (0.5–1 mg/kg) protects horses for 2–4 moths against *T. vivax* and *T. congolense.* The injection must be given deeply intramuscularly and

the dosage should be split over several injection sites. Quinapyramine prosalt (7.4 mg/kg, sc.) may be used to prevent *T. brucei* but also *T. evansi*. The prophylactic effect lasts for 3–4 months.
Insecticides, used as toxicants or as repellents may reduce the attacks by tsetse flies. At the time of high insect activity the use of insecticides may also reduce the general fly-annoyance in the environment of horses. Insecticides may be used as whole-body sprays or as sponge-on, smear-on, etc.
(Figures 440, 441, 442, Table 17)

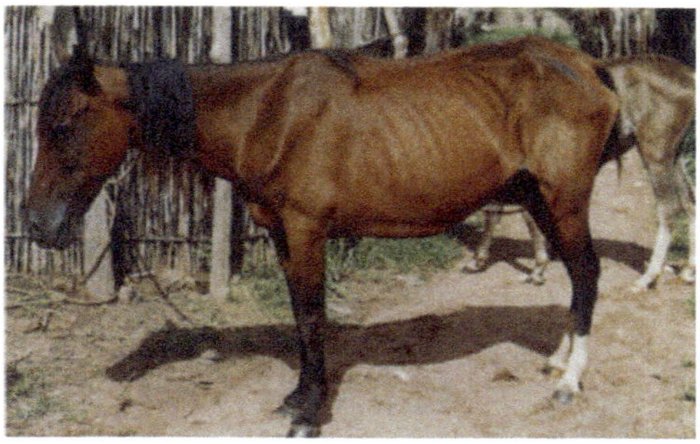

Fig. 440 Horse infected with *Trypanosoma congolense* showing oedema on the lower thorax

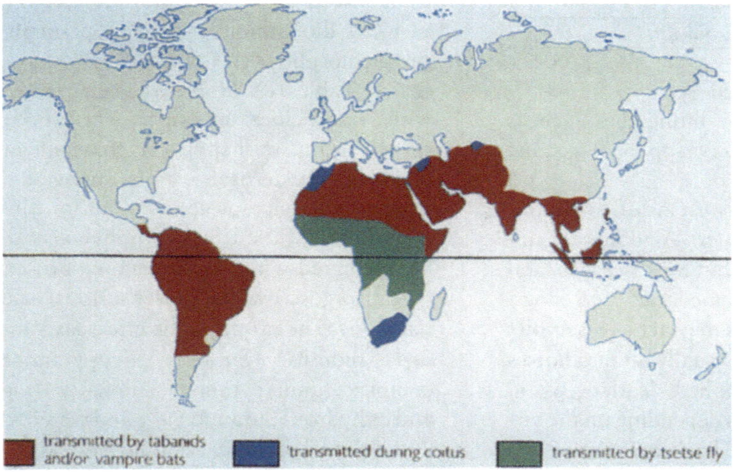

Fig. 441 Geographic distribution of equine trypanosomosis [37]

Table 17 Trypanocidal drugs to be used in equines

Generic name	Dose (mg/kg) and Route	Suscetible Trypanosomes
Quinapyramine dimethyl sulfate or chloride	5, subcut.	*T. brucei, T. congolense, T. equiperdum T. evansi, T. simiae , T. vivax*
Homidium chloride or bromide	1, IM	*T. brucei, T. congolense, T. vivax*
diminazene aceturate	3.5–7, IM	*T. brucei, T. congolense, T. evansi, T. vivax*
Isometamidium chloride	0.5–2, IM	*T. congolense, T. vivax*
Pyrithidium bromide	2, IM	*T. congolense, T. vivax*
Suramin	7–10. IV	*T. brucei, T. equiperdum, T. evansi*

Diminazene aceturate should not be administered to equines if possible. If there are no other compounds available, the daily dosage should be split into 2–3 aliquots and administered 4 h apart. Suramin is no longer commercially available [39]

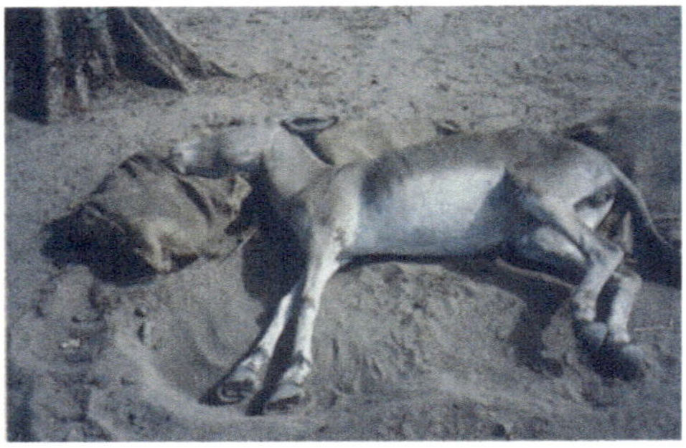

Fig. 442 Donkey with heavy *Trypanosoma brucei* infection

Trypanosoma evansi "Surra", "El Debab", "Dioufar", "Thaga", "Doukane"

Hosts: Horse and dromedary

Vector: Transmission by biting flies such as *Tabanus* spp., *Stomoxys* spp., *Chrysozona* spp. and *Lyperosia* spp.

Species description: *T. evansi* is difficult to differentiate from *T. brucei*. All domestic animals are susceptible but the disease is fatal only in horses, dromedaries and dogs. Other animal species may act as reservoirs of infection. Surra is usually fatal to horses if treatment is not applied, death occurs in a few days or months depending on the virulence of the strain. The disease progress is slower in Africa than in Asia.

Geographic distribution: Northern and Sahelian Africa, Asia, Central and South America

Symptoms: Progressive weakness, emaciation and oedema are the most common clinical signs. Oedema varying from urticarial plaques on the neck and the flanks to extended oedema of the legs and the lower parts of the body. Fever attacks, difficulties in walking, lacrimation, conjunctivitis, hypertrophy of the superficial lymph nodes and ascites may occur. Nervous signs only occur in the terminal stage.

Significance: *T. evansi* is a dangerous disease for horses and dromedaries in Africa north of latitude 15° and many other parts of the world.

Diagnosis: Emaciation and oedema. Trypanosomes are found in bloodsmears but the typical form is morphologically indistinguishable from the slender and intermediate forms of *T. brucei*.

Therapy: The most effective but often poorly tolerated compound against *T. evansi* is quinapyramine (5 mg/kg, sc.). The dosage should be split in three portions and administered at 6-hour intervals. Suramin sodium (7–10 mg/kg, im. or iv.) has also be used successfully but this compound is no longer commercially available.

Prophylaxis: Transmission by flies (but also fly annoyance in general) can be reduced by using insecticides (coumaphos, malathion, carbaryl, dioxathion, pyrethrins, permethrin, dichlorphos ☞ HORSES AND DONKEYS, ■ 5.1, Table 18). Horses may be treated with insecticides in dips, whole-body sprays, or fine mist sprays; as toxicants or repellents in aerosols or as sponge-on, smear-on, or wipe-on applications for control of biting flies. Chemoprophylaxis can be attempted with quinapyramine prosalt (7.4 mg/kg, sc.) which causes serious local reactions. The prophylactic effect lasts for 3–4 months. Suramin-quinapyramine complex (quinapyramine sulphate 10 g and anhydrous Suramin 8.4 g and water ad 200 ml of solution; administered at 10 mg/kg, sc.) protects horses against *T. evansi* for 6 months.

(Figure 443)

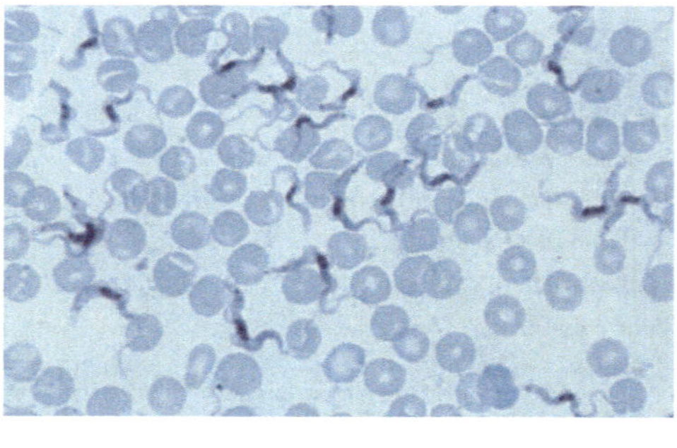

Fig. 443 *Trypanosoma evansi* (15–34 µm, mean: 24 µm long); stained bloodsmear

Trypanosoma equiperdum "Dourine"

Species description: Dourine is venereal disease of horses and donkeys, transmitted mechanically by coitus and rarely by biting flies. Demonstration of the trypanosomes from the urethral or vaginal discharges, the skin plaques or the peripheral blood is difficult and centrifugation of these fluids may help to find the pathogens (☞ HORSES AND DONKEYS, ■ 3).

(Figure 444)

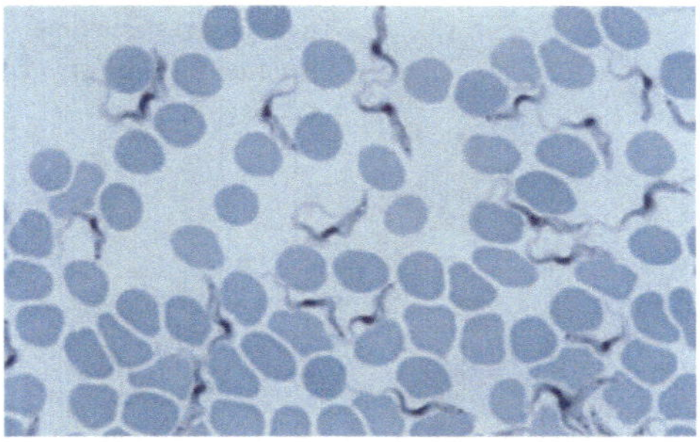

Fig. 444 *Trypanosoma equiperdum* (25 µm); stained bloodsmear (mouse)

Babesia equi (syn. *Nuttallia equi)*
Equine babesiosis

Hosts: Horse, mule, donkey and zebra

Vector: Vectors are *Rhipicephalus bursa* in the Mediterranean basin and *Rhipicephalus evertsi* in tropicoequatorial Africa. *Dermacentor* spp. and *Hyalomma* spp. may also play a role in other parts of Africa.

Species description: *B. equi* is a small *Babesia* species (2 µm in length) in horses and generally more pathogenic than *B. caballi.* It characteristically divides into four daughter organisms which form a Maltese cross. In endemic areas the course may be chronic. In the peracute course of the disease death may occur within 2 days after the onset of the disease and in the acute course the disease process lasts for 8–10 days after which the animal recovers and becomes a carrier. Special attention should be paid to previously non-exposed horses entering enzootic areas. Zebras may act as reservoirs. There is generally no transovarian transmission.

Geographic distribution: Tropical and subtropical areas

Symptoms: Around 10 days after the tick bite fever may occur (up to 41°C). *B. equi* organisms start to occur at this time in the circulating blood. Anaemia and haemoglobinuria may occur and there is listlessness, depression and inappetence. Oedema of the head, limbs and ascites occur and petechial haemorrhage and icterus of the mucous membranes of the eyes are seen. The symptoms are similar to Equine Infectious Anaemia, African Horse Sickness, leptospirosis and trypanosomosis. Intercurrent infections occur and *Babesia* spp. superimposed on a chronic horse sickness or trypanosomosis are often seen.

Significance: *B. equi* infections are of great importance as a primary cause of disease but also as secondary infections in many of the warmer parts of the world and all over the African continent.

Diagnosis: This is made by the demonstration of the parasites (Maltese cross forms) in stained bloodsmears during the period of fever. Petechiae of the mucous membranes of the eyes are characteristic of babesiosis but not specific.

(Figures 445, 446, 447, 448)

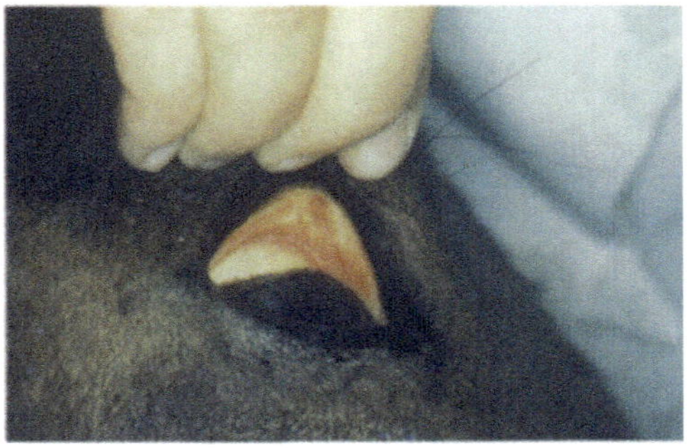

Fig. 445 Icterus due to *Babesia equi* infection |4|

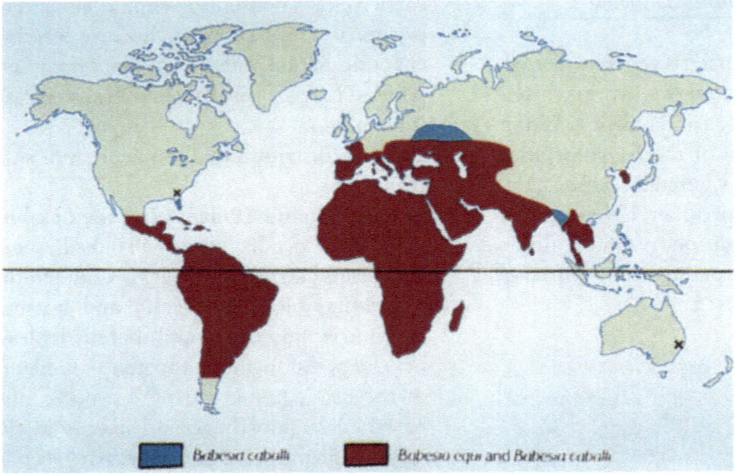

Fig. 446 Geographic distribution of equine babesiosis. The crosses mark localities where isolated outbreaks occur [37]

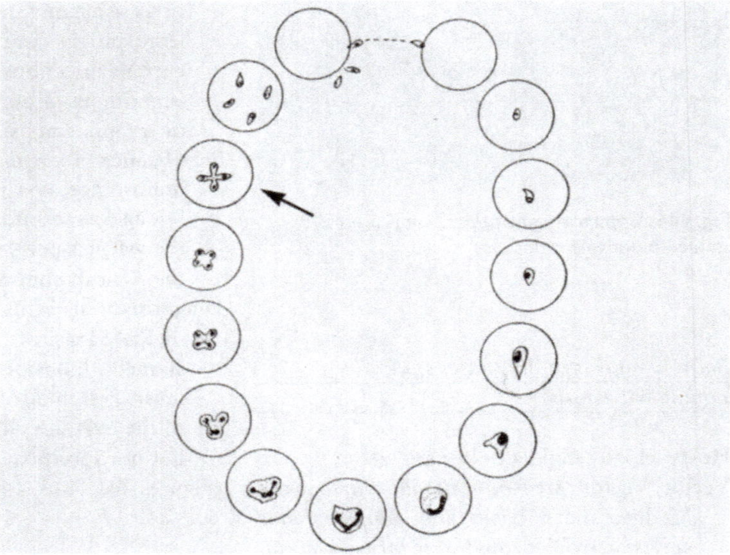

Fig. 447 Various erythrocytic forms of *Babesia equi* found in the red cells (maximum length of 2.5 µm). The *Maltese cross* (arrow) is typical of the species but not always seen at the examination of a bloodsmear [3]

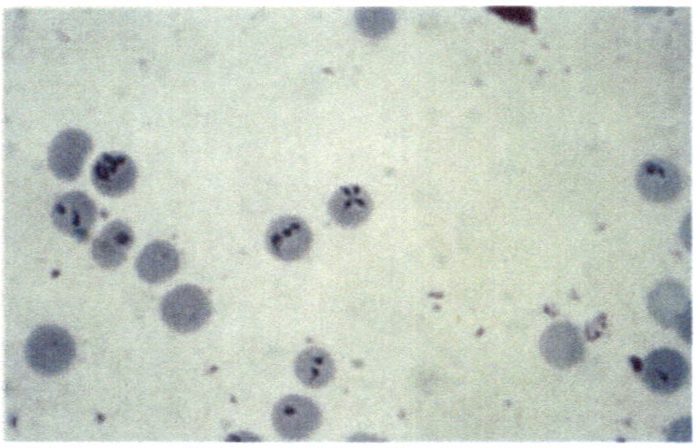

Fig. 448 *Babesia equi*; stained bloodsmear [36]

Babesia caballi (syn. *Piroplasama caballi*)
Equine piroplasmosis

Hosts: Horse, donkey and mule

Vector: *Hyalomma* spp. in North Africa and the Mediterranean basin, *Dermacentor marginatus* (Mediterranean macchia) and *Rhipicephalus* spp. Transovarian transmission occurs regularly.

Species description: *B. caballi* is a large species, resembling *B. bigemina*. Parasites commonly occur as pairs, are pyriform and measure 2.5–4 µm. The course of *B. caballi* infections is characterized by a great variation of the clinical manifestations. It may be acute or chronic, mild or severe and end in death.

Geographic distribution: The Americas, Asia, Europe

Symptoms: Although anaemia and icterus occur, haemoglobinuria is rare. Paralysis as a result of central nervous disorders is common. Incoordination, restlessness and walking in circles may be found during infection.

Significance: *B. caballi* is a widespread infection of horses and may cause significant losses in horse populations where it is prevalent.

Diagnosis: Demonstration of the parasites, preferably in peripheral blood (skin vessels of the ear). The clinical signs and the presence of tick vectors may be of additional help. Serodiagnostic tests (IFAT, CFT) are available for both equine *Babesia* species. However, the indirect fluorescent antibody test (IFAT, ☞ METHODS, 5.2) is more sensitive than the complement fixation test (-CFT, ☞ METHODS, 5.5).

(Figures 449, 450)

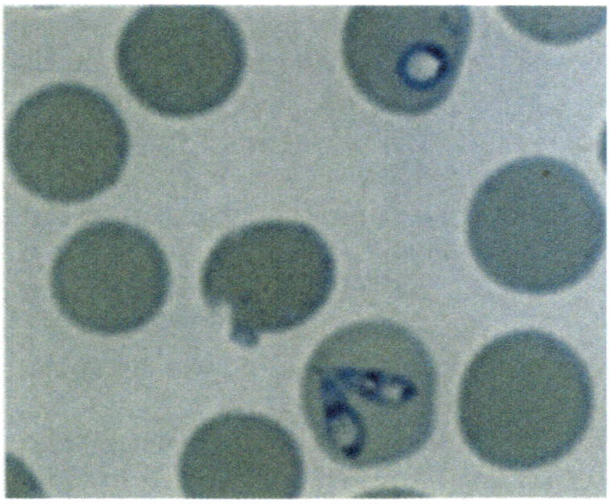

Fig. 449 *Babesia caballi*; stained bloodsmear

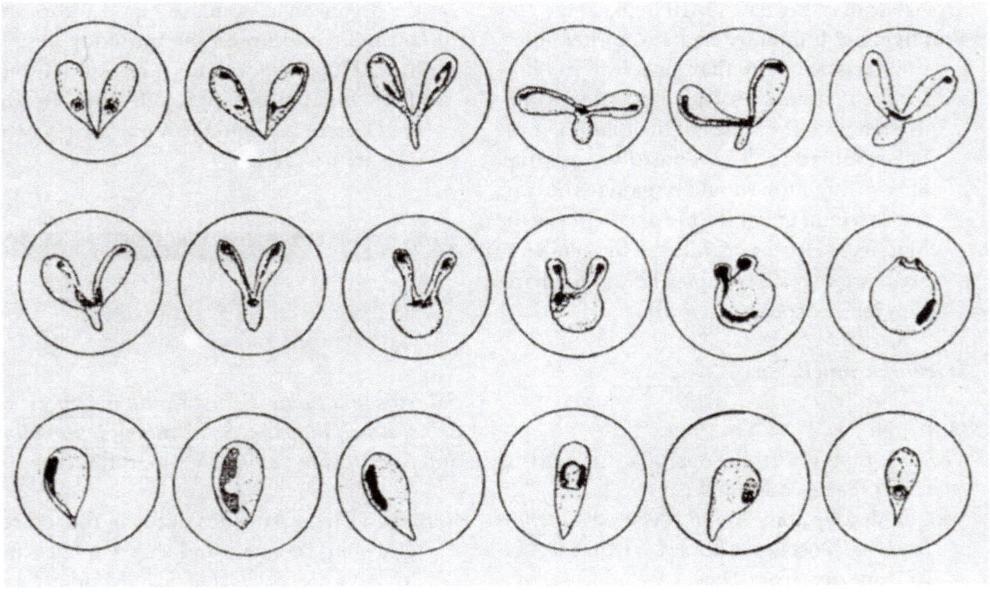

Fig. 450 Various erythrocytic forms of *Babesia caballi* found in the red cells (length: 2.5–4 µm) [3]

• Trematoda found in the blood and circulatory system

Therapy: Most of the babesiacidal drugs used in other animal species are effective against *B. caballi* but only a few are effective against *B. equi* and often in markedly increased dosage rates (*Cave:* Side effects!). Imidocarb dipropionate (and dihydrochloride) administered once is used successfully against *B. caballi* (1 × 4.8 mg/kg, im. or sc.) and *B. equi* (2 × 4.8 mg/kg, sc. or im.). Side effects (extreme restlessness, sweating and abdominal pain), especially at 4.8 mg/kg, can be avoided by pretreatment with atropin sulfate (1%, 1 ml/100 kg) and dividing the dosage in two injections 3 hours apart.
B. caballi is susceptible to diminazene aceturate at 5 mg/kg, given twice at 24-hour intervals, but 6–12 mg/kg is required for *B. equi*.
The following compounds are effective against *B. caballi* but not against *B. equi*: trypan blue (2–3 mg/kg, iv.), quinoronium sulfate (2 × 0.3 mg/kg, sc., at 6-hour intervals), phenamidine (8–10 mg/kg, im.) and amicarbalide diisethoanate (5–10 mg/kg, im.).

Prophylaxis: Immunity in horses after infection lasts for more than one year and horses are therefore protected in enzootic areas even with the seasonal fluctuation of the tick population. Tick control is essential. Special attention should be paid to the ears, to the region under the tail and between the hind legs. Horses introduced into endemic areas are very susceptible and should therefore receive special attention.

Haemobartonella sp.

Hosts: Horse

Vector: Blood sucking ectoparasites (lice, ticks; species not known)

Species description: An unspecified *Haemobartonella* occurs in horses in tropical Africa (reported from Niger)

Geographic distribution: Tropical Africa

Symptoms: Anaemia, epistaxis, progressive weakening, locomotory disorders with painful joints and wasted muscles

Significance: As resurgent parasites in immunosuppressed animals *Haemobartonella* sp. may be of some importance.

Diagnosis: Coccoid (0.1–1 µm) or bacilliform (1–5 µm × 0.7–1.5 µm) parasites appear on the surface of erythrocytes.

Therapy: Oxytetracycline (5–15 mg/kg, iv.) and diminazene (3.5 mg/kg, im.)

Prophylaxis: ☞ THERAPY AND PROPHYLAXIS OF ECTOPARASITES, p. 257

Ehrlichia equi

Remarks: An infectious, non-contagious seasonal disease seen in California and other parts of the USA. This rickettsial organism is found in cytoplasmatic vacuoles of neutrophils, and occasionally eosinophils during the acute stage. The organisms may be demonstrated in Giemsa-stained bloodsmears as morulae or inclusion bodies of 1.5–5 µm in diameter. The symptoms of the disease are fever, depression, ataxia, limb oedema, petechiation and icterus. The diagnosis is based on the demonstration of the organism in standard bloodsmears and an indirect fluorescent antibody test is available. Tetracycline (7 mg/kg, iv. once daily for 8 days) is highly effective. Recovered horses are immune for at least 2 years and are no carriers.

HELMINTHS

• Nematoda larvae and microfilariae found in the blood

Schistosoma bovis, *Schistosoma mattheei*, *Schistosoma indicum*, *Schistosoma japonicum* and *Schistosoma spindale* Blood flukes

Remarks: These parasites occur in the mesenteric veins of cattle and sheep, horses and donkeys. *S. bovis* (Africa, Middle East, western Asia), *S. mattheei* (Central and Southern Africa), *S. indicum* (India subcontinent), *S. japonicum* (East Asia), *S. spindale* (India, Southeast Asia, East Asia). The major clinical signs associated with the intestinal and hepatic forms develop after the onset of the egg excretion and consist of enteritis and intestinal atony, anaemia and progressive emaciation in heavily infected animals.

Significance: Schistosomosis is primarily an infection of ruminants and only causes problems in horses when heavy burdens are acquired.

Diagnosis: Spindle shaped eggs occur in the faeces (☞ CATTLE, ■ 1)

Therapy: ☞ CATTLE, ■ 2

Prophylaxis: ☞ CATTLE, ■ 1

Remarks: *Schistosoma nasale* parasitizes in the veins of the nasal mucosa and occurs in India and Southeast Asia. The eggs are found in the nasal discharge.

- **Nematoda larvae and microfilariae found in the blood**

Strongylus vulgaris

Location: Larvae congregate during their migration in the cranial mesenteric artery, causing thrombosis, embolism and intestinal infarction (☞ HORSES AND DONKEYS, ■ 1).

Remarks: The problems (colic, intestinal infarcts) associated with *S. vulgaris* are not caused by the adult parasites in the caecum but almost exclusively by the migratory activities of the larvae.

Setaria equina

Remarks: The sheathed microfilariae can be demonstrated in peripheral blood samples. (Figures 451, 452)

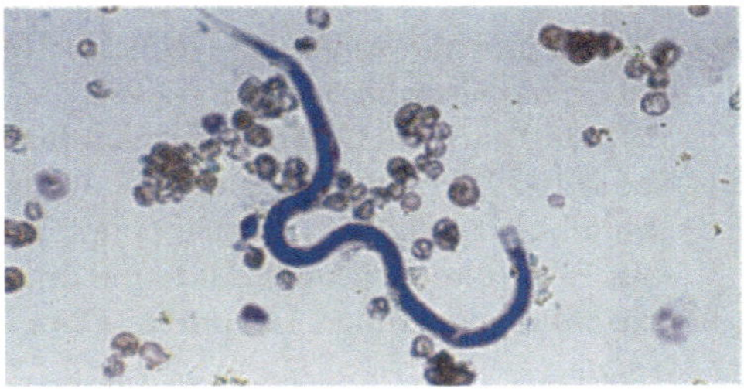

Fig. 451 *Setaria* sp. microfilaria (190–256 µm); stained bloodsmear

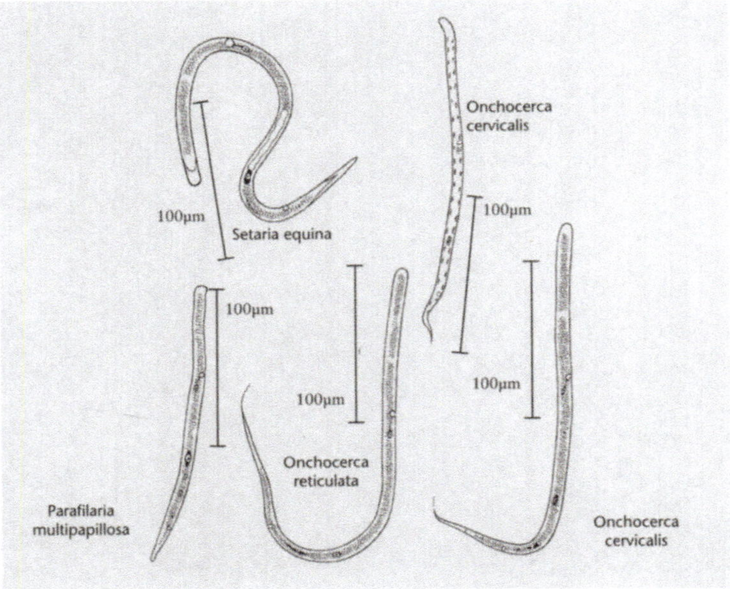

Fig. 452 Microfilariae of filariid parasites of horses [38]

Parafilaria multipapillosa

"summer bleeding"

Remarks: Microfilariae can be demonstrated in blood discharged from "summer bleeding"nodules, caused by adult female parasites. They are less than 200 µm long and have a rounded posterior extremity.

Onchocerca cervicalis and *Onchocerca reticulata*

Remarks: Microfilariae of these two nematodes may be demonstrated by excising a small piece of skin from the linea alba and placing it in physiological saline solution. Microfilariae usually migrate out of the dermis into the solution (overnight). *O. cervicalis* microfilariae are slender and 207–240 µm long. *O. reticulata* microfilariae are 330–370 µm long and have a long, whip-like tail ending in a fine point. The distance from the genital cell to the tip of the tail is greater than 140 µm for *O. reticulata*.

PROTOZOA

Neospora caninum

Remarks: *N. caninum* can be transmitted transplacentally in equines. Abortion and weakness with paralysis in newborn foals may occur. Tachyzoites of *N. caninum* were found in sections of lung of an equine fetus aborted 2 month before term. Individual tachyzoites were approximately 3–5 × 2–3 µm, divided by endodyogeny, and stained positively with anti-*N. caninum* serum but not with anti-*Toxoplasma gondii* serum. *T. gondii* antibody was not found in the mare's serum (☞ CATTLE, ■ 4.6).

Trypanosoma equiperdum Dourine

Hosts: Horse and donkey

Vector: Generally transmitted by coitus and very rarely by biting flies

Species description: Dourine is a venereal disease of horses, transmitted mechanically by coitus and rarely by biting flies. *T. equiperdum* occurs in donkeys but the disease is asymptomatic. Oedema on the genitals are not obvious and skin plaques only occur in less than 10% of infected donkeys. The sperm and the vaginal discharge are very virulent and donkeys therefore are a continuous reservoir of the pathogen.

Geographic distribution: North (Mediterranean coast) and South Africa, Middle East and South America.

Symptoms: Clinical signs develop over weeks or months. Early signs include mucopurulent discharge from the urethra in stallions and from the vagina in mares, followed by oedema of the genitalia. Later characteristic circular, raised, itching plaques 2–10 cm in diameter appear on the skin and infected horses become progressively emaciated. Paralysis occurs in the terminal phase, accompanied by intense emaciation and oedema of the lower parts of the body. Mortality in untreated cases is 50–70%.

Significance: *T. equiperdum* causes the most important venereal disease in horses and is responsible for great losses wherever it occurs.

Diagnosis: Demonstration of the trypanosomes from the urethral or vaginal discharges, the skin plaques or the peripheral blood is generally not possible, although centrifugation of these fluids may help to find the pathogens. The clinical disease is typical in endemic areas to allow diagnosis. Infected animals can be detected with the complement fixation test but cross reaction with *T. evansi* and *T. brucei* are common. In endemic areas infected horses should be treated.

Therapy: Quinapyramine sulfate (3–5 mg/kg, sc.) is one of the few compounds effective against *T. equiperdum*. In many countries chemotherapy is prohibited and strict border controls are required before introducing equines.

Prophylaxis: In endemic areas effective prophylaxis is not feasible. Infected horses transmit the disease during coitus. Donkeys act as reservoir hosts without clinical signs. Eradication is only possible if a strict control of all imported horses and breeding can be carried out and stray horses can be eliminated.

(Figures 103, 444, 453, 454, Table 6)

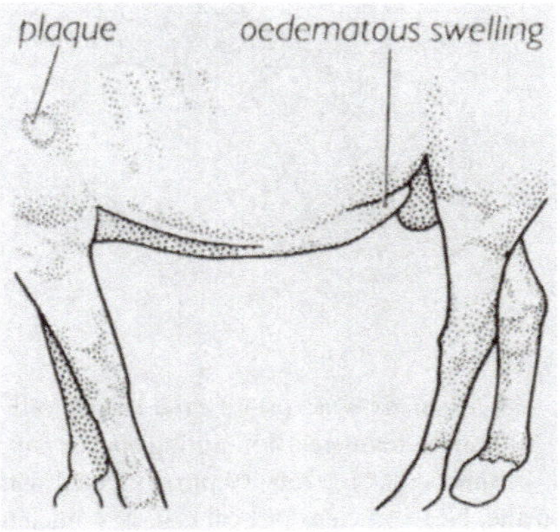

Fig. 453 Oedema of the genitalia and skin plaques associated with Dourine (*Trypanosoma equiperdum* infection) [37]

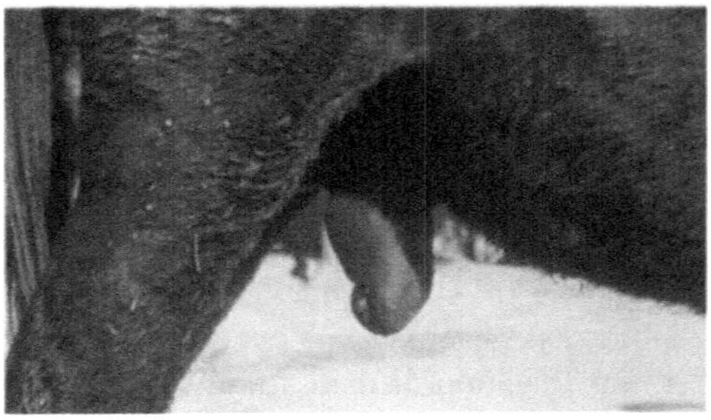

Fig. 454 Oedematous swellings of the praeputium due to *Trypanosoma equiperdum* infection (donkey) [4]

Klossiella equi

Remarks: This species occurs world-wide in the kidneys of horses, donkeys and zebras. Thin-shelled oocysts (50–100µm in diameter) may incidentally be found in the epithelial cells of the loop of Henle. These oocysts contain 40–60 sporocysts (4–6 × 6–10 µm) with 10–15 sporozoites each. Sporocysts are passed in the urine and may be discovered in the sediment. *K. equi* are generally regarded as nonpathogenic.
(Figure 455)

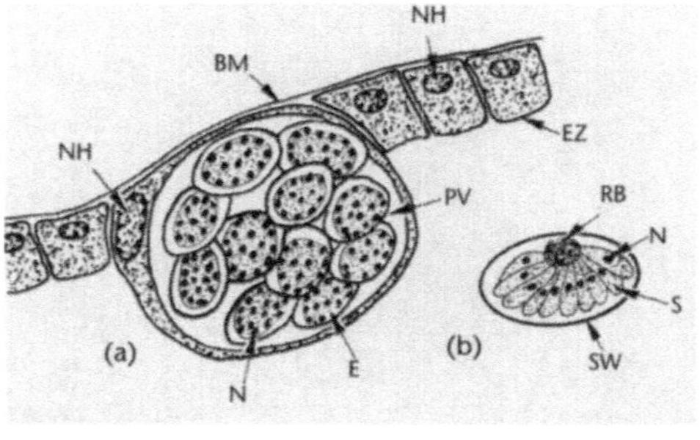

Fig. 455 *Klossiella equi*: (a) infected kidney cell (50–100 µm in diameter) containing sporocysts and (b) sporocyst (4–6 × 6–10 µm) excreted with the urine, NH = nucleus of host cell, N = nucleus of parasite, E = developing sporocyst, EZ = endothelial cell, SW = wall of the sporocyst, RB = residual bod, BM = basal membrane, PV = parasitophorous vacuole and S = sorozoite [7]

4 Stages in internal organs

4.1 Locomotory system

4.1.1 Muscles

PROTOZOA

Sarcocystis bertrami, S. equicanis and *S. fayeri*

Location: Sarcocysts are found in the heart, diaphragm and other muscles

Hosts: Horse and donkey

Species description: *S. bertrami*, *S. equicanis* and *S. fayeri* are described as equine species and it seems that the dog acts as final host. The origin and general life cycle of *Sarcocystis* spp. is imperfectly understood. *S. neurona* is a recently described new species the life cycle of which is still unknown.

Geographic distribution: World-wide

Symptoms: *Sarcocystis* spp. of horses are only mildly pathogenic. Slight fever, anaemia may occur in the acute phase of infection while chronic infection may cause a multifocal granulomatous myositis.

Significance: *Sarcocystis* spp. in horses is very common and compared to those species found in cattle and small ruminants only mildly pathogenic (☞ CATTLE, ■ 4.1.1).

Diagnosis: Muscle cysts (up to 10 mm in length) may be found. These whitish streaks are embedded in the muscles and divided into compartments, packed with banana-shaped parasitic cells.

Therapy: Unknown

Prophylaxis: Uncooked horse meat fed to dogs and probably to other carnivores closes the life cycle of equine *Sarcocystis* spp.

Toxoplasma gondii

Remarks: *T. gondii* can infect virtually all warm-blooded animals. Only Felidae can act as definite hosts. Infection takes place by ingestion of sporulated oocysts. Horses can become infected by eating herbage contaminated with cat faeces or by accidentally ingesting tissues of infected rodents. The prevalence of infection is usually high (> 30%) but clinical disease attributable to this parasite is rare. However, in the muscle cells of horse tissue cysts of *T. gondii* are found (☞ SWINE, ■ 4.1).

4.1.2 Tendons

HELMINTHS

- Nematoda larvae and adult nematodes found in the tendons

Onchocerca cervicalis
Nuchal ligament worm

Location: Ligamentum nuchae
Hosts: Horse and donkey
Species description: The male is 6–7 cm long and the female up to 30 cm. The microfilariae are 200–240 µm in length and 4–5 µm in diameter, unsheathed and with a short tail. Microfilariae are found in the skin of the ventral midline. Intermediate hosts are biting midges (*Culicoides nubeculosus* and other *Culicoides* spp.).
Geographic distribution: World-wide
Significance: Adult *O. cervicalis* parasites are non-pathogenic and cause little reaction. Microfilariae may cause dermatitis.
(Figures 452, 456, 457)

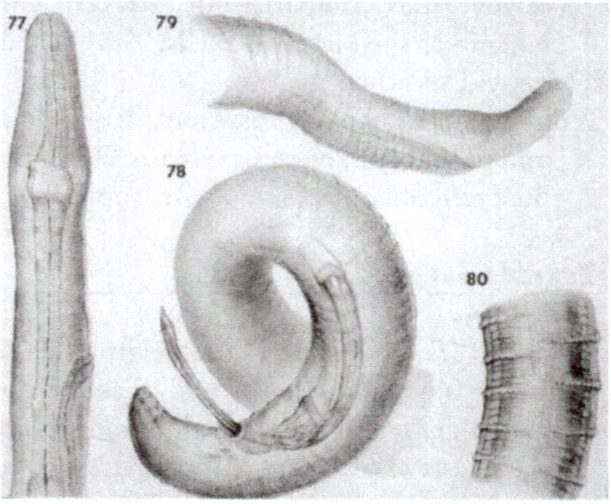

Fig. 456 *Onchocerca cervicalis*; anterior end (77), tail end of a male (78), posterior end of a female (79), cuticular striation (80); males are 6–7 cm long, and females are up to 50 cm long [40]

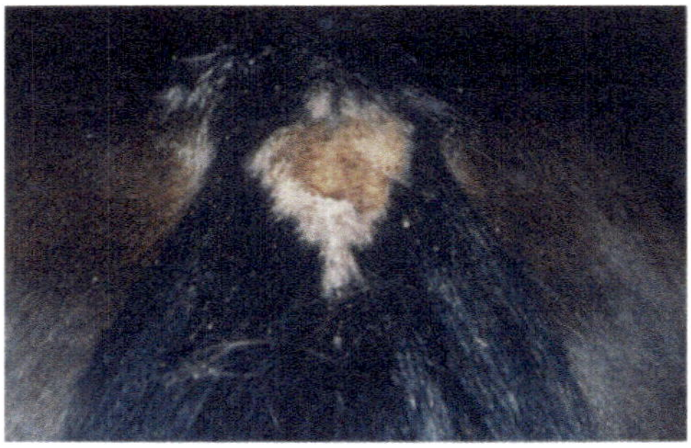

Fig. 457 Moist dermatitis and loss of tail hair due to *Onchocerca cervicalis*

Onchocerca reticulata Ligament worm

Location: Connective tissue of the flexor tendons and the suspensory ligament of the fetlock, mainly the foreleg.
Hosts: Horse and donkey
Species description: Microfilariae occur in the skin on either side of the linea alba and cause a dermatitis during the activity period of the intermediate host (*Culicoides nubeculosus* and other *Culicoides* spp.). They measure 330–370 µm and possess a long whiplash-like tail.
Geographic distribution: World-wide
Significance: Chronic inflammations and calcifications may cause lameness. Microfilariae may cause dermatitis.
(Figures 452, 458, 459)

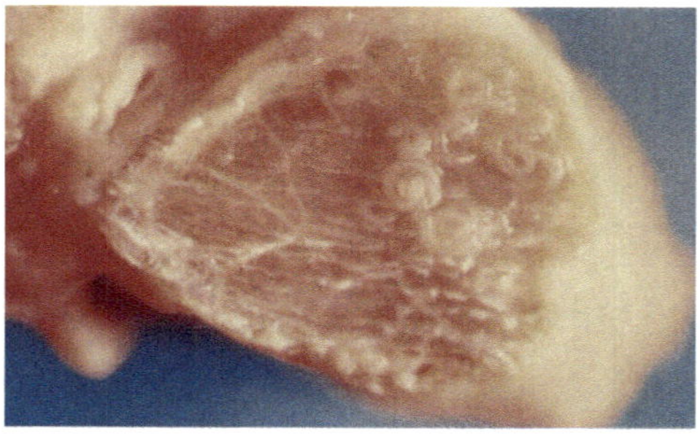

Fig. 458 *Onchocerca reticulata*; adult worms in the tissue of the flexor tendons and associated tissue [15]

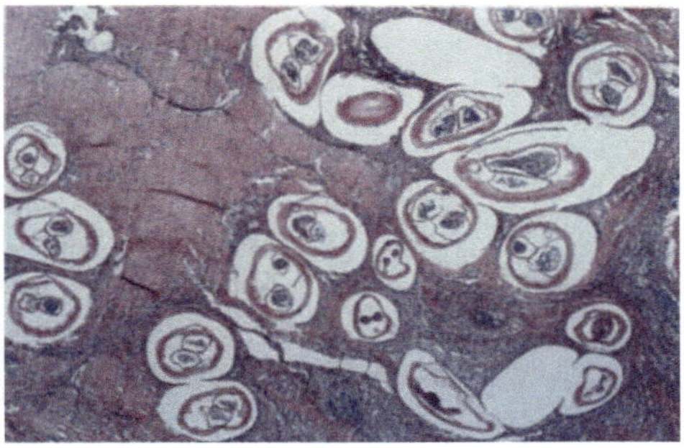

Fig. 459 *Onchocerca reticulata*; tendon of the musculus interosseus with multiple sections of the adult worms (histological section)

Onchocerca raillieti

Location: Adults occur in the cervical ligament, subcutaneous cysts on the penis and in the perimuscular connective tissue.

Hosts: Donkey

Species description: Very little is known about this parasite.

Geographic distribution: Africa

Significance: Adult parasites are non-pathogenic.

- **General features of O. *cervicalis*, O. *reticulata* and O. *raillieti***

Significance: Adult parasites of O. *cervicalis* and O. *raillieti* are non-pathogenic and cause few problems. However, O. *reticulata* infections in the flexor tendons and suspensory ligament may be associated with lameness. A seasonal, sporadic dermatitis is known to occur in many parts of the world due to the presence of microfilariae. The reaction may be induced by both the microfilariae (dead and dying ones) in the dermis and the bites of the insects (hypersensitivity to midge bites). Microfilariae also accumulate in the eyes of horses but there is still some debate about their role in the pathogenesis of equine uveitis. *Onchocerca* infections are often accompanied by depigmentation of the bulbar conjunctiva. Other lesions of onchocercosis involve the cornea and include oedema and punctate or streaking types of opacities of the stroma, superficial erosions and sclerosing keratitis.

Symptoms: Adult parasites cause little symptoms. Calcifications in the connective tissue (caused by dead parasites) may be found without clinical symptoms. Lameness due to O. *reticulata* infections may occur.

Papular or exudative dermatitis with alopecia and pruritus due to microfilariae ("summer mange", allergic "dermatitis") is a well-known entity associated with *Onchocerca* infections.

Diagnosis: The diagnosis of *Onchocerca*-associated dermatitis may be based on the good responsiveness to microfilaricidal treatment. Microfilariae can be found by a full-thickness skin biopsy > 6 mm. The tissue is macerated in isotonic saline for several hours. Microfilariae are concentrated and stained with methylene blue after removal of skin pieces. Microfilariae can be differentiated microscopically from *Setaria* spp. which occur in the blood and possess a sheath around the larvae.

Therapy: No treatment is effective against the adults. Ivermectin (200 µg/kg, sc.) is efficacious (> 99%) against microfilariae and produces marked clinical improvement in horses with onchocercal dermatitis. A single oral dosage of ivermectin showed marked clinical improvement within 1–2 weeks after treatment and the *Onchocerca* spp. microfilariae disappeared within this time. The presence of O. *cervicalis* microfilariae in the skin of horses is not always associated with dermatitis, but where dermatitis occurs, it can be treated successfully with ivermectin. Diethylcarbamazine (5–8 mg/kg, sc.) for 21 days is effective against microfilariae.

Prophylaxis: Generally not indicated. Insecticidal sprays and repellents may reduce the attacks by biting midges.

(Figures 452, 460, 461, 462, 463)

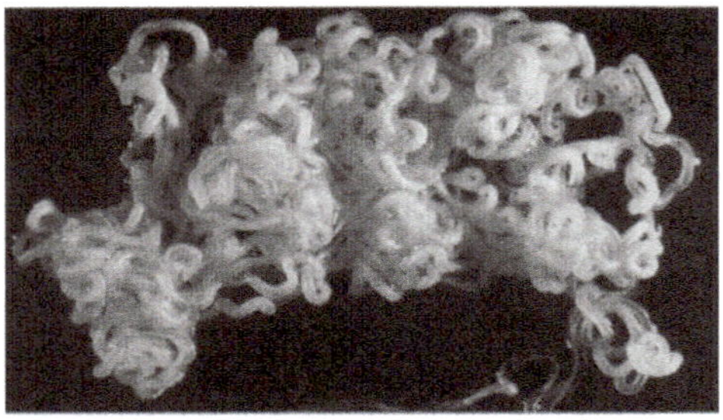

Fig. 460 *Onchocerca* sp.; adult convoluted parasite. The worm is up to 30 cm long and found interwined through the connective tissues and can be isolated by artificial digestion [37]

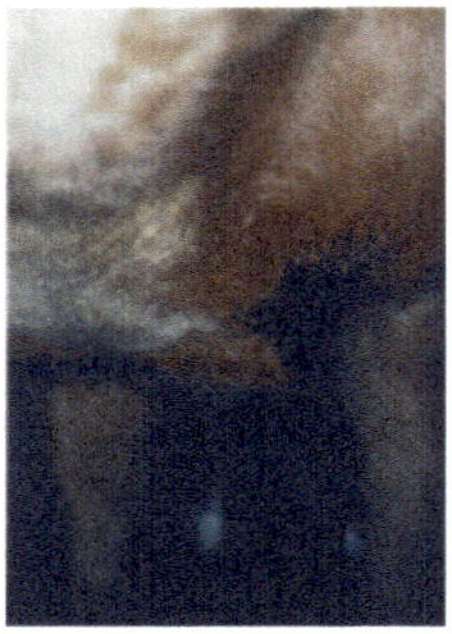

Fig. 461 *Onchocerca* sp. associated moist dermatitis (horse)

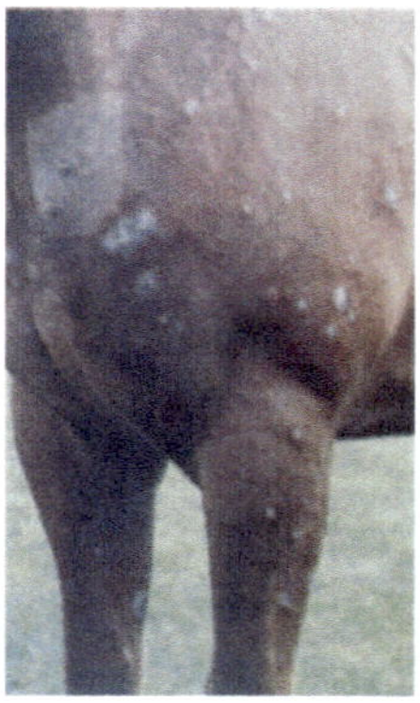

Fig. 462 *Onchocerca* sp. associated dermatitis [41]

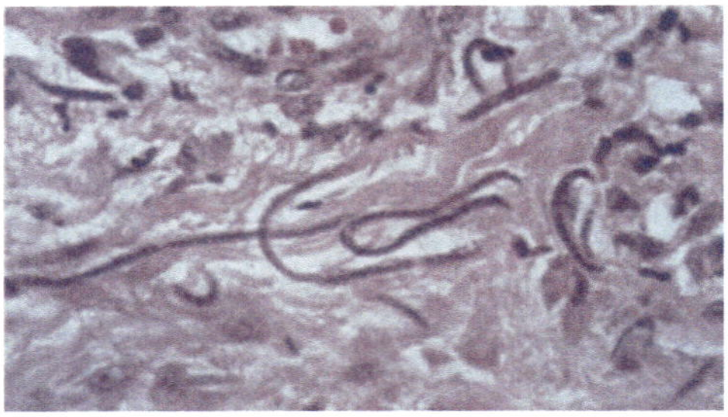

Fig. 463 Microfilariae of *Onchocerca* sp. found in the subcutaneous tissue of a horse (histological section) [41]

4.2 Liver

HELMINTHS

- Trematoda found in the liver

Fasciola gigantica ☞ CATTLE, ■ 4.2
Fasciola hepatica ☞ CATTLE, ■ 4.2
Dicrocoelium dendriticum ☞ CATTLE, ■ 4.2

- Cestoda found in the liver

Remarks: Larvae of the canine tapeworm *Taenia hydatigena* occasionally also occurs in equines (☞ CATTLE, ■ 4.2 and 4.4 and SHEEP AND GOATS, ■ 4.2 and 4.4).
Hydatid cysts (larvae) of the canine tapeworm *Echinococcus granulosus* are often found in the liver of horses (☞ CATTLE, ■ 4.2).
(Figure 464)

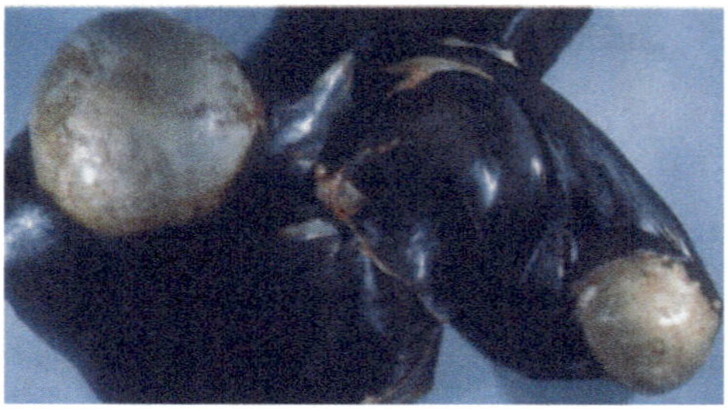

Fig. 464 Hydatid cysts of *Echinococcus granulosus* found in the liver of a horse

• Nematoda found in the liver

Capillaria hepatica

Remarks: Occasionally the parasite is found in the liver of horses. It deposits its eggs in the liver parenchyma where they produce granuloma and fibrosis. *C. hepatica* is common in rodents but may occur from time to time in a variety of other hosts including horse and man. *C. hepatica* very rarely causes disease in horses.

Parascaris equorum

Remarks: Larvae are transient visitors in the liver during their migration from the intestine to the heart. They may cause "white spots" which are seen at necropsy (☞ HORSES AND DONKEYS, ■ 1)

Strongylus edentatus and *Strongylus equinus*

Remarks: Fourth-stage larvae of these nematodes may cause nodules and tracts during their migratory period in the liver (☞ HORSES AND DONKEYS, ■ 1)

4.3 Respiratory system

HELMINTHS

• Cestoda found in the respiratory system

Echinococcus granulosus

Remarks: Larvae (hydatid cysts) of the canine tapeworm *E. granulosus* may also be found in the lungs of equines (☞ CATTLE, ■ 4.2 and ☞ HORSES AND DONKEYS, ■ 4.2)

• Nematoda found in the respiratory system

Dictyocaulus arnfieldi Equine lungworm

Location: Bronchi and bronchioles
Hosts: Donkey and horse

Species description: *D. arnfieldi* has a direct life cycle. The ingested larvae penetrate the intestine and reach the lungs via the circulatory system. In the lungs they break through the blood vessels into the bronchi and develop to adults. The prepatent period is 5–6 weeks. *D. arnfieldi* is very prevalent in donkeys and other equines and relatively rare in horses. Donkeys are often carriers and thus a risk for horses kept in the same environment.

Geographic distribution: World-wide, particularly in areas with heavy rainfall

Symptoms: Severe coughing, loss of appetite, chronic pneumonia, pulmonary oedema, secondary bacterial infections. Heavy infections may cause death, particularly in foals.

Significance: Donkeys are common hosts and symptomless carriers who constitute a reservoir of infection for horses. *D. arnfieldi* does no damage if only a few are present, but large numbers can cause death.
Problems arise when horses and donkeys are kept together, especially in warm, humid areas and where hygiene is poor.

Diagnosis: Identification of embryonated eggs in fresh or larvae in older faeces and tracheal mucus; clinical signs in the infected horses.

Therapy: Levamisole (1×5 mg/kg, im.) twice, 3 weeks apart, mebendazole (20 mg/kg, po.) on five consecutive days, fenbendazole (50 mg/kg, po.) are effective against *D. arnfieldi*. Ivermectin oral paste (0.2 mg/kg) is highly effective against *D. arnfieldi* adults and fourth-stage larvae.

Prophylaxis: Regular treatment of both horses and donkeys if they are kept together. The treatment scheme against the other "horse strongyles" is also effective against *D. arnfieldi*. If possible, horses and donkeys should be kept on different pastures. Removal of faeces at the feeding place is important.

(Figure 432, 465)

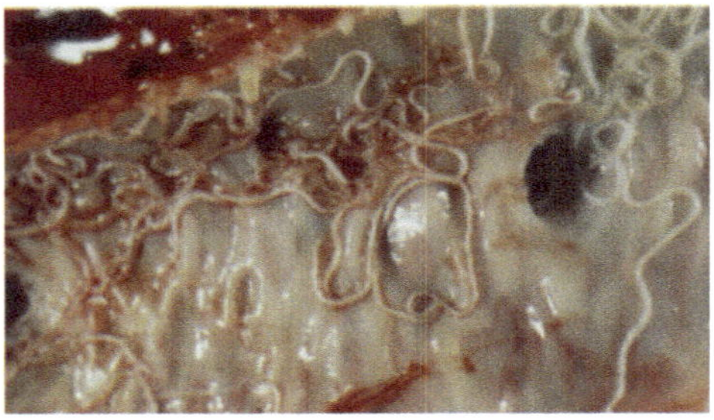

Fig. 465 *Dictyocaulus arnfieldi*; adult parasites in the trachea female: 3.8–8.5 cm, male: 2.6–4.3 cm [4]

Habronema spp.

Remarks: Larvae may occasionally occur in the lungs (☞ HORSES AND DONKEYS, ■ 1).

ARTHROPODS

• Insecta larvae found in the respiratory system

Rhinoestrus purpureus

Remarks: Life cycle similar to those of the genus *Oestrus*. Larval stages are obligatory parasites of horses and mules in tropical Africa. Larvae are deposited by the adult fly in batches of 8–40 into the nostrils or eyes. The larvae crawl into the nasal cavity where they remain for several months before moving to the sinuses where they mature. They cause obstruction, irritation and sneezing (☞ SHEEP AND GOATS, ■ 4.3 p. 183, Figure 489).

4.4 Abdominal cavity

HELMINTHS

• Cestoda found in the abdominal cavity

Cysticercus tenuicollis

Remarks: The larval stage of the canine tapeworm *Taenia hydatigena* may sometimes be found as long-necked cysts attached to the omentum, intestinal mesentery and serosal surface of abdominal organs (☞ SHEEP AND GOATS, ■ 4.4).

• Nematoda found in the abdominal cavity

Setaria equina Equine abdominal worm

Location: Adult worms in the abdominal cavity and very rarely as aberrant worms in other parts of the body (lungs, eyes). Microfilariae occur in the blood.

Hosts: Horse and donkey

Species description: Microfilariae produced by adult worms are ingested by mosquitoes (*Aedes* spp. and *Culex* spp.) where they develop within two weeks. When mosquitoes feed again on horses the infective larvae are re-injected. Adult males reach 8 cm in length and females 13 cm. The head end shows typical peribuccal prominences. Microfilariae are sheathed and 190–256 µm in length (Figure 452).

Geographic distribution: World-wide

Symptoms: Generally no symptoms are seen except when worms (mainly microfilariae) are present in the eyes causing blindness.

Significance: Adult *Setaria equina* in the abdominal cavity are non-pathogenic. Very rarely larvae may migrate to the anterior chamber of the eyes or to the brain and spinal cord where they cause damage.

Diagnosis: Detection of sheathed microfilariae in the bloodsmear.

Therapy: Is generally not indicated. There is no therapy yet against adult *Setaria*. Diethylcarbamazine (40 mg/kg, po.) given for 1–3 days or ivermectin (0.2 mg/kg, sc.) are partially effective against microfilariae.

Prophylaxis: *Setaria* control is closely associated to mosquito control. Topical insecticides may be useful to reduce mosquito bites.

(Figures 466, 467, 468)

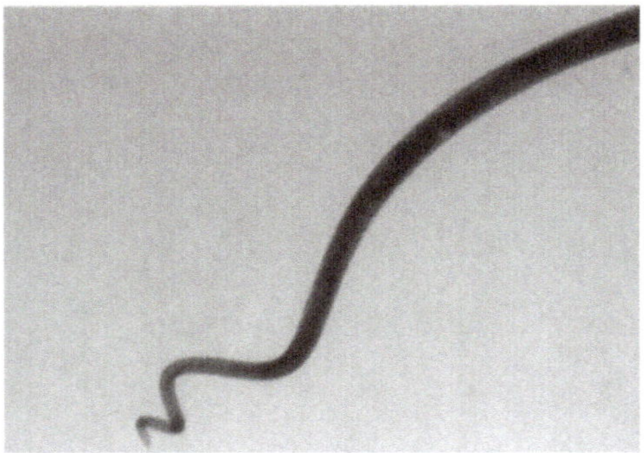

Fig. 466 *Setaria* sp.; coiled tail end (males reach 8 cm in length and females 13 cm)

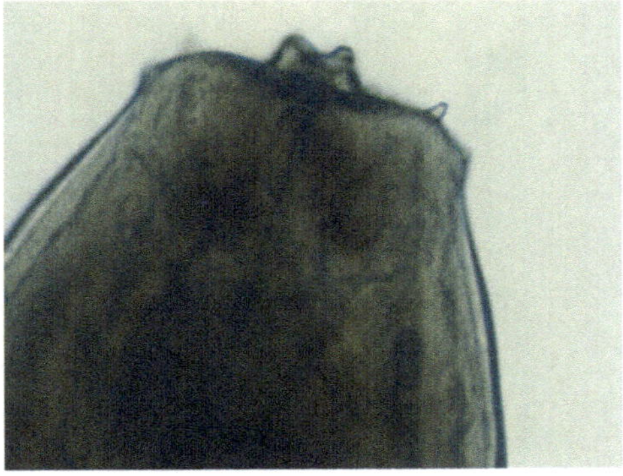

Fig. 467 *Setaria equina*; adult; anterior end with typical peribuccal prominences

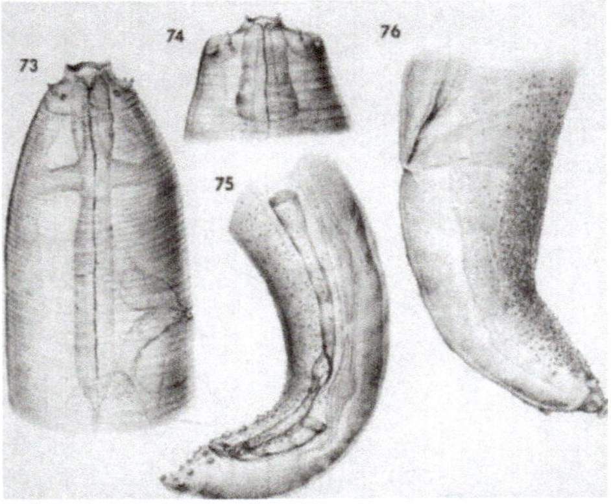

Fig. 468 *Setaria equina*; anterior end (73 and 74) and posterior end of a male (75), posterior end of a female (76) [40]

Strongylus edentatus* and *Strongylus equinus

Remarks: Fifth-stage larvae may occasionally be found during their migration subserous or within the abdominal cavity (☞ HORSES AND DONKEYS, ■ 1).

4.5 Central nervous system

PROTOZOA

Sarcocystis neurona

Remarks: This is an apicomplexan parasite which is associated with myeloencephalitis in horses. Only asexual stages of this parasite presently are known, and they are found within neuronal cells and leukocytes of the brain and spinal cord. The parasite is located in the host cell cytoplasm, does not have a parasitophorous vacuole, and divides by endopolygeny. Schizonts are 5–35 µm × 5–20 µm and contain 4–40 merozoites arranged in a rosette around a prominent residual body. Merozoites are approximately 4 × 1 µm, have a central nucleus, and lack rhoptries. Schizonts and merozoites react with *Sarcocystis cruzi* antiserum but not with *Caryospora bigenetica, Toxoplasma gondii, Hammondia hammondi* or *Neospora caninum* antisera in an immunohistochemical test.

Toxoplasma gondii

Remarks: *T. gondii* tissue cysts may also be found in the brain and spinal cord of horses. Infection is acquired by ingesting sporulated oocysts (☞ HORSES AND DONKEYS, ■ 4.1.1 and ☞ SWINE, ■ 4.1)

Neospora caninum

Remarks: *N. caninum* tissue cysts were also found in the central nervous system of equines (☞ HORSES AND DONKEYS, ■ 3 and ☞ CATTLE, ■ 4.6)

HELMINTHS

- Cestoda cysts found in the central nervous system

Echinococcus granulosus

Remarks: Larvae (hydatid cysts) of the canine tapeworm *E. granulosus* may also be found in the brain of equines (☞ CATTLE, ■ 4.2 and ☞ HORSES AND DONKEYS, ■ 4.2).

Coenurus cerebralis

Larvae of the canine tapeworm *Taenia multiceps* may also be found in the brain of equines (☞ SHEEP AND GOATS, ■ 4.6).

5.1 Skin and coat

PROTOZOA

Besnoitia bennetti

Location: The cysts of this parasite occur in subdermal connective tissue of horses.
Hosts: Horse and donkey
Species description: The morphology and life-cycle is essentially the same as for *B. besnoiti* of cattle, although the definitive host is unknown.
Geographic distribution: Africa, southern Europe, South America
Symptoms: General thickening of the skin, loss of hair and scurfy appearance. The disease has a chronic course (7–8 weeks) and progressive weakness in infected animals may occur.
Significance: *B. bennetti* may account for a chronic, depleting skin disease of horses in some parts of Africa.
Diagnosis, Therapy and Prophylaxis: (☞ CATTLE, ■ 5.1 *B. besnoiti*)
(Figure 469)

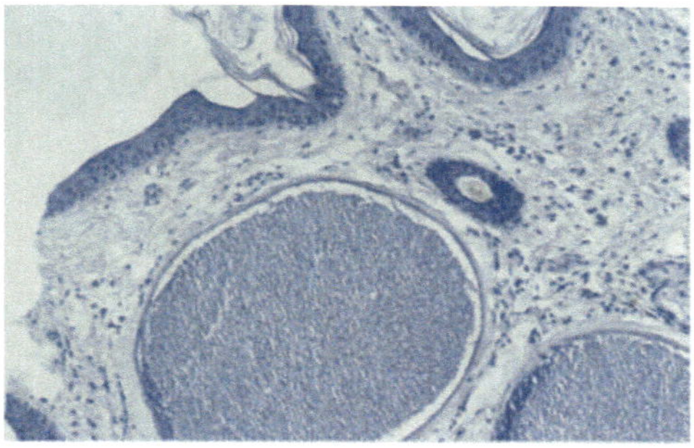

Fig. 469 *Besnoitia bennetti*; subcutaneous cyst (up to 600 µm in diameter) with several thousands of cystozoites (histological section)

HELMINTHS

• Nematoda found in the skin

Third-stage larvae of ***Draschia megastoma*** (syn. *Habronema megastoma*) **and *Habronema* spp.** Larvae of equine stomach worms; summer sores, cutaneous or ocular habronemosis

Location: Third-stage larvae of *Habronema* spp. are found in non-healing skin wounds. Adult worms are found in the stomach (☞ HORSES AND DONKEYS, ■ 1).
Species description: Larvae of the spiruroid worms *Habronema* spp. which are deposited in existing wounds by infected flies (*Musca domestica* and *Stomoxys calcitrans*) cause a granulomatous dermatits which delays healing. Larvae deposited in the wounds migrate and feed, extending the wound and preventing healing. If licked by the host the larvae mature in the stomach.
Geographic distribution: World-wide
Symptoms: Typical skin wounds (ocular and cutaneous habronemosis) which are not healing and which contain larvae. These

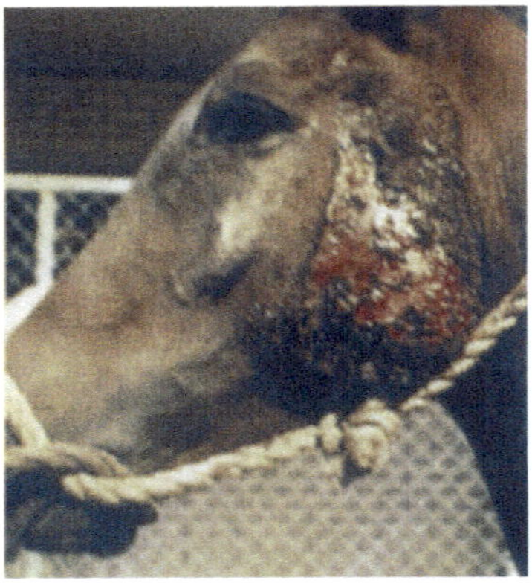

Fig. 470 Cutaneous habronemosis (summer sores) [36]

wounds tend to heal spontaneously during the period when flies are inactive (winter, dry season) but often recur in subsequent seasons when fly activity starts again (summer, wet season).

Diagnosis: Adult worms may be found during postmortem examinations (☞ HORSES AND DONKEYS, 1). Ova or larvae in the faeces are diagnostic but are easily overlooked. Non-healing, reddish brown, greasy skin granuloma that contain rice-grain-sized, calcified material is indicative for cutaneous habronemosis. Larvae are recognized by their spiny knobs on their tails, in lesion scrapings are indicative of ocular or cutaneous habronemosis.

Therapy: Two injections of ivermectin (200 µg/kg, im.) cured the cutaneous lesions caused by third-stage larvae of *Habronema* spp.. A insecticide (lindane) ointment should afterwards be applied to the wound to prevent reinfection.
Trichlorfon (25 mg/kg, iv.) administered in 1 l isotonic saline solution cured summer sores within 30 days. Premedication with atropin was necessary. Organophosphates (coumaphos, dichlorvos, crotoxyphos + dichlorvos, lindane) applied topically to the abraded surface may kill the larvae. Insect repellents may reduce transmission by flies.

Prophylaxis: Fly prevention by stacking manure and using insecticides. Skin wounds should be treated with fly repellents (citronella oil, diethyltoluamide and diethyl phtalate). Cypermethrin (0.1% solution, using 150–250 ml per animal) and pyrethrins (0.01%) are highly effective to control flies on horses.
(Figures 470, 471)

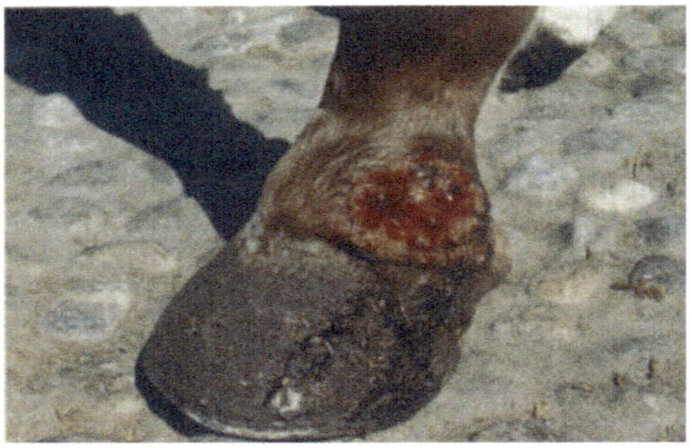

Fig. 471 Cutaneous habronemosis; typical lesions on the coronary border

Parafilaria multipapillosa

"summer bleeding"

Location: Adult worms are found in subcutaneous nodules. The haemorrhagic exudates of these nodules contain eggs and larvae.

Species description: Subcutaneous nodules, containing 3–7 cm long filarial worms, which break open and ooze blood. Blood-sucking flies (*Haematobia atripalpis* and other *Haematobia* spp.) act as intermediate hosts.

Geographic distribution: North Africa, eastern and southern Europe, Asia and South America

Symptoms: Subcutaneous nodules, particularly on the head and upper forequarters, which appear suddenly, break open, bleed and then heal up during the winter or dry season to re-appear the following season.

Significance: The nodules may interfere with the harness of working horses but are generally of little consequence.

Diagnosis: Nodules in the skin, transient haemorrhage with eggs and unsheathed microfilariae in the exudate. The microfilariae are less than 200 µm long and have a rounded posterior extremity.

Therapy: No satisfactory treatment is available. Metrifonate (4–6 × 35 mg/kg, daily) and diethylcarbamazine (10–20 × 6–8 mg/kg, daily) but also fenbendazole (5 × 50 mg/kg, po.) are described to be used for treatment but with a moderate success.

Prophylaxis: Fly control may reduce the incidence.

(Figures 452, 472, 473, 474, 475)

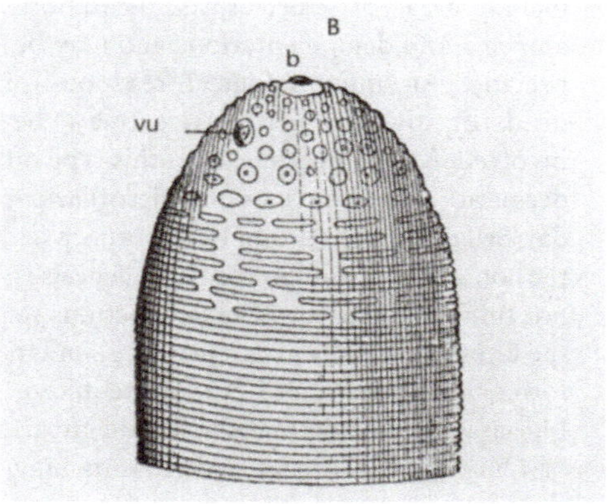

Fig. 474 *Parafilaria multipapillosa*; anterior end with vulva (vu) and buccal opening (b) [9]

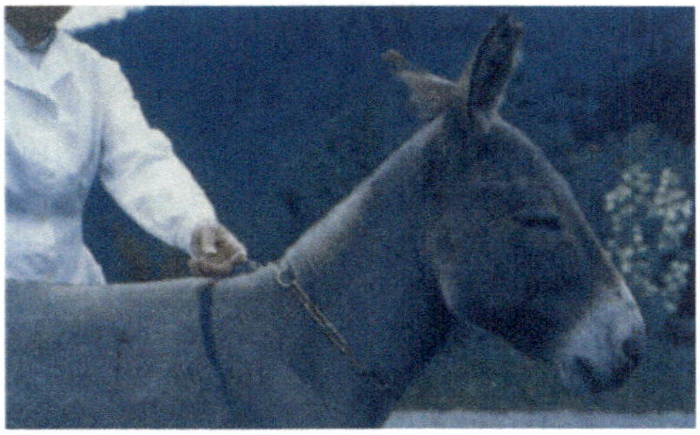

Fig. 472 "Summer bleeding" due to *Parafilaria multipapillosa*; bleeding wound on the withers

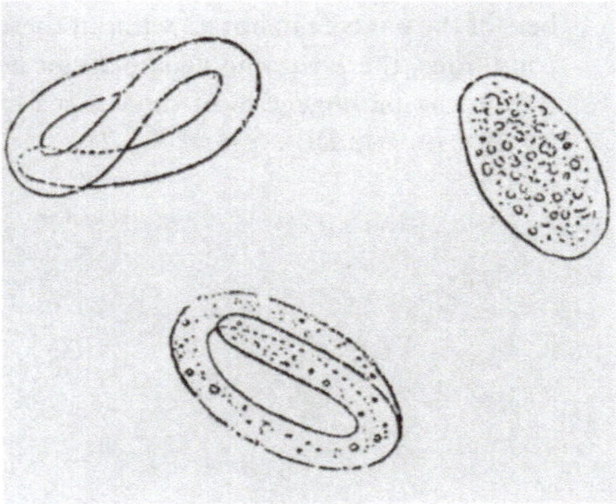

Fig. 475 *Parafilaria multipapillosa*; eggs (52–58 × 24–33 µm) containing a microfilaria [9]

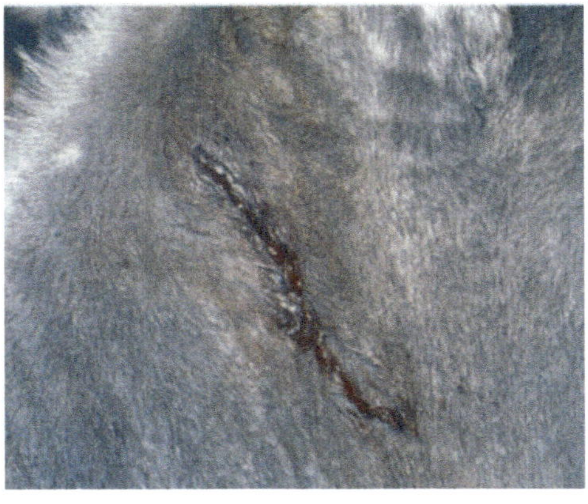

Fig. 473 "Summer bleeding" due to *Parafilaria multipapillosa*; bleeding wound

Onchocerca cervicalis Nuchal ligamen worm
Onchocerca reticulata Ligament worm

Remarks: The adult worms in ligaments cause swelling, calcification and pain, and the microfilariae may affect the cornea of the eye. Microfilariae concentrate in skin of the ventral midline, along the linea alba. Microfilariae can be found in horses with dermatitis of the face, neck, chest, withers, forelegs and abdomen. These lesions often include areas of scale, crusts, ulceration, alopecia and depigmentations and may be pruritic. An immunological reaction to dead or dying microfilariae may be involved in the pathogenesis of this type of dermatitis. Treatment with microfilaricidal drugs usually dramatically improves the condition, although the pathogenesis is not fully understood. Allergic reactions to the bites of small flies may produce similar forms of dermatitis and exacerbate microfilaria-associated dermatitis. The diagnosis of *Onchocerca*-associated dermatitis may therefore be based on responsiveness to microfilaricidal treatment. Large numbers of microfilariae can also be found in horses without dermatitis.

O. cervicalis has been associated with poll evil, fistulous withers and equine uveitis, but because of the presence of large numbers of the parasite in horses without these conditions, there is some debate about its role in the pathogenesis of these diseases (☞ HORSES AND DONKEYS, ■ 4.1.2).

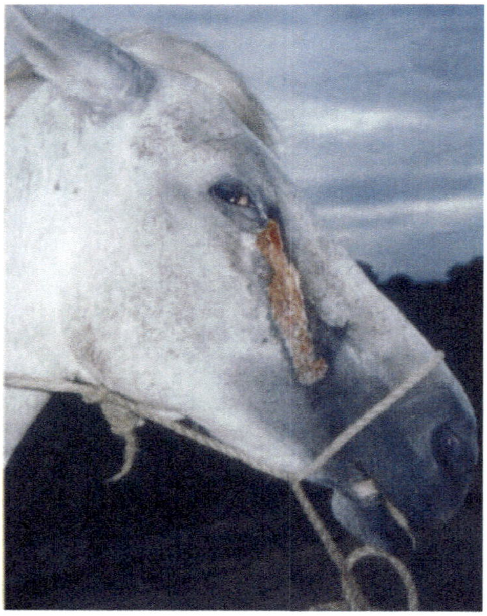

Fig. 476 Moist dermatitis associated with the lacrimal duct. Masses of microfilariae were found in the wound [58]

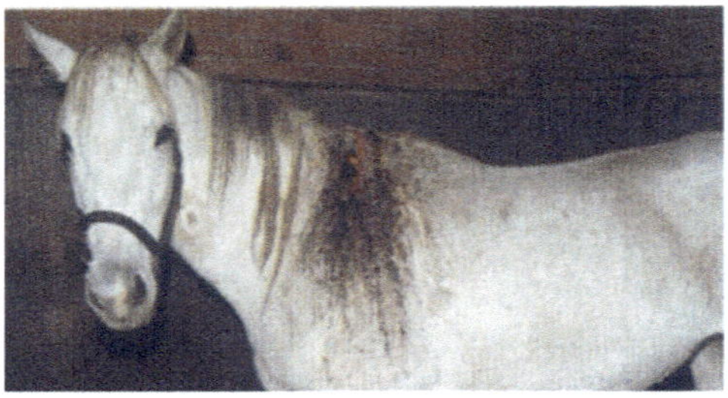

Fig. 477 Fistulous withers may be caused by *Onchocerca cervicalis* [37]

Diagnosis, Therapy and Prophylaxis: ☞ HORSES AND DONKEYS, ■ 4.1.2
(Figures 452, 476, 477)

ARTHROPODS

Arthropods are divided into two main groups:

Arachnida (arachnids) including:
- *Ticks*
- *Mites*

Insecta including:
- *Lice*
- *Fleas*
- *Dipterida*

• Arachnida found in/on the skin

– Ticks

(☞ CATTLE, ■ 5.1)

Ticks may provoke disease in three different ways:

- **Direct noxious effects**

Heavy tick infestations cause irritation of the skin with subsequent ulceration and secondary infection. The wounds are attracted by screwworms and other flies and myiasis may develop. The presence of large numbers of ticks is associated with anaemia and annoyance and animals become anxious and restless.

In horses ticks of the following genera have a direct noxious effect:

IXODIDAE ("hard ticks")

Amblyomma spp. (*A. variegatum* and *A. cohaerens*)
Boophilus spp.
Dermacentor spp.
Hyalomma spp.
Ixodes spp.
Rhipicephalus spp. (*R. appendiculatus*, *R. evertsi*, *R. bursa*, *R. parvus* and *R. pulchellus*)

ARGASIDAE ("soft ticks")

Otobius megnini Spinose ear tick

- **Transmission of diseases**

One of the most damaging effects of ticks is their ability to transmit diseases to their hosts. Some of these diseases are serious with fatal consequences. Transovarian transmission from one tick generation to another via the eggs is possible and aids to spread out the disease.

Babesia equi Equine biliary fever

Remarks: *B. equi* is transmitted by *Rhipicephalus evertsi* (South Africa), *R. sanguineus* (North Africa) and *R. pulchellus* (East Africa), *Hyalomma dromedarii* and *H. detritum* (North Africa). *Otobius megnini* is suspected to transmit *B. equi* in Madagascar (☞ Horse and Donkeys, ■ 2).
(Figure 478)

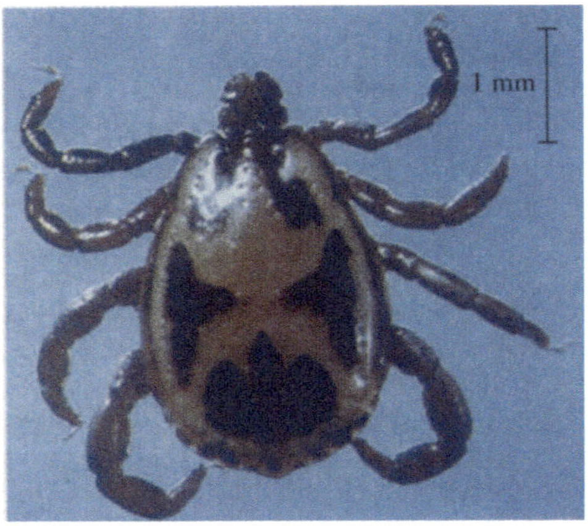

Fig. 478 *Rhipicephalus pulchellus*; male [8]

Babesia caballi

Remarks: *B. caballi* is transmitted by *Rhipicephalus evertsi* and *R. bursa* (South Africa), *R. sanguineus*, *H. dromedarii* and *H. excavatum* (North Africa) and *H. marginatum* rufipes (Africa south of the Sahara).

Borrelia theileri Spirochaetosis

Remarks: *B. theileri* is transmitted in South Africa by *Boophilus decoloratus* (the common blue tick) and *Rhipicephalus evertsi* (the red-legged tick) and *Hyalomma dromedarii* (North Africa).

- **Tick Toxicoses**

Tick paralysis

43 tick species belonging to 10 genera are known to induce tick paralysis in man and a variety of mammals. These ticks are capable of releasing a toxin into the host which causes a condition associated with progressive, ascending, afebrile, symmetrical paralysis, with hind legs being affected first followed by the forelegs. Animals may die. Paralysis is relieved if ticks are removed in time. Most of domestic animals appear to be susceptible to tick paralysis.

Amblyomma spp., *Ixodes* spp. and *Dermacentor* spp. in particular are capable of causing tick paralysis in horses.

Sweating sickness

An acute, febrile tick-borne toxicosis characterized by a profuse and moist eczema hyperaemia of the skin and visible mucous membranes. Watering of the eyes and nose, salivation and an extremely sensitive skin with a sour odour are other typical signs of sweating sickness. Eventually the skin becomes cracked and predisposed to secondary infections (incl. screwworm and myiasis). Often the course is acute and death may occur within a few days. In less acute cases recovery may occur.
Sweating sickness is mainly a disease of young calves but also sheep in eastern, central and

southern Africa. The causative agent are certain strains of *Hyalomma truncatum* which produce an epitheliotropic toxin. Calf mortality may reach 70%.

Symptoms: Generalized hyperaemia with subsequent desquamation of the superficial layers of the mucous membranes of the upper respiratory, gastrointestinal and external genital tracts and profuse moist dermatitis. For diagnosis it is essential to determine the presence of the vector. Clinical signs appear 4–11 days after the tick bite.

Prophylaxis: Control of tick infestations is the only effective measure. Removal of ticks, symptomatic treatment and good nursing are indicated.

General toxicosis

Tick toxicosis is a general aggravation of the toxic effect of the parasite's saliva. Certain toxins have a suppressive effect on the immune system of the host and occasionally this may reactivate chronic infections (e.g. *Babesia* spp. and *Anaplasma* spp. during *Rhipicephalus appendiculatus* (brown ear tick) infections). Toxicosis, associated with general disorders occurs with *Ornithodorus savignyi* (sand tampan) in young calves and lambs, especially when there are many bites. Animals show cutaneous oedema, haemorrhage, rapidly progressing weakness and prostration. Death can occur within 6 hours. Toxicosis may occur in recumbent animals, during rest.

- **Description of ticks affecting equines**

IXODIDAE (**"hard ticks"**)

Amblyomma spp.
Boophilus spp.
Dermacentor spp.
Hyalomma spp.
Ixodes spp.
Rhipicephalus spp.

A general description of each genus is made in CATTLE, ■ 5.1

- **General features of horse tick infestations**

Significance: Members of these genera are important for horses. Ticks are of high economic significance for horses in tropical and subtropical regions. Heavy infestations cause great debilitation. Some species transmit diseases one of which is equine babesiosis which is accompanied by high mortality. Wounds left from tick bites are susceptible to additional attacks by various biting and calliphorine flies (myiasis).

Symptoms: Infested horses itch, bite and scratch, causing other skin wounds (self-trauma) which become infected. Anaemia, loss of appetite and weight loss are observed in heavy infestations. Tick paralysis caused by certain tick species (*see* above) can be fatal within several days if the parasites are not removed.

Diagnosis: Identification of adult ticks found on the host animal.

Therapy and Prophylaxis: ☞ below THERAPY AND PROPHYLAXIS OF ECTOPARASITES, p. 257.

ARGASIDAE ("**soft ticks**")

Otobius megnini Spinose ear tick

Location: Larvae and nymphs feed deep in the external ear canal. Adults are non-parasitic and live on the ground.

Hosts: Horse, donkey, mule, cattle, sheep and goat

Species description: One-host tick. Free-living adult females lay eggs on the ground which hatch within 3 weeks. Larvae and nymphs live and feed on one host for up to 7 months. Infestations of this species usually build up in kraals and stables, where the host densities are high. *O. megnini* can persist in empty kraals and stables for more than 2 years.

Geographic distribution: Arid and semi-arid areas of South Africa, and South West Africa

Symptoms: Infested horses continuously shake their heads. Loss of appetite, debilitation and anaemia may be present. Irritation in the ear associated with secondary infections (incl. myiasis) may dominate the clinical picture. Rarely the middle and inner ear are also affected after perforation of the tympanic membrane.

Significance: Heavy infestations cause otitis externa, great annoyance and blood loss. *O. megnini* is an important tick of horses in some parts of Africa.

Diagnosis: Ticks may be found by swabbing the ear or by direct inspection of heavily infected ears.

Therapy and Prophylaxis: ☞ below THERAPY AND PROPHYLAXIS OF ECTOPARASITES, p. 257 and ☞ CATTLE, ■ 5.1.

– Mites

Chorioptes equi Itchy leg mite

Location: Lower legs and feet, especially on the hind legs; horses with long hairs on the fetlocks are particularly susceptible.

Hosts: Horse, donkey and mule

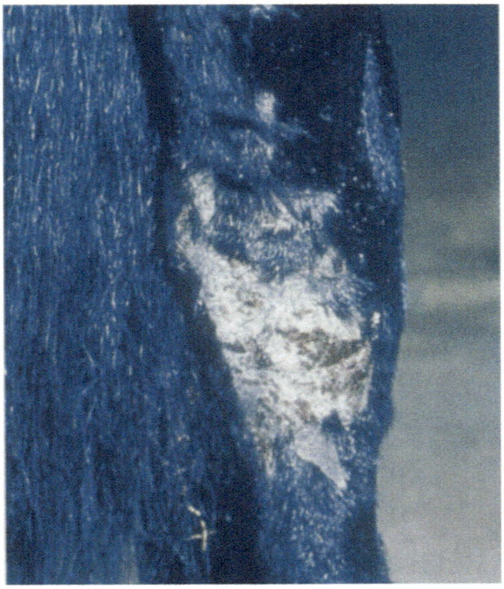

Fig. 479 *Chorioptes equi*; affected leg (posterior view) [15]

Species description: *Chorioptes* mites puncture the skin and suck lymph fluid. The mites can survive off the host for about 3 weeks.

Geographic distribution: World-wide

Symptoms: Chorioptic mange mites irritate the skin. The serum oozes and dries to crusts and scabs. These lesions are itching and infested horses bite, scratch and stamp.

Significance: Infestations are not usually severe but may persist for a long time.

Diagnosis: Demonstration of mites in skin scrapings taken from the edge of the lesions.

Therapy and Prophylaxis: ☞ CATTLE, ■ 5.1 and below THERAPY AND PROPHYLAXIS OF ECTOPARASITES, p. 257

(Figure 479)

Psoroptes equi Scab mite, equine body mite

Location: Areas of thick hair such as neck and base of the tail of horses are preferred by *Psoroptes equi*. Although infections may spread over the entire body surface the disease is not as serious as in sheep.

Hosts: Horse, donkey and mule

Species description: *Psoroptes* mites puncture the skin and suck lymph fluid and can survive off the host for about 2–3 weeks.

Geographic distribution: World-wide

Symptoms: Intense itching, and scratching, followed by hair loss and skin trauma which may be secondarily infected. Severe infestations cause anorexia, emaciation and anaemia.

Significance: Psoroptic mange is rarely observed. Heavy infestations cause severe debilitation.

Diagnosis: Demonstration of mites in skin scrapings taken from the edge of the lesions.

Therapy and Prophylaxis: ☞ below THERAPY AND PROPHYLAXIES OF ECTOPARASITES, p. 257

Psoroptes hippopotis

Remarks: *Psoroptes hippopotis* occurs in ears of horses and mules. Its own significance is still under discussion.

Sarcoptes equi Common mange mite, sarcoptic mange

Location: *Sarcoptes* mites prefer the head, the neck and the shoulders. Untreated infestations may spread over the entire body surface.

Hosts: Horse, donkey and mule

Species description: These mites can only survive a few days off the host, as they are highly susceptible to dryness. All stages occur in skin tunnels which may be extended over the entire skin of the host. The feeding and burrowing of *Sarcoptes* mites cause great irritation and itching, producing lesions with exudate which may become crusts.

Geographic distribution: World-wide

Symptoms: Infected horses bite and scratch. Chronic infestations cause thickened, wrinkled skin as a result of progressive proliferation of subcutaneous connective tissue.

Significance: Sarcoptic mange in horses is the most severe type but not very common, but it can cause much damage if allowed to spread out within a population.

Diagnosis: Demonstration of mites in skin scrapings collected from the damaged areas until the moist layers of skin are reached.

Therapy and Prophylaxis: ☞ below THERAPY AND PROPHYLAXIS OF ECTOPARASITES, p. 257 (Figure 480)

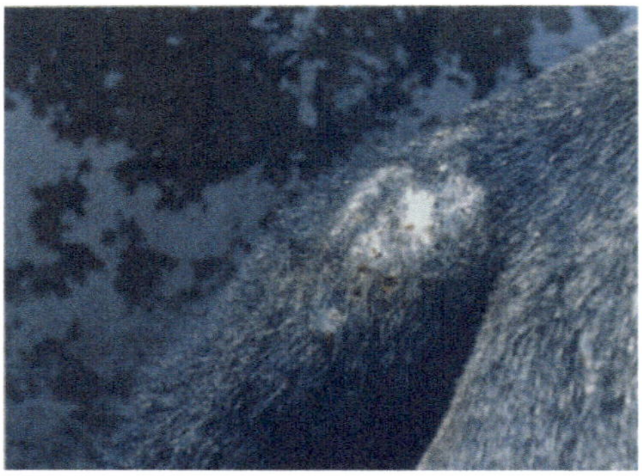

Fig. 480 *Sarcoptes equi* infestation [4]

Demodex equi Demodectic mange

Location: The mites live in the hair follicles and the sebaceous glands

Hosts: Horse

Species description: *Demodex* mites are cigar-shaped organisms which are known to be able to live on their host in harmony. Only if the host's immune system is affected they may cause severe skin lesions.

Geographic distribution: World-wide

Symptoms: *D. equi* infestations produce papules and ulcers, particularly around the eyes and on the forehead. Subsequently the lesions spread to the shoulders and finally over the entire body. The affected body is covered with scales. There is no pruritus.

Significance: *D. equi* is seldom diagnosed in horses.

Diagnosis: Demonstration of the mites in the hair follicles and the sebaceous glands.

Therapy and Prophylaxis: There is no satisfactory treatment. Prophylaxis is unknown.

- **Control of mite infestations in horses**

Most organophosphates are effective against mange mite infections in horses. Acaricides are applied by spraying, rubbing or dipping (for application mode, *see* below). For groups of animals dipping is the most convenient and effective method. Permethrin spray (0.05%) but also other pyrethroids are effective. Flumethrin (0.005%) is effective against chorioptic mange in horses. Ivermectin (0.2 mg/kg, sc.) is highly effective against *Sarcoptes* mange and to a lesser extent against *Psoroptes* mange. All the tools (e.g. curry-combs, etc.) in infested stables should also be washed with an acaricide to avoid transmission.

• Insecta found on the skin

– Lice

MALLOPHAGA Chewing Lice

Werneckiella equi equi (syn. *Damalinia equi)* Biting louse of horses

Werneckiella equi asini Biting louse of donkeys

Location: *Werneckiella* spp. are usually found on the neck and the base of the tail. In heavy infestations the parasite covers the whole body.

Hosts: Horse, donkey and mule

Species description: Adults are 1–2 mm long. The head is broad and flat. The body is wingless and flattened dorsoventrally. *Werneckiella* spp. feed on skin and hair. Development occurs exclusively on the host, within 3–4 weeks. Eggs are attached to the hair, hatch to nymphs which moults 3 times before reaching adulthood. *Werneckiella* spp. are specific for equines.

Geographic distribution: World-wide

Symptoms: Infested horses rub, scratch and bite themselves. This is accompanied by rough coat, skin infections, myiasis and loss of hair. Unthriftiness and weight loss are commonly seen in heavy infestations.

Significance: *Werneckiella* spp. bites cause mange-like skin irritations and itching. *Werneckiella* spp. may act as vectors of the Equine Infectious Anaemia.

Diagnosis: Identification of lice found on the coat.

Therapy and Prophylaxis: ☞ below *Haematopinus asini*

(Figures 481, 482)

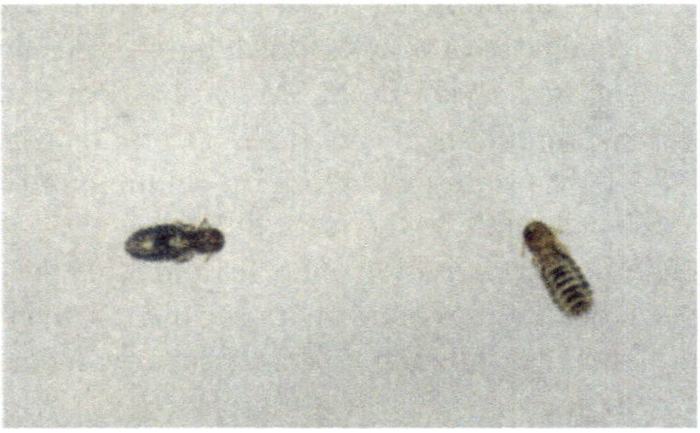

Fig. 481 *Werneckiella equi*; equine chewing lice (up to 1.8 mm long)

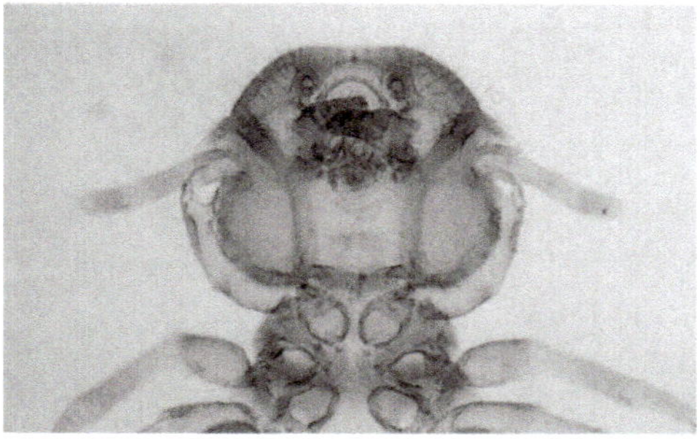

Fig. 482 *Werneckiella* sp.; head [15]

ANOPLURA Blood sucking lice

Haematopinus asini Sucking louse of horses

Location: *H. asini* is predominantly found around the head, neck, on the back and brisket and between the legs.

Hosts: Horse, donkey and mule

Species description: *H. asini* is 3–3.5 mm long, with 3 pairs of legs and a long narrow head with piercing mouth parts to suck blood and tissue fluids. Development occurs exclusively on the host, within 3–4 weeks. Eggs are attached to the hair and hatch to nymphs which moult 3 times before reaching adulthood. *H. equi* is specific for equines.

Geographic distribution: World-wide

Symptoms: Anaemia due to heavy blood loss, lowered condition and weight loss and increased susceptibility to other diseases may occur. Heavy infestations cause loss of appetite and vitality, particularly in foals.

Significance: *H. equi* is more dangerous than *D. equi* because of its blood sucking activity.

Diagnosis: Identification of lice found on the coat.

Therapy: Because lice do not leave the host, treatment of the horse with an insecticide is necessary. Organophosphates, carbamates (carbaryl) but also pyrethrins and pyrethroids are effective against lice.

Prophylaxis: Frequent grooming helps to reduce the parasite numbers.

(Figures 483, 484, 485)

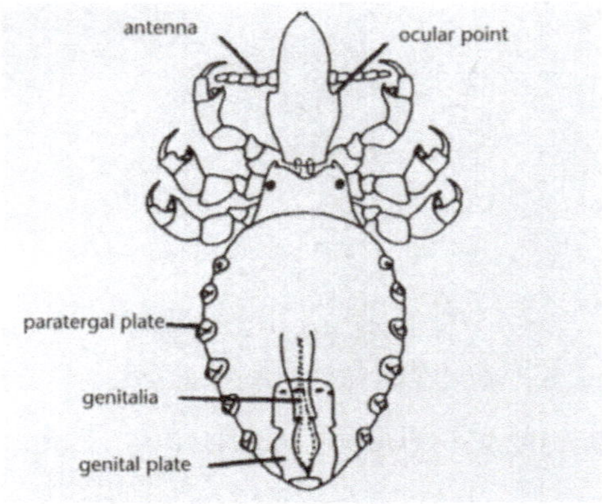

Fig. 483 *Haematopinus asini*; dorsal view (schematic) [29]

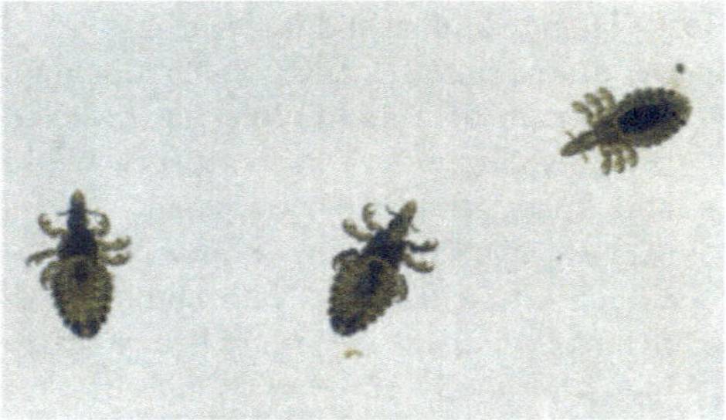

Fig. 484 *Haematopinus asini* (male is up to 2.4 mm long; female is up to 3.5 mm long)

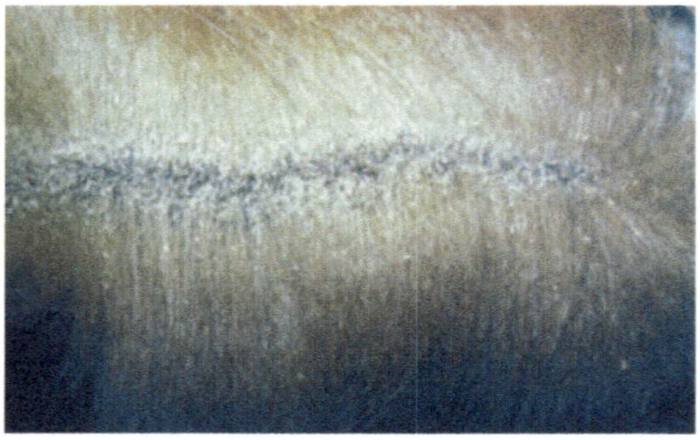

Fig. 485 *Haematopinus asini* infestation

– Fleas

Fleas are not found on horses.

– Dipterida

CULICIDAE Mosquitoes

They belong, like flies, to the order Dipterida, with a single pair of wings. The main genera are *Anopheles*, *Culex* and *Aedes*.
Females are capable of sucking blood which appears to be necessary for the laying of eggs. Eggs are laid either on water or on vegetation floating on the surface of water, therefore mosquitoes are found near stagnant pools (☞ CATTLE, ■ 5.1).

Significance: Mosquitoes can cause considerable distress to livestock but their main importance is their ability to act as intermediate hosts or vectors of equine encephalomyelitis, African Horse Sickness (not the main vector) and *Setaria equina*.

SIMULIIDAE

Simulium **spp.** Black flies, midges

Remarks: Small size (1–5 mm), found in swarms near free-running well-aerated streams. Simulids cause severe irritation to horses and other livestock when they occur in large numbers. Herds and flock will stampede, often with disastrous results. Bites are inflicted on all parts of the body, giving rise to vesicles which burst exposing the underlying flesh. Skin wounds caused by simulids heal very slowly. Certain areas of the tropics are rendered uninhabitable by simulids (☞ CATTLE, ■ 5.1).

Significance: Irritation of horses and other livestock. Skin wounds with secondary myiasis. Transmission of *Onchocerca volvulus* in man.

CERATOPOGONIDAE

***Culicoides* spp.** Biting midges, seasonal dermatitis, sweet itch

Remarks: Very small size (1–3 mm long). Adult female midges attack horse, man and other species (☞ CATTLE, ■ 5.1), causing marked irritation by penetration of the skin with their proboscis. The bites cause intense itching. Only the females suck blood mainly during the twilight periods and at night. *Culicoides* occur often in large swarms a few hundred metres around the breeding sites. These are moist areas such as fresh or brackish water or seepages from decaying vegetable or dung heaps.

Significance: 1) Massive irritation of livestock, itching, allergic skin reactions in horses (sweet-itch, seasonal dermatitis).
2) Transmission of *Onchocerca gibsoni* and other *Onchocerca* spp. in cattle and horses; African Horse Sickness, blue tongue of sheep.

Therapy and Prophylaxis: It has been reported that horses, stabled from one hour before sunset until the dew has disappeared the following morning, are protected from attacks by biting midges and thus from transmission of African Horse Sickness. Insecticides to be used ☞ THERAPY AND PROPHYLAXIS OF ECTOPARASITES, p. 257. Permethrin (0.05%), is especially used to control *Culicoides* spp. on horses.
(Figure 486)

TABANIDAE

***Tabanus* spp., *Haematopota* spp. and *Chrysops* spp.** Horse flies

Significance: Female tabanids attack mammals to suck blood. They cause deep, painful, irritating bites. They generally bite several times for one blood meal because they are disturbed by the host's defense. A number of diseases (besnoitiosis, anaplasmosis, trypanosomosis and anthrax, equine infectious anaemia) are mechanically transmitted by tabanids. This is especially important when horseflies are numerous among a crowded livestock population.

Therapy: ☞ THERAPY AND PROPHYLAXIS OF ECTOPARASITES, p. 257 and CATTLE, ■ 5.1).

Prophylaxis: Insecticidal spraying also against the larval stages on the ground (e.g. wet soil, vegetation, etc.).

MUSCIDAE

***Musca* spp., *Lyperosia* spp. and *Haematobia* spp.**

Significance: Muscid flies annoy horses, especially during the summer or rainy season. They swarm around horses and other farm livestock. The resulting irritation is incessant and much of the energy of the animals is lost to defend against fly attacks. In addition to the nuisance the flies often carry pathogens on their feet and bodies. Some

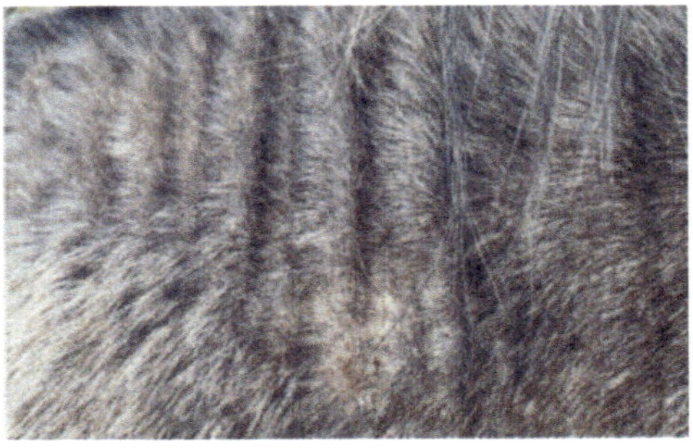

Fig. 486 Sweet-itch lesions ("seasonal dermatitis") due to *Culicoides* spp. [37]

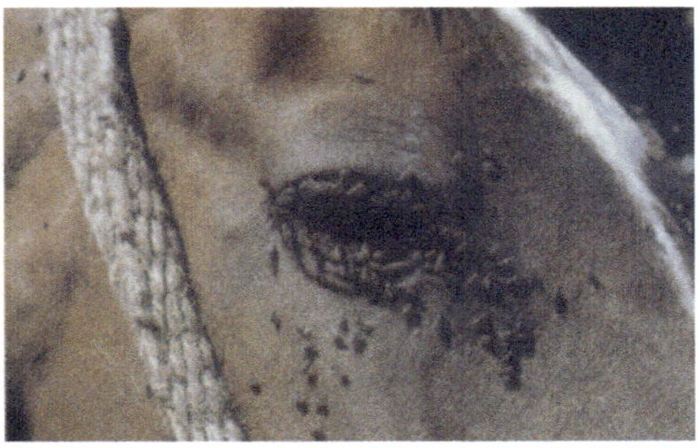

Fig. 487 "Fly worry" due to muscid flies (e.g. *Musca autumnalis*) [37]

also act as intermediate host for other parasites. *Musca domestica* (non-biting muscid) is attracted to wounds and moist parts of the body, especially the eyes where they may provoke an ulcerative dermatitis. *M. domestica* also act as vector of *Habronema* spp. (*H. muscae* and *H. megastoma*), *Thelazia* spp. and *Haematobia* spp. The horn flies are biting muscids and vectors of the filarial worm *Parafilaria multipapillosa* (☞ CATTLE, ■ 5.1).
(Figure 487)

Stomoxys calcitrans The stable fly

Significance: *S. calcitrans* also belongs to the muscids. It attacks a wide variety of mammals including horses. It is a biting muscid and occurs world-wide. Both sexes of this fly are bloodsuckers and can become extremely irritating pests of man and domestic animals. *S. calcitrans* acts as intermediate host of *Habronema microstoma* which lives in the stomach of horses and causes intense worry and irritation to animals, toxic reactions and immunosuppression (☞ CATTLE, ■ 5.1).

GLOSSINIDAE

***Glossina* spp.** Tsetse flies

Significance: Both sexes suck blood and are equally capable or transmitting trypanosomes. Tsetse flies, especially in great numbers can significantly contribute to the fly-worry in horse populations (☞ CATTLE, ■ 5.1).

CALLIPHORIDAE
The blow flies and their allies

They are highly important in many domestic animal species and man. The adults are free-

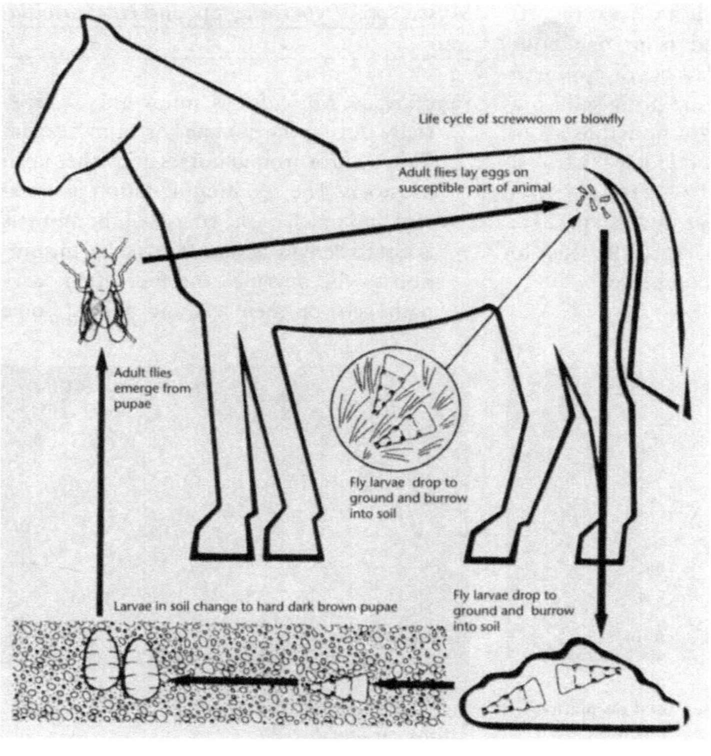

Fig. 488 Life cycle of screwworm or blowfly [36]

living and the larvae are parasitic maggots which develop in the tissue of their host, causing a condition called myiasis. The larvae may be laid into pre-existing wounds. Myiasis is often a secondary skin problem.

The family of Calliphoridae can be divided into 2 groups: ***metallic-* and *non-metallic flies***

Metallic flies are green, blue or purplish coloured and belong to the genera *Chrysomya, Lucilia* and *Calliphora*.

Lucilia and *Chrysomya* are the most important genera responsible for sheep myiasis (☞ SHEEP AND GOATS, 5.1).

Chrysomya bezziana The cattle screwworm

Remarks: *C. bezziana* infests cattle but also horses, sheep, dogs and sometimes man. It occurs in tropical and southern Africa. *C. bezziana* causes severe myiasis and toxins produced by the larvae result in retarded healing of wounds. Death may occur in severe cases (☞ CATTLE, ■ 5.1).
(Figure 488)

Callitroga (syn. *Cochliomyia*) ***hominivorax***
The "American screwworm"

Remarks: *C. hominivorax* occurs since recently also in North Africa. Cattle, pigs and equines suffer most frequently, but other animals, including fowls and even man may also be affected. Pathology is essentially the same as in *C. bezziana* (☞ CATTLE, ■ 5.1).

Non-metallic flies are dull grey, yellow-brown or black and belong to the genera *Wohlfartia* and *Sarcophaga*.

Sarcophaga haemorrhoidalis
The red-tailed flesh-fly

Remarks: *S. haemorrhoidalis* sometimes causes myiasis in man and animals (☞ CATTLE, ■ 5.1).

Wohlfartia magnifica
The Old World flesh fly

Remarks: *W. magnifica* may cause myiasis (☞ CATTLE, ■ 5.1).

OESTRIDAE

Rhinoestrus purpureus

Remarks: Life cycle similar to those of the genus *Oestrus*. Larval stages are obligatory parasites of horses and mules in tropical Africa. Larvae are deposited by the adult fly in batches of 8–40 into the nostrils or eyes. The larvae crawl into the nasal cavity where they remain for several months before moving to the sinuses where they mature. They cause obstruction, irritation and sneezing (☞ HORSES AND DONKEYS, ■ 4.3).
(Figure 489)

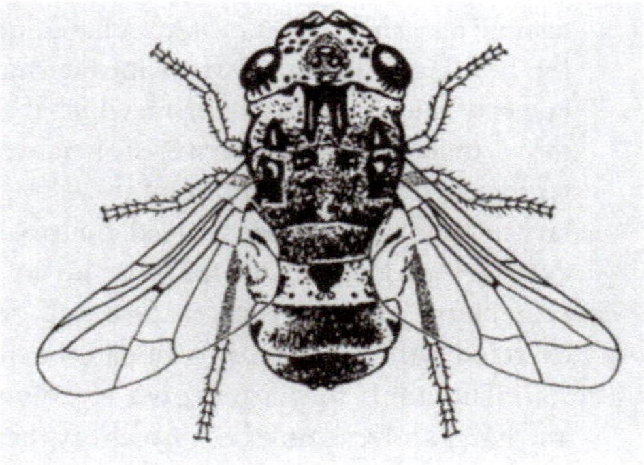

Fig. 489 *Rhinoestrus purpureus*; adult fly (8–11 mm long) [33]

Hypoderma bovis Cattle grub, warble fly

Remarks: *Hypoderma bovis* is of minor significance in horses, except where horses are kept within cattle populations in areas which are heavily infested with *H. bovis*. The adult flies constitute serious annoyance for horses. Subcutaneous larvae damage the skin and underlying tissue. Allergic reactions to these grubs may occur. The back of

infested horses becomes irritated, thickened and disfigured and the breathing holes are visible in the skin (☞ CATTLE, ■ 5.1).
(Figure 490)

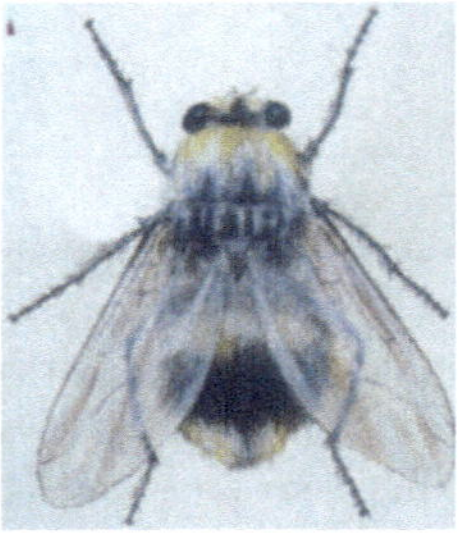

Fig. 490 *Hypoderma bovis*; adult fly (15 mm long) is of minor significance in horses, except where horses are kept within cattle populations in areas with a high *H. bovis* density [19]

GASTROPHILIDAE Bot flies

Gasterophilus (syn. *Gastrophilus*) **spp.**
Horse bot flies

Remarks: The larvae of these flies are gastrointestinal parasites of equines. After hatching, the first larval instars burrow into dermal layers of the mouth cavity, from which they move to either the pharynx, stomach or rectum, where the second- and third-stage larvae attach. The larvae feed on tissue exudates and remain in the host up to 1 year before they become mature and are excreted with the faeces to pupate in the soil. The adult flies are brown in colour and hairy and resemble bees which lay their eggs onto the skin of their host (☞ HORSES AND DONKEYS, ■ 1).

Gasterophilus intestinalis (syn. *G. equi*)
Common horse bot fly

Remarks: *G. intestinalis* occurs in horse and donkeys global. Female flies deposit their eggs mainly on forelegs, between the knee and the hoof but also in the scapular region where they are licked by the host which stimulates hatching (8–18 mm).
(Figure 491)

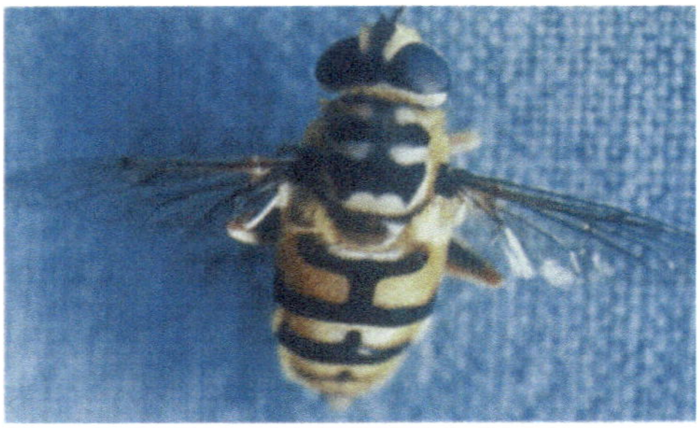

Fig. 491 *Gasterophilus* sp.; adult fly

Gasterophilus nasalis Throat bot fly

Remarks: *G. nasalis* eggs are laid in the intermandibulary space up to 500 and usually 1 per hair.

Gastrophilus pecorum

Remarks: *G. pecorum* eggs are laid on the leaves of plants and its larvae are ingested by grazing animals.

Gasterophilus haemorrhoidalis
The nose or lip bot fly

Remarks: *G. haemorrhoidalis* eggs are laid on hairs of the lips and around the mouth. The third-stage larvae attach in the hosts rectum, sometimes in great numbers.

- **General features of Gasterophilus spp.**

Significance: 1) The adult flies distress their equine host markedly up to the point of causing stampeding.
2) Irritation by the larvae during migration, e.g. dermatitis, inflammation of the pharynx, oesophagus, stomach or rectum (rectum prolapse).
3) Large numbers in the pyloric region may interfere with the sphincter function.

Therapy and Prophylaxis: ☞ HORSES AND DONKEYS, ■ 1

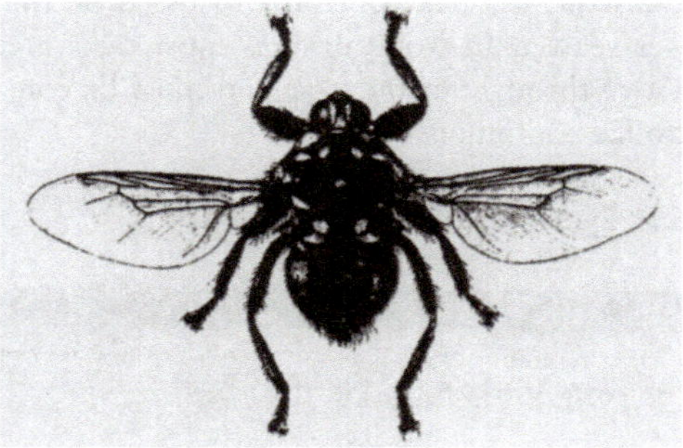

Fig. 492 *Hippobosca equi* (up to 8 mm long) [29]

HIPPOBOSCIDAE

Hippobosca **spp.** Louse flies
(Figure 492)
Hippobosca equina The horse louse fly

Hosts: Horse and cattle
Geographic distribution: World-wide
(Figure 493)

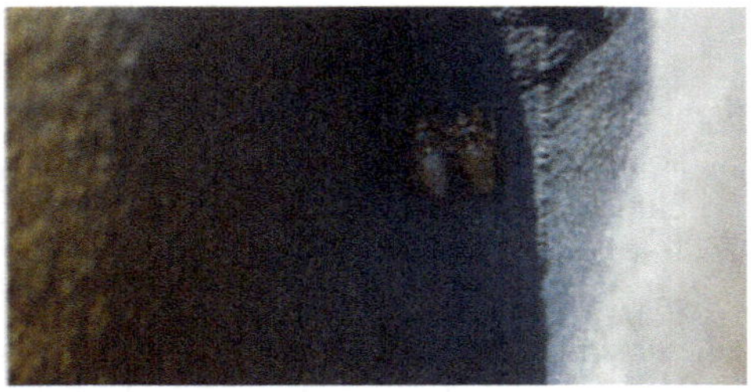

Fig. 493 *Hippobosca equina* (up to 8 mm long); attached to the skin

Hippobosca variegata

Hosts: Horse and cattle
Geographic distribution: Afrotropical and Oriental regions

Hippobosca rufipes The cattle louse fly

Hosts: Wild and domestic Bovidae, less frequent in horses
Geographic distribution: Afrotropical regions (warm arid and semi arid areas of Africa)

Hippobosca maculata
Horse and cattle louse fly

Hosts: Horse and cattle
Geographic distribution: Tropical and subtropical areas of Africa

- **General features of *Hippobosca* spp.**

Location: The adult louse flies remain for long periods on their host and cluster in the perineal region, between the hind-legs to the pubic region, but may also bite on other parts of the body.
Species description: The flies live permanently on their host and feed on blood. Mainly cattle and horses are affected. They rarely fly and usually not more than a few metres. They spend their whole time on the host and are strongly attached to the hairs of their host and therefore difficult to dislodge. When disturbed they can quickly move sideways.
Symptoms: Infested animals scratch and rub and skin-trauma is often seen as a consequence of heavy infestations.
Significance: These flies are a source of great irritation.
Diagnosis: Identification of flies located under the tail and between the hindlegs.
Therapy: Infested animals should be treated topically with insecticides (☞ THERAPY AND PROPHYLAXIS OF ECTOPARASITES).
Prophylaxis: Regular grooming may be helpful to reduce louse fly infestations.

- **Therapy and prophylaxis of ectoparasites (arachnids and insects)**

A great number of acaricides and insecticides is used to control both arachnids and insects. Methods of application include whole-body sprays, dips, dusts and topical application to the dermis and ears. Dips are more effective for ticks. Thorough treatment of the infested area is required, especially when ticks infest the ears or underside of the tail or when mites infest localized patches on the skin. Elimination of parasites or stages in the environment is difficult because

Table 18 Acaricides or insecticides approved for the control of ticks, flies and lice in horses (☞ Table 11, CATTLE, ■ 5.1)

Organophosphates	
	Bromocyclene
	Coumaphos
	Crotoxyphos + dichlorvos
	Diazinon
	Dichlorvos
	Malathion
	Phoxim
	Propoxur
	Stirofos
	Trichlorfon (metrifonat)
Carbamates	
	Carbaryl
Chlorinated Hydrocarbons	
	Lindane
	Methoxychlor
Pyrethrins and Pyrethroids	
	Flumethrin
	Cypermethrin
	Fenvalerate
	Permethrin
	Pyrethrin
Avermectins	
	Ivermectin

many ectoparasites are capable of surviving in the environment for prolonged periods (e.g. some ticks can live on the ground for more than 300 days without feeding). In areas where many ticks exist reinfection of the host occurs continuously and treatment therefore must be repeated regularly. Some ticks are not strictly species-specific and ticks normally adapted to horses can occasionally also affect cattle or other animals and they must be treated, too, if attempts are made to reduce overall tick infestations.
In subhumid areas the period of highest tick activities is the wet season and only few ticks are found on animals during the dry season. Consequently tick control is focussed on the wet season. In tropical areas most ticks are active throughout the year and must be controlled continuously.

5.2 Eyes

HELMINTHS

- Nematoda found in the eyes

Thelazia lacrymalis Eyeworm

Location: Tear ducts and conjunctival sacs
Hosts: Horse
Species description: Viviparous female sheds larvae into the tear secretions. Larvae are picked up by the intermediate hosts which are several species of muscid flies. Transmission occurs when flies feed on the eyes of horses.
Geographic distribution: World-wide
Symptoms: Chronic conjunctivitis, lacrimation, swollen eyes, covered with exudate and pus. Kertatitis, opacity of the cornea and in severe cases ulceration of the cornea.
Significance: *T. lacrymalis* is very common in some areas but only heavy infections cause clinical problems. Irritation of the eyes followed by bacterial secondary infections may occur.
Diagnosis: Detection of adult worms in the conjunctival sacs. Examination of the lacrimal secretion may reveal first-stage larvae.
Differential Diagnosis: Infective larvae of *Habronema* spp. may produce ulcerative granulomas near the medial canthus of the eyelid. *Onchocerca* spp. larvae invade the eye and may also cause conjunctivitis. Small (< 1 mm), raised, white nodules in the pigmented conjunctiva are pathognomonic for *Onchocerca* infections.
Therapy: Fenbendazole (10 mg/kg, po.) administered for 5 days is efficacious against *T. lacrymalis*. Ivermectin (200 µg/kg, sc.) or levamisole (5 mg/kg., po.) or directly into the conjunctival sac have limited effect against *T. lacrymalis*. Mechanical removal with forceps following instillation of a local

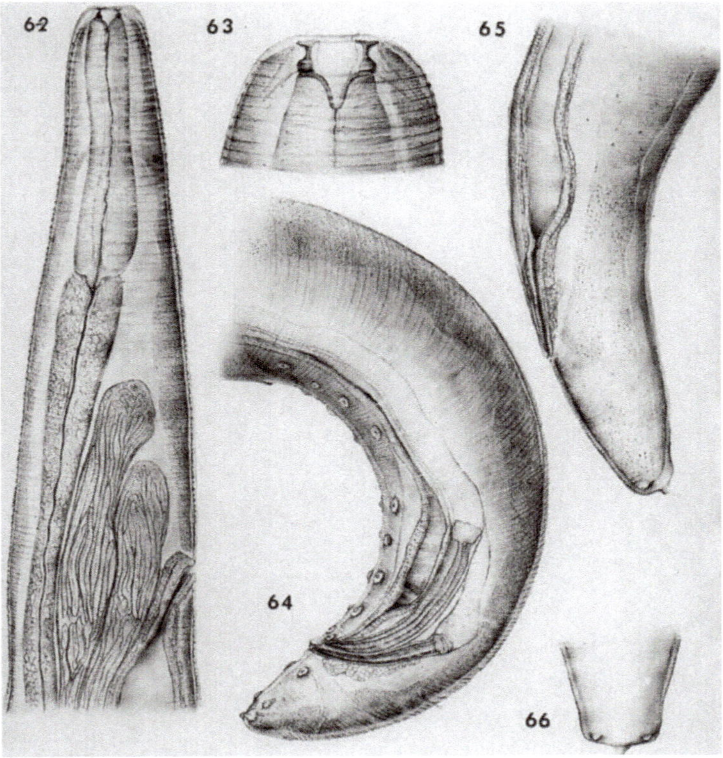

Fig. 494 *Thelazia lacrymalis*; anterior end with typical cuticular striation (62 and 63), posterior end of a male (64), posterior end of a female (65) and tip of the tail (66); females are up to 18 mm long and males are up to 11 mm long [40]

anaesthetic may be helpful. Concurrent use of an antibiotic suspension against secondary invaders is recommended.

Prophylaxis: Fly control measures, directed especially against the face fly, may help to control thelaziosis.

(Figure 494)

Setaria equina

Remarks: Microfilariae may occasionally be found in the eyes (☞ HORSES AND DONKEYS, ■ 4.4).

Rhinoestrus purpureus

Remarks: Larvae are often deposited in batches of 8–40 at a time into and around the eyes and may occasionally cause "ophtalmomyiasis". Larvae may be found in the eye exudates (☞ HORSES AND DONKEYS, ■ 4.3).

V

Parasites of Dromedaries*

CONTENTS

* In this chapter main emphasis is given to the description of the parasites of the one-humped camel (*Camelus dromedarius*). Some remarks will be made to parasites which are also important for the two-humped camel (*Camelus bactrianus*).

1 Stages in the gut and faeces

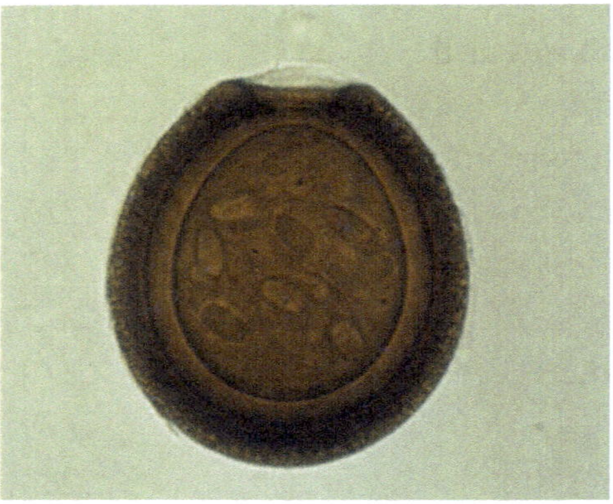

Fig. 495 Oocyst of *Eimeria cameli* (80–100 × 62–94 µm) [4]

PROTOZOA

Eimeria spp. Coccidiosis of camels

Eimeria cameli

Location: Small intestine, rarely caecum
Hosts: Dromedary and Bactrian camel
Species description: This is the most frequently encountered *Eimeria* species in camels in North Africa. The oocysts are large and measure 80–100 × 62–94 µm. A large micropyle (10–27 µm wide) is characteristic. Developmental stages occur in the small intestine. Giant schizonts up to 350 µm in diameter may be seen. Inflammatory lesions of the small intestine have been associated with this species.
Geographic distribution: World-wide (Figures 495, 496)

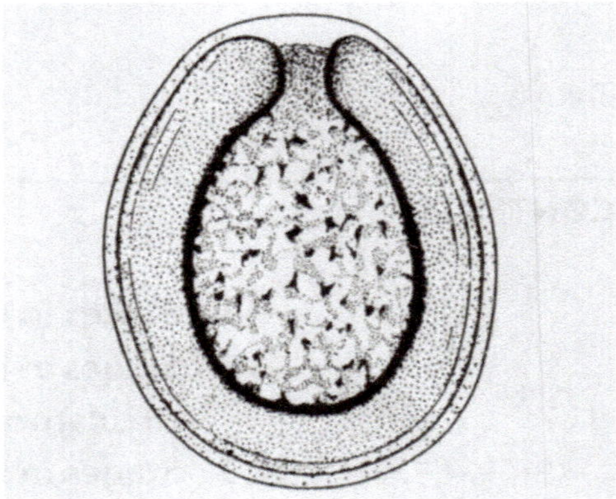

Fig. 496 Oocyst of *Eimeria cameli* (schematic) [42]

Eimeria dromedarii

Location: Small intestine
Hosts: Dromedary and Bactrian camel
Species description: This species is found frequently, often together with *E. cameli*. The oocysts are much smaller than those of *E. cameli*, measuring 23–33 × 20–25 µm.
Geographic distribution: World-wide, especially Iraq, Pakistan, India

- **General features of coccidiosis in camels**

Symptoms: Inappetence and severe enteritis due to *Eimeria* spp. have been observed. Progressive rapid weight loss and emaciation may result. Watery diarrhoea sometimes containing blood has been found in heavy infections. Dehydration and secondary infections may severely aggravate the disease and cause mortalities in young camels.

Significance: Coccidiosis in camels may cause high mortalities especially in young camels.

Diagnosis: This is based on the clinical signs and the demonstration of high numbers of oocysts in the diarrhoeic faeces. Cystic structures containing immature oocysts occur in the intestinal mucosa.

Therapy and Prophylaxis: ☞ CATTLE, ■ 1; COCCIDIOSIS OF CATTLE, p. 24 ff.

Remarks: Young camels are much more susceptible to infections. Watering devices should be protected from faecal contamination.

Other *Eimeria* species harboured by camels (one- and two-humped camels) are: *Eimeria bactriani* (oocysts: 21–34 × 20–28 µm, CIS), *Eimeria rajasthani* (34–39 × 25–27 µm, India) and *Eimeria nölleri*. Two species of *Isospora* occur in camels: *Isospora orlovi* (27–35 × 15–20 µm) and *Isospora cameli*. In this genus oocysts contain 2 sporocysts, each of which contains 4 sporozoites. The pathogenic role of *Isospora* spp. in camels is unknown.

Cryptosporidium parvum (syn. *C. bovis*)

Remarks: Cryptosporidiosis may affect young camels. Severe diarrhoea, emaciation, dehydration and death may occur (☞ CATTLE, ■ 1). This protozoan parasite is often superimposed on a primary immunosuppression. Diagnosis is based on the demonstration of oocysts in carbol-fuchsin stained smears of fresh faeces (☞ CATTLE, ■ 1).

Balantidium coli

Remarks: Cases of clinical balantidiosis have been reported from camels. Diarrhoea and emaciation and faeces containing 300 cysts per gram were found. However, it is likely that *Balantidium* spp. play a secondary role, superimposed on a massive irritation of the intestinal mucosa by other pathogens or following immunosuppression. Therapy is rarely indicated. Oxytetracycline (5–10 mg/kg, im. or iv.) may support recovery (☞ Swine, ■ 1 p. 295).

HELMINTHS

- Trematoda eggs found in the faeces and adult trematodes living in the gastrointestinal tract

Paramphistomatidae Rumen flukes

Remarks: Various species of *Paramphistomum* which also occur in other domestic and wild ruminants (☞ CATTLE, ■ 1) have been found in camels. Rumen flukes normally do not cause clinical signs unless masses of immature worms attach to the intestinal mucosa.

- Trematodes whose eggs may appear in the faeces

Fasciola hepatica Liver flukes

Large liver fluke of temperate areas and high altitude regions in East Africa. This is one of the trematodes most frequently encountered in camels in Africa and Asia (☞ CATTLE, ■ 1 and ■ 4.2 and DROMEDARIES, ■ 4.2).

Fasciola gigantica Giant liver fluke

Tropical large liver fluke; this species also occurs in camels in Asia and Africa (☞ CATTLE, ■ 1 and ■ 4.2 and DROMEDARIES, ■ 4.2).

Dicrocoelium spp. Liver flukes

Location: Adult liver flukes in biliary ducts; eggs in the faeces

Remarks: This genus is very seldom found in camels.

Eurytrema pancreaticum Pancreas fluke

Location: Adult pancreas flukes in pancreatic ducts; eggs in the faeces
Remarks: Camels are rarely affected by this trematode (☞ CATTLE, 1 and 4.5; SHEEP AND GOATS, 4.5 and DROMEDARIES, 4.5).

Schistosoma bovis and *Schistosoma mattheei* Blood flukes

Location: Adult blood flukes in mesenteric veins; eggs in the intestinal wall and faeces (☞ CATTLE 1 and 2 and DROMEDARIES, 2).

- Cestoda eggs found in the faeces and adult cestodes living in the gastrointestinal tract

Seven species of cestodes, all belonging to the family Anoplocephalidae, have been identified in the small intestine of camels.

Moniezia expansa and *Moniezia benedeni* Common tapeworms

Remarks: *Moniezia expansa* is a cosmopolitan parasite which has been found in camels in Africa and Asia. *Moniezia benedeni* has been found in camels only in Africa (☞ CATTLE, 1).

Stilesia globipunctata

Remarks: This is mainly a parasite of small ruminants. It also occurs in camels and is widespread in Africa. This parasite also has been reported from Pakistan and India. (☞ SHEEP AND GOATS, 1)

Stilesia vittata

Remarks: This parasite is similar to *S. globipunctata*. It is 18–23 cm long and ≤ 1 mm wide. The scolex is 0.5–0.6 mm in size and the number of testicles is 10–14. Pathology and significance is the same as with *S. globipunctata*.
(Fig. 497, 498)

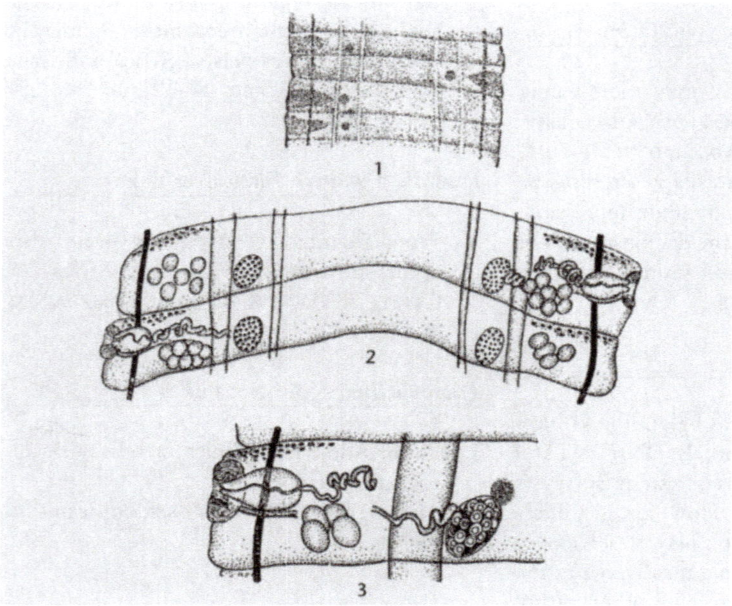

Fig. 497 *Stilesia vittata*; details of segments: (1) immature segment, (2) mature segments and (3) details of genitals [43]

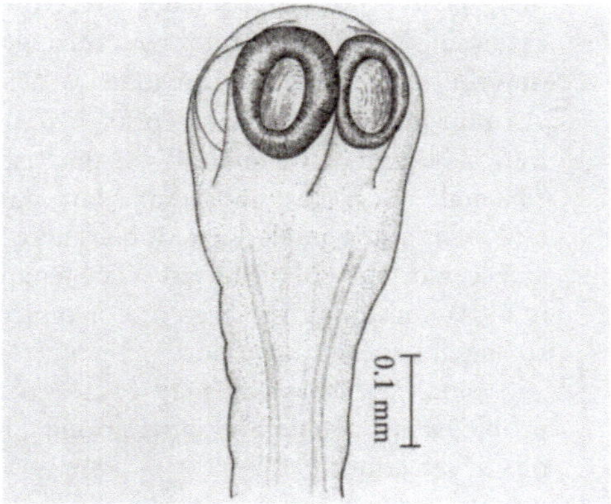

Fig. 498 *Stilesia vittata*; scolex [43]

Avitellina centripunctata* and *Avitellina woodlandi

Remarks: *A. centripunctata* is widespread in camels in Africa and Asia (☞ CATTLE, ■ 1 and SHEEP AND GOATS, ■ 1). *Avitellina woodlandi* has only been described in dromedaries from Africa.
(Figure 499)

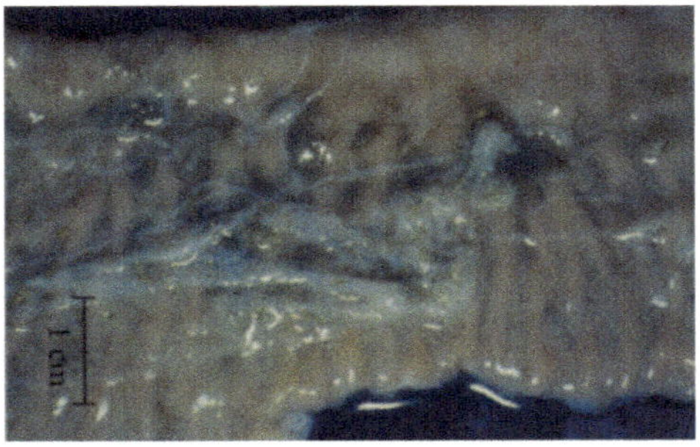

Fig. 499 Tapeworms (*Avitellina* spp.) in the small intestine of a dromedary [13]

Thysaniezia ovilla (syn. *T. giardi*)

Remarks: This species has been found in dromedaries in Chad (☞ CATTLE, ■ 1 and SHEEP AND GOATS, ■ 1).

- **Therapy and prophylaxis of intestinal tapeworms of dromedaries**

Most of the drugs used against tape worm infections in cattle may be used for dromedaries (☞ CATTLE, ■ 1).

- Nematoda eggs found in the faeces, adult nematodes living in the gastrointestinal tract and first-stage larvae of *Dictyocaulus filaria*

Gongylonema pulchrum Gullet worm

Location: Oesophagus
Remarks: ☞ CATTLE, ■ 1

Gongylonema verrucosum
Rumen gullet worm

Location: Rumen
Remarks: ☞ CATTLE, ■ 1

Parabronema skrjabini

Location: Abomasum
Remarks: This spirurid nematode occurs usually in small and large ruminants (☞ CATTLE, ■ 1 and SHEEP AND GOATS, ■ 1). In Africa it has been found in dromedaries in many countries.

Haemonchus longistipes

Location: Abomasum
Remarks: This species is specific to camels and occurs in Africa and Asia. In general, *H. longistipes* is very similar to *H. contortus* (☞ SHEEP AND GOATS, ■ 1). The male is 18–28 mm long. The spicules are 534–664 µm long. The gubernaculum is 250–380 µm long. The female is 26–39 mm long, with a vulva which is not covered by a linguiform flap. The eggs are 60–80 × 69–50 µm. *H. longistipes* is an important parasite of camels, causing great losses, especially in young animals. It occurs mostly in mixed infections with other gastrointestinal nematodes. (Figure 500)

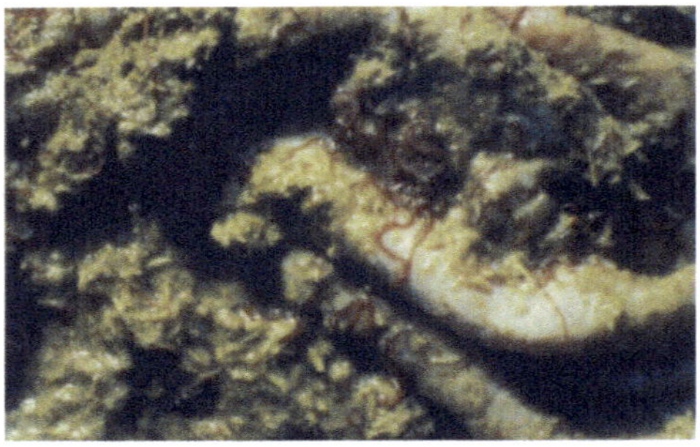

Fig. 500 *Haemonchus longistipes* in the abomasum of a dromedary [13]

Haemonchus contortus Twisted wire worm

Location: Abomasum
Remarks: This nematode is frequently found in camels which have shared grazing with sheep (☞ CATTLE, 1 and SHEEP AND GOATS, 1).

Camelostrongylus mentulatus

Location: Abomasum
Remarks: This trichostrongylid is commonly found in camels in the north of the African continent and is rare elsewhere. This genus resembles *Ostertagia* except that the spicules have peculiar denticular structures extending in a longitudinal row throughout the entire length. The male is 6.5–7.5 mm long, with spicules 600–730 μm long. The gubernaculum is 68–82 μm long. The male bursa is composed of 2 large lateral lobes and a small dorsal lobe. There is an accessory bursal membrane. The female is 8–10 mm long. The eggs are of typical strongyle-type and measure 75–85 × 40–50 μm. *C. mentulatus* may cause great problems in camels and often occurs in mixed infections.
(Figure 501)

Ostertagia circumcincta* and *Ostertagia trifurcata

Location: Abomasum
Remarks: These two species are cosmopolitan parasites and best adapted to sheep and goat (☞ SHEEP AND GOATS, 1). However, they are also found in camels.

Impalaia tuberculata* and *Impalaia nudicollis

Location: Abomasum and sometimes small intestine

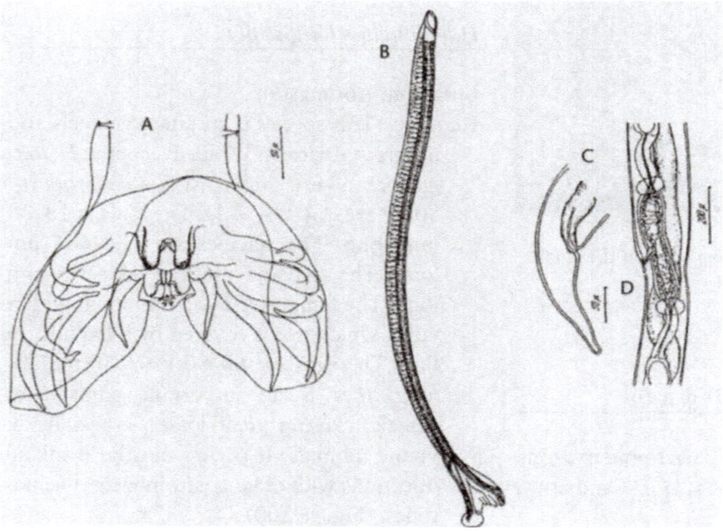

Fig. 501 *Camelostrongylus mentulatus;* bursa copulatrix (A), spicule (B), tail end of female (C) and vulva region (D) [9]

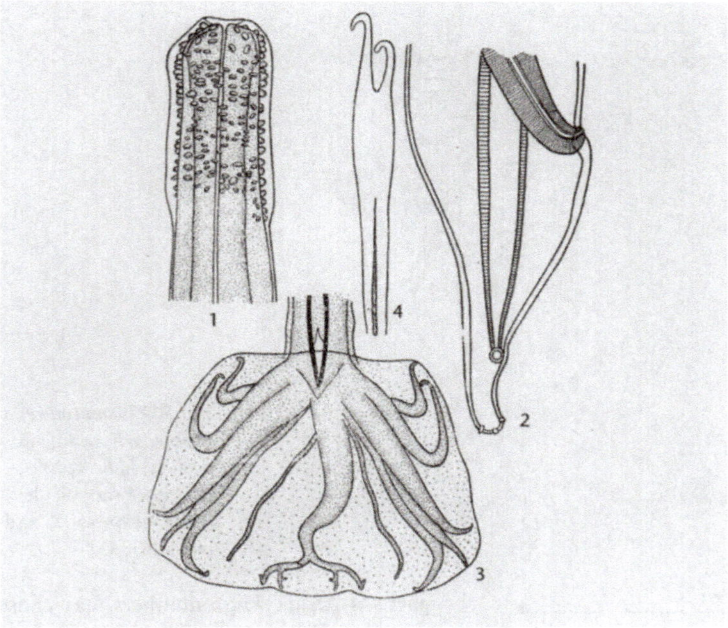

Fig. 502 *Impalaia tuberculata*; anterior end (1), posterior end of female (2), male bursa (3) and spicule (4) [44]

Remarks: These parasites belong to the Nematodirinae and have both been identified in dromedaries throughout Africa. *I. tuberculata* males are 7–9 mm long, with spicules about 600 µm long and a gubernaculum 9 µm long. The cervical cuticle is studded with small papillae. The female is 14–18 mm long. The eggs measure 60 × 32 µm. The males of *I. nudicollis* are 7.5–8.2 mm long, with spicules 910–980 µm long and a gubernaculum which is 94–100 µm long. The female is 14.8–16.7 mm long. The eggs are 63–74 × 39–46 µm. *I. aegyptiaca* has been found only in Egypt.

(Figure 502)

Nematodirus spp. (_N. dromedarii, N. spathiger, N. mauritanicus, N. abnormalis_ and _N. helvetianus_)

Location: Small intestine

Remarks: *N. spathiger* is the most prevalent species found in dromedaries (☞ CATTLE, 1 and SHEEP AND GOATS, 1). The males of *N. mauritanicus* are 13–15 mm long, with spicules 4.5–5.5 mm long, joined for a part of their length, with their tip enclosed in a thin, lanceolate membrane. The females are 21–24 mm long. The eggs measure 220–280 × 110 × 115 µm.

(Figure 503)

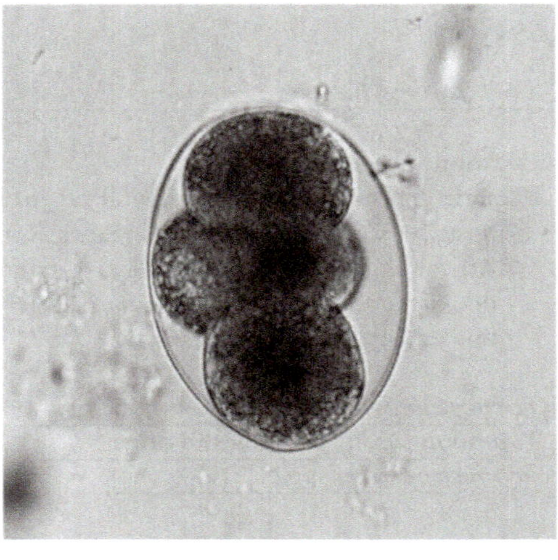

Fig. 503 Egg of *Nematodirus* sp. (220–280 × 110–115 µm)

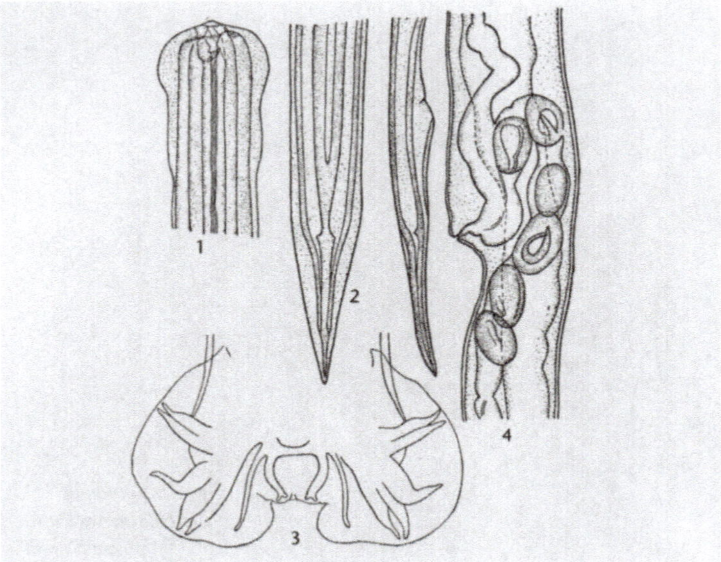

Fig. 504 *Nematodirella dromedarii*; head end with cephalic vesicle (1), tip of the spicule (2), male bursa (3) and vulva (4) [45]

Nematodirella dromedarii

Location: Small intestine

Remarks: This genus resembles *Nematodirus* but differs in that the vulva is in the anterior third of the body and the anterior branch of the female genital system is atrophied and sterile. The male is 10–15 mm long, with spicules 5.0–5.4 mm long. The female is 10–29 mm long. The eggs measure 230–260 × 100–120 µm.

(Figure 504)

Trichostrongylus axei

Location: Abomasum

Remarks: This species occurs in a wide range of hosts (☞ Cattle, 1), including camels in Africa. High numbers cause massive irritation of the abomasal mucosa, reduced digestion and absorption of nutrients.

Trichostrongylus spp. *(T. colubriformis, T. probolurus, T. vitrinus* and other *Trichostrongylus* spp.*)*

Location: Small intestine

Remarks: *Trichostrongylus* spp. may occur in the small intestine of dromedaries in all parts of Africa. High numbers may cause massive inflammation and irritation of the duodenum, associated with diarrhoea which may be fatal in young camels. For therapy and control ☞ Cattle, 1 and Sheep and Goats, 1.

Cooperia oncophora

Location: Small intestine

Remarks: *C. oncophora* may occasionally occur in dromedaries. Infections are often mixed with other trichostrongylids. *Cooperia* spp. have an extensive geographic distribution. For therapy and control ☞ Cattle, 1 and Sheep and Goats, 1.

Lungworms whose first-stage larvae may be found in the faeces of the dromedary

DICTYOCAULIDAE

Dictyocaulus filaria Common lungworm

(☞ Sheep and Goats, 4.3 and Dromedaries, 4.3)

Dictyocaulus cameli Camel lungworm

(☞ Dromedaries, 4.3)

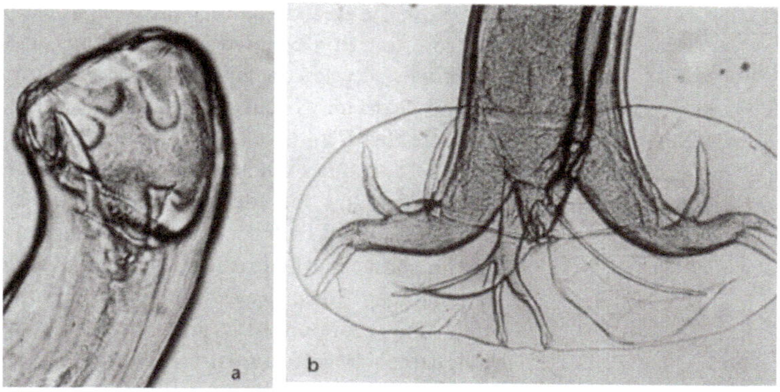

Fig. 505 *Bunostomum trigonocephalum*; anterior end (a) and male bursa (b) [4]

Bunostomum trigonocephalum Hookworm

Location: Small intestine

Remarks: This is essentially a parasite of small ruminants (☞ SHEEP AND GOATS, ■ 1), but it has been found in dromedaries in Africa and Asia. The male is 12–18 mm, and the female 22–25 mm long. It is a highly pathogenic species and may cause anaemia when present in high numbers.

(Figure 505)

Oesophagostomum columbianum
Nodular worm

Location: Large intestine

Remarks: This is essentially a parasite of sheep and goats (☞ SHEEP AND GOATS, ■ 1) but it has also been found in dromedaries in Africa. Extensive nodule formation in the entire gastrointestinal tract is the predominant sign of this parasite.

Oesophagostomum venulosum
Nodular worm

Location: Large intestine

Remarks: This is another nematode which occurs predominantly in small ruminants (☞ SHEEP AND GOATS, ■ 1). However, it may also be found in dromedaries in Africa and Asia.

Oesophagostomum vigintimembrum
(syn. *O. venulosum*)

Location: Large intestine

Remarks: This species seems to be specific for dromedaries, but its frequency of occurrence is low.

Chabertia ovina "Large-mouthed bowel worm"

Location: Colon

Remarks: This is a parasite of ruminants, particularly sheep, encountered rarely in dromedaries (☞ SHEEP AND GOATS, ■ 1).

Trichuris ovis* and *Trichuris globulosa
Whipworm

Location: Caecum

Remarks: *T. globulosa* is the commonest and most widespread trichurid of camels, reported from Africa and Asia. *T. ovis* is a cosmopolitan parasite of sheep, occasionally encountered in camels (☞ SHEEP AND GOATS, ■ 1). A number of other *Trichuris* spp. occur in camels elsewhere in the world: *T. cameli* and *T. raoi* (India), *T. skrjabini* (CIS), *T. affinis* (Asia). *Trichuris* spp. cause irritation and inflammation of the caecum and colon which often results in impaired water absorption and dehydration in heavy infections. For therapy and control ☞ below and SHEEP AND GOATS, ■ 1.

Strongyloides papillosus

Location: Small intestine

Remarks: This nematode has been found frequently in dromedaries in Africa. Only the parthenogenetic females are parasitic and infection may be acquired by percutaneous penetration of infective larvae (☞ CATTLE, 1 and SHEEP AND GOATS, 1).

(Figure 506)

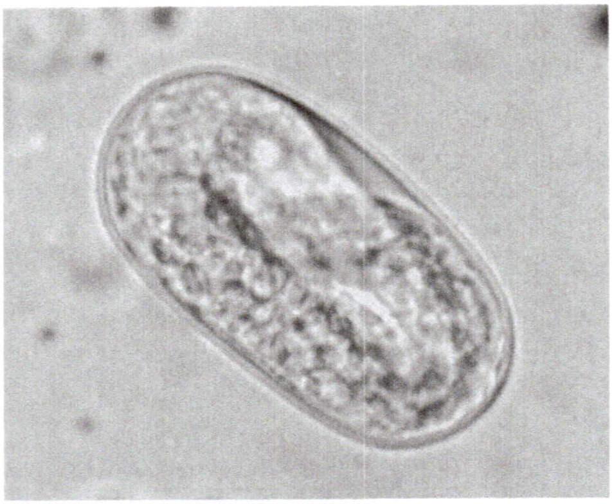

Fig. 506 Egg of *Strongyloides* sp. (47–65 × 25–26 µm)

- **General features of gastrointestinal nematode infections in dromedaries**

Although it seems that the environment in which camels live is conducive to the development and transmission of helminths, the helminth fauna is very rich and losses due to helminths play an important role in camel rearing. Under natural conditions camels are practically never infected with just a single species of gastrointestinal helminths; multiple parasitism is the rule. It is practically impossible to distinguish the diseases produced by different helminths with the exception of an acute haemonchosis which may cause a distinct disease entity. Haemonchosis caused by *H. longistipes* and/or *H. contortus* is the most severe gastrointestinal helminth infection of camels. Heavy infections occur more often in young camels and cause general weakness, anaemia, oedema of the hollow above the eyes, the sides of the sternal cushion (resulting in a characteristic swelling) and sometimes between the jaws. Progressive wasting and death may occur. Heavy infections are associated with a low PCV, albumin, calcium, phosphate, magnesium and copper level. Pathological findings include emaciation, ascites, hydrothorax and hydropericardium. The abomasum shows marked oedema, petechiae and sometimes erosions. However, clinical signs are often more pronounced in adult compared to adult camels (reverse age susceptibility), a phenomenon which was also described in context with ovine haemonchosis. Other helminth infections cause retarded growth, progressive wasting, alternation of constipation and diarrhoea. Anaemia only develops in a chronic stage of infection. *Oesophagostomum* spp. cause multiple nodule formation and *Trichuris* spp. cause a catarrhal enteritis.

Diagnosis: It is often possible to establish a diagnosis from the clinical signs of severe infections. By contrast, diagnosis can prove difficult in less severe cases. However, haemonchosis has to be distinguished from acute trypanosomosis which causes febrile episodes and a somnolent attitude, both normally absent from haemonchosis and infections with other gastrointestinal helminths. Faecal examination for worm eggs is usually helpful, although sometimes in peracute infections eggs are not present in the faeces. During the dry season some helminths undergo hypobiosis and cannot be detected by coprological methods during this period.

Therapy and Prophylaxis: Helminth infections are seasonal and usually concentrated to the rainy season when the preparasitic development may take place (☞ CATTLE, 1). Anthelmintic treatments during the rains may reduce the worm load and increase the growth rate which may be of vital importance for animals to survive the dry season. Most of the anthelmintics used in cattle and small ruminants for the treatment of gastrointestinal helminths may also be used in camels. Thiabendazole

(100–150 mg/kg, po.), tetramisole (10 mg/kg, sc. or 15 mg/kg, po.), levamisole (7.5 mg/kg, sc.), morantel tartrate (3–5 mg/kg, po.) and pyrantel (25 mg/kg, po.) are effective against adult nematodes including *Dictyocaulus* spp. but they are not effective against hypobiotic larvae which occur during the dry season. For dry season treatments the modern benzimidazoles (albendazole, fenbendazole, mebendazole, netobimin, etc., ☞ CATTLE, ■ 1) or ivermectin (200 µg/kg, sc.) may be used in order to eliminate also the hypobiotic larvae. A monthly treatment during the rainy season and an early dry season treatment with a larvicidal compound may markedly reduce the problems associated with helminth infections. Special attention should be paid to the weaned animals. Development of infective larvae on the ground may be reduced by keeping the ground around watering points as dry as possible and by using clean water for drinking purposes.
(Figure 507)

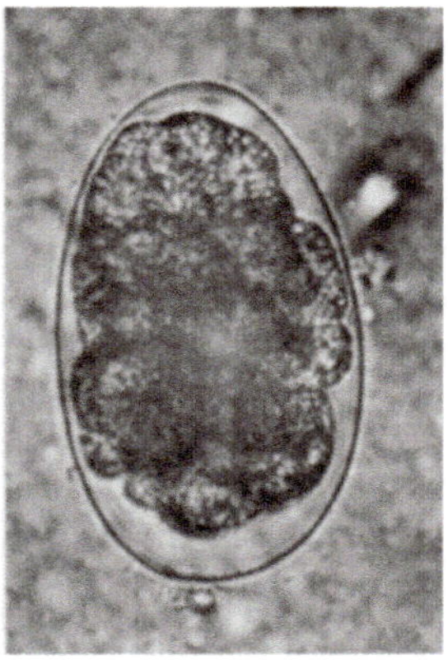

Fig. 507 Strongyle-type egg (70–100 × 30–45 µm) [13]

2 Stages in the blood and circulatory system

PROTOZOA

TRYPANOSOMATIDAE

Trypanosoma evansi (syn. *T. brucei evansi*)
Surra, tahaga, djaffa, dbab

Hosts: Dromedary, equine, buffalo, carnivore and many other mammal species

Vector: Blood-sucking flies such as *Tabanus* spp., *Haematopota* spp., *Atylotus* spp., *Philoliche* spp. and occasionally *Stomoxys* spp., *Lyperosia* spp. and *Haematobia* spp.

Species description: *T. evansi* is not transmitted by tsetse flies. Several species of blood sucking flies act as vectors. No developmental stages have been demonstrated in the vectors which differentiate the parasite from *T. brucei*. *T. evansi* is 15–35 µm long and 1.5–2.5 µm wide. *T. evansi* is morphologically identical with *T. brucei* and other members of the subgenus *Trypanozoon*. It can be distinguished from *T. brucei* by isoenzyme electrophoresis and DNA probes. *T. evansi* is not restricted to the bloodstream and may enter the joint fluids and other tissue compartments. It may cross the blood-brain barrier. These extravascular trypanosomes are less accessible to chemotherapy. Surra can attack camels at any age. There is a hig incidence of infection in juvenile camels shortly after weaning.

Geographic distribution: Africa north of the Sahara desert, Asia, CIS

Symptoms: In a typical case the dromedary loses weight, develops drooping hump, is unable to walk long distances and may develop oedema of the feet, brisket, underbelly and eyelids. The coat becomes rough. During the initial attack of fever there may be lacrimation, shivering, reduced appetite and mild diarrhoea. The animal always shows progressive anaemia and fluctuating body temperature with initial peaks of fever up to 41 °C. Later, in the chronic stage of infection the appetite is relatively unimpaired and the temperature may become normal or slightly elevated. The mucous membranes are pale and the PCV (particular cellular volume) drops below 25%, sometimes as low as 10%. The herders may notice a characteristic odour of the camel's urine and may identify infected animals by this sign alone. Abortion in all stages of pregnancy is common. Infected calves may be born alive but weak with parasitaemia. Death of the newborn calf is common. Reduced milk production, cases of blindness and central nervous lesions have been reported. The herd eventually reaches an endemic disease situation. Some animals may carry the trypanosomes for years, whereas others remain free of infection. Within such a group there are all forms and stages of surra, from new infections to subclinical and chronic conditions. Some animals live for up to 4 years with subclinical infections, some animals suddenly die due to other, superimposed infections and some eventually undergo self-cure. Numerous environmental and host factors influence the course of the disease, such as other infections, nutritional constraints, age, pregnancy, previous exposure or immunosuppression by other diseases and stress.

Significance: This trypanosome species causes the most widespread and most important disease in dromedaries. The overall productivity of a camel herd regarding calves, milk and weight gains is greatly impaired. Mortality may reach 20%.

Diagnosis: Trypanosomosis is diagnosed by demonstrating the parasite. However, dromedaries are usually far away from laboratory facilities. A tentative diagnosis can be reached by taking into account the owners observations such as weight loss, weakness, blindness, abortions, change of the odour of the urine and the clinical examinations of camels in the field. The predominant sign is anaemia, the mucous membranes being pale or white. Tachycardia may result. Postmortem examination reveals no absolutely typical signs. The carcass is pale and there are signs of dehydration, hypoproteinaemia, enlarged lymph nodes and splenomegaly. The direct methods of trypanosome detection utilize a wet blood film, a stained thick drop of blood and a thin bloodsmear. Concentration techniques such as the buffy coat technique under dark ground illumination provide both information about the level of anaemia (PCV) and the level of parasitaemia at the same time. For mass screening of dromedary herds there are numerous indirect tests. An immunofluorescent antibody test and ELISA tests have been successfully used for epidemiological surveys. A card agglutination test set has been introduced for the serodiagnosis of *T. evansi* infection in camels.

Therapy: Two drugs are recommended for the treatment of *T. evansi* infections in dromedaries: Quinapyramine as prosalt and Cymelarsan.

Cave: Most of the drugs for cattle trypanosomosis are either not curative (e.g. homidium bromide = Ethidium; pyrithidium bromide = Prothidium) or are too toxic for camels (e.g. diminazene aceturate = Berenil). Suramin and quinapyramine sulfate were successfully used but are no longer commercially available. Suramin (12 mg/kg or about 5 g/adult camel, given by slow intravenous injection) may cure infections and due to its slow elimination it has also a prophylactic effect for 6–12 weeks.

Cave: Suramin may cause phlebitis when administered paravenously. It is well tolerated up to 3-times the recommended dosage.

Quinapyramine methylsulfate (3–5 mg/kg, sc.) is used as a curative drug, whereas quinapyramine methylsulfate and quinapyramine chloride at a ratio of 3:2 (5–8.3 mg/kg, sc.) are applied for prophylactic purposes (duration 4–6 months). This compound is easier to dissolve and its subcutaneous application is easier.

Cave: Severe overdosing causes salivation and muscle tremor. Numerous *T. evansi* strains with a dual resistance to suramin and quinapyramine exist widely nowadays. In such cases isometamidium chloride (Samorin or Trypamidium, 0.5–0.7 mg/kg, iv., administered as a 2% solution) may be used. Unfortunately it has only a moderate effect against *T. evansi* and its use should be restricted to emergencies where dual resistance occurs. Isometamidium is only curative in acute cases when trypanosomes are still intravascular but it fails when they are extravascular. A recently developed arsenical (Cymelarsan®, 0.25 mg/kg, im.) is highly effective against *T. evansi* which are resistant to other drugs. It may be used for the treatment of acute and chronic *T. evansi* infections in camels.

Prophylaxis: There is no vaccine and vector control is difficult. Therefore, the control of *T. evansi* in camels relies entirely on drug therapy.

(Figures 508, 509, 510, Table 6)

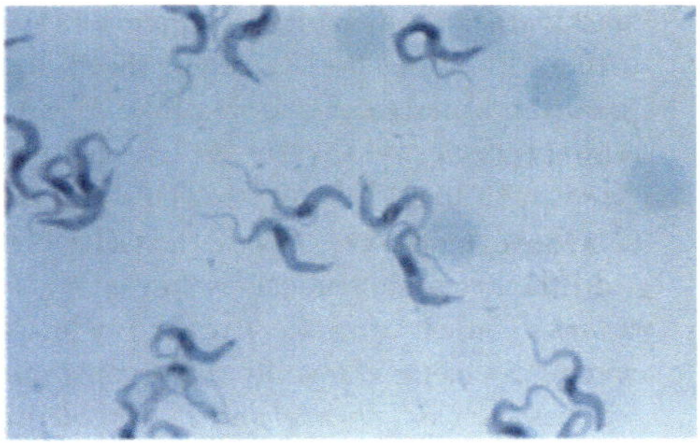

Fig. 508 *Trypanosoma evansi;* stained bloodsmear (15–35 × 1.5–2.5 μm) [4]

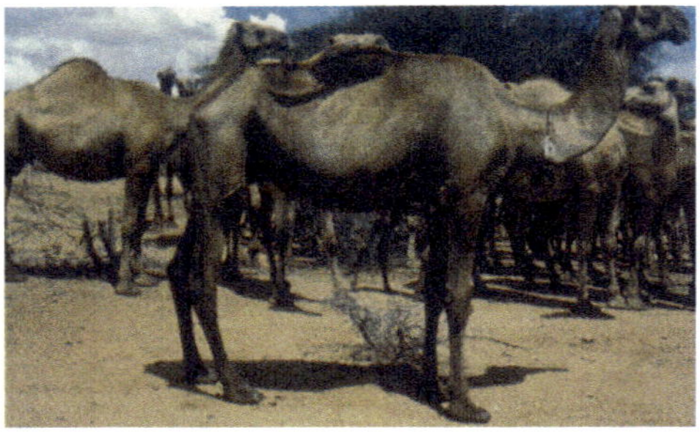

Fig. 509 Weight loss and emaciation due to a chronic *Trypanosoma evansi* infection [46]

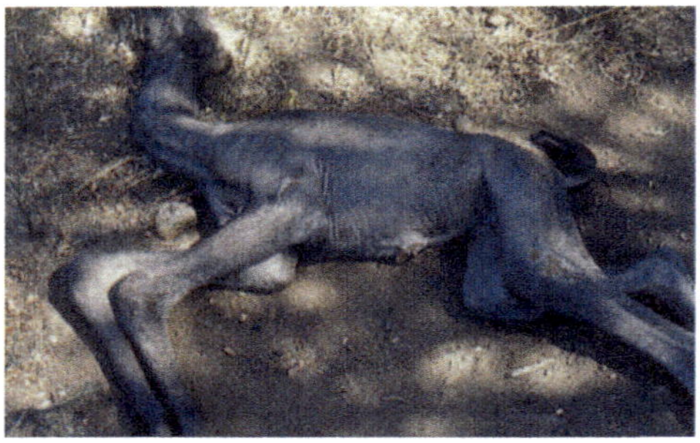

Fig. 510 Weakness of a newborn dromedary due to *Trypanosoma evansi* infection of the dam [46]

Trypanosoma congolense, Trypanosoma vivax and *Trypanosoma brucei*

Nagana, sleeping sickness

Remarks: Tsetse-transmitted trypanosomosis occurs in cattle, horse, camel, sheep and goat, and many other domestic and wild animal species (☞ CATTLE, ■ 2, SHEEP AND GOATS, ■ 2 and HORSES AND DONKEYS, ■ 2). Most camels live outside the tsetse belt and their trypanosomosis is caused by *T. evansi*. Camels are also affected to a lesser extent by tsetse-transmitted trypanosome species such as *T. brucei* and *T. congolense* which cause an acute disease with very high mortalities. Tsetse flies may have prevented the movement of camels into central Africa. Reports on the pathogenicity of *T. vivax* and *T. simiae* in camels are contradictory. For diagnosis ☞ CATTLE, ■ 2. For therapy and prophylaxis ☞ *T. evansi*.

THEILERIIDAE

Theileria camelensis

Remarks: This is a non-pathogenic *Theileria* species found in erythrocytes of camels in Egypt and Eritrea. The vector is *Hyalomma dromedarii* (☞ CATTLE, ■ 2)
(Figures 511, 512)

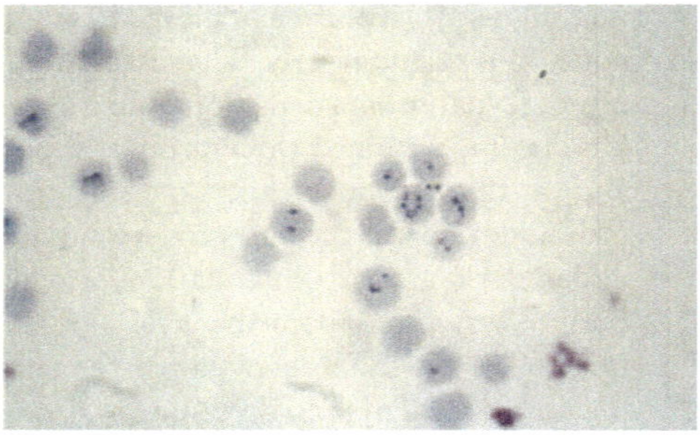

Fig. 511 *Theileria camelensis*; erythrocyte forms [15]

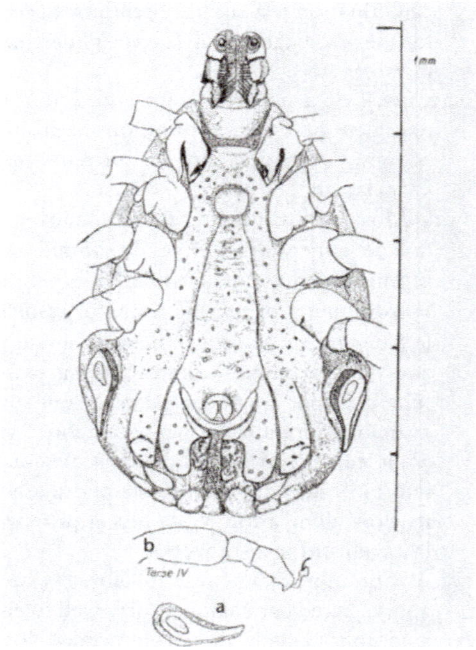

Fig. 512 *Hyalomma dromedarii*, the vector of *Theileria camelensis*; ventral view of a male, stigmata (a) and tarsus of leg IV (b) [9]

RICKETTSIALES

ANAPLASMATACEAE

Anaplasma marginale

Remarks: *A. marginale* may also be found in camels. Little is known about the pathogenic role in camels. It may be important in immunosuppressed animals (☞ CATTLE, ■ 2).

Cowdria ruminantium Heartwater

Remarks: *Amblyomma lepidum* and *A. gemma* are the vectors of the disease in East Africa (☞ CATTLE, ■ 2 and DROMEDARIES, ■ 5.1).

HELMINTHS

- Trematoda found in the blood and circulatory system

Schistosoma bovis* and *Schistosoma mattheei
Blood flukes, bilharziosis

Remarks: S. bovis occurs in the portal and mesenteric veins of cattle, sheep and goats, equines and dromedaries in central, eastern and western Africa. The eggs are spindle-shaped and partially passed in the faeces. The size of the eggs is 132–247 by 38–60 µm. S. mattheei occurs in the portal and mesenteric veins and less frequently in cystic and lung veins of cattle, sheep, goats, wild ruminants, equines and dromedaries in northern and Central Africa. There are usually no specific clinical signs of infection (☞ Cattle, ■ 2 and Sheep and Goats, ■ 2).

- Nematoda found in the blood and circulatory system

Dipetalonema evansi
(syn. *Deraiophoronema evansi*)

Remarks: This filarial nematode is specific for camels. It develops in the heart and in hepatic, pulmonary and spermatic arteries as well as in lymph nodes and lymph vessels. It has been found in eastern and northern Africa. The vectors are mosquitos of the genus *Aedes*. The males are 8–11 cm long and the females 14.5–18.5 cm. The microfilariae are ensheathed and measure 200–315 µm and occur in the peripheral blood. Light infections are inapparent. However, massive infections cause emaciation, apathy and sometimes orchitis and nervous symptoms. Filarial nematodes within arteries cannot be detected clinically. Any clinical manifestation can be confused with trypanosomosis, although the latter is accompanied by febrile episodes which are absent from filarial infections. Fouadin (stibophen, 0.5 mg/kg, iv.) was effective for both therapeutic and prophylactic purposes as prevention during the period of activity of the mosquito's intermediate hosts. Ivermectin (200 µg/kg, sc.) may eliminate the microfilariae.
(Figure 513)

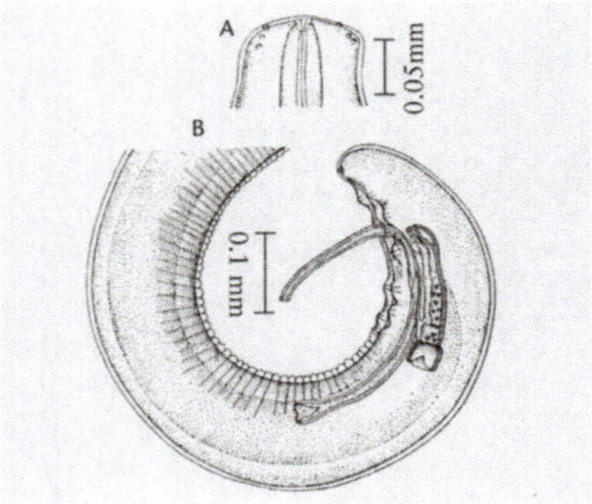

Fig. 513 *Dipetalonema evansi;* anterior end (A) and male posterior end (B) [9]

Onchocerca armillata Aortic filariosis

Remarks: This species develops within the aorta, particularly in cattle (☞ CATTLE, ■ 2). It has been found in this location in dromedaries in Nigeria. This infections is difficult to diagnose and usually does not cause clinical signs. Therapy is usually not indicated.

3 Stages in the urogenital system

No pathogenic parasites have been found so far in the urogential system of dromedaries

4.1 Locomotory system

4.1.1 Muscles

PROTOZOA

Sarcocystis cameli

Remarks: This species occurs commonly in North Africa (Egypt, Morocco, Sudan). The parasite is widespread, a high percentage of camels investigated at slaughter being infected. However, the pathogenic role of *S. cameli* is uncertain. Myocardial lesions have been attributed to *Sarcocystis* spp. in camels. In another study almost 50% of emaciated camels killed at Cairo abattoir showed sarcocysts. The definitive host is the dog. The prepatent period in dogs is 10–14 days, the patent period 69–73 days. The sarcocysts are up to 12 mm long and 2 mm in diameter. The bradyzoites are banana shaped, 15–20 × 4–6 µm. General life cycle of *Sarcocystis* spp. ☞ CATTLE, ■4.The antemortem diagnosis is difficult and therapy is usually not indicated. Infected, raw meat of camels is the only source of infection for dogs. If the overall incidence of sarcosporidiosis is to be reduced, the life cycle has to be interrupted at the stage where the definitive host (dog) has access to infected meat of the intermediate host (camel).

Toxoplasma gondii

Remarks: Tissue cysts of *T. gondii* may also occur in camels. A diagnosis based on clinical signs is not possible. Cysts may be seen in histopathological examinations. The chronic stage of infection is usually inapparent. The infection has recently been detected in camels by means of serological tests such as the Sabin-Feldman dye test, complement fixation, indirect immunofluorescence and indirect haemagglutination. The prevalence ranged from 3% to 67%. A heavy infection with a virulent strain may cause severe, fatal illness. Inappetence, lacrimation and polypnoea may be seen during the course of infection. For the general life cycle of *Toxoplasma gondii* ☞ SWINE, ■4.1. Felidae act as definitive hosts and many mammal species including man may be intermediate hosts. Raw, infected meat of camels may also be a source of infection for man and certainly for cats. Prevention is based on the interruption of this complex life cycle.

HELMINTHS

• Cestoda larvae found in the muscles

The following two cysticerci are found in the muscles of dromedaries.

Cysticercus dromedarii (syn. *C. cameli*)

Remarks: The larvae (*Cysticercus dromedarii*) of a hyena tapeworm (*Taenia hyaenae*) are frequently found in the muscles of the dromedary, cattle and goats. Antelopes are the usual intermediate hosts. They are rarely found in sheep. *C. dromedarii* cysts are twice as large as those of *C. bovis*, measuring

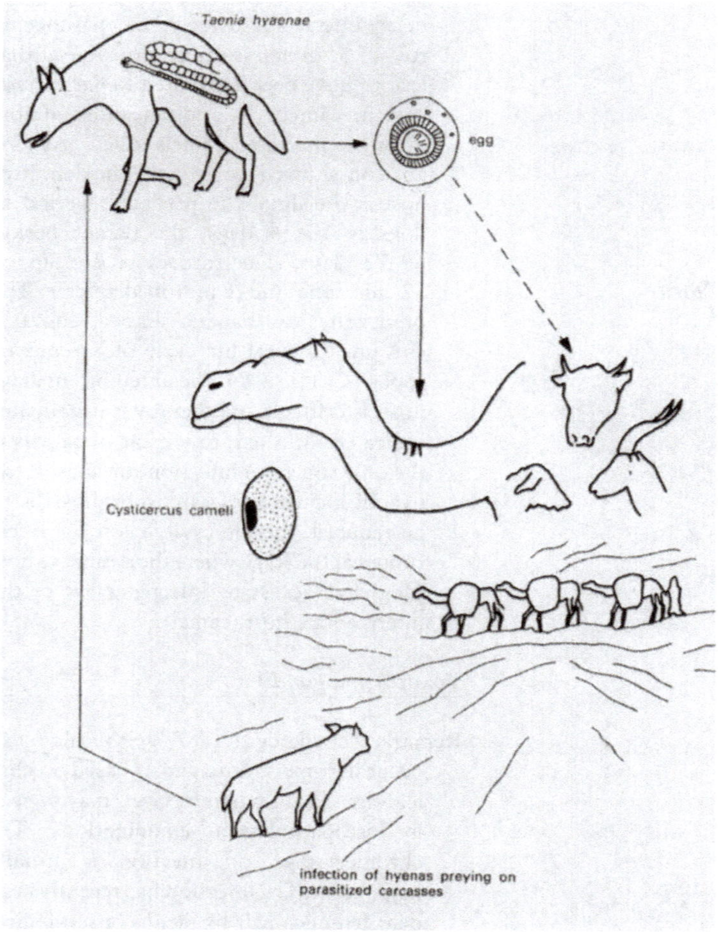

Fig. 514 Life cycle of *Cysticercus dromedarii*; hyena infected with the tapeworm *Taenia hyaenae* act as final host. Excreted eggs cause the development of cysticerci in the dromedary [16]

12–18 mm in length. They are pearly white and the lateral invaginated protoscolex has a double row of hooks. Although not dangerous to man, their presence is repugnant, and parasitized meat has to be condemned. (Figure 514)

Cysticercus bovis

Remarks: This is the larval stage of *Taenia saginata*, a tapeworm of man. Bovines are the usual intermediate hosts (☞ CATTLE, ■ 4.1.1), and infections of camels are very rare.

- **Prophylaxis of *Cysticercus* spp. infections in camels**

Infections of muscles with cysticerci are usually not associated with any detectable clinical signs. Prevention is based on the interruption of the life cycle which is in case of *C. cameli* almost impossible. In case of *C. bovis* the prevention of infection in camels may be achieved by anthelmintic treatments of infected human beings. Human infection is acquired by eating infected camel meat as well as beef. This may be prevented by a rigourous meat inspection, directed to the heart, masseter, muscles and tongue. Carcasses infected with cysticerci must be cooked sufficiently to destroy the cysticerci. Abattoir waste should be destroyed and not be given to dogs or left for wild carnivores.

4.1.2 Tendons

HELMINTHS

- Nematoda larvae and adult nematodes found in the tendons

Two species of filarial nematodes of the genus *Onchocerca* have been identified in camels (☞ CATTLE, ■ 5.1).

Onchocerca fasciata

Remarks: This parasite is specific for camels and occurs in the subcutaneous connective tissue and the nuchal ligament. It has been reported from Sudan, Ethiopia, Kenya and Mauritania. There is only fragmentary knowledge of the structure of this worm. The microfilariae are 200–285 µm long and 35–50 µm wide (mean 255 × 40 µm).

Onchocerca gutturosa

Remarks: This nematode develops in subcutaneous connective tissue, the nuchal ligament and other tissues, such as the scapular cartilage. It is mainly a parasite of cattle (☞ CATTLE, ■ 4.1.2), but it has also been found in camels.

- **General features of filarial nematode infections**

Affected animals have skin nodules on various parts of the body, particularly on the head and neck. The nodules are firm, not sensitive to the touch, and range from 0.5–4 cm in diameter. Microfilariae may be found in the surrounding skin or within the nodules. They are rarely found in the peripheral blood. The nodules have a fibrous capsule. The filaria can be seen when a nodule is cut open, perhaps accompanied by pus. The animals seem to tolerate these infections without clinical signs. Allergic skin reactions due to microfilariae may occur. Therapy is usually not indicated. Allergic dermatitis may successfully be treated with ivermectin (0.2 mg/kg, sc.).

4.2 Liver

HELMINTHS

- Trematoda found in the liver

Four species of trematodes parasitize the liver of camels.

Fasciola hepatica Common liver fluke

Remarks: This trematode is frequently encountered in camels in Africa and Asia in those regions where *F. hepatica* is very prevalent in the cattle population (☞ CATTLE, ■ 4.2).

Fasciola gigantica Giant liver fluke

Remarks: This species is often found in camels in Africa and Asia. *F. gigantica* is common in cattle in many parts of Africa (☞ CATTLE, ■ 4.2).

Dicrocoelium **spp.** (*D. dendriticum* and *D. hospes*) Lancet flukes

Remarks: Lancet flukes are found very seldom in camels. In many parts of the world this parasite is very prevalent among cattle and small ruminants (☞ CATTLE, ■ 4.2).

Eurytrema pancreaticum Pancreas fluke

Remarks: This trematode normally occurs in the pancreatic ducts and less often in the bile ducts of ruminants (☞ CATTLE, ■ 4.5). Camels may also become infected.

- **General features of trematode infections of the liver**

Hepatic infections are generally subclinical in camels, with the exception of heavy *Fasciola* spp. infections. Chronic fasciolosis is the most common form in camels and other hosts (☞ CATTLE, ■ 4.2). The symptoms of chronic fasciolosis are generally associated with hepatic fibrosis and hyperplastic cholangitis. Anaemia, oedema (bottle jaw), digestive disturbances (constipation, diarrhoea) and cachexia develop gradually. Acute fasciolosis is less common than the chronic disease and occurs mainly in sheep (☞ SHEEP AND GOATS, ■ 4.2). It is basically a hepatitis caused by the simultaneous migration of large numbers of immature flukes. Sudden death may occur in acute fasciolosis.

Diagnosis: The oval, operculated, golden-brown eggs (130–150 × 65–90 µm) appear in the sediment of the faeces (☞ CATTLE, ■ 1). The detection of the adult flukes in the liver at necropsy or slaughter is the most reliable method to confirm fasciolosis.

Therapy: Treatment is indicated in those rare cases when fasciolosis is diagnosed or expected to cause problems in camel herds. Several fasciolicidal drugs are currently available (☞ CATTLE, ■ 4.2) and may be used, although few publications refer to their use in camels. Triclabendazole (12 mg/kg, po.) is highly effective in cattle. Nitroxynil (10 mg/kg, sc.) and rafoxanide (7.5 mg/kg, po.) are drugs recommended for camels. These two anthelmintics are also effective, in the same dosage, against myiasis of the nasal cavity, particularly *Cephalopina titillator,* and bloodsucking nematodes. Albendazole (10 mg/kg, po.) is also effective against *Fasciola* spp.

- Cestoda found in the liver

Stilesia hepatica

Remarks: This cestode occurs occasionally in the bile ducts of camels. It is common in small ruminants in many parts of Africa (☞ SHEEP AND GOATS, ■ 4.2). Infections are usually inapparent. Heavy burdens were associated with cholangitis and cirrhosis. Therapy is not indicated.

Echinococcus granulosus
(syn. *E. polymorphus, E. unilocularis*)
Hydatid tapeworm, hydatidosis

Remarks: Larvae (hydatid cysts) of *E. granulosus* are found in the liver and the lungs of dromedary, cattle, sheep, goat, swine, horse, and other domestic animals and man (= intermediate hosts). Adult tapeworms are found in the small intestine of the dog, hyena and other related carnivores (= final hosts). Hydatids are localized mainly in the liver and lungs, but also in other organs of camels (☞ CATTLE, ■ 4.2 and ■ 4.3, and DROMEDARIES, ■ 4.3). The incidence of hydatidosis in camels is highest in North and East Africa. It also occurs in Central and West Africa with a rather low incidence, although in Nigeria infection rates of 50% have been reported. Both liver and lung hydatidosis in camels are usually asymptomatic. The diagnosis is based on postmortem findings. Therapy is usually not indicated. Although infections with hydatids do not have serious consequences for camels, echinococcosis is a major helminthosis with regard to the public health. It is therefore necessary to limit the threat to human health by excluding dogs from places where camels are slaughtered and by seizure and destruction of any organ bearing hydatid cysts at slaughter.

Prophylaxis: ☞ CATTLE, ■ 4.2 and ■ 4.3

Cysticercus tenuicollis

Remarks: This is the larval stage of *Taenia hydatigena*, a tapeworm which occurs in the small intestine of domestic and wild canidae. In camels these larvae develop on the liver surface and serosal surface of the abdominal cavity as they do in the preferred hosts sheep and cattle (☞ CATTLE, ■ 4.4 and SHEEP AND GOATS, ■ 4.4). *C. tenuicollis* may be found occasionally in camels at the abattoir. The infection is asymptomatic unless a large number of larvae migrate through the liver parenchyma. Blood loss and death may then occur (☞ SHEEP AND GOATS, ■ 4.4).

4.3 Respiratory system

HELMINTHS

- Cestoda found in the lungs and trachea

Echinococcus granulosus
Hydatid tapeworm, hydatidosis

Remarks: Hydatid cysts of *E. granulosus* are found in the liver and the lungs of dromedary and other domestic animals and man (= intermediate hosts). Lungs harbouring hydatid cysts near the surface show protuberances. Within the lung tissue they can be felt as hard lumps, not very mobile. (☞ DROMEDARIES, ■ 4.2 and CATTLE, ■ 4.2).

- Nematoda found in the lungs and trachea

Dictyocaulus filaria Parasitic bronchitis

Remarks: This lungworm is encountered most frequently in the respiratory tract of camels in Africa. It is also prevalent in Asia and Europe. Severe infections with *Dictyocaulus* spp. are accompanied by general depression, cough, and polypnoea, dyspnoea and rapid loss of condition. Apathy and anorexia may occur. The adult worms occur in the bronchi and bronchioles. The life cycle is direct. First-stage larvae are passed in the faeces and their demonstration is essential, together with the respiratory signs for the diagnosis (☞ SHEEP AND GOATS, ■ 4.3). The following anthelmintics are recommended to treat *D. filaria* infections in camels: albendazole (2.5 mg/kg, po.), febantel (7.5 mg/kg, po.), fenbendazole (10–15 mg/kg, po.), oxfendazole (7 mg/kg, po.), ivermectin (0.2 mg/kg, sc.) tetramisole (10 mg/kg, sc. or 15 mg/kg, po.) and levamisole (7.5 mg/kg, sc.). All of these compounds are also effective against the most important gastrointestinal nematodes of camels.

Dictyocaulus viviparus* and *Dictyocaulus cameli (syn. *D. viviparus*)

These species may rarely occur in camels (☞ CATTLE, ■ 4.3).

ARTHROPODS

- Insecta larvae found in the respiratory system

Cephalopina *(Cephalopsis)* ***titillator***
Camel nasal botfly

Remarks: The adult fly occurs in subsaharan

Africa, Middle East and Asia. The larvae migrate into the nasal cavity, frontal sinus and pharynx of camels. The larvae are similar to those of *Hypoderma bovis* and measure 25–35 × 8–9 mm. The larvae irritate and damage the mucosa markedly. Infestations may be associated with extensive sneezing, restlessness and head shaking. Severe conditions must be differentiated from central nervous disorders. Ivermectin (0.2 mg/kg, sc.) has shown variable efficacy against the larvae of *C. titillator*. Rafoxanide (7.5–10 mg/kg, po.) as a drench or bolus, trichlorfon (75 mg/kg, po. or as a drench) and nitroxynil (10–15 mg/kg, sc.) have been reported to be effective.
(Figures 515, 516, 517)

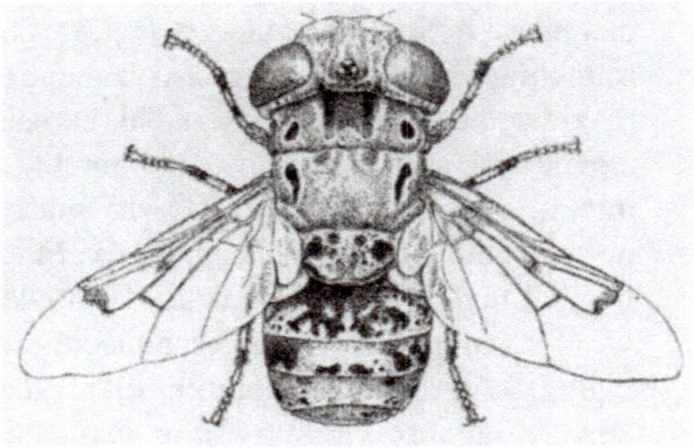

Fig. 515 *Cephalopina titillator* (camel nasal bot fly); adult [47]

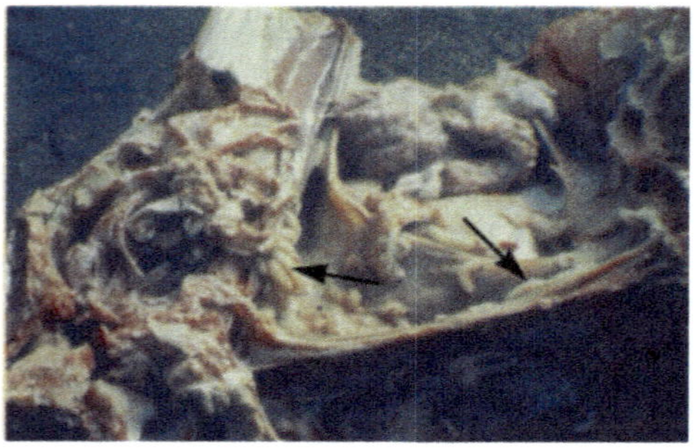

Fig. 516 Masses of nasal bot fly larvae (arrows) in the nasal cavity of a dromedary [13]

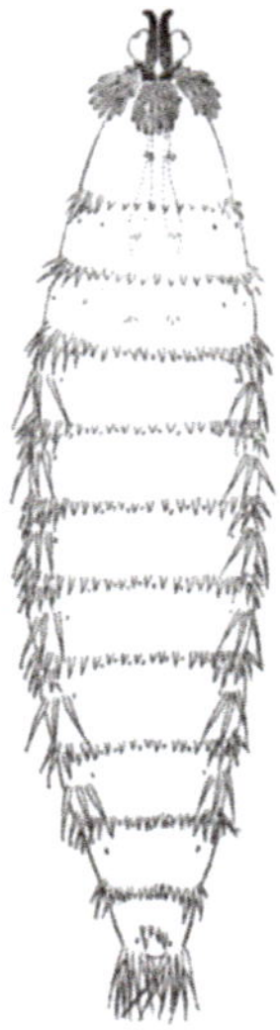

Fig. 517 *Cephalopina titillator*; larva [48]

Oestrus ovis

Remarks: *O. ovis* infestations in camels have been reported from Egypt (☞ Sheep and Goats, ■ 4.3).

4.4 Abdominal cavity

HELMINTHS

• Cestoda found in the abdominal cavity

Cysticercus tenuicollis Larval stage of the canine tapeworm *Taenia hydatigena*

Remarks: Cysticerci are found attached to the omentum, the intestinal mesentery and to the serosal surface of abdominal organs, especially the liver. Adult tapeworms occur in the small intestine of dogs and other Canidae. Infections in camels and other intermediate hosts are usually inapparent (☞ Dromedaries, ■ 4.2 and Sheep and Goats, ■ 4.4).

4.5 Pancreas

HELMINTHS

- Trematoda found in the pancreas

Eurytrema pancreaticum Pancreas fluke

Remarks: This trematode normally occurs in the pancreatic ducts and less often in the bile ducts of ruminants. Camels may also become infected (☞ DROMEDARIES, ■ 4.2 and SHEEP AND GOATS, ■ 4.5).

4.6 Central nervous system

HELMINTHS

- Cestoda cysts found in the central nervous system

Coenurus cerebralis Larval stage of the canine tapeworm *Taenia multiceps* (syn. *Multiceps multiceps*); "gid", "stuggers", sturdy"

Remarks: The intermediate stage, a coenurus, develops in the brain and spinal cord of sheep and goat and sometimes camel. Adult *Taenia multiceps* occurs in the small intestine of the dog, fox, coyote, hyena and other Canidae (☞ SHEEP AND GOATS, ■ 4.6). *Coenurus* cysts cause increased intracranial pressure which is the cause of the neurological symptoms. Development of coenurus in the nervous system produces noticeable changes in behaviour, with diminution of appetite, even anorexia, depression, unwillingness to move or difficulty in walking. Animals may make circling in movements. Clinical diagnosis has to be distinguished from myiasis of the respiratory passages caused by *Cephalopina titillator* (☞ DROMEDARIES, ■ 4.3) and from rabies. The latter produces excitement, sneezing, snorting and sometimes abnormal behaviour. No drug therapy is available. Prophylaxis consists of destroying any coenurus cysts at slaughter, although this applies mainly to sheep, because the skull of camels is not usually opened at slaughter. The adult tapeworm in dogs can be controlled by using one of the cestodicidal anthelmintics such as praziquantel (5 mg/kg, po. or 5.7 mg/kg, sc. or im.), bunamidine hydrochloride (25–50 mg/kg, po.), nitroscanate (50 mg/kg, po.) or the combination of febantel/praziquantel/pyrantel (☞ SHEEP AND GOATS, ■ 4.6).
(Figure 518)

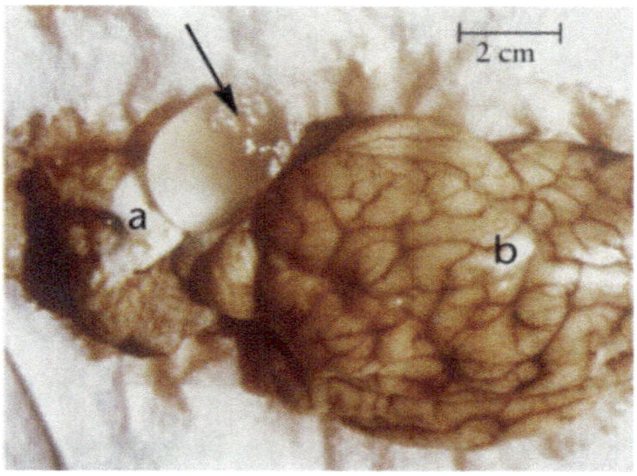

Fig. 518 Cyst of *Coenurus cerebralis* (arrow) located between the cerebellum (a) and cerebrum (b) [8]

5 Stages on the body surface

5.1. Skin and coat

HELMINTHS

- Nematoda found in the skin and subcutis

Onchocerca fasciata

Remarks: This parasite is specific for camels and occurs in the subcutaneous connective tissue and the nuchal ligament. Skin nodules may appear but clinical signs are usually absent.

Onchocerca gibsoni

Remarks: The adult worms are found in subcutaneous nodules on the brisket, shoulders and external surfaces of the hindlimbs of cattle (☞ CATTLE, ■ 5.1) and occasionally of dromedaries. Microfilariae are found intradermally around the nodules with a predilection to the brisket region. Adult worms cause nodular swellings in the skin but infected animals are not clinically ill. The intermediate hosts are members of the genus *Culicoides* (e.g. *C. pungens* and other *Culicoides* spp.).

***Stephanofilaria* sp.**

Remarks: *Stephanofilaria* spp. are small filarial parasites (family: Filariidae) which are responsible for circumscribed dermatitis (☞ CATTLE, ■ 5.1). Several genera of the order Dipterida act as intermediate hosts. (Figure 519)

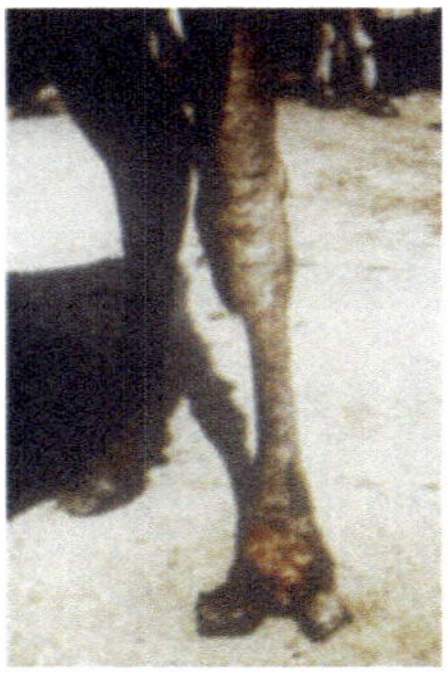

Fig. 519 *Stephanofilaria* sp. infection, causing a moist dermatitis on the leg of a camel [8]

ARTHROPODS

Arthropods are divided into two main groups:

Arachnida (arachnids) including:
- *Ticks*
- *Mites*

Insecta including:
- *Lice*
- *Fleas*
- *Dipterida*

- Arachnida found in/on the skin

– **Ticks**

The role of ticks as disease vectors (bunyaviruses, rickettsiae) in camels is minor. Routine prophylactic tick control is therefore not as widely practised in camel herds as it is done in cattle rearing systems. Nevertheless ticks suck blood and can cause severe anaemia and debil-

ity in camels as well as paralysis (☞ CATTLE, ■ 5.1). Tick infestations are seasonal, occurring predominantly during the wet season. Heavy infestations should be treated with an acaricide. When animals bear a high number of ticks and, at the same time, show signs of paralysis or other non-specific clinical signs, acaricidal treatment should be applied. *Cowdria ruminantium* is transmitted by *Amblyomma lepidum* and *Amblyomma gemma* in East Africa. The non-pathogenic *Theileria camelensis* is transmitted by *Hyalomma dromedarii* (☞ DROMEDARIES, ■ 2).
(Figures 520, 521, 522, 523)

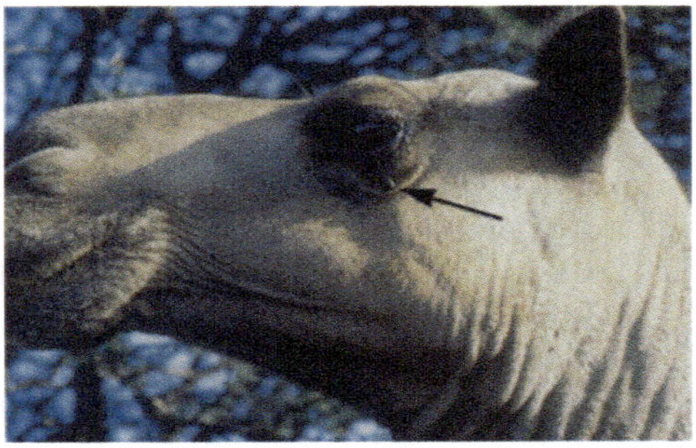

Fig. 520 Ticks affecting the eyelid of a dromedary [46]

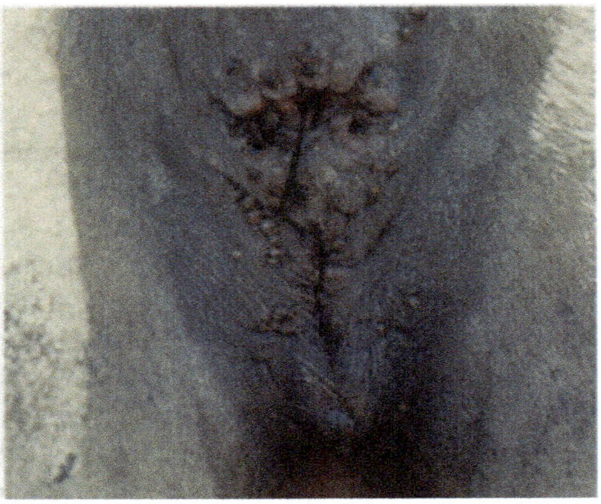

Fig. 521 Ticks affecting the vulva and perineal region of a dromedary [46]

The following ticks are commonly found on camels:

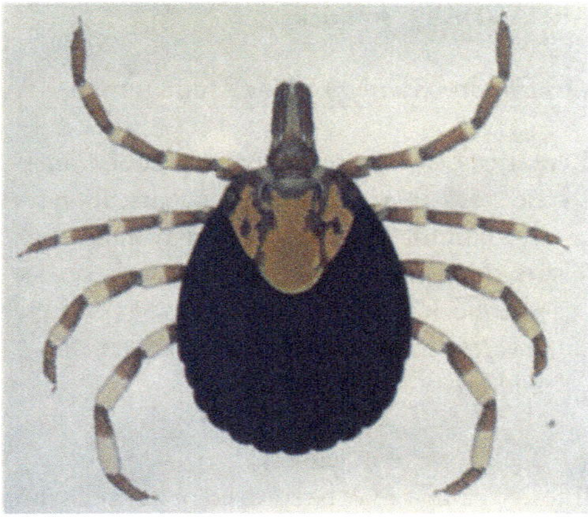

Fig. 522 *Amblyomma gemma*; female (2-5 mm × 4 mm) [13]

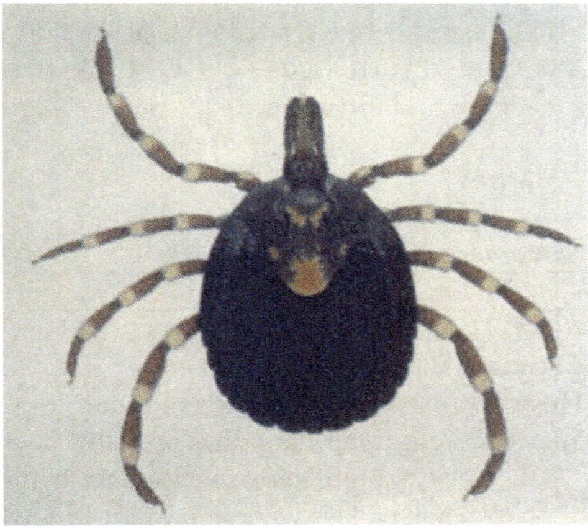

Fig. 523 *Amblyomma lepidum*; female (5 mm × 4 mm) [13]

IXODIDAE ("hard ticks")

Hyalomma dromedarii
Hyalomma rufipes and other *H.* spp. (*H. anatolicum, H. detritum, H. impressum* and *H. plumbeum)*
Amblyomma lepidum, A. gemma, A. variegatum
Boophilus decoloratus
Rhipicephalus pulchellus, R. appendiculatus, R. sanguineus

A general description of each genus is made in CATTLE, ■ 5.1

ARGASIDAE ("soft ticks")

Ornithodoros savignyi The sand tampan

Remarks: *O. savignyi* is a major pest of domestic stock in areas where it occurs. Its bites are painful and the saliva may cause tick toxicosis. The sand tampan may also cause allergic dermatitis in man. *O. savignyi* may severely irritate camels (☞ CATTLE, ■ 5.1 and SHEEP AND GOATS, ■ 5.1).

- **Tick control in camels**

Infested camels may be sprayed or doused with lindane (Gammatox) which has proved to be a highly effective and well-tolerated acaricide for camels. However, many of the modern ectoparasiticides recommended for cattle may also be used in camels. ☞ CATTLE ■ 5.1 THERAPY AND PROPHYLAXIS OF ECTOPARASITES (arachnids and insects) p. 141

– **Mites**

Sarcoptes scabiei var. *cameli*
Camel mange, "Jarab"

Location: Skin
Hosts: Dromedary and Bacterian camel
Species description: Mange has probably been the most common disease of camels. In the past when camels were important for civil and military transport, mange was regarded as a major disease. Animals were usually in poor condition and fatigued by long journeys and poor feeding. Unsatisfactory hygienic condition favoured the development and transmission of mange. Camel mange is caused by *S. scabiei* var. *cameli*, a mite almost exclusively confined to the genus *Camelus*. However, it has been reported that human beings may also be infected by this mite. The life cycle of the mite lasts for 4–5 weeks. Fertilized females burrow into the epidermis, causing inflammation and intense pruritus. Direct transmission occurs between animals. Infestations can also be transmitted indirectly via objects (e.g. harness, tents, luggage, etc.) which have been in contact with an infested camel or via soil (resting place). The mites survive off the host for a maximum of 2 weeks. The development and spread of camel mange may be favoured by factors such as poor nutrition, poor hygiene, stress (long journeys) and other diseases (trypanosomosis). Mange may be more acute during the cold season and during rainy periods. Both very young and very old camels are particularly susceptible.
Geographic distribution: Sarcoptic mange occurs wherever camels are kept.
Symptoms: Skin reactions start on the head, base of the neck, mammary gland, prepuce and flank. The head is almost always affected since camels use their teeth to scratch affected areas. First clinical signs such as erythema, vesicles and intense pruritus occur 2–3 weeks after infection. About 2 weeks after the first signs, the affected skin has lost its hair and becomes reddened and moist. The lesions may become generalized after 20–30 days. Later the skin becomes dry and hard, with folds (hyperkeratosis) forming in the neck region, around joints and on the thighs. Itchiness is less pronounced in this stage. Intense itching, scratching and rubbing distract the affected animal from eating, and progressive weight loss and emaciation result. Decubitus sores develop rapidly and secondary infections, particularly with pyogenic bacteria may aggravate the condition.
Significance: Sarcoptic mange in camels is one of the most important diseases of camels, causing weight loss, emaciation and severe secondary skin infections. Direct transmission from camel to man is common and causes a condition termed pseudoscabies.
Diagnosis: Mange is easy to diagnose clinically. Intense itching, pruritus, depilation and encrusted plaques are characteristic for the mange. These signs must be differentiated from tick-associated skin reactions, eczema (rare in camels), depilation due to malnutrition and poxvirus infections in young camels. The chronic stage is characterized

by extensive hyperkeratosis, showing thickened skin and folds around joints, hind limbs and neck. Laboratory diagnosis is not easy. Deep skin scrapings (until the skin starts to bleed) may reveal the mite. Pseudoscabies in man is transmitted during milking and is therefore seen in the interdigital space of the hands, the flexor surface of the wrists, the forearms, the elbows and the axillary folds. Camel riders show lesions between the thighs.

Therapy: The most commonly used acaricide is lindane (0.05%). However, most of the acaricides recommended for cattle mange (organophosphates and pyrethroids) may also be used for camels, except malathion (0.75%) which does not seem to be very effective. The acaricides are applied by brushing the affected regions and/or as sprays. Spray treatment must be applied thoroughly to all parts of the body and treatment must be repeated after 8–15 days. Once a herd is infected, continuous reinfection of both man and camels occurs and it is therefore essential to treat both. The recommended treatment for man is hexachlorcyclohexane. Ivermectin (0.2 mg/kg, sc., twice at 2-week-intervals) proved to be highly effective against camel mange. It is also effective against the most important gastrointestinal nematodes (*Haemonchus* spp.).

Prophylaxis: The entire herd should be treated at the same time. Freshly introduced animals must be treated. Attention must be paid to the indirect transmission of mange via harness and other equipment. These should also be treated with an acaricide. Dietary supplements would help to improve the general condition and thus reduce the susceptibility to mange.

(Figures 220, 524, 525, 526)

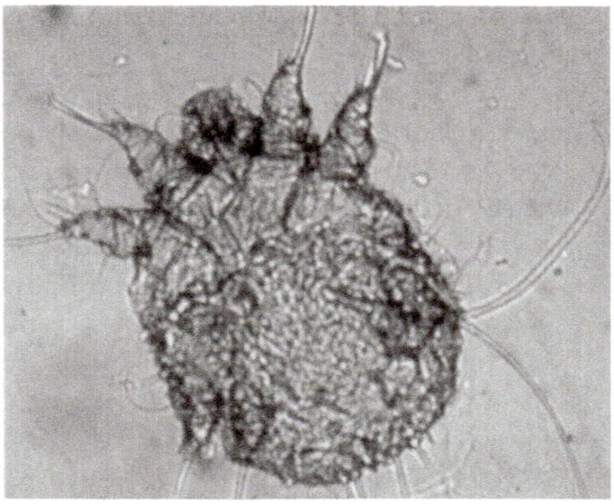

Fig. 524 *Sarcoptes scabiei* var. *cameli* (syn. *camelensis*); adult mite (female up to 0.6 mm long, male up to 0.3 mm long) with long unjointed pedicels [13]

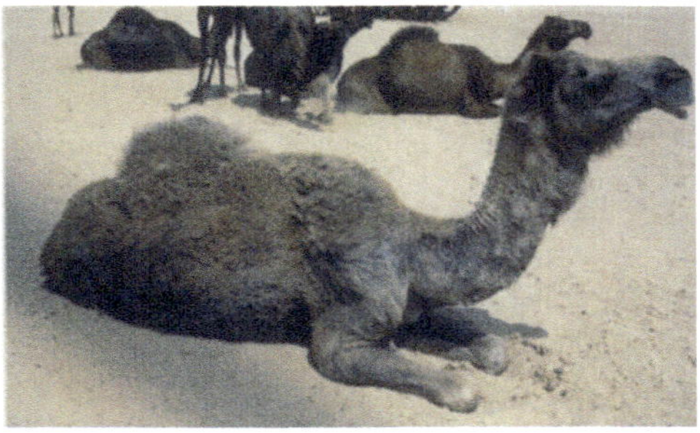

Fig. 525 Dromedary with generalized sarcoptic mange [46]

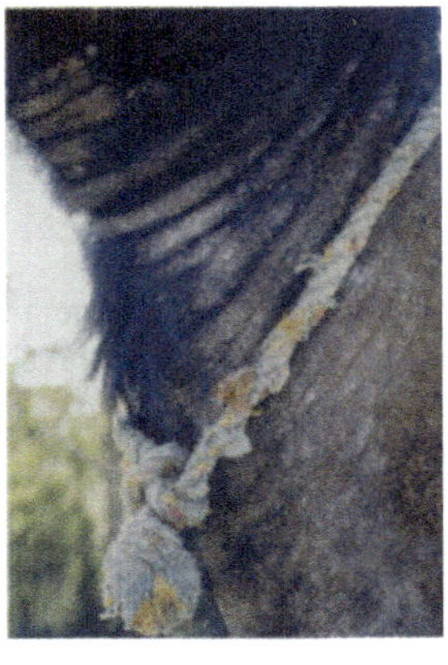

Fig. 526 Hairless, rough skin due to sarcoptic mange [46]

Chorioptes **spp.** Chorioptic mite, foot mange, leg mite

Remarks: Chorioptic mange occurs mainly on the legs, base of tail and upper rear surface of the udder. Chorioptic mange has been found repeatedly in dromedaries kept in zoos. For diagnosis, therapy and prophylaxis ☞ above *Sarcoptes scabies* and CATTLE, ■ 5.1.
(Figure 527)

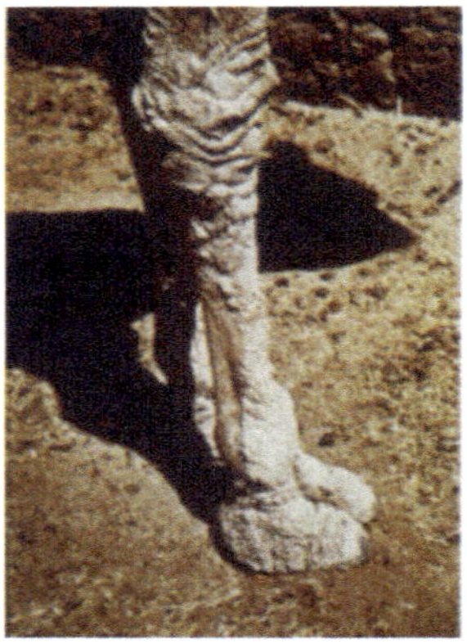

Fig. 527 Hyperkeratosis, dry and hard skin due to Chorioptic mange [8]

• Insecta found on the skin

– **Lice**

ANOPLURA
Blood sucking lice of camels

Microthoracius cameli (syn. *Haematopinus cameli*)

Remarks: This species is closely related to members of the genus *Linognathus* (☞ CATTLE, ■ 5.1). It is the only blood-sucking louse of camels. Animals in poor conditions carry high numbers of lice. Louse worry is characterized by licking, scratching and rubbing. Heavy infestations may cause anaemia, particularly in young animals. The coat becomes rough and secondary bacterial infections may occur. Most of the insecticides recommended for cattle may be used for louse infestations in camels.
(Figure 528)

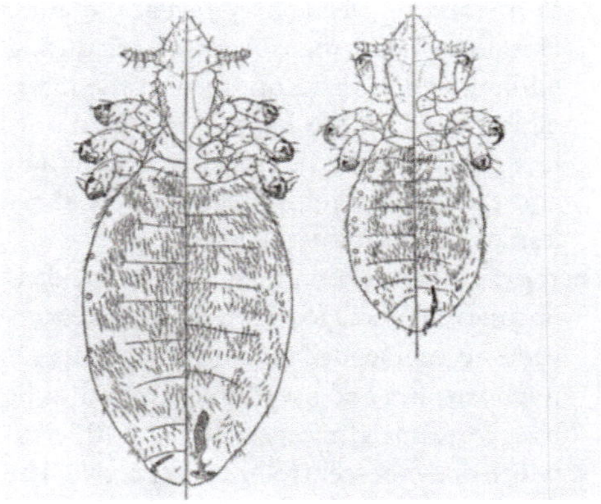

Fig. 528 *Microthoracius cameli*; female (4 mm long) dorsal and ventral view (left); male (2 mm long) dorsal and ventral view (right) [9]

– **Fleas**
No fleas have been found on the body surface of dromedaries

– **Dipterida**

Many of the dipteran flies which attack cattle may also affect camels, when they enter the habitat of these flies. Fly worry is particularly a problem around watering places, in oases and along well aerated streams. For symptoms, therapy and prophylaxis ☞ CATTLE, ■ 5.1.

CALLIPHORIDAE
The blowflies and their allies

They are highly important in many domestic animal species and man. The adults are free-living and the larvae are parasitic maggots which develop in the tissue of their host, causing a condition called myiasis. The larvae may be laid into pre-existing wounds. Myiasis is often a secondary skin problem. Many of the species found on cattle and small ruminants may occasionally occur in camels (☞ CATTLE, ■ 5.1 and SHEEP AND GOATS, ■ 5).

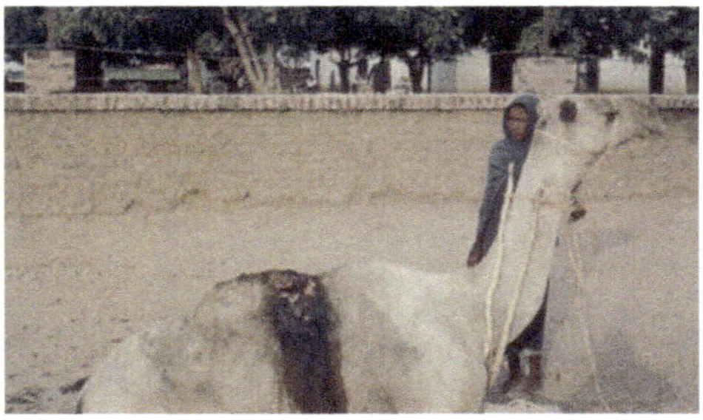

Fig. 529 Saddle wounds are often invaded by blowflies [15]

In camels larvae of the following flesh flies often cause myiasis.
(Figure 529)

Wohlfahrtia magnifica

The Old World flesh fly
(☞ Cattle, ■ 5.1)

Wohlfahrtia nuba

Remarks: This larviparous flesh fly occurs in man and dromedaries in Sudan and Ethiopia, Senegal and probably in many other countries of North Africa and the Middle East. Primary skin wounds are often infested by larvae of this fly. This myiasis (mainly vaginal myiasis) is currently a severe problem in two-humped camels in Mongolia.

Sarcophaga dux

Remarks: This fly lays its larvae in decomposing flesh, wounds and ulcers. It has been found in skin lesions of camels in India.

HIPPOBOSCIDAE
The louse flies

Hippobosca camelina Camel louse fly

Remarks: This blood sucking louse fly occurs on camel and horse and occasionally cattle wherever camels are present, mainly in the northern part of eastern Africa and the Mediterranean region. These flies are a source of great irritation and occur in clusters in the perineal region, between the hindlegs to the pubic region, but may also bite on other parts of the body. Infested animals scratch and rub and skin-trauma is often seen as a consequence of heavy infestations. ☞ CATTLE, ■ 5.1; THERAPY AND PROPHYLAXIS OF ECTOPARASITES, p. 141.

5.2 Eyes

***Thelazia* spp.** (*Thelazia rhodesi* and *Thelazia leesei*) Eye worms

Remarks: *T. rhodesi* (☞ CATTLE, ■ 5.2) may occasionally occur in camel. *T. leesei* is specific for camels and transmitted by *Musca lucidala*. This spirurid nematode develops in the conjunctival sacs of camels in Africa and Asia. One or both eyes may be affected often without clinical signs. Heavy infections may cause irritation and keratitis with marked discharges. Eggs or first-stage larvae may be found in the lacrimal secretions. Therapy (☞ CATTLE, ■ 5.2) is only indicated when intense lacrimal secretion and secondary infections occur. This condition is rather rare.

VI

Parasites of Swine

CONTENTS

1 Stages in the gut and faeces

PROTOZOA

Eimeria spp. and *Isospora suis*

Coccidiosis in pigs

Location: Jejunum and ileum

Hosts: Pig

Species description: Coccidiosis in swine is caused by eight species of the genus *Eimeria* and one of *Isospora*. Coccidiosis is caused by intracellular parasites that inhabit the intestinal tract, particularly the small intestine. The life cycles of coccidia are complex and include both sexual (gametogony) and asexual (schizogony) cycles within the host. Some development (sporogony) also takes place outside the host. The host cells are destroyed by schizogony, gametogony and the release of oocysts. Each oocyst that is ingested has the potential of destroying thousands or even millions of intestinal epithelial cells since each schizont contains numerous merozoites and several generations of schizonts may be produced. Multiplication of coccidia depends on a continuous ingestion of oocysts. The severity of coccidiosis therefore depends on the number of oocysts ingested and the pathogenicity of the particular species. Some species of coccidia are more pathogenic (*I. suis, E. debliecki, E. scabra, E. polita, E. spinosa*) than others (*E. neodebliecki, E. perminuta, E. porci, E. suis*). Usually mixed coccidia infections occur. Unsporulated oocysts are passed in the faeces but infection is only transmitted if the oocysts are sporulated. Coccidiosis (especially caused by *I. suis*) as a disease entity occurs mainly in newborn piglets (3–21 days of age); however, older pigs may act as carriers. Morbidity is usually high (50–75%) but the mortality varies markedly due to differences in the pathogenicity of a particular species, or in the environment (poor hygiene, lack of milk supply, etc.) and the presence of other coexisting diseases (colibacillosis and rotavirus infections, transmissible gastroenteritis, etc.).

Geographic distribution: World-wide

Symptoms: Diarrhoea which persists for 4–6 days, in neonatal piglets, is the predominant clinical sign. The faeces are generally yellow-white in colour but rarely bloody. In cases where the diarrhoea stops itself, stunting and emaciation are the only clinical signs.

Significance: Several coccidia species (especially caused by *Isospora suis*) may be important among the pathogens causing diarrhoea in neonatal piglets.

Diagnosis: Oocysts may not be shed during the diarrhoeal phase, so faecal flotation examination is of little value for diagnosing swine coccidiosis during the acute phase. The presence of fibrino-necrotic membranes (macroscopic), shortened villi and necrosis of epithelial cells (microscopic) in the jejunum and ileum are found at necropsy. The endogenous forms of coccidia (merozoites, small schizonts) are revealed in the villous epithelial cells by histopathological techniques or stained impression smears of the jejunum and ileum. The characteristic oocysts are most easily detected in the faeces of recovered litter-mates but generally not during the diarrhoeic period. Postmortem examination of the intestine of previously ill pigs for endogenous forms is the preferred diagnostic method.

Therapy: Coccidia infections are often self-limiting and end spontaneously within a few weeks unless reinfection occurs. Medication usually does not cure but slows or inhibits the development of stages resulting from reinfection and thus shortens the length of illness, reduces discharge of oocysts and lessens the incidence of secondary infections. Reduction of the oocyst excretion of clinically ill piglets can be achieved with sulfaguanidine (0.22 mg/kg, po.), sulfamethazine or sulfamerazine. Amprolium (25–65 mg/kg, po.) is beneficial for prevention but treatment of scouring piglets has minimal effect. Supportive treatment with antibiotics and rehydration may also be very important.

Prophylaxis: Good sanitation (removal of faeces, disinfection of farrowing facilities) is of utmost importance if the coccidia life cyle should be broken, since the previous litters may be the source of infection. Amprolium (8 days before until 8 days after birth) prevented cocciodiosis in piglets. Salinomycin sodium (60 ppm for body weight < 50 kg, 25 ppm for > 50 kg) and halofuginone hydrobromide (3 ppm) reduced *Eimeria* spp. and *I. suis* oocyst excretion.

(Figures 530, 531, 532, 533, Table 19)

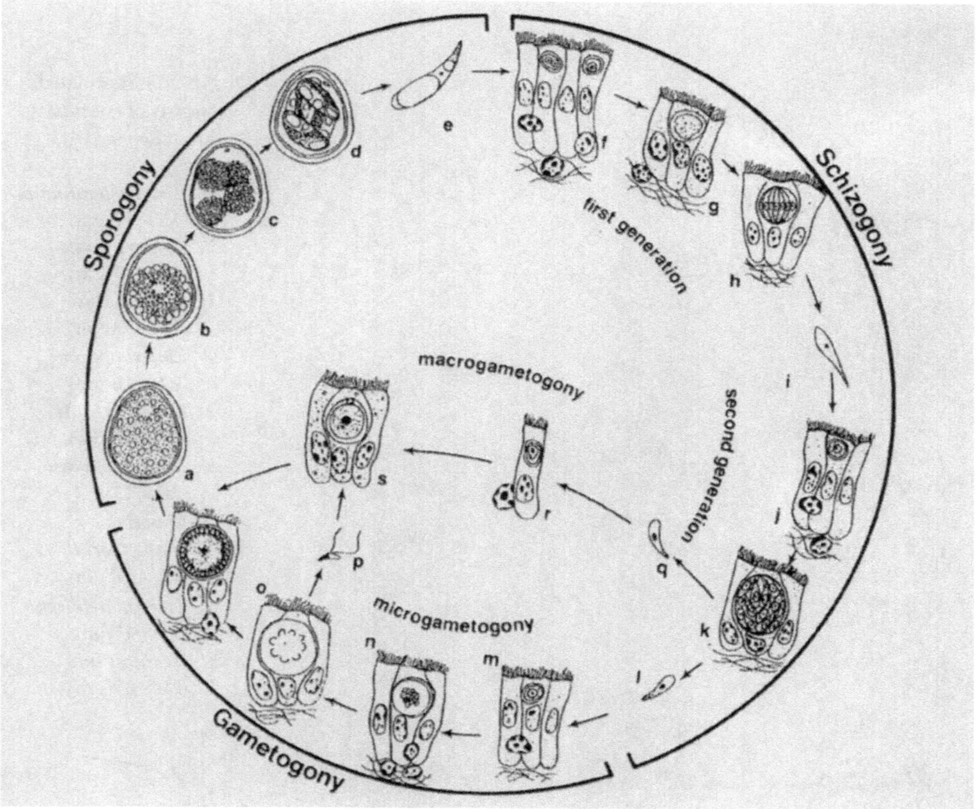

Fig. 530 Life cycle of *Eimeria debliecki*; oocyst sporulation (a–d), isolated sporozoite (e), schizogony with first and second generation of merozoites (f–k), second generation of merozoites (l and q), formation of microgametes (m–o), microgamete (p) and formation of macrogametes (r–s). The cycle ends with the formation of a zygote [14]

Table 19 Coccidia of pigs [1]

Species	Average dimensions (microns)	Shape	Morphology
E. debliecki	25 × 17	Ellipsoidal	Wall smooth, colourless, asymmetrical sporocysts
E. neodebliecki	21 × 16	Ellipsoideal	Wall smooth, colourless
E. perminuta	13 × 12	Spherical, subsperical	Wall rough, yellow
E. polita	27 × 21	Ellipsoideal	Wall rough, yellow to colourless
E. porci	22 × 16	Ovoid	Wall smooth, colourless, broad sporocysts
E. scabra	32 × 23	Ovoid	Wall rough with radial striations, yellow to brown
E. spinosa	20 × 13	Ovoid	Wall rough, spined, brown
E. suis	17 × 13	Ellipsoidal, subsperical	Wall smooth, colourless
Isospora suis	20 × 17	Spherical, subspherical	Wall smooth, colourless, thin

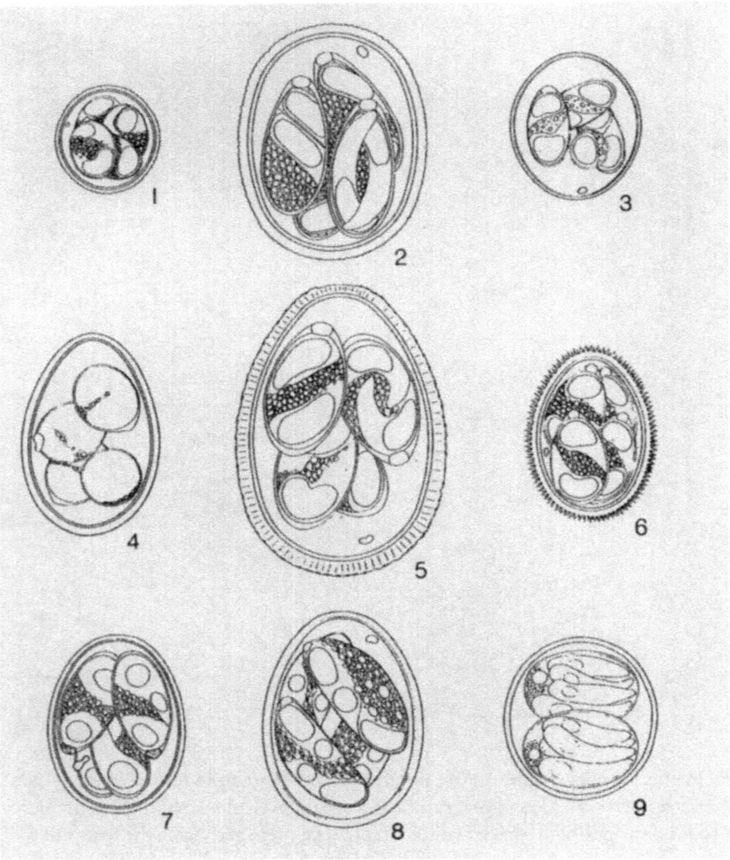

Fig. 531 Sporulated oocysts of coccidia from the pig [14]:

1 *Eimeria perminuta* (13 × 12 μm)
2 *Eimeria polita* (27 × 21 μm)
3 *Eimeria suis* (17 × 13 μm)
4 *Eimeria porci* (22 × 16 μm)
5 *Eimeria scabra* (32 × 23 μm)
6 *Eimeria spinosa* (20 × 13)
7 *Eimeria neodebliecki* (21 × 16 μm)
8 *Eimeria debliecki* (25 × 17 μm)
9 *Isospora suis* (20 × 17 μm)

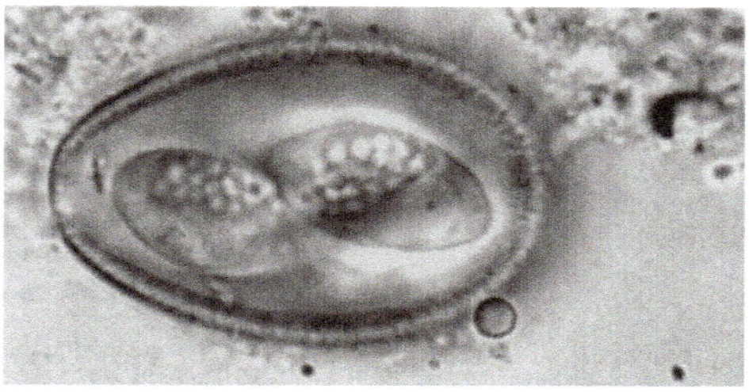

Fig. 532 Oocyst of *Eimeria scabra*; sporulated (32 × 23 μm) [4]

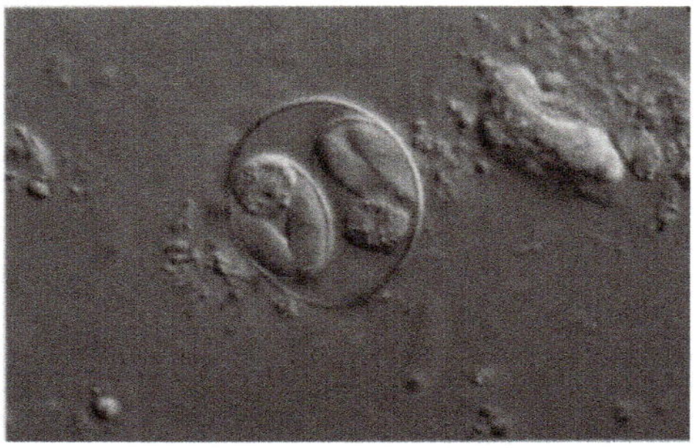

Fig. 533 Oocyst of *Isospora suis*; sporulated (20 × 17 μm) [4]

Cryptosporidium parvum

Remarks: Little is known about *C. parvum* in piglets. It is thought to be prevalent but usually of low morbidity and mortality. Infection may result in non-haemorrhagic diarrhoea (☞ CATTLE, 1).

Balantidium coli (syn. *B. suis*)

Location: Caecum, colon

Hosts: Pig, occasionally in peccary, man, dog and rat

Species description: The motile trophozoites are ovoid and variable in size, 30–150 × 25–120 μm. Cilia cover the entire body. The cyst form is spherical and measures 45–65 μm in diameter. *B. coli* reproduces in the lumen of the large intestine by binary fission where it is a commensal. Under normal conditions *B. coli* cannot penetrate intact intestinal mucosa. If another pathogen initiates a lesion, then *B. coli* may act as a secondary invader.

Geographic distribution: World-wide

Symptoms: Enteritis, diarrhoea, dysentery, colitis, anaemia, retarded growth and emaciation in young piglets

Significance: *B. coli* almost exclusively plays a role as a secondary invader in the large intestine of pigets. *B. coli* is much more pathogenic to man than to swine. It causes severe colitis, with ulcers of the mucosa and watery diarrhoea.

Diagnosis: *B. coli* can be easily recognized by microscopic examination of intestinal contents or by histologic examination of intestinal lesions.

Therapy: No treatment is necessary in pigs. Treatment of the primary infection is indicated.

Prophylaxis: Prevention of *B. coli* infections of swine is not indicated since it is a permanent inhabitant. General health care and good hygiene prevent primary infections which are necessary for *B. coli* to become pathogenic. Control of the transmission from pig to man depends on good sanitation.

(Figures 534, 535, 536)

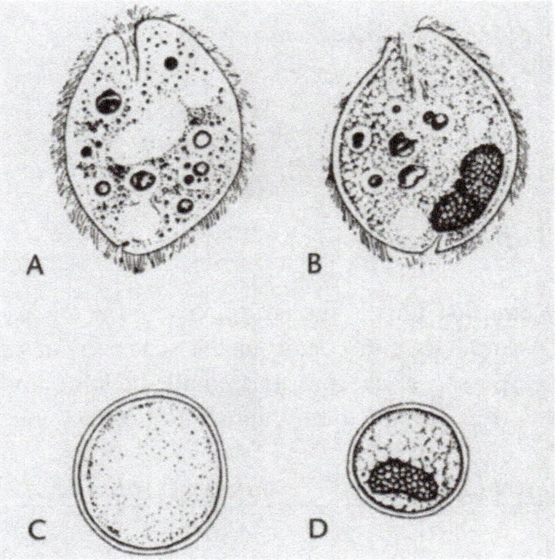

Fig. 534 *Balantidium coli* (schematic); living trophozoite (A), stained trophozoite (B), fresh cyst (C) and stained cyst (D) [14]

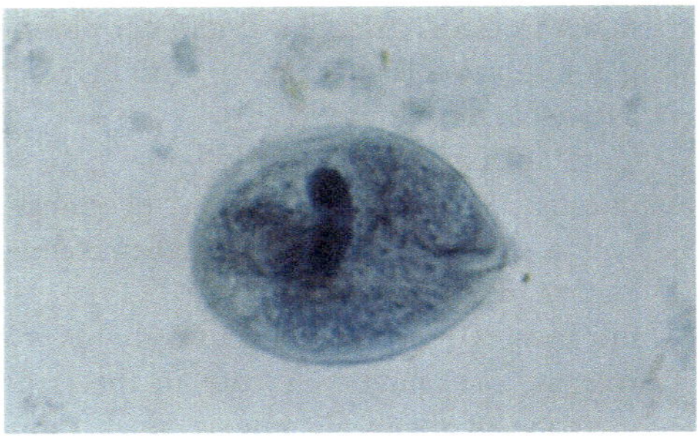

Fig. 535 *Balantidium coli*; trophozoite stained (50–150 µm) [4]

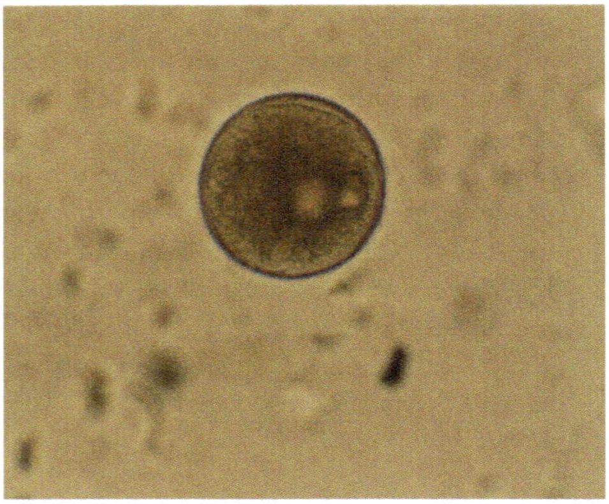

Fig. 536 *Balantidium coli*; cyst (50–100 µm in diameter)

Tritrichomonas suis

Remarks: This is the largest of the pig trichomonads and occurs in the stomach, nasal passages, caecum and small intestine and occasionally in the vagina; non-pathogenic.

Trichomonas (syn. *Trichomitus*) *rotunda*

Remarks: It occurs in the caecum and colon of swine; non-pathogenic.

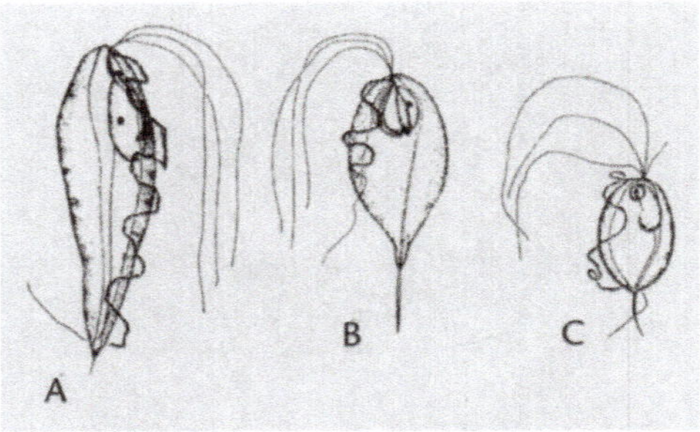

Fig. 537 Trichomonads of swine; (A) *Tritrichomonas suis* (11 × 3 µm), (B) *T. rotunda* (9 × 6 µm) and (C) *Tetratrichomonas buttreyi* (6 × 3 µm) [14]

Tetratrichomonas buttreyi

Remarks: It is the smallest of the pig trichomonads. It occurs in the caecum and colon; non-pathogenic.
(Figure 537)

Giardia lamblia

Remarks: It occurs in the duodenum, jejunum and ileum of man, primates (highly pathogenic) and many other mammals including swine where it is non-pathogenic (☞ SHEEP AND GOATS, 1).

Entamoeba suis (syn. *E. polecki*)

Remarks: It occurs in the caecum and colon of swine and is generally non-pathogenic. Occasionally enteritis and diarrhoea may be found but the pathogenic role of *E. suis* is in debate.

HELMINTHS

(Figure 538)

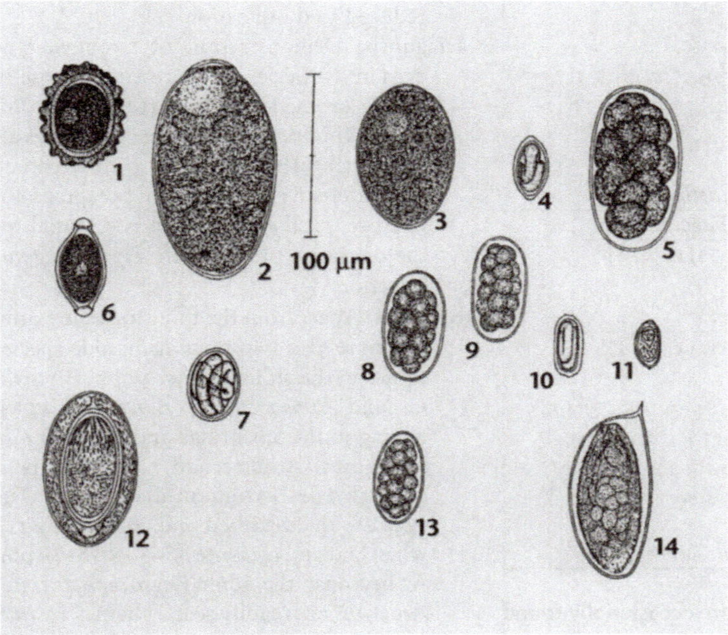

Fig. 538 Eggs of helminths found in swine [3]

1 *Ascaris suum*
2 *Fasciola hepatica*
3 *Paragonimus* sp.
4 *Ascarops strongylina*
5 *Stephanurus dentatus*
6 *Trichuris suis*
7 *Metastrongylus apri*
8 *Oesophagostomum dentatum*
9 *Hyostrongylus rubidus*
10 *Physocephalus sexalatus*
11 *Brachylaemus* sp.
12 *Macracanthorhynchus hirundinaceus*
13 *Globocephalus* sp.
14 *Schistosoma suis*

- Trematoda eggs found in the faeces and adult trematodes living in the gastrointestinal tract

Gastrodiscus aegyptiacus Intestinal fluke

Remarks: It occurs in the small and large intestine of equines, pig and warthog in Africa and India. If present in high numbers the parasite can significantly affect pigs (☞ HORSES AND DONKEYS, 1).
(Figure 539)

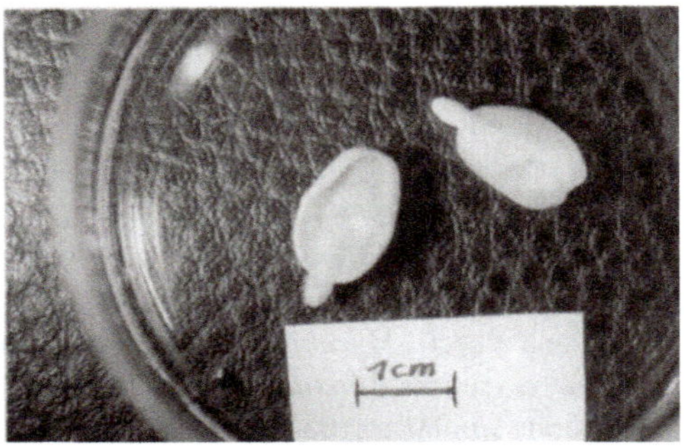

Fig. 539 *Gastrodiscus aegyptiacus*; ventral view (right) and dorsal view (left)

Gastrodiscoides hominis

Remarks: This is a common trematode found in the caecum and colon of pigs in South and East Asian countries.

Postharmostomum suis

Remarks: It has been reported from Tunisia where it was found in the small intestine of pigs. Intermediate hosts are land snails of the genus *Xerophila*. It is not very pathogenic (☞ POULTRY, 1).

- Eggs of the following trematodes may occasionally be found in the faeces of pigs

Schistosoma bovis, S. mattheei, *Dicrocoelium* spp. and *Fasciola* spp.

(☞ SWINE, 4.2 and CATTLE, 1)

Eurytrema pancreaticum

(☞ SWINE, 4.5 and CATTLE, 1)

- Nematoda eggs found in the faeces, adult nematodes living in the gastro-intestinal tract and first-stage larvae of lungworms (*Metastrongylus* spp.)

Gongylonema pulchrum Gullet worm

Remarks: *G. pulchrum* are occasionally found at necropsy in the oesophageal mucosa of swine but they are of little or no clinical significance (☞ CATTLE, 1).

Hyostrongylus rubidus Red stomach worm

Location: Stomach
Hosts: Pig
Species description: *H. rubidus* belongs to the trichostrongylids, is 4–10 mm long, bright red (blood sucker) and has a direct nematode life cycle. *H. rubidus* is found under a heavy catarrhal exudate and produces lesions similar to those of *Ostertagia* spp. in ruminants, except that hyperaemia of the mucosa is more common. Inhibition of larvae during periods of adverse environmental conditions (winter, dry season) occurs. In sows these inhibited larvae resume their development prior to parturition with the result that the environment of the piglets is contaminated.
Geographic distribution: World-wide
Symptoms: Variable appetite, anaemia, gastritis, diarrhoea associated with weight loss.
Significance: Moderate by contributing to mixed worm infections, resulting in reduced feed utilization.
Diagnosis: Demonstration of strongyle-type eggs in the faeces which resemble those of other strongyle worms (*Oesophagostomum, Globocephalus, Trichostrongylus*). Faecal culture is required to differentiate the different eggs. Mucosal scrapings for microscopical examination is essential for the detection of immature *Hyostrongylus* infection.
Remarks: Apart from the thin stomach worm, there are also two thick nematode species found in the stomach: *Ascarops strongylina* and *Physocephalus sexalatus* which belong to the Spiruridae and are > 12 mm long, much stouter and have coprophageous beetles as intermediate hosts. The eggs are thick-shelled and contain a larva when laid and measure 35–40 × 15–20 µm. At necropsy the adult *Physocephalus* and *Ascarops* are readily seen, whereas *H. rubidus* is more difficult to recognize. The stomach worms are more common in grazing pigs.
Therapy: Most modern benzimidazoles and probenzimidazoles and ivermectin (300 µg/kg, sc.) are highly effective against adult and immature stages (including hypobiotic larvae) of the stomach worms. Pyrantel (12.5 mg/kg, po.) and levamisole (5 mg/kg, im. or sc.) are effective against the adult stomach worms (Table 20).
Prophylaxis: Frequent removal of faeces and provision of dry quarters effectively reduce the infection risk.
(Figures 540, 541, 542, 543, 544, 545, 546)

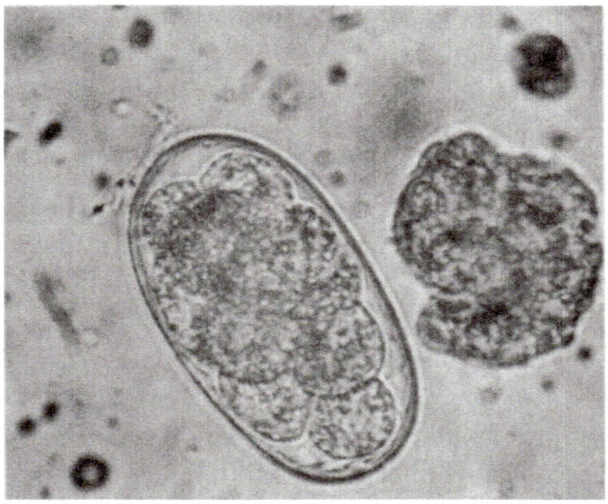

Fig. 540 Egg of *Hyostrongylus rubidus* (69–85 × 39–45 µm; typical strongyle-type egg) [11]

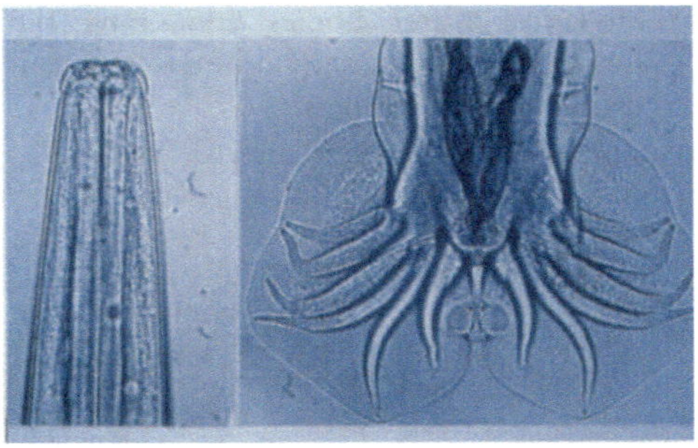

Fig. 541 *Hyostrongylus rubidus*; anterior end (left) and male bursa (right); males are 4–7 mm long, females are 5–10 mm long [4]

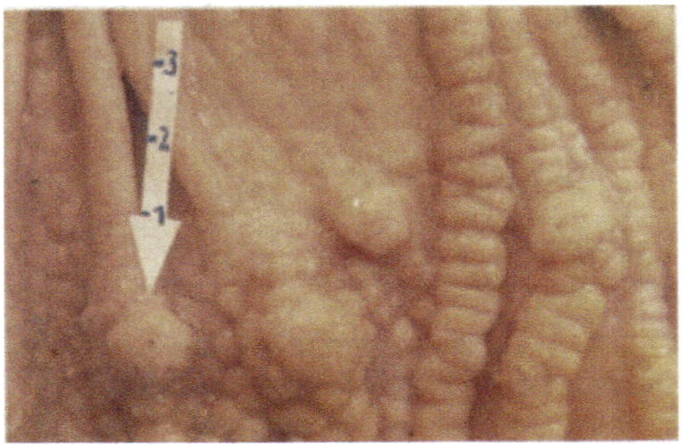

Fig. 542 Nodule formation in the gastric mucosa caused by *Hyostrongylus rubidus* [4]

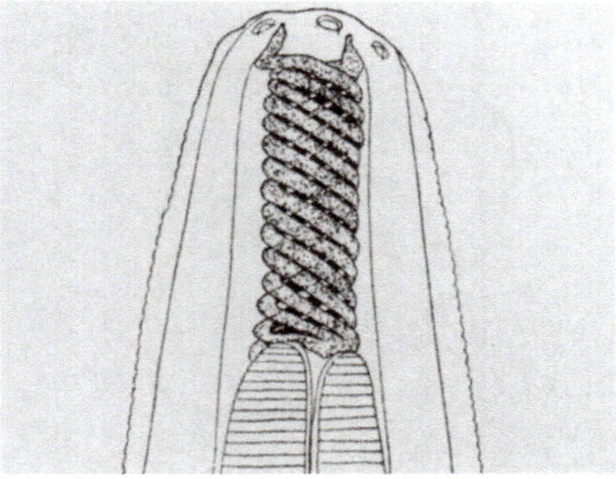

Fig. 543 *Ascarops strongylina*; anterior end; males are 10–15 mm long, females are 16–22 mm long [3]

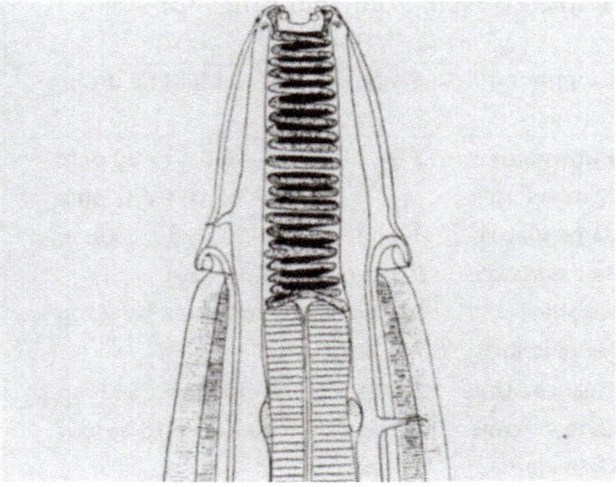

Fig. 544 *Physocephalus sexalatus*; anterior end; males are 6–13 mm long, females are 13–22.5 mm long [3]

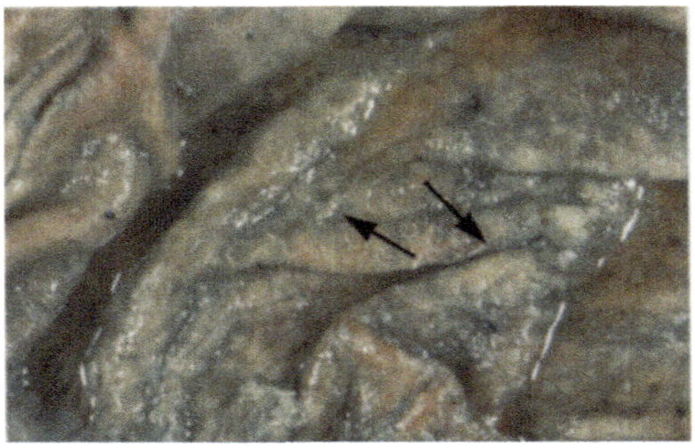

Fig. 545 *Physocephalus sexalatus* on the gastric mucosa [4]

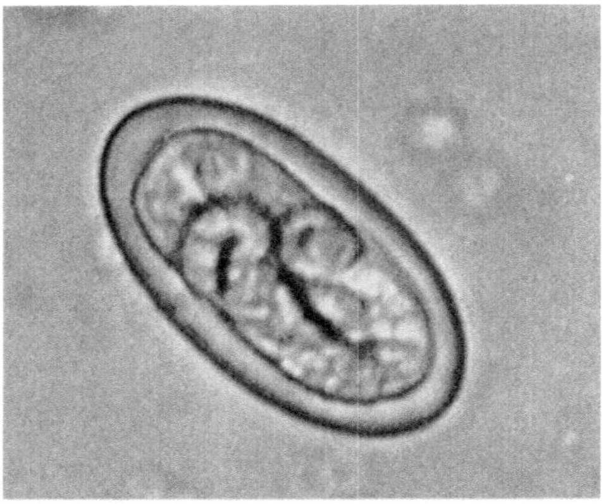

Fig. 546 Egg of *Physocephalus sexalatus* (34–39 × 15–17 µm) [11]

Table 20 Nematodicidal drugs for swine

Compound	Single dosing[1]	Multiple dosing[1]
Flubendazole	5.0	5–10 days x 30 ppm
Mebendazole	–	5–10 days x 30 ppm
Parbendazole	30, po.	7–10 days x 3000 ppm
Fenbendazole	5.0, po.	6–15 days
Febantel	5.0, po.	5 days x 0.5–0.7 mg/kg
Netobimin	7.5, po.	–
Thiabendazole	500, po.	5–10 days x 500 mg/kg
Oxibendazole	15, po.	10 days x 1g/kg/day
Oxfendazole	4.5, po.	–
Dichlorvos	30–40, po.	–
Levamisol	5–7.5, po.	–
Piperazine	250–312, po.	–
Pyrantel tartrate	12.5, po.	–
Thiabendazole	50–100, po.	–

[1]mg/kg body weight; po = orally

Gnathostoma hispidum

Location: Stomach

Hosts: Pig, warthog and man (exceptionally)

Species description: Males are 15–25 mm and females 22–45 mm long. The whole body is covered with spines. The eggs measure 73 × 40 µm. Eggs develop in water to second-stage larvae before hatching. Larvae develop to third-stage larvae when ingested by the intermediate hosts which are members of *Cyclops* spp. and related Crustacea. Infection of pigs by ingesting infected *Cyclops* or paratenic hosts (e.g. fish, birds, small mammals). Migration of larvae through the liver. Adults are embedded deeply in the gastric mucosa, producing cavities which contain reddish fluid and are surrounded by inflamed areas.

Geographic distribution: Europe, Asia, Africa (Zaire)

Symptoms: Inappetence, gastritis, weight loss in heavy infections. Mild infections are inapparent.

Significance: Severe infections cause gastritis.

Diagnosis: Demonstration of eggs in the faeces

Therapy: ☞Therapy of *Hyostrongylus rubidus*

Prophylaxis: Water bodies containing the intermediate hosts should be avoided as a drinking place for pigs.

(Figures 547, 548)

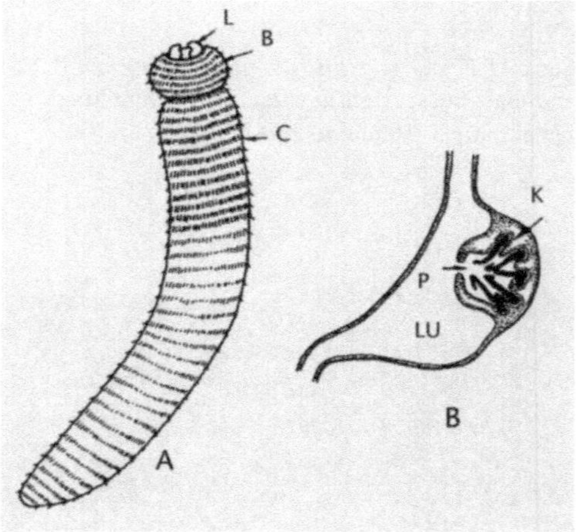

Fig. 547 *Gnathostoma hispidum*; adult parasite (males are up to 25 mm long, females are up to 45 mm long) covered with cuticular spines (A) and adults embedded in cyst-like cavities (B); L = lips, B = bulbus, C = cutucular spines, K = cyst wall, P = porus and LU = gastric lumen [33]

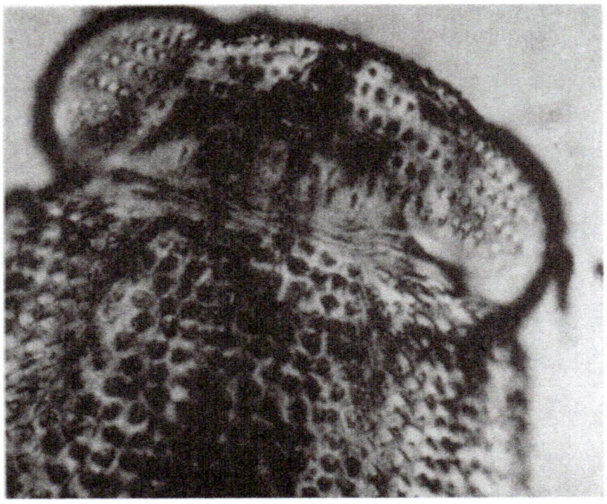

Fig. 548 *Gnathostoma hispidum*; anterior end with cuticular spines [49]

Trichostrongylus axei Stomach hair worm

Remarks: *T. axei* may occasionally be found in the stomach of pigs. It is of minor importance in pigs (☞ CATTLE, 1).

Ascaris suum Large roundworm of swine

Location: Small intestine
Hosts: Pig
Species description: *A. suum* is a large, white worm, 15–40 cm in length. The life cycle is direct. Infective larvae develop within 10–15 days and remain in the egg. After ingestion, the larvae are released in the intestine and burrow into the wall of the gut. The majority of the larvae pass to the liver via the hepatoportal bloodstream. Destruction of hepatic tissue and haemorrhage occurs, signs of which appear as "milk-spots" after the healing of these tracks. Larvae are carried in the blood to the lungs where they penetrate the blood vessels to enter alveoli to proceed to the pharynx to be finally swallowed. Further development to the adult stage occurs in the small intestine. Adult females are known to produce an enormous number of eggs (up to 200,000/day) which are very resistant to adverse climatic conditions and may be infective for years in the environment.
Geographic distribution: World-wide, widespread throughout the tropics
Symptoms: Damage caused by migrating larvae is of principal importance. Migration through the liver causes the white scar-like "milk-spots" which are the major reason for swine liver condemnation. Massive migration through the lungs may cause pneumonia followed by bacterial infections. Death may occur following heavy infections. Repeated infections, accompanied by lung haemorrhage and oedema and emphysema may result in a chronic, asthma-like condition characterized by unthriftiness. Adult ascarids in moderate numbers are relatively non-pathogenic but compete with their host for food and can therefore markedly reduce feed efficiency. High numbers of adult worms can sometimes "ball up" causing intestinal obstruction, perforation and peritonitis. Obstruction of the bile ducts and icterus may also occur.
Significance: *A. suum* is the most important swine endoparasite, causing heavy economic losses due to weight loss, mortality and condemnation of livers. *A. suum* infections can exacerbate swine influenza and endemic pneumonia and secondary bacterial infections.
Diagnosis: Demonstration of thick shelled eggs (60 × 45 µm) which are uneven in outline during the patent period. Young pigs often show signs (especially respiratory) during the prepatent period. A presumptive diagnosis can be made based on the history and signs and the demonstration of migrating larvae, especially in the lungs and liver at necropsy. Adult worms are found at necropsy and occasionally within the faeces of pigs.
Therapy: Piperazine preparations are cheap but effective only against adult worms. The benzimidazoles and probenzimidazoles, dichlorvos, ivermectin, levamisole and pyrantel are effective against immature and adult stages and have a broader spectrum of activity than piperazine. Pyrantel and ivermectin (300 µg/kg, sc.) are effective against migratory larvae.
Prophylaxis: Since the destruction of migrating

immature larvae is difficult, control measures should prevent or reduce the ingestion of eggs by pigs. Apart from a good basic hygiene in pig quarters control is based on anthelmintics. In intensive pig rearing systems a simple anthelmintic program is as follows: treat sows 10–14 days before breeding and again before farrowing; treat weaners before entering clean pens; treat boars at 6-month intervals. In traditional pig rearing systems where pigs are kept freely around the compounds no effective prophylaxis is possible. Regular treatment is required.
(Figures 549, 550, 551, 552, Table 20)

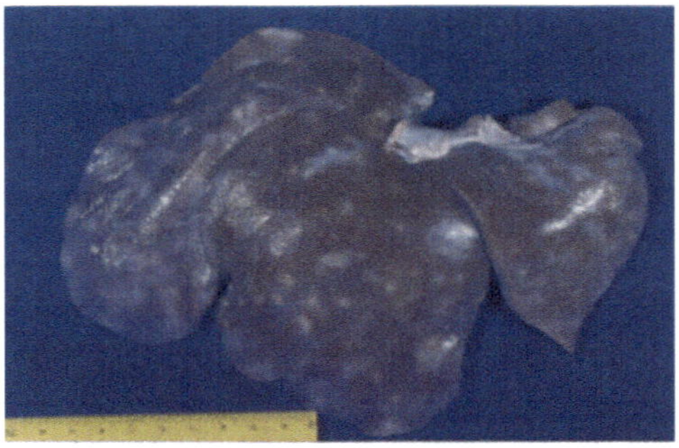

Fig. 550 "Milkspots" in the liver of a pig

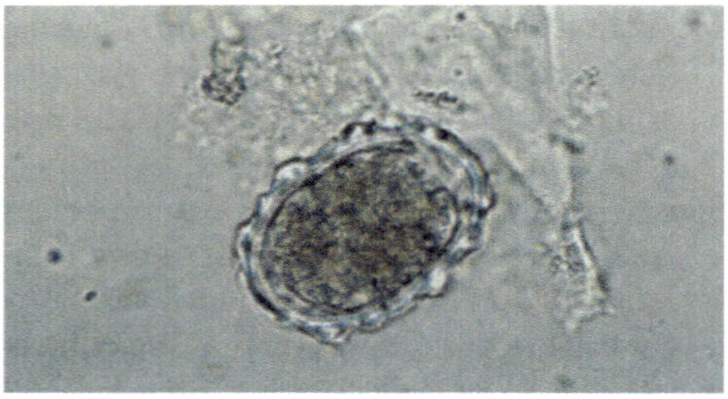

Fig. 549 Egg of *Ascaris suum* (50–70 × 40–60 µm)

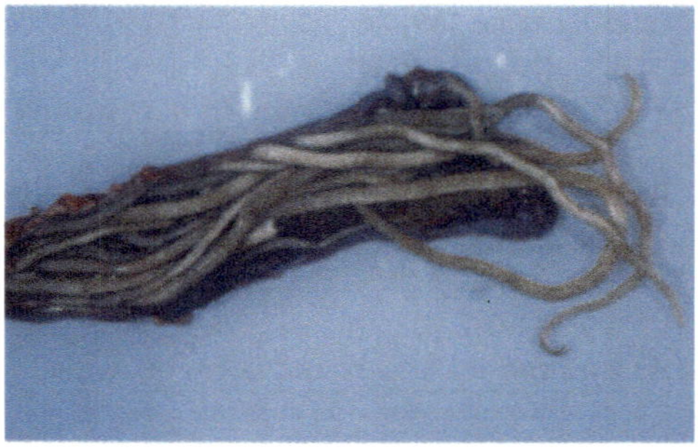

Fig. 551 *Ascaris suum*; adult worms found in the small intestine

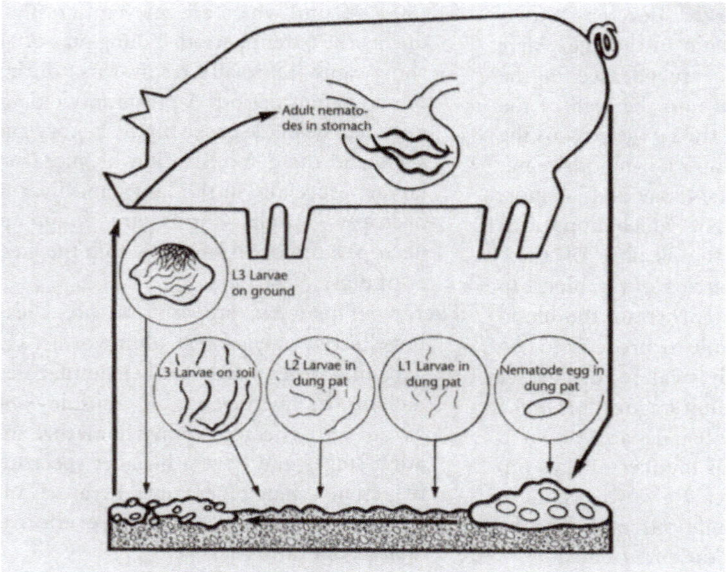

Fig. 552 Life cycle of a roundworm. Adult *Ascaris suum* worms are found in the small intestine. The larvae migrate from the intestine via liver, heart to the lungs [50]

Globocephalus urosubulatus and other *Globocephalus* spp. Pig hookworms

Location: Small intestine
Hosts: Domestic pig and wild boar
Species description: Very little is known about the life cycle which is probably direct. Adults are 6–8 mm long and have a typical hookworm-like buccal capsule to suck blood. Eggs are passed in the faeces and develop to infective third-stage larvae within 8–12 days. Infection occurs by ingesting third-stage larvae or by transcutaneous penetration. Migration of larvae through heart, lungs, trachea, oesophagus, intestines.
Geographic distribution: World-wide
Symptoms: Anaemia, hypoproteinaemia, progressive weight loss and emaciation may occur in heavy infections.
Significance: *Globocephalus* spp. infections are generally of little significance although, if the parasite occurs within a particular population it may cause severe losses. Piglets are generally most severely affected.
Diagnosis: Strongyle-type eggs occur in the faeces. Adult worms are found at necropsy.
Therapy: ☞ *Hyostrongylus rubidus*
Prophylaxis: ☞ *Hyostrongylus rubidus*
(Figures 553, 554, 555)

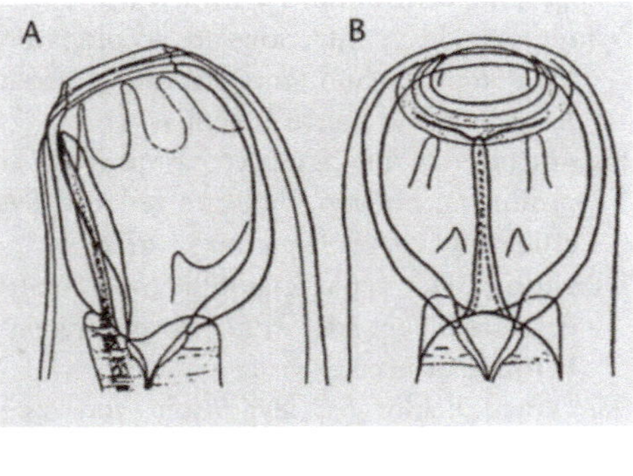

Fig. 553 *Globocephalus urosubulatus*; lateral view of anterior end (A) and dorsal view of anterior end (B) [34]

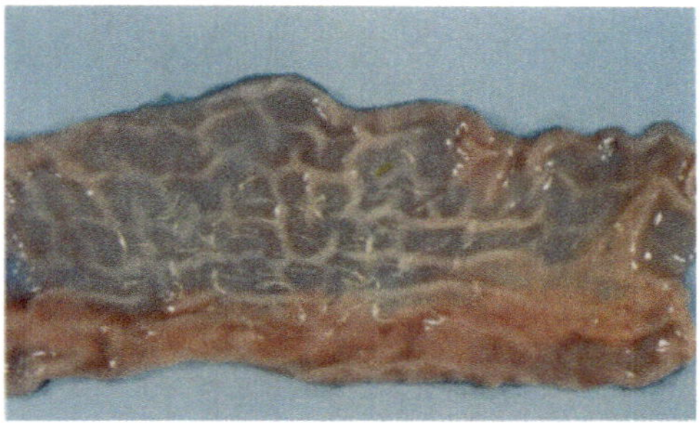

Fig. 554 *Globocephalus urosubulatus* in the small intestine of a pig

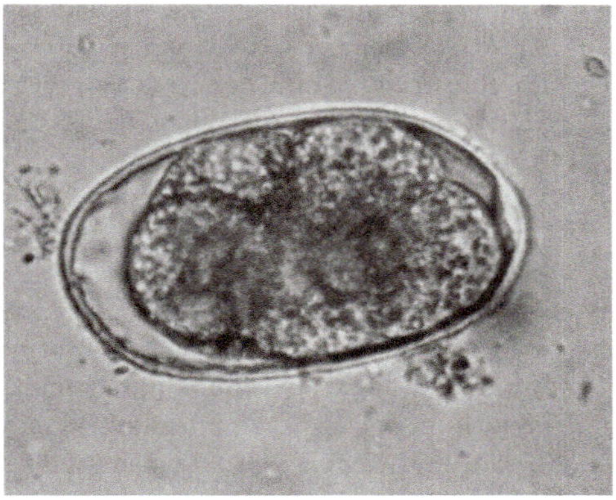

Fig. 555 Egg of *Globocephalus urosubulatus* (50–56 × 26–35 µm) [11]

Strongyloides ransomi Intestinal threadworm

Location: Small intestine
Hosts: Pig
Species description: The life cycle is similar to that of *S. papillosus* (☞ Cattle, 1). Transmission of larvae in the colostrum is the most common route of infection of nursing piglets. The adult worms which are exclusively female, burrow into the intestinal wall and cause irritation and inflammation. Infection of the host can occur by both skin penetration and ingestion of infective larvae. Prepatent period is 6–9 days. Adult breeding stock may be infected with dormant larvae in their subcutaneous fat. Pregnancy and farrowing appear

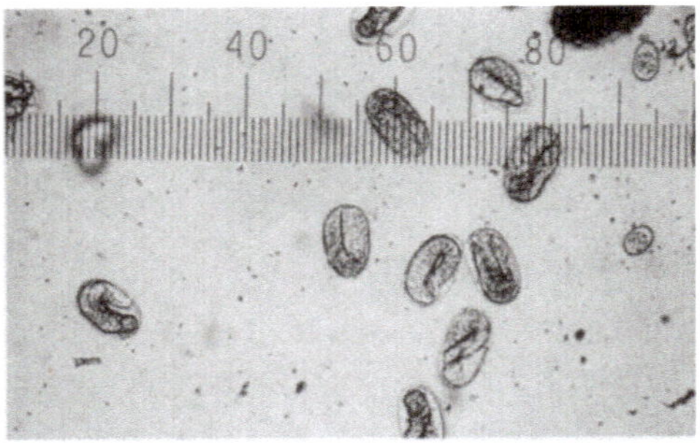

Fig. 556 Eggs of *Strongyloides ransomi* (40–55 × 20–35 µm) contain a first-stage larva

to stimulate the re-emergence of these larvae which then may infect the piglets via the colostrum. In only one week after birth piglets may pass eggs in their faeces that can develop within 24 hours to infective larvae. Consequently a quick rise in worm burdens is typical for threadworm infections.

Geographic distribution: World-wide, particularly common in warm climates

Symptoms: In light infections the animals show no signs. In heavy infections bloody diarrhoea, anaemia, emaciation and sudden death (especially in piglets) may occur. During the migratory phase of infection coughing, muscle soreness, abdominal pain and vomitus can be observed.

Significance: Highly significant for neonatal piglets

Diagnosis: Demonstration of thin-shelled, embryonated eggs in the faeces or the adults in scrapings from the intestinal mucosa is diagnostic. Eggs must be differentiated from the larger *Metastrongylus* eggs. At necropsy immature worms may be recovered from minced tissues placed in a Baermann isolation funnel.

Therapy: Infections in suckling piglets can only be reduced by treating the sows before farrowing. The benzimidazoles, febantel and levamisole are effective against intestinal infections. Ivermectin (300 µg/kg, sc.) is effective against adults and if administered 1–2 weeks before farrowing, controls the milk borne infection.

Prophylaxis: Cleaning the pig's living quarters can reduce free-living larvae and thus the infection risk. Wherever this is not feasible, anthelmintic treatment of sows prior to parturition and close observation of neonatal piglets (incl. treatment) is required.

(Figure 556)

Trichinella spp. (*T. spiralis, T. britovi, T. nativa, T. nelsoni* and *T. pseudospiralis*)
Trichina worm

Remarks: Adult worms occur in the small intestine. Encysted larvae are found in the diaphragm and masseter, lingual and intercostal muscles of pig and many other mammals. These cysts are found by microscopical examination of infected muscles (☞ SWINE, ■ 4.1).

Trichuris suis Whipworm

Location: Caecum and colon

Hosts: Pig and wild boar

Species description: *T. suis* is 5–8 cm long and has a typical whip-like tail. Direct life cycle. Infection occurs by ingesting infective eggs (containing first-stage larvae). *Trichuris* eggs may remain viable for several years. After being ingested *T. suis* larvae hatch and enter the intestinal wall and develop further to the second-stage larvae and finally proceed to the large intestine for final maturation. Prepatent period is 6 weeks.

Geographic distribution: World-wide

Symptoms: Heavy infections are accompanied by diarrhoea and unthriftiness. Chronic infections may cause anaemia.

Significance: *T. suis* causes economic losses by producing poor growth and reduced feed efficiency wherever pigs are reared.

Diagnosis: The typical, double operculated eggs are diagnostic. Adult worms are easily found at necropsy.

Therapy: Dichlorvos, levamisole and some benzimidazoles generally at increased dosage rates are effective. Ivermectin (300 µg/kg, sc.) resulted in a 80% reduction of the adult worm population (Table 21).

Prophylaxis: Removal of the faeces from the quarters reduces the infection risk drastically. Eradication is difficult because *Trichuris* eggs may be infective for 6 or more years on soil.
(Figures 94, 557, Table 21)

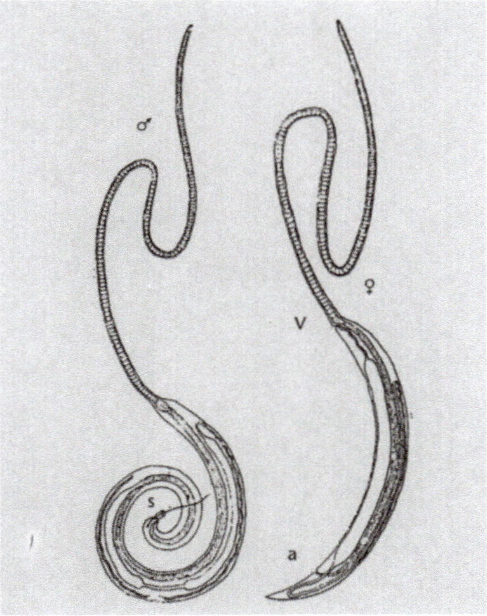

Fig. 557 *Trichuris suis* (4.5–5.5 mm long); male (left) and female (right); s = spicule, a = anus and v = vulva [9]

Table 21 Compounds to be used against *Trichuris suis* infections

Compound	Single dosing	Multiple dosing
Flubendazole	5.0, po.	5-10 days x 30 ppm
Mebendazole	–	10 days x 30 ppm
Oxibendazole	15.0, po.	10 days x 1 g/100 kg/day
Fenbendazole	30.0, po.	6-15 days x 16-20 ppm
Febantel	20.0, po.	
Levamisole	7.5, sc.	

po. = orally, sc. = subcutaneous

Oesophagostomum dentatum and other *Oesophagostomum* spp. Nodular worms

Location: Adult worms are found in the lumen of the large intestine. Larvae occur in the mucosa of the small and large intestine.
Hosts: Pig and wild boar
Species description: Adults are 8–14 mm long, white and have a shallow buccal capsule. The life-cycle is direct and infection results from ingestion of infective third-stage larvae. After ingestion the larvae moult and burrow into the intestinal mucosa anywhere between the pylorus and the rectum. After 5–7 days the larvae moult to fourth-stage larvae within the nodule and emerge into the intestinal lumen, where they mature and start to excrete eggs about 40–50 days after infection. Sows may have a periparturient rise in *Oesophagostomum* egg output, which is an important source of infection in newborn piglets.
Geographic distribution: World-wide
Symptoms: Diarrhoea, weight loss and anorexia may be observed in heavy infection.
Significance: The nodular worm is highly prevalent and among the most significant nematodes in pigs. It causes extensive nodule formations associated with decreased feed utilization, disturbed water and electrolyte metabolism and progressive weight loss.
Diagnosis: Typical strongyle eggs (75 × 40 µm) are found in the faeces. These can be differentiated from *Hyostrongylus* by larval culture. Adult worms are found sometimes in great numbers at necropsy. Multiple nodules, seen from the serosa side, may be found at slaughter (☞ CATTLE, 1).
Therapy: The benzimidazoles, levamisole, dichlorvos, pyrantel tartrate and ivermectin are effective (☞ *Hyostrongylus rubidus*).
Prophylaxis: Anthelmintic treatment does not always affect the larvae within the nodules. Therefore, repeated treatments several weeks apart are necessary to reduce the nodular worm incidence within a population.
Remarks: *O. quadrispinulatum* is similar to *O. dentatum* but does not occur in Africa.
(Figures 558, 559, 560, Table 22)

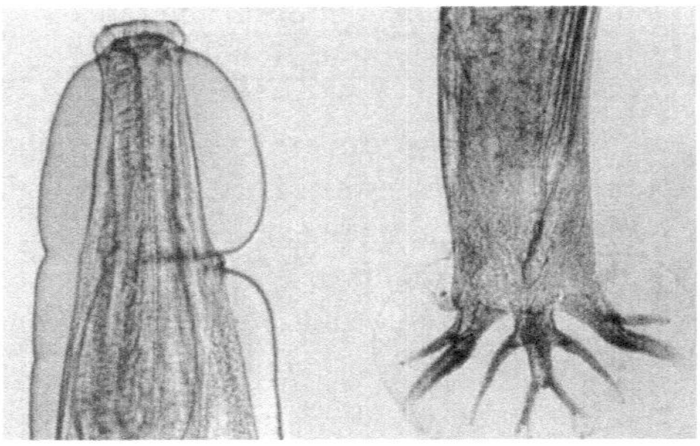

Fig. 558 *Oesophagostomum dentatum* (10–14 mm); anterior end (left) and posterior end of a male (right) [4]

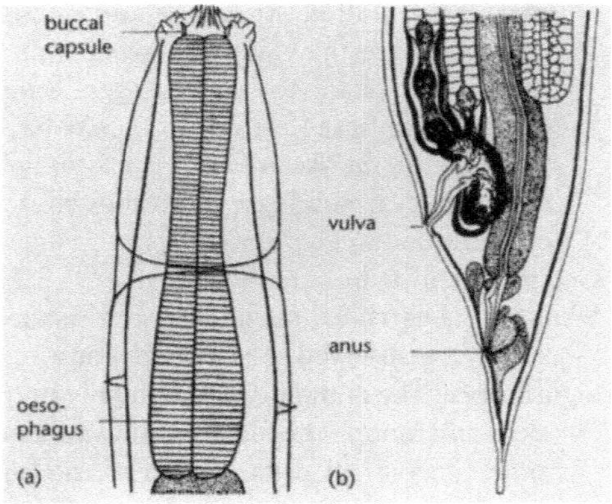

Fig. 559 *Oesophagostomum dentatum*; anterior end (a) and female tail end (b) [5]

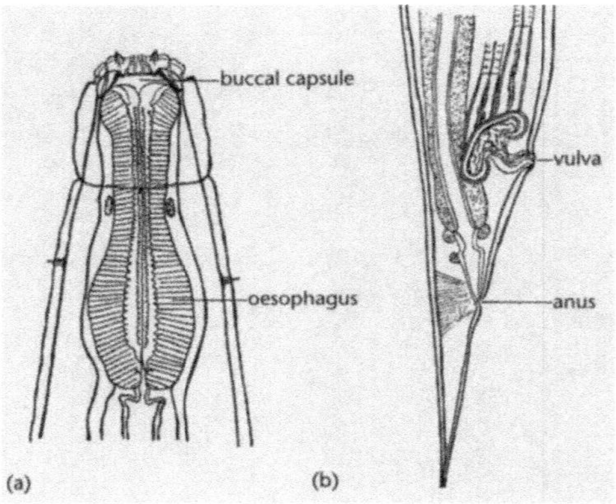

Fig. 560 *Oesophagostomum quadrispinulatum*; anterior end (10–15 mm) (a) and female tail end (b) [5]

Table 22 Comparison of the morphology of *Oesophagostomum dentatum* and *Oesophagostomum quadrispinulatum*

	Oesophagostomum quadrispinulatum	***Oesophagostomum dentatum***
Buccal capsule	Sides not parallel, diverging posteriorly	Sides papallel, not diverging
Oesophagus	Vase-shaped, swollen at anterior end	Club-shaped, not swollen at anterior end
Spicules	0.9–0.95 mm long	1.15–1.3 mm long
Female: posterior end	Long, tapering tail; distance between vulva and anus and tip of tail longer than that of *O. dentatum*	Relatively short tail; distance between vulva and anus and anus and tip of tail shorter than that of *O. quadrispinulatum*

Metastrongylus **spp.** Lungworms

Remarks: Eggs of the lungworms occur in the faeces (☞ SWINE, ■ 4.3).
(Figures 561, 562)

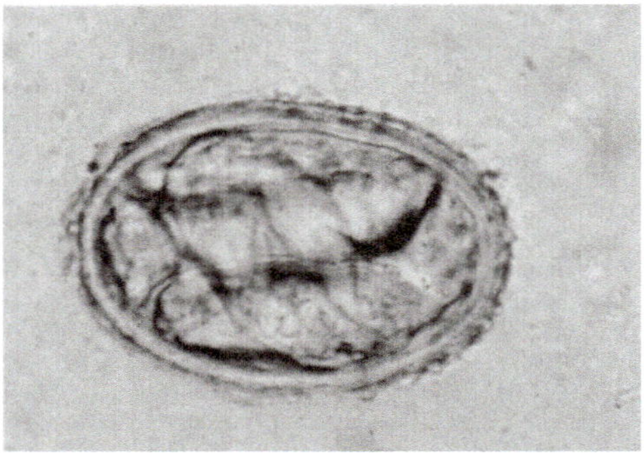

Fig. 561 Egg of *Metastrongylus apri* (51–63 × 33–42 µm) [11]

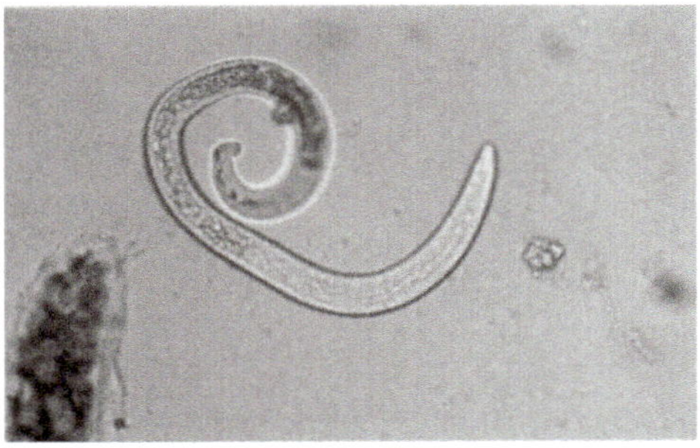

Fig. 562 First-stage larva of *Metastrongylus* spp.

ACANTHOCEPHALA

Macracanthorhynchus hirudinaceus
"Thorny headed worm"

Location: Small intestine
Hosts: Domestic and wild pig
Species description: *M. hirudinaceus* belongs to the Acanthocephala, a group of parasitic worms closely allied to the nematoda. Adults are 10–35 cm long, with reddish, transversely wrinkled bodies. The anterior end shows a spiny, retractable proboscis (rostellum) which anchors each worm to the intestinal wall. The eggs (67–110 × 40–65 µm) are ingested by the grubs of various beetles that serve as intermediate hosts.
Geographic distribution: World-wide, except western Europe (common in Madagascar).
Symptoms: Signs are not specific. Heavy burdens may cause diarrhoea, reduced weight gain and emaciation.
Significance: Mild infections are inapparent, heavy infections may cause irritation of the intestines, accompanied by weight loss. The site of the attachment often shows a necrotic center surrounded by a zone of inflammation. These lesions can usually be seen through the serosa. Perforation of the intestinal wall followed by peritonitis may occur.
Diagnosis: Eggs with four shells appear in the faeces. They do not reliably float in salt solutions and should therefore be looked for in the sediment. *M. hirudinaceus* is attached to the intestinal wall which is in contrast to *Ascaris suum* which lies freely within the small intestine.
Therapy: Levamisole (5–7.5 mg/kg, sc.) and fenbendazole (5 × 20 mg/kg, po.) at daily intervals are effective.
Prophylaxis: Control is only feasible if the use of contaminated hog lots can be avoided.
(Figures 563, 564, 565)

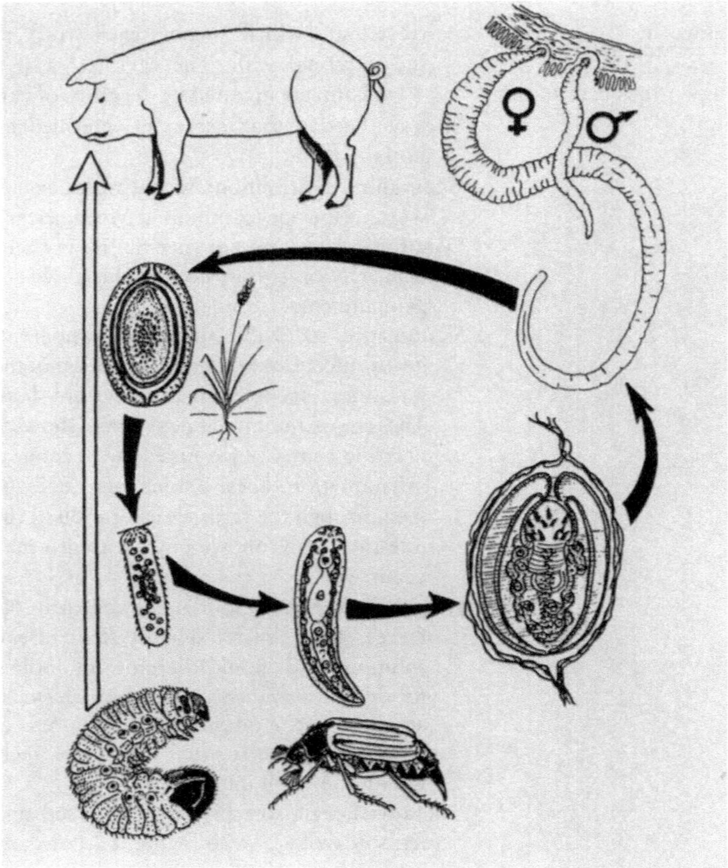

Fig. 563 Life cycle of *Macracanthorhynchus hirudinaceus*
Larvae of different beetles act as intermediate hosts [51]

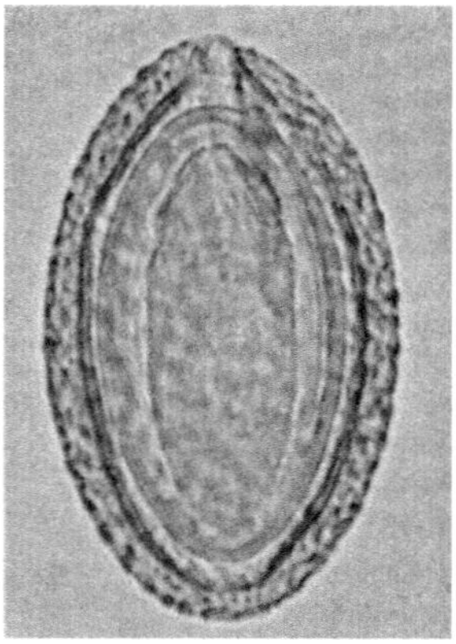

Fig. 564 Egg of *Macracanthorhynchus hirudinaceus* (70–110 × 40–65 µm) [50]

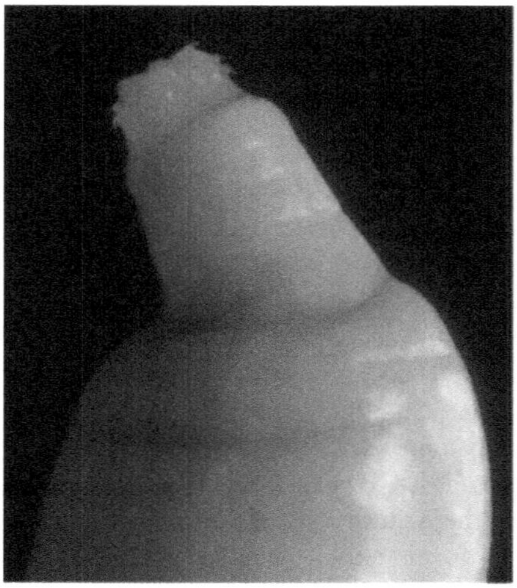

Fig. 565 *Macracanthorhynchus hirudinaceus*; anterior end with the typical spiny rostellum [10]

PROTOZOA

TRYPANOSOMATIDAE

Trypanosoma congolense simiae (syn. *T. porci, Nannomonas simiae*)

Hosts: Warthog, pig and camel

Vector: *Glossina brevipalpis* and *Glossina morsitans*.

Species description: This is a polymorphic form resembling *T. congolense*. Its natural host is the warthog and it is highly pathogenic for pig and camel. *Glossina* flies introduce *T. congolense simiae* to domestic pigs but thereafter mechanical transmission by *Stomoxys* spp. and tabanids is also possible. *T. congolense simiae* differs from *T. congolense* in that it is polymorphic instead of monomorphic. It is 12–24 µm long. About 90% of its forms are long and stout with a conspicuous undulating membrane, about 7% are long and slender with an inconspicuous undulating membrane and about 3% are short with an inconspicuous undulating membrane. A free flagellum is usually absent. The disease is characterized by disseminated intravascular coagulation, haemorrhage in the heart, lungs and meninges (☞ CATTLE, ■ 2 p. 55)

Geographic distribution: Tropical East and Central Africa

Symptoms: Hyperthermia, inappetence, depression, polypnoea and death within a few hours

Significance: *T. congolense simiae* is the most important trypanosome of domestic swine and causes a very acute and fatal disease in pigs.

Diagnosis: This is based on the peracute course, clinical signs of the disease and the demonstration of large numbers of organisms in the peripheral blood.

Therapy: Isomethamidium chloride (12.5–35 mg/kg, im.) at increased dosage rates or a combination of quinapyramine (7.5 mg/kg, sc.) and diminazene aceturate (5 mg/kg, im.) can be used to treat *T. congolense simiae* infections.

Prophylaxis: The suramin-quinapyrimidine complex (4 ml solution/5 kg, ☞ HORSES AND DONKEYS, ■ 2) protects piglets against *T. congolense simiae* for a period of 3 months and adults for 5 months. Insecticide application to avoid bites by tsetse flies may be necessary in endemic areas, where losses due to *T. congolense simiae* and other trypanosomes are high.

Trypanosoma (syn. *Pycnomonas*) *suis*

Hosts: Pig

Vector: *Glossina brevipalpis* (savannah regions) and Glossina vanhoofi (forest)

Species description: This suid specific trypanosome is poorly known. It is monomorphic, 14–19 µm in length, stout and with a short free flagellum. *T. suis* causes a chronic infection in adults and a more acute disease with death in less than 2 months in young pigs. It cannot be transmitted to sheep, goat and other domestic animals.

Geographic distribution: Central Africa (Zaire, Tanzania, Burundi)

Symptoms: Fever, apathy, progressive weakness and death in suckling piglets; unthriftiness in adult pigs

Significance: *T. suis* may cause great losses in suckling pigs.

Diagnosis: Clinical signs and the demonstration of the organisms in the blood

Therapy and Prophylaxis: ☞ *T. congolense simiae* and ☞ CATTLE, ■ 2

Trypanosoma congolense

Remarks: *T. congolense* occurs in swine but may regress spontaneously. Once the disease sets in it develops a chronic course associated with emaciation, progressive anaemia, weakness and ataxia (☞ CATTLE, ■ 2).

Trypanosoma brucei

Remarks: *T. brucei* is not very pathogenic for pigs and develops as a chronic, usually mild or asymptomatic disease (☞ CATTLE, ■ 2).

Trypanosoma vivax

Remarks: *T. vivax* is generally non-pathogenic for pigs (☞ CATTLE, ■ 2).

Trypanosoma evansi

Remarks: *T. evansi* affects a wide range of hosts, including pig. The most severe disease occurs in camels, horses and dogs. The transmission is mechanical by biting flies (☞ HORSES AND DONKEYS, ■ 2). *T. evansi* infections in pig are chronic in nature and the clinical signs are unspecific (apathy, weakness) and often overlooked.

BABESIIDAE

Babesia (syn. *Piroplasma*) ***trautmanni***
Porcine piroplasmosis

Vector: *Rhipicephalus sinus, R. appendiculatus, R. sanguineus, Boophilus decoloratus* and *Dermacentor* spp.

Species description: The morphology of *B. trautmanni* is similar to that of *B. bigemina*. It is the large porcine babesia species (2.5–4 µm long and 1.5–2 µm wide), characteristically long and narrow. It occurs frequently in pairs, but the infected cells may also contain up to 6 organisms. Oval, amoeboid and ring forms may occur. Babesiosis of swine is seasonal, according to the vector. Wild boar and wart hogs may serve as natural reservoir. Mortality may reach 50%. Pigs of all age are affected.

Geographic distribution: Southern Europe, equatorial Africa

Symptoms: Fever, anaemia, haemoglobinuria, jaundice, oedema and incoordination. Abortion may occur in pregnant sows.

Significance: *B. trautmanni* infections may cause severe losses in pig farms in endemic areas. These losses are seasonal.

Diagnosis: Clinical signs, especially haemoglobinuria and icterus and demonstration of the parasites in Giemsa-stained blood smears.

Therapy: Diminazene aceturate (3.5 mg/kg, im.), trypan blue, phenamidineand quinuronium are also effective. (☞ CATTLE, ■ 2).

Prophylaxis: Regular tick control (☞ SWINE, ■ 5.1)

(Figure 566)

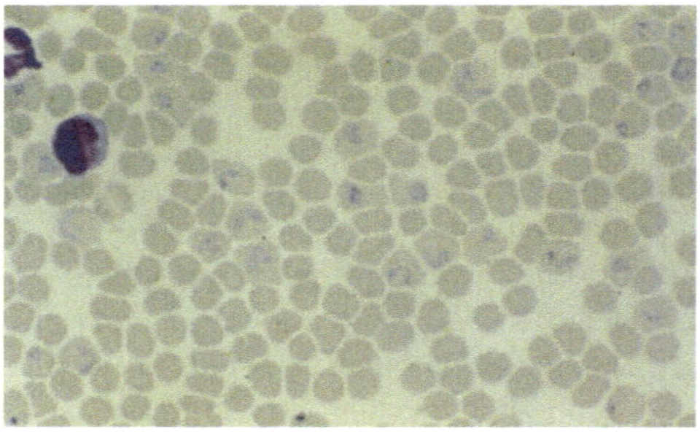

Fig. 566 *Babesia trautmanni* (2.5–4 × 2 µm); stained bloodsmear [4]

Babesia perroncitoi Porcine babesiosis

Vector: *Rhipicephalus sinus, R. appendiculatus, R. sanguineus, Dermacentor reticulatus* and other tick species to be established.

Species description: The morphology of *B. perroncitoi* is similar to that of *B. bovis*. It is the small porcine *Babesia* species, a small rounded form (0.7–2 µm in diameter). Oval to pyriform forms may occur (1.2–2.6 µm long and 0.7 –1.9 µm wide).

Geographic distribution: Mediterranean basin, West and Central Africa

Symptoms: Comparable to *B. trautmanni*. For significance, diagnosis, therapy and prophylaxis ☞ *B. trautmanni*

(Figure 567, 568)

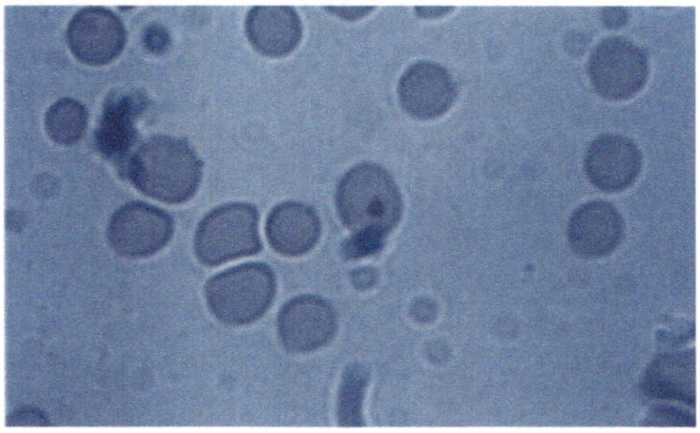

Fig. 567 *Babesia perroncitoi* (0.7–1.8 µm in diameter); stained bloodsmear [8]

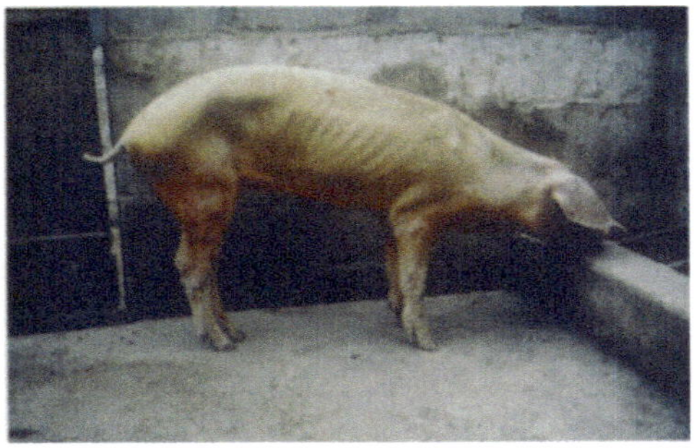

Fig. 568 Babesiosis in pigs; emaciation and icterus [8]

RICKETTSIALES

Eperythrozoon spp.

Eperythrozoon suis

Vector: *E. suis* is transmitted by parenteral routes. *Haematopinus suis* and probably other arthropods may transmit the infection. Mechanical transmission by surgical instruments (e.g. hypodermic needles) may also occur.

Species description: *E. suis* and *E. parvum* (☞ below) occur in pigs on the surface of erythrocytes. Severe cases generally occur in young pigs. Transplacental transmission may occur. *E. suis* is generally not very pathogenic but may assume increased significance together with other concomitant infections (babesiosis, trypanosomosis, etc.).

Geographic distribution: America, Europe, Asia and equatorial Africa

Symptoms: Varying degrees of haemolytic anaemia, icterus (yellow belly), fever, anorexia, weakness. Anaemia is the predominant clinical sign of *E. suis* infections in neonatal piglets. Abortion may occur in infected sows.

Significance: *E. suis* is of great economic significance in suckling pigs wherever it occurs.

Diagnosis: Acute eperythrozoonosis may be diagnosed by demonstrating large numbers of rickettsiae in Giemsa-stained bloodsmears (☞ METHODS, 3.1). The parasites may be found free in the plasma, surrounding platelets, or on the surface of erythrocytes as rings (2–3 µm in diameter). Serological tests, e.g. indirect haemagglutination, IFAT and ELISA are available and most useful for epidemiological studies. *E. suis* infection should be differentiated from *Anaplasma* infections.

Therapy: Oxytetracycline (6.6 mg/kg, im.) and other tetracyclines are effective in single dosages against *E. suis*. Haematinic drugs (e.g. iron dextran) may support recovery. If required, oral application of oxytetracycline is an effective herd treatment.

Prophylaxis: Control of ectoparasites (especially *Haematopinus suis* and *Sarcoptes suis*) may reduce *E. suis* infections (☞ SWINE, ■ 5.1 and CATTLE, ■ 2)

Eperythrozoon parvum

Remarks: *E. parvum* is smaller than *E. suis* (0.5–0.8 µm in diameter) and non-pathogenic. It also occurs on the surface of erythrocytes.

(Figure 569)

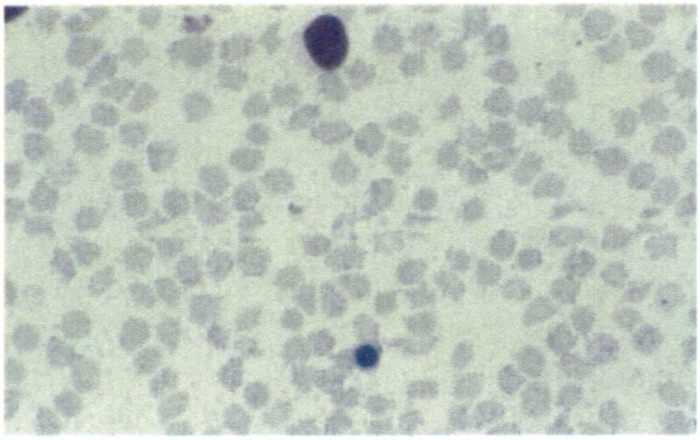

Fig. 569 *Eperythrozoon parvum* (0. 4–1 µm); stained bloodsmear [4]

HELMINTHS

- Nematoda larvae (microfilariae) found in the blood and circulatory system

Setaria congolensis

Remarks: Microfilariae occur in the peripheral blood and are ingested by mosquitoes (☞ SWINE, ■ 4.4 and CATTLE, ■ 2). The adult worms occur in the abdominal cavity of pigs.

3 Stages in the urogenital system

HELMINTHS

• Nematoda found in the urogenital system

Stephanurus dentatus "Kidney worm"

Location: Adult *S. dentatus* worms are found in the kidneys, walls of the ureters and perirenal fat. Immature larvae may be found in the liver and peritoneal cavity and occasionally in other tissues or organs (e.g. thoracic organs or spinal cord, etc.)

Hosts: Pig

Species description: Adult *S. dentatus* worms (2– 4 cm long and about 2 mm in diameter) are usually found in pairs within cysts (up to 4 cm in diameter) in the kidney or nearby fat. It is mainly a parasite of pigs raised outdoors. Eggs pass out with the urine and hatch in 2 days. Infective third-stage larvae develop within 4 days and may infect pigs percutaneously or by being ingested. In addition earthworms may ingest and accumulate larvae. Consequently pigs may acquire heavy infections by eating earthworms. The larvae then migrate via blood vessels to the liver, where they wander for 3 months or more. The larvae proceed to migrate through the peritoneum to the kidney, where cysts are formed. Eggs do not appear in the urine until 9–16 months after infection. Patent infections in piglets < 5 months old were acquired prenatally. Female worms live as long as 3 years and produce up to 1 million eggs per day. The principal economic loss results from condemnation of organs affected by migrating larvae. The liver is usually most severely affected, showing cirrhosis, scar formation, extensive thrombosis of the portal vessels. Kidney and lung damage is also common.

Geographic distribution: Tropical and subtropical regions

Symptoms: Heavy infections result in reduced growth. Pleuritis and peritonitis are common. Inappetence, emaciation, ascites due to cirrhosis. The infection is a herd problem and lack of growth and wasting in the pig herd are the predominant signs.

Significance: The kidney worm causes great losses due to poor growth and condemnation of damaged organs (mainly liver) and tissues at slaughter.

Diagnosis: During the long prepatent period clinical signs may be present but no eggs can be found in the urine. Prepatent infections are therefore very difficult to diagnose and a definite diagnosis depends on the demonstration of the worms at necropsy.

Therapy: Ivermectin (300 µg/kg, sc.), fenbendazole (3 mg/kg/day for 3 days), oxfendazole (3–4.5 mg/kg, po.) and levamisole (8 mg/kg) are effective against *S. dentatus*.

Prophylaxis: This is largely a matter of hygiene. Indoor housing and rigorous outdoor sanitation (provision of a concrete platform under the feeding troughs) reduces the kidney worm incidence drastically. In traditional pig rearing systems control relies on regular treatment of young pigs and the elimination of old (inapparent but egg-excreting) animals.

(Figures 570, 571, 572, 573)

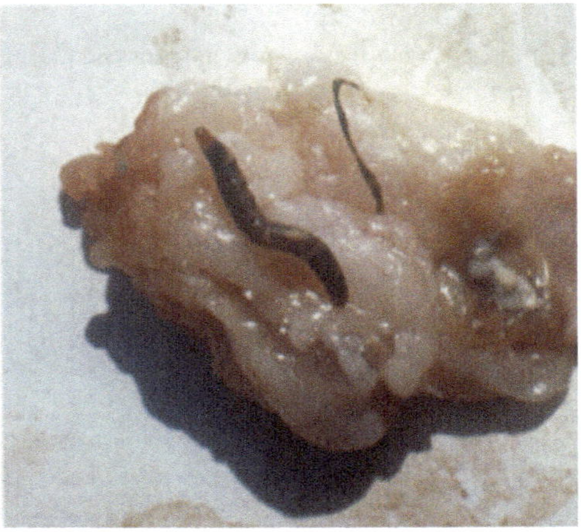

Fig. 570 *Stephanurus dentatus* (male: 20–30 mm; female: 30–45); adult worms found in a kidney cyst [8]

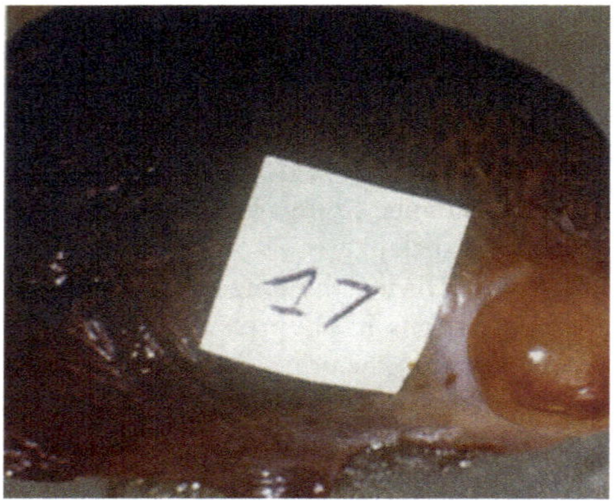

Fig. 571 Liver damage associated with *Stephanurus dentatus* is often an important cause of disease [8]

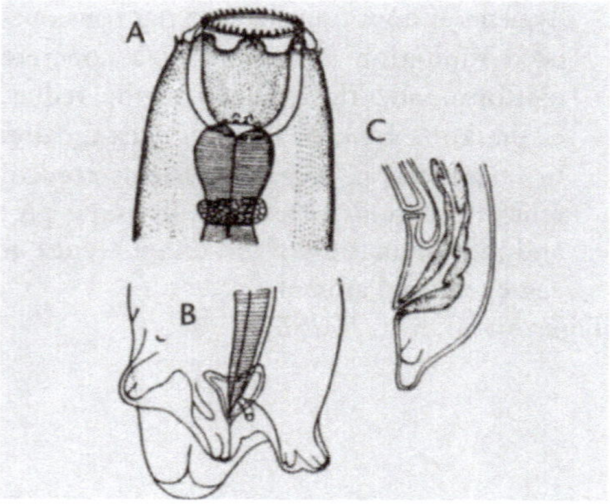

Fig. 572 *Stephanurus dentatus*; anterior end (A), posterior end of a male (B) and tail end of a female (C) [34]

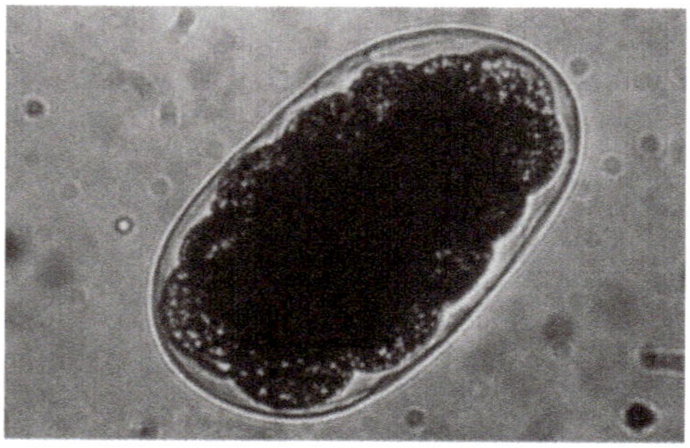

Fig. 573 Egg of *Stephanurus dentatus* (90–114 × 53–70 µm) appears in the urine [8]

Dioctophyma renale

Remarks: *D. renale* occurs most commonly in mink, dog and many other species. It may occasionally be found in pig. The females are the largest nematodes known (75–100 cm long and > 1 cm in diameter). The adults live in the renal tissue and destroy the renal parenchyma gradually as they grow. Pitted, thick shelled eggs with bipolar plugs are passed in the urine. Oligochaete annelids act as intermediate hosts. Infection is acquired by ingesting larvae or transport hosts (e.g. fish, frogs) which contain encysted larvae. After ingestion larvae migrate from the stomach to the peritoneal cavity and liver before maturing in the kidneys. Diagnosis is made on demonstration of eggs in the urine and mature parasites in the kidneys at necropsy. *D. renale* infections are incidentally found at necropsy and are something of a curiosity. Most modern benzimidazoles are expected to be effective. Surgical removal may often be necessary.

(Figures 574, 575, 576)

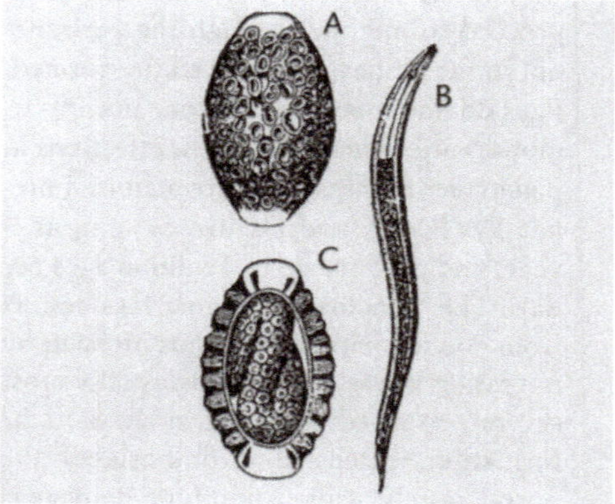

Fig. 574 *Dioctophyma renale*; (A) egg (71–84 × 46–52 µm); (B) embryonated egg and (C) larva after hatching [9]

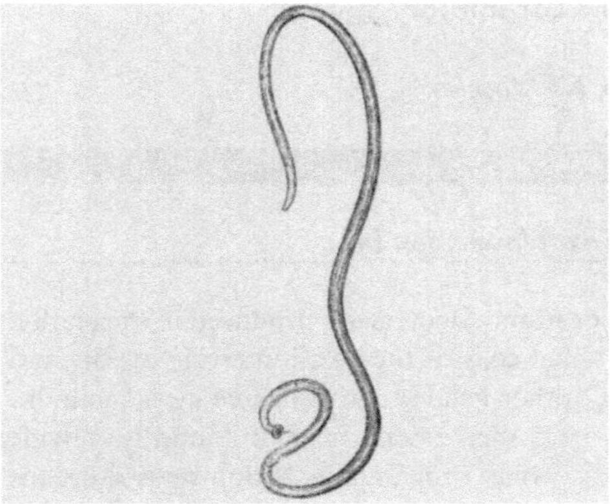

Fig. 575 *Dioctophyma renale*; male (35 cm × 3–4 mm long) [9]

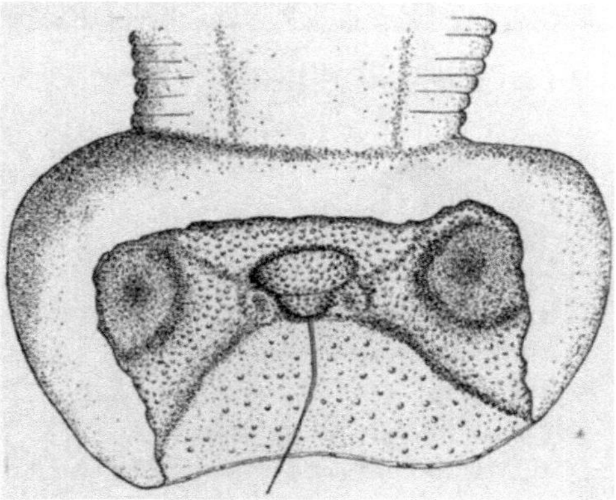

Fig. 576 *Dioctophyma renale*; male bursa (schematic) [9]

4 Stages in internal organs

4.1 Locomotory System

4.1.1 Muscles

PROTOZOA

Toxoplasma gondii

Location: Oocysts are produced in the epithelial cells of the small intestine of cats and other Felidae. *Toxoplasma* cysts (containing merozoites) may be found in a wide variety of mammals and in several organs (including brain).

Hosts: Felidae are definitive hosts, many mammal species (including all domestic animals) and man act as intermediate hosts.

Species description: Infection of intermediate hosts by ingesting sporulated oocysts or infected meat or infected animals. The definitive host can also be the intermediate host. After infection parasitaemia (trophozoites or tachyzoites, crescent-shaped, 4–8 × 2–4 µm) occurs and susceptible tissues all over the body are invaded and the parasites multiply. The parasites finally remain in cysts (bradyzoites) and only in the most receptive tissues. In general, the parasite cysts appear in the brain, eye, lungs, liver, skeletal and cardiac musculature. *T. gondii* cysts in muscles are 100 µm in diameter, the tachyzoites in the cysts are 6–8 µm long. Infection of the intermediate hosts occurs by ingestion of sporulated oocysts from the faeces of the final host (cat) or *Toxoplasma* cysts by raw meat from infected intermediate hosts (horse, swine, sheep and other species). Transplacental infection is common (☞ Sheep and Goats, ■4.1.1). In carnivores, infection is acquired by ingestion of fresh, infected meat or carcasses of a wide range of intermediate hosts. In herbivores, most infections are thought to result from ingestion of herbage contaminated by *Toxoplasma* oocysts derived from cat faeces. In omnivores, including man, infection seems to result both from ingestion of undercooked meat and from accidental ingestion of oocysts.

Cave: Raw meat of pigs is an important source of infection for humans. Populations at risk are serologically negative pregnant women and immunosuppressed persons.

Geographic distribution: World-wide

Symptoms: The majority of infections is subclinical. Fever, apathy, diarrhoea, respiratory distress (coughing, dyspnoea) and CNS symptoms may occur during the acute phase. Pregnant sows may abort or farrow weak or stillborn pigs.

Significance: *T. gondii* is one of the most common parasites in animals and probably also in man. Uncooked meat of swine is the major source of infection for man. Toxoplasmosis is an important cause of abortion and stillbirths in sheep, goats and sometimes in pigs.

Diagnosis: Demonstration of *Toxoplasma* cysts in stained biopsy sections or in artificially digested tissue. The diagnosis should be supported by immunohistochemistry (using mono- or polyclonal antibodies), isolation of the organisms and serological testing. Isolation may be based on intraperitoneal injection of suspected material into mice free of natural *Toxoplasma* infections in order to detect cysts in mouse brain after 4–6 weeks. Isolation may also be carried out by inoculation of the suspected material onto a tissue culture (e.g. Vero cells). Several serological tests are available (also as kits) for the detection of *Toxoplasma* antibodies (Sabin-Feldman dye test, Indirect Fluorescent Antibody Test, indirect haemagglutination, ELISA (☞ METHODS, 5). The B1 gene-derived PCR provides a highly sensitive tool for the diagnosis of *T. gondii* in clinical material. As little as one tachyzoite may be detected with this method.

Therapy: Specific treatment is not recommended for domestic animals. Sulfadiazine (73 mg/kg, po.) acts synergistically with pyrimethamine (0.44 mg/kg, po.) in laboratory animals and man. Clindamycin (10–40 mg/kg, po.; 25–50 mg/kg, im.) is the drug of choice for treatment of *Toxoplasma* infections in dogs and cats.

Prophylaxis: Raw meat of pigs is the main source of infection in man. Prevention is based on the interruption of the complex life cycle. Cats and pigs should not be kept together. Control of rodents is an essential part of the prevention of *Toxoplasma* infection in domestic animals, especially pigs, since rodents attract cats but can also be a source of infection if they are eaten by pigs. Feeding of uncooked garbage should be eliminated.

(Figures 577, 578, 579, 580)

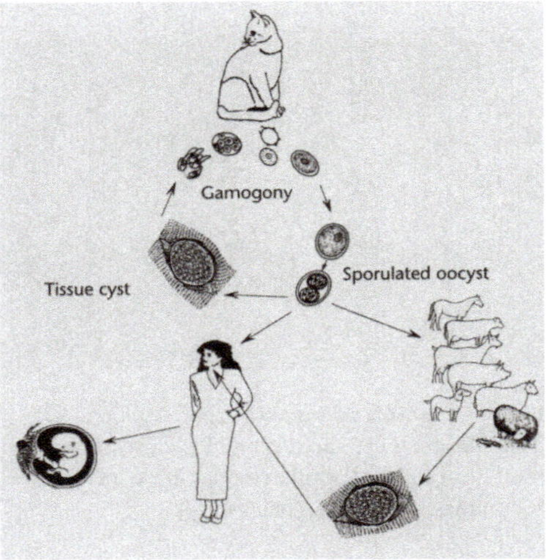

Fig. 577 Transmission cycle of *Toxoplasma gondii* Gamogony occurs in the final host (cat) and oocysts are excreted which infect domestic animals and man where tissue cysts are formed. *T. gondii* is of great importance when seronegative pregnant women become infected. The parasite may then affect the fetus [10]

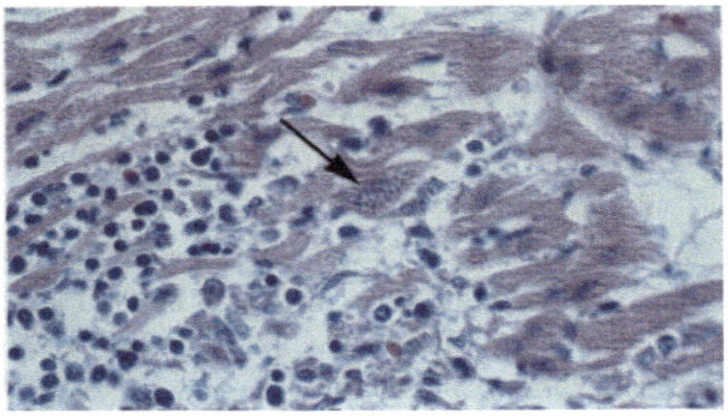

Fig. 578 *Toxoplasma gondii*; muscle cysts

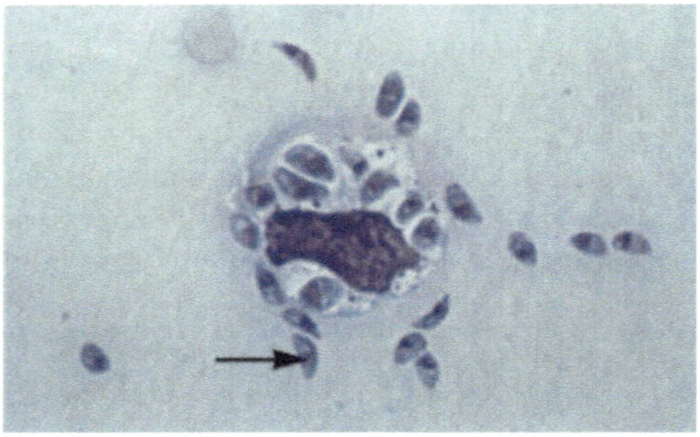

Fig. 579 *Toxoplasma gondii*; tachyzoites (6–8 µm long) [4]

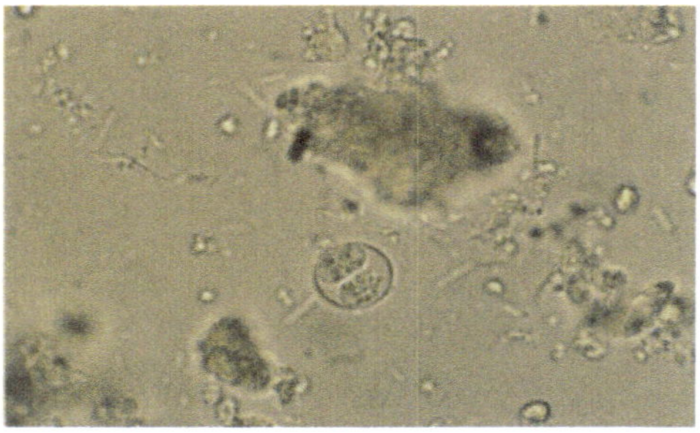

Fig. 580 Sporulated oocyst (12.4 × 10.5 µm) of *Toxoplasma gondii* are excreted exclusively in the faeces of Felidae. Sporulated oocyst are infectious for animals and human beings [10]

Sarcocystis spp.

Cysts of the following three species are found in swine: *S. suihominis*, *S. suicanis* (syn. *S. miescheriana*) and *S. porcifelis*.

Location: Cysts (Sarcocysts) are found in the muscles of swine. Infective sporocysts are passed in the faeces of the final host.

Hosts: The pig is the intermediate host of all three species is the pig. Definitive hosts of *S. suihominis* are man and primates, of *S. suicanis* the dog, wolf, fox and of *S. porcifelis* the cat.

Species description: *Sarcocystis* spp. develop in a 2-host cycle consisting of an intermediate host (prey) and the final host (predator). *S. suihominis* (common), *S. suicanis* (common) and *S. porcifelis* (uncommon) are the three species found in swine. In all three species swine acts as intermediate host, where the asexual part of the *Sarcocystis* life cycle takes place and cysts are formed in striated or cardiac muscles. These cysts contain infective, banana-shaped merozoites 60 days after infection. The sexual cycle is found in intestinal epithelial cells of the final hosts where gametogony occurs. Infection is acquired by ingestion of infective sporocysts of the final host.

Geographic distribution: World-wide

Symptoms: Most infections are asymptomatic and the parasite (cysts) is discovered only at slaughter. Intensity of clinical signs depends on the number of ingested sporocysts. More than 1 million is lethal. Acute sarcocystosis shows a biphasal fever between 5–9 days and 11–15 days after infection. During the second phase apathy, dyspnoea, anaemia and cyanosis (skin, ears, tail), muscle spasms, hyperexcitability and prostration are predominant. Abortion following heavy infection is reported in cows and may also occur in pregnant sows.

Significance: *Sarcocystis* infections are very common and generally asymptomatic in swine. However, when high numbers of sporocysts are ingested they may cause a severe disease condition.

Diagnosis: Generally not possible with the naked eye. Demonstration of muscle cysts in histological sections or following artificial digestion of infected muscles. Acute cysticercosis in swine may be diagnosed by Giemsa-stained bloodsmears taken from the surface of organs at necropsy or by stained histological sections. Serological techniques may be employed to discover chronic infections (important is the presence of cysts).

Therapy: Therapy is generally not indicated. Halofuginone (0.5 mg/kg, po.) may be used.

Prophylaxis: Dogs and other carnivores should not be allowed to eat raw meat, offal or dead animals. Also, man should not consume uncooked meat. Supplies of grain and feed should be kept covered. Dogs and cats

should be kept away from buildings, used to store feed or house animals. Amprolium (100 mg/kg, po.) daily for 30 days and Halofuginone 3 ppm) may be used for prophylaxis in heavily infected herds.
(Figures 581, 582, 583)

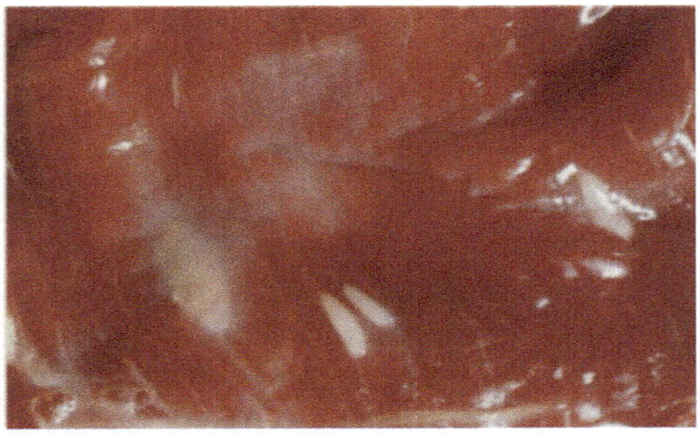

Fig. 581 Cysts of *Sarcocystis suicanis* in diaphragm (up to 1.5 mm long)

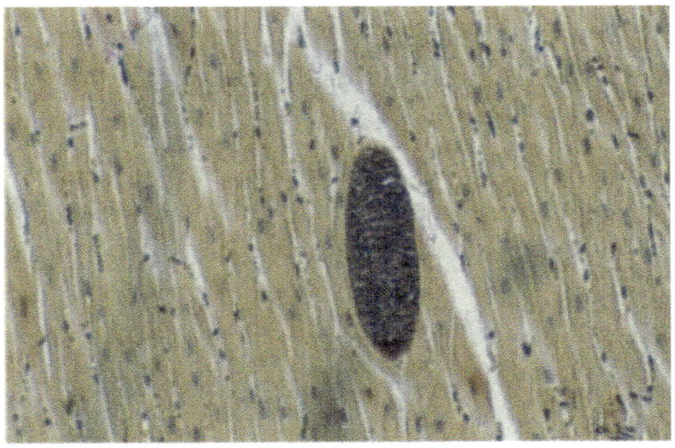

Fig. 582 Cysts of *Sarcocystis* sp. in the musculature

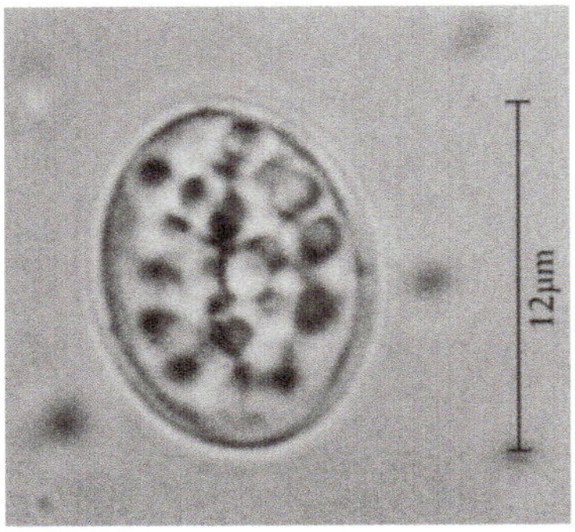

Fig. 583 Sporocyst of *Sarcocystis suicanis*; excreted by the dog [4]

HELMINTHS

• Cestoda larvae found in the muscles

Cysticercus cellulosae Cyst of the human tapeworm *Taenia solium*

Location: *C. cellulosae* cysts are found in the skeletal and cardiac muscles of pigs and man. Adult tapeworms (*T. solium*) are found in the small intestine of man.

Hosts: Pig is an intermediate host of the human tapeworm *T. solium*. Man can be both final and intermediate host of *T. solium*.

Species description: Cysts (cysticerci) are white, 5–18 mm in diameter and contain one protoscolex with a hook collar. Infection of pigs occurs by ingesting gravid proglottids or eggs which are passed in the faeces of infected man. These proglottids contain embryophores, releasing oncospheres which migrate to skeletal muscle and the heart via blood stream. Cysticerci develop within 2–3 months after the ingestion of the eggs and remain infective up to 2 years. Man acquires infection by eating infective pig muscle. Cysticerci are released in the human small intestine where the scolices evaginate and attach to the intestinal wall. The prepatent period is 7–8 weeks.

Geographic distribution: World-wide

Symptoms: Cysticercosis in swine is generally asymptomatic.

Significance: Cysticercosis in swine is not associated with pathology or clinical disease. Pathology in man is related to the number and localization of cysticerci. Neurocysticercosis in humans is a serious condition often with fatal consequences. Adult tapeworms produce no significant pathological changes in man.

Diagnosis: Antemortem diagnosis is based on the detection of specific antibodies (e.g. ELISA). Cysticercosis in swine is diagnosed at slaughter where macroscopic cysts may be discovered.

Therapy: Therapy of cysticercosis in swine is generally not indicated. *T. solium* can be treated with niclosamide or praziquantel, the latter is also effective against cerebral cysts of *T. solium* in man. Fenbendazole (5 mg/kg, po.) administered for 7 days and mebendazole (25 mg/kg, po.) for 5 days were described to be effective against cysticercosis in swine.

Prophylaxis: Man should not consume raw meat of pigs. Freezing for one week destroys the larvae that are a source of human infection. Improved sanitation (e.g. separation of human excrements and pig feeding ground) reduces the incidence of autochthonous infection and the infection of swine.

(Figures 154, 584, 585)

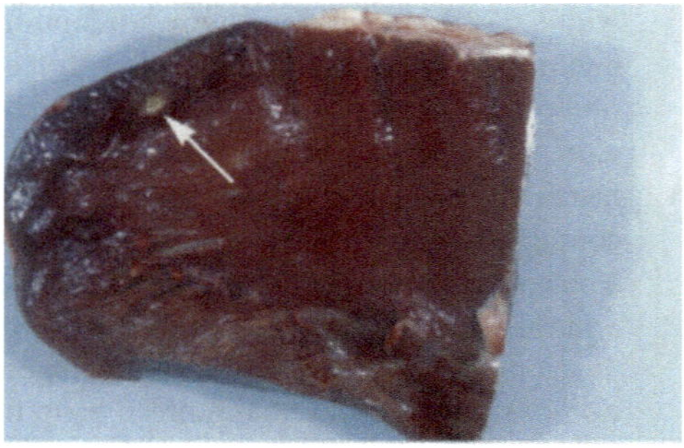

Fig. 584 *Cysticercus cellulosae* in muscle tissue (0.5–2 cm in diameter)

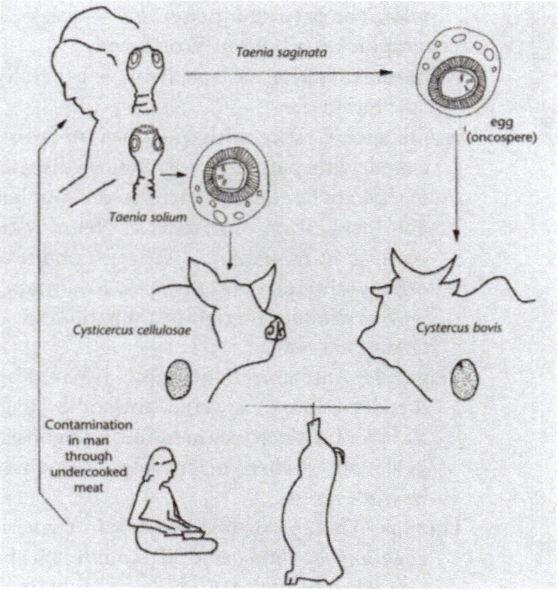

Fig. 585 Transmission cycle of *Taenia solium* (larval stage: *Cysticercus cellulosae* in swine) and *Taenia saginata* (larval stage: *Cysticercus bovis* in cattle) [16]

• Nematoda larvae and adult nematodes found in the muscles

***Trichinella* spp. (*T. spiralis, T. britovi, T. nativa, T. nelsoni* and *T. pseudospiralis*)**

Trichina worm

Location: Adult worms occur in the small intestine. Encysted larvae are found in muscles.

Hosts: Pig, wild boar, rat, man and many other mammals

Species description: Adult trichina worms are very small nematodes, 2–4 mm long. A females produces several hundreds of larvae which penetrate the intestinal wall and migrate via the lymph and blood vessels to the muscles where they encyst and remain viable for years. Further development only occurs if the infected tissue is ingested by another host, often a rat, man, or pig. Swine may therefore be both intermediate and principal host for trichina worms. After the ingestion of trichina cysts the larvae are liberated and mature in several days. The adult worms copulate in the small intestine and the females penetrate the mucosa to produce larvae for 2 weeks.

Geographic distribution: World-wide

Symptoms: Infection of the intestines may cause diarrhoea and fever but is generally not typical to allow diagnosis. Infection of the muscles may cause myositis, muscle pain, stiffness, polypnoea, oedema, eosinophilia and in severe cases death.

Significance: *Trichinella* spp. are less pathogenic in swine than in man. The larvae accumulate in the diaphragm and jaw muscles of pigs. Adults cause few problems in swine whereas in man they cause nausea, diarrhoea and abdominal pain. 4–6 days after infection death may occur in humans and is usually caused by paralysis of the respiratory muscles but also infection of the brain.

Diagnosis: At necropsy, encysted larvae may be found in muscles (diaphragm) which are squeezed in a compressorium for subsequent microscopic examination. Muscles may also be artificially digested to detect trichina larvae (☞METHODS, 2.1 and 2.2). Serological tests (ELISA, IFAT) are available to detect infections in domestic animals and man (☞METHODS, 5.2 and 5.3).

Therapy: *Trichinella*-infected pigs are generally not treated. Their meat should be condemned!

Prophylaxis: To prevent infection of pigs, garbage must be cooked before being fed to pigs. Human infections can be controlled by thorough cooking or freezing of pork and game animals before consumption.

Cave: T. nativa and related species may survive freezing.

(Figures 586, 587, 588)

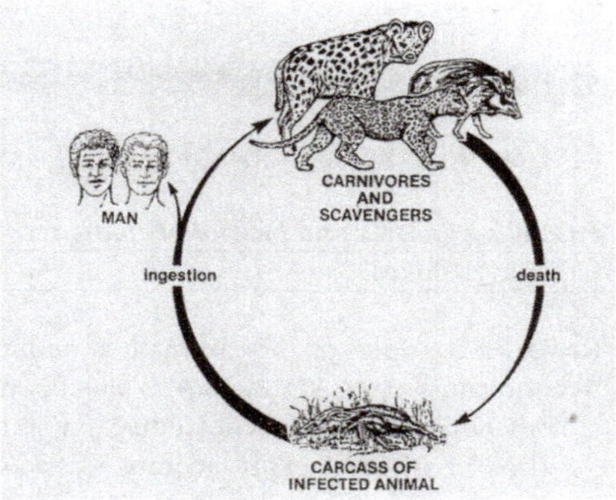

Fig. 586 Transmission cycle of *Trichinella* spp. in tropical Africa; the bushpig and other wild suids are the principal source of infection for man [21]

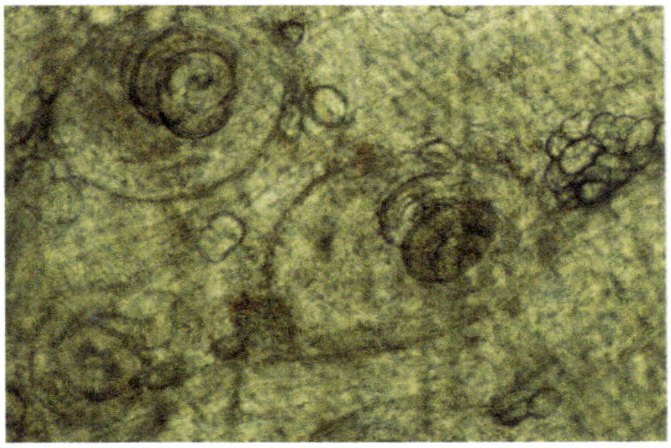

Fig. 587 Muscle cyst containing a *Trichinella spiralis* larva (0.4–0.6 × 0.25 mm)

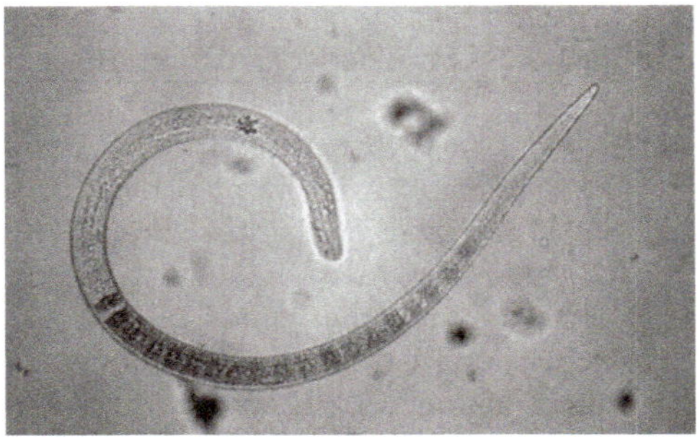

Fig. 588 *Trichinella spiralis* larva (800–1000 µm long) obtained from a digested muscle cyst

4.2 Liver

HELMINTHS

• Trematoda found in the liver

Fasciola gigantica and *Fasciola hepatica*
Large liver flukes

Remarks: *Fasciola* spp. are normally found in ruminants (☞ CATTLE, ■ 4.2) but many other mammal species including pig can also be affected. Pigs acquire *Fasciola* infections especially if they are grazing in swampy areas where the intermediate hosts are present. Fasciolosis in swine is generally asymptomatic. Losses occur by liver condemnation at slaughter.

***Dicrocoelium* spp.** Small liver flukes

Remarks: *Dicrocoelium* spp. are normally found in ruminants but many other mammal species including pig can also be affected (☞ CATTLE, ■ 4.2).

Eurytrema pancreaticum Pancreatic fluke

Remarks: *E. pancreaticum* is a parasite of the pancreatic ducts and occasionally of the bile ducts of sheep, pigs and cattle. There are no obvious clinical signs and *Dicrocoelium*-like eggs can be demonstrated in the faeces (☞ SHEEP AND GOATS, ■ 4.5).

• Cestoda found in the liver

Echinococcus granulosus Hydatid cysts

Location: Larvae (hydatid cysts) of *E. granulosus* are found in the liver and the lungs of swine and other intermediate hosts. Adult tapeworms are found in the small intestine of the dog and other canids.

Hosts: Canids are the final hosts of *E. granulosus*. Intermediate hosts are herbivores, swine, humans and many other domestic animals.

Species description: Pigs are known to be intermediate hosts in many countries but generally there are only little data available about the role of pigs as intermediate hosts in African countries. Intermediate hosts acquire infection by eating eggs shed in the faeces of canids. Eggs develop to hydatid cysts which may reach the size of an orange over the period of several months. These cysts are infective for canids.

Geographic distribution: World-wide

Symptoms: Generally inapparent infections in pigs. Pressure atrophy of the liver, digestive disturbances and ascites may be found in heavy infections. Dyspnoea and coughing may be observed when lungs are greatly affected.

Significance: Hydatid cysts generally cause no clinical disease in swine.

Diagnosis: Demonstration of hydatid cysts at necropsy or at slaughter. Cysts containing "*Echinococcus* sand" which is composed of thousands of typical protoscolices with a hook collar. Antemortem diagnosis is difficult. Serological tests are available and of great importance for epidemiological studies.

Therapy: Therapy is generally not indicated. Most of the modern benzimidazoles applied orally over the period of 10–20 days at doubled dosage rates may be used to reduce the number and size of hydatid cysts.

Prophylaxis: In endemic areas a strict separation of dogs from pigs is necessary to reduce the incidence of hydatidosis in swine.

(Figure 589)

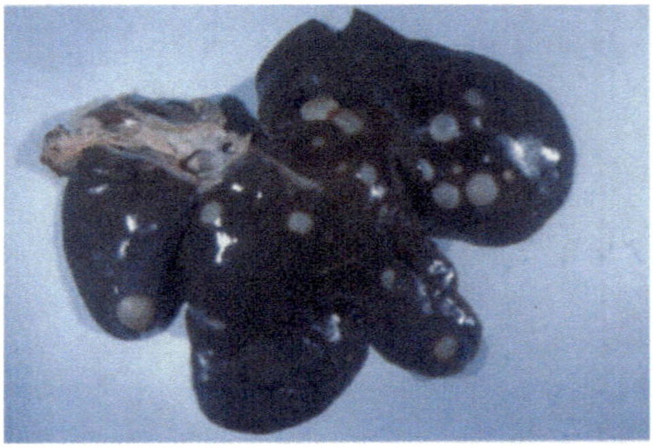

Fig. 589 Hydatid cyst of *Echinococcus granulosus* found in the liver of a pig

Cysticercus tenuicollis

Cysts of *Taenia hydatigena*

Remarks: Larvae of the canine cestode *Taenia hydatigena* may also be found in swine. Larval migration through the liver may produce haemorrhagic tracks and masses of larvae may cause a severe condition associated with anaemia, fever, inappetence and death (hepatitis cysticercosa). Larvae wander under the liver capsule and form thin-necked cysts. These cysts are always covered by a layer of serosa, and therefore they seem to be attached to the peritoneum. Preferred serosal sites of cysticerci are the omentum and mesentry although they may also be found attached to the serosa of the liver. Cysticerci are up to 8 cm in diameter and cause no pathology. Diagnosis is made at necropsy or slaughter (☞ CATTLE, ■ 4.4).
(Figure 590)

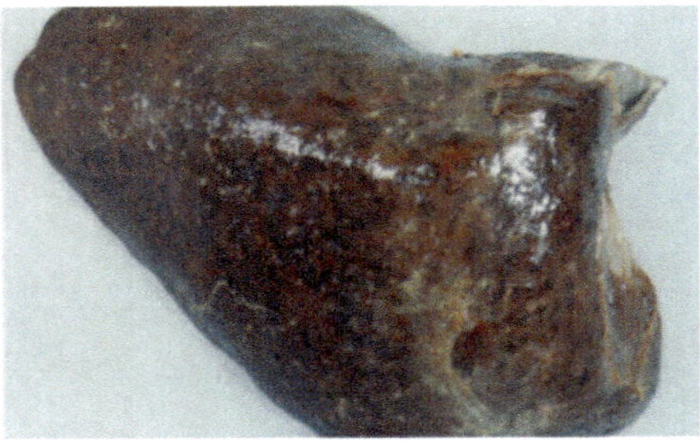

Fig. 590 Haemorrhagic tracks in the liver parenchyma due to a high number of migrating *Cysticercus tenuicollis* larvae

- Nematoda found in the liver

Ascaris suum

Remarks: Migration of larvae through the liver causes haemorrhage, necrosis and fibrosis that appears as white spots ("milk-spots") under the capsule after healing. Condemnation of livers at slaughter is one of the major losses due to *A. suum* infections in pig farming (☞ SWINE, ■ 1).
(Figure 591)

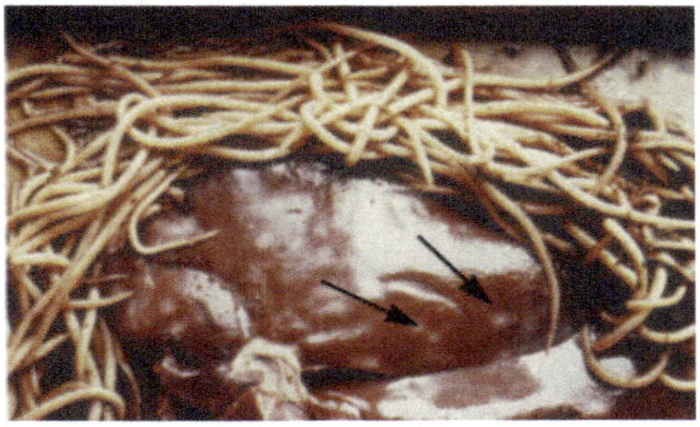

Fig. 591 Liver of swine with "milk spots" (arrows) and masses of adult *Ascaris suum* found in the small intestine [10]

4.3 Respiratory system

HELMINTHS

- Nematoda found in the lungs and trachea

***Metastrongylus* spp. (*M. apri*, syn. *M. elongatus, M. pudendotectus, M. salmi* and *M. madagascariensis*)** Porcine lungworms

Location: Bronchi and bronchioles
Hosts: Pig and wild boar
Species description: The adult parasites are slender and white, with males measuring up to 25 mm in length and females up to 48 mm. *Metastrongylus* spp. have an indirect life cycle in which most earthworms may serve as intermediate hosts. Eggs are laid in the bronchi, coughed up and passed in the faeces. After the ingestion by earthworms the eggs hatch and within 10 days infective third-stage larvae develop within the earthworms. Pigs become infected by ingesting earthworms. The third-stage larvae penetrate small intestine of the pig and proceed via lymph and blood vessels to the lungs. The prepatent period is 2–4 weeks. *M. elongatus* is the most common species.

Natural infections may involve one or more *Metastrongylus* species.

Geographic distribution: World-wide, with the exception of *M. madagascariensis* which has only been found in Madagascar.

Symptoms: Bronchitis, coughing, pneumonia, retarded growth in pigs kept on permanent pastures

Significance: Lungworms cause considerable economic losses due to reduced weight gain, respiratory disturbances following secondary infections. *Metastrongylus* spp. were also suspected to carry the virus of swine influenza and classical swine fever (hog cholera). Lungworms primarily cause clinical disease in young pigs, whereas older pigs show very few signs.

Diagnosis: Characteristic eggs are found in the faeces. At slaughter, the adult worms can be demonstrated. Serodiagnostic tests may also be used to detect the infections.

Therapy: For individual therapy ivermectin (300 µg/kg, sc.) and levamisole (7.5 mg/kg, sc.) are highly effective against adult lungworms. The broad spectrum anthelmintics such as fenbendazole (5 mg/kg, over 5– 15 days), flubendazole (30 ppm, over 10 days) are also effective when administered orally for several days. Febantel (20 mg/kg, po.) and mebendazole (30 ppm) are effective against *Metastrongylus* spp. at increased dosage rates.

Prophylaxis: Lungworm control is closely associated with earthworm control. Pigs kept clear of soil, especially during the rains may reduce disease incidence. Young pigs (< 6 months) should not come in contact with earthworms. If swine are not housed in clean quarters, nose rings will prevent pigs from rooting for earthworms

(Figures 538, 561, 562, 592, 593, 594)

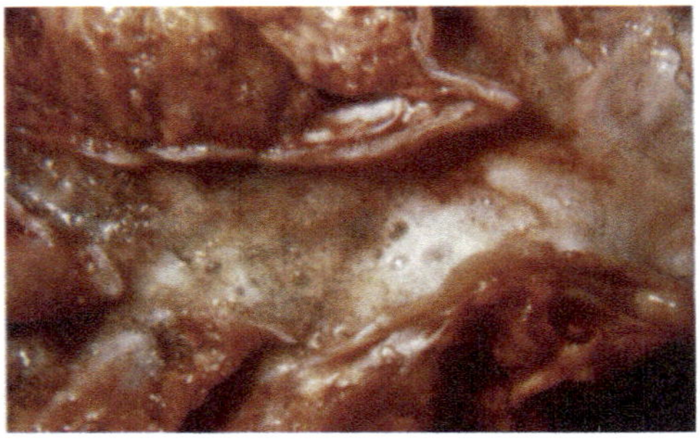

Fig. 592 *Metastrongylus apri* in the trachea of a pig (males: 11–26 mm long; females: 28–60 mm long) [8]

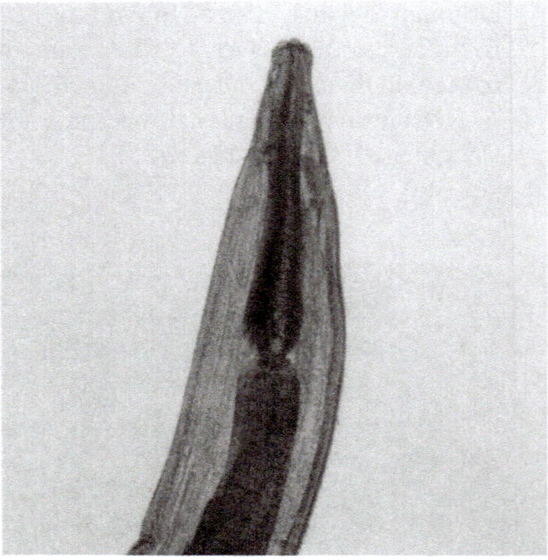

Fig. 593 *Metastrongylus apri*; anterior end

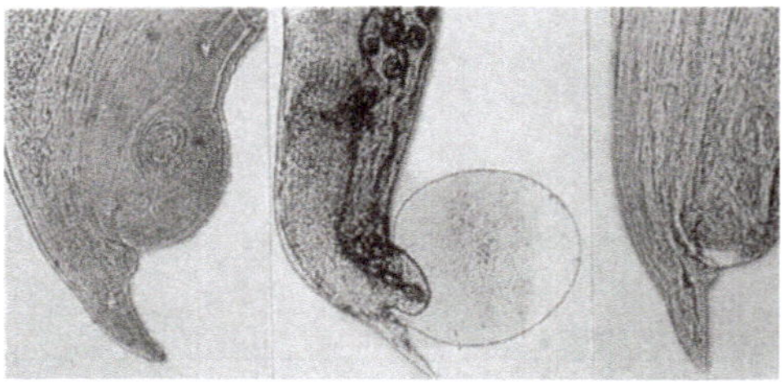

(a) (b) (c)

Fig. 594 Posterior end of female lungworms of pigs: (a) *Metastrongylus apri*, (b) *M. pudendotectus* and (c) *M. salmi* [4]

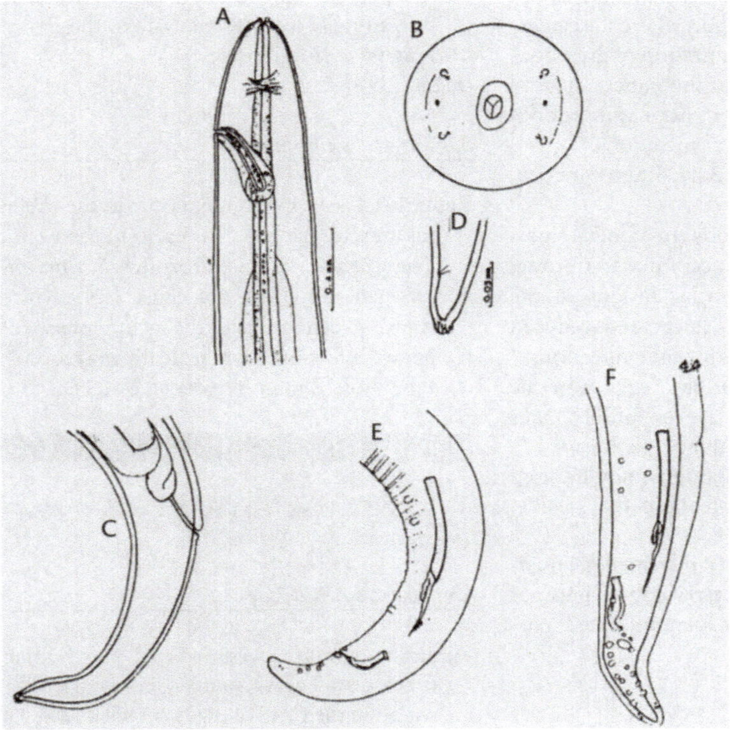

Fig. 595 *Setaria congolensis*; female anterior end (A), anterior end frontal view (B), female posterior end (C), female posterior end (D), male posterior end lateral (E) and male posterior end ventral (F) [34]

4.4 Abdominal cavity

HELMINTHS

• Nematoda found in the abdominal cavity

Setaria congolensis

Remarks: *S. congolensis* occurs in the peritoneal cavity of pigs in Africa (Zaire). Microfilariae occur in the blood and are ingested by mosquitoes (*Aedes* spp., *Culex* spp. and *Anopheles* spp.) which act as vectors. The exact life cycle of *S. congolensis* is unknown. Adult worms in the abdominal cavity are non-pathogenic. Pathogenic effects may occur when microfilariae migrate into the eye or the CNS or other organs. Little is known about *Setaria* infections in pigs and it seems that the worms are occasionally discovered at slaughter without pathological alterations or previous clinical signs. If therapy and prophylaxis are required ☞ *Setaria equina* (☞ HORSES AND DONKEYS, ■ 4.4 and *Setaria labiato-papillosa* (☞ CATTLE, ■ 4.4).
(Figure 595)

4.5 Pancreas

HELMINTHS

• Trematoda found in the pancreas

Eurytrema pancreaticum Pancreatic fluke

Location: It occurs in the pancreatic ducts and occasionally the bile ducts (☞ SHEEP AND GOATS, ■ 4.5 and CATTLE ■ 4.5).

Hosts: Pigs, sheep and cattle

Species description: These flukes are 8–16 mm long, 6 mm wide and belong to the Dicrocoeliidae. The first intermediate hosts are terrestrial snails (*Bradybaena* spp.) and the second intermediate hosts are grasshoppers (*Conocephalus* spp.) where the cercariae encyst. After the ingestion of grasshoppers larvae migrate to the pancreatic and bile ducts where they mature and produce eggs 11–14 weeks after infections.

Geographic distribution: Asia, South America, East Africa

Symptoms: There are no obvious clinical signs.

Significance: Losses may occur due to fibrotic, necrotic and degenerative lesions of the pancreas and biliary ducts and reduced growth in animals with heavy infections.

Diagnosis: *Dicrocoelium*-like eggs can be demonstrated in the faeces, adult flukes may be seen at slaughter or necropsy.

Therapy: The same compounds may be used as in *Dicrocoelium* infections (☞ CATTLE, ■ 4.2).

Prophylaxis: The control of intermediate hosts may not be feasible, especially if pigs are kept permanently on contaminated pastures or soil.

4.6 Central nervous system

PROTOZOA

Toxoplasma gondii

Remarks: *Toxoplasma* cysts may occur also in the brain of pigs (☞ also SWINE, ■ 4.1). Fever, weakness, and incoordination, associated with a high mortality in neonatal piglets may indicate the brain invasion by the parasite in the acute phase. Chronic infections (*Toxoplasma* cysts in the brain) may be asymptomatic.
(Figure 596)

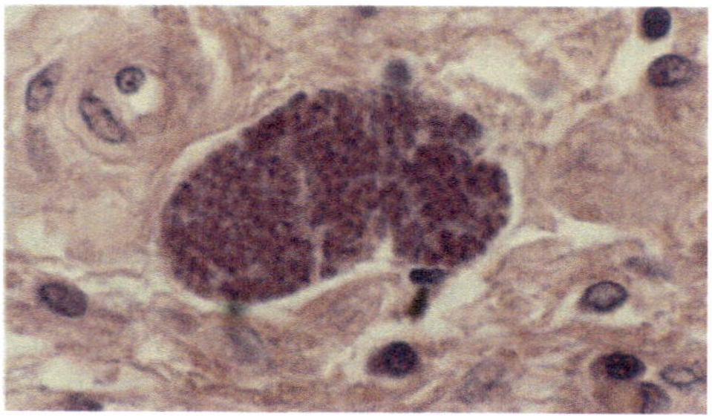

Fig. 596 *Toxoplasma gondii*; thin-walled cyst in the brain (25 × 50 µm)

Sarcocystis suihominis

Remarks: Tissue cysts may occur in the skeletal muscle, the heart and also in the brain. These cysts contain merozoites. *S. suihominis* generally does not cause CNS symptoms, except during the acute phase of heavy infections, when death may occur. Final host is man (☞ SWINE, ■ 4.1).

HELMINTHS

- Cestoda cysts found in the central nervous system

Cysticercus cellulosae

Remarks: Larvae (cysticerci) of the human tapeworm *Taenia solium* are occasionally found in the CNS of pigs (☞ SWINE, ■ 4.1).

- Nematoda found in the central nervous system

Trichinella spp.

Remarks: Larvae may sometimes be found in the CNS of pigs (☞ SWINE, ■ 1)

Stephanurus dentatus

Remarks: Larvae may occasionally invade the CNS of pigs (☞ SWINE, ■ 3)

5.1. Skin and coat

5.1 Skin and coat

HELMINTHS

- Nematoda found in the skin

Suifilaria suis

Location: Subcutaneous and intermuscular connective tissue
Host: Pig
Species description: The adult parasites are difficult to see. Males are 17–25 mm long and the female worms are 32–40 mm long and 0.15–0.17 mm wide. The hind end of the male is spirally coiled and bears two unequal spicules. The tail of the female shows a number of small tubercles. The life cycle is not known. The female worms lay eggs in the skin.
Geographic distribution: Southern Africa
Symptoms: Numerous small vesicular eruptions on the skin
Significance: This filaroid worm produces skin vesicles, containing eggs, which may burst and become secondarily infected. Apart from producing nodules *S. suis* does not affect the health of pigs.
Diagnosis: Multiple, whitish nodules in the skin and connective tissues. These nodules contain eggs which measure 51–61 x 28–32 µm. The hard, white nodules of *S. suis* should be distinguished from *Cysticercus cellulosae* (larval stage of *Taenia solium*) larvae which contain fluid and a scolex.
Therapy and Prophylaxis: Unknown and generally not indicated

ARTHROPODS

Arthropods are divided into two main groups:

Arachnida (arachnids) including:
- *Ticks*
- *Mites*

Insecta including:
- *Lice*
- *Fleas*
- *Dipterida*

- Arachnida found in/on the skin

– Ticks
(Figure 597)

Ticks are found on a wide variety of host animals and are generally not very host-specific. They are not considered to be common parasites of pigs. The economic importance of ticks is considerable because of the annoyance to the host (direct noxious effects, tick worry), transmission of diseases (Babesioses) and the fatal tick toxicoses (paralysis, sweating sickness, general toxicosis). In intensive pig production systems, ticks are seldom a problem because animals are raised in close confinements. If pigs are kept in free range systems, tick infestations may assume increased significance (☞ SWINE, ■ 2).

Significance: Heavy tick infestations cause blood loss and skin wounds. Infested pigs itch, bite and scratch, causing self-inflicted skin trauma, susceptible to secondary infections and myiasis. Anaemia and weight loss may also occur. Ticks of potential importance to pigs belong to two families: the Ixodidae ("hard ticks") and the Argasidae ("soft ticks").

Fig. 597 Life cycle of a 3-host tick [50]

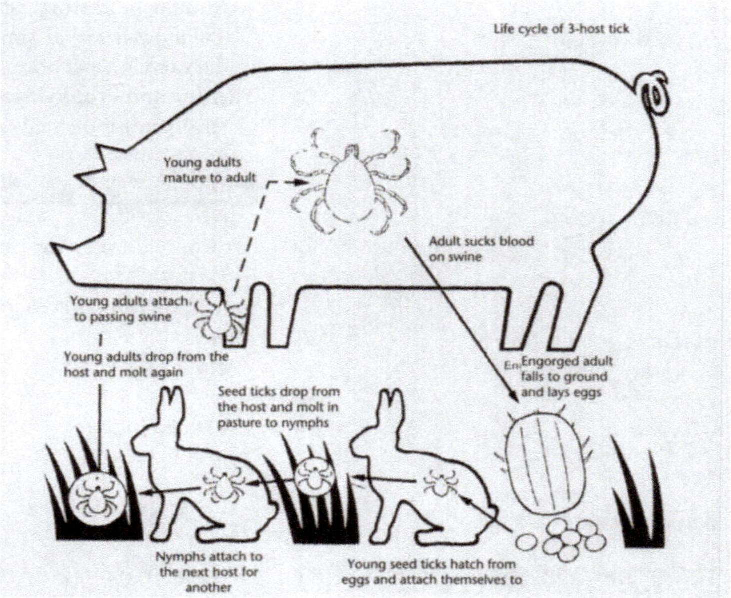

IXODIDAE (**"hard ticks"**)

Boophilus decoloratus The blue tick

Remarks: This is a one-host tick and known to be a vector of *Babesia trautmanni* in East Africa. It occurs in Africa south of the Sahara.
(Figure 598)

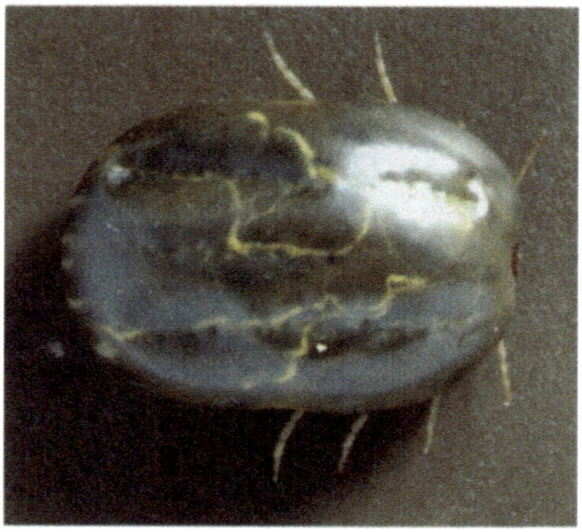

Fig. 598 *Boophilus* sp.; vector of *Babesia trautmanni* adult engorged female [10]

Rhipicephalus* spp. *(R. sinus, R. appendiculatus* and *R. sanguineus)

Remarks: These species (mainly ticks of cattle) are vectors of *Babesia trautmanni* and *Babesia perroncitoi* in pigs.

***Dermacentor* spp.**

Remarks: One-host or three-host ticks. Some species of this genus are suspected to be vectors of *Babesia trautmanni* and *B. perroncitoi* in pigs. Some species are associated with tick paralysis.

***Amblyomma* spp.**

Remarks: This are three-host ticks. Several species of *Amblyomma* ticks are found on pigs in central and southern Africa. Apart from skin irritation at the site of attachment they may also cause tick paralysis.
(Figure 599)

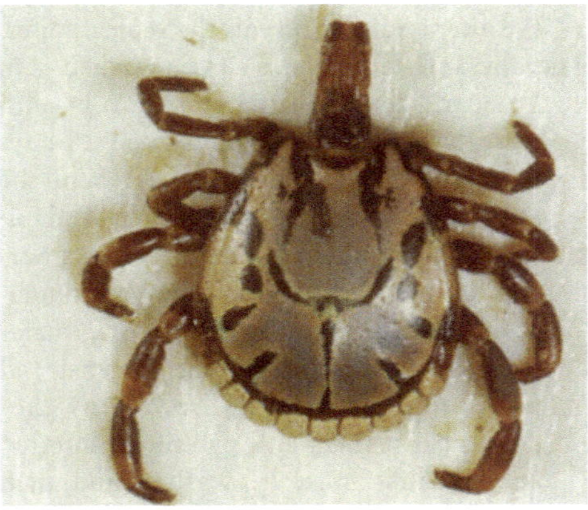

Fig. 599 *Amblyomma* sp.; adult male; members of this genus may cause severe irritation and tick paralysis in pigs [10]

Ixodes spp.

Remarks: *Ixodes* spp. are three-host ticks and occur on pigs and other animals in Europe, North America and South Africa and may cause tick paralysis in domestic animals (☞ CATTLE, ■ 5.1).

ARGASIDAE ("soft ticks")

Ornithodorus moubata The eyeless tampan

Remarks: This tick lives in the native huts and in the sand under trees where animals and human beings frequently seek shelter. In huts they live in cracks in the floor or under loose soil, from which they emerge at night to feed. In burrows they bury themselves in the earth lining, coming out to feed when a suitable host is available. Adult females lay batches of about 100 eggs and broods over the eggs in the sand. Development includes a larval stage which remains quiescent until it has moulted to the nymphal stage. Several nymphal stages are passed through and the nymphs, like the adults, attack their host for short periods to feed. This tampan sucks blood from its hosts. It is extremely resistant to both starvation and desiccation (survival time off the host up to 5 and more years). *O. moubata* constitutes the main reservoir host for the virus of African Swine Fever. It is also an important vector of the virus among domestic and wild *Suidae* (warthogs, bush pigs, etc.; ☞ SHEEP AND GOATS, ■ 5.1, Figure 371).

Ornithodoros moubata porcinus
(syn. *O. porcinus*)

Remarks: This subspecies infests the burrows of warthogs and acts as the reservoir and vector of African Swine Fever. So does *O. erraticus* (syn. *marocanus*) in Spain and *O. puertoricensis* on the Caribbean islands. *O. coriaceus* transmits the virus of epizootic bovine abortion, blue tongue and possibly African Swine Fever. *O. turicata* and *O. talaje* are vectors of Mexican and American Relapsing Fever.

Otobius megnini The spinose ear tick

Remarks: Its larval and nymphal stages are parasites of the ears of dog, sheep, horse, cattle, pig and many other domestic and wild animals. The nymphs bear numerous spine-like processes. The body colour is bluish-grey and the legs, mouth parts and sines are pale yellow. Adult ticks are not parasitic and live in cracks and crevices in walls and woodwork, under stones or under the bark of trees. *O. megnini* may severely affect the ears of its hosts. Animals become restless, do not feed well and rapidly lose condition. The affected ears become filled with masses of ticks, wax and debris and are liable to be invaded by secondary organisms. These organisms may perforate the ear drum and set up infections in the middle and inner ears and death may occur from meningitis (☞ CATTLE, ■ 5.1).

- **Tick control in swine**

A number of acaricides is available as sprays or dips. Toxaphene (chlorinated hydrocarbone) as a 0.5% spray protects against reinfestations for more than 2 weeks. Other effective acaricides include coumaphos, dioxathion and malathion and the pyrethrinoids. A 5% coumaphos dust applied to the ears effectively controls the spinose ear tick (☞ CATTLE, ■5.1).

– Mites

Sarcoptes suis Mange mite, itch mite

Location: Skin of the head, ears, shoulders, neck, legs and tail. In heavy infestations skin lesions may occur all over the body.
Hosts: Pig and wild boar
Species description: *S. suis* is a tiny mite, 0.3–0.5 mm long with a round body, blunt mouthparts and 8 stumpy legs with an unsegmented pedicel. The legs end in bell-shaped suckers (caruncles). Female mites burrow tunnels in skin and lay eggs which develop within 17 days in a cycle of incomplete metamorphosis (eggs, nymphs, adults) in adult mites. 4–5 days after mating the new generation of adult mites starts to lay eggs. The burrowing of *Sarcoptes* mites causes great irritation, itching and lesions with exudates which become crusts. Chronic skin inflammation, accompanied by proliferation of the subcutaneous connective tissue results in thickened skin that may crack and leave wounds which may become secondarily infected. In temperate zones *S. suis* mites can survive for a few weeks off the host. In dry areas the mites die within a few days after leaving the pig. *S. suis* is transmitted directly via skin contact of infested pigs.
Geographic distribution: World-wide
Symptoms: Infested pigs are restless, and continually scratch and rub. The annoyance caused by *S. suis* distracts pigs from feeding, resulting in reduced weight gain.
Significance: Sarcoptic mange is of great economic importance wherever pigs are raised.
Diagnosis: Restlessness, continuous scratching and rubbing. Crusts and barks on the skin, especially on the inside of the ears, which are inflamed and scabby. Microscopical investigation of skin scrapings, taken from the alterated skin reveals the typical mites.
Therapy: Infested animals can be washed with an acaricide or treated systemically with ivermectin (300 µg/kg, sc., 2 × at 28 days interval). It is recommended to treat all the animals of a herd at the same time. The following acaricides are effective against Sarcoptic mange: Organophosphates (coumaphos, crotoxyphos + dichlorvos, malathion, trichlorfon, diazinon, phosmet and phoxin), chlorinated hydrocarbons (lindane), permethrin and pyrethrin. Infested animals first must be washed and then treated (spray) thoroughly twice at 3-week-intervals. Washing with acaricides results in a reduction of skin lesions and symptoms but animals generally remain infested. Treatment with ivermectin seems to kill all the mites and animals are free of infestation as long as no infected pig is introduced to the treated herd.
Prophylaxis: Infested pigs should not be introduced to the herd to avoid reinfection. Elimination of predisposing factors (e.g. malnutrition, intestinal parasites and other chronic infections).
(Figures 216, 217, 220, 221, 600, 601, 602, 603)

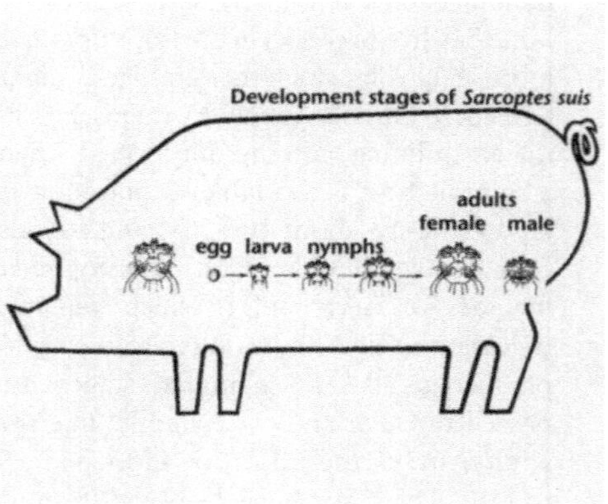

Fig. 600 Life cycle of *Sarcoptes suis* [10]

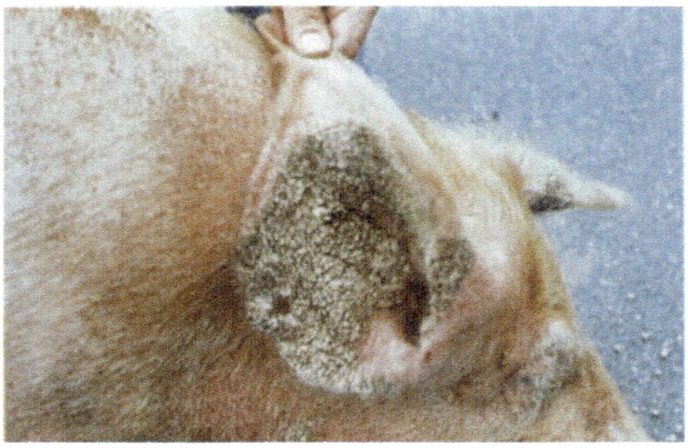

Fig. 601 Chronic *Sarcoptes suis* infestation results in thickened skin and crusts in the ears

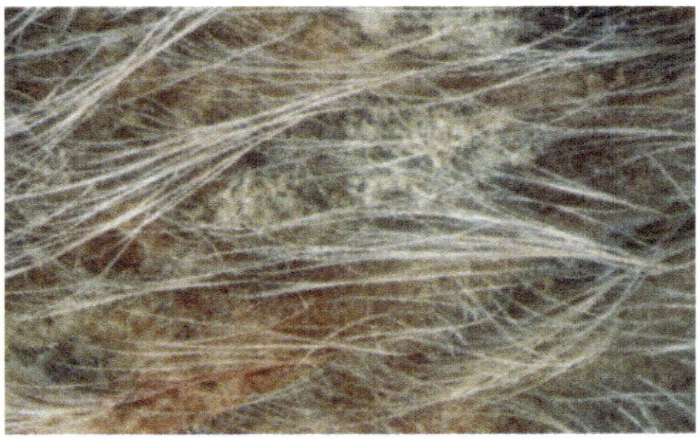

Fig. 602 Crusts and barks on the skin of a pig due to Sarcoptic mange

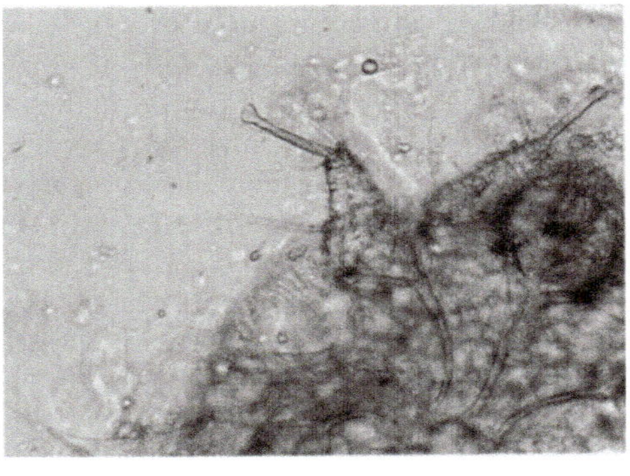

Fig. 603 Details of the *Sarcoptes suis* mite; tarsal suckers have long, unjointed pedicels

Demodex suis Follicle mite

Location: Within the hair follicles and the sebaceous glands

Hosts: Pig

Species description: The follicle mite is about 0.25 mm long, with a cigar-shaped body and 8 stubby legs. Several *Demodex* species which are morphologically identical occur on many other host species. *Demodex* spp. are regarded as distinct species and are host-specific. The entire life cycle is spent on the host and completed in about 3 weeks.

Geographic distribution: World-wide

Symptoms: Infested pigs scratch and rub, and large pustules may occur. Loss of hair, thickened and wrinkled skin may be seen.

Significance: Follicle mite in pigs cause great irritation which may develop to large abscesses. The exact prevalence of follicle mite infestations is unknown.

Diagnosis: Mites may be demonstrated by microscopic examination of deep skin scrapings.

Therapy: The same treatment may be applied to *Demodex* infestations as to *Sarcoptes suis*, although available treatments are less effective for *Demodex* infestations.

Prophylaxis: There is no effective prophylaxis because inapparent carriers may transmit the infestation.

• Insecta found on the skin

– Lice

ANOPLURA

Haematopinus suis Swine louse

Location: Lice may be found all over the body surface

Hosts: Pig

Species description: The swine louse is easily seen with the naked eye. It is 5–6 mm long. It has a long narrow head, long mouthparts adapted for sucking blood, and large claws on each of the six legs. *H. suis* is the only louse found on pigs. The pig louse spends its entire life cycle on the pig. Eggs are glued to the hairs and the development is completed in 2–3 weeks. Lice cannot survive off the host. Heavy infestations may cause severe anaemia, discomfort and annoyance. Lice are blood suckers. Self trauma of the skin as a result of the excessive scratching results in excoriation, thickening and soreness of the skin. Infested pigs are more susceptible to other diseases.

Geographic distribution: World-wide

Symptoms: Infested animals rub and scratch vigorously on any convenient object. They have a reduced weight gain. Anaemia may occur in heavy infestations.

Significance: Louse infestation is one of the most important diseases in pigs. *H. suis* transmits the swine pox virus, *Eperythrozoon suis* (☞ SWINE, ■ 2) and probably swine fever.

Diagnosis: Presence of these large insects on pigs

Therapy: A number of insecticides is recommended for use as sprays to control swine lice. Thorough applications are necessary and usually 1–2 l/mature animal are required. The following insecticides are effective against the pig louse: organophosphates (coumaphos, crotoxyphos + dichlorvos, malathion, stirofos, trichlorfon, diazinon, phosmet and phoxin), chlorinated hydrocarbons (lindane, methoxychlor) and permethrin. Dips, overall body treatment (dust) or spraying are the possible methods of treating infected animals. Fenthion (3%) pour-on is a ready-to-use formulation for lice control. Insecticidal treatment should be repeated 1 week after the initial treatment since eggs may survive. Ivermectin (300µg/kg, sc.) provides an effective lice control.

Prophylaxis: Regular treatment is required. In particular, sows should be treated prior to farrowing to prevent lice from moving onto the piglets.

(Figures 604, 605)

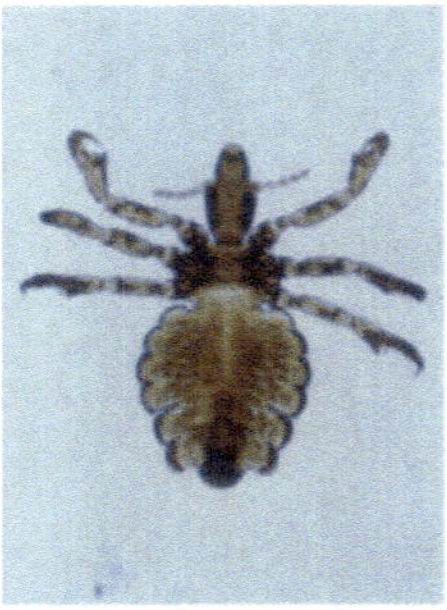

Fig. 604 *Haematopinus suis*; the swine louse (5–6 mm long) [4]

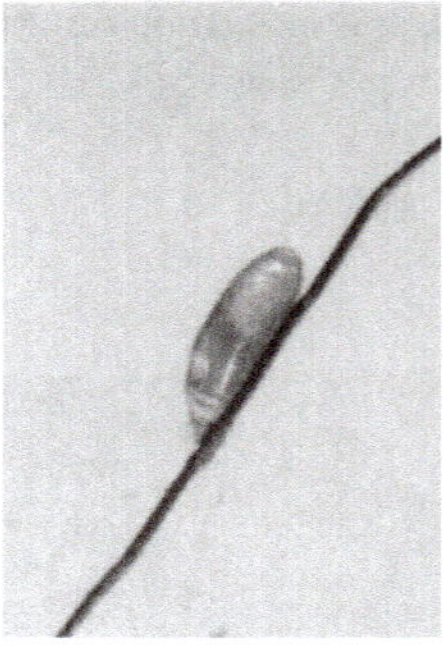

Fig. 605 *Haematopinus suis*; louse egg attached to the hair

– Fleas

SIPHONAPTERA

Remarks: Fleas are not host-specific and may attack any convenient mammal or bird for a blood meal. The two fleas most commonly found on swine are *Pulex irritans*, the human flea and *Echidnophaga gallinacea*, the stickfast flea. *Ctenocephalides felis,* the cat flea, may occasionally be found on young piglets. *Tunga penetrans*, the jigger or chigger flea occurs in Africa.

Fleas are wingless insects 2–4 mm long, have a thick brown chitinous exoskeleton and powerful legs. Female fleas lay eggs which drop off the host into the animal bedding. Larvae hatch in 2–16 days and feed on organic material such as dry blood, faeces, etc. Larvae mature in 1–2 weeks and pass through a pupal stage of varying length, depending on environmental conditions. Only the adult flea is parasitic and requires periodic blood meals. Fleas can survive for many months (*Pulex irritans* up to 2 years) in the absence of a host.

Symptoms: Restlessness, stampeding when masses attack animals. Allergic dermatitis may be seen, but should be differentiated from other similar conditions (e.g. sarcoptic mange).

Significance: Fleas are generally of minor significance in pig production, but when masses of fleas occur in sheds they may severely irritate and debilitate pigs. An allergic dermatitis, similar to that of dogs may occur in pigs, and its signs resemble those of sarcoptic mange. Fleas are also capable of transmitting Classical Swine Fever. Masses of *Tunga penetrans* were found to produce agalactia in sows (in Zaire) and death of piglets. Ovigerous females (chiggers) were localized in the teats and obstructed the ducts.

Diagnosis: It is not easy, as adult fleas may leave the host and eggs and larvae are difficult to find. The bites are similar to those of mosquitoes, lice and mites.

Therapy and Prophylaxis: These are based on locating the flea-breeding area. Both the surrounding and the animals should be sprayed with an insecticide (organophosphates, chlorinated hydrocarbons or pyrethrinoids). Infested litter, bedding and manure should be burned and removed from the pig quarters. Housing can be sprayed with malathion (2.5%) and the pigs dusted with rotenone (1%) powder, lindane (1%) or malathion (6%) powder. Insecticidal sprays combined with growth regulators (e.g. deflubenzuron, fenoxycarb, methoprene) eliminate the adult fleas and interrupt larval development of fleas for several months.

(Figures 606, 607, 608, 609, 610)

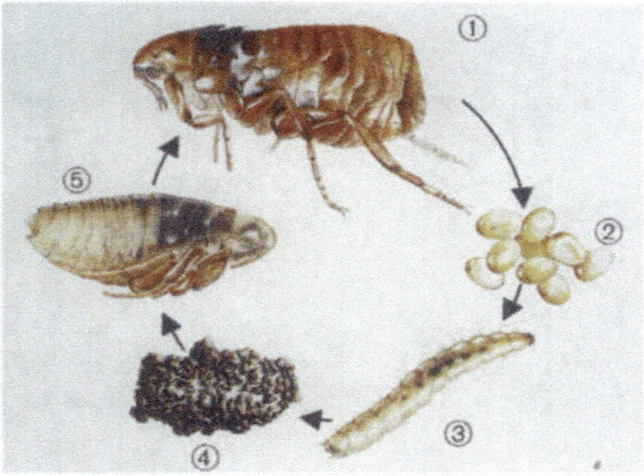

Fig. 607 Life cycle of fleas
Adult females (1) deposit around 100 eggs (2) after a blood meal, 4–12 days later spiny larvae develop (3) which develop in a pupal stage (4) from which adult fleas (5) hatch after a period varying from 3 weeks to several months [52]

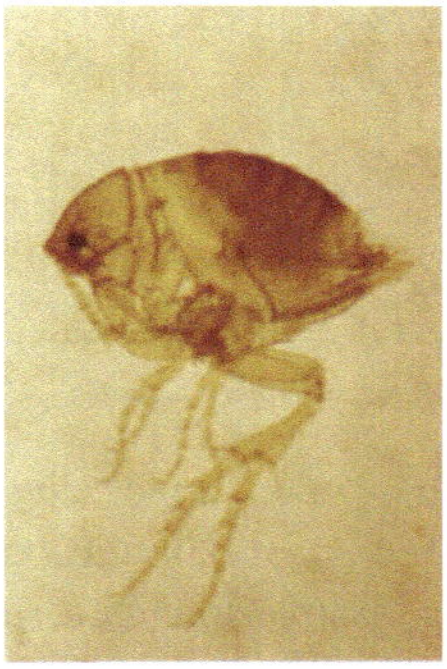

Fig. 608 *Tunga penetrans*; the jigger flea (1 mm long) [4]

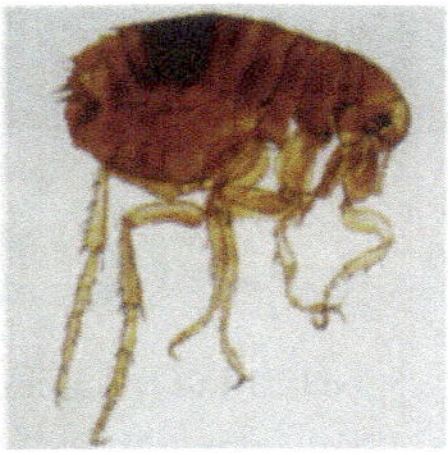

Fig. 606 *Pulex irritans*; the human flea (male: 2–2.5 mm long, female: 2–3.3 mm long) [52]

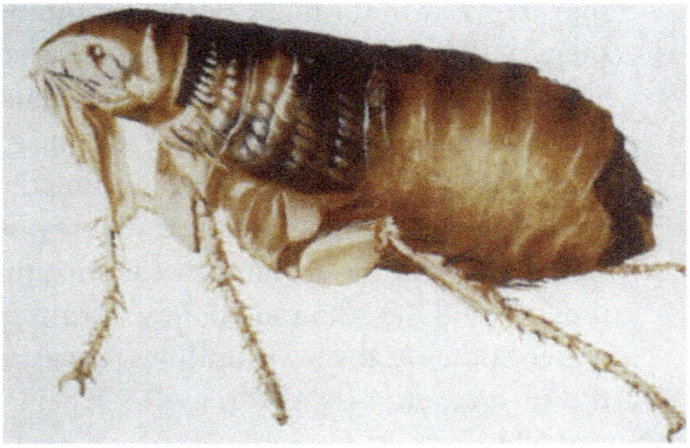

Fig. 609 *Ctenocephalides felis*; the cat flea (male: 2–2.5 mm long, female: 2–3.2 mm long) [52]

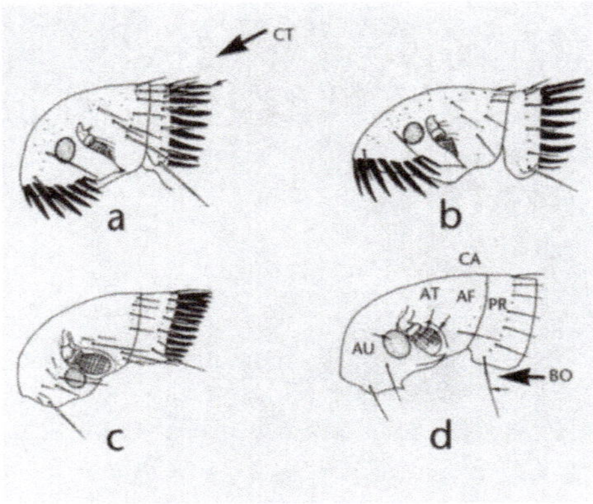

Fig. 610 Heads of some flea species which may affect domestic animals including pigs: (a) *Ctenocephalides canis*, (b) *C. felis*, (c) *Ceratophyllus gallinae* and (d) *Pulex irritans*; CT = ctenidia, AU = ommatidium, PR = pronotum, AT = antennae and CA = caput (head) [33]

– Dipterida

CULICIDAE Mosquitoes

***Aedes* spp., *Anopheles* spp., *Culex* spp. and others**

Remarks: Mosquitoes may also attack livestock, causing discomfort and irritation. Massive attacks cause skin lesions in form of raised, oedematous swellings (a few mm in diameter) on the legs and abdomen which tend to disappear within 1–2 days but this can make pigs unacceptable for marketing at that time. Control within the piggery is possible by using diazinon aerosol spray in the late evening as a regular procedure. Mosquito screening and insect repellants are also helpful in minimizing mosquito troubles in piggeries. Where possible, the breeding ground of the mosquitoes should be eliminated (e.g. draining water bodies in the surroundings, covering the surface, etc.) (☞ CATTLE, ■ 5.1.). (Figure 611)

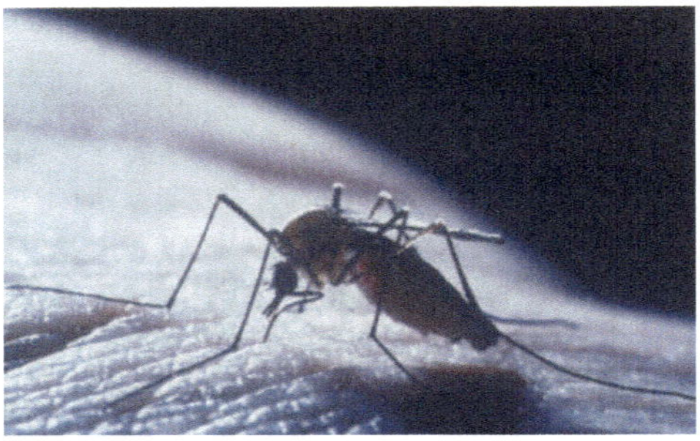

Fig. 611 *Aedes* sp. in feeding position (5–6 mm long)

Flies are of importance in pig production world-wide. They may annoy animals by their painful bite while others transmit diseases. The larvae of some species invade pre-existing skin wounds and cause myiasis which may cause severe losses.

SIMULIIDAE

***Simulium* spp.** Black flies, midges or buffalo gnats

Remarks: This small fly occurs world-wide and is found in swarms near free-running well-aerated streams. Simulids cause severe irritation to livestock, including pigs when they occur in large numbers. Bites are inflicted on all parts of the body, giving rise to vesicles which burst exposing the underlying flesh. Skin wounds caused by simulids heal very slowly. Certain areas of the tropics are rendered uninhabitable by simulids (☞ CATTLE, ■ 5.1). (Figure 612)

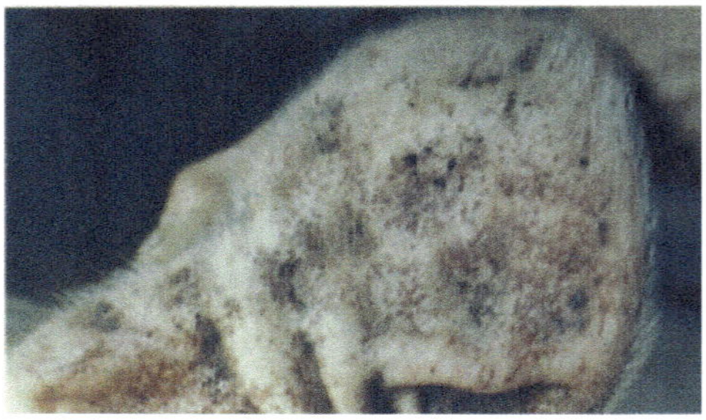

Fig. 612 Massive skin irritation on the ears of a pig due to *Simulium* sp. bites [30]

TABANIDAE Horse flies

Remarks: These robust flies have powerful wings and breed on leaves of plants in the vicinity of water. They attack pigs and other large animals by biting in different places and then taking blood, frequently on the back, head, ears and the udder of sows. They are capable of transmitting infectious diseases, including hog cholera (☞ CATTLE, ■ 5.1).

MUSCIDAE

Musca domestica The common house fly

Remarks: Apart from being attracted to organic material this non-biting muscid fly may also be attracted to wounds and other moist parts of the body. *M domestica* is known to transfer pathogenic bacteria mechanically from one wound to another. It is also capable to spread hog cholera, eggs of nematodes and cestodes, stages of protozoa and several viruses. The preferred breeding place is in the faeces of animals or in decaying organic matter (☞ CATTLE, ■ 5.1).

Stomoxys calcitrans The stable fly

Remarks: It is a biting muscid and occurs world-wide. Both sexes of this fly are bloodsuckers and can become extremely irritating pests of man and domestic animals, including pigs. Its preferred breeding ground is in decaying vegetable matter or in moist straw or hay. This fly prefers strong light rather than dark stables. It can be a carrier of hog cholera and possibly other infectious pathogens (☞ CATTLE, ■ 5.1).

GLOSSINIDAE

Glossina spp. Tsetse flies

Remarks: Both sexes suck blood and are equally capable or transmitting trypanosomes. Tsetse flies, especially in great numbers can severely annoy and debilitate pig populations (☞ CATTLE, ■ 5.1).

CALLIPHORIDAE The blow flies and their allies

Callitroga (syn. *Cochliomyia*) *hominivorax* The "American screwworm"

Remarks: *C. hominivorax* is a primary blowfly and has recently been found to occur also in North Africa. Pigs and many other domestic animals may be affected. The larvae of the screwworm fly (maggots) penetrate into pre-existing wounds and extend the lesions considerably (☞ CATTLE, ■ 5.1). The life cycle differs from other flies in that breeding takes place in the wounds of the live animal and not in carcasses.

Chrysomya bezziana: The cattle screwworm in Africa and Asia

Remarks: Cattle are commonly infested (☞ CATTLE, ■ 5.1)) but also horses, sheep, dogs, sometimes man and rarely pigs. *C. bezziana* is also a primary blowfly.

Calliphora spp.

Remarks: Blowflies of the subfamily *Calliphorinae* differ from screwworm flies in that they are secondary blowflies which deposit their eggs in necrotic wounds which have been previously struck by screwworms (primary blowflies).

The disease condition commonly referred to as "myiasis"
Most cases of myiasis occur in rainy weather. Maggots penetrate the wound tissue, which they liquefy and thus extend the lesions. There is a foul-smelling exudate and death from screwworm infections is frequent.

Prophylaxis: To prevent myiasis, surgical wounds should be avoided during the fly season (e.g. rainy season, summer) and attention should be given to skin wounds and injuries. Wounds can be protected from myiasis by the application of a wound dressing containing an insecticide (e.g. organophosphates such as coumaphos or chlorinated hydrocarbons such as lindane) and an antiseptic. After wounds are invaded by larvae they may effectively be treated with pressurized aerosols containing coumaphos, lindane or ronnel (korlan). These are very effective in killing the larvae in wounds but they will not protect the wounds from re-invasion.

- **Control of Flies**

Fly control in piggeries is a continuing exercise during the months of fly activity (summer, rainy season). Breeding of flies can be prevented if dung is removed regularly or liquefied. Manure should be removed at least weekly (complete life cycle of the housefly takes 15 days) and spread thinly on soil so that fly eggs and larvae are killed by desiccation. Destruction of flies within pig sheds can be carried out in a number of ways. Insecticides are applied in form of sprays, baits or impregnated strips. Malathion, trichlorfon, tetrachlorvinphos can be used to spray buildings (ceiling, wall spaces, etc.). Feed or water should be covered for spraying to avoid contamination. Space or aerosol sprays (foggers) used daily with knockdown insecticides are also effective and less prone to resistance development than are long-term acting pyrethroids. Baits applied to clean concrete surfaces and pen divisions are effective and usually contain insecticides such as ronnel, diazinon, malathion, trichlorfon and dichlorvos. Fly electrocutors and adhesive papers offer a non-chemical method of controlling flies. Screen doors reduce the number of flies entering the buildings where livestock is kept. Insect growth regulators (deflubenzuron, cyromazine and others) may be used as larvicides.

VII

Parasites of Poultry

CONTENTS

1 Stages in the gut and faeces

PROTOZOA

Histomonas meleagridis

Infectious enterohepatitis or "Blackhead"

Location: Caecum and liver

Hosts: Turkey, less frequently chicken and guineafowl

Species description: *H. meleagridis* is the cause of enterohepatitis or "blackhead" in turkeys but also in chicken, guineafowl and other gallinaceous birds. Chickens appear to act as reservoirs of the parasite for the main susceptible host, the turkey. The caecal worm *Heterakis gallinarum* and its eggs can carry *H. meleagridis*. Turkeys may therefore acquire *H. meleagridis* by ingestion of infected *Heterakis* eggs. Blackhead is not transmitted through the egg of the turkey.

Geographic distribution: World-wide; in Africa: East, North, parts of West and Central Africa

Symptoms: Histomonosis is mainly a disease of young turkeys. The chicken is more resistant to the infection, although it may occasionally also become infected. Symptoms are weakness, inappetence, listlessness, standing for long periods in a dejected attitude with eyes closed, dropped and ruffled feathers. Especially characteristic is the appearance of sulphur-yellow faeces. Birds become progressively weaker and death occurs within a week of first symptoms. The term "blackhead" is derived from the cyanotic (blue-violet) appearance of the comb and the wattles but it is not a constant or pathognomonic feature of *H. meleagridis* infection. The caeca and liver show marked lesions. The caeca are enlarged, thickened, intensively inflamed and the mucosa is replaced by areas of necrosis. Casts may occupy the lumen of both caeca. The liver is enlarged and shows necrotic areas (0.5–2 cm in diameter), dark brown in colour often with a yellowish perimeter. The surface of necrotic areas is almost always depressed. The caecal lesions may be confused with those due to *Eimeria tenella* but this infection is accompanied by characteristic stages of the parasite in the casts.

Significance: The disease is known to affect primarily turkeys. However, it also affects chickens around 12 weeks of age. The disease in chickens involves mainly the caeca. Mild liver lesions occur occasionally. Mortality in chickens is low but the morbidity can be high in young animals.

Diagnosis: This is often based on necropsy findings. Necrotic lesions of the liver at postmortem are pathognomonic. Detection of the parasites is difficult. The organisms are polymorphic and the morphology depends on the organ location and the stage of the disease. Histological examination of stained sections of the liver shows necrosis and colonies of the organisms. (In a few cases confirmation may be obtained by demonstration of *H. meleagridis* from direct smears of the affected liver or caeca contents).

Therapy: Dimetridazole at 0.0125% (100–200 ppm) in the feed or in the drinking water at 0.63 g/l and for prevention 0.315 g/l. Aminonitrothiazole at 0.5% is curative or at 0.01% preventive in the feed. It should be administered for 14 days.

Ronidazole at 0.0045–0.006% (60–90 ppm) in water given for 3 days prevents mortality.

Ipronidazole (50–85 ppm) is highly effective. For short-term therapy 0.025% in the

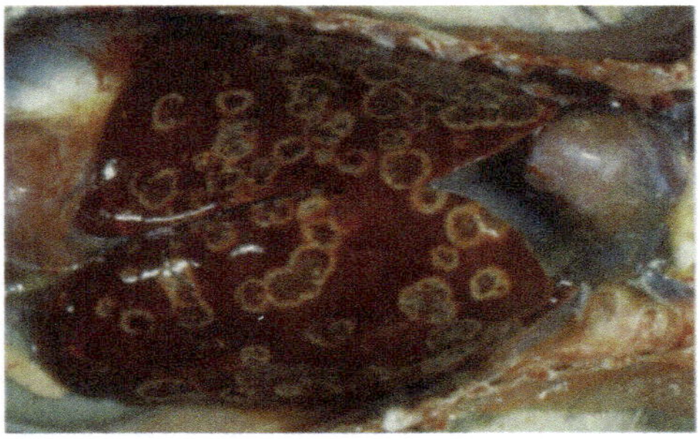

Fig. 613 *Histomonas meleagridis*; typical necrotic lesions in the liver of a turkey [53]

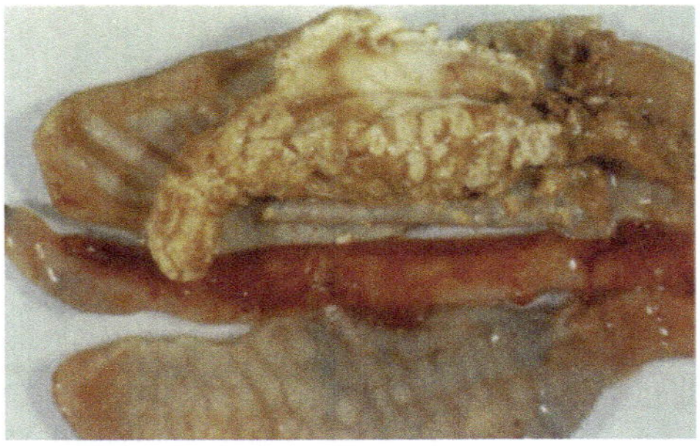

Fig. 614 *Histomonas meleagridis*; necrotic lesions in the caeca of a turkey. Casts occupy parts of the caecal lumen [53]

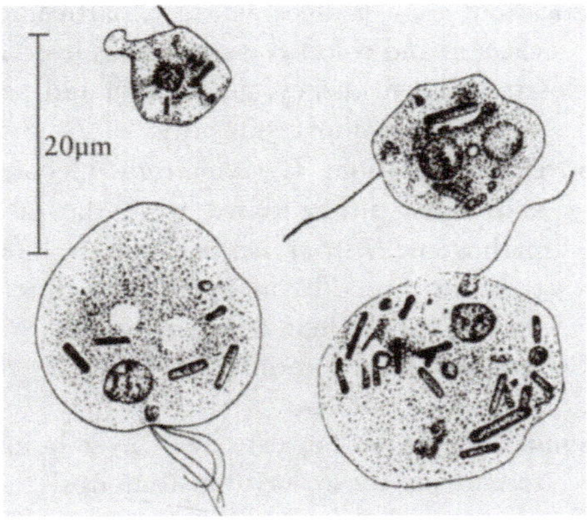

Fig. 615 Various forms of *Histomonas meleagridis* (schematic). The organism is pleomorphic, the morphology depends on the organ location, stage of infection and probably other factors [3]

feed or 0.0125% in the drinking water. For prevention continuous administration at the dosage of 0.00625% in the feed is suggested.

Prophylaxis: It is essential to avoid contact between turkeys and domestic chicken and where the two are kept on the same farm a separate area should be allocated to each of them. Regular treatment with anthelmintics to reduce *Heterakis gallinarum* infections is of benefit to reduce the overall incidence of histomonosis. Continuous administration of the above-mentioned drugs in prophylactic dosages may prevent outbreaks in populations at risk.

Remarks: *Parahistomonas wenrichi* is a non-pathogenic species resembling *H. meleagridis* and occurs in the liver. The most important difference is the size: *P. wenrichi* is about 1.5 times as large as *H. meleagridis* and has four flagella instead of one or two in the latter species.

(Figures 613, 614, 615)

Trichomonas gallinae

Location: Upper digestive tract (crop, oesophagus, pharynx, proventriculus) and liver

Hosts: Pigeon, turkey and chicken

Species description: *T. gallinae* is the cause of avian trichomonosis found particularly in pigeons but also in turkeys and chickens. It is basically a disease of young birds with inflammation and ulceration in the oesophagus, crop and proventriculus. Contaminated drinking water is the main source of infection. The incubation period is 3–14 days.

Geographic distribution: World-wide; in the Central African Republic, Zaire and southern Africa

Symptoms: Drowsiness, a pendulous crop and a foul odour from the mouth are usually observed in infected chickens. Primary lesions in the oropharyngeal mucosa, followed by parasite invasion into the pharyngeal glands and progressive penetration of the underlying tissue. Infection of the liver with multiple abscesses is considered as an important cause of death in infected birds.

In pigeons suffocation and impaired feeding due to the massive lesions is often found to be an important cause of death.

Significance: *T. gallinae* causes a condition in chicken termed "canker". Turkeys, chicken and a wide variety of wild birds are parasitized with varying degrees of pathogenicity.

Diagnosis: At necropsy, yellowish necrotic lesions are evident in the mouth, crop and oesophagus with extension to the bones of the skull, the liver and elsewhere. Parasites are usually very numerous in the mouth and crop contents. A smear from crop or oesophagus lesions will usually demonstrate the parasite. This material or the carcass should be fresh for a successful identification of the trichomonads.

Therapy: In chickens treatment is generally not indicated. In pigeons metronidazole (60 mg/kg, po.) and dimetridazole (50 mg/kg, po.) in the feed or in drinking water (0.05%, during 5–6 days) may be used to suppress the disease.

Prophylaxis: Wild pigeons and other birds play an important role in introducing the infection to domestic birds. The drinking places should therefore be shielded to prevent the introduction of infection.

(Figures 616, 617, 618)

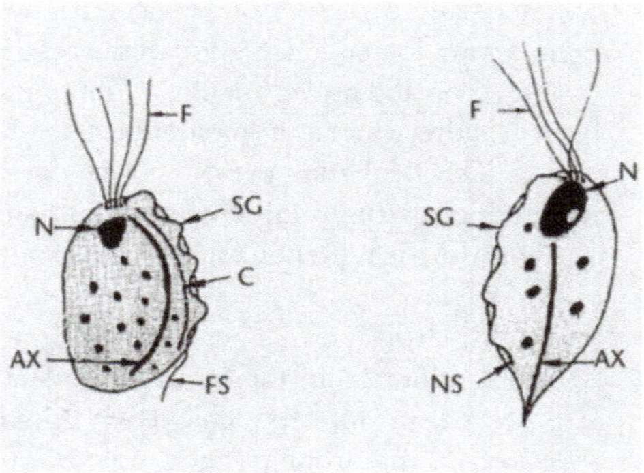

Fig. 616 *Trichomonas* species affecting birds; *T. gallinarum* (a), *T. gallinae* (b); AX = axostyl, C = costa, SG = recurrent flagellum, FS = free end of SG and F = flagellum [33]

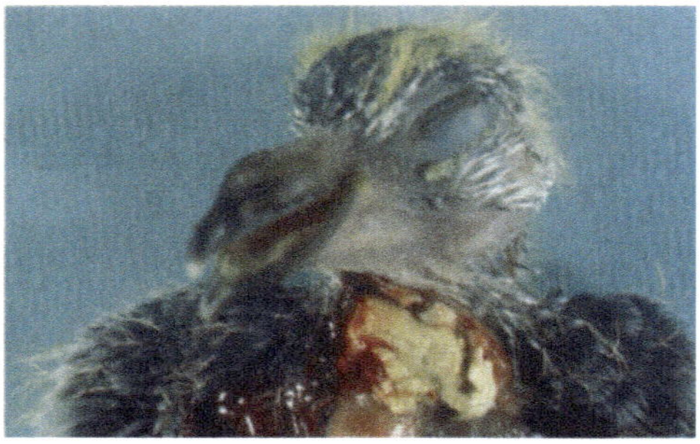

Fig. 617 *Trichomonas gallinae*; caseous necrotic material in the crop of a young pigeon [4]

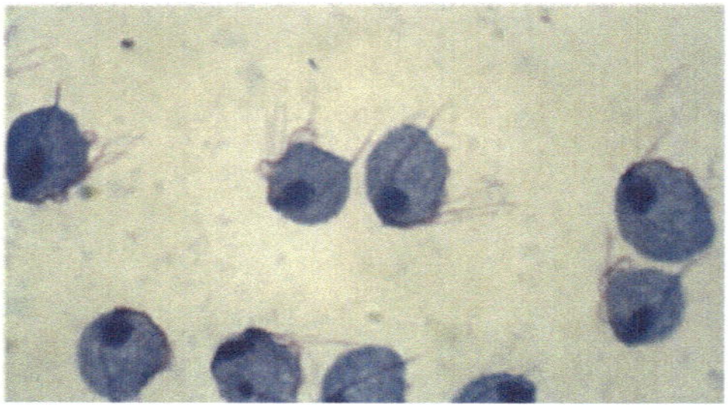

Fig. 618 *Trichomonas gallinae* (6–18 µm); stained [15]

Tetratrichomonas gallinarum

(syn. *Trichomonas gallinarum*)

Location: Lower digestive tract, particularly caecum and colon and sometimes liver

Hosts: Chicken, turkey, guineafowl and possibly other gallinaceous birds

Species description: *T. gallinarum* infections should be differentiated from the more pathogenic *Histomonas meleagridis*. Infection is acquired by ingestion of trichomonads in contaminated feed or water.

Geographic distribution: World-wide, the same as *T. gallinae*

Symptoms: Enterohepatitis with liver lesions resembling those due to histomonosis.

Significance: This is a common parasite which probably cannot cause disease by itself, although infected birds have been reported to show blackhead-like lesions of the Caecum and liver. Often a watery, slimy inflammation of the caecum is observed.

Diagnosis: This is based on the demonstration of the organisms (up to 8 µm) in smears of the large intestinal mucosa.
Therapy: ☞ *T. gallinae*
Prophylaxis: ☞ *T. gallinae*

- **Coccidiosis in Chicken**

Coccidiosis in chicken is, following bacterial diseases, the second largest problem worldwide, wherever poultry is reared in crowded conditions. The following characteristics of Coccidia may be responsible for their great significance: short life cycle (5–7 days); no intermediate host is required and *Eimeria* spp. have a very high reproductive capacity.

In chickens six different species are important:

Eimeria tenella

It is very pathogenic, causes bloody caecal coccidiosis and often mortality.

Eimeria necatrix

It is very pathogenic, causes bloody intestinal coccidiosis and often mortality.

Eimeria maxima

It can be responsible for high morbidity and sometimes high mortality. It often causes subclinical coccidiosis associated with marked weight loss.

Eimeria acervulina

It is even less pathogenic than maxima, but reduces weight gain and feed conversion and impairs absorption of nutrients and pigments (subclinical coccidiosis).

Eimeria mitis

It is difficult to diagnose; in case of heavy infections, symptoms like *E. acervulina*.

Eimeria brunetti

It may be very pathogenic, causes weight loss and mortality. Difficult to diagnose because of the indistinct lesions in the lower intestinal tract. Sometimes necrosis in the lower small intestine and the large intestine.

- **General features of *Eimeria* spp. in chicken**

Species description: The life cycle of all *Eimeria* spp. involves two or more generations of an asexual development known as schizogony, followed by a sexual phase termed gametogony which results in the formation of oocysts. Oocysts are excreted in the faeces and become infective in the litter only after sporulation during which sporozoites are produced. Some *Eimeria* spp. cause clinical coccidiosis (e.g. *E. tenella*, *E. necatrix*), associated with bloody diarrhoea, weakness and death while other species cause subclinical coccidiosis (e.g. *E. maxima*, *E. acervulina*). The overall losses due to subclinical infections are enormous and result in markedly reduced production (growth and egg production). Immunosuppressive diseases may act in concert with coccidiosis to produce a more severe disease. Marek's disease may interfere with immunity to coccidiosis, and infectious bursal disease may exacerbate coccidiosis, placing a heavier burden on anticoccidial drugs.
Geographic distribution: World-wide
Diagnosis: This is based on both clinical observations and laboratory investigations. An outbreak of coccidiosis is often associated with the following signs: signs of illness in the flock, abnormal faeces, birds that have a moribund appearance with lethargy, ruffled feathers and loss of skin pigmentations. Coccidiosis may be followed by diarrhoea which may be bloody in case of *E. tenella* and *E. necatrix* or contain mucus in case of *E. acervulina* or *E. maxima*. Oocyst counting may contribute additional infor-

mation about the overall herd situation but this cannot be used alone to identify outbreaks or species involved in outbreaks. Coccidiosis can best be diagnosed from birds killed for immediate necropsy. Many stages of Coccidia can be seen in smears taken from suspected intestinal lesions. Mucosal scrapings may be diluted with saline on a slide, covered with a coverslip and then examined with a microscope. Oocysts or macrogametes are most easily seen, but in many cases the lesions are caused by maturing schizonts. The presence of clusters of large schizonts in the midgut area is pathognomonic for *E. necatrix*, while a similar finding in the caecum indicates *E. tenella*.

In warm, moist areas the development of Coccidia is even more facilitated. Coccidiosis in chickens is exclusively represented by species of the genus *Eimeria*. For simplicity reasons the *Eimeria* infections found in domestic fowls are distinguished as 1) those causing marked haemorrhage in the intestinal tract and 2) those without marked haemorrhagic lesions.

(Figures 619, 620, 621)

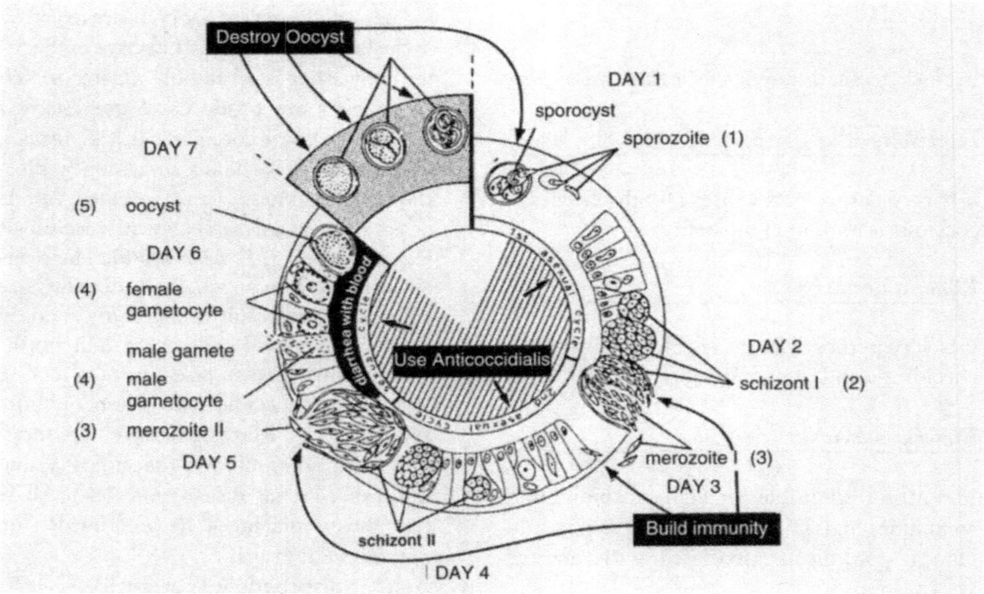

Fig. 619 Coccidia have a very definite pattern of development. There are two or more generations of an asexual development known as schizogony, followed by a sexual phase (gametogony) which results in the formation of oocysts. Oocysts are excreted in the faeces and become infective in the litter only after sporulation during which sporozoites are produced [54]

Development stages of coccidia: (1) sporozoites (motile infective stages), (2) schizonts (multiplying asexual reproductive stage), (3) merozoites (lst to 3rd-generation motile infective stage), (4) gametocytes (sexual reproductive stages, female non-motile macrogametocyte and male motile microgametocyte) and (5) oocysts (zygotes formed by the sexual union of gametocytes)

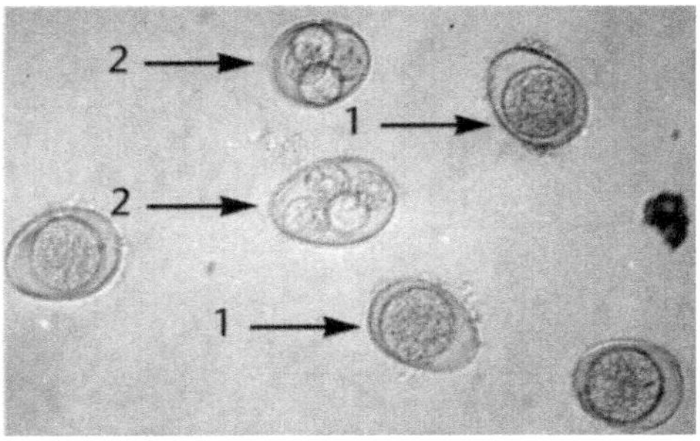

Fig. 620 Unsporulated (1) and sporulated (2) oocysts of *Eimeria maxima* (30 × 20 µm) [15]

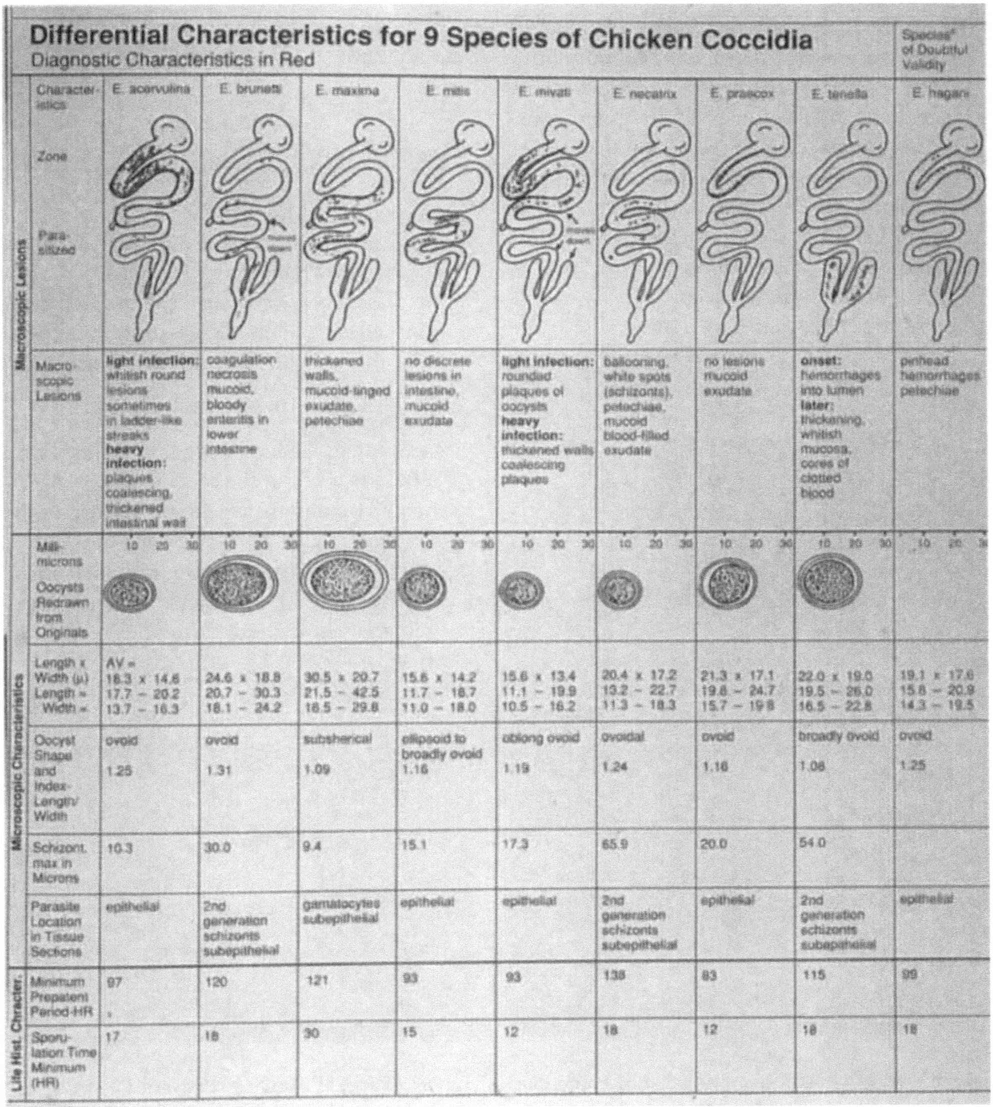

Differential Characteristics for 9 Species of Chicken Coccidia
Diagnostic Characteristics in Red

	Characteristics	E. acervulina	E. brunetti	E. maxima	E. mitis	E. mivati	E. necatrix	E. praecox	E. tenella	Species* of Doubtful Validity: E. hagani
Macroscopic Lesions	Zone Parasitized									
	Macroscopic Lesions	**light infection:** whitish round lesions sometimes in ladder-like streaks **heavy infection:** plaques coalescing, thickened intestinal wall	coagulation necrosis mucoid, bloody enteritis in lower intestine	thickened walls, mucoid-tinged exudate, petechiae	no discrete lesions in intestine, mucoid exudate	**light infection:** rounded plaques of oocysts **heavy infection:** thickened walls coalescing plaques	ballooning, white spots (schizonts), petechiae, mucoid blood-filled exudate	no lesions mucoid exudate	**onset:** hemorrhages into lumen **later:** thickening, whitish mucosa, cores of clotted blood	pinhead hemorrhages petechiae
Microscopic Characteristics	Millimicrons / Oocysts Redrawn from Originals	10 20 30	10 20 30	10 20 30	10 20 30	10 20 30	10 20 30	10 20 30	10 20 30	10 20 30
	Length x Width (µ) Length = Width =	AV = 18.3 x 14.6 17.7 – 20.2 13.7 – 16.3	24.6 x 18.8 20.7 – 30.3 18.1 – 24.2	30.5 x 20.7 21.5 – 42.5 16.5 – 29.8	15.6 x 14.2 11.7 – 18.7 11.0 – 18.0	15.6 x 13.4 11.1 – 19.9 10.5 – 16.2	20.4 x 17.2 13.2 – 22.7 11.3 – 18.3	21.3 x 17.1 19.8 – 24.7 15.7 – 19.8	22.0 x 19.0 19.5 – 26.0 16.5 – 22.8	19.1 x 17.6 15.8 – 20.9 14.3 – 19.5
	Oocyst Shape and Index-Length/Width	ovoid 1.25	ovoid 1.31	subsherical 1.09	ellipsoid to broadly ovoid 1.16	oblong ovoid 1.19	ovoidal 1.24	ovoid 1.16	broadly ovoid 1.08	ovoid 1.25
	Schizont, max in Microns	10.3	30.0	9.4	15.1	17.3	65.9	20.0	54.0	
	Parasite Location in Tissue Sections	epithelial	2nd generation schizonts subepithelial	gamatocytes subepithelial	epithelial	epithelial	2nd generation schizonts subepithelial	epithelial	2nd generation schizonts subepithelial	epithelial
Life Hist. Chracter.	Minimum Prepatent Period HR	97	120	121	93	93	138	83	115	99
	Sporulation Time Minimum (HR)	17	18	30	15	12	18	12	18	18

Fig. 621 Differential characteristics for nine *Eimeria* species of chicken [54]

- **Coccidiosis with marked haemorrhage**

Eimeria tenella

Location: Caecum

Significance: *E. tenella* is highly pathogenic. This acute infection occurs most commonly in young chicks. Heavy infections are characterized by the presence of blood in the droppings and by high morbidity and mortality.

Diagnosis: At postmortem in the acute phase, the caecum are distended by blood following erosion of the mucosa. Large second-generation schizonts and free merozoites can be detected in smears from the caecum mucosa. Caecal cores are composed of necrotic debris, gametocytes and oocysts may be found during the recovery period of the host. Acute deaths without the presence of oocysts may occur.

(Figures 622, 623, 624)

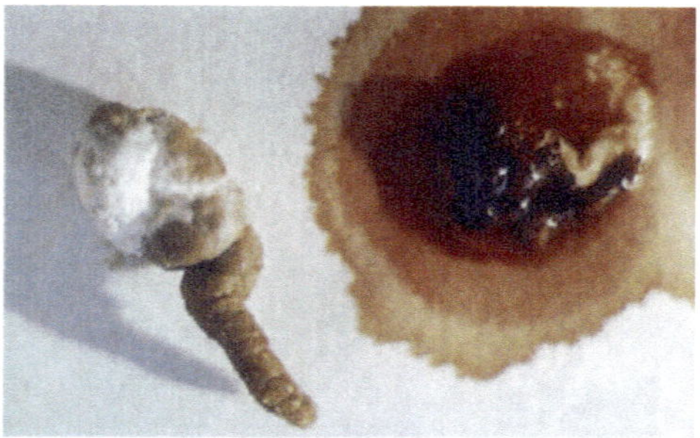

Fig. 622 Bloody faeces 4–6 days after infection with *Eimeria tenella* (right) and normal faeces (left) [54]

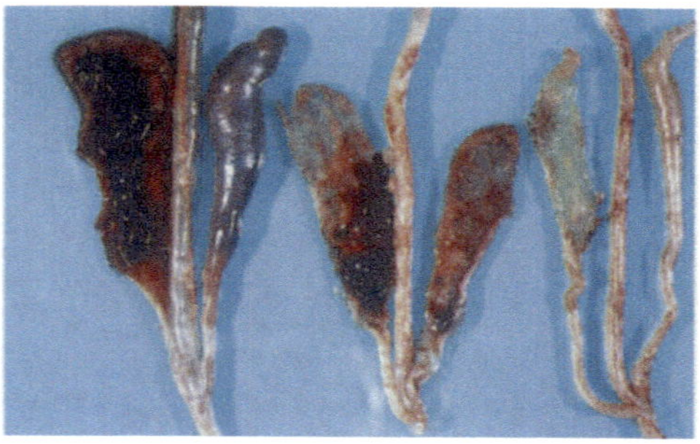

Fig. 623 Caeca of chicken, distended by blood due to *Eimeria tenella* infection (left and middle) and normal caecum (right) [53]

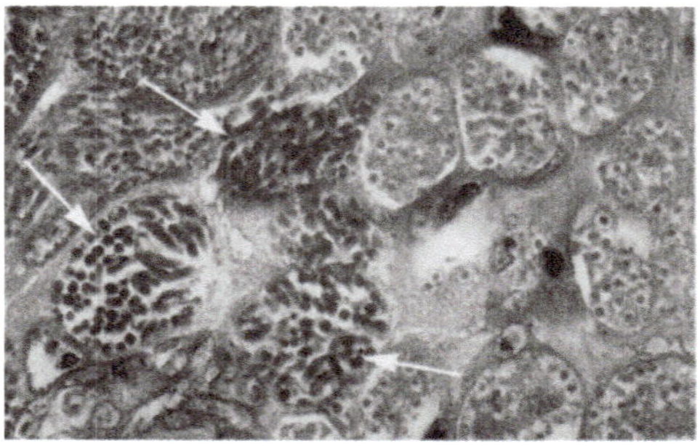

Fig. 624 Schizonts of *Eimeria tenella* in caecal mucosa (arrows) (60–70 μm in diameter) [54]

Eimeria necatrix

Location: Small intestine

Significance: *E. necatrix* is a highly pathogenic species which may cause heavy mortality. Lesions are confined to the small intestine where haemorrhage accompanies the maturation of the deeply penetrating schizonts.

Diagnosis: White spots (colonies of schizonts) are often visible in the intestinal wall. Oocysts occur in the caecum where macroscopic lesions are absent, an important distinction between this species and the *E. tenella*. It may be distinguished from *E. maxima* by the presence of very large schizonts in scrapings from the small intestine.

(Figure 625, 626)

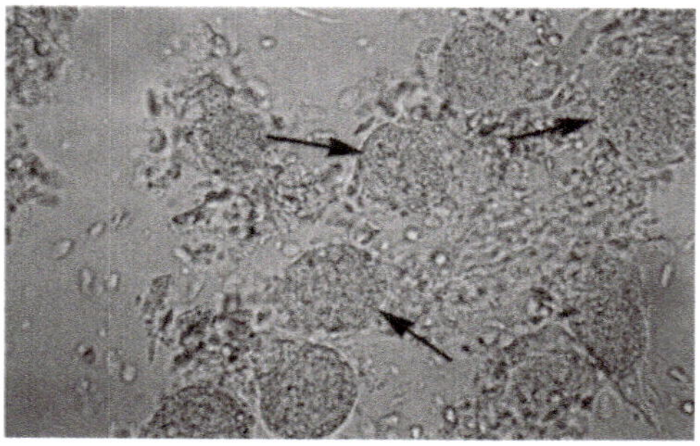

Fig. 625 Large schizonts (arrows) of *Eimeria necatrix* in the scraping of small intestinal mucosa (60–70 μm in diameter) [53]

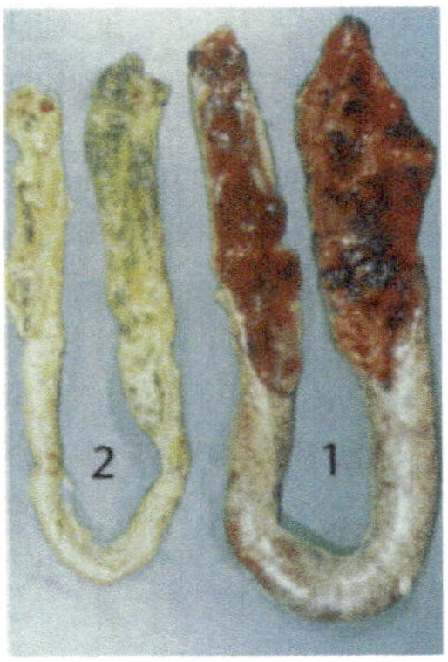

Fig. 626 *Eimeria necatrix* causes haemorrhage and necrosis in the mucosa of the small intestine (1); normal intestine (2) [53]

- **Coccidiosis without marked haemorrhage**

Eimeria maxima

Location: Mid-small intestine

Significance: *E. maxima* can be responsible for high morbidity and sometimes high mortality. *E. maxima* often causes subclinical coccidiosis associated with marked weight loss. Lesions occur most frequently in the mid-small intestine although the whole of the small intestine may be involved.

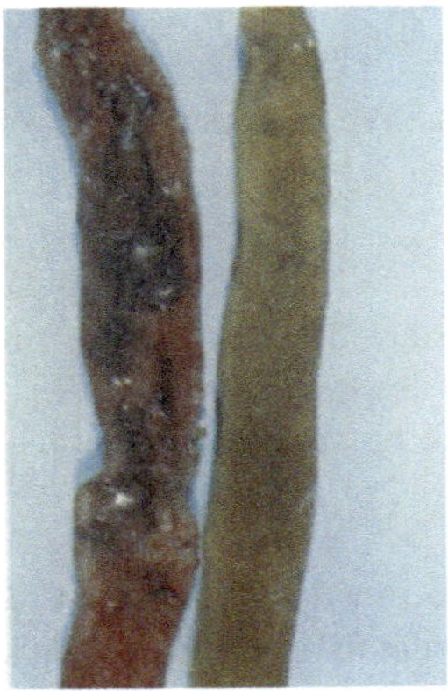

Fig. 627 Mucoid exudate and haemorrhage in the mid small intestine due to *Eimeria maxima* (left); normal intestine (right) [53]

Diagnosis: Typically the intestine appears thickened with pink mucoid exudate. Haemorrhage may be pronounced in heavy infections. Gametocytes or large yellowish oocysts may be seen in smears from the intestinal mucosa.

(Figure 627)

Eimeria brunetti

Location: Lower small intestine, caecum

Significance: The pathogenicity of this species is high. In heavy infections numerous small haemorrhages may occur in the mucosa with blood-stained exudates.

Diagnosis: This is difficult due to the indistinct lesions in the lower intestinal tract. Yellowish-white caseous material may be found in the lumen of the lower intestine and rectum. Rounded oocysts with a variable size occur throughout the intestine. Stained smears from the intestinal mucosa should be made to differentiate from *Clostridium perfringens* infections.

The following species are regarded as less pathogenic although they might cause weight loss in heavy or concomitant infections:

Eimeria mivati

Remarks: This species occurs in the upper small intestine. Heavy infections may produce mortalities of up to 10%. Light infections cause weight loss.

Eimeria acervulina

Remarks: This species occurs in the upper small intestine and is not very pathogenic but reduces weight gain and feed conversion and impairs the absorption of nutrients. It generally causes a subclinical coccidiosis.

(Figure 628, 629)

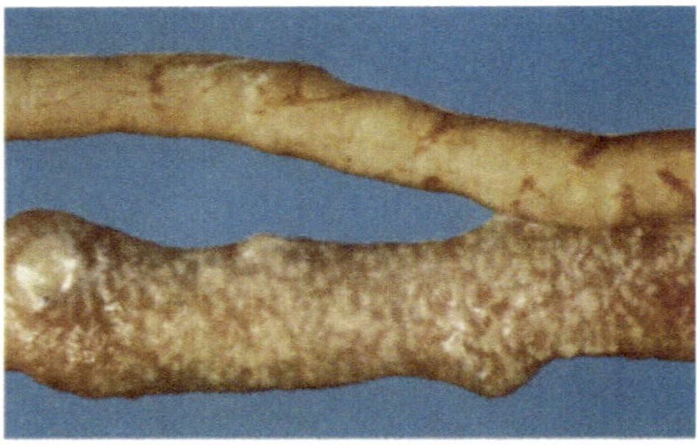

Fig. 628 *Eimeria acervulina* infection cause typical striation and thickening of the mucosa [55]

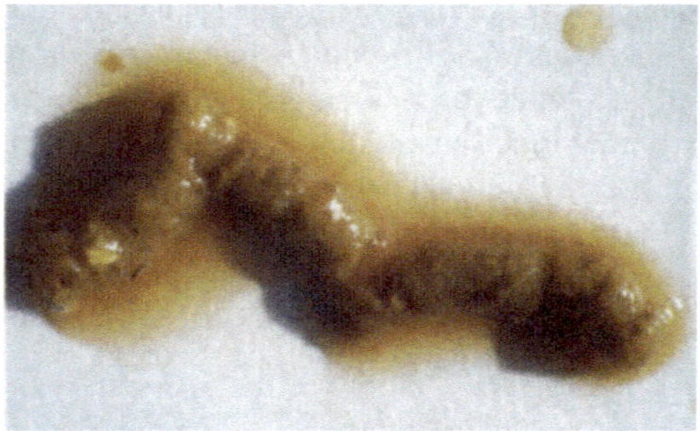

Fig. 629 Mucoid faeces due to *Eimeria acervulina*, *Eimeria mivati* and *E. maxima* [54]

Eimeria mitis

Remarks: This species is difficult to diagnose and heavy infections cause lesions similar to those of *E. acervulina.*

Eimeria praecox

Remarks: This species occurs in the upper third of the small intestine. It is of low pathogenicity.

- **Control of Coccidiosis**

In the past chemotherapy was used to treat outbreaks after signs of infection and losses were apparent. Soon the concept of preventive medication emerged with the realization that most of the damage is done once signs of coccidiosis occur. Today, almost all broiler flocks in intensive poultry systems receive preventive medication, and treatment is used as a last resort.

If layers are kept permanently in battery cages, the replacement flocks can be raised under permanent coccidiostatica application. If layers are kept in systems with direct contact to faeces, the coccidiostatica application to the replacement flocks should be stopped at the 11th–13th week of age, in order to achieve immunization. The contact to the contaminated faeces should then be maintained.

Therapy: Sulfachlorpyrazine (300 ppm in drinking water), sulfadimethoxine combined with ormetoprine (125 and 75 ppm in feed), sulfaquinoxaline combined with pyrimethamine (14 ppm and 45 ppm, in drinking water), nicarbazine (125 ppm in feed), amprolium (125 ppm in feed or via drinking water), amprolium combined with ethopabate (125 and 8 ppm via drinking water) or toltrazuril (25–75 ppm via drinking water during two consecutive days). Other combinations may also be used. Therapy should be continued until the symptoms have disappeared (3–6 days).

Prophylaxis: Anticoccidial drugs represent a wide variety of chemicals including one group of antibiotics (ionophores). The demand on control of coccidia in broilers, turkeys and replacement pullets is very different.

Different programs have been developed and are as follows:

Continuous feeding

A common program with 1 drug only, which is mainly used where coccidiosis one does not seem to be a major problem.

Shuttle programs

One drug is used in the starter feed (2–3 weeks) and another in the grower feed. Several shuttle programs using various drugs are practiced throughout the world. The drugs used should be complementary in spectrum of activity.

Rotation programs

In these programs the same anticoccidial is used for several grow outs, and then replaced by another.

There are other programs which may also be useful in practice. General rules cannot be made for such a choice but it is necessary to change products every now and then. A wide variety of anticoccidials is currently available (Tables 23–25). Depending on the product used, the withdrawal periods and the indications should be strictly considered. Anticoccidials should not be administered to laying hens. Toltrazuril (7 mg/kg, po.) is a modern anticoccidial and not related to any other drug currently in use. It is effective against all the pathogenic *Eimeria* spp. of chicken and may be used for both therapy and prophylaxis of coccidiosis. Since toltrazuril does not interfere with the development of immunity it may be used for prevention of coccidiosis in replacement chickens. A strategic use every 3 to 4 weeks during rearing will provide reliable protection. Usually a 2-day treatment every 3 to 4 weeks up to 18 weeks of age will be sufficient. It is well established that outbreaks of coccidiosis are often related to stress (e.g. vaccination, debeaking, handling of birds, heat stress, change of diet). In all these cases a strategic administration of toltrazuril at these times will protect birds from coccidiosis.

Note: Even at recommended dosage anticoccidials demonstrate side effects such as depressed growth, toxicity in layers, interactions with minerals, immunosuppression. It is therefore essential to concentrate anticoccidial drugs correctly. Coccidial resistance has been reported with almost all commercially available drugs. Resistance of Coccidia against drugs may be expressed by decreasing weight gains, reduced utilization of nutrients and rather rarely by clinical coccidiosis and mortality.

(Tables 23, 24, 25)

Table 23 Therapeutic anticoccidial drugs, applied in drinking water

Generic names	Dosage (mg/kg body weight) in drinking water
Amprolium (1) + Ethopabate (2)	0,012-0,024% (1) + 0,0076-0,0152% (2) during 5-7 days
Diaverdin (1) + Sulfaquinoxaline (2)	0,00192% (1) + 0,00768% (2) during 3 days, 2 days break, and 3 days treatment again
Pyrimethamin (1) + Sulfaquinoxaline (2)	0,0015% (1) + 0,0045% (2) during 6 days or during 3 days, 2 days break, and 3 days treatment again
Sulfaclozin.natric.monohydrate	0,03% for 3 days, 2-3 days break, 3 days treatment or treatment on day 1.-3.-5.-7. and 9 or 1.-2.-5.-6. and 9.

Table 24 Combined prophylactic anticoccidial drugs for poultry

Generic names	Dosage (mg/kg) in feed
Amprolium (1) +	250-400(1) +
Ethopabate (2)= Acetaminoethoxy-methylbenzoat	20-32 (2)
Metichlorpindol (1), Methylbenzoquat (2)	100 (1) + 8,35 (2)
25% Aklomide (1) + 20% Sulfanitran (2)	250 (1) + 200 (2)
Amprolium (1) + Sulfaquinoxaline (2) + Ethopabate (3)	80 (1), + 60 (2) + 5(3)
Pancoccin (1) + Pyrimethamin (2)	145 (1) + 5 (2)
Sulfadimethoxine (1) + Ormetoprim (2)	125 (1) + 75 (2)
Bithionol (1) + Methiotriaziamin (2)	500 (1) + 100 (2)
Nitromide (1) + Sulfanitran (2) + Roxarsone (3)	250 (1) + 300 (2) + 50 (3)

Table 25 Prophylactic anticoccidial drugs for poultry (applied in feed)

Generic names	Dosage (mg/kg) in feed
Aklomide (Chloro-Nitrobenzamid)	250
Amprolium (Amino-propyl-pyridinyl-methyl-picoloniumchlorid)	125-250
Arprinocid (9-(2-chloro-6-fluorobenzyl)-adenin)	70
Arsanilic acid or sodium-arsanilate	400
Beclotiamin (drug closly related to Amprolium)	40-125
Buqinolate (Alkyl-hydroxy-isobutoxy-chinolincarboxyl)	82,5
Clopidol; Meticlorpindol; Clopindol (Dichlor-dimethyl-pyridinol)	125-250
Decoquinate (Hydroxychinolin-derivate)	30
Diclazuril (2,6 dichloro-a (4-chlorophenyl)-4-(4,5-dihydro-3,5 dioxo-1,2,4-triazin-2 (3H)-yl)benzenacetonitril	1
Dinitrotolmid (Dinitro-ortho-toluamid)	40-250
Furazolidone (Nitrofuraldehyd-amino-oxazolidon)	55
Glycarbylamid (Imidazolcarboxamid)	30
Halofuginone (extract from *Dichroa febrifuga*)	3
Lasolocid (from *Streptomyces lasaloliensis*)	75-125
Madurimicin (from Actinomadura yumaensis)	5
Methylbenzoquat (Methyl-benzyloxy-butyl-dihydroxychinolin carboxylat	10-30
Monensin (from *Streptomyces cinnamonensis*)	100-120
Narasin (from *Streptomyces aureofaciens*)	60-70
Nicarbazin (Dinitrocarbanil-hydroxi-dimethyl-pyrimidin)	100-200
Nihydrazon (Nitrofuraldehyd-acetylhydrazon)	110
Nitrofurazone (Nitro-furfurylidin-semicarbazon)	55
Nitromide (Nitrobenzamid)	250
Nitrophenid (Dinitrophenyl-disulfid)	125
Robenidine (Chlorobenzyl-amino-guanidin)	33
Roxarsone (Hydroxy-nitrobenzen-arson-acid)	5
Salinomycin (from *Streptomyces albus*)	50-70

Cryptosporidium spp. (*C. baileyi* and *C. meleagridis*)

Location: Epithelial cells of respiratory and gastrointestinal tract and bursa. Predilection sites are caecum, posterior parts of colon, and bursa.

Hosts: *C. baileyi* occurs in chicken and *C. meleagridis* in fowls.

Species description: In chicken and turkeys *Cryptosporidium* spp. are primary pathogens that can produce respiratory and intestinal disease resulting in morbidity and mortality. The life cycle differs from that of *Eimeria* spp. in that the intracellular stages are confined to the microvillus region of the host cell and the oocysts which sporulate within the host cell are infective when released in the faeces. Another feature of *Cryptosporidium* spp. is the establishment of infections in the mucosal epithelium of a variety of organs. For example, *C. baileyi* can infect the cloaca, bursa of Fabricius, the upper and lower respiratory tracts and the eye lids.

Geographic distribution: World-wide

Symptoms: Disease associated with enteric infection is rare. By contrast, respiratory infections may produce a variety of clinical signs, depending on the particular sites involved. There may be inflammation of the air sacs, pneumonia, sinusitis or conjunctivitis with coughing, dyspnoea, nasal discharges and mortality.

Significance: Cryptosporidia are often found in healthy birds, although reduced weight gain and severe clinical signs were found following infection of the respiratory tract. An interaction between Cryptosporidia and viral infections (Marek, Turkey Viral Hepatitis) has repeatedly been reported in the sense that one infection may favour the other.

Diagnosis: This is done by demonstration of oocysts in the faeces (☞ CATTLE, 1) or by histological examination of infected tissue at necropsy. Smears of the tracheal mucosa may reveal the parasites after staining with carbol-fuchsin. An ELISA test may be used for epidemiological studies.

Therapy: There is no specific therapy. Cryptosporidia are unsusceptible to all tried anticoccidial agents.

Prophylaxis: This is based on strict disinfection of the chicken quarters. *Cryptosporidium* oocysts are very resistant to most of chemical agents, except ammonia, 10% formalin or hydrogen peroxide (☞ CATTLE, 1).

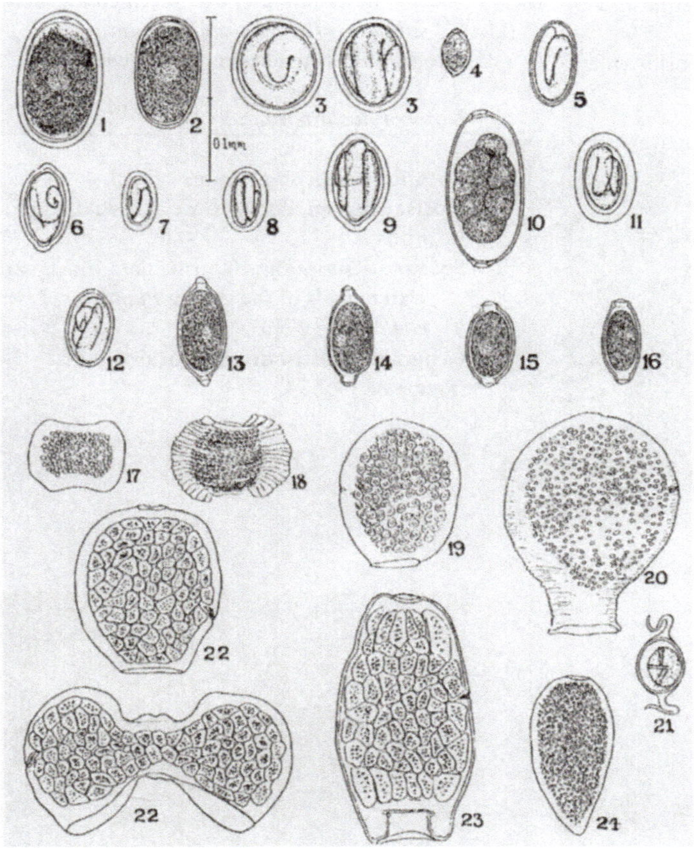

Fig. 630
Helminth eggs and segments of cestodes found in chicken [3]

1 *Ascaridia galli*
2 *Heterakis gallinarum*
3 *Subulura brumpti*
4 *Prosthogonimus* sp.
5 *Strongyloides avium*
6 *Tetrameres americana*
7 *Acuaria spiralis*
8 *Acuaria hamulosa*
9 *Gongylonema ingluvicola*
10 *Syngamus trachea*
11 *Hartertia gallinarum*
12 *Oxyspirura mansoni*
13 *Capillaria annulata*
14 *Capillaria retusa*
15 *Capillaria columbae*
16 *Capillaria longicollis*

Ripe segments of tapeworms (not drawn to scale)
17 *Amaebotaenia sphenoides*, 18 *Hymenolepis carioca*, 19 *Raillietina cesticillus*, 20 *Choanotaenia infundibulum*, 21 single egg of *C. infundibulum*, 22 *Raillietina echinobothrida* and 23 *R. tetragona*

HELMINTHS

(Figure 630, ☞ p. 349)

- Trematoda eggs found in the faeces and adult trematodes living in the gastrointestinal tract

Echinostoma revolutum

Location: Rectum, caecum
Hosts: Duck, goose and other water birds and rarely chicken and turkey
Species description: The first intermediate host can be one of a variety of species of water snails. The second intermediate host can be the same or another water snail species or tadpoles of *Rana esculenta* and of other frogs.
Geographic distribution: World-wide
(Figure 631, 632)

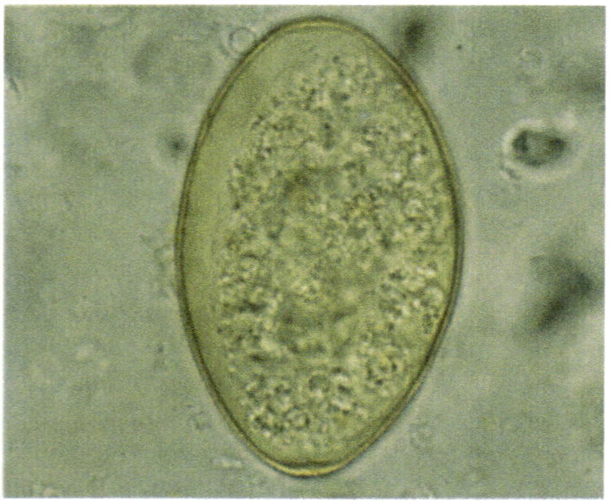

Fig. 631 Egg of *Echinostoma* sp. (97–126 × 60–70 µm) [4]

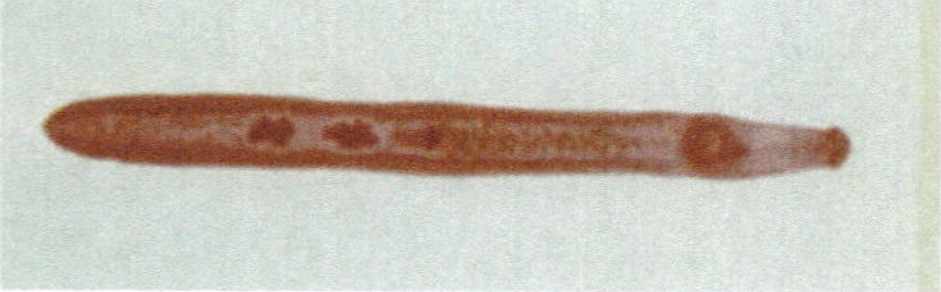

Fig. 632 *Echinostoma* sp., stained (10–22 × 2 mm) [4]

Echinoparyphium recurvatum

Location: Small intestine, especially duodenum
Hosts: Duck, goose, rarely chicken, pigeon and turkey
Species description: Two intermediate hosts similar to *Echinostoma revolutum*
Geographic distribution: World-wide, especially Asia, North Africa

Hypoderaeum conoideum

Location: Posterior part of the small intestine
Hosts: Duck, goose and other water birds, chicken, turkey and pigeon
Species description: Two intermediate hosts similar to *Echinostoma revolutum*
Geographic distribution: World-wide

Notocotylus attenuatus

Location: Caecum, rectum
Hosts: Chicken, duck, goose and wild aquatic birds
Species description: Intermediate hosts are water snails of the genera *Planorbis*, *Lymnaea* and *Bulinus*.
Geographic distribution: World-wide
(Figures 633, 634)

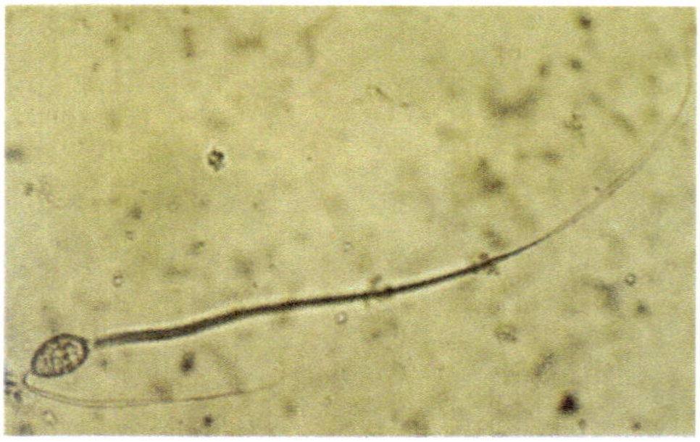

Fig. 633 Egg of *Notocotylus attenuatus* (20 × 10 µm) with two long filaments (up to 200 µm long) [11]

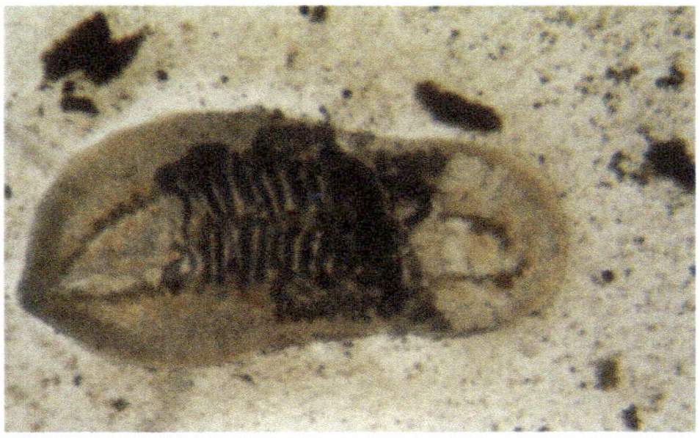

Fig. 634 *Notocotylus attenuatus* (2–5 × 0.6–1.4 mm) [53]

Catatropis verrucosa

Location: Caecum

Hosts: Chicken, duck, goose and wild aquatic birds

Species description: Intermediate hosts are water snails (Planorbis). Cercariae leave the snail and encyst on water plants which are ingested by the final host.

Geographic distribution: World-wide (Figure 635)

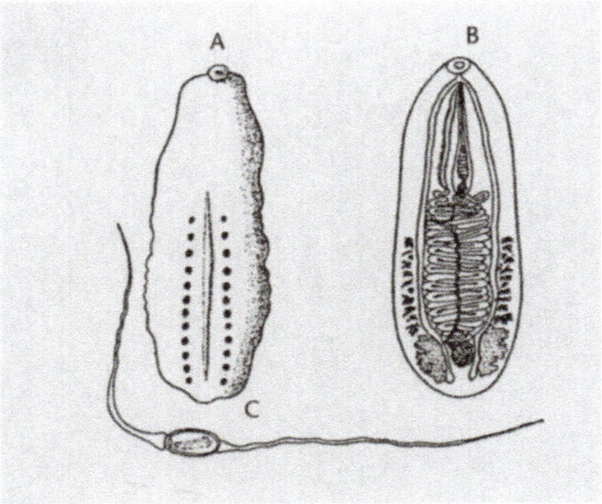

Fig. 635 *Catatropis verrucosa* (1–6 × 0.75– 2 mm); ventral view (A), dorsal view (B); egg (18–28 µm long; (C) with two filaments (160–200 µm long) [9]

Postharmostomum commutatum (syn. *P. gallinarum*)

Location: Caecum

Hosts: Chicken, pheasant, turkey, pigeon and guinea-fowl

Species description: First intermediate hosts are snails of the genera *Eulota, Subulina, Euhadra* and *Philomycus*. After liberation Cercariae may encyst in the same or other species of snails.

Geographic distribution: Southern Europe, Asia

- **General features of avian intestinal trematodes**

Symptoms: High numbers may cause marked irritation of the intestinal mucosa, enteritis, diarrhoea, emaciation. Secondary infections with other pathogens (e.g. *Eimeria* spp.) may cause high mortality rates.

Significance: Infections with trematodes may assume increased significance wherever birds have access to habitats where the snails live. Most of these trematodes are primarily parasites of aquatic birds. Chickens may also acquire infections when infected intermediate hosts are ingested. High mortalities may occasionally occur in young ducks, geese and chickens.

Diagnosis: This is based on the demonstration of trematode eggs in the faeces (sedimentation). Adult worms may be found at necropsy where a catarrhal, haemorrhagic enteritis may be seen in heavy infections.

Therapy: Niclosamide (60 mg/bird) is effective against Echinostomatidae. Niclosamid should not be used in geese. Fenbendazole (40 mg/kg, po.) was effective against *Echinostoma* spp. in geese. Praziquantel (20–25 mg/kg, po. during several days) and flubendazole (10–50 mg/kg, po. during 5 days) may be used in aquatic birds.

Prophylaxis: Chickens should be kept away from contaminated water bodies.

- Cestoda eggs and proglottids found in the faeces and adult cestodes living in the gastrointestinal tract

Davainea proglottina

Location: Duodenum
Hosts: Chicken
Species description: This is a small tapeworm 1.5–4 mm long with only 4–7 whitish, transparent proglottids. The eggs are round and have embryonal hooks; they measure 55 × 36 µm. The suckers are armed with 3–6 rows of hooks. The intermediate hosts are various species of gastropod molluscs (e.g. *Limax, Arion, Cepaea, Agriolimax* spp.). The chicken acquires infection after ingestion of the infected mollusc. This microscopic tapeworm may be recognized in the duodenal mucosa by protrusion of the gravid proglottids above the villi if the open intestine is floated in water.
Significance: This species is highly pathogenic. (Figures 636, 637, 638, 639, 640)

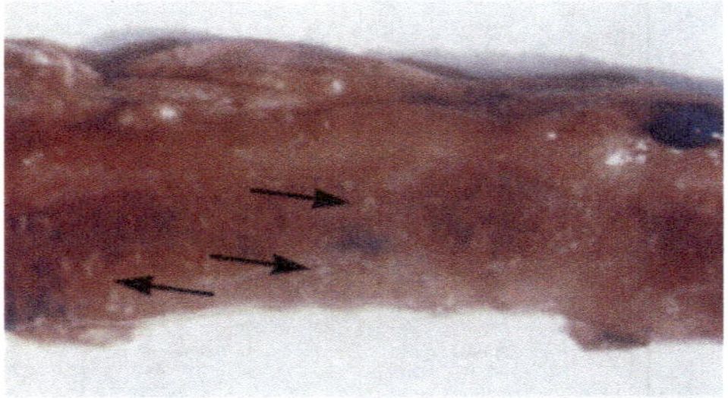

Fig. 636 *Davainea proglottina* (1.5–4 mm × 0.4–0.6 mm) attached to the intestinal mucosa [8]

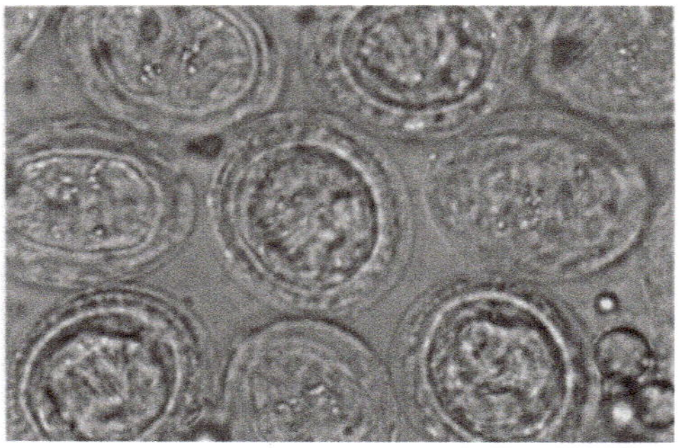

Fig. 637 Eggs of *Davainea proglottina* (55 × 36 µm) containing embryonal hooks

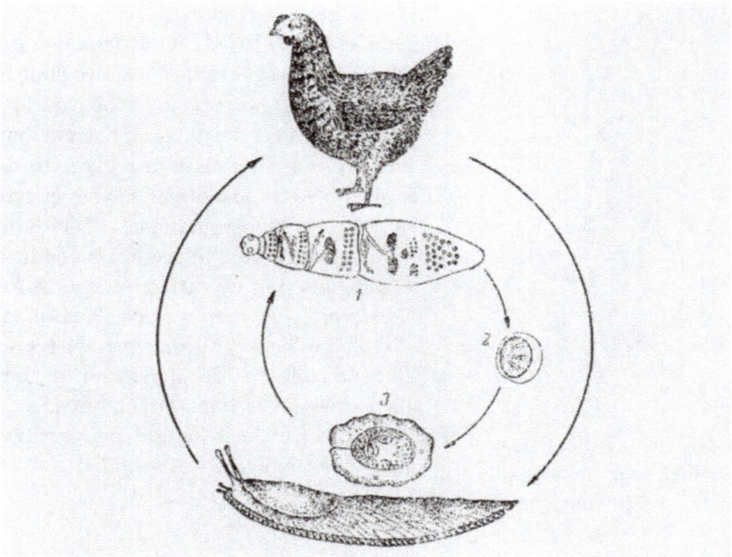

Fig. 638 Life cycle of *Davainea proglottina*; adult worm (1), eggs (2) and larval stage in the intermediate host (3)

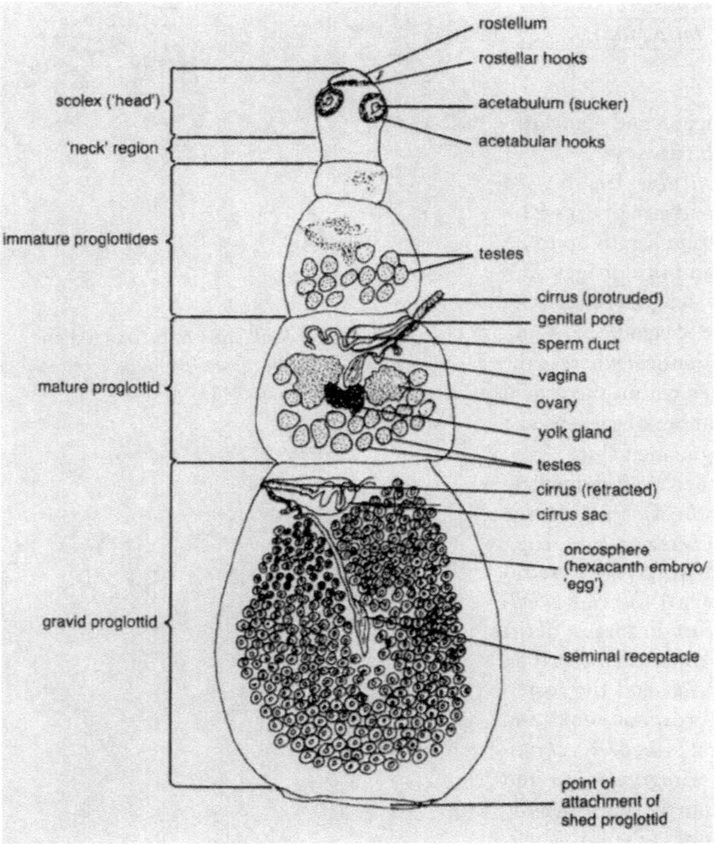

Fig. 639 *Davainea proglottina*; scolex and proglottids (schematic) [5]

	Davainea proglottina	*Raillietina (Raillietina) tetragona*	*Raillietina (Raillietina) echinobothrida*	*Raillietina (Skrjabinia) cesticellus*	*Houttuynia struthionis*	*Amoebotaenia sphenoides*	*Choanotaenia infundibulum*
Length	0,5–3 mm	25 cm	13 cm	4–13 cm	60 cm	4 mm	0,5–20 cm
Suckers	Armed, oval	Armed	Armed, circular	Unarmed	Unarmed	Unarmed	Unarmed
Scolex hooks:							
Shape	Hammer	Hammer	Hammer	Hammer	Hammer	Rosethorn	Rosethorn
Number	80–94	100	200	400–500	160	12–14	16–20
Size	7–8 μm	6–8 μm	10–30 μm	7–12 μm	Large 77,6 μm; Small 63 μm	—	25–30 μm
Eggs	One per capsule	6–12 per capsule	8–12 per capsule	One per capsule	15–25 per capsule	One per capsule	One per capsule *Musca* spp. other arthropods
Intermediate hosts	Slugs	*Musca* spp. ants	Ants	*Musca* spp. beetles	Unknown	Earthworms	

Fig. 640 Description of the morphology of cestode species of poultry [5]

Raillietina spp. (*R. cesticillus, R. echinobothrida* and *R. tetragona*)

Location: Small intestine

Hosts: Chicken, turkey, pigeon and many other domestic and wild birds

Species description: *R. cesticillus*: length 9–13 cm, width 1.5–3 mm and size of eggs 93 × 74 µm; *R. echinobothrida* length up to 25 cm, width 1.2–4 mm and size of eggs 93 × 74 µm; *R. tetragona* length 10–25 cm, width 1–4 mm and size of eggs 93 × 74 µm. The size of the eggs is identical whereas the number of egg capsules within the gravid proglottids and the number of eggs in each capsule may be of diagnostic value.

Ants (Hymenoptera) act as intermediate hosts for *R. echinobothrida*; flies (*Musca domestica*) or ants (*Tetramorium* spp.; *Orthophagus* spp. and others) for *R. tetragona*; beetles (Coleoptera) for *R. cesticillus*. *R. tetragona* is one of the largest of the fowl tapeworms, the scolex is smaller than that of *R. echinobothrida* and the rostellum is armed with 1–2 rows of hooks and the suckers are oval and armed. *R. echinobothrida* resembles *R. tetragona* in size and shape but the rostellum is more heavily armed (two rows of hooks) than in *R. tetragona*. *R. cesticillus* is smaller and has a large scolex with a wide rostellum armed with 400–500 small hooks.

Significance: The pathogenicity of *R. echinobothrida* and *R. tetragona* is moderate to severe. *R. cesticillus* is mild or harmless.

(Figures 641, 642, 643, 644)

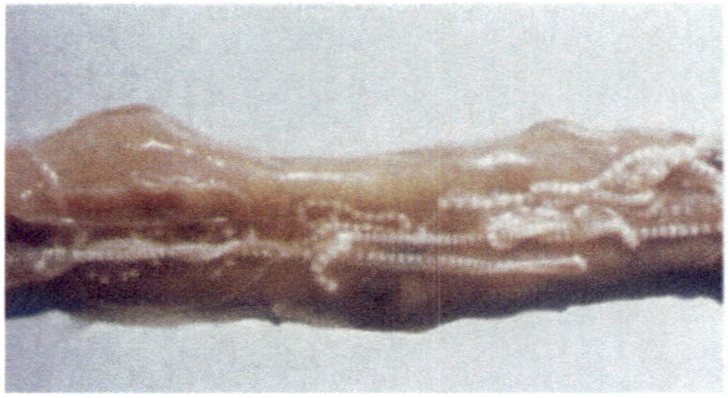

Fig. 641 *Raillietina* sp. (up to 25 cm long and 4 mm wide) in the small intestine [8]

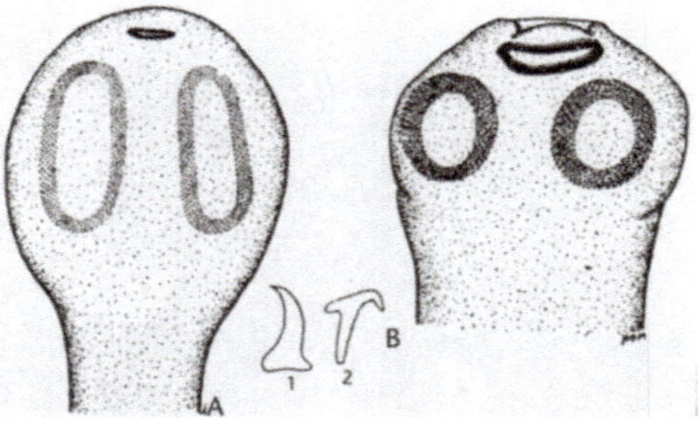

Fig. 642 Scolex of *Raillietina tetragona* (A) and scolex of *R. echinobothrida* (B); hook from sucker (1) and from rostellum (2) [3]

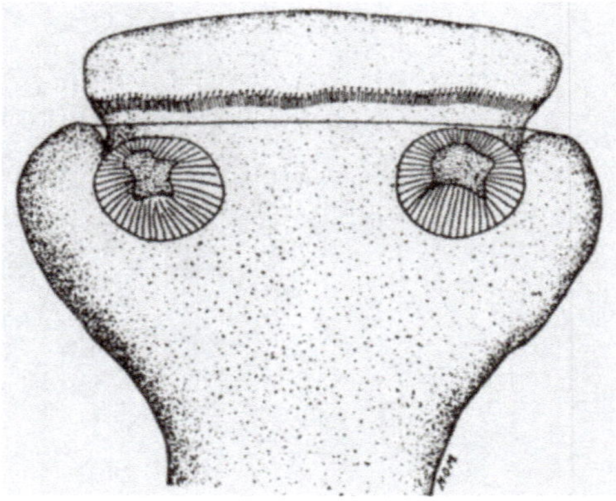

Fig. 643 Scolex of *Raillietina cesticellus* [3]

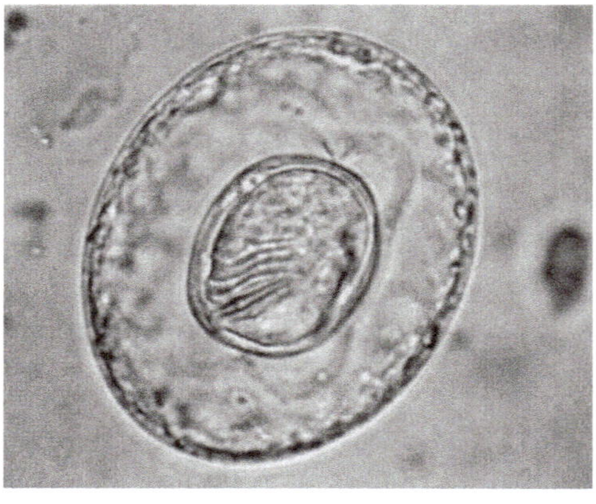

Fig. 644 Egg of *Raillietina* spp. (90–95 × 70–75 µm) [11]

Amoebotaenia cuneata (syn. *A. sphenoides*)

Location: Small intestine
Hosts: Chicken
Species description: This is a short tapeworm (< 4 mm) and may be recognized as whitish projections among the villi of the duodenum. A triangular anterior end with a pointed scolex gives the entire worm a wedge-shaped anterior. The suckers are unarmed and the rostellum is armed with a single row of 12–14 hooks. The eggs are round and measure 47 × 42 µm. The intermediate hosts are earthworms (several genera).
Significance: This species is mildly pathogenic.
(Figures 630, 645)

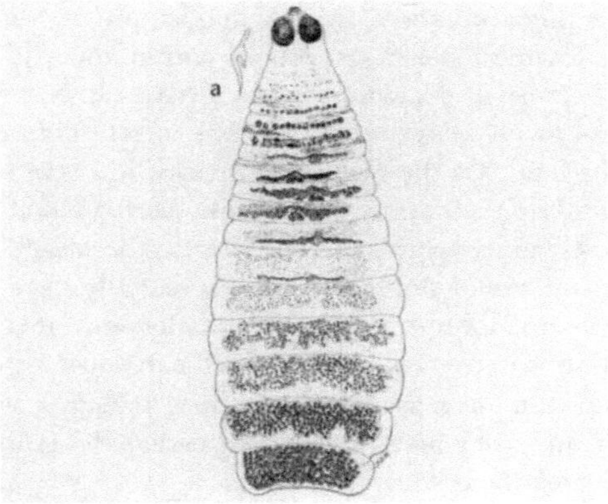

Fig. 645 *Amoebotaenia* spp. (2–4 mm long) rostellar hook (a) [3]

Choanotaenia infundibulum

Location: Small intestine
Hosts: Chicken
Species description: The worms are up to 23 cm long and 1.5–3 mm wide. Eggs measure 54 × 47µm with a distinctive elongated filament. The segments are markedly wider posteriorly than anteriorly, giving the worm a characteristic shape. The intermediate hosts are the house fly (*Musca domestica*) and beetles of several genera.
Significance: This species is moderately pathogenic.
(Figures 630, 646)

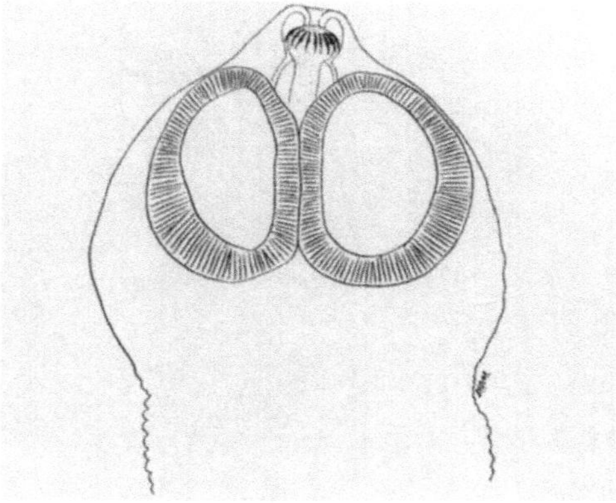

Fig. 646 Scolex of *Choanotaenia infundibulum* (up to 23 cm long and 1.5–3 mm wide) [3]

Hymenolepis spp. (*H. cantaniana, H. carioca*)

Location: Small intestine
Hosts: Chicken
Species description: The intermediate hosts are stable flies or dung beetles for *H. carioca* and other beetles for *H. cantaniana*. *H. cantaniana* is a short tapeworm with a maximum length of 2 cm. It resembles *H. carioca* which is much longer. The latter is about 1 mm in diameter and the proglottids look more like a thread than a worm.
Significance: The pathogenicity of these species is mild.
(Figure 647, 648)

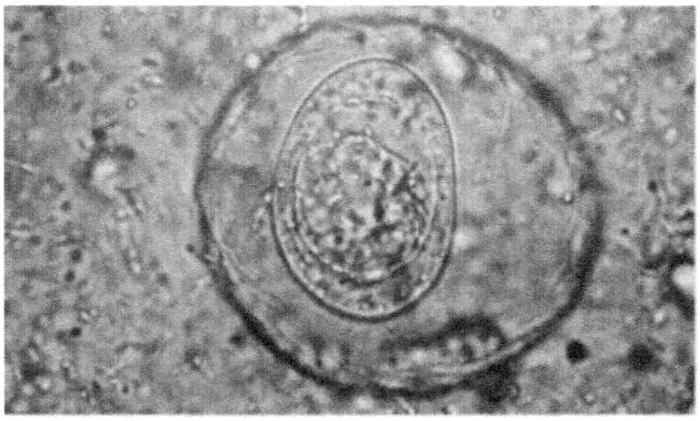

Fig. 647 Egg of *Hymenolepis* spp. (76 × 62 µm) [8]

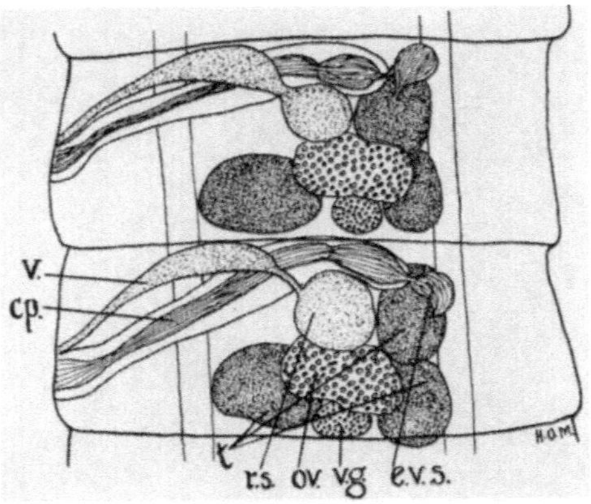

Fig. 648 Mature segments of *Hymenolepis carioca*; v = vagina, cp = cirrhus pouch, ov = ovary, t = testes, r.s. = receptabulum seminis, v.g. = vitelline gland and e.v.s = external vesiculum seminalis [3]

Fimbriaria fasciolaris

Location: Small intestine

Hosts: Chicken

Species description: The anterior portion of the body of this cestode forms a folded expansion or "pseudoscolex" by which the parasite attaches itself. The cestode is 40 cm long and 1.5 mm wide. Copepods (*Diaptomus* spp. and *Cyclops* spp.) act as intermediate hosts.

Significance: The pathogenicity of this species is mild.

(Figure 649)

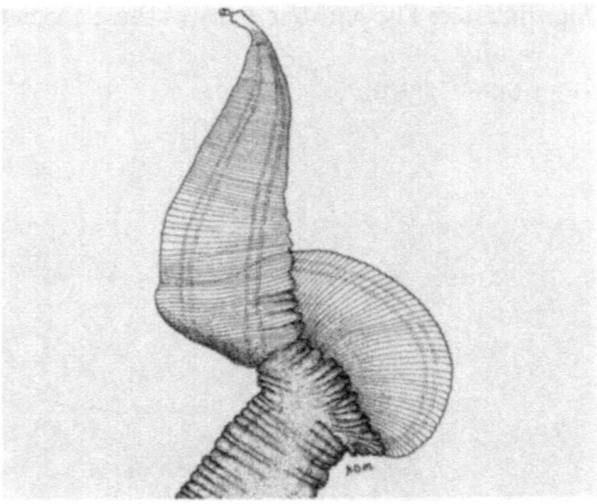

Fig. 649 Scolex and pseudoscolex of *Fimbriaria fasciolaris* (up to 40 cm long and 1.5 mm wide) [3]

- **General features of avian cestode infections**

Chickens kept in free range systems on pastures are often infected with tapeworms (Cestoda). In many African and Asian countries a high percentage of chickens are infected with tapeworms. In contrast, tapeworm infections are very rarely encountered in intensive poultry rearing systems.
D. proglottina is the most important species and highly pathogenic. The parasite may occur in high numbers in the duodenum and is known to penetrate deeply within the villi. Necrosis and haemorrhagic enteritis can occur following heavy infections. The infection may be fatal. Of the *Raillietina* species *R. echinobothrida* is the most pathogenic. Multiple nodules and hyperplastic enteritis at the attachment site of the scolex can occur. Other species are not normally harmful unless the infection is extremely heavy, which can cause significant decrease of production. Infection is acquired by ingestion of intermediate hosts in which the cysticercoids occur.

Symptoms: Chronic infections are characterized by reduced growth rate, emaciation, paralysis and weakness.

Diagnosis: Although proglottids are passed in the faeces, diagnosis is usually made at necropsy. Representative members of the flock should be examined and mucosal scrapings should be examined microscopically to detect the small cestode species. It is difficult to make a reliable diagnosis of all the individual species and also not necessary for chemotherapy.

Therapy: Praziquantel (1 × 10 mg/kg, po.) is highly effective against adult cestodes of chickens. Niclosamid (20 mg/kg, po. during 2–6 days) is effective against most of the chicken tapeworms. A single application of niclosamid (50–200 mg/kg, in drinking water; water should be consumed within 3–4 hours) may also be an efficient way of controlling cestode infections. Fenbendazole (100 ppm. via feed, during 4 days), mebendazole (60 ppm via feed, during 7 days), flubendazole (60 ppm, during 7 days), oxfendazole (10 mg/kg, po.) and febantel (30 mg/kg, po.) may be used to control tapeworms in chickens.

Cave: Niclosamid is toxic for geese! The combination of praziquantel and pyrantel tartrate is toxic for chickens and may cause severe neurological problems.

Prophylaxis: Control measures should be directed against the intermediate hosts which is normally impossible. Insecticides may be used for flies and ants in the chicken house. Beetles and earthworms are difficult to control but alternation of ranges may be helpful. The use of insecticides on the pastures is not justifiable.

- Nematoda eggs found in the faeces and adult nematodes living in the gastrointestinal tract

- **Nematodes of primary importance**

Ascaridia galli

Location: Small intestine

Hosts: Chicken, turkey, geese, duck

Species description: The males are 50–76 mm and the females are 72–116 mm long. The eggs are elliptical, thick-shelled and 77–94 × 43–55 µm in size. The head has 3 large lips and the tail of the male shows a typical circular preanal sucker. The life cycle is direct. Earthworms can ingest the eggs and when they are swallowed by the final host can transmit the infection mechanically. The eggs hatch in the intestine of the host and live for the first ten days in the lumen after which larval development continues within the mucosa of the intestines until 17 days after infection. Subsequently the larvae re-enter the lumen and reach maturity in 6 to 8 weeks. The incubation period is 3–5 days (clinical symptoms following invasion of the larvae) and the prepatent period is 6–8 weeks.

Geographic distribution: World-wide

Symptoms: Marked lesions may be produced when large numbers of young parasites penetrate into the duodenal mucosa. They cause haemorrhage and enteritis and the birds become anaemic and suffer from diarrhoea. Chickens become unthrifty, emaciated and weak.

Significance: *A. galli* may be a serious nematode for young chickens 3–4weeks old. The egg production may seriously be impaired and yield pale egg yolk.

Diagnosis: Detection of eggs in the faeces (*cave: Heterakis* eggs [see below] look very similar!) or of the adult worms in the intestine at autopsy.

Therapy: A wide variety of compounds may be used to treat *Ascaridia* infections in chickens. These are cambendazole (70 mg/kg, po.), febantel (60 ppm via feed over 6 days or 15 mg/kg, po. over 2 days), fenbendazole (60 ppm, over 3 days), flubendazole (30 ppm, over 7 days), levamisole (30 mg/kg, po. or 300 ppm via feed), mebendazole (60 ppm, over 7 days), piperazine (200–300 mg/kg, po.) and pyrantel tartrate (10–40 mg/kg po. over 2 days).

Prophylaxis: Special attention should be paid to the young birds. Eggs develop in moist environment. Therefore, litter should be removed regularly and kept dry.

(Figures 650, 651)

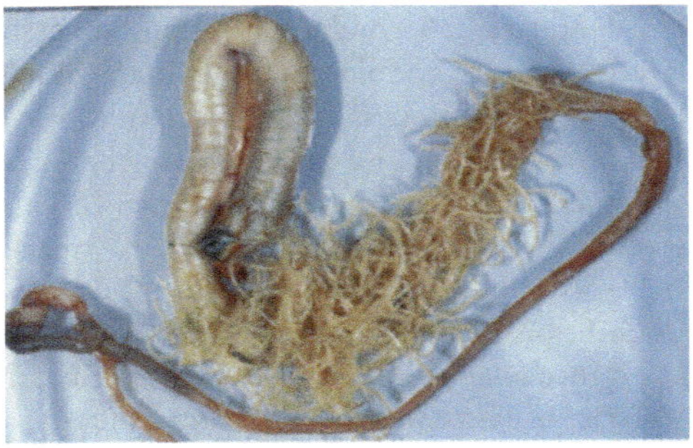

Fig. 650 *Ascaridia galli*; masses in the small intestine [53]

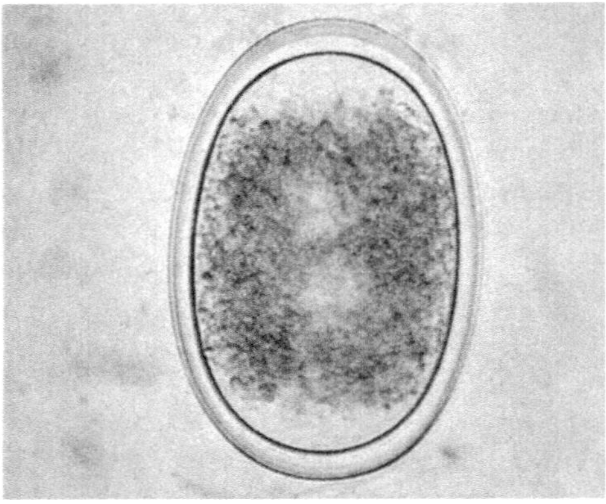

Fig. 651 Egg of *Ascaridia galli* (77–94 × 43–55 µm) [11]

Heterakis gallinarum Caecal worm

Location: Caecum

Hosts: Chicken, turkey and guineafowl

Species description: The male is 7–13 mm and the female is 10–15 mm long. There are large lateral alae extending some distance down the sides of the body. The life cycle is direct. Earthworms may also ingest the eggs of the *Heterakis* and may be the means of causing infections in poultry. The larval development in the egg to the infective second larval stage (eggs are infective !) in the environment depends on the temperature and takes 2–4 weeks at 27°C.

Geographic distribution: World-wide

Symptoms: Primary infections are usually inapparent. Secondary infections are associated with nodule formation in the mucosa and submucosa of the caecum. Marked inflammation and thickening of the intestinal wall may occur in heavy infections. Heavy infections in laying hens may markedly reduce the egg production.

Significance: The principal economic importance of *H. gallinarum* lies in its role as carrier of *Histomonas meleagridis*, the causal pathogen of enterohepatitis ("blackhead") of turkeys. The protozoan remains viable in the egg of *H. gallinarum*.

Diagnosis: Detection of eggs in the faeces (flotation). The eggs have thick, smooth shells; they measure 65–77 × 35–48 µm. The eggs are similar to those of *Ascaridia galli* but they are generally smaller than 77 µm. Adult worms may be found in the caecum at necropsy.

Therapy: Most of the compounds effective against *Ascaridia galli* may also be used to control *Heterakis gallinarum* (☞ above), except piperazine and pyrantel tartrate which are not effective against this parasite.

Prophylaxis: Preventive control of *H. gallinarum* is indicated in flocks where histomonosis occurs.

(Figures 652, 653, 654)

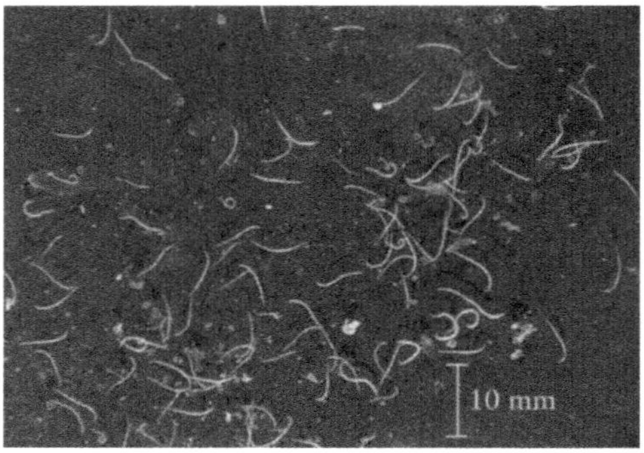

Fig. 652 *Heterakis* sp. in a petri dish; males are 7–13 mm and females 10–15 mm long

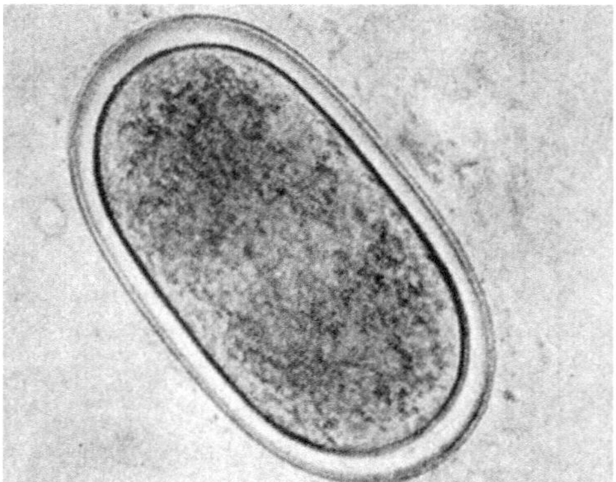

Fig. 653 Egg of *Heterakis gallinarum* (66–79 × 41–48 µm) [11]

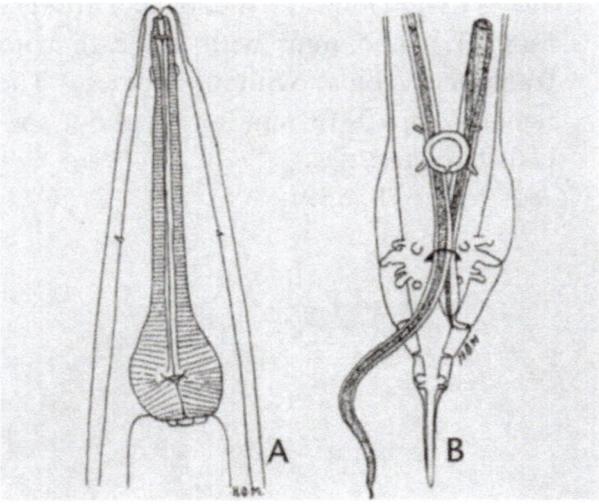

Fig. 654 *Heterakis gallinarum*; anterior end (A) and posterior end (B) of a female [3]

Capillaria annulata (syn. *Eucoleus annulatus*) **and _Capillaria contorta_** (syn. *Eucoleus contortus*) Crop capillariosis

Location: Mucosa of the crop and oesophagus

Hosts: Chicken, turkey, guineafowl and wild birds

Species description: The intermediate hosts for *C. annulata* are earthworms. *C. contorta* has a direct life cycle although earthworms may act as intermediate hosts. *C. annulata* can easily be identified by a cuticular swelling just back of the head. The male is 18–26 mm long and 52–74 µm wide. The spicules are 1.12–11.6 mm long and the spicule sheath is covered with fine spines. The female is 25–60 mm long and 77–120 µm wide. The eggs are operculated and measure 55–66 × 25 µm. *C. contorta* males are 8–17 mm long and 60–70 µm wide. The spicules are slender and about 800 µm long and the spicule sheath is covered with fine hair-like processes. Females are 15–60 mm long and 120–150 µm wide. The vulva is prominent and circular.

Symptoms: Heavy infections are characterized by marked thickening of the crop and oesophageal wall, a marked catarrhal or croupous inflammation and sloughing of the mucosa. The birds are emaciated and weak.

Significance: The *Capillaria* species of the crop and oesophagus are highly pathogenic and deaths may occur in heavy infections.

(Figures 630, 655, 656, 657)

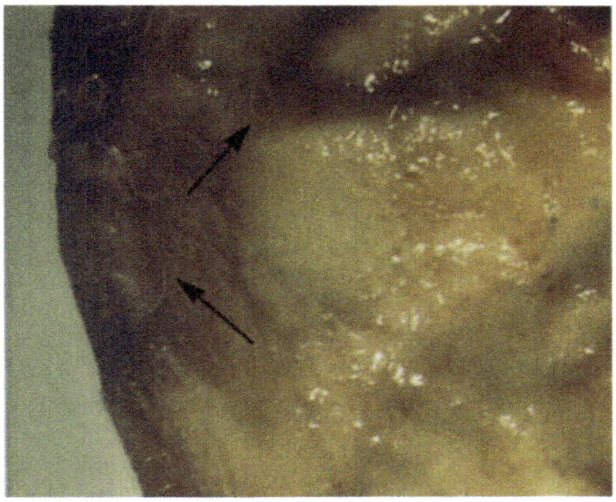

Fig. 655 *Capillaria* (syn. *Eucoleus*) *annulatus* in the crop of a turkey; males are 14–16 mm and females are 20–26 mm long [8]

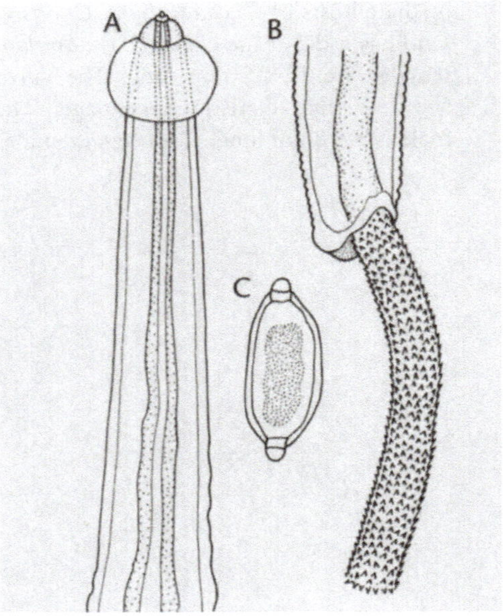

Fig. 656 *Capillaria* (syn. *Eucoleus*) *annulatus*; anterior end (A) and posterior end (B) of male with spiny spicule sheath and egg (C) [56]

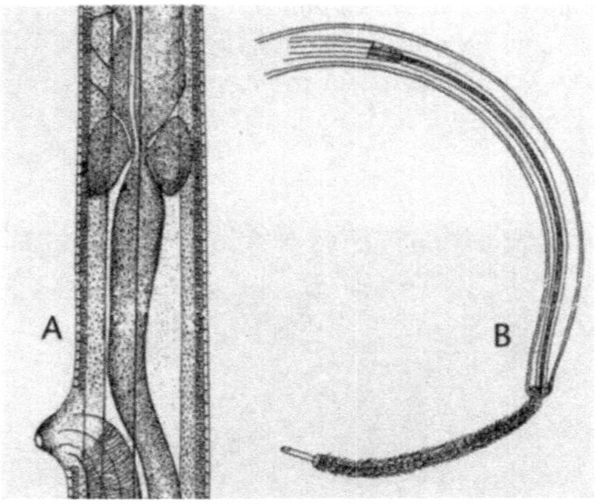

Fig. 657 *Capillaria contorta* (syn. *Thomix contorta, Eucoleus contorta*); female vulva (A) and posterior end of male with spiny spicule sheath (B) [56]

Capillaria caudinflata, Capillaria obsignata and other *Capillaria* spp.

Small intestinal capillariosis

Location: Small intestine, sometimes caecum

Hosts: Chicken, turkey and guineafowl

Species description: Earthworms are the intermediate hosts of *C. caudinflata*. *C. obsignata* has a direct life cycle. *C. caudinflata* females are 12–25 mm long. The vulva shows a characteristic appendage. The male is 9–18 µm long. *C. obsignata* males are 7–13 mm long and the spicules are very long (1.1–1. 5 mm) with a sheath with transverse folds without spines. The females are 10–18 mm long without special characteristics.

(Figures 630, 658, 659)

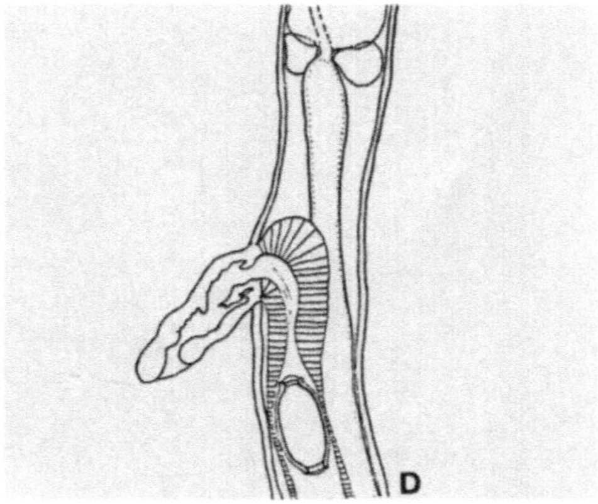

Fig. 658 *Capillaria caudinflata*; vulva with typical appendage [56]

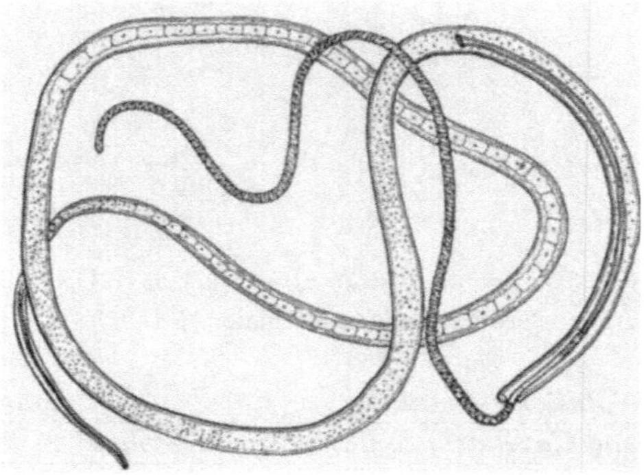

Fig. 659 *Capillaria obsignata*; male with spicule sheath without spines but with transverse folds [56]

Capillaria anatis Caecal capillariosis

Location: Caecum, rarely small intestine

Hosts: Duck, goose, chicken, turkey and guineafowl

Species description: Males are 8–15 mm and the spicules are 0.7–1.9 long. Females are 11–28 mm long. The eggs measure 46–67 × 22–29 µm. This is commonly a parasite of water birds but may also occur in chickens. The life cycle is direct.

Symptoms: The intestinal capillariosis (*C. caudinflata, C. obsignata* and *C. anatis*) is seen in birds of all ages. Older birds may act as carriers of the infection. Disease may occur during the prepatent period. There is emaciation, diarrhoea associated with a slimy, stringy mucous. Chronically infected birds have thickened intestinal walls covered with a catarrhal exudate.

Significance: Intestinal *Capillaria* infections cause marked losses due to reduced weight gains.

- **General features of *Capillaria* spp. infections**

Diagnosis: Usually made at necropsy when large numbers of parasites can be found in the crop or in the intestine after an intestinal lavage. The lemon-shaped eggs may also be detected in large numbers in the faeces.

Therapy: The same compounds as for *Heterakis gallinarum* may be used to treat *Capillaria* infections (☞ above).

Prophylaxis: Regular investigations of faeces may provide information about the level of infection in intensive poultry systems. Regular anthelmintic control may reduce disease incidence. The control of earthworms on the pastures is not feasible.

(Figures 660, 661)

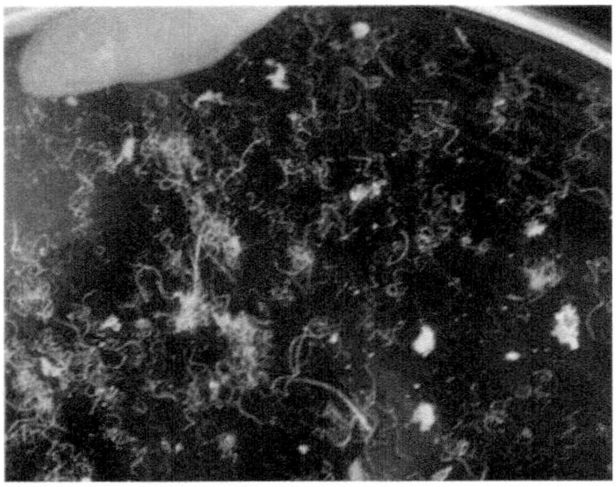

Fig. 660 *Capillaria* sp.; adult worms in a petri dish [53]

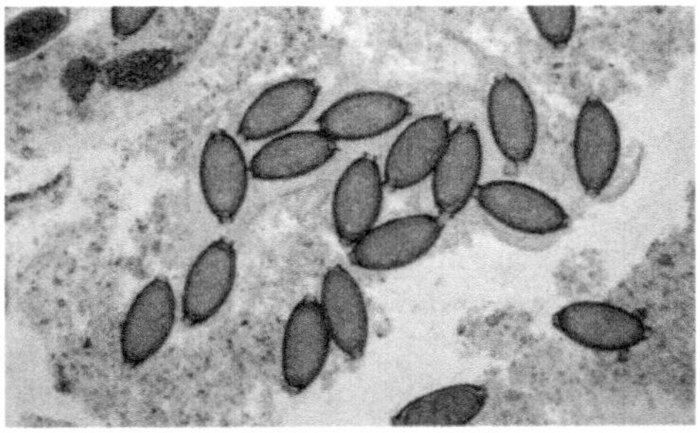

Fig. 661 Eggs of *Capillaria* sp. (43–65 × 20–35 µm) [53]

Trichostrongylus tenuis

Location: Caecum, sometimes small intestine

Hosts: Chicken, turkey, duck and other game birds

Species description: Excretory pore at the head end. Males are 5.5–9 mm and females 6.5–11 mm long. The spicules are dark and unequal in length (the longer 120–164 µm and the shorter 104–150 µm long) both much twisted and provided with an ear-like structure on the proximal end. The eggs are thin-shelled and measure 65–75 × 35–42 µm. The life cycle is direct and infective third-stage larvae develop in 2 weeks.

Geographic distribution: World-wide

Symptoms: Heavy infections cause weight loss, anaemia, inappetence, progressive emaciation. The faeces may be slimy, liquid and bloody.

Significance: This is a very pathogenic species. Heavy infections may cause severe losses especially in floor-reared birds and backyard flocks. *T. tenuis* may be fatal for young goslings.

Diagnosis: Typical strongyle-type eggs appear in the faeces. Adult parasites may be found at necropsy.

Therapy: Febantel (60 ppm via feed over 6 days or 15 mg/kg, po. over 2 days), fenbendazole (60 ppm, over 3 days), flubendazole (30 ppm, over 7 days) and mebendazole

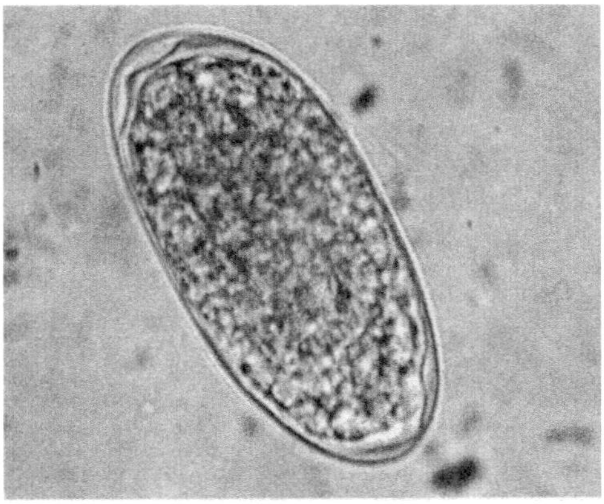

Fig. 662 Egg of *Trichostrongylus tenuis* (65–75 × 35–42 µm) [11]

(60 ppm, over 7 days) are highly effective against *T. tenuis* in chickens.

Prophylaxis: Contaminated pastures should be avoided in flocks where the parasite causes problems. Regular anthelmintic treatments are indicated.

(Figure 662)

- **Nematodes of secondary importance**

Dispharynx spiralis (syn. *D. nasuta, Acuaria spiralis*)

Location: Proventriculus

Hosts: Chicken, turkey, pigeon and guinea-fowl

Species description: The body of this parasite is usually rolled in a spiral and four wavy cuticular cordons on the anterior end are typical. Males are 7–8 mm and females 9–10 mm long. Embryonated eggs are produced by the females. Intermediate hosts are the pillbug (*Armadillidium vulgare*) and the sowbug (*Porcellio scaber*) and probably other isopods. These roundworms are usually found with their heads buried deep in the mucosa. *D. spiralis* has been considered as the main cause of "grouse disease" in the USA.

Geographic distribution: Africa, Asia, the Americas

Symptoms: Deep ulcers may occur in the proventriculus and the wall may markedly be thickened in heavy infections. Affected birds rapidly loose weight and become weak and anaemic.

Significance: This parasite may cause severe losses in young birds.

Diagnosis: This is based on the demonstration of embryonated eggs in the faeces or the adult parasites at necropsy. The parasites are often completely concealed beneath the proliferating tissue.

Therapy and Prophylaxis: ☞ PREVENTION AND CONTROL OF INTESTINAL NEMATODE INFECTIONS, p. 366

(Figures 630, 663)

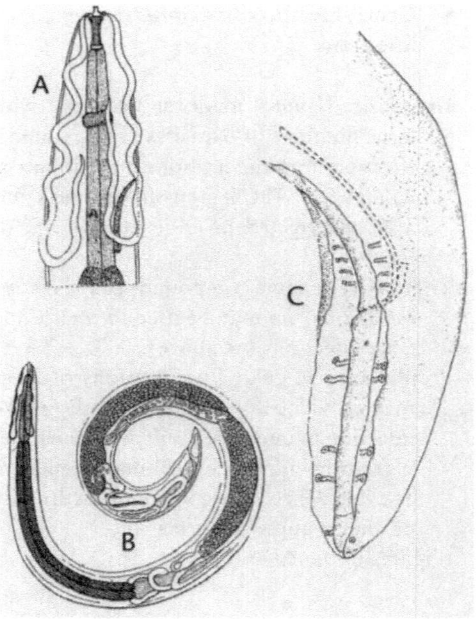

Fig. 663 *Dispharynx spiralis*; anterior end with wavy cuticular cordons (A), total female parasite (B; up to 10 mm long) and male posterior end (C) [56]

Tetrameres spp. (*T. americana* and *T. fissispina*)

Location: Proventriculus, oesophagus and rarely intestine

Hosts: *T. americana* occurs in chicken, turkey, duck and other birds; *T. fissispina* occurs most commonly in duck and goose and rarely in other poultry. It may occur in chicken.

Species description: There is a marked sexual dimorphism. The females of this species are globular, blood red with four longitudinal furrows. Females of *T. americana* measure 3.5–4.5 mm by 3 mm. Males are 5–5.5 mm long. Eggs measure 42–50 × 24 µm and are embryonated when laid. Two double rows of posteriorly directed spines extend throughout the whole body length. The spicules are unequal in length and measure 100 µm and 290–312 µm. *T. fissispina* is similar in appearance to *T. americana.*

Females are 1.7–6 mm long and 1.3–5 mm wide. Males are 3–6 mm long with 4 longitudinal rows of spines along the median and lateral lines. Eggs measure 48–56 × 26–30 μm and are embryonated when laid. Intermediate hosts include grasshoppers, cockroaches for *T. americana* and amphipods, grasshoppers, earthworms and cockroaches for *T. fissispina*.

Geographic distribution: *T. americana* has been reported from USA and South Africa. *T. fissispina* occurs world-wide.

Symptoms: Emaciation and anaemia may result in heavy infections. The wall of the proventriculus may be thickened so that the lumen is almost obliterated.

Significance: Heavy infections may cause severe digestive disturbances, weight loss and death.

Diagnosis: Embryonated eggs appear in the faeces and adult worms may be found at necropsy as black or red spots in the opening of the glands.

Therapy and Prophylaxis: ☞ PREVENTION AND CONTROL OF INTESTINAL NEMATODE INFECTIONS, p. 366

(Figures 664, 665, 666, 667)

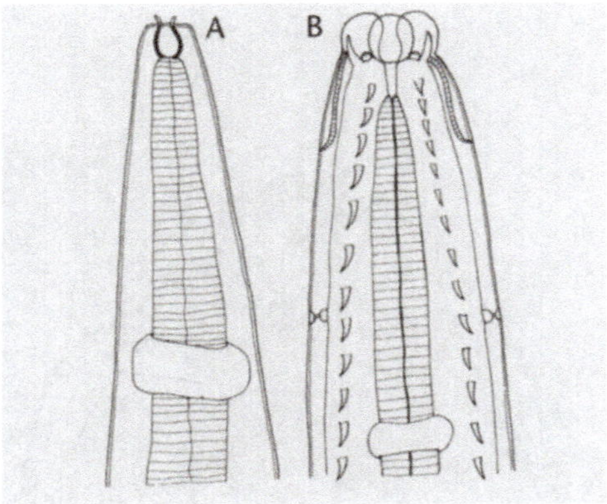

Fig. 664 Anterior ends of *Tetrameres americana* (A) and *T. fissispina* (B) [56]

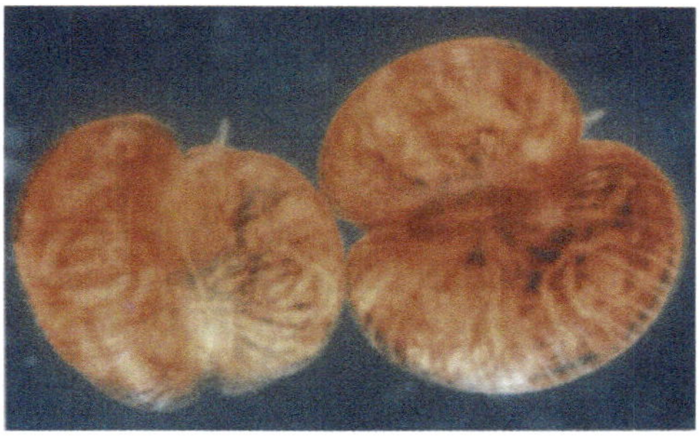

Fig. 665 *Tetrameres fissispina*; females (2.5–4 mm long and up to 2 mm wide) [4]

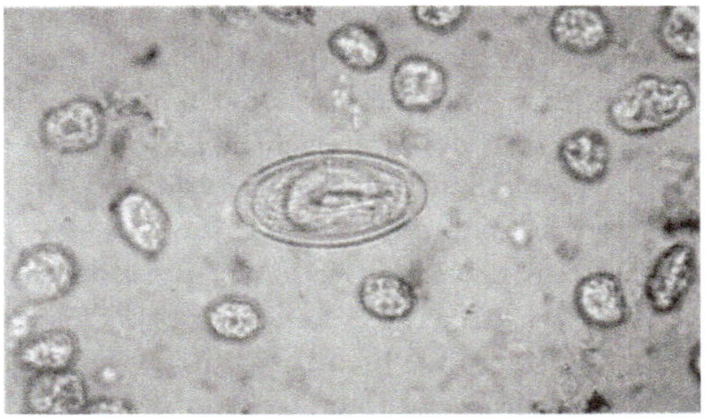

Fig. 666 Egg of *Tetrameres fissispina* (45–57 × 25–32 μm) [11]

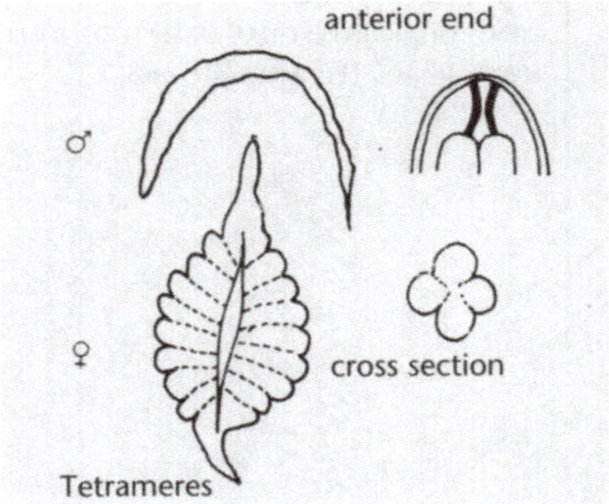

Fig. 667 Details of *Tetrameres* sp. [16]

Acuaria (syn. *Cheilospirura*) ***hamulosa***

Location: Gizzard

Hosts: Chicken, turkey and game birds

Species description: Intermediate hosts are grasshoppers and beetles. Males are 10–14 mm and females 16–29 mm long, with two large triangular lateral lips. The cuticle of the anterior part of the body is ornamented with four "cordons" which are epaulette-like thickenings and extending at least 2/3 of the length of the body. The male has four pairs of pre-cloacal and 6 pairs of post-cloacal papillae. The eggs measure 40–45 × 24–27 μm and are embryonated when passed in the faeces.

Geographic distribution: World-wide

Symptoms: Light infections are inapparent. Heavy infections cause inappetence, weakness, progressive emaciation and anaemia.

Significance: Low numbers of these worms are relatively non-pathogenic. Heavy infections cause massive alterations of the gizzard.

Diagnosis: Embryonated eggs are passed in the faeces. Several species of Spiruridae may occur in the faeces and the eggs are very similar and difficult to differentiate. The worms may be found after the horny lining of the gizzard has been removed. They may be found in soft, yellowish-red nodules in the thinner parts of the wall (Figure 630).

Therapy and Prophylaxis: ☞ PREVENTION AND CONTROL OF INTESTINAL NEMATODE INFECTIONS, p. 366 (Figures 630, 668)

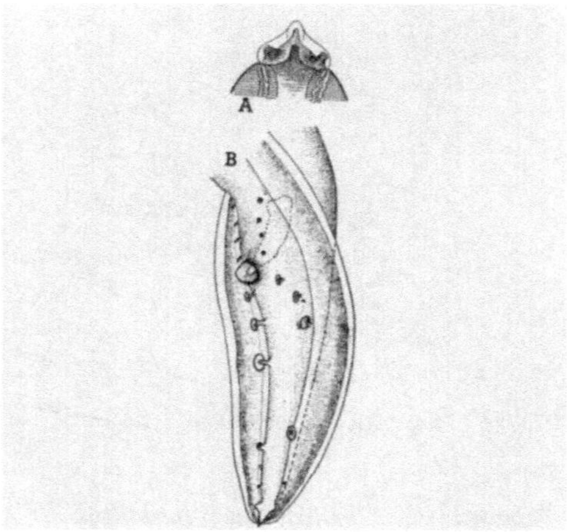

Fig. 668 *Acuaria hamulosa*; anterior end (A) and female posterior end (B) [56]

Hartertia gallinarum

Location: Small intestine

Hosts: Chicken

Species description: This worm resembles closely *Ascaridia galli*. The male is 28–40 mm long and the female is 60–100 mm long. The eggs are thick shelled and measure 45–53 × 27–33 μm and contain a fully developed embryo when laid. Intermediate hosts are termites and chickens become infected when eating infected termites.

Geographic distribution: South and West Africa, Asia

Symptoms: Diarrhoea, weight loss and decreased egg production, emaciation and weakness.

Significance: This parasite may cause losses of chickens kept in free range systems in Africa.

Diagnosis: This can be made by finding the eggs in the faeces but it is often difficult to distinguish them from eggs of other nematodes of chickens. Diagnosis should therefore be confirmed by autopsy of selected cases (Figure 630).

Therapy: ☞ *Ascaridia galli*, p. 357

Prophylaxis: Chickens should be kept away from termites when losses due to *H. gallinarum* occur. ☞ PREVENTION AND CONTROL OF INTESTINAL NEMATODE INFECTIONS, p. 366
(Figures 630, 669, 670)

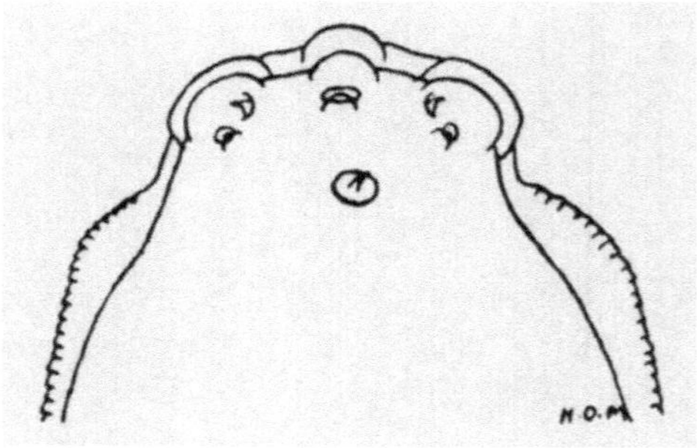

Fig. 669 *Hartertia gallinarum*; anterior end [3]

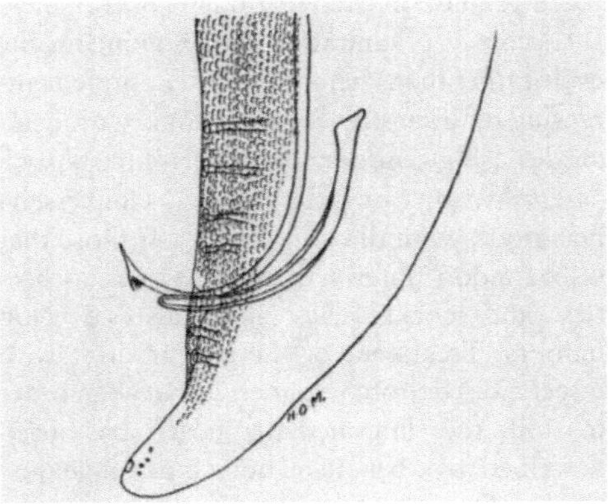

Fig. 670 *Hartertia gallinarum*; male posterior end, lateral view [3]

Subulura brumpti

Location: Caecum

Hosts: Chicken, turkey, duck, guineafowl and other birds

Species description: This is a small nematode with anterior end curved dorsally and an oesophagus dilatated posteriorly, followed by a bulb. The males are 6.9–10 mm long and the females 9–17.5 mm. The eggs measure 52–64 × 41–49 µm and have a smooth shell. The eggs contain a fully developed embryo when laid. The intermediate hosts are various beetles and cockroaches.

Geographic distribution: Africa, the Americas, Asia

Symptoms: There are generally no marked clinical signs.

Significance: This parasite seems to be relatively non-pathogenic.

Diagnosis: This is based on the demonstration of the eggs in the faeces and the identification of adult worms at necropsy.

Therapy: Levamisole (30 mg/kg, po.) has been used for therapy.

Prophylaxis: This is difficult since the intermediate hosts are difficult to remove or destroy in the environment of chickens. Modern confinement rearing of poultry may greatly reduce the incidence of parasitic infections where this type of ground-living intermediate host occurs.

(Figures 630, 671)

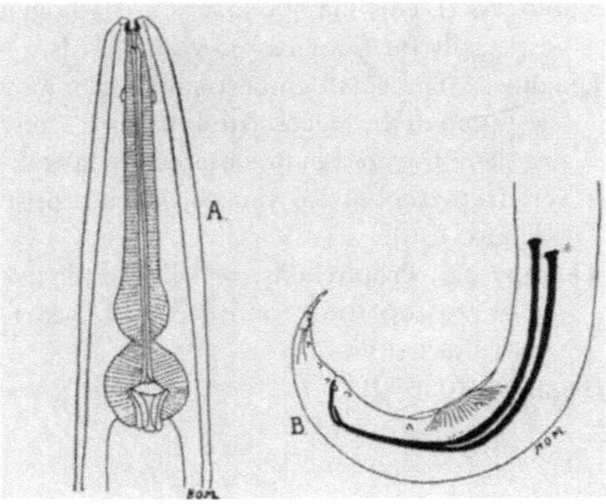

Fig. 671 *Subulura brumpti*; anterior end (A) and male posterior end, lateral view (B) [3]

Subulura suctoria and *Subulura differens*

Remarks: *S. suctoria* occurs in the caecum of chickens, turkeys, guinea fowls in Africa and South America. It is larger than *S. brumpti*: males are 11.8–13.8 mm and females 20–33 mm long. The eggs measure 51–70 × 45–64 µm. Intermediate hosts are beetles. The pathogenicity seems to be low although heavy infections may cause losses due to reduced performance. *S. differens* is similar to *S. brumpti* and occurs in chickens and guinea-fowls in southern Europe, Africa and Brazil. For therapy and prophylaxis ☞ PREVENTION AND CONTROL OF INTESTINAL NEMATODE INFECTIONS, p. 366.

Strongyloides avium

Location: Caecum, sometimes small intestine

Hosts: Chicken, turkey and goose

Species description: Only the females are parasitic. Parasitic adults are 2.2 mm long and the size of the eggs is 52–56 × 36–40 µm. Direct life cycle; percutaneous infections may occur.

Geographic distribution: World-wide

Symptoms: Acute heavy infections cause weakness, emaciation and bloody, slimy diarrhoea. Young birds suffer more from infections.

Significance: This may be a serious pathogen especially for floor-reared young birds.

Diagnosis: The small embryonated eggs may be found in the faeces. Adult parasites may be demonstrated in mucosa scrapings taken from the caecal mucosa at necropsy (Figure 130).

Therapy and Prophylaxis: ☞ below PREVENTION AND CONTROL OF INTESTINAL NEMATODE INFECTIONS

(Figures 630, 672)

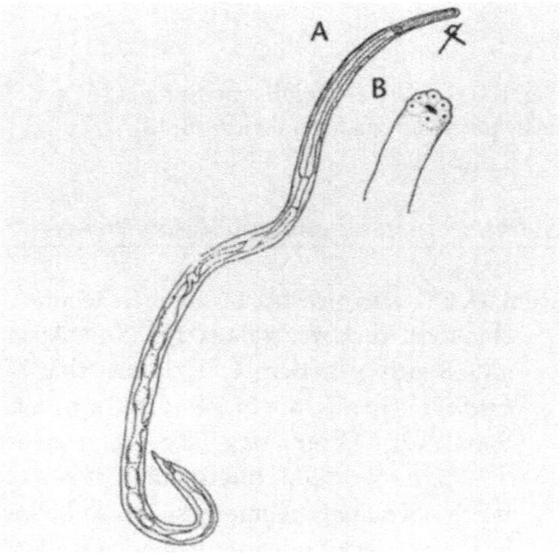

Abb. 672 *Strongyloides avium*; parasitic female (A) and head of female (B) [56]

- **Prevention and control of intestinal nematode infections**

Modern poultry management practices, especially confinement-rearing of chickens have greatly reduced the prevalence and spectrum of nematode infections in poultry. Many nematodes that caused extensive problems in "backyard" flocks are seldom seen in commercial poultry systems. However, nematode infections are still of great significance wherever chickens are reared on pens or on pastures. For most nematodes control measures consist of sanitation and breaking the life cycle rather than chemotherapy. Confinement-rearing on litter prevents infections with nematodes using outdoor intermediate hosts such as earthworms or grasshoppers. Conversely, nematodes with direct life cycles or those that utilize indoor intermediate hosts such as beetles and cockroaches may also develop indoors. Treatment of the soil or litter with insecticides (stirofos, ronnel, carbaryl) in order to kill the intermediate hosts has been described to be beneficial but it is no longer justifiable. Extreme care should be taken to insure that feed and water are not contaminated. To control beetles, the floor may be sprayed with permethrin after the old litter has been removed. Raising different bird species and/or different ages together or in close proximity is a dangerous procedure as regards parasitism. In many situations nematodes can only be controlled effectively by means of chemotherapy. A wide variety of drugs is available and the poultry producers should only use drugs which are approved for birds that will produce eggs or meat for human consumption. The withdrawal periods should strictly be respected. Anthelmintics may be administered via feed or drinking water. The drugs listed under therapy of *Ascaridia galli* (p. 357) infections may be used to control the most important nematode infections in poultry. Tetramisole may be used to control *Subulura brumpti* and *Strongyloides avium*. Tetramisole is not effective against *Dispharynx spiralis* which can partially be controlled with mebendazole. Apart from the modern benzimidazoles piperazine may also be used to treat *Tetrameres* spp. infections. Ivermectin (0.2–0.4 mg/kg, po.) has been reported to be highly effective against *Ascaridia* and *Capillaria* and probably other intestinal nematodes.

PROTOZOA

Trypanosoma spp. Avian trypanosomosis

Remarks: Several species of trypanosomes occur in avian hosts. They are usually not a problem in commercial flocks but widespread in wild birds. Avian trypanosomosis is reported to be seasonal in temperate zones, being discovered only during summer times. Bloodsucking arthropods, including mosquitoes, simuliids, red mites and hippoboscids are the vectors. Bird trypanosomes persist during periods of adverse environmental conditions (e.g. winter), are more or less restricted to the bone marrow, and reappear in the peripheral blood in spring. Avian trypanosomes are presumably non-pathogenic. *T. avium* occurs in Europe and *T. gallinarum* has been described from the chicken in central Africa. Avian trypanosomes are very polymorphic, sometimes attaining great size. They may be 26–69 µm long or even longer. There is a free flagellum and the body often appears to be striated.

Toxoplasma gondii

Remarks: Chickens kept on pastures, pens or in free range systems are often infected with *T. gondii* because of their continuous ingestion of oocysts with infected faeces of cats. The infection in adult birds is often inapparent although free merozoites may be seen in bloodsmears or in leucocytes. These merozoites are 6–7 µm long. Young chickens may seriously be affected during these acute stage of infection, showing weakness, emaciation, diarrhoea, atactic gait and even death (☞ POULTRY, ■ 4.1 and SWINE, ■ 4.1).

Sarcocystis spp. Sarcosporidiosis

Remarks: Chickens kept in free range systems often harbour cysts of *Sarcocystis* spp. in their muscles. The examination of blood within 14 days after infection may reveal free merozoites which are about 9 µm long (☞ POULTRY, ■ 4.1). These merozoites develop within the epithelial cells of the blood vessels.

Plasmodium spp. Avian malaria

Location: Gamonts are found in the erythrocytes and endothelial cells of birds.

Hosts: A wide variety of birds may be affected, including chicken, turkey, guineafowl and wild birds.

Vector: Mosquitoes (mainly *Culex* and *Aedes*)

Species description: The avian malaria is caused by several species of *Plasmodium*. Species with round or irregular gamonts which displace the nucleus of the host erythrocytes are *P. gallinaceum* and *P. juxtanucleare*.

Species with elongate gamonts which do not usually displace the nucleus of the host erythrocytes are *P. durae, P. fallax* and *P. lophurae*. The pathologic effects in avian hosts range from no apparent signs to severe anaemia. Zoo penguins are very susceptible and succumb very quickly. Infected mosquitos introduce sporozoites into the host.

Geographic distribution: World-wide

Symptoms: Affected birds are droopy and weak. Severely affected birds have a protruding abdomen and the liver and spleen are enlarged and discoloured (dark-brown to black). Birds become progressively weak and apathetic. Coma and death may occur in heavy infections after a short period.

Ocular haemorrhage may occur. Severe anaemia may also be observed. Central nervous dysfunction may result from blockage of capillaries by exoerythrocytic stages of *P. gallinaceum*.

Significance: Infections occur world-wide with high frequencies. *P. gallinaceum, P. juxta-*

nucleare and *P. durae* are the most pathogenic species for chickens and may cause mortalities of up to 90%.

Diagnosis: Giemsa-stained bloodsmears usually reveal numerous organisms (gamonts and meronts) in the erythrocytes. Infected cells also have dark pigment granules (digested haemoglobin). As liquid blood samples cool, microgamonts produce microgametes that enter the plasma. Microgametes of *Plasmodium* spp. and related *Haematozoa* can be mistaken for *Borrelia spirochaetes*, when moving in wet smears.

Therapy: Affected animals or flocks may be treated with chloroquine (1 mg/kg, im., daily during 5 days; 250 mg/120 ml of drinking water) can be used. Grape or orange juice may be used to disguise the drug's bitterness. Quinacrine (1.6 mg/kg, im., daily during 5 days) and primaquine (100 mg/kg, po.) and sulfonamids combined with trimethoprime may be used. In penguins, 5 mg/kg daily in fish may be used for prevention. Pyrimethamine, chlorguanil or trimethoprime may also be used. Pyrimethamine is reported to be the best suppressive drug. Any antimalarial drug may be tried, but strain differences in drug susceptibility are found.

Prophylaxis: Mosquito screening of the chicken houses may prevent transmission by the vector.

(Figure 673)

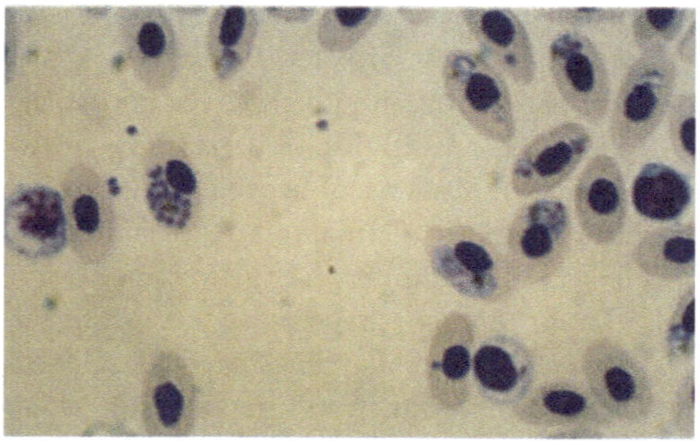

Fig. 673 *Plasmodium gallinaceum*; schizont and macrogametocyte; stained bloodsmear (1000 ×) [15]

Haemoproteus spp. (*H. columbae* and *H. danilewskii*)

Remarks: Over 120 species of *Haemoproteus* have been reported mostly from wild waterfowl, passerine birds and some other orders of birds. Chickens are not affected by this parasite. Vectors are hippoboscid flies and biting midges (*Culicoides* spp.) for some species. Gamonts may be demonstrated in stained bloodsmears and schizonts in the endothelial cells of the blood vessels of the lungs. Schizonts may be found in the liver, spleen and kidneys. Antimalarial drugs may be used for treatments (☞ above *Plasmodium* spp.).

(Figure 674)

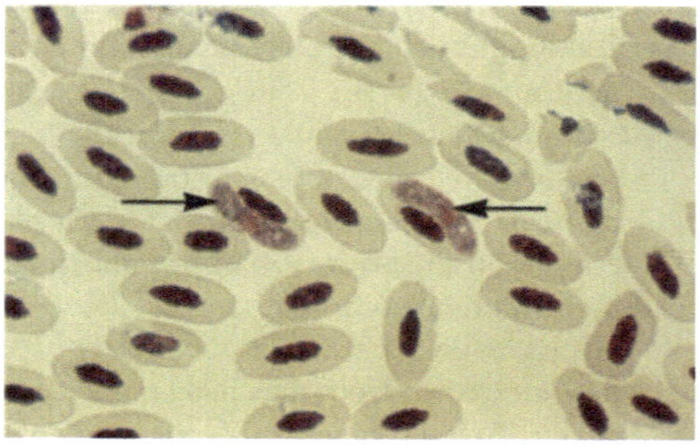

Fig. 674 *Haemoproteus* sp.; gamonts (arrows); stained bloodsmear (1000 ×) [4]

Leucocytozoon spp. (*L. caulleryi* and *L. sabrazesi*)

Location: Gamonts occur in the red blood cells and white blood cells which are often distorted by the large size of the organism.

Hosts: Many wild and domestic birds are affected by these parasites.

Species description: Parasites of this genus undergo schizogony in the endothelial cells and parenchymatous cells of the liver, heart, kidney and other organs of avian hosts. Large schizonts are produced. The gamonts occur in the circulating blood, and the infected host cells become grossly distorted and assume a spindle-shape. The vectors are black flies (*Simulium* spp.) or biting midges (*Culicoides* spp.). Of the numerous *Leucocytozoon* species many are restricted to a certain group or order of birds.

Geographic distribution: *Leucocytozoon* spp. occur world-wide. *L. caulleryi* and *L. sabrazesi* were reported from chickens and guinea fowls in Asia.

Symptoms: Some strains of *L. caulleryi* are non-pathogenic and others are highly pathogenic, killing a high percentage of chickens in a flock. Affected chickens are anaemic, listless, diarrhoeic, have pallid combs and wattles and have marked haemorrhage in their lungs, livers and kidneys. There may be gross haemorrhage from the kidney lesions into the peritoneal cavity. *L. sabrazesi* causes a disease in chickens characterized by anaemia, pyrexia, diarrhoea, paralysis of the legs and a ropy discharge from the mouth.

Significance: *Leucocytozoon* spp. may cause considerable losses in infected flocks.

Diagnosis: In stained bloodsmears (Giemsa or Brilliant-cresyl blue) gamonts may be seen. The shape of the gamont varies with the species, some are elongated while others are rounded. There are no pigment granules. Haemorrhages, splenomegaly and hepatomegaly are seen at necropsy. Grossly visible white dots in many organs are the meronts.

Therapy: Treatment usually is not effective. Pyrimethamine (1 ppm) and sulfadimethoxine (10 ppm) administered simultaneously may prevent but not cure infections of *L. caulleryi*. Pyrimethamine (25 ppm) was recommended for therapy. Furazolidone (150 ppm, po.) may be used to avoid clinical symptoms.

Prophylaxis: Control requires eliminating the arthropod vector from the environment of the host. Insecticidal sprays and repellents sprayed within houses may be used to reduce the insect populations.

(Figure 675)

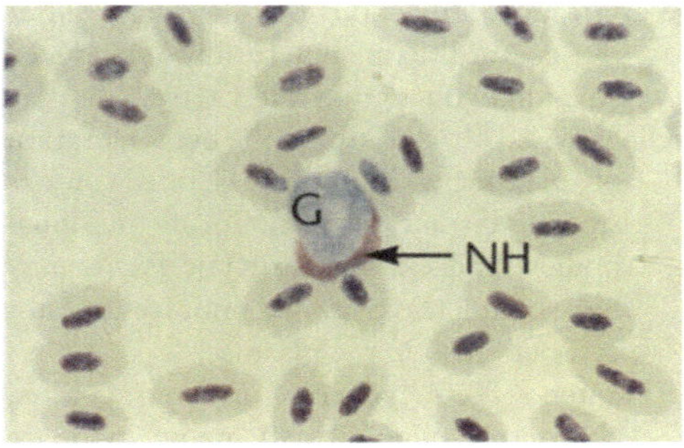

Fig. 675 *Leucocytozoon* sp.; gamont (G) in an erythrocyte (1000 ×). The nucleus of the host cell (NH) is peripheral; stained bloodsmear [4]

RICKETTSIALES

Aegyptianella spp. (*A. pullorum* and *A. moshkovskii*)

Location: The pathogens occur as initial bodies followed by development forms and marginal bodies in the cytoplasm of erythrocytes ("signet-ring").

Hosts: Chicken, turkey, duck, goose and other birds

Species description: The organisms are transmitted by *Argas persicus* and probably other tick species. Transmission by blood inoculation is possible. The incubation period is 12–15 days. The early trophozoites or initial bodies occur in erythrocytes, are small (0.5–1.0 µm) and round to oval. Spherical bodies up to 4 µm may occur, containing up to 25 small granules. The clinical condition is often complicated by fowl spirochaetosis which is also transmitted by *Argas persicus*.

Geographic distribution: North and South Africa, Asia, southern Europe, UIS

Symptoms: Ruffled feathers, anorexia, droopiness, diarrhoea and hyperthermia may be found. Anaemia, jaundice, enlargement of the liver and the spleen, yellow-green kidneys and punctiform haemorrhage of the serosa may be seen at necropsy.

Significance: Indigenous poultry rarely suffer the acute disease, but freshly introduced stock may die within a few days.

Diagnosis: This is based on the demonstration of organisms in Giemsa-stained blood-smears. Intraerythrocytic forms (marginal bodies) and extraerythrocytic forms may be seen in leucocytes, lymphocytes, monocytes but also in the plasma.

Therapy: Tetracyclines (oxytetracycline, chlortetracycline, 15–30 mg/kg, po.) are effective.

Prophylaxis: ☞ POULTRY, ■ 5.1 TICK CONTROL

(Figure 676)

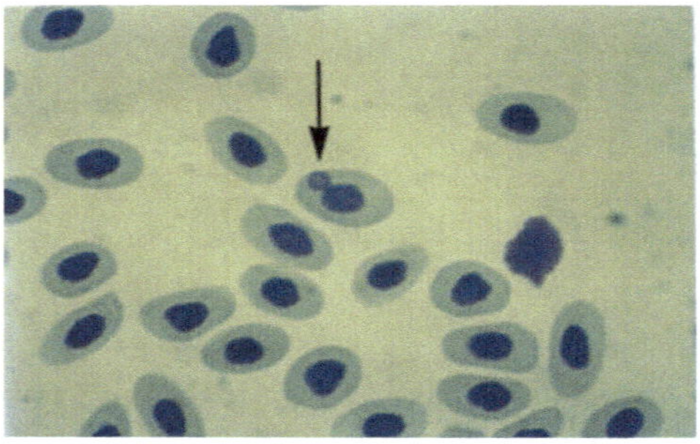

Fig. 676 *Aegyptianella pullorum*; the organism forms a marginal body in the cytoplasm of erythrocytes (arrow) (1000 ×) [13]

3 Stages in the urogenital system

HELMINTHS

- Trematoda found in the urogenital system

***Prosthogonimus* spp. (*P. pellucidus* (syn. *cuneatus*), *P. ovatus* and other *Prosthogonimus* sp.)** Oviduct fluke

Location: Bursa of Fabricius, oviduct, posterior intestine

Hosts: Chicken, duck, goose and many species of wild birds

Species description: The adult flukes are 8–12 mm long and bear two suckers. The eggs measure 22–27 × 13–18 µm, are operculated and bear a small spine opposite to the operculum. They are passed in the faeces. The first intermediate hosts are aquatic snails and the second are the nymphal stage of various species of dragonflies. Metacercariae may persist in the insect until the final host is infected by eating either the adult dragonfly or the nymphal stage. In the final host the liberated immature trematodes migrate to the cloaca and the bursa of Fabricius where they become adult. In the mature chicken the parasites enter the oviduct.

Geographic distribution: World-wide

Symptoms: The disease usually occurs seasonally (spring and summer in temperate areas). Several hens begin to lay eggs with soft shells or no shells at all. There is marked discharge from the cloaca, consisting chiefly of lime and the feathers around the cloaca are soiled with albumen which may contain the parasites. The birds become listless, the abdomen is pendulous and the legs are held widely apart during walking. Laying is suspended and the birds are obviously ill. If peritonitis develops, the comb and wattles become cyanotic and the birds die. The trematodes may also occur within the deposited eggs.

Significance: *Prosthogonimus* spp. are among the most pathogenic trematodes of poultry. Chickens are mainly affected but occasionally also ducks. The fluke causes marked inflammation of the oviduct, the production of abnormal eggs and discharges of albumen from the cloaca. Peritonitis often develops by retroperistaltic movements of the oviduct.

Diagnosis: Large numbers of parasite eggs may be found in the discharges from the cloaca. Sometimes the parasites may be found in the abdominal cavity at necropsy.

Therapy: Praziquantel (5–10 mg/kg, po.) and mebendazole (10–50 mg/kg, po.) may be used to control *Prosthogonimus* infections.

Prophylaxis: Affected flocks should be kept away of the intermediate hosts. Fencing in chicken flocks prevents access to lake shores where chickens may acquire infection by eating dragonfly naiads.

(Figures 630, 677, 678, 679)

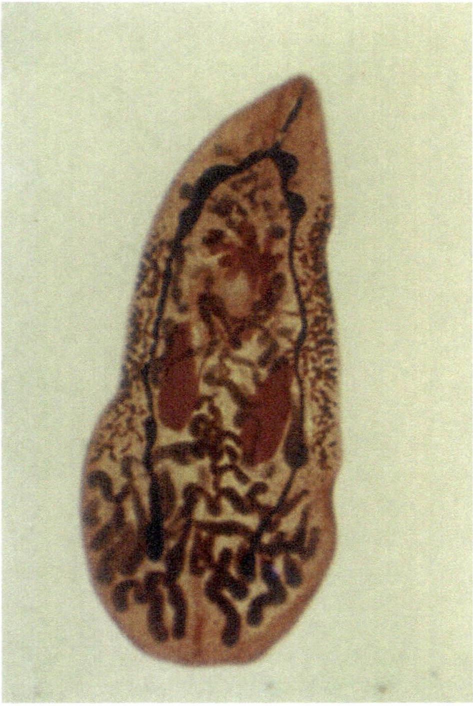

Fig. 677 *Prosthogonimus cuneatus* (syn. *P. pellucidus*); stained [4]

Fig. 678
Prosthogonimus macroorchis (8–12 mm long) [56]

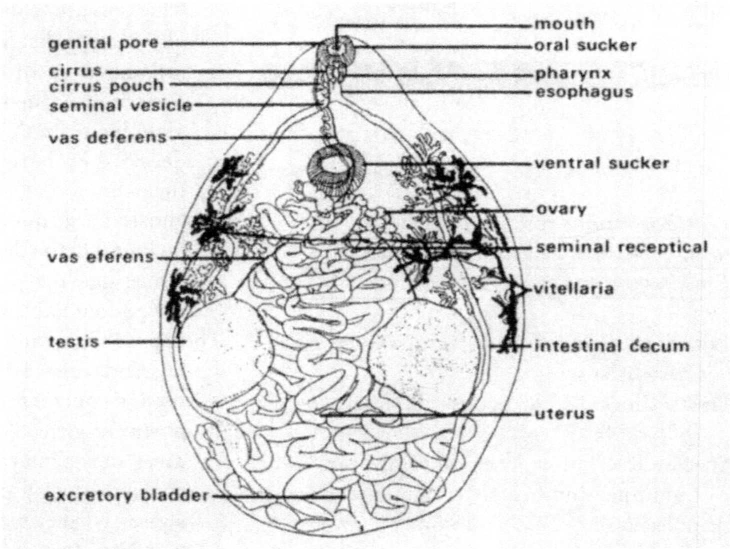

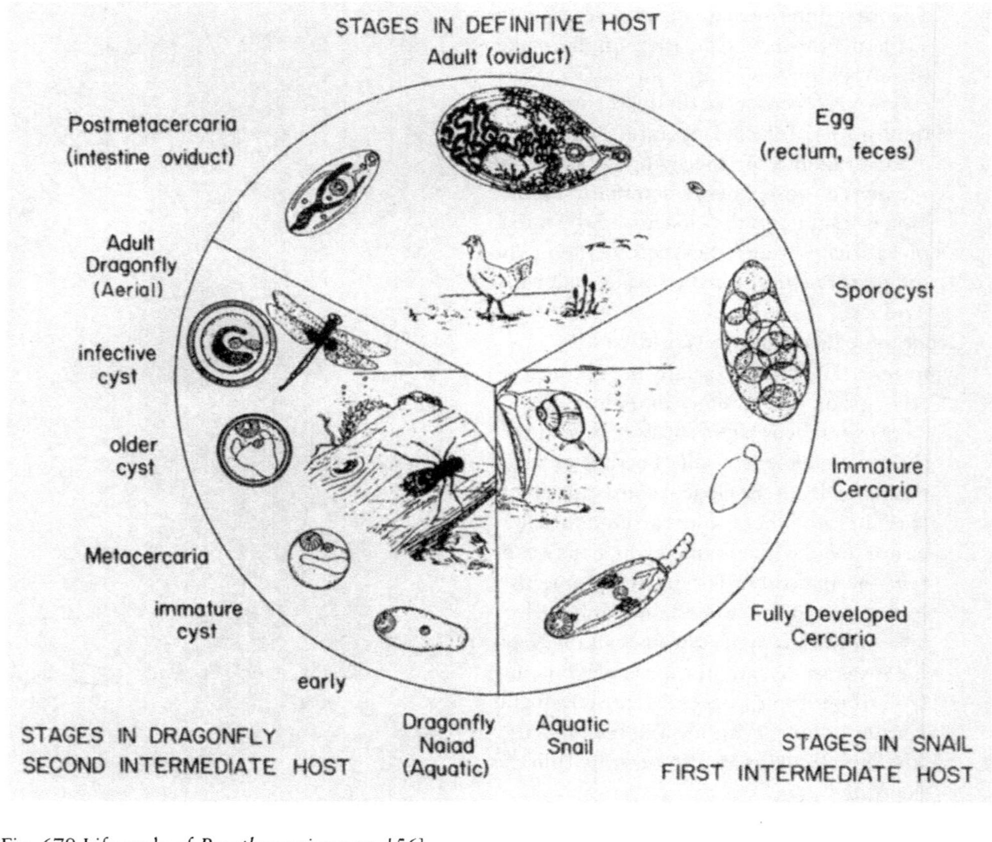

Fig. 679 Life cycle of *Prosthogonimus* sp. [56]

4.1 Locomotory system

4.1.1 Muscles

PROTOZOA

Toxoplasma gondii

Location: Intracellular cysts with a diameter of 50 µm occur in muscles and several other tissues of chickens.

Hosts: Cats and other members of the Felidae are definitive hosts. Many mammals including all domestic animals act as intermediate hosts (☞ SWINE, ■ 4.1).

Species description: Infection is acquired orally by ingestion of sporulated oocysts from faeces of the final host (☞ SWINE, ■ 4.1).

Geographic distribution: World-wide

Symptoms: Natural infections are often clinically inapparent. The chicken is quite resistant to *T. gondii* but disease has been observed from both natural and experimental infections. Clinical signs in chickens include anorexia, paleness, emaciation, reduced egg production, diarrhoea, incoordination, ataxia, trembling, opisthotonus, torticollis and blindness. Mortality may be as high as 50%.

Significance: In chickens only sporadic outbreaks of *T. gondii* have been reported.

Diagnosis: This is usually difficult and based on finding the cysts in the muscle using the artificial digestion method. It is also possible to employ serological tests (complement fixation, haemagglutination or indirect immunofluorescent antibody tests) but the most convincing diagnosis is the isolation of the parasite by inoculation of suspect material into mice. Impression smears of peritoneal fluids or tissues stained with Giemsa, or tissue sections of brain, liver, spleen, lungs and lymph nodes may reveal the organisms by direct microscopic examination.

Therapy: This is generally not indicated.

Prophylaxis: Prevention of avian toxoplasmosis requires management practices that eliminate the source of infected tachyzoites and oocysts, by preventing exposure to cats and coprophageous arthropods. The destruction of oocysts which are disseminated throughout the premises is impossible.

***Sarcocystis* spp. (*S. horvathi, Sarcocystis* sp. and *S. rileyi*)** Sarcosporidiosis

Location: Muscles of the breast, thigh, neck and oesophagus

Hosts: Chicken, duck and many other domestic and wild birds

Species description: Two species occur in chickens: *S. horvathi* and *Sarcocystis* sp. *S. rileyi* mainly occurs in ducks but it has also been reported from chickens. Sarcocysts of *S. rileyi* are elongate, with their long axis parallel to the muscle fibres. They are whitish and appear spindle-shaped when removed from the musculature. Sarcocysts are divided into compartments, each of which contains numerous banana-shaped cystozoites (bradyzoites). Cystozoites are 8–15 µm long and 2–3 µm wide. The life cycle is not completely known but dogs and cats may act as final hosts. Chickens are infected by ingesting oocysts or sporocysts via faeces of the final hosts (cats or dogs).

Sarcocystis spp. found in chickens: *S. horvathi:* sarcocyst: 1–10 mm, cystozoites: 9–12 × 2.5–3 µm and final host: unknown; *Sarcocystis* sp. sarcocyst: 1–10 mm, cystozoites: 14–17.5 × 2–2.5 µm and final host: dog and cat; *S. rileyi* sarcocyst: 3–5 mm, cystozoites: 8–15 × 2–3 µm and final host: unknown.

Geographic distribution: World-wide

Symptoms: Infections with *Sarcocystis* spp. in chickens are generally inapparent. Muscular dystrophy may occasionally occur.

Significance: Sarcosporidiosis may be prevalent in traditional poultry rearing systems. The pathogenicity and significance of this parasite seems to be low.

Diagnosis: This is based on demonstrating the Sarcocysts or cystozoites in artificially digested muscles and other organs at necropsy.

Therapy: Unknown and not indicated

Prophylaxis: This is difficult in extensive husbandry systems with free ranging. Intensive poultry rearing avoids the ingestion of oocysts and sporocysts of the final hosts (possibly dogs, cats and other carnivores).

4.2 Liver

PROTOZOA

Histomonas meleagridis "Blackhead"

Remarks: Extensive liver lesions may occur. These are circular, yellowish green, and characteristically depressed. In turkeys they may be up to 4 cm in diameter. The liver and caecal lesions together are pathognomonic. However, the liver lesions must be differentiated from those of tuberculosis, leukosis, avian trichomonosis and mycosis, which are raised and greyish or grey-yellow (☞ POULTRY, ■ 1).

4.3 Respiratory system

PROTOZOA

Remarks: The following parasites may also be found in the tissue of the lungs:

Trichomonas gallinae (☞ POULTRY, ■ 1)
Toxoplasma gondii (☞ SWINE, ■ 4)
Cryptosporidium spp. (☞ POULTRY, ■ 1)
Schizonts of the following Protozoa:
Sarcocystis spp. (☞ POULTRY, ■ 4.1)
Haemoproteus spp. (☞ POULTRY, ■ 2)
Leucocytozoon spp. (☞ POULTRY, ■ 2)
Plasmodium spp. (☞ POULTRY, ■ 2)

HELMINTHS

- Nematoda found in the respiratory system

Syngamus trachea "Gapeworm"

Location: Trachea and lungs

Hosts: Chicken and many other domestic and wild birds

Species description: The parasite is bright red in colour and found permanently in copulation. The male is 2–6 mm long and the female 5–20 mm. The mouth opening is wide, without leaf-crowns, and the buccal capsule is cup-shaped. The eggs measure 70–100 × 43–46 µm and have a thickened operculum at either pole. Infection may occur directly by ingestion of infective eggs or larvae. However, it is well established that severe field infections are associated with the ingestion of transport hosts such as earthworms, snails, slugs, and arthropods (e.g. flies). Gapeworm larvae may encyst and survive for years within an invertebrate host. Range infections occur seasonally, e.g. when great numbers of earthworms appear on the surface by rains in spring or at the onset of the rainy season, etc. *Cyathostoma bronchiale* is the causative agent of the disease in geese and ducks.

Geographic distribution: World-wide

Symptoms: Sudden death and verminous pneumonia characterize early outbreaks. Signs of gasping, choking, shaking of the head, inanition, emaciation and suffocation may follow.

Significance: This may be of great economic significance in range-reared chickens. Young birds are affected most severely. Gapeworms are not a problem in confinement-reared poultry but cause serious losses in range-reared chickens, turkeys and other birds.

Diagnosis: This is based on the demonstration of the typical eggs in the faeces and the clinical signs. At necropsy adult gapeworms may be found to obstruct the lumina of the trachea and bronchi. The blood-red female gapeworm is usually found in copulation with a much smaller, paler male with its head embedded deep in the host tissue. The joined pair has a "Y"-shaped appearance.

Therapy: Febantel (60 ppm via feed over 6 days or 15 mg/kg, po. over 2 days), fenbendazole (100 ppm, over 4 days), flubendazole (30 ppm, over 7 days) and mebendazole (60 ppm, over 7 days) are effective against gapeworms in chickens. Ivermectin may be used orally at a dosage of 200 µg/kg. Thiabendazole (300 mg/kg, po., 1 ×) is also effective.

Prophylaxis: The control of gapeworm infections in range-reared chickens is almost impossible since the transport hosts are difficult to be eliminated. To prevent wild birds from introducing infection, pens should be isolated by overhead and lateral screening. The control of the transport hosts by soil treatments with chemicals is unsafe and not justifiable.

(Figures 680, 681, 682, 683)

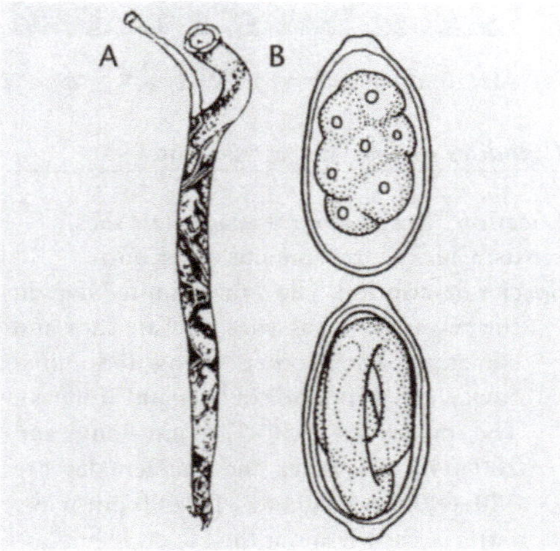

Fig. 681 *Syngamus trachea*; male and female worms in permanent copulation (A); eggs (B) [56]

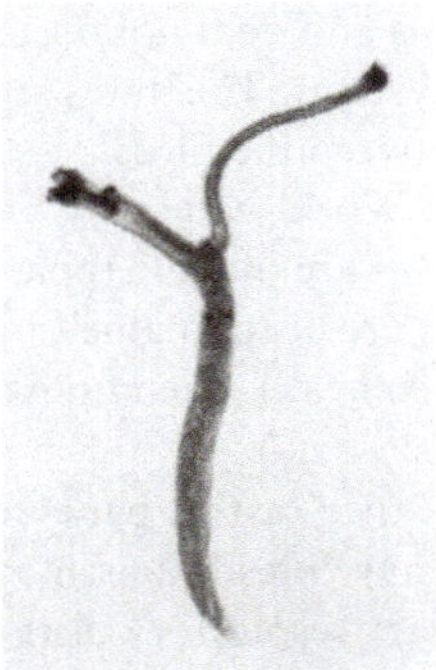

Fig. 682 *Syngamus trachea*; a joined pair with a Y-shaped appearance [8]

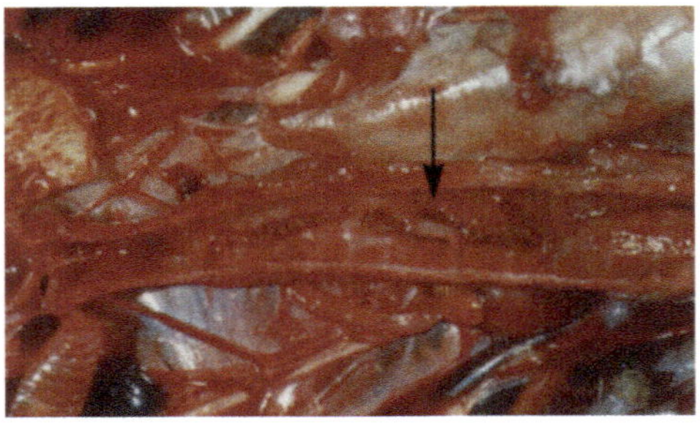

Fig. 680 *Syngamus trachea*; adult parasites in the trachea. Males are 2–6 mm and females are 15–30 mm long [53]

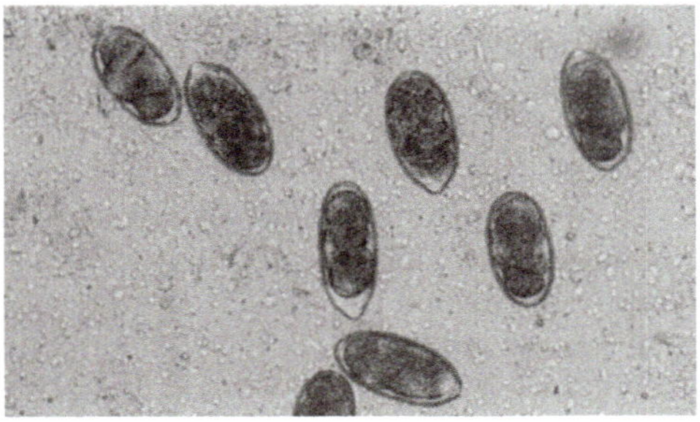

Fig. 683 Eggs of *Syngamus trachea* (74–95 × 39–44 µm)

ARTHROPODS

- Arachnida found in the respiratory system

Cytodites nudus The "air sac mite"

Location: Respiratory passages (air sacs)
Hosts: Chicken, pigeon and other birds
Species description: The "air sac mite" lives in the respiratory passages and air sacs and sometimes also in other organs (abdominal cavity, e.g. serosa side of liver and kidneys). The males are 450–575 µm long and 280–340 µm wide, and the females are 480–600 µm long and 315–400 µm wide. Little is known about the life cycle but larvae (not eggs!) are produced by the female. Parasites are spread by respiratory mucus. The parasite has a moderate pathogenicity. It occurs mainly in range-reared small holder poultry systems and does not occur in intensive rearing systems. The mites are easily transmitted between the birds.
Geographic distribution: World-wide
Symptoms: Light infections are often inapparent. Heavy infections are accompanied by cough, dyspnoea (open beak), pneumonia, bronchitis, peritonitis.
Significance: The significance of this parasite is still in debate. Heavy infestations may predispose to secondary respiratory disorders.
Diagnosis: This is based on the demonstration of the mites on smears taken from the respiratory system at necropsy. The mites may be seen macroscopically as little white dots on the surface of the air bags.
Therapy: The elimination of affected or exposed birds has been the recommended method of control. Ivermectin was effective in golden pheasants only at very high doses (50 mg/kg, sc.).
Prophylaxis: Unknown
(Figures 684, 685, 686)

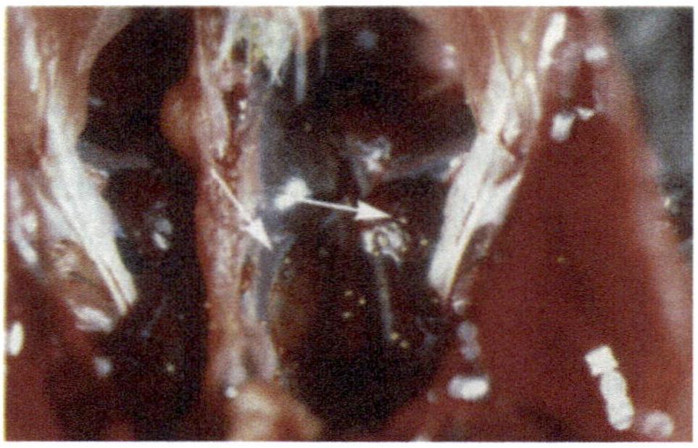

Fig. 684 *Cytodites nudus*; adult mites (450–600 µm) found in the air sacs (arrows) [53]

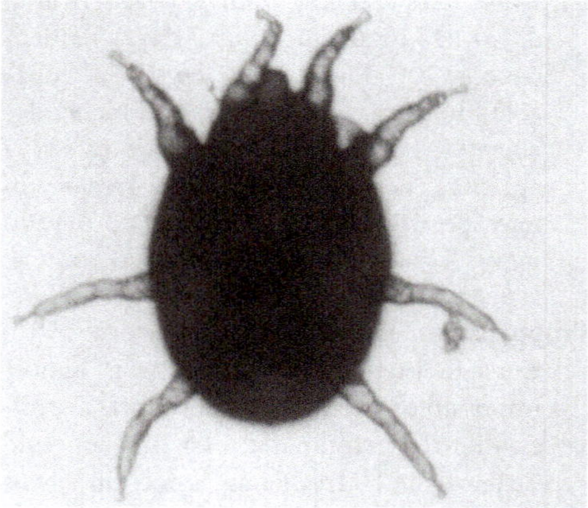

Fig. 685 *Cytodites nudus;* adult mite [53]

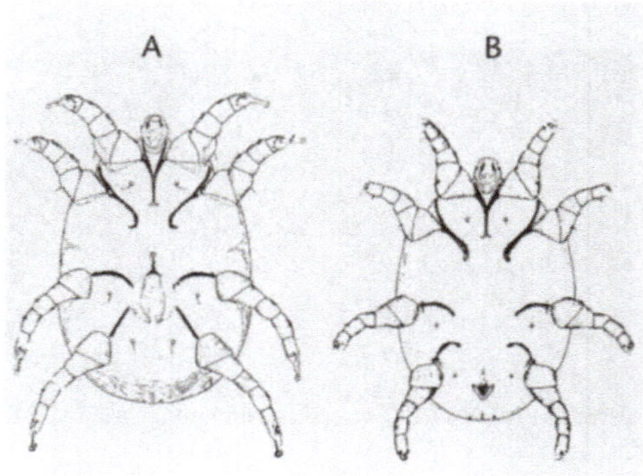

Fig. 686 *Cytodites nudus*; ventral view of adult female (A) and male (B) [29]

5.1 Skin and feathers

HELMINTHS

• Trematoda found in the subcutaneous tissue

Collyriclum faba

Location: These trematodes appear anywhere on the body as subcutaneous cysts.
Hosts: Chicken, turkey and other bird species
Species description: The subcutaneous cysts are 4–6 mm in diameter, usually containing two adults and occur most frequently near the vent of the host. The worms measure 3–5 × 4.5–5.5 mm. They are flattened ventrally, convex dorsally and have a spiny tegument. The eggs measure 19–21 × 9–11 µm. The cysts ooze exudate which attracts flies and predisposes to bacterial infections. The life cycle is unknown but probably involves snails and insects such as dragonflies and mayflies as intermediate hosts. Only birds with access to marshy places become infected.
Geographic distribution: Asia, Europe, the Americas, Africa
Symptoms: Young birds show locomotory difficulties, inappetence, anaemia, emaciation and even death.
Significance: Infections with this trematode may be frequent in flocks which have access to marshy places. The presence of the cysts decreases the value of the carcass.
Diagnosis: Typical cysts are found around the cloacal opening and also along the abdomen and thorax. Each cyst has a central opening and contains a pair of worms. The cysts also contain a black fluid and the eggs which are discharged through the pore.
Therapy: Chemotherapy is unknown. The parasites should be removed surgically followed by an antiseptic treatment of the wound.
Prophylaxis: Prevention requires restricting birds from areas frequented by aquatic insects.

ARTHROPODS

The ectoparasites (Arthropods) are divided into two main groups:

Arachnida (arachnids) including:
– *Ticks*
– *Mites*

Insecta including:
– *Lice*
– *Heteroptera*
– *Fleas*
– *Dipterida*

• Arachnida found in/on the skin

– Ticks

Losses caused by ticks are threefold: 1) loss of blood (anaemia), 2) transmission of other diseases (avian spirochaetosis, rickettsial diseases, viruses, etc.) and 3) tick toxicosis (e.g. paralysis)(☞ CATTLE, 1).

IXODIDAE ("hard ticks")

Hard ticks are not a primary problem in chickens. Birds are preferred hosts of larvae and nymphs of some species of *Hyalomma* and *Amblyomma* ticks that are common in the adult stage on mammals. *Haemaphysalis cinnabarina*, *H. leporispalustris*, *H. chordeilis*, *Amblyomma haebraeum* and other hard ticks of many species will feed on poultry as well as wild ground birds. Hard ticks are likely to be found only on birds that have access to range (bushy pastures and pens are preferred sites of hard tick stages). Mainly young birds are affected. Extreme emaciation, progressive weakness, restlessness and swollen eyelids may be seen in young chickens. Control is based on the use of contact-acaricides, (☞ *Argas persicus*, below) and preventingchickens from entering breeding areas of the ticks.

ARGASIDAE ("soft-ticks")

Argas persicus, A. walkerae, A. reflexus hermanni and other *Argas* spp. Fowl ticks

Location: Skin

Hosts: Chicken, turkey, pigeon, duck, goose and many other domestic and wild birds; man may also be affected.

Species description: *Argas persicus* is the most important poultry ectoparasite in many tropical and subtropical countries, being a limiting factor in successful rearing of standard breeds of poultry.

Unfed ticks are relatively easily recognized by their flattened ovoid shape and the reddish-brown colour.

The fowl tick is capable of transmitting *Borrelia anserina*, *Aegyptianella pullorum*, fowl cholera (*Pasteurella multocida*) and possibly other diseases. These ticks are particularly active in poultry houses during warm and dry weather. All stages may be found hiding in cracks and crevices during the day. Larvae can be found on the birds since they remain attached and feed for 2–7 days. Nymphs and adults feed at night in 15–30 min. Nymphs feed and moult several times before reaching the adult stage. Adults feed repeatedly and the females lay 50–100 eggs after each feeding. Adult females may live for more than 4 years without a blood meal. *A. persicus* and *A. reflexus hermanni* are found in chickens in West Africa. *A. reflexus hermanni* in Egypt is suspected of transmitting West Nile and *Chenuda* virus and the *Quaranfil* virus group.

Geographic distribution: *A. persicus* occurs world-wide in tropical and subtropical countries. *A. walkerae* occurs in sub-Saharan Africa.

Symptoms: In addition to transmitting avian spirochaetosis, aegyptianellosis and fowl cholera, *Argas* spp. produce anaemia (most important). Loss of blood may reach proportions of fatal anaemia. Low numbers may cause emaciation, weakness, slow growth and lowered production. Since the ticks are nocturnal, the birds may show some uneasiness when roosting. *A. persicus* and *A. walkerae* may cause tick paralysis, a flaccid, afebrile motor paralysis. A specific paralytic toxin is suspected to be transmitted by the sucking tick.

Significance: Soft-bodied ticks of the genus *Argas* are the most important ticks of poultry.

Diagnosis: Red spots may be seen on the skin where the ticks have fed. Larvae may be found in the feathers. The adult parasites may be found in cracks of the woodwork or in the walls of the fowl house.

Therapy and Prophylaxis: This requires treatment of premises because adult and nymphal ticks are on their hosts for only a short time and then hide in the surroundings. After houses are cleaned, walls, ceilings, cracks, and crevices should be treated thoroughly with carbaryl, coumaphos, malathion, stirofos or a mixture of stirofos and dichlorvos. The efficiency may be increased by using high pressure sprayer (☞ Table 27, p. 389).

(Figures 687, 688, 689, 690)

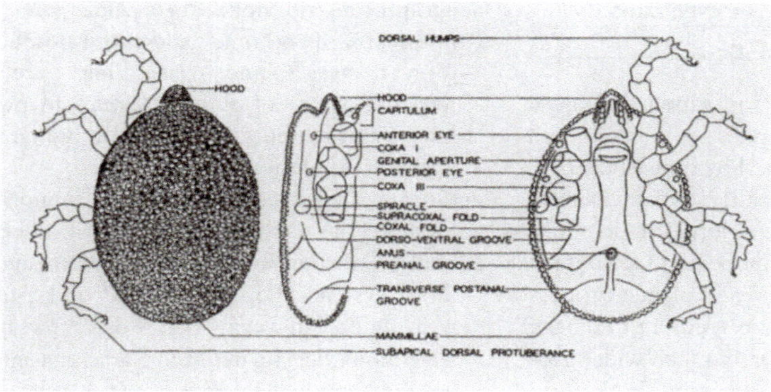

Fig. 687 *Argas* sp.; dorsal (left), lateral (middle) and ventral view (right) [24]

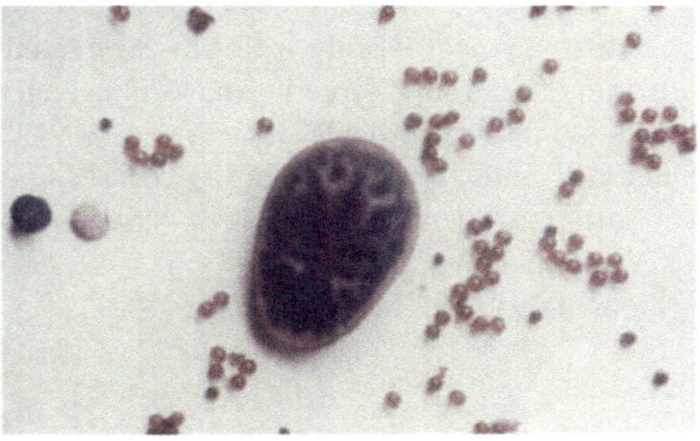

Fig, 688 *Argas reflexus*; adult female (5.5–11 mm long) and eggs [8]

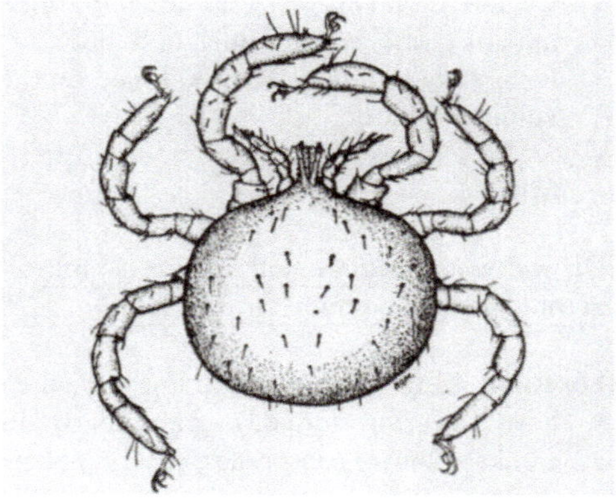

Fig. 690 *Argas persicus*; larva [3]

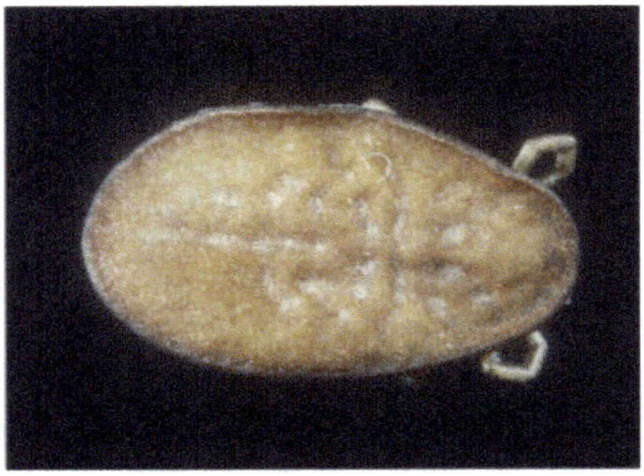

Fig. 689 *Argas persicus*; dorsal view (males are 4–5 mm and females are 7–10 mm long) [8]

Ornithodoros moubata The eyeless tampan of Africa

Remarks: *O. moubata* is widely distributed throughout East Africa and northern South Africa, extending into drier parts of Central Africa. *O. moubata* and *O. savignyi* have become associated with man and his domestic animals. These ticks live in the native huts and in the sand under trees where animals and human beings frequently seek shelter. The significance is based on the irritation of the host and transmission of *Borrelia anserina* and *Aegyptianella pullorum* to fowl. *O. moubata* is also the vector of *Borrelia duttoni* (relapsing fever of man) and African Swine Fever (☞ SHEEP AND GOATS, ■ 5.1).

Ornithodoros savignyi The eyed tampan, the sand tampan

Remarks: It buries itself in sandy and loose clayey soils, under trees, near wells and shady spots frequented by domestic stock, particularly camels, cattle, mules, chickens and man on which it feeds. It does not occur in huts. The numbers of *O. savignyi* in infested localities reach plague proportions. The biology is very similar to that of *O. moubata*, but is has a much wider geographic distribution occurring in the arid parts of Africa, the Near East, India and Ceylon. *O. savignyi* is not known to transmit any pathogen but camels and cattle suffer greatly and may even be killed by the volume of blood lost.

– Mites

Dermanyssus gallinae Red mite, roost mite, poultry or chicken mite

Location: Mites may be found in the chicken houses during the day, particularly in cracks or where roost poles touch supports or on birds during the night.

Hosts: Chicken, turkey and other domestic and wild birds

Species description: The nymphs and adults periodically visit the host to suck blood (preferably during the night) and between the meals hide in cracks and crevices in the quarters of the birds. Under favourable conditions the mites reproduce rapidly and may become a serious pest causing irritation and anaemia due to loss of blood. A house may remain infested for 6 months after birds are removed. Mites may be transmitted by mite dispersion (egg flats, crates, persons going from farm to farm) or by direct bird contact. The chicken mite can be identified by the shape of the dorsal plate and by the long whip-like chelicerae that appear to be stylets. The adult females measure 0.7 × 0.4 mm, varying in colour from gray to deep red, depending on their blood content.

Geographic distribution: World-wide

Symptoms: Birds become listless, egg production decreases and deaths may occur because of loss of blood. *D. gallinae* may occur as a temporary parasite on humans, causing skin lesions.

Significance: Chicken mites may be found at pest level in traditional, small farm flocks and are rare in modern commercial cage-layer systems. Populations may build up very quickly in warm areas. Losses may be enormous due to irritation, anaemia and markedly reduced performance.

Diagnosis: This is based on finding the mites in the environment of the birds (nest, litter, crevices). The mites can be seen with the naked eye, especially when they are red after a recent blood meal. Masses of mites may be found in the naso-pharyngeal system of dead birds.

Therapy and Prophylaxis: ☞ CONTROL OF CHICKEN MITES AND TROPICAL-FOWL MITES INFESTATIONS, p. 382

(Figures 691, 692, 693, 694)

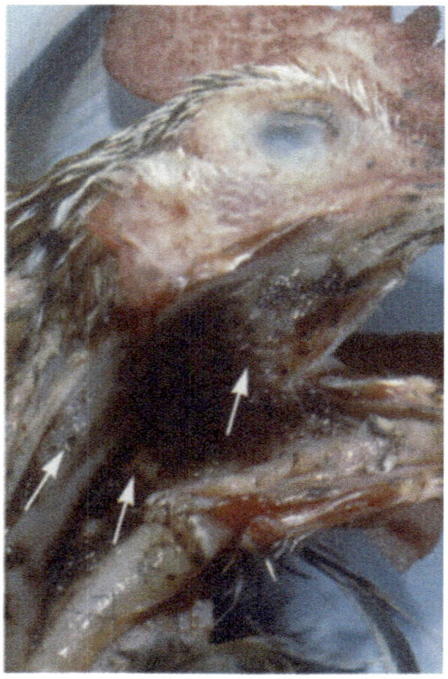

Fig. 691 *Dermanyssus gallinae*; masses of mites are often found in the naso-pharyngeal system of dead birds (arrows) [53]

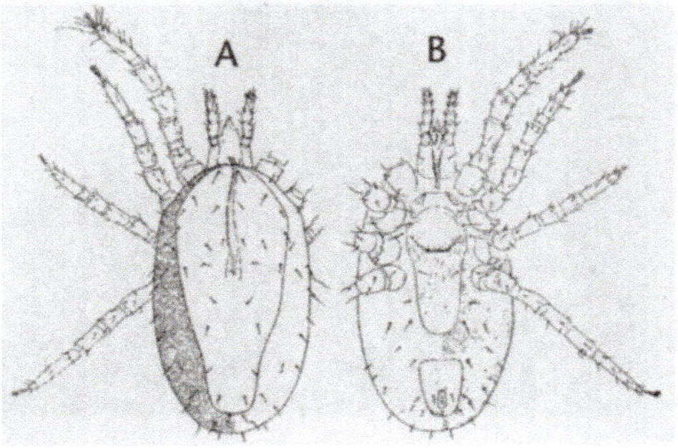

Fig. 692 *Dermanyssus gallinae*; dorsal view (A)

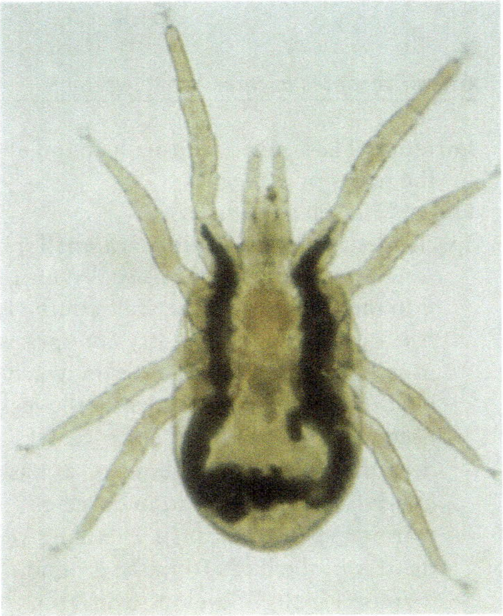

Fig. 693 *Dermanyssus gallinae*; adult mite (600–1000 μm long) [4]

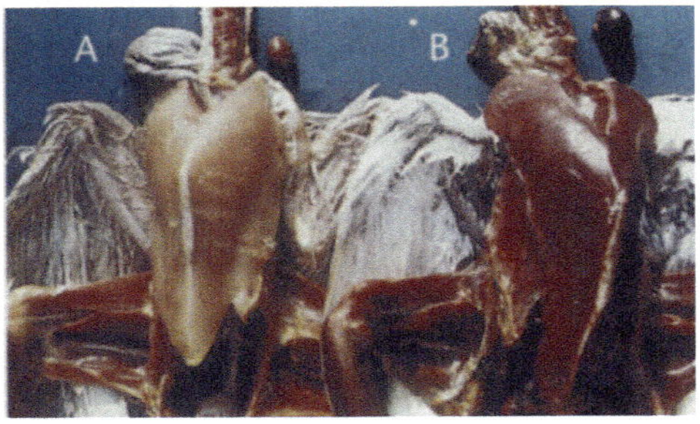

Fig. 694 Anaemia due to heavy *Dermanyssus gallinae* infestation (A); not-infested control animal (B) [54]

Ornithonyssus (syn. *Bdellonyssus, Liponyssus*) ***bursa*** Tropical fowl mite

Location: *O. bursa* occurs either on the bird or in its nest.

Hosts: Chicken, turkey, duck, pigeon and other birds

Species description: The tropical fowl mites are found on the fluff of the feathers, especially on those around the vent. These mites can pass their entire life cycle on chickens. They tend to be present on few feathers, giving them a dirty appearance. The life cycle is not yet completely known. *O. bursa* can also affect man but only temporarily because it is unable to survive away from its bird host. Only the adults, the protonymphs and the deutonymphs feed on the hosts blood. *O. bursa* replaces *O. sylviarum* (northern fowl mite) in warmer parts of the world.

Geographic distribution: Tropical and subtropical regions

Symptoms: Irritation, loss of weight, reduction in egg production, anaemia and death

Significance: Apart from irritating the birds and causing anaemia these two mites may transmit infections (e.g. fowlpox, Newcastle disease, *Pasteurella* spp., etc.). This might be of fundamental importance in intensified poultry rearing systems.

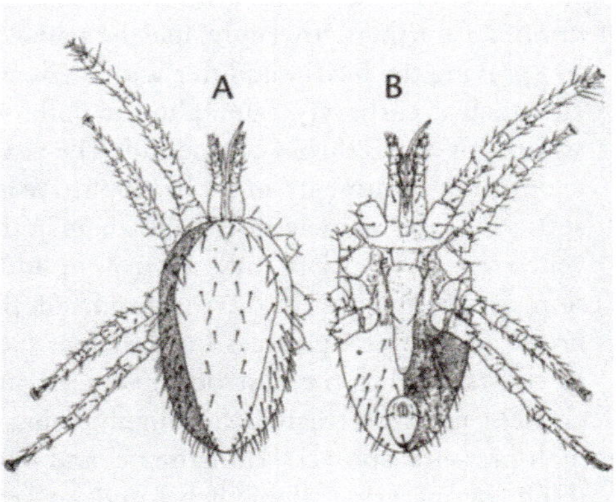

Fig. 695 *Ornithonyssus bursa*; dorsal view (A) and ventral view (B) [56]

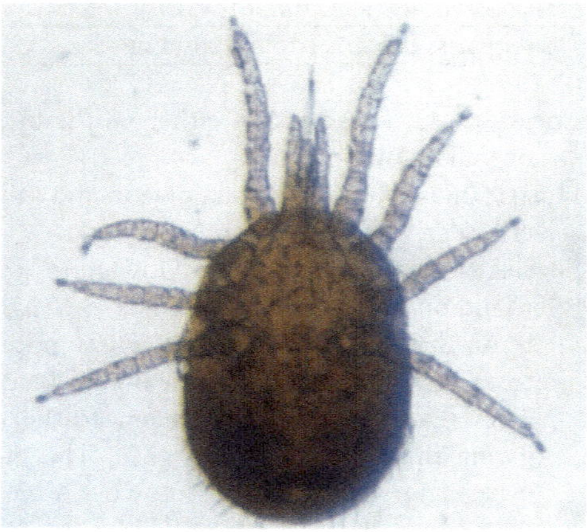

Fig. 696 *Ornithonyssus bursa*; adult (450–650 µm long) [53]

Diagnosis: This is determined by finding them on the feathers of affected birds. The distribution of the mites on the birds may be patchy, hundreds being found in small areas.

Therapy and Prophylaxis: ☞ CONTROL OF CHICKEN MITES AND TROPICAL-FOWL MITES INFESTATIONS.

(Figures 695, 696)

- **Control of chicken mites and tropical-fowl mites infestations**

Control of chickens infested with the tropical fowl mite (and also with *Ornithonyssus sylviarum*, the northern fowl mite) may be achieved by spraying the birds and litter with an acaricide such as carbaryl, coumaphos, malathion, stirofos or a pyrethroid compound. The acaricide spray treatments must be applied with sufficient force to penetrate the feathers in the vent area. For chicken mite control, in addition to treating the birds, the inside of the house and all hiding places for the mite, such as roosts, behind the nest boxes, cracks and crevices must be treated thoroughly using a high-pressure sprayer. Dimethoate and fenthion, permethrine, flumethrine and amitraz may be used as residual house sprays when poultry is not present (☞Table 27, p. 389).

(Figure 697)

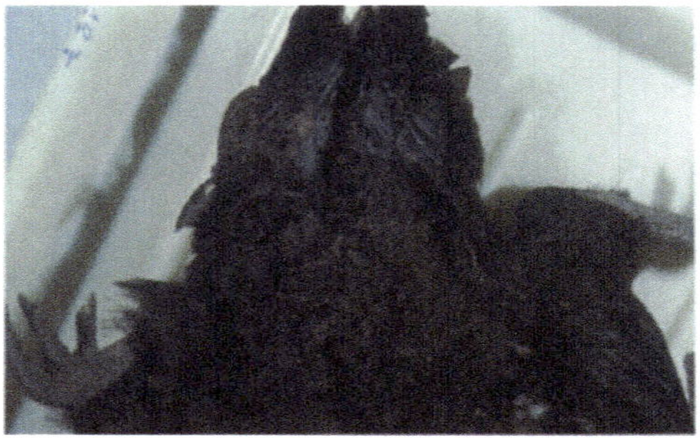

Fig. 697 Heavy infestation with unfed *Dermanyssus gallinae*

Cnemidocoptes mutans Scaly leg mites

Location: These mites are usually found under the scales of the legs.

Hosts: Chicken and turkey

Species description: *C. mutans* is a small spherical, sarcoptic mite that usually burrows into the tissue under the scales of the legs. It is rare in modern poultry enterprises. It usually occurs on older birds on which the irritation and exudation cause the legs to become thickened, encrusted and deformed. This is the result of a massive hypertrophy of the stratum corneum (dermatitis hypertrophicans). The mites reach the feet of the birds from the ground. The lesions usually develop from the toes upwards. The parasites pierce the skin underneath the scales, causing an inflammation with exudate that hardens on the surface and displaces the scales. The entire life cycle is spent on the skin and mites are transmitted by direct contact.

Geographic distribution: World-wide

Symptoms: Thickened scaly skin leading to lameness and malformation of the feet

Significance: This may be a serious problem in traditionally reared chickens.

Diagnosis: This is based on the typical deformation of the legs (scaly legs) and the demonstration of mites in skin scrapings.

Therapy: If individual birds are to be treated, the affected legs may be dipped twice (10-

day interval) in kerosene, mineral oil or linseed oil, or coated with vaseline. It is important that the crusts are carefully removed or soaked with a detergent prior to acaricidal treatment. The legs may also be dipped in acaricides.

Prophylaxis: Affected birds should be culled or isolated and houses cleaned and sprayed as recommended for chicken mite infestations.

(Figures 698, 699)

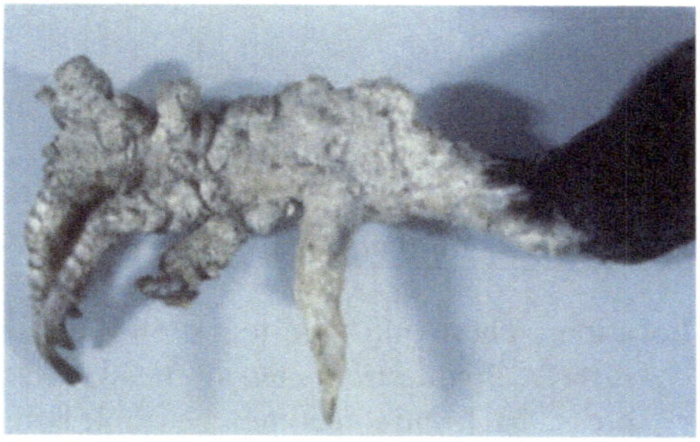

Fig. 698 Deformed legs due to *Cnemidocoptes mutans* infestation [53]

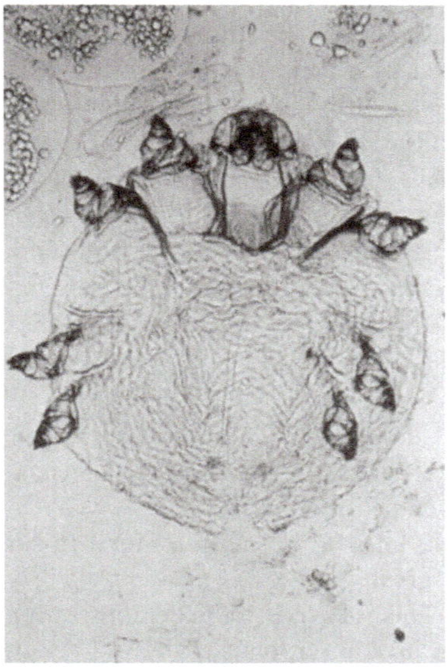

Fig. 699 *Cnemidocoptes mutans*, the scaly leg mite; males are 170–250 μm and females are 370–495 μm long [4]

Cnemidocoptes gallinae (syn. *Mesocnemidocoptes laevis gallinae*) Depluming mite or depluming itch

Location: The mites burrow into the skin alongside the shafts of the feathers on the back, head, neck, around the vent and on the breast and tights.

Hosts: Chicken, pheasant, pigeon and goose

Species description: These mites resemble the scaly leg mite in general structure although they are smaller, the adult females measuring about 0.3 mm in diameter. The mites occur more frequently in summer when infestations are spread rapidly by contact. Infestations cause inflammation and itching. The feathers break off and they are pulled out by the birds.

Geographic distribution: World-wide

Symptoms: The intense irritation induces the host to pull out body feathers. Infested birds show reduced weight gains and lowered production.

Significance: Heavy infestations are associated with great irritation and reduced performance of affected flocks. This infection is rare in modern poultry-rearing systems.

Diagnosis: Demonstration of the mites at the base of the feathers. This can be made by pulling out a few feathers at the edge of the lesions and searching for mites. (10% KOH-solution). The legs and pedicels are stumpy. All legs of the male possess suckers, while none of the female do so.

Therapy and Prophylaxis: Affected birds should be isolated and dipped in an acaricide (malathion, carbaryl, permethrin, stirofos). Disinfection of houses as recommended for chicken mites is important (☞ Table 27, p. 389).

Laminosioptes cysticola Cyst mite, subcutaneous mite

Location: Subcutaneous tissue

Hosts: Chicken and turkey

Species description: The parasites are found in the subcutaneous tissue where they cause calcified nodules around dead parasites.

The life cycle is unknown.

Geographic distribution: World-wide

Symptoms: Infestations are usually inapparent.

Significance: These mites are non-pathogenic but large numbers of nodules may reduce the value of the carcass.

Diagnosis: Examination of the skin and subcutis under a dissecting microscope usually reveals the mites.

Therapy and Prophylaxis: This is unknown. Destroying affected birds is indicated to reduce the infestations within the flocks.

(Figures 700, 701)

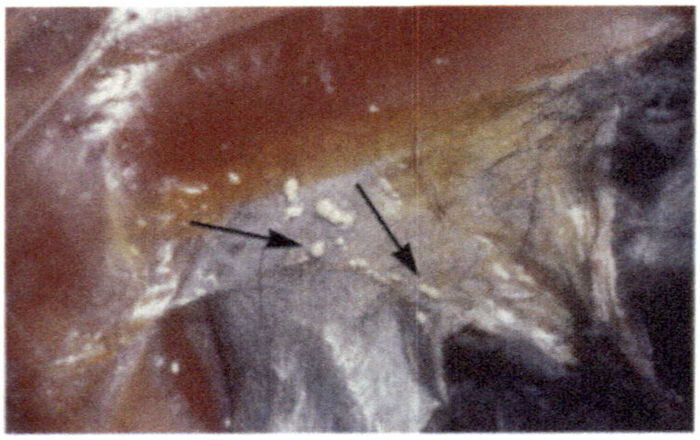

Fig. 700 *Laminosioptes cysticola*; calcified nodules in the subcutaneous tissue (arrows) [53]

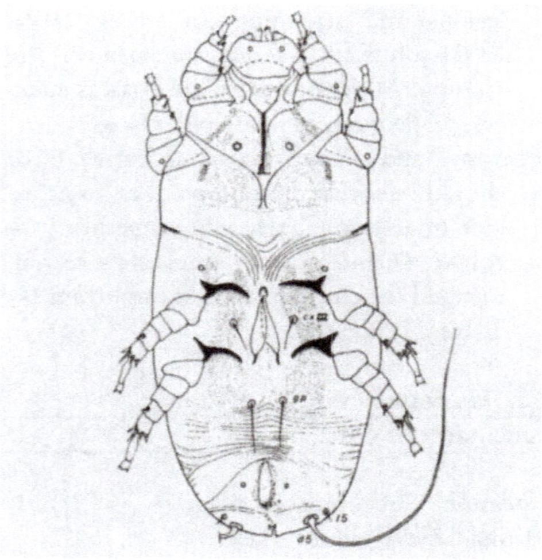

Fig. 701 *Laminosioptes cysticola*; ventral view of a female (250–270 μm long) [29]

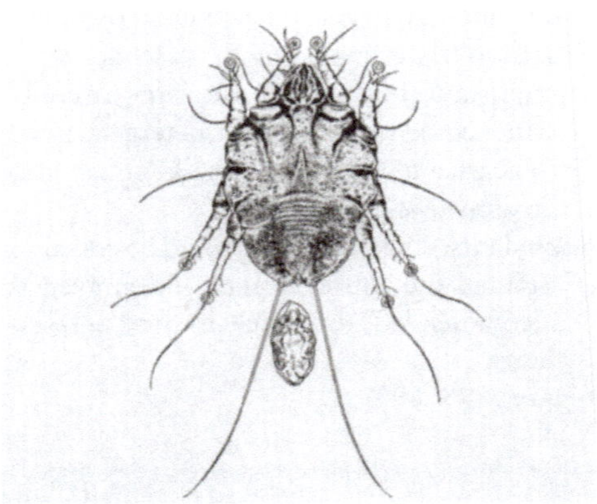

Fig. 702 *Epidermoptes bilobatus*; skin mite (160–270 μm long) [56]

Epidermoptes bilobatus Skin mite

Location: These mites are found on the skin surface. Predilection sites are head, neck, breast, back and sometimes the whole body surface.

Hosts: Chicken

Species description: These mites are very small, the females measuring 0.17–0.22 mm. This is a common skin parasite of chicken and can cause a scaly skin disease. It has been described as a cause of pityriasis. It may produce lesions such as a fine scaly dermatitis, followed by a formation of thick, brownish, sharply edged scabs. Concomitant fungus infection by *Lophophyton gallinae* may aggravate the disease. Birds with *E. bilobatus* infection often have depluming mites at the same time. Bacterial infections may develop after the primary skin lesions.

Geographic distribution: World-wide

Symptoms: Pruritus, featherlessness, emaciation, even death

Significance: Losses in heavily infested flocks may be great.

Diagnosis: This is based on the demonstration of mites in skin scrapings.

Therapy: The following acaricides may be used to dip or spray infested chickens: Pyrethroids (fenvalerate, flumethrine, permethrine), organophosphates (trichlorfon, cythionate) and carbamates (carbaryl, propoxur) (☞ Table 27, p. 389).

Prophylaxis: All the animals of a flock must be treated at the same time and the chicken quarters should also be disinfected.

(Figure 702)

Hypodectes propus Nest-inhabiting mites

Remarks: This is a free living nest-inhabiting mite which produces eggs which develop directly into hypopodes. These stages invade transiently the subcutaneous tissue of birds and grow markedly in size. By the time the hypopodes leave the host they have increased tenfold in length. After leaving the host the hypopodes moult directly into the adult stage.

Symptoms: Itching, feather loss, restlessness

Diagnosis: By finding the adults in the nest or the nymphes II in alterated tissue

Therapy and Prophylaxis: Nests should be treated with acaricides and infested birds should be eliminated.

(Figure 703)

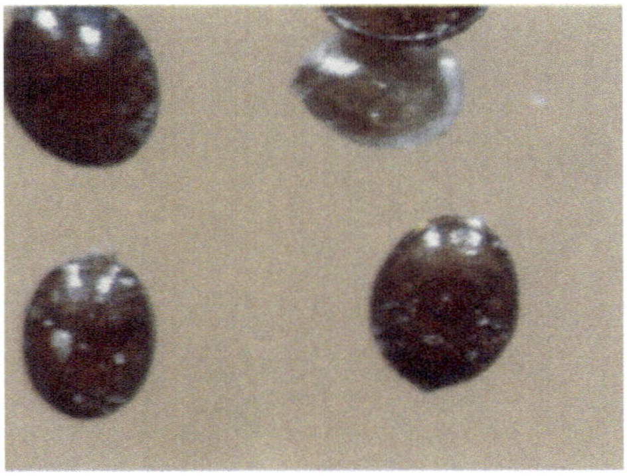

Fig. 703 *Hypodectes propus*; environmental stage of nest-inhabiting mites

- Insecta found on the skin

– **Lice**

MALLOPHAGA Chewing lice, chicken lice

Location: Skin and feathers

Hosts: Chicken

Species description: All chicken lice belong to the order Mallophaga, the chewing lice. More than 40 species of Mallophaga have been reported from domestic chickens. Chewing lice are characterized by possession of broad, chewing-type mandibles located ventrally on the head, incomplete metamorphosis, no wings, dorsoventrally flattened body and short antennae with 3–5 segments. Birds frequently harbour several species at the same time. All the various lice species are controlled by the same methods. Cross contamination is possible, e.g. lice from guinea fowl may occur on chicken and turkeys if these birds have physical contact. Pigeon lice are frequently found on domestic fowl if the pigeons nest above the fowl. Lice spend the entire life cycle on the birds. Eggs are attached to the feathers, often in clusters, and require 4–7 days to hatch. The more common louse species of chickens are listed in Table 26. Lice normally eat feather products but *Eomenacanthus stramineus* may consume blood and is regarded as the most common and most destructive louse of birds, world-wide. It is up to 3.5 mm long and deposits its eggs in masses at the base of feathers, especially around the vent. As a rule, lice are not very pathogenic to mature birds but louse-infested chicks may die. Lousiness frequently accompanies manifestations of poor health such as internal parasitism, infectious disease, malnutrition as well as poor sanitation.

Geographic distribution: World-wide

Symptoms: Restlessness, emaciation, feather damage, anaemia, markedly reduced performance

Significance: Lice infestation in chickens is a very important cause of production losses in traditional and intensive poultry rearing systems.

Diagnosis: Lousiness (pediculosis) is diagnosed by finding the straw-coloured lice on skin or feathers of birds. Lice of domestic birds vary in size from less than 1 mm to over 6 mm. Masses of eggs may be found attached to the bases of the feathers.

Therapy: Lice are best controlled by spraying with

pyrethroids, carbaryl, coumaphos, dichlorvos, malathion and stirofos (☞ Table 27, p. 389).

Prophylaxis: To avoid cross-contamination, lice must be controlled on all the birds in the environment of chickens at the same time. Wild galliform or birds should never be allowed to contact poultry flocks. If treatment is required, the birds should be treated 2 times on a 10-day interval. Only the mature forms will be controlled as most of the available insecticides do not kill the eggs. Spraying of the birds is generally the most efficient way of controlling lice. Dipping is also possible when the flocks are small. Egg-laden feathers will remain a source of reinfestation and therefore thorough clean-up of all the facilities and the environment should be carried out. (Figures 704, 705)

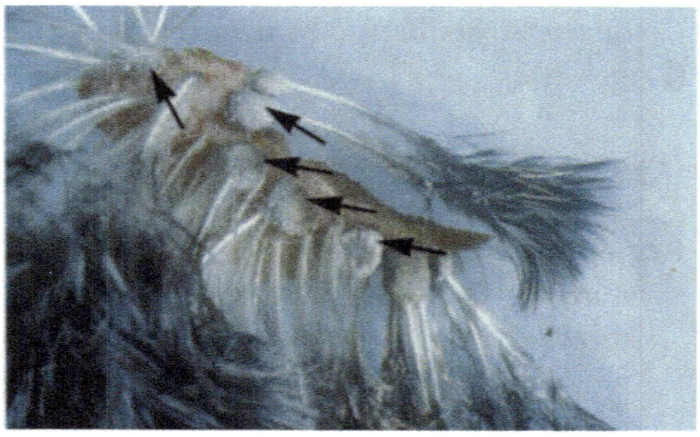

Fig. 705 Eggs of *Eomenacanthus stramineus* at the base of feathers (arrows) [53]

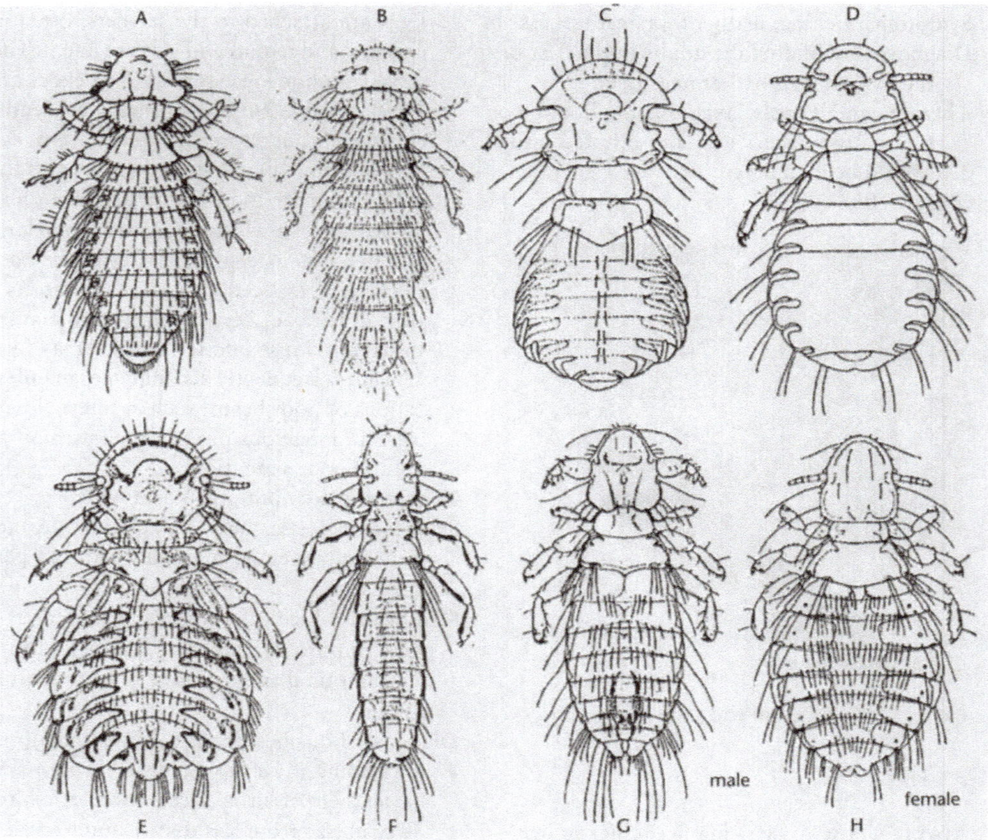

Fig. 704 Chewing lice (Mallophaga) of chicken; *Menopon gallinae* (A), *Eomenacanthus stramineus* (B), *Goniodes* (syn. *Oulocrepis*) *dissimilis*, the brown chicken louse (C), *Goniocotes gallinae* (D), *Goniodes* (syn. *Stenocrotaphus*) *gigas* (E), *Lipeurus caponis* (F) and *Cuclotogaster heterographus* (G and H) [35]

Table 26 Mallophaga of chickens, guinea fowls and pigeons

Scientific name	Common name	Host
Menoponidae		
Eomenacanthus stramineus	Body louse	Chickens
Menopon gallinae	Shaft louse	Chickens
Lipeurus caponis	Wing louse	Chickens
Numidilipeurus tropicalis	Tropical wing louse	Chickens
Philopteridae		
Cuclotogaster heterographus	Head louse	Chickens
Goniocotes gallinae	Fluff louse	Chickens
Goniodes dissimilis	Brown chicken louse	Chickens
Goniodes gigas	Tropical brown chicken	Louse
Goniodes numidae	Feather louse	Guinea fowl
Lipeurus numidae	Slender louse	Guinea fowl
Campanulotes bidentatus	Small pigeon louse	Pigeons
Columbicola columbae	Slender pigeon louse	Pigeons

(Figures 706, 707, 708, 709, 710, 711, 712)

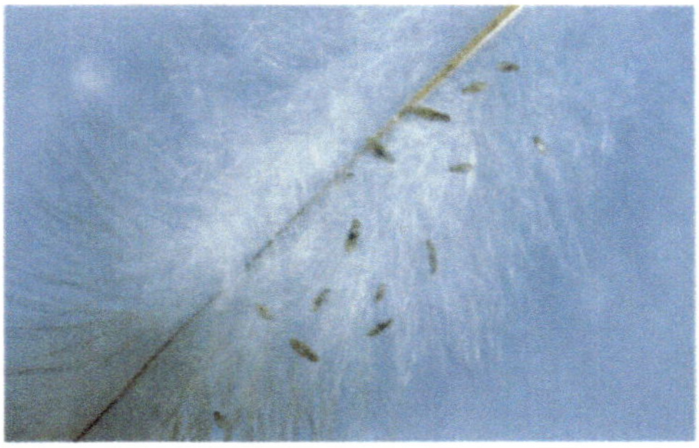

Fig. 707 Mallophaga found in a feather

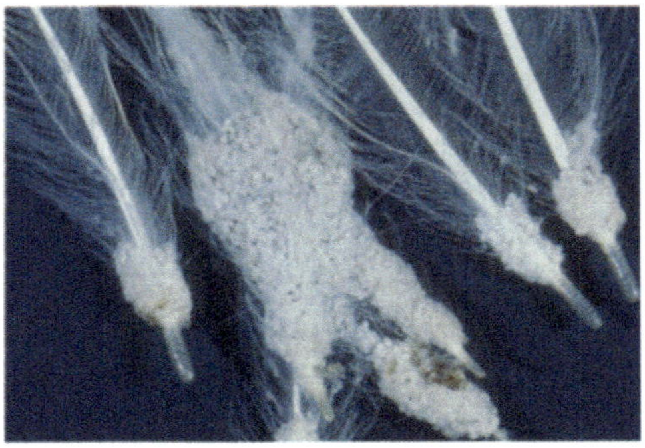

Fig. 708 Masses of eggs of *Menopon gallinae* at the base of feathers

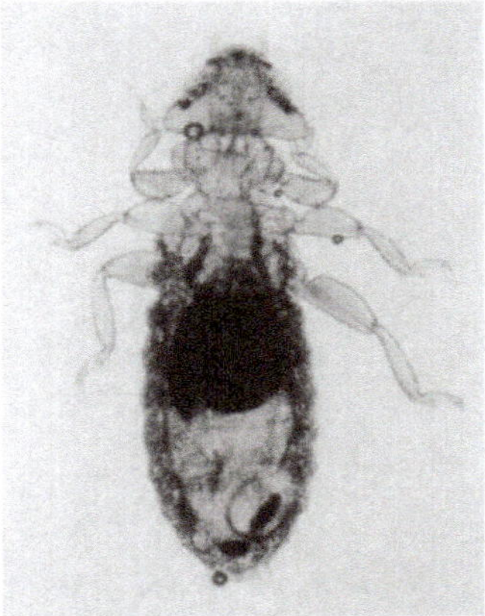

Fig. 706 *Eomenacanthus stramineus*, the body louse (2.9–3.2 mm long) [4]

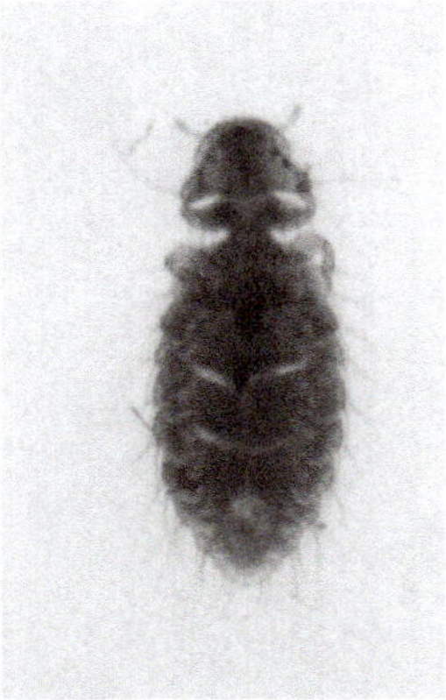

Fig. 709 *Menopon gallinae*, the shaft louse (1.5–1.9 mm long) [8]

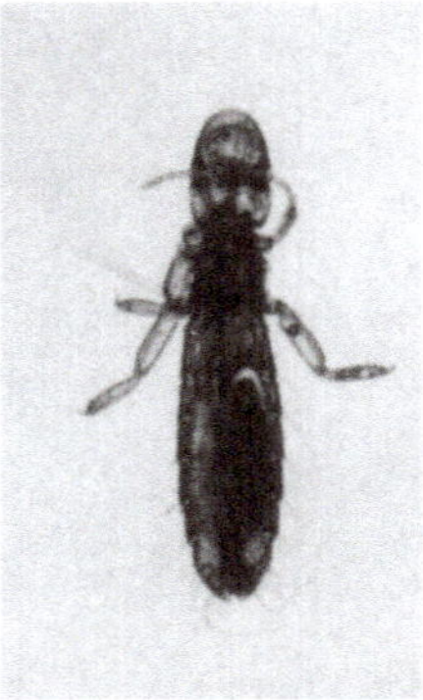

Fig. 710 *Lipeurus caponis*, the wing louse (2.0–2.5 mm long) [8]

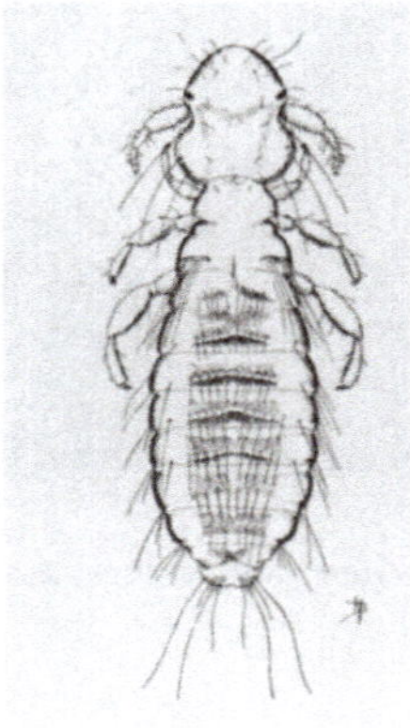

Fig. 711 *Cuclotogaster heterographus*, the head louse (2.4–2.5 mm long) [56]

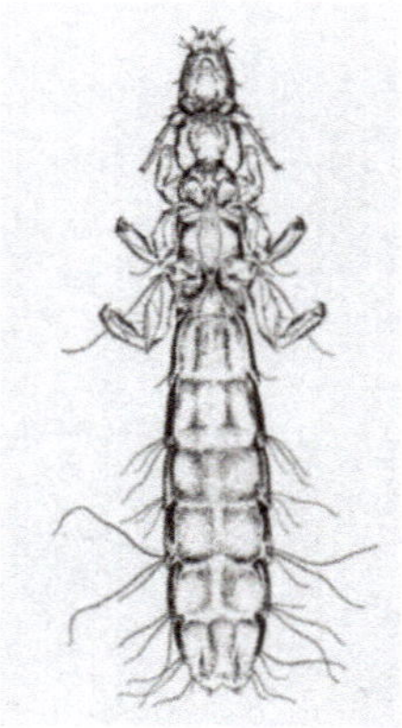

Fig. 712 *Columbicola columbae*, the slender pigeon louse (2.0–2.8 mm long) [56]

– Heteroptera

Cimex lectularius Common bedbug

Remarks: The bedbug is a common blood-sucking parasite in temperate and subtropical climates that attacks poultry, most mammals, including man. Feeding usually occurs at night. The bugs become engorged within 10 minutes, then hide in cracks and crevices. If attacked by large numbers of bugs, birds may become anaemic and performance is severely reduced (decreased egg production, high feed consumption). Heavily infested nests are abandoned. Bites are usually followed by swelling and itching. Bedbugs are rare in modern laying operations, but traditional poultry systems are often heavily affected. Control is based on thorough cleaning of the houses and quarters and the reduction of hiding places for the bugs. A thorough high-pressure spraying of the houses as for the control of fowl ticks is effective. Pyrethroids, organophosphates, carbamates and combinations are highly effective against Heteroptera (☞ Table 27 p. 389).
(Figure 713)

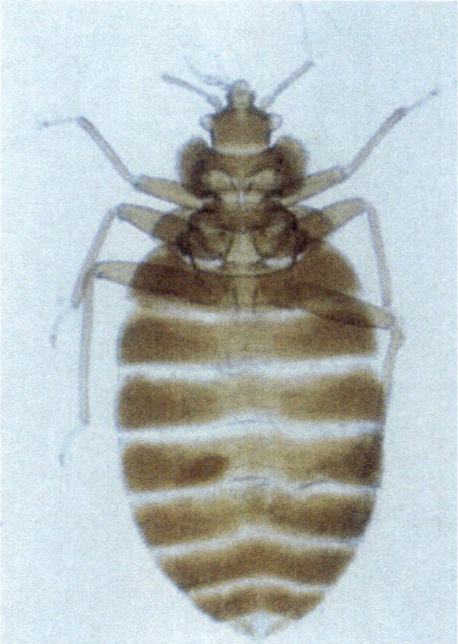

Fig. 713 *Cimex lectularius*, the common bed-bug (3–6 × 3 mm) [4]

Table 27 Some insecticides for external parasite control on poultry

Lice, mites, fleas	
Dusts	
Malathion (4–5%)	Ready-to-use
Permethrin (0.25%)	Ready-to-use
Rabon	Ready-to-use
Carbaryl (5%)	Ready-to-use
Sprays	
Malathion	0.5% spray
Permethrin	0.05% spray
Tetrachlorvinphos*	0.5% spray
Stirofos (23%) and dichlorvos (5.7%)	0.5% spray
Fowl ticks, bedbugs	
Sprays	
Malathion	0.3% spray
Tetrachlorvinphos*	1.0% spray
Carbaryl	0.2% spray

* not directly on poultry

– Fleas

SIPHONAPTERA

Fleas are parasites in the adult stage but free-living as larvae. Adults vary in size from 1.5–5 mm, and possess a tough, laterally compressed body, piercing-sucking mouthparts and long legs for leaping. They are cosmopolitan in distribution but more abundant in temperate and warm climates. Females develop several eggs per day which roll off the host into surrounding litter where they incubate. Dampness and warmth is essential for further development. Larvae develop within 1–2 weeks which feed on organic matter. The larvae then pupate and the inactive pupal stage varies from 1 week to several months.
(Figure 714 and p. 332 ff.)

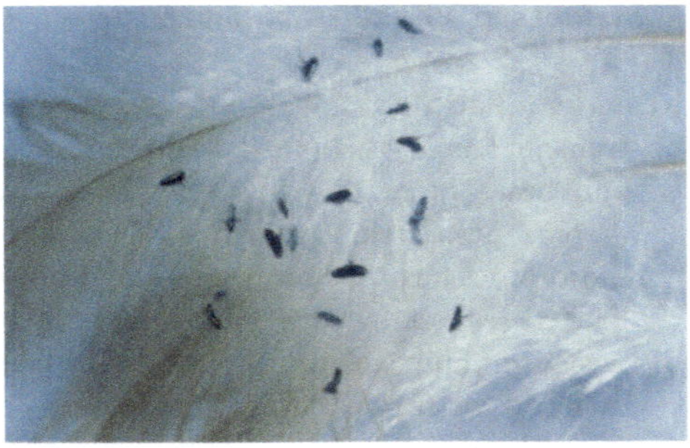

Fig. 714 *Ceratophyllus gallinae* in situ

Echidnophaga gallinacea Sticktight flea

Remarks: The sticktight flea is common on chickens and many other bird and mammal species in tropical and subtropical areas of the world. Adults usually attach to the skin of the head for days or weeks. The sessile adults often occur in clusters of 100 or more. The adults forcibly eject their eggs so that they reach surrounding litter. The larvae best develop in sandy, well-drained litter. Irritation and blood loss cause anaemia, reduced performance and death, particularly in young birds.
(Figure 715)

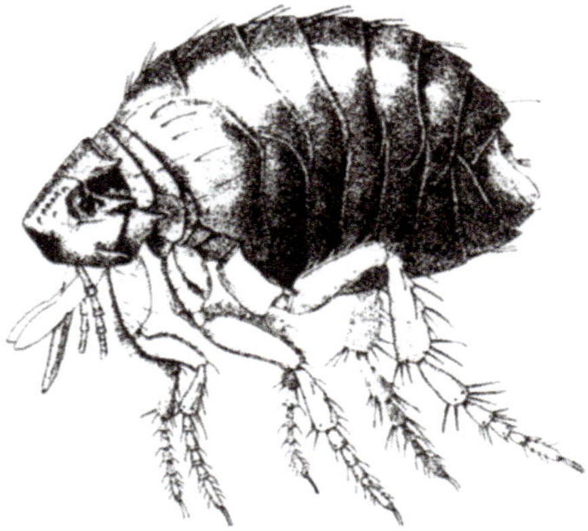

Fig. 715 *Echidnophaga gallinacea*, the sticktight flea (about 1 mm long) [56]

Ceratophyllus gallinae Common chicken flea, European chicken flea

Remarks: This is the common chicken flea with a world-wide distribution. It occurs on chickens, many other bird species, rodents, dog and man. It breeds in nests and litter, and only goes on the birds to feed.
(Figure 716)

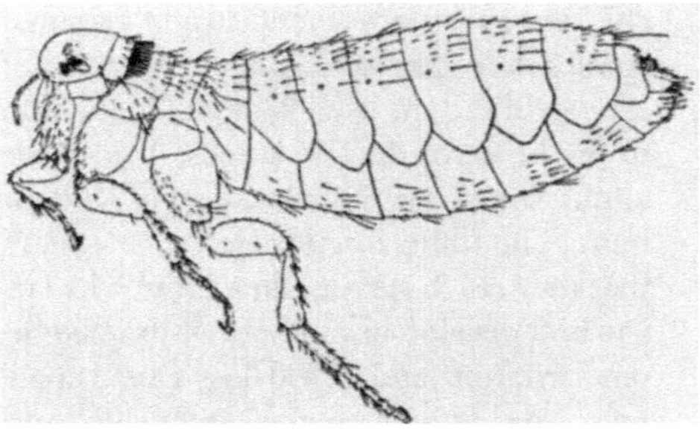

Fig. 716 *Ceratophyllus gallinae*, the common chicken flea (2.0–3.5 mm long) [56]

Ceratophyllus columbae

Remarks: This flea occurs on domestic pigeon and chickens.

Ctenocephalides felis

Remarks: It has been found in poultry houses at pest levels. Most of these houses are using cats as rodent control and it appears that the cats introduce the fleas in the house and these then move to the birds. Pulex irritans, the human flea, may occasionally also attack chickens.

- **Control of fleas**

The most important control measures are removing infested litter and dusting the litter surface with carbaryl, coumaphos or malathion to kill immature fleas.

– Dipterida

The order Dipterida includes several families whose members annoy or suck blood from birds (Table 28).

CULICIDAE Mosquitoes

Aedes spp., *Anopheles* spp. *and Culex* spp.

Remarks: A great number of mosquitoes is known to feed on poultry. Only females suck blood. Adults are most active towards the evening and at night. Poultry production facilities that utilize lagoons can have problems with mosquitoes breeding in the lagoon. Masses of mosquitoes may attack poultry and numerous deaths within a flock may occur. Several viruses are known to be transmitted by mosquitoes, e.g. fowl pox virus by *Aedes* spp. The best control is prevention of mosquito development in the environment of the chicken. Mosquitoes breed in swamps, ponds, stagnant pools and water-filled containers of all types. Such breeding grounds should be covered or eliminated (e.g. draining swampy areas). For housed poultry residual wall sprays and fogging within poultry houses may reduce the mosquitoes markedly. Screening to prevent mosquito entry may aid in control. Poultry in open houses or on range are most difficult to protect from mosquitoes (☞ CATTLE, ■ 5.1; Table 28).

SIMULIIDAE

Simulium spp. Blackflies, buffalo gnats

Remarks: Blackflies are bloodsuckers and transmit leucocytozoonosis to duck, turkey and other birds. Many species occur in tropical areas. They are similar in size to mosquitoes but are dark, short, and humpbacked with short legs. They often attack in swarms and cause great irritation, anaemia and death of birds either directly or through disease transmission. Blackfly control is extremely difficult since immature stages are restricted to running, well-aerated water, which is often some distance from the poultry farm. Screening may aid to control attacks. Measures recommended for mosquito control are applicable to blackfly control (☞CATTLE, ■ 5.1; Table 28).

CERATOPOGENIDAE

Culicoides spp. Biting midges

Remarks: Many species of *Culicoides* attack chickens. These are extremely small although they can easily be seen as small blackish specks moving on the skin. Their bites cause marked irritation and intense itching. Some species transmit diseases (e.g. avian infectious synovitis, *Haemoproteus nettionis* to duck, possibly also fowl pox). Control is extremely difficult since the midges will pass through ordinary screen mesh, but screens treated with malathion (6%) solution have eliminated midges for 3 weeks. Fogging with mosquito or fly sprays and residual deposits applied for fly control will help to reduce the problem. Since the habitats where these species develop are so variable, it is difficult to destroy the midges on the breeding ground (☞ CATTLE, ■ 5.1; Table 28).

MUSCIDAE

Musca domestica Housefly and its relatives

Remarks: These non-biting flies are readily produced on poultry farms and are a health and sanitation problem for both the poultry producers and neighbours. These flies do not bite or attack birds directly, but their significance is associated with the transmission of diseases. Many species may be involved. So-called filth flies are a world-wide problem on poultry farms with many other species of *Musca* and indigenous blowflies (Calliphoridae) and flesh flies (Sarcophagidae) involved. Filth flies lay their eggs in manure (some sarcophagids deposit living larvae), in moist spilled feed or on dead bird carcasses. Larvae of the housefly may develop in manure and then move to drier areas for pupation. Flies are suspected to be vectors of many mammalian as well as avian gastrointestinal diseases. Newcastle disease virus was found in flies. Houseflies and maggots may act as intermediate hosts for the tapeworm *Choanotaenia infundibulum*. Common houseflies and blowflies are capable of carrying eggs of the caecal worm *Heterakis gallinae*, which may contain the protozoan agent of histomonosis of turkeys. Certain fly larvae feed on decomposing cadavers and may ingest the toxin of the bacterium *Clostridium botulinum*. If poultry eat such maggots, botulism ("Limberneck") may occur. Prompt burial, burning or the use of disposal pits for animal cadavers will prevent botulism from such sources. Houseflies may also transmit fowl cholera, tuberculosis (*Mycobacterium avium*) when ingested by chickens and turkeys. Myiasis is not as common as in mammals. The black blowfly (*Phormia regina*) can deposit eggs in wounds in chickens, turkeys and geese and the maggots may destroy living tissue. Fly control is based on preventing breeding of flies in manure. Flies cannot breed in dry manure (moisture < 60%). Sufficient air flow should be provided over the manure. Water leaks may support fly breeding and should therefore be avoided. Insecticides may be used in several ways: as space sprays, fogs and mists (temporary control of adult flies), surface sprays (residual effect of insecticides on surfaces), baits (insecticide granules combined with fly attractants, e.g. muscamone are placed in protected areas and are highly effective). The use of larvicidal insecticides on manure is unsafe and detrimental to predators and other organisms in the manure. Insect growth regulators (cyromazine) are highly effective and may circumvent this problem (☞ CATTLE, ■ 5.1; Table 28).

Stomoxys calcitrans Stable fly

Remarks: The stable fly attacks mammals and birds. This fly is similar in size and appearance to the common housefly, but possesses a piercing beak. Both sexes suck blood and cause intense irritation and anaemia when present in high numbers. It develops in manure with high fibre content or in wet crop refuse such as straw left in the field or other crop residues. Control is by the same measures used against houseflies. Prevention requires clean-up of crop residues and proper manure management to prevent mixing of moist manure with spilled feed. The stable fly acts as intermediate host of *Hymenolepis carioca* (☞ CATTLE, ■ 5.1).

Table 28 Fly control in poultry facilities

Residual and bait sprays	
Permetrin	0.25% spray
Stirofos	1% spray
Tetrachlorvinphos*	1% spray
Contact sprays	
Dibrom	0.25%
Pyrethrin (0.75%) and piperonylbutoxide (0.5–3.75%)	Ready-to-use oil spray
Dichlorvos	0.5% spray
Dry sugar baits	
Dibrom	Ready-to-use bait
Trichlorfon (1%)	Ready-to-use bait
Dichlorvos (1%)	Ready-to-use bait
Methomyl (Golden malrin, 1%)	Ready-to-use bait
Bomyl (True Grit Blue, 1%)	Ready-to-use bait

* not directly on poultry

HIPPOBOSCIDAE

Pseudolynchia canariensis The pigeon fly

Remarks: This is an important parasite of pigeons in warm or tropical areas. It may transmit *Haemoproteus columbae*, which causes pigeon malaria. Larvae mature inside the female and pupate immediately upon being ejected. The adult fly is dark brown and about 6 mm in length. The adult fly moves rapidly through the feather and sucks blood. The fly may also bite humans, inflicting a painful skin wound that persists for several days. Infested birds suffer from blood loss and irritation.
(Figure 717)

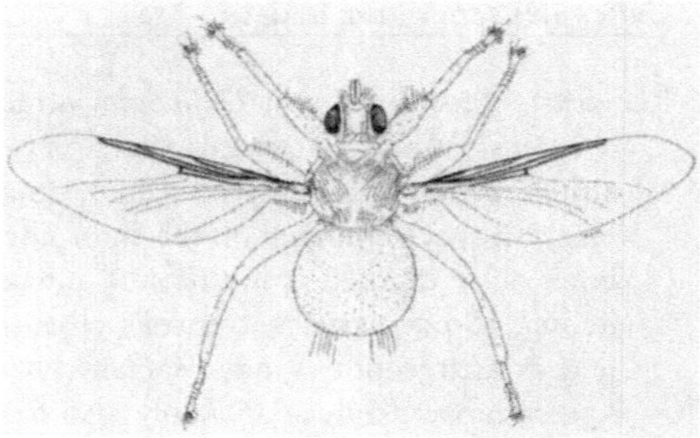

Fig. 717 *Pseudolynchia canariensis*, the pigeon fly (up to 6 mm long) [3]

5.2 Eyes

HELMINTHS

• Nematoda found in the eyes

Oxyspirura spp. (*O. mansoni, O. parvorum* and *O. petrowi*) Manson's eyeworm

Location: This worm occurs under the nictitating membrane and in the conjunctival sacs and nasolacrimal ducts.

Hosts: Chicken and guineafowl

Species description: This slender nematode is 12–18 mm long. The eggs pass down the lacrimal ducts and out in the faeces of the birds. The intermediate stages develop in the cockroach (*Phycnoscelus surinamensis*). The fowls acquire the parasite by ingesting infected cockroaches. Larvae migrate along the oesophagus, pharynx, and lacrimal ducts to the eye.

Geographic distribution: Tropical and subtropical regions

Symptoms: Infected birds show a peculiar ophthalmia. They appear uneasy and continuously scratch at the eyes, which are usually watery and show severe inflammation. The nictitating membrane becomes swollen, projects slightly beyond the eyelids at the corners of the eyes. It is usually kept in continual motion. The eyelids are sometimes stocked together and a white cheesy material collects beneath them. Severe ophthalmia may develop and the eyeball may be destroyed. The worms are seldom found in severely affected eyes.

Significance: *Oxyspirura mansoni* is rarely found but may severely affect individual birds.

Diagnosis: Embryonated eggs (50–65 × 45 µm) are passed in the droppings. Adult worms may be found under the nictitating membrane and in the conjunctival sacs.

Therapy: Some drops of a 10% solution of levamisole (applied topically) kill the parasites as does levamisole (30 mg/kg, po.). Topical application of ivermectin (0.05 mg/kg) may also be effective against the parasites.

Prophylaxis: Strict sanitary measures, including the use of insecticides on cockroach-infested premises, provide efficient control. (Figure 718)

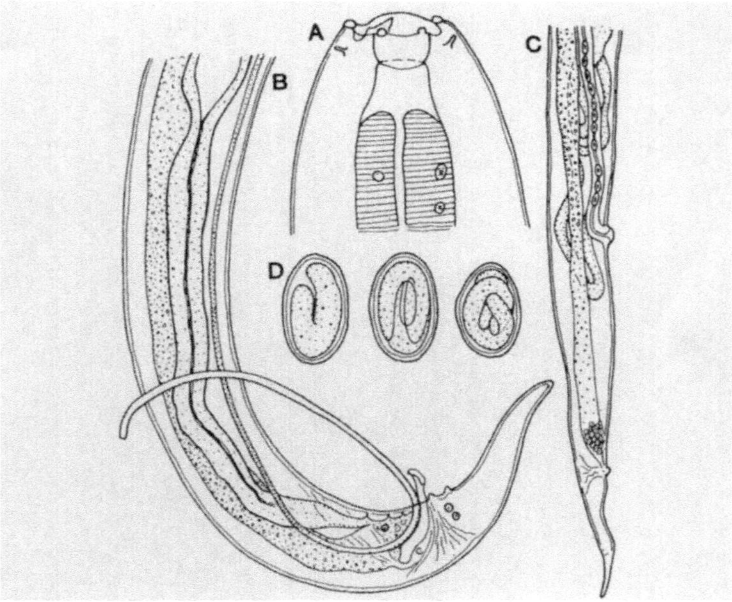

Fig. 718 *Oxyspirura mansoni*, anterior end (A), posterior end (B) of male, posterior end of female (C) and eggs (D) [56]

Bibliography

[1] Manual of Veterinary Parasitological Laboratory Techniques, Reference Book 418 (1987); HMSO Copyright Unit, Norwich, UK

[2] Current Veterinary Therapy 3: Food Animal Practice/J.L. Howard (1993); W.B. Saunders Company, Philadelphia, Pennsylvania, USA

[3] Helminths, Arthropods and Protozoa of Domesticated Animals/E.J.L. Soulsby (1982); Ballière Tindall, Division of Cassell Ltd.; London, UK

[4] F. Hörchner, A.O. Heydorn, E. Schein, D. Mehlitz, Institut für Parasitologie und Tropenveterinärmedizin, Berlin, Germany

[5] Veterinary Helminthology/R.K. Reinecke (1983); Blackwell Wissenschafts-Verlag, Berlin, Germany

[6] Parasites of Cattle (1981); Merck & Co., Inc., Rahway N.J., USA

[7] Diagnose und Therapie der Parasiten von Haus-, Nutz- und Heimtieren/H. Mehlhorn, D. Düwel und W. Raether (1986); Gustav Fischer Verlag, Stuttgart, Germany

[8] S. Geerts, Prince Leopold Institute of Tropical Medicine, Antwerp, Belgium

[9] Traité d'Helminthologie Médicale et Vétérinaire (1936)/ Traité d'Entomologie Médicale et Vétérinaire/ M. Neveu-Lemaire (1938); Édition Vigot, Paris, France

[10] Allcom Advertising AG, Allschwil, Switzerland

[11] Diagnose von Helminthosen durch koproskopische Untersuchung/D. Thienpont, F. Rochette und O.F.J. Vanparijs (1979); Janssen Pharmaceutica, Beerse, Belgium

[12] Magen-Darmnematoden des Rindes: Diagnostischer Atlas/D. Barth unter Mitarbeit von M. Visser (1991); Ferdinand Enke Verlag, Stuttgart, Germany

[13] G. Uilenberg; Centre de coopération internationale en recherche agronomique pour le développement (CIRAD) et Departement d'Élevage et de Medicine Vétérinaire (EMVT), Maison-Alfort Cedex, France

[14] Veterinary Protozoology/N.D. Levine (1985); The Iowa State University Press, Ames, Iowa, USA

[15] Utrecht University, Department of Parasitology and Tropical Veterinary Medicine, Utrecht, The Netherlands

[16] Manual of Tropical Veterinary Parasitology/translated by M. Shah-Fischer and R.R. Say (1989); CAB International, Oxon, UK

[17] ILRAD (1989) Annual Report of the International Laboratory for Research on Animal Diseases; International Laboratory for Research on Animal Diseases, Nairobi, Kenya

[18] Helminthes et Helminthoses des Ruminants Domestiques d'Afrique Tropicale/M. Graber et C. Perrotin (1983); Les Éditions du Point Vétérinaire, Maisons-Alfort, France

[19] Veterinary Parasitology/G.M. Urquhart, J. Armour, J.L. Duncan, A.M. Dunn and F.W. Jennings (1987); Blackwell Scientific Publications Ltd., Oxford, UK

[20] G. Wahl, Thesis; Institut für Tropenmedizin, Tübingen, Germany

[21] Parasitic Helminths and Zoonoses in Africa/ C.N.L. Macpherson and P.S. Craig (eds) (1991); Academic Division of Unwin Hyman Ltd., London, UK

[22] J.P. Dubey; United States Department of Agri-

culture, Animal Parasitology Institute, Beltsville, USA
[23] A. Renz; Universität Hohenheim, Fachbereich Parasitologie, Stuttgart, Germany
[24] Manual on Livestock Ticks for Animal Disease (1965); Animal Disease Eradication Division, Agricultural Research Service, U.S. Department of Agriculture, Hyattsville, Maryland, USA
[25] Pictorial Keys to Arthropods, Reptiles, Birds and Mammals of Public Health Significance (1967); U.S. Department of Health, Education, and Welfare, Public Health Service, Bureau of Disease and Environmental Control, National Communicable Disease Center, Atlanta, Georgia, USA
[26] Parasitology in Focus: Facts and Trends/H. Mehlhorn (1988); Springer-Verlag GmbH & Co. KG, Berlin, Germany
[27] Ticks, mites and insects infesting domestic animals in South Africa: Part 1. Descriptions and biology/C.J. Howell, J.B. Walker and E.M. Nevill (Science Bulletin No. 393, 1978); Division of Agricultural Information, Department of Agricultural Technical Services, Pretoria, South Africa
[28] A Manual of Parasitic Mites of Medical or Economic Importance/E.W. Baker, T.M. Evans, D.J. Gould, W.B. Hull and H.L. Keegan (1956); U.S. Department of Health Education and Welfare, Public Health Service, Bureau of Disease Prevention and Environmental Control, National Communicable Disease Center, Atlanta, Georgia, USA
[29] Medical and Veterinary Entomology/D.S. Kettle (1984); Croom Helm Ltd., Kent, UK
[30] Prof. Gräfner, Schwerin, Germany
[31] Manual for the Control of the Screwworm Fly *Cochliomyia hominivorax*, Coquerel; Food and Agriculture Organization of the United Nations, Animal Production and Health Division, Rom, Italy
[32] Parasites of Sheep (1981); Merck & Co., Inc., Rahway NJ, USA
[33] Diagnose und Therapie der Parasitosen von Haus-, Nutz- und Heimtieren/H. Mehlhorn, D. Düwel und W. Raether (1993); Gustav Fischer Verlag, Stuttgart, Germany
[34] Nematode Parasites of Domestic Animals and of Man/N.D. Levine (1980); Burgess Publishing Company, Minneapolis, Minnesota, USA
[35] Bestimmungstabellen der Vorratsschädlinge und des Hausungeziefers Mitteleuropas/H. Weidner (1982); Gustav Fischer Verlag, Stuttgart, Germany
[36] Parasites of Horses (1981); Merck & Co., Inc., Rahway N.J., USA
[37] A Colour Atlas of Equine Parasites/D. E. Jacobs (1986); Gower Medical Publishing Ltd., London, UK
[38] Parasitology for Veterinarians/J.R. Georgi (1985); W.B. Saunders Company, Philadelphia, USA
[39] The Merck Veterinary Manual/C.M. Fraser (1991); Merck & Co., Inc., Rahway, N.J., USA
[40] Helminths of Domestic Equids/J.R. Lichtenfels (1975); Helminthological Society of Washington, USA
[41] Atlas der Hauterkrankungen des Pferdes: Diagnose und Behandlung von Hautkrankheiten/L.F. Montes und J.T. Vaughan (1985); Munksgaard, International Publishers Ltd., Copenhagen, Denmark
[42] Coccidia and Coccidiosis/ László P. Pellérdy (1974); Blackwell Wissenschaft, Berlin, Germany
[43] Grundlagen der Zestodenkunde. Anoplocephalata der Haus- und Wildtiere (1951), in: *Osnovy nematodologii*, Vol. 3/ A.A. Spasskii; Publishing House of the Academy of Sciences of the USSR, Moscow, Russia
[44] Strongylata, in: Key of parasitic nematodes, Vol. 3/ K.J. Skrjabin, N.P. Shikhobalova, R.S. Shults, T.J. Popova, S.N. Boev, S.L. Deljamure (1952); Publishing House of the Academy of Sciences of the USSR, Moscow, Russia
[45] Trichostrongylids of animals and of man (1954), in: *Osnovy nematodologii*, Vol. 3/ K.J. Skrjabin, N.P. Shikhobalova, R.S. Shults; Publishing House of the Academy of Sciences of the USSR, Moscow, Russia
[46] D. Schillinger, MSD AGVET, Grünwald, Germany
[47] Nasopharyngeal botflies (Oestridae) (1957), in: Fauna USSR, No. 68/K.J. Grunin; Publishing House of the Academy of Sciences of the USSR, Moscow, Russia
[48] Larvae of the nasal botfly of domestic animals in USSR (1953), in: Fauna USSR, No. 51/ K.J. Grunin; Publishing House of the Academy of Sciences of the USSR, Moscow, Russia
[49] J.A. Euzéby; École Nationale Veterinaire de Lyon, Charbonnieres Cedex, Lyon, France
[50] Parasites of Swine (1981); Merck & Co., Inc., Rahway, N.J., USA
[51] Atlas de Parasitologie: Schémas explicatifs d'épidémiologie/ Y.J. Golvan; Édition-Librairie „Le Léopard d'Or" S.A.R.L., Paris, France
[52] Die Ektoparasiten; Bayer AG, Leverkusen, Geschäftsfeld Tiergesundheit, Germany
[53] R. Morgenstern; Institut für Tierpathologie, Bern, Switzerland

[54] Baycox Manual, Coccidiosis in Poultry; Bayer AG, Geschäftsfeld Tiergesundheit, Leverkusen, Germany
[55] Cogicitial lesion scoring standards for chickens; Dow Chemical Europe, Horgen, Switzerland
[56] Diseases of Poultry/B.W. Calnek, H.J. Barnes, C.W. Beard, W.M. Reid and H.W. Yoder, Jr. (1991); The Iowa State University Press Ames, IA., USA
[57] Labordiagnostik für die tierärztliche Praxis/H. Plonait (1980); Blackwell Wissenschaft Kurfürstendamm 57, Berlin, Germany
[58] International Trypanotolerance Center (ITC), Banjul, The Gambia

Further Reading

Laboratory diagnosis of parasites

Barth, D. (1991) Magen-Darmnematoden des Rindes; Ferdinand Enke Verlag, Stuttgart

Irvin, A.D., Cunningham, M.P. and A.S. Young (1981) Advances in the Control of Theileriosis. Current Topics in Veterinary Medicine and Animal Sciences Vol. 14; Martinus Nijhoff Publishers, The Hague, Boston, London

Manual of recommended diagnostic techniques and requirements for biological products for list A and B diseases (1989) Volume I; Office International des Epizooties, Paris

Manual of recommended diagnostic techniques and requirements for biological products for list A and B diseases (1990) Volume II; Office International des Epizooties, Paris

Manual of Veterinary Parasitological Laboratory Techniques. Reference Book 418. (1987) Ministry of Agriculture, Fisheries and Food; Her Majesty's Stationery Office, London

Murray, M., Trail, J.C.M., Turner, D.A. and Y. Wissocq (1983) Livestock Productivity and Trypanotolerance; Network Training Manual; ILCA, Addis Ababa

Nansen, P., Jørgensen, R.J. and E.J.L. Soulsby (1981) Epidemiology and Control of Nematodiasis in Cattle. Current Topics in Veterinary Medicine and Animal Sciences. Vol. 9; Martinus Nijhoff Publishers, The Hague, Boston, London

Thienpont, D., Rochette, F. and O.F.J. Vanparijs (1979) Diagnose von Helminthosen durch koproskopische Untersuchung; Janssen Research Foundation, Beerse

Immunology

Grange, J.M., Fox, A. and N.L. Morgan (eds) (1987) Immunological techniques in microbiology; Blackwell Scientific Publications, Oxford, London, Edinburgh, Boston, Palo Alto, Melbourne

Roitt, I., Brostoff, J. and D. Male (1993) Immunology. Third edition; Mosby, London

Walls, K.W. and P.M. Schantz (eds) (1986) Immunodiagnosis of parasitic diseases. Vol. 1 Helminthic diseases; Academic Press, Inc. Ltd., London

Molecular biology

Blancou, J. (coordinator) (1990) Biotechnology and veterinary science. Scientific and Technical Review; Office International des Epizooties Paris

Parasitic diseases of domestic animals

General

Barret, M.A. and P.J. Larkin (1974) Milk and beef production in the tropics; Oxford University Press, London

Camus, E. and N. Barré (1988) Heartwater. A review; Office International des Epizooties, Paris

Closas, A.S.G., Meulemans, G. and J.L. Lancaster (1988) Update on avian diseases. Technical series No. 8; Office International des Epizooties, Paris

Diseases of camels. Scientific and Technical Review (1987) Vol. 6, No. 2; Office International des Epizooties, Paris

Eckert, J., Kutzer, E., Rommel, M., Bürger, H.-J., und W. Körting (1992) Veterinärmedizinische Parasitologie. Vierte Auflage; Verlag Paul Parey, Berlin und Hamburg

Fraser, C.M. (ed) (1991) The Merck Veterinary Manual. Seventh Edition; Merck & Co. Inc., Rahway, N.J.

Georgi, J.R. (1985) Parasitology for Veterinarians. Fourth edition. W.B. Saunders Company, Philadelphia, Pennsylvania

Golvan, Y.J. (1990) Atlas de parasitologie; Le Léopard d'Or, Paris

Hall, H.T.B. (1977) Diseases and Parasites of Livestock in the Tropics; Longman Group Ltd., London

Jacobs, D.E. (1986) A colour atlas of equine parasites; Baillière Tindall, London

Mehlhorn, H. (1988) Parasitology in Focus. Facts and Trends; Springer Verlag, Berlin, Heidelberg

Mehlhorn, H., Düwel, D. and W. Raether (1993) Diagnose und Therapie der Parasitosen von Haus-, Nutz- und Heimtieren. Second edition; Gustav Fischer Verlag, Stuttgart

Miller, H.R.P. (coordinator) (1990) Immunity to and diagnosis of internal parasitism. Scientific and Technical Review; Office International des Epizooties, Paris

Pictorial keys to arthropods, reptiles, birds and mammals of public health significance (1967) U.S. Department of Health, Education and Welfare; Public Health Service, Atlanta

Reinecke, R.K. (1983) Veterinary Helminthology; Butterworths, Durban, Pretoria

Ristic, M. and I. McIntyre (1981) Diseases of cattle in the tropics. Current Topics in Veterinary Medicine and Animal Sciences. Vol. 6; Martinus Nijhoff Publishers, The Hague, Boston, London

Robertson, Sir A. (1976) Handbook on animal diseases in the tropics; British Veterinary Association, London

Schwabe, C.W. (1969) Veterinary medicine and human health. Second edition; The Williams & Wilkins Company, Baltimore

Seifert, H.S.H. (1992) Tropentierhygiene; Gustav Fischer Verlag, Jena, Stuttgart

Soulsby, E.J.L. (1982) Helminths, arthropods and protozoa of domesticated animals. Seventh Edition; Baillière Tindall, London

Troncy, P.M., Itard, I. and P.C. Morel (1989) Manual of Tropical Veterinary Parasitology; CAB International, Wallingford

Uilenberg, G. (1992-1995) Cowdria Newsletter; CIRAD-EMVT, Paris, France

Urquhart, G.M., Armour, J., Duncan, J.L., Dunn, A.M. and F.W. Jennings (1985) Veterinary Parasitology; Longman Scientific & Technical, Essex

World Animal Health, Year books, List A disease outbreaks statistics (1988-1994); Office International des Epizooties, Paris

World Animal Health, Year books, Animal health status and disease control methods (1988-1994); Office International des Epizooties, Paris

Protozoa

Adam, K.M.G., Paul, J. and V. Zaman (1979) Medical and Veterinary Protozoology. An illustrated guide; Churchill Livingstone, Edinburgh & London

Gardiner, C.H., Fayer, R. and J.P. Dubey (1988) An atlas of protozoan parasites in animal tissue. Agricultural Research Service. Agriculture Handbook Number 651; United States Department of Agriculture, Beltsville

Koch, H.T. Aspects of the epidemiology of January Disease (*Theileria parva bovis* infection) in Zimbabwe. Proefschrift; University of Utrecht, Utrecht

Levine, N.D. (1985) Veterinary Protozoology. First edition; Iowa State University Press, Ames

Long, P.L. (ed) (1990) Coccidiosis of man and domestic animals; CRC Press, Inc., Boca Raton, Ann Arbor, Boston

Olubayo, R.O. (1991) Expression of trypanotolerance by African wild bovidae with special reference to the buffalo (*Syncerus caffer*); Proefschrift, University of Utrecht, Utrecht

Ristic, M. (ed) (1988) Babesiosis of domestic animals and man; CRC Press, Inc., Boca Raton, Florida

Tenter, A.M. (1984) Serodiagnose experimenteller und natürlicher Piroplasmeninfektionen der Pferde. Vet. med. Diss.; Hannover

Theileriasis. Scientific and Technical Review (1989) Vol. 8, No. 1; Office International des Epizooties, Paris

Helminths

Dunn, A.M. (1969) Veterinary helminthology; William Heinemann Medical Books Ltd., London

Euzéby, J. (1961) Les maladies vermineuses des animaux domestiques et leurs incidences sur la pathologie humaine. Tome premier. Maladies dues aux némathelminthes. Fascicule premier; Vigot frères éditeurs, Paris

Euzéby, J. (1963) Les maladies vermineuses des animaux domestiques et leurs incidences sur la pathologie humaine. Tome premier. Maladies dues aux némathelminthes. Fascicule deuxième; Vigot frères éditeurs, Paris

Euzéby, J. (1966) Les maladies vermineuses des animaux domestiques et leurs incidences sur la pathologie humaine. Tome II. Maladies dues aux plathelminthes. Fascicule premier; Vigot frères éditeurs, Paris

Graber, M. and C. Perrotin (1983) Helminthes et helminthoses des ruminants doméstiques d'-Afrique tropicale; Éditions du Point Vétérinaire, Maisons-Alfort

Levine, N.D. (1979) Nematode parasites of domestic animals and man. Second Édition; Burgess Publishing Company, Minneapolis, Minnesota

Lichtenfels, J.R. (1975) Helminths of domestic equids. Special issue. Vol. 42. Proceedings of the Helminthological Society of Washington

Macpherson, C.N.L. and P.S. Craig (1991) Parasitic helminths and zoonoses in Africa; Unwin Hyman, London

Norval, R.A.I., Perry, B.D. and A.S. Young (1992) The epidemiology of theileriosis in Africa. Academic Press, Inc. Ltd., London

Round, M.C. (1968) Check list of the helminth parasites of African mammals. Technical communication No. 38 of the Commonwealth Bureau of Helminthology, St. Albans, CAB, Farnham Royal, Bucks

Wahl, G. (1991) Die Onchocerca-Arten der Rinder in Nord-Kamerun und ihre Bedeutung für die Epidemiologie der menschlichen Onchocercose. Biol. Diss.; Tübingen

Arthropods

Hoogstraal, H. (1988) Bibliography of ticks and tickborne diseases. Vol. 8; United States Medical Research Unit Number Three, Cairo

Howell, C.J., Walker, J.B. and E.M. Newill (1978) Ticks, mites and insects infesting domestic animals in South Africa. Part 1. Descriptions and biology; Department of Agricultural and Technical Services, Pretoria

Kettle, D.S. (1984) Medical and Veterinary Entomology; Croom Helm, London & Sydney

Manual on Livestock Ticks (1965) Agricultural research service; U.S. Department of Agriculture, Hyattsville

Therapy

Campbell, W.C. (ed) (1989) Ivermectin and abamectin; Springer-Verlag New York, Berlin, Heidelberg

Doherty, T.J. and J.P. Mulville (1992) Diagnosis and Treatment of Large Animal Diseases. W.B. Saunders Company, Philadelphia, Pennsylvania

Howard, J.L. (1993) Current Veterinary Therapy. Food animal practice. Third edition; W.B. Saunders Company, Philadelphia, Pennsylvania

Acknowledgement

The author would like to thank all those who helped in so many ways to make this publication possible

Support in fund raising and financing

Ciba-Geigy Foundation for Cooperation with Developing Countries, Prof. Dr. K. Leisinger and F. Nicolier; Basle, Switzerland

Ciba-Geigy Ltd. Animal Health Division, Basle, Switzerland

University of Berne, Prof. Dr. H. Luginbühl and Prof. Dr. B. Gottstein; Berne, Switzerland

Swiss Development Cooperation, Dr. F. von Sury and Dr. P. Egger; Berne, Switzerland

Dr. J.F. Graf; Centre de Recherche Agricole, St. Aubin, Switzerland

Prof. Dr. K. Pfister; Department of Parasitology, Institute of Animal Pathology, University of Berne, Switzerland

Main contributors and advisors

Prof. Dr. G. Uilenberg; IEMVT, Paris, France

Prof. Dr. B. Hörning, Dr. J.L. Charbon and Dr. M. Kunz; Department of Parasitology, Institute of Animal Pathology, University of Berne, Switzerland

Dr. R. Morgenstern, Dr. A. Tontis, Dr. W. Meier, Dr. H. Häni, PD Dr. D. Dobbelaere, G. Di Lullo and H. Muff; Institute of Animal Pathology, University of Berne, Switzerland

Dr. N. Müller, Dr. P. Jacquier, Dr. A. Hemphil and Dr. R. Felleisen; Institute of Parasitology, University of Berne, Switzerland

Prof. Dr. A. Friess; Institute of Animal Anatomy, University of Berne, Switzerland

Prof. Dr. S. Geerts, Prof. Dr. V. Kumar, Prof. Dr. P. Kageruka and Dr. R. De Deken, Prince Leopold University of Tropical Medicine; Antwerp, Belgium

Prof. Dr. F. Hörchner, Prof. Dr. E. Schein, Prof. Dr. D. Mehlitz and Prof. Dr. A.-O. Heydorn; Institute of Parasitology and Tropical Veterinary Medicine, University of Berlin, Germany

Dr. D. Schillinger; MSD AG VET, Grünwald, Germany

Dr. I. Roditi; Institute of General Microbiology, University of Berne, Switzerland

Dr. K. Bairden; Institute of Veterinary Parasitology, University of Glasgow, UK

Dr. J. Zinsstag; Centre Suisse de Recherches Scientifiques, Abidjan, Côte d'Ivoire

Dr. T. Fritsche; Appenzell, Switzerland

Dr. M. Eysker; Institute of Parasitology, Utrecht, The Netherlands

Prof. Dr. I. McIntyre, Dr. P. Ankers, Dr. B. Touray, Dr. R. Dwinger, Dr. P. Rawlings, Dr. W. Snow, Dr. D. Clifford, Dr. P. Leperre, J. Faye, A. Kaufmann, Dr. J. Claxton, and G. Zürcher; International Trypanotolerance Centre, Banjul, The Gambia

Dr. B. Loum and Dr. M'bake; Department of Livestock Services, Yundum, The Gambia

Dr. R.O. Olubayo; Kenya Agricultural Research Institute, Kabete, Kenya

Prof. Dr. C.D. Ezeokoli; Department of Animal Production and Aquaculture, Abakaliki, Nigeria

Dr. J.Y. Chollet; Laboratoire National Vétérinaire de Boklé, Garoua, Cameroun

Dr. E. Otupiri; Upper Region Agricultural Development Programme, Bolgatanga, Ghana

Prof. Dr. R.A. Ogunsusi; Federal University of Technology, Akure, Nigeria

Dr. D. Mostafa; Laboratoire de Recherches et d'Analyses des Services Vétérinaires, Casablanca, Maroc

P.T. Oberem; Coopers Animal Health (Pty) Ltd, Kempton Park, South Africa

Dr. T.D. Gunter; Pfizer South Africa, Johannesburg, South Africa

Dr. F. Oussaid; Service de Parasitologie E.N.V. Algier, Algier

Dr. D.T. de Waal and Dr. R.M.R. Alves; Department of Agricultural Development, Onderstepoort, South Africa

Prof. Dr. A.M. Makumyaviri; Faculté de Médecine Vétérinaire, Lubumbashi, Zaire

Dr. A. N'Depo; Laboratoire Nationale de Pathologie Animale, Bingerville, Cote d' Ivoire

Dr. S.N. Appiah; Animal Health and Production Department, Kumasi, Ghana

Dr. S. Mamadou and Dr. M. Salambere; Laboratoire Nationale D'Élevage, Ouagadougou, Burkina Faso

Dr. S. Asres; University of Agriculture, Dire Dawa, Ethiopia

Dr. P.G. Sinyangwe; Central Veterinary Research Institute, Lusaka, Zambia

Dr. R. Bohrmann; Central Veterinary Laboratory, Windhoek, Namibia

Dr. R.C. Chhabra; Paraclinical Veterinary Studies, University of Harare, Zimbabwe

Dr. K. Adomefa; Centre de Recherche et d'Elevage, Avetonou, Togo

Dr. W. Godana; Veterinary Service Department, Addis Ababa, Ethiopia

Dr. W. Amanfou; Animal Health and Production Department, Accra, Ghana

Prof. Dr. W.K. Munyua; Division of Veterinary Parasitology, University of Nairobi, Kenya

Dr. C.O. Nwosu; Department of Veterinary Microbiology and Parasitology, University of Ibadan, Nigeria

Dr. P. Gerlach, K. Metzger, M. Bussmann, C. Baer and S. Lotrovsky; Birkhäuser Verlag, Basle, Switzerland

Special thanks are due to my family Angela, Andrea, Simon, Thomas and Philippe for all their support and understanding during the preparation of the present manual.

Index

C

N

GPSR Compliance

The European Union's (EU) General Product Safety Regulation (GPSR) is a set of rules that requires consumer products to be safe and our obligations to ensure this.

If you have any concerns about our products, you can contact us on ProductSafety@springernature.com

In case Publisher is established outside the EU, the EU authorized representative is:

Springer Nature Customer Service Center GmbH
Europaplatz 3
69115 Heidelberg, Germany

Batch number: 10726322

Printed by Printforce, the Netherlands